£100.00

£100.00

INFERTILITY AND ASSISTED REPRODUCTION

Infertility and Assisted Reproduction presents, in detail, the techniques and philosophies behind medical procedures of infertility and assisted reproduction. Assisted reproductive technology is available to two-thirds of the world's population, and world-class experts in their field, representing research from 18 different countries, have contributed to this groundbreaking textbook. This is one of the most rapidly changing and hotly debated fields in medicine. Different countries have different restrictions on the research techniques that can be applied to this field, and, therefore, experts from around the world bring varied and unique authorities to different subjects in reproductive technology. This comprehensive textbook encompasses the latest research into the physiology of reproduction, infertility evaluation and treatment, and assisted reproduction and concludes with perspectives on the ethical dilemmas faced by clinicians and professionals. This book is designed to be a definitive resource for those working in the areas of reproductive medicine the world over.

Dr. Botros R. M. B. Rizk is Professor of Obstetrics and Gynecology, Head of the Division of Reproductive Endocrinology and Infertility, and Medical and Scientific Director of USA ART program at the University of South Alabama, College of Medicine, Alabama, USA.

Dr. Juan A. Garcia-Velasco is an Assistant Professor of Obstetrics and Gynecology at Rey Juan Carlos University School of Medicine, Madrid, Spain, and the Director of the Instituto Valenciano de Infertilidad in Madrid.

Dr. Hassan N. Sallam is Professor in Obstetrics and Gynecology, Vice-Dean and Director of Research in the Faculty of Medicine, and the Director of the Suzanne Mubarak Regional Center for Women's Health and Development at the University of Alexandria, Egypt.

Dr. Antonis Makrigiannakis is Professor of Obstetrics and Gynecology at the University of Crete Medical School.

INFERTILITY AND ASSISTED REPRODUCTION

EDITED BY

BOTROS R. M. B. RIZK
University of South Alabama, College of Medicine

JUAN A. GARCIA-VELASCO
Rey Juan Carlos University School of Medicine

HASSAN N. SALLAM
University of Alexandria

ANTONIS MAKRIGIANNAKIS
University of Crete

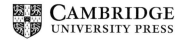
CAMBRIDGE
UNIVERSITY PRESS

CAMBRIDGE UNIVERSITY PRESS
Cambridge, New York, Melbourne, Madrid, Cape Town, Singapore, São Paulo, Delhi

Cambridge University Press
32 Avenue of the Americas, New York, NY 10013-2473, USA

www.cambridge.org
Information on this title: www.cambridge.org/9780521873796

First published 2008

Printed in the United States of America

A catalog record for this publication is available from the British Library.

Library of Congress Cataloging in Publication Data
Infertility and assisted reproduction / edited by Botros Rizk ... [et al.].
p. ; cm.
Includes bibliographical references and index.
ISBN 978-0-521-87379-6 (hardback)
1. Infertility. 2. Human reproductive technology. I. Rizk, Botros.
[DNLM: 1. Infertility – therapy. 2. Reproductive Techniques, Assisted. 3. Fertilization – physiology. WP 570 I4315 2008]
RC889.I5612 2008
616.6'92–dc22   2008005761

ISBN 978-0-521-87379-6 hardback

■ CONTENTS ■

CONTRIBUTORS

EDITORS

Botros R. M. B. Rizk, M.D., M.A., F.R.C.O.G.,
F.R.C.S.(C), H.C.L.D., F.A.C.O.G., F.A.C.S.
Professor and Head, Division of Reproductive
Endocrinology and Infertility,
Department of Obstetrics and Gynecology,
University of South Alabama, Medical and
Scientific Director USA ART program,
Mobile, Alabama, USA

Juan A. Garcia-Velasco, M.D., Ph.D.
Director, IVI-Madrid, Assistant Professor,
Rey Juan Carlos University, Madrid, Spain

Hassan N. Sallam, M.D., F.R.C.O.G., Ph.D. (London)
Director, The Suzanne Mubarak Regional Centre
for Women's Health and Development,
Professor, Obstetrics and Gynaecology,
and Vice Dean, University of Alexandria,
Alexandria, Egypt

Antonis Makrigiannakis, M.D.
Professor of Obstetrics and Gynecology,
Laboratory of Human Reproduction,
Department of Obstetrics and Gynecology,
University of Crete, Crete, Greece

AUTHORS

Michel Abou Abdallah, M.D.
Executive Director, Middle East Fertility Society,
Beirut, Lebanon

Mohamed Aboulghar, M.D.
Professor, Department of Obstetrics and Gynaecology,
Cairo University, Medical Director,
Egyptian IVF-ET Centre, Cairo, Egypt

Mostafa Abuzeid, M.D., F.A.C.O.G., F.R.C.O.G.
Director of the Division of Reproductive Endocrinology,
Department of Obstetrics and Gynecology,
Hurley Medical Center, Flint, Michigan, USA

Practice Director, IVF Michigan,
Rochester Hills, Michigan, USA
Professor, Department of Obstetrics and Gynecology,
Michigan State University College of Human Medicine,
East Lansing, Michigan, USA

G. David Adamson, M.D., F.R.C.S.C., F.A.C.O.G., F.A.C.S.
Director, Fertility Physicians of Northern California,
Palo Alto, California, USA
Director, Fertility & Reproductive Health Institute
of Northern California, San Jose, California, USA
Clinical Professor, Stanford University,
Associate Clinical Professor,
U.C. San Francisco School of Medicine,
San Francisco, California, USA

Ashok Agarwal, Ph.D., H.C.L.D.
Professor and Director,
Reproductive Research Centre,
Glickman Urological Institute,
The Cleveland Clinic Foundation,
Cleveland, Ohio, USA

Claudio Alvarez
Instituto Valenciano de Infertilidad, Santiago, Chile

Amutha Anpananthar, M.B.B.S., B.Sc.
University College London,
Department of Community Child Health,
London, UK

Aydin Arici, M.D.
Associate Professor and Head, Division of Reproductive
Endocrinology & Infertility, Department of Obstetrics
and Gynecology, Yale University School of Medicine,
New Haven, Conneticut, USA

Alicia Armstrong, M.D., M.H.S.C.R.
Reproductive Biology and Medicine Branch, National
Institute of Child Health & Human Development,
Bethesda, Maryland, USA

Cem S. Atabekoglu, M.D.
Department of Obstetrics and Gynecology, Ankara
University School of Medicine, Ankara, Turkey

Nabil Aziz, M.B., Ch.B., M.R.C.O.G., M.D.
Consultant Gynecologist, Liverpool Women's Hospital,
Lecturer, The University of Liverpool, Liverpool, UK

Shawky Z. A. Badawy, M.D.
Professor and Chair, Department of Obstetrics and
Gynecology, Division of Reproductive Endocrinology
and Infertility, State University of New York, Upstate
Medical University, Syracuse, New York, USA

Susan Baker
Associate Professor, Division of Maternal Fetal Medicine,
Department of Obstetrics and Gynecology,
University of South Alabama, Mobile, Alabama, USA

Juan Balasch, M.D.
Professor and Chairman, Institute Clinic Gynecology,
Obstetrics and Neonatology,
Hospital Clinic-Institut d'Investigacions
Biomediques August Pi I Sunyer (IDIBAPS),
Faculty of Medicine – University of Barcelona,
Barcelona, Spain

Theodore A. Baramki, M.D., F.A.C.O.G.
Department of Gynecology and Obstetrics,
Johns Hopkins University School of Medicine,
Baltimore, Maryland, USA

Alberto Barros
Centre for Reproductive Genetics, Porto, Portugal

Mohamed A. Bedaiwy, M.D.
Department of Obstetrics and Gynecology, The Cleveland
Clinic Foundation, Cleveland, Ohio, USA

Bulent Berker, M.D.
Ankara University School of Medicine, Department of
Obstetrics & Gynecology, Division of Reproductive
Endocrinology & Endoscopic Surgery, Ankara, Turkey

O. Bern
Infertility and IVF Unit, Assaf Harofeh Medical Center,
Zerifin, Sackler School of Medicine, Tel-Aviv
University, Tel-Aviv, Israel

C. M. Boomsma, Ph.D. Student
Division Perinatology and Gynaecology,
University Medical Center Utrecht,
Utrecht, The Netherlands

E. Bosch
Instituto Universitario IVI, Madrid, Spain

Gurkan Bozdag, M.D.
Hacettepe University Faculty of Medicine, Department of
Obstetrics and Gynecology, Ankara, Turkey

Hyacinth N. Browne, M.D.
Reproductive Biology and Medicine Branch,
National Institute of Child Health & Human
Development, Bethesda, Maryland, USA

Cristiano E. Busso
Instituto Valenciano de Infertilida, Valencia, Spain

Rafael A. Cabrera, M.D.
HOUSTON IVF,
Memorial Hermann Memorial City Hospital,
Houston, Texas, USA

Robert F. Casper, M.D., F.R.C.S.(C)
Professor, Division of Reproductive Sciences, Fran and
Lawrence Bloomberg Department of Obstetrics &
Gynecology, Senior Scientist, Samuel Lunenfeld
Research Institute, Mount Sinai Hospital,
The University of Toronto, Toronto,
Ontario, Canada, President, CAREM
(Canadian American Reproductive Medicine),
Windsor, Ontario, Canada

Charles Chapron, M.D.
Reproductive Endocrinology and Infertility,
Department of Obstetrics and Gynecology,
Hôpital Cochin, Paris, France

Ri-Cheng Chian, Ph.D.
McGill University, Department of Obstetrics and
Gynecology, Royal Victoria Hospital, Montreal,
Quebec, Canada

Patrizia Maria Ciotti, B.Sc.
Infertility and IVF Centre, University of Bologna,
Bologna, Italy

Mel Cohen, Ph.D.
Executive Director, Reproductive Medicine & Fertility
Centers, Colorado Springs, Colorado, USA
Corona Institute for Reproductive
Medicine & Fertility, Corona, California, USA
New Mexico Gynecology & Fertility Institute,
Santa Fe, New Mexico, USA

Frank Comhaire, M.D., Ph.D.
Professor Emeritus, Endocrinology-Andrology,
Ghent University Hospital, Gent, Belgium

Nieves Cremades
IVF Lab, Department of Gynecology and Obstetrics,
Academic Hospital of Alicante, Spain

Diane K. Cridennda, L.Ac.
Owner/Director, East Winds Acupuncture, Inc.,
Colorado Springs, Colorado, USA

Giuseppe Damiano, M.D.
Infertility and IVF Centre, University of Bologna,
Bologna, Italy

Alan H. DeCherney, M.D.
Branch Chief of Reproductive Biology and
Medicine Branch, National Institute of
Child Health & Human Development,
Bethesda, Maryland, USA

Aygul Demirol, M.D.
    Medical Director, CLINIC Women Health,
        Infertility and IVF Center, Ankara, Turkey

Ezgi Demirtas, M.D.
    McGill University,
        Department of Obstetrics and Gynecology,
        Royal Victoria Hospital, Montreal, Quebec, Canada

Martine De Rycke, Ph.D.
    Research Centre for Reproduction and Genetics,
        Academisch Ziekenhuis, Vrije Universiteit Brussel,
        Brussels, Belgium

Petra De Sutter, M.D., Ph.D.
    Center for Reproductive Medicine,
        Research Fellow of the Flemish Foundation for
        Scientific Research (FWO), Women's Clinic,
        Ghent University Hospital, Ghent,
        Belgium

Paul Devroey, M.D., Ph.D.
    Clinical Director,
        Research Centre for Reproduction and Genetics,
        Academisch Ziekenhuis, Vrije Universiteit Brussel,
        Brussels, Belgium, The Center for Reproductive
        Medicine, Brussels, Belgium

Dominique de Ziegler
    Joint Division of Reproductive Endocrinology and
        Infertility, Department of Obstetrics and Gynecology,
        University Hospitals of Geneva and Lausanne,
        Switzerland

Richard Palmer Dickey, M.D., Ph.D., F.A.C.O.G.
    Section of Reproductive Endocrinology,
        Department of Obstetrics and Gynecology,
        Louisiana State University School of Medicine,
        New Orleans, Louisiana, USA, Medical Director,
        The Fertility Institute of New Orleans,
        Mandeville, Louisiana, USA

Maria Dirodi, M.D.
    Infertility and IVF Centre, University of Bologna,
        Bologna, Italy

J. Domingo
    Instituto Universitario IVI, Spain

F. Domínguez
    Fundacion IVI, Instituto Universitario IVI, Universidad
        de Valencia, Valencia, Spain

Shai Elizur, M.D.
    McGill University, Department of Obstetrics and
        Gynecology, Royal Victoria Hospital, Montreal,
        Quebec, Canada

John Erian, M.B., B.Ch., F.R.C.O.G.
    Consultant Gynaecologist and Minimal Access Surgeon,
        Kent, UK

Ibrahim Esinler, M.D.
    Hacettepe University Faculty of Medicine,
        Department of Obstetrics and Gynecology,
        Ankara, Turkey

Tommaso Falcone, M.D.
    Professor and Chair,
        Department of Obstetrics & Gynecology,
        The Cleveland Clinic Foundation,
        Cleveland, Ohio, USA

Valeria Farfalli, M.D.
    S.I.S.Me.R., Reproductive Medicine Unit, Bologna, Italy

Bart C. J. M. Fauser, M.D., Ph.D.
    Professor of Reproductive Medicine, Chair,
        Department of Reproductive Medicine & Gynecology,
        Head, Division of Perinatology & Gynecology,
        University Medical Center, Utrecht, The Netherlands

Anna Pia Ferraretti, M.D., Ph.D.
    Scientific Director, S.I.S.Me.R. Reproductive Medicine
        Unit, Bologna, Italy

Gordon Lucas Fifer, M.D.
    Department of Urology, Tulane University, School of
        Medicine, New Orleans, Louisiana, USA

Timothee Fraisse, M.D.
    Joint Division of Reproductive Endocrinology and
        Infertility, Department of Obstetrics and Gynecology,
        University Hospitals of Geneva and Lausanne,
        Switzerland

S. Friedler, M.D.
    Infertility and IVF Unit, Assaf Harofeh Medical Center,
        Zerifin, Sackler School of Medicine,
        Tel-Aviv University, Tel-Aviv, Israel

Juan A. Garcia-Velasco, M.D.
    Director, IVI Madrid,
        Assistant Professor of Obstetrics and Gynecology,
        Rey Juan Carlos University, Madrid, Spain

David K. Gardner, Ph.D.
    Chair of Zoology, University of Melbourne, Australia,
        Scientific Director, Colorado Center for
        Reproductive Medicine, Englewood, Colorado, USA

Tarek A. Gelbaya, M.D.
    Department of Obstetrics and Gynaecology,
        Royal Bolton Hospital, Bolton, UK

Jan Gerris, M.D., Ph.D.
    Professor, Division of Gynecology,
        Center for Reproductive Medicine,
        Women's Clinic, University Hospital,
        Ghent, Belgium

Luca Gianaroli, M.D.
    S.I.S.MeR. Centre, Bologna, Italy

Yariv Gidoni, M.D.
McGill University, Department of Obstetrics and
Gynecology, Royal Victoria Hospital, Montreal,
Quebec, Canada

Raúl Gomez, M.D.
Universidad de Valencia, Valencia, Spain

Alfredo Guillén
IVI-Madrid, Spain

Timor Gurgan, M.D.
Professor, Hacettepe University,
Department of OB/GYN, Reproductive Endocrinology
and IVF Unit, Academic Director,
CLINIC Women Health, Infertility and IVF Center,
Ankara, Turkey

Levent Gurkan, M.D.
Department of Urology, Tulane University,
School of Medicine, New Orleans,
Lousiana, USA

Julie Hazelton
Division of Reproductive Endocrinolgy and Infertility,
Department of Obstetrics and Gynecology,
University of South Alabama, Mobile,
Alabama, USA

Wayne J. G. Hellstrom, M.D., F.A.C.S.
Professor, Department of Urology, Tulane University,
School of Medicine, New Orleans, Lousiana, USA

Ahmet Helvacioglu, M.D., F.A.C.O.G.
Obstetrics and Gynecology, Fairhope, Alabama, USA

Timothy N. Hickman, M.D.
Medical Director, Houston IVF, Memorial Hermann
Memorial City Hospital, Houston, Texas, USA

James Hole, D.O., F.A.C.O.G.
Division of Maternal Fetal Medicine,
Department of Obstetrics and Gynecology,
University of South Alabama, Mobile, Alabama, USA

Scherri B. Holland, R. N.
Division of Reproductive Endocrinolgy and Infertility,
Department of Obstetrics and Gynecology,
University of South Alabama, Mobile,
Alabama, USA

Hananel Holzer, M.D.
McGill University, Department of Obstetrics and
Gynecology, Royal Victoria Hospital, Montreal,
Quebec, Canada

Amjad Hossain, Ph.D., H.C.L.D.
Assistant Professor and Director, Andrology and ART
Laboratory Services, Division of Reproductive
Endocrinology and Infertility, Department of
Obstetrics and Gynecology, University of Texas
Medical Branch, Galveston, Texas, USA

Ziad R. Hubayter, M.D.
Department of Gynecology and Obstetrics,
Division of Reproductive Endocrinology and Infertility,
The Johns Hopkins University, Baltimore,
Maryland, USA

Chris A. Huff
Division of Reproductive Endocrinology and Infertility,
Department of Obstetrics and Gynecology,
University of South Alabama, Mobile,
Alabama, USA

Hesham Al Inany, M.D.
Department of Obstetrics and Gynaecology,
Cairo University, Egyptian IVF-ET Centre,
Cairo, Egypt

Howard W. Jones, Jr.
Emeritus Professor, Eastern Virginia Medical School,
Founder of the Jones Institute,
Norfolk, Virginia, USA

Nadia Kabli, M.D.
Fellow of Reproductive Endocrinology and Infertility,
McGill University, Montreal, Quebec, Canada

E. Kasterstein
Infertility and IVF Unit,
Assaf Harofeh Medical Center, Zerifin,
Sackler School of Medicine, Tel-Aviv
University, Tel-Aviv, Israel

Ruth Kennedy, C.R.N.P.
IVF Coordinator, Division of Reproductive
Endocrinology and Infertility,
Department of Obstetrics and Gynecology,
University of South Alabama, Mobile,
Alabama, USA

Alexis H. Kim
Fertility Physicians of Northern California, Palo Alto,
California, USA

D. Komarovsky
Infertility and IVF Unit, Assaf Harofeh Medical Center,
Zerifin, Sackler School of Medicine, Tel-Aviv
University, Tel-Aviv, Israel

T. F. Kruger, M.D.
Reproductive Biology Unit, Department of
Obstetrics and Gynecology,
University of Stellenbosch and TygerBerg Hospital,
TygerBerg, South Africa

Michela Lappi
Medicine via pazzani, Bologna, Italy

Mariano Lavolpe, M.Sc.
Associate Director IVF Laboratory,
Center for Studies in Gynecology and
Reproduction (CEGYR), Buenos Aires,
Argentina

N. S. Macklon, M.B.Ch.B., M.D.
Department of Reproductive Medicine and Gynecology,
University Medical Center, Utrecht, The Netherlands

Paul C. Magarelli, M.D., Ph.D.
Owner/Medical Director, Reproductive Medicine &
Fertility Centers, Colorado Springs, Colorado, USA
Associate Professor, University of New Mexico,
Department of Obstetrics & Gynecology,
Albuquerque, New Mexico, USA

M. Cristina Magli, M.Sc., S.I.S.Me.R.
Reproductive Medicine Unit, Bologna, Italy

Ahmed Mahmoud, M.D., Ph.D.
Laboratory of Andrology, Ghent University Hospital,
Gent, Belgium

Antonis Makrigiannakis, M.D.
Professor of Obstetrics and Gynecology,
Laboratory of Human Reproduction,
Department of Obstetrics and Gynaecology,
University of Crete, Crete, Greece

Suketu M. Mansuria, M.D.
Assistant Professor of Obstetrics, Gynecology and
Reproductive Sciences, Division of Minimally Invasive
Gynecologic Surgery, University of Pittsburgh Medical
Center, Magee-Womens Hospital, Pittsburgh,
Pennsylvania, USA

Claire Mazoyer, M.D.
Laboratory of Hormonology and Tumor Markers,
Department of Clinical Chemistry/Anatomopathology,
University Hospital Free University Brussels,
Brussels, Belgium

Laurie J. McKenzie, M.D., F.A.C.O.G
Houston IVF, Houston, Texas, USA

Ioannis E. Messinis
Department of Obstetrics and Gynecology,
University of Thessalia, Larissa, Greece

Sameh Mikhail, M.D.
Department of Medicine, Rochester General Hospital,
Rochester, New York, USA

Mohamed F. M. Mitwally, M.D.
Clinical Assistant Professor,
Division of Reproductive Endocrinology & Infertility,
Department of Obstetrics and Gynecology,
University of New Mexico, Albuquerque,
New Mexico, USA
Reproductive Endocrinologist,
RMFC (Reproductive Medicine and Fertility Center),
Colorado Springs, Colorado, USA

David Mortimer, Ph.D.
President, Oozoa Biomedical, Inc.,
West Vancouver, British Columbia,
Canada

Sharon T. Mortimer
Oozoa Biomedical, Inc., West Vancouver,
British Columbia, Canada

Hany F. Moustafa, M.D.
Fellow, Division of Reproductive Endocrinology
and Infertility, Department of Obstetrics
and Gynecology, University of South Alabama,
Mobile, Alabama, USA,
Alabama Lecturer, Suez Canal University,
Ismailia, Egypt

Suheil J. Muasher, M.D.
Department of Gynecology and Obstetrics,
Division of Reproductive Endocrinology and Infertility,
Johns Hopkins University,
Baltimore, Maryland, USA, Director,
The Muasher Center for Fertility and IVF,
Fairfax, Virginia, USA, Department of Obstetrics and
Gynecology, Johns George Washington University,
Washington, DC, USA, Department of Obstetrics and
Gynecology, Virginia Commonwealth University,
Richmond, Virginia, USA

Santiago Munnè, Ph.D.
Reprogenetics, Paramus, New Jersey, USA

Manubai Nagamani, M.D.
Professor and Chief, Division of Reproductive
Endocrinology and Infertility,
Department of Obstetrics and Gynecology,
University of Texas Medical Branch,
Galveston, Texas, USA

Zsolt Peter Nagy, M.D., Ph.D., H.C.L.D.
Scientific and Laboratory Director,
Reproductive Biology Associates, Atlanta,
Georgia, USA

Luciano G. Nardo, M.D.
Department of Reproductive Medicine, St Mary's Hospital,
Division of Human Development,
University of Manchester, Manchester, UK

Mary George Nawar, M.D., M.R.C.Oph.
Department of Obstetrics and Gynecology,
University of South Alabama, Mobile,
Alabama, USA

Camran Nezhat, M.D., F.A.C.O.G., F.A.C.S.
Fellowship Director,
Center for Special Minimally Invasive Surgery,
Past President, Society of Laparoendoscopic Surgeons,
Clinical Professor of OB/GYN(Adj),
Clinical Professor of Surgery(Adj), Stanford
University Medical School, Stanford University,
Palo Alto, California, USA

Florencia Nodar, M.Sc.
Director, IVF Laboratory, Center for Studies in
Gynecology and Reproduction (CEGYR),
Buenos Aires, Argentina

Anastasios Pachydakis, M.D., D.F.F.P., M.R.C.O.G.
    Specialist Registrar Obstetrics and Gynaecologist,
        Princess Royal University Hospital UK,
        Sidcup, UK

Antonio Pellicer
    Professor, IVI, Instituto Valenciano de Infertilidad,
        Valencia, Spain

M. E. Poo, C., M.D.
    Spanish Stem Cell Bank, Prince Felipe Research Center,
        University of Valencia, IVI Foundation, University of
        Valencia, Valencia, Spain

Eleonora Porcu, M.D.
    Director, Infertility and IVF Center, University of Bologna,
        Bologna, Italy

Kathy B. Porter, M.D., M.B.A.
    Professor and Chair, Department of Obstetrics and
        Gynecology, University of South Alabama, Mobile,
        Alabama, USA

Marc Princivalle, Ph.D.
    Target Validation, Ferring Research Ltd, Southampton, UK

Guillermo Quea
    IVI-Madrid, Spain

Caroline Ragheb
    University of Alabama, School of Medicine, Birmingham,
        Alabama, USA

Nasir Rana, M.D., M.P.H., F.A.C.O.G.
    Associate Director, Oak Brook Institute of Endoscopy,
        Oak Brook, Illinois, USA, Assistant Professor,
        Rush Medical College, Chicago, Illinois, USA

Vanesa Y. Rawe, M.Sc., Ph.D.
    Director, Basic Research Laboratory,
        Center for Studies in Gynecology and Reproduction
        (CEGYR), Buenos Aires, Argentina

A. Raziel
    Infertility and IVF Unit, Assaf Harofeh Medical Center,
        Zerifin, Sackler School of Medicine, Tel-Aviv
        University, Tel-Aviv, Israel

Robert W. Rebar, M.D.
    Executive Director, American Society for Reproductive
        Medicine, Volunteer Professor, Department of
        Obstetrics and Gynecology, University of Alabama,
        Birmingham, Alabama, USA

S. Reis
    Instituto Universitario IVI, Madrid, Spain

J. Remohí
    Instituto Universitario IVI, Madrid, Spain

Antonio Requena
    IVI-Madrid, Spain

Botros R. M. B. Rizk, M.D., M.A., F.R.C.O.G., F.R.C.S.(C),
    H.C.L.D., F.A.C.O.G., F.A.C.S.
    Professor and Head, Division of Reproductive
        Endocrinology and Infertility,
        Department of Obstetrics and Gynecology,
        University of South Alabama,
        Medical and Scientific Director, USA
        ART program, Mobile, Alabama, USA

Christine B. Rizk
    John Emory Scholar, Emory University, Atlanta,
        Georgia, USA

Christopher B. Rizk
    Rice University, Houston, Texas, USA

David B. Rizk
    Research Assistant, Department of Obstetrics and
        Gynecology, University of South Alabama,
        College of Medicine, Mobile,
        Alabama, USA

A. Rolaki
    Laboratory of Human Reproduction,
        Department of Obstetrics and Gynaecology,
        Medical School, University of Crete, Crete,
        Greece

R. Ron-El, M.D.
    Professor and Head of Fertility and IVF Unit,
        Assaf Harofe Medical Center, Tel-Aviv University,
        Zerifin, Israel

Carlos Rotman, M.D., F.A.C.O.G.
    Director, Oak Brook Institute of Endoscopy,
        Oak Brook, Illinois, USA,
        Associate Professor, Rush Medical College,
        Chicago, Illinois, USA

Rosália Sá
    Lab Cell Biology, ICBAS, University of Porto,
        Porto, Portugal

Jean Clair Sadeu, M.D.
    Follicle Biology Laboratory, Vrije Universiteit Brussel
        (VUB), Brussels, Belgium

Hassan N. Sallam, M.D., F.R.C.O.G., Ph.D. (London)
    Director, The Suzanne Mubarak Regional Centre for
        Women's Health and Development, Professor,
        Obstetrics and Gynaecology, University of Alexandria,
        Alexandria, Egypt

Joseph S. Sanfilippo, M.D., M.B.A.
    Professor of Obstetrics,
        Gynecology and Reproductive Sciences,
        Division of Reproductive Endocrinology &
        Infertility & Minimally Invasive Gynecologic Surgery,
        Vice Chairman, Division of Reproductive Sciences,
        University of Pittsburgh Medical Center,
        Magee-Womens Hospital, Pittsburgh,
        Pennsylvania, USA

Jonathan G. Scammell, Ph.D.
  Professor, Pharmacology and Chair Comparative
    Medicine, University of South Alabama
    College of Medicine, Mobile, Alabama, USA

M. Schachter
  Infertility and IVF Unit,
    Assaf Harofeh Medical Center,
    Zerifin, Sackler School of Medicine,
    Tel-Aviv University, Tel-Aviv, Israel

A. Michele Schuler, D.V.M., Ph.D.
  Department of Comparative Medicine,
    University of South Alabama, Mobile, Alabama, USA

Gamal I. Serour, F.R.C.O.G., F.R.C.S.
  Professor of Obstetrics and Gynecology,
    Director, International Islamic Center of Population
    Studies and Research, Al-Azhar University, Former
    Dean of Al-Azhar University, Clinical Director,
    The Egyptian IVF & ET Center, Maadi, Cairo, Egypt

Françoise Shenfield, L.R.C.P., M.R.C.S., M.A.
  Reproductive Medicine Unit,
    University College Hospital,
    London, UK

Jennifer Shinners, M.D.
  Department of Obstetrics and Gynecology,
    State University of New York,
    Upstate Medical University, Syracuse,
    New York, USA

Frances Shue, M.D.
  Department of Obstetrics and Gynecology,
    State University of New York,
    Upstate Medical University, Syracuse,
    New York, USA

Sherman J. Silber, M.D.
  Infertility Center of St. Louis, St. Luke Hospital,
    St. Louis, Missouri, USA

Joaquina Silva
  Centre for Reproductive Genetics, Porto, Portugal

Carlos Simón, M.D.
  Spanish Stem Cell Bank, Prince Felipe Research Center,
    University of Valencia, IVI Foundation,
    University of Valencia, Valencia, Spain

Johan Smitz, M.D., Ph.D.
  Laboratory of Hormonology and Tumor Markers,
    Department of Clinical Chemistry/Anatomopathology,
    University Hospital Free University Brussels,
    Brussels, Belgium

Jonathan Y. Song, M.D., F.A.C.O.G.
  Oak Brook Institute of Endoscopy, Oak Brook,
    Illinois, USA, Assistant Professor,
    Rush Medical College, Chicago,
    Illinois, USA

Mário Sousa, M.D., Ph.D.
  Specialist of Laboratorial Medicine of Reproduction,
    Director, Lab Cell Biology,
    Inst. Biomedical Sciences Abel Salazar,
    University of Porto, Porto,
    Portugal

Samuel J. Strada, Ph.D.
  Dean, College of Medicine,
    Professor of Pharmacology
    University of South Alabama,
    Mobile, Alabama, USA

D. Strassburger
  Infertility and IVF Unit,
    Assaf Harofeh Medical Center,
    Zerifin, Sackler School of Medicine,
    Tel-Aviv University, Tel-Aviv, Israel

Carlos E. Sueldo, M.D., F.A.C.O.G.
  Clinical Professor, University of California
    San Francisco-Fresno, Fresno,
    California, USA
    Senior Consultant,
    Oak Brook Institute of Endoscopy,
    Oak Brook, Illinois, USA
    Center for Studies in Gynecology and Reproduction,
    Buenos Aires, Argentina, USA

Eric S. Surrey, M.D.
  Medical Director,
    Colorado Center for Reproductive Medicine,
    Englewood, Colorado, USA

Alastair Sutcliffe, M.D., M.R.C.P., F.R.C.P.C.H.
  Senior Lecturer in Child Health,
    Honorary Consultant, Institute of Child Health,
    Royal Free and University of Medical School,
    University of College London,
    Department of Community Child Health,
    London, UK

Seang Lin Tan, M.D., M.B.B.S., F.R.C.O.G., F.R.C.S.C.,
    M.med. (O&G), M.B.A.
  Professor and Chair, McGill University,
    Department of Obstetrics and Gynecology,
    Royal Victoria Hospital Montreal, Quebec, Canada

Biljana Popovic Todorovic
  The Center for Reproductive Medicine, Brussels,
    Belgium

Togas Tulandi, M.D., M.H.C.M.
  Professor of Obstetrics and Gynecology,
    Milton Leong Chair in Reproductive Medicine,
    McGill University, Montreal, Quebec, Canada

Evert J. P. Van Santbrink, M.D., Ph.D.
  Division of Reproductive Medicine,
    Department of Obstetrics and Gynecology,
    Dijkzigt Academic Hospital, Rotterdam,
    The Netherlands

Stefano Venturoli, M.D.
    Infertility and IVF Centre,
        University of Bologna,
        Bologna, Italy

A. Watrelot, M.D.
    CRES (Centre de Recherche et d'Etude de la Sterílíte),
        Lyon, France

Hakan Yarali, M.D., Ph.D.
    Hacettepe University Faculty of Medicine,
        Department of Obstetrics and Gynecology,
        Ankara, Turkey

Edgardo Yordan
    Oak Brook Institute of Endoscopy, Oak Brook,
        Illinois, USA

■ FOREWORD ■

Howard W. Jones, Jr.

This text on infertility and assisted reproduction is truly international. There are authors from 18 nations. This reflects the widespread availability of assisted reproductive technology (ART) and indicates that experts are found worldwide. Indeed, in a compilation of legislation and guidelines concerning ART, sponsored by the International Federation of Fertility Societies and published as a supplement to *Fertility and Sterility* in 2007 under the title "Surveillance 07," it was noted that two-thirds of the world's population lived in countries where ART is available. To be sure, it needs to be added that accessibility within various countries varies widely.

"Surveillance 07" also found that there was a wide variation among nations in what society really wished to survey and control. Indeed, this variation has had some interesting and unexpected consequences. For example:

■ In Italy, cryopreservation of fertilized eggs is prohibited. This has stimulated investigation into the improvement of cryopreservation or vitrification for oocytes (see chapter by Porcu).

■ In Belgium, among those qualified for insurance coverage provided by the government, no more than a single fertilized egg can be transferred in the first IVF attempt, provided the patient is younger than 36 years of age. This has provided and given stimulus to the evaluation of elective single embryo transfer (eSET). It turns out that eSET offers a good pregnancy rate and largely eliminates multiples (see chapter by Gerris).

The complete physician does not practice medicine like a cook who depends on a cookbook to prepare a special dish.

To be sure, the physician needs practical knowledge, but the complete physician also must know the underlying physiology and pathology of the problem at hand in order to select the best solution. Thus, this new text can make the physician complete. For example, as to the matter of implantation after transfer of a fertilized egg, this text addresses the practical (see chapter by deZiegler) aspects and the molecular aspect (see chapter by Simon).

To understand controlled ovarian hyperstimulation prior to IVF, it is necessary to understand the basic physiology (see chapters by Makrigiannakis and Messinis). Only with this information can one understand the ins and outs of the various types of stimulation and the response thereto (see chapters by Fauser, Macklon, Aboulghar, and Nardo).

Reproductive medicine in contrast to other subspecialties deals with hot-button ethical and public policy issues simply because it deals with reproduction, which society regards as special and different. The complete physician must understand the patient's concerns in this area (see chapter by Shenfeld).

All in all, the physician can become complete by having this text at hand.

◼ PREFACE ◼

Samuel J. Strada, Ph.D.

The readers of this text will encounter a comprehensive and perspicacious view of the discipline of reproductive medicine as revealed by leaders in their respective fields. The editors have assembled a talented group of authors spanning six geographic continents. Some sections of the book – for example, its second section on infertility – are comprehensive enough to stand on their own. The section begins with the evolution of the female and covers in detail the roles of endoscopy, hysteroscopy, and laparoscopy in the management of infertility. The following section deals with ultrasonography of both the female and male, which is followed by a cutting-edge section on the evaluation of the infertile male, beginning with standards of current clinical management and ending with future implications for developing DNA technology. Subsequent sections focus on the physiology of ovulation and the pharmacological agents prescribed by gynecologists today, in addition to a discussion of future pharmacological advances that have the potential to significantly alter treatment strategies. Other clinical areas discussed include the medical management of endometriosis, the relationship of polycystic ovaries to infertility, and the status of premature ovarian failure. A comprehensive assessment on the state of the art in assisted reproduction is detailed in the third section of the book. This is the expertise of one of its editors, Dr. Botros R. M. B. Rizk, so it is perhaps not too surprising that this topic did receive significant attention. More esoteric topics, or at least topics that are not usually found in texts of this genre, include cryobiology, herbal Chinese medicine and assisted reproductive technology (ART), various congenital malformations and chromosomal abnormalities associated with ART, and a concluding section entitled "Ethical Dilemmas in Fertility and Assisted Reproduction," which evaluates stem cell research from scientific, legal, and religious perspectives. In other words, there is something in this textbook for everyone interested in reproductive biology, whether a novice or an expert in the field.

■ INTRODUCTION ■

Botros R. M. B. Rizk, Juan A. Garcia-Velasco, Hassan N. Sallam, Antonis Makrigiannakis

The past three decades have witnessed a transformation in reproductive medicine from science fiction to one of the most advanced medical disciplines. Our textbook is a confirmation of the tremendous achievements in scientific research that changed the course of our clinical practice. Thirty years of in vitro fertilization (IVF) was celebrated this year in Alexandria, honoring Robert Edwards specifically. More than four million IVF babies have been born worldwide. The doors that were opened by Robert Edwards and Patrick Steptoe lead to many miracles. Intracytoplasmic sperm injection, in vitro maturation, oocyte vitrification, pre-implantation genetic diagnosis, and ovarian transplantation are dreams that were fulfilled. Many couples still have no hope of having their own families and demand us to keep moving forward.

The authors of the chapters of this book have lead the world for the three decades. They contributed their finest and most advanced research. We find in every one of them a sincere desire to uphold the ethics and the respect in our society. The friendship and cordiality between them has been amazing. They represented the six continents truly, and many of them have worked in more than one continent. It is not surprising that they worked together in such an elegant and a unique way. The different chapters are individualized in style, but the spirit of the book has united them. From reproductive physiology to surgery and assisted reproduction, the authors move with great elegance. The ethical and moral issues have been thoughtfully considered. To every author we acknowledge his or her expertise and admire and enjoy their friendship. We place in your hands, our readers, a text that covers the present state of the art and gives you a glimpse of the future, confirming your instincts and stimulating your desire for knowledge. We hope that you enjoy reading it as we have enjoyed editing it.

PART I

PHYSIOLOGY OF REPRODUCTION

FOLLICULOGENESIS: FROM PREANTRAL FOLLICLES TO CORPUS LUTEUM REGRESSION

Antonis Makrigiannakis, A. Rolaki

INTRODUCTION

The most common function of the female gonad is to produce gametes, the oocytes, and sex hormones, such as estrogens and progesterone, which control the development of the female secondary sexual characteristics and support pregnancy. These two functions are exerted cyclically between puberty and the menopause, and they are regulated by diverse endocrine and paracrine factors acting on many cell types situated in the ovary. Ovarian functions result from the evolution of a morphological unit, the ovarian follicle, which consists of a central oocyte surrounded by granulosa cells and other layers of somatic theca cells (1). The maturation of the follicle proceeds through primordial, primary, and secondary stages of development and is controlled by various factors produced in the ovary. The main physiological stimulants for differentiation and luteinization of granulosa cells, which are a main cellular component of the follicle, are the gonadotropin hormones, follicle-stimulating hormone (FSH), and luteinizing hormone (LH). Throughout the reproductive life span of the female, only limited number of follicles will reach the stage of Graafian follicle and will ovulate, whereas the vast majority is gradually eliminated through a process called atresia. In every menstrual cycle, only one follicle, named the dominant follicle, is destined to complete maturation and ovulate, and thus, the formation of the multiple embryos during pregnancy is prevented.

Degeneration of the old corpus luteum is a process essential for maintaining the normal production of progesterone in every menstrual cycle. The complexity of the interrelation of the events that control oocyte growth and ultimate acquisition of developmental competence is under continuous investigation (2). It is generally believed that follicular atresia and luteolysis occur by mechanisms that accompany a highly organized type of cell death, called programmed cell death or apoptosis (3). The present review reports a variety of factors involved in the different stages of follicular development. Elucidation of the mechanisms that regulate follicular development may lead to the prevention of female reproductive disorders or other pathological conditions and to the development of new culture methods for oocytes for in vitro fertilization.

PREOVULATORY FOLLICLE

The development of preantral follicles involves oocyte enlargement, zona pellucida formation, extensive granulosa cell proliferation, formation of a basal lamina, condensation of stromal cells around the basal lamina to form the theca layer, and the development of fluid-filled spaces that gradually coalesce to form the antral cavity (4, 5). In the absence of appropriate gonadotropic stimulation, follicles develop until the early antral stage and atresia occurs.

The early stages of follicular development, including the early antral follicle, are independent of the FSH and the luteinizing hormone (LH). In agreement with these findings is the study of Touraine et al., which shows that inactivation of FSH receptor does not disrupt the follicular growth to the large preantral stages (6). The low responsiveness of antral follicles to gonadotropins results presumably by the low number of gonadotropin receptors on follicle cells at this stage of development, although it is believed that anti-Mullerian hormone (AMH) reduces the FSH responsiveness of preantral and small antral follicles (7). However, the preantral follicle is affected by other nongonadotropic factors, such as members of the TGF-β family, estrogens, androgens, insulin, and insulin-like growth factor-1 (6, 1). The follicles at the preantral stage are shown to produce very low amounts of progesterone, and androstenedione and no estradiol production is detectable (8) and possesses only faint aromatizing capacity.

A Graafian or antral follicle measures 0.4–2.3 mm in diameter and is characterized by a cavity of antrum containing a fluid termed follicular fluid. The development of the antral cavity begins with the formation of a cavity on the one pole of the oocyte. After antrum formation, the development of the follicle precipitates, and in sixty days, the follicle reaches the preovulatory stage. The size of an antral follicle is mainly determined by the size of the antral cavity and the proliferation rate of the follicle cells. In a dominant follicle, for example, extremely rapid proliferation of granulosa and theca cells occurs, and therefore, the dominant follicle is correlatively bigger in size than any other follicle during the follicular phase of the cycle.

During antrum development, the follicles acquire capillary networks, located in the theca interna and externa. The blood vessels increase in number and size as follicular development proceeds but do not penetrate the basal membrane (9). It is believed that VEGF, a mitogenic factor, is involved in angiogenesis process and thus in antral cavity formation, through VEGF receptors. It has been shown that inhibition of VEGF results in decreased follicle angiogenesis, reduced recruitment, and growth of antral follicles in the primate. VEGF is also thought to be involved in the ovulatory process, as other studies correlate the VEGF with local factors involved in ovulation (10). Furthermore, suppression of VEGF in the developing follicle is associated with inhibition of follicular angiogenesis and antral follicular development, which results in the inhibition of ovulation (11, 12).

FSH is considered to be the fundamental driver of folliculogenesis. During the normal menstrual cycle, elevated FSH levels in the early follicular phase stimulate recruitment and growth of preantral and small antral follicles. In the mid- and late follicular phases, however, the decline of FSH concentrations and a progressive rise of LH levels are associated with the selection and growth of the dominant follicle destined for ovulation. Gonadotropins are even used in controlled ovarian stimulation (COS), which is an important component of assisted reproduction technology (ART). Particularly, exogenous FSH administration, alone or with variable amounts of LH activity, causes a rise of FSH concentrations throughout the follicular phase, so that the development of multiple ovarian follicles and oocytes is achieved (13). However, recent studies have shown that selective addition of LH activity, in the form of low-dose hCG, can replace mid- or late follicular phases' FSH administration (14).

CORPUS LUTEUM

Following ovulation, under the influence of luteogenic hormones, the corpus luteum (CL) develops from the remnants of the ovulated ovarian follicle. This process called luteinization and the stimulus for its initiation, the preovulatory LH surge, are common among species. The morphological events underlying this process involve intense reorganization of constituent cells, particularly granulosa cells, phenomena that includes varying cell-matrix interactions. These events, however, are poorly characterized. After expulsion of the oocyte, the blood capillaries of the theca rapidly invade the granulosa, thereby provoking the transformation of these cells (luteinization) and the formation of the CL. The blood vessels completely traverse the granulosa and open up in the follicular cavity. The granulosa cells are transformed into large luteal cells whose ultrastructure is the same as that of steroidogenic cells. The main hormone product of the CL is progesterone, which induces the necessary endometrial modifications required for the acquisition of a receptive state, an anticipation of embryo implantation. The life span of the CL is limited. In a nonfertile cycle, corpora lutea regress at the end of the menstrual cycle and are eliminated by a process called luteolysis. If pregnancy does occur, regression must be inhibited since the CL is the main source of steroidogenesis, supporting the establishment and maintenance of a successful pregnancy. Although some of the biochemical and endocrine events characterizing the formation and regression of CL have been well established, the molecular aspects underlying luteinized granulosa cell (GC) migration and survival and the endocrine/paracrine mechanisms by which LH and hCG act on GCs to transform the ruptured follicle into the CL are not well characterized. A number of studies have shown that cell-cell adhesion is strongly correlated with maturation and integrity of CL (15). It is also believed that VEGF and its receptor Flt-1, which is expressed on luteinizing GCs (Figure 1.1), are involved in CL development. Recent studies, in a rat model, have shown that suppression of VEGF resulted in nearly complete

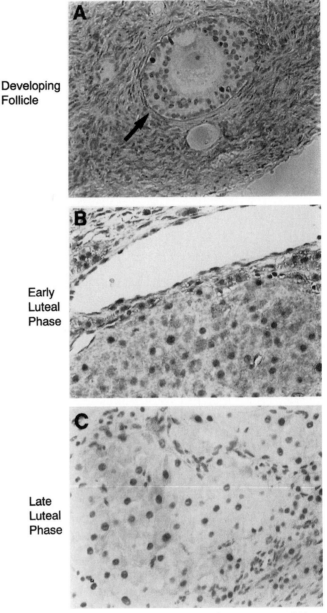

Developing Follicle

Early Luteal Phase

Late Luteal Phase

Figure 1.1. In situ staining of ovarian tissue for expression of Flt-1. Ovarian tissue was stained with antibodies against Flt-1 to determine its expression in developing follicles and during CL formation and regression. Flt-1 was not detected in developing follicles (A, arrows) but was present on the GCs of early luteal phase (B), expression that was not evident during the late luteal phase (C). (magnification: ×400).

suppression of CL formation (16). Our unpublished data extend these observations and support the idea that hCG promotes the migration and survival of human luteinized GCs, through a VEGF-dependent mechanism. Particularly, the following model is proposed (Figure 1.2): The binding of luteogenic hormone (LH or hCG) to GCs triggers their release of VEGF and induces the surface expression of VEGFR on these cells. The released VEGF (and possibly VEGF from other sources) in turn binds to the newly expressed VEGFR on the GCs, stimulating the secretion of FN into the surrounding matrix and upregulating the surface expression of at least two FN-binding

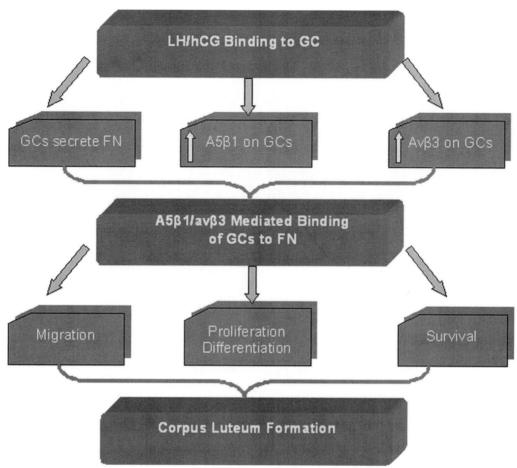

Figure 1.2. Proposed mechanism for the involvement of fibronectin and two of its integrin ligands in CL formation and their regulation by hCG through VEGF in this process.

integrins, $\alpha_5\beta_1$ and $\alpha_v\beta_3$. Subsequent interactions between FN and these integrins trigger adhesive events and intracellular signaling cascades involved in promoting the migration, survival, and differentiation of GCs, activities that contribute ultimately to the formation and/or persistence of the CL. Relative to atresia, little is known about luteolysis and the mechanisms that are involved in this process. Apoptosis seems to be the mechanism of CL regression in humans (17). While apoptosis is present already in the early CL, it is significantly increased in the late CL when luteal regression takes place (18). The Bcl-2 family members have been shown to play a central role in this process (19, 20).

Apoptosis and Apoptosis-Related Genes

It has been mentioned before that apoptosis or programmed cell death is an essential process in maintaining ovarian homeostasis in mammals and plays a prominent role in the development of fetal ovaries and in the postnatal ovarian cycle (21). It ensures that in every estrus/menstrus cycle, only one or very few follicles will ovulate. This process minimizes the possibility of multiple embryos during pregnancy. The rest of the follicles are gradually eliminated during the fertility period of the female. The apoptotic process of the old corpora lutea is essential for preserving the cyclicity and for ensuring the release of progesterone during the estrus/menstrus cycle (22). Furthermore,

recent studies have shown that apoptosis of granulosa cells affects the conception in ovulation induction cycle (23) and that might explain the etiology of unexplained infertility (24). As is the case with other major organ systems, an evolutionarily conserved framework of genes and signaling pathways has been implicated in determining whether or not ovarian germ cells and somatic cells will die in response to either developmental cues or pathological insults. Therefore, it has been suggested that some apoptosis-related genes may have a role in ovarian follicular growth and atresia. The p53 gene is one of the most highly investigated tumor suppressor genes, and it seems to be a key player in apoptosis (25). The basic action of p53 is to protect the cellular genome from a variety of deleterious stimuli, such as reactive oxygen species and ionizing radiation. p53 is a transcriptional factor, which has the ability to alter the activity of target genes, an action that can be modulated by another antioncogenic protein, the product of the Wilms' tumour suppressor gene (WT1) (26). Regarding p53, nuclear accumulation of this tumor suppressor protein has been documented in GCs of follicles destined for atresia in the rat ovary, whereas in vivo gonadotropin priming inhibits granulosa cell apoptosis with a concomitant suppression of p53 immunoreactivity (27). These initial investigations have since been confirmed and extended by a number of laboratories, collectively supporting the hypothesis that nuclear translocation of p53 in GCs heralds their demise during follicular atresia (28).

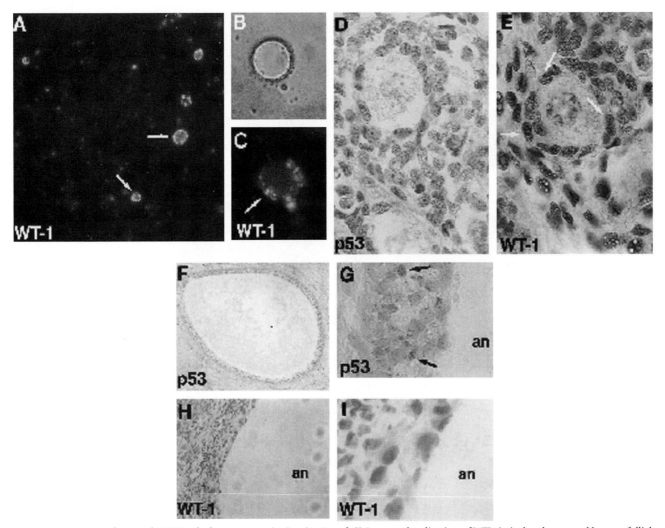

Figure 1.3. Expression of p53 and WT1 in the human ovary in situ. (A, B, and C) Immunolocalization of WT1 in isolated preantral human follicles. Human preantral follicles were isolated from ovarian biopsy specimens and immunostained for WT1. Under low magnification (A), multiple preantral follicles of varying sizes *(arrow*s) can be seen surrounded by WT1-positive GCs. Under high magnification (B, phase contrast), remaining adherent GCs stain intensely for WT1 (C, *arrow*). Immunohistochemical detection of p53 (D) and WT1 (E) in fetal human ovary in situ. Note that p53 staining is absent (D) in contrast to the very strong staining of WT1 in almost all GCs (E, *arrow*s). Immunohistochemical detection of p53 in an atretic follicle (F) and at a higher magnification (G); WT1 staining (H) and at a higher magnification (I) in an atretic follicle. Note that in the representative atretic follicle, p53 nuclear staining and some cytoplasmic staining were present in many GCs (G, *arrow*) in contrast to the absence of WT1 (H and I) in an antrum. Magnification: A and F, ×3100; B and C, ×3600; D, E, G, and I, ×3400; H, ×3200.

That p53 serves a similar function in the human ovary is suggested by the findings of p53 expression in the human ovary and isolated granulosa cells (29), as well as by recent studies on the ability of overexpressed p53 to induce apoptosis in transformed human granulosa cell lines (30). However, the spatial localization of p53 in the human ovary during follicular development and the regulation of tumor suppressor gene expression in nontransformed human GCs remain to be determined. Evidence linking these two important members of the tumor suppressor gene family, p53 and WT1, to ovarian follicular growth and atresia has been provided (31). It was shown that the p53 gene is expressed in GCs and is closely related to their survival. This apoptosis-inducing gene is reduced by treatment with exogenous gonadotropin in vivo (27), suggesting that p53 may play an important role in regulating follicular survival during gonadotropin-dependent stages of follicular life or maintenance of luteal cells during pregnancy. WT1, a known transcriptional regulator of p53, is also expressed in human GCs (31). Data that we have published indicate that this gene is constitutively expressed in human granulosa cells and its expression remains strong during early stages of development but progressively declines during gonadotrophin-dependent follicular maturation. These data suggest a possible implication of WT1 in the mechanisms responsible for the maintenance of a quiescent state in follicles during gonadotropin-independent stages of follicular life (31) (Figure 1.3). Many p53-regulated target genes have been identified, including the *bcl-2* prosurvival gene, the *bax* proapoptotic gene, and several reduction-oxidation genes. In particular, it is believed that interaction among pro- and antiapoptotic members of the bcl-2 family in the mitochondrion determines whether or not the apoptotic pathways are activated. This interaction regulates release of cytochrome *c* from the mitochondrion into the cytosol, which activates caspase-9 and downstream caspases, including caspase-3 (32). Bcl-2 gene was first discovered by its involvement in B-cell malignancies. A growing number of studies have implicated this proto-oncogene in apoptotic events of ovarian follicles in the different developmental stages. In the recent years, it has been demonstrated that Bcl-2 is an important factor in regulating apoptosis of human GCs (33), but the role of Bcl-2 in ovarian function remains to be fully elucidated. Bax gene is another member of the bcl-2 gene family, which can induce apoptosis through inactivation of bcl-2 in cells. Targeted disruption of the bax gene in mice leads to a defect in the ability of GCs to undergo apoptosis during follicular atresia (34), while a reduction in bax levels was correlated with gonadotropin-mediated follicular survival in rat GCs (27). Bax has also been detected in human apoptotic GCs, but not in healthy follicles (29), even though its precise role in the development and apoptosis of human follicles is not yet understood.

Role of Steroids

Sex steroids play an important role in the development of the ovarian follicle and in the preservation of fertility in women (35). In the ovary, steroids are produced by theca and granulosa cells, and this process is induced by gonadotropins. The well-known "two-cell, two-gonadotrophin" theory emphasizes the fact that stimulation of both theca cells by LH and granulosa cells by FSH is required for estradiol synthesis. Progesterone (P4) is one of the major steroids secreted by the ovary, and it is synthesized by preantral follicles. The rate of secretion is increased while follicular development proceeds, and many studies have shown the importance of these high P4 levels in regulating ovulation (36). It has been suggested that progesterone, and other ovarian steroids, may act upon the ovary in part through influences on cGMP concentrations (37). Progesterone production is induced by LH as it has been shown in rat and porcine cultured GCs, whereas progesterone antagonist, RU486, inhibits luteinization of GCs coming from preovulatory follicles (38). Moreover, it has recently been indicated that progesterone is involved in stimulating ovulation in human ovarian follicles (39), probably by inducing production of proteolytic enzymes, important for ovulating process. Progesterone also acts through the progesterone receptor to inhibit GC/luteal cell apoptosis (40). We have also shown that RU486 triggers apoptosis in human GC. Androgens are produced by theca cells in response to LH and exert their actions via receptors localized to secondary and dominant follicles in human. Prenatal testosterone treatment in ewes indicates an enhancement in follicular development (41), whereas treatment with androgens in primate ovaries led to an increased number of small antral and preantral follicles (42). Moreover, androgens are thought to play a role in oocyte maturation by enhancing granulosa cells' differentiation (43). In PCOS patients, abnormal androgen production, by theca cells, leads to hyperandrogenism, which is thought to be responsible for anovulation (44). This hypothesis is supported by reports from therapies with the antiandrogens, flutamide, or cyproterone acetate, where ovulation was restored and the rates of pregnancy were extremely higher (45). However, the precise mechanisms that lead to anovulation in a large number of PCOS patients are very complex and need

to be elucidated in the future. Estrogens are also produced in the ovary by aromatization of androgens. In particular, androgens are the substrate of P450 aromatase, an enzyme that mediates the conversion to estrogens. Estradiol exerts its actions via two forms of receptors, ERa and ERb. Both isoforms are important for the female reproductive ability, but ERb receptor has shown to be implicated in follicular growth (46). In normal ovaries, increased estrogen production by the dominant follicles leads to a decrease in FSH serum concentration due to negative feedback effects of estradiol on the hypothalamipituitary axis. The reduction in FSH levels inhibits the development of less mature follicles, but whether estrogens are essential for follicular growth and oocyte maturation remains unclear yet.

Role of Adhesion Molecules

Follicular development is established by gap junctions and adhesion-type junctions between GCs. The degeneration of the follicles and the CL regression are associated with the loss of adherence between GC. Previous studies have also revealed that a single large GC is twice as likely to be apoptotic after culture, as an aggregated GC (47). This observation implies that cell contact may inhibit GC apoptosis. Despite the fact that aggregated GCs are more steroidogenic, there is evidence that progesterone production is not associated with the mechanism by which cell contact prevents apoptosis of GCs. It was also been found that gap junctions are not involved with the survival of GCs, and this observation supported the idea that the adhesion-type junctions convey the protective effects of cell contact. Cell-to-cell contact is mediated by a great diversity of cell adhesion molecules including some integrins, the immunoglobulin supergene family, selectins, and cadherins. The expression of these adhesion molecules is cell specific, with cadherins involved in mediating calcium-dependent cell-to-cell adhesion in virtually all solid tissues of multicellular organisms (48). Cadherins are a rapidly expanding family of calcium-dependent CAMs and have been shown to regulate epithelial, endothelial, neural, and cancer cell adhesion, with different CADs expressed on different cell types. The adhesion junctions are formed between adjacent cells through a homophilic interaction of N-cadherin molecules, which is expressed in primordial, primary, and early secondary follicles, as well as in healthy antral follicles (47) and is located at the junctional interface between aggregating cells. Luteal cells are also strongly positive for N-cadherin in the early luteal and midluteal phase, whereas there is only weak N-cadherin staining during late luteal phase. As the follicle degenerates, the expression of N-cadherin decreases, and GCs ultimately dissociate (47). In addition, apoptosis does not occur in preantral follicles and is very low in the early luteal phase, whereas it increases significantly in the late luteal phase (47). These observations suggest (a) that the expression of N-cadherin is regulated in human GCs in vivo during follicular maturation and CL formation and (b) that there is a direct correlation between the presence of the N-cadherin molecule and the absence of features characteristic of cellular apoptosis. The mechanism through which N-cadherin exerts the survival effects on GCs is not yet completely understood. Recent studies have shown that N-cadherin interacts with the FGF receptor, which is required for cell contact to prevent apoptosis (49). Additionally, bFGF induces the tyrosine phosphorylation of its own receptor by inducing PKC activity, a process that is involved in stimulating calcium uptake into the cytoplasmic stores (50). Taking these data together, it is likely that N-cadherin interaction with FGF receptor promotes cell survival by enhancing the activity of PKC and thereby maintaining calcium homeostasis (51). Moreover, it have been demonstrated that cell-cell aggregation promotes survival of GCs and that loss of N-cadherin from the cell surface induces apoptosis in these cells, supporting a major role of this adhesion molecule in the GC life cycle. N-cadherin possesses an extracellular domain with five tandemly arranged repeats. The N-terminal repeat contains the adhesive domain that is involved in cadherin-specific adhesions. Cleavage of the extracellular domain by metalloproteinases (MMP) is followed by loss of the adhesive ability of N-cadherin and cell death. It has been shown that inhibition of cleavage by MMP inhibitor decreases the rate of apoptosis in granulosa cells (47). Other studies have indicated cAMP-dependent pathways that induce downregulation of N-cadherin in a dose-dependent manner.

E-cadherin is also an important member of the cadherin superfamily, and it is expressed in spontaneously immortalized granulosa cells (SIGC) (52). E-cadherin connects adjacent cells, and a disruption in calcium-dependent cell contacts, with EGTA or an E-cadherin antibody, results in an increase in caspase-3 activity, in both the cytoplasm and nuclei of SIGCs. There have been detected cleavage products of β-catenin, which is an E-cadherin-associated protein, in apoptotic SIGCs. Previous studies have revealed that β-catenin and E-cadherin are substrates for caspase-3. These findings strengthened the idea that the increase of the cytoplasmic caspase-3 activity is associated with the degradation of β-catenin and E-cadherin. It is thus presumed that promotion of cell survival by E-cadherin is regulated by a signal transduction pathway that inhibits the activation of caspase-3.

CONCLUSIONS

Follicular development and CL formation and regression in human ovaries are strongly correlated with female reproductive capacity. Production of steroids and apoptosis of ovarian cells seems to play an active and important role in ovarian physiological functions. Disruption of the normal activity of the ovary may lead to reproductive disorders or even malignancies. Therefore, the mechanisms that control the normal life cycle of the dominant follicle, from folliculogenesis to luteolysis, must be elucidated.

KEY POINTS

■ Development of multiple ovarian follicles and oocytes is achieved in controlled ovarian stimulation, which is an important component of assisted reproduction technology.

■ The main hormone product of the CL is progesterone, which induces the endometrial modifications required for embryo implantation.

■ Progesterone is also involved in stimulating ovulation in human ovarian follicles.

■ In PCOS patients, abnormal androgen production, by theca cells, leads to hyperandrogenism, which is thought to be responsible for anovulation.

■ Estrogen production by the dominant follicle leads to a decrease in FSH levels, which inhibits the development of less mature follicles.

■ Apoptosis or programmed cell death ensures that in every estrus/menstrus cycle, only one or very few follicles will ovulate. This process minimizes the possibility of multiple embryos during pregnancy.

REFERENCES

1. McGee EA, Hsueh AJ. 2000. Initial and cyclic recruitment of ovarian follicles. *Endocr Rev* 21:200–14.
2. Fair T. 2003. Follicular oocyte growth and acquisition of developmental competence. *Anim Reprod Sci* 15:203–16.
3. Markström E, Svensson EC, Shao R, et al. 2002. Survival factors regulating ovarian apoptosis—dependence on follicle differentiation. *Reproduction* 123:23–30.
4. Zeleznik JA. 2004. The physiology of follicle selection. *Reprod Biol Endocrinol* 2:31–7.
5. Rizk B (Ed.). 2008. Ultrasonography in reproductive medicine and infertility. Cambridge, UK: Cambridge University Press, (in press).
6. Touraine P, Beau I, Gougeon A, et al. 1999. New natural inactivating mutations of the follicle-stimulating hormone receptor: correlations between receptor function and phenotype. *Mol Endocrinol* 13:1844–54.
7. Visser JA, Themmen AP. 2005. Anti-Mullerian hormone and folliculogenesis. *Mol Cell Endocrinol* 234:81–6.
8. Roy SK, Treacy BJ. 1993. Isolation and long-term culture of human preantral follicles. *Fertil Steril* 59:783–90.
9. Barboni B, Turriani M, Galeati G, et al. 2000. Vascular endothelial growth factor production in growing pig antral follicles. *Biol Reprod* 63:858–64.
10. Kaczmarek MM, Schams D, Ziecik JA. 2005. Role of the vascular endothelial growth factor in ovarian physiology—an overview. *Reprod Biol* 5:111–36.
11. Waltenberger J, Claesson-Welsh L, Siegbahm A, et al. 1994. Different signal transduction properties of KDR and Flt-1, two receptors for vascular endothelial growth factor. *J Biol Chem* 269:26988–95.
12. Filicori M, Cognigni EG. 2001. Roles and novel regimens of luteinizing hormone and follicle stimulating hormone in ovulation induction. *J Clin Endocrinol Metab* 86:1437–41.
13. Rizk B. 2006. Genetics of ovarian hyperstimulation syndrome. In Rizk B (Ed.), *Ovarian Hyperstimulation Syndrome*. Cambridge, New York: Cambridge University Press, Chapter 4, pp. 79–91.
14. Filicori M, Cognigni EG, Tabarelli C, et al. 2002. Stimulation and growth of antral ovarian follicles by selective LH activity administration in women. *J Clin Endocrinol Metab* 87:1156–61.
15. Mohri H. 1996. Fibronectin and integrins interactions. *J Invest Med* 44:429–41.
16. Senger DR, Claffey KP, Benes JE, et al. 1997. Angiogenesis promoted by vascular endothelial growth factor: regulation through $\alpha_1\beta_1$ and $\alpha_2\beta_1$ integrins. *Proc Natl Acad Sci USA* 94:13612–17.
17. Vaskivuo TE, Ottander U, Oduwole O, et al. 2002. Role of apoptosis, apoptosis-related fectors and 17beta-hydroxysteroid dehydrogenases in human corpus luteum regression. *Mol Cell Endocrinol* 30:191–200.
18. Vaskivuo TE, Tapanainen JS. 2003. Apoptosis in the human ovary. *Reprod BioMed Online* 6(1):24–35.
19. Rodger FE, Fraser HM, Krajewski S, et al. 1998. Production of the proto-oncogene Bax does not vary with changing in luteal function in women. *Mol Hum Reprod* 4:27–32.

20. Sugino N, Suzuki T, Kashida S, et al. 2000. Expression of Bcl-2 and Bax in the human corpus luteum during the menstrual cycle and in early pregnancy: regulation by human chorionic gonadotropin. *J Clin Endocrinol Metabol* 85:4379–86.

21. Rolaki A, Drakakis P, Millingos S, et al. 2005. Novel trends in follicular development, atresia and corpus luteum regression: a role for apoptosis. *Reprod Biomed Online* 11:93–103.

22. Amsterdam A, Gold RS, Hosokawa K, et al. 1999. Crosstalk among multiple signaling pathways controlling ovarian cell death. *Trends Endocrinol Metabol* 10:255–62.

23. Oosterhuis GJE, Michgelsen HW, Lambalk CB, et al. 1998. Apoptotic cell death in human granulosa-lutein cells: a possible indicator of in vitro fertilization outcome. *Fertil Steril* 4:747–9.

24. Idil M, Cepni I, Demirsoy G, et al. 2004. Does granulosa cell apoptosis have a role in the etiology of unexplained infertility? *Eur J Obstet Gynecol Reprod Biol* 112:182–4.

25. Kaelin WG Jr. 1999. Cancer. Many vessels, faulty gene. *Nature* 399:203–4.

26. Davies R, Moore A, Schedl A, et al. 1999. Multiple roles for the Wilms' tumor suppressor, WT1. *Cancer Res* 59:1747–50.

27. Tilly JL, Tilly KI. 1995. Inhibitors of oxidative stress mimic the ability follicle-stimulating hormone to suppress apoptosis in cultured rat ovarian follicles. *Endocrinology* 136:242–52.

28. Kim JM, Yoon YD, Tsang BK. 1999. Involvement of the Fas/Fas ligand system in p53-mediated granulosa cell apoptosis during follicular development and atresia. *Endocrinology* 140:2307–17.

29. Kugu K, Ratts VS, Piquette GN, et al. 1998. Analysis of apoptosis and expression of bcl-2 gene family members in the human and baboon ovary. *Cell Death Differen* 5:67–76.

30. Hosokawa K, Aharoni D, Dantes A, et al. 1998. Modulation of Mdm2 expression and p53-induced apoptosis in immortalized human ovarian granulosa cells. *Endocrinology* 139:4688–700.

31. Makrigiannakis A, Amin K, Coukos G, et al. 2000. Regulated expression and potential roles of p53 and Wilms' tumor suppressor gene (WT1 during follicular development in the human ovary. *J Clin Endocrinol Metab* 85:449–59.

32. Quirk MS, Cowan GR, et al. 2003. Ovarian follicular growth and atresia: the relationship between cell proliferation and survival. *J Anim Sci* 82:40–52.

33. Sasson R, Winder N, Kees S, Amsterdam A. 2002. Induction of apoptosis in granulosa cells by TNFα and its attenuation by glucocorticoids involve modulation of Bcl-2. *Biochem Biophys Res Com* 294:51–9.

34. Knudson CM, Tung KSK, Tourtellotte WG, et al. 1995. Bax-deficient mice with lymphoid hyperplasia and male germ cell death. *Science* 270:96–99.

35. Drummond EA. 2006. The role of steroids in follicular growth. *Reprod Biol Endocrinol* 4:16–26.

36. Robker RL, Russell DL, Espey LL, et al. 2000. Progesterone-regulated genes in the ovulation process: ADAMTS-1 and cathepsin L proteases. *Proc Natl Acad Sci USA* 97:4689–94.

37. La Polt SP, Leung K, et al. 2002. Roles of cyclic GMP in modulating ovarian functions. *Reprod Biomed Online* 6:15–23.

38. Natraj U, Richards JS. 1993. Hormonal regulation, localisation and functional activity of the progesterone receptor in granulosa cells of rat preovulatory follicles. *Endocrinology* 133:761–9.

39. Zalanyi S. 2001. Progesterone and ovulation. *Eur J Obstet Gynecol Reprod Biol* 98:152–9.

40. Makrigiannakis A, Coukos G, Christofidou-Solomidou M, et al. 2000. Progesterone is an autocrine/paracrine regulator of human granulosa cell survival *in vitro*. *Ann N Y Acad Sci* 900:16–25.

41. Steckler T, Wang J, Bartol FF, et al. 2005. Fetal programming: prenatal testosterone treatment causes intrauterine growth retardation, reduces ovarian reserve and increases ovarian follicular recruitment. *Endocrinology* 3185–93.

42. Vendola KA, Zhou J, Adesanya OO, et al. 1998. Androgens stimulate early stages of follicular growth in the primate ovary. *J Clin Investig* 101:2622–9.

43. Hillier SG, De Zwart FA. 1981. Evidence that granulosa cell aromatase induction/activation by follicle-stimulating hormone is an androgen receptor-regulated process in-vitro. *Endocrinology* 109:1303–5.

44. Abbott DH, Dumesic DA, Franks S. 2002. Developmental origin of polycystic ovary syndrome—a hypothesis. *J Endocrinol* 174:1–5.

45. De Leo V, Lanzetta D, D'Antona D, et al. 1998. Hormonal effects of flutamide in young women with polycystic ovary syndrome. *J Clin Endocrinol Metab* 83:99–102.

46. Hegele-Hartung C, Seibel P, Peters O, et al. 2004. Impact of isotype-selective oestrogen receptor agonists on ovarian function. *Proc Natl Acad Sci USA* 101:5129–34.

47. Makrigiannakis A, Coukos G, Christofidou-Solomidou M, et al. 1999 N-cadherin mediated human granulosa cell adhesion prevents apoptosis: a role in follicular atresia and luteolysis? *Am J Pathol* 154:1391–406.

48. Knudsen KA, Soler AP, Johnson KR et al. 1995. Interaction of a-actinin with the cadherin cell-cell adhesion complex via acatenin. *J Cell Biol* 130:67–77.

49. Trolice MP, Pappalardo A, Peluso JJ. 1997. Basic fibroblast growth factor and N-Cadherin maintain rat granulosa cell and ovarian surface epithelial cell viability by stimulating the tyrosine phosphorylation of the fibroblast growth factor receptors. *Endocrinology* 138:107–13.

50. Fewtrell C. 1993. Ca$^+$ oscillations in non-excitable cells. *Annu Rev Physiol* 55:427–54.

51. Peluso JJ. 1997. Putative mechanism through which N-Cadherin-mediated cell contact maintains calcium homeostasis and thereby prevents ovarian cells from undergoing apoptosis. *Biochem Pharmacol* 54:847–53.

52. Peluso JJ, Pappalardo A, Fernandez G. 2001. E-Cadherin-mediated cell contact prevents apoptosis of spontaneously immortalized granulosa cells by regulating Akt kinase activity. *Biol Reprod* 65:94–101.

MECHANISMS OF FOLLICULAR DEVELOPMENT: THE ROLE OF GONADOTROPHINS

Ioannis E. Messinis

INTRODUCTION

Folliculogenesis in women is a dynamic and uninterrupted process from fetal life until menopause. Following pubertal maturation of the reproductive axis, all types of follicles from the primordial to the preovulatory stage are present in the human ovary. Over the past twenty years, it has become clear that these follicles represent sequential forms of the developmental process classified into eight categories, based on the size and the number of the granulosa cells (Gougeon, 1986). For example, class 1 corresponds to a secondary preantral follicle and class 8 to a large preovulatory follicle.

Folliculogenesis is a lengthy process (Figure 2.1). Based on the calculation of the doubling time of granulosa cells, it is estimated that the time spent from the primordial to the preovulatory stage is approximately one year (Gougeon, 1986). However, maturation of a follicle from class 1 to class 8 is achieved within eighty-five days (Gougeon, 1986). At the beginning, proliferation of the granulosa cells on several layers takes place and the primordial follicle becomes preantral. Following this, the theca interna develops and the antral cavity is formed. The rate at which follicles leave the primordial pool is not known. However, it seems that the departure follows an ordered sequence, so that follicles formed first leave the pool earlier (Hirshfield, 1991).

It remains unclear which factors are responsible for the initiation of maturation of a primordial follicle or what is the trigger for the passage of a follicle from the preantral to the antral stage (Figure 2.1). In humans, this part of folliculogenesis is gonadotrophin independent. The growth of a follicle from class 1 to class 5 is to some extent affected by gonadotrophins, while from class 5 to class 8, that is, during the last fifteen days of follicle maturation that correspond to the follicular phase of the normal menstrual cycle, gonadotrophins are the only determinants of follicle growth (Gougeon, 1986). In other words, follicle maturation to the preovulatory stage is not feasible without the presence of follicle-stimulating harmone (FSH) and luteinizing harmone (LH).

INITIAL RECRUITMENT: PREANTRAL FOLLICLE GROWTH

The term "recruitment" refers to a cohort of follicles that leave a particular developmental stage for further growth (Figure 2.1). At the primordial stage, the term "initial recruitment" has been proposed (McGee and Hsueh, 2000). Similarly, the term "cyclic recruitment" has been proposed for the cohort of antral follicles from which "selection" of the dominant follicle takes place during the early follicular phase of the cycle (McGee and Hsueh, 2000). It has been established that FSH is the principal hormone that promotes follicle maturation, especially at more advanced stages of development. Although receptors of FSH are expressed in the granulosa cells of preantral follicles (Roy et al., 1987), evidence has been provided that in humans this hormone is not required for follicle maturation up to the antral stage. A logical explanation is that primordial follicles are located in an avascular part of the ovary, and therefore, they can be easily reached by locally produced but not by systemic factors (van Wezel and Rodgers, 1996). There are several examples of follicle maturation up to the early antral stage in women either in the presence of negligible amounts of FSH in the circulation, such as before puberty (Peters et al., 1978), during pregnancy (Westergaard et al., 1985), and in cases of hypogonadotrophic hypogonadism (Rabin et al., 1972), or in the absence of FSH activity, such as in mutations of FSHβ (Matthews et al., 1993) and inactivating mutations of the FSH receptor (Touraine et al., 1999).

The situation is different in certain species in which FSH participates in the control of preantral follicle development, although it is still unclear whether this hormone is involved in the mechanism that triggers initial recruitment. In vitro data have demonstrated that FSH is a growth and differentiation factor for rat preantral follicles in the presence of a cGMP analog that suppresses apoptosis (McGee et al., 1997). However, FSH alone did not prevent apoptosis in these follicles. Also, preantral follicle growth, number of cells, and cell differentiation were promoted by FSH, and these effects were enhanced by the addition of antimullerian hormone (AMH or MIS) or activin (McGee et al., 2001). In contrast to rats, in mice, AMH, produced by preantral follicles, inhibited initial recruitment as well as the stimulatory effect of FSH on the growth from the primary to the early antral stage (Visser and Themmen, 2005). Although still unclear, species variability may account for these opposite actions of AMH. Recently, AMH was able to inhibit initiation of human primordial follicle growth in vitro (Carlsson et al., 2006).

Several genes encoding specific proteins and growth factors are expressed in the granulosa cells of small follicles. These factors including epidermal growth factor (EGF), transforming growth factor-α (TGF-α), TGF-β and insulin-like growth factor-1 (IGF-1) may be involved in the initiation of growth

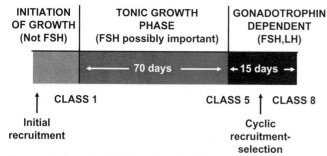

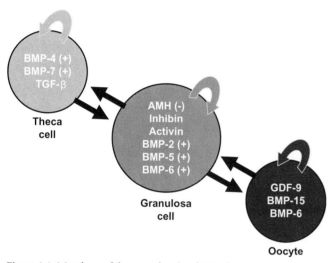

Figure 2.1. Growth of follicles through different stages and duration of follicle maturation. Class 1 corresponds to the secondary preantral follicle and class 8 to the large preovulatory follicle. The period from class 5 to class 8 corresponds to the follicular phase of the normal menstrual cycle and is gonadotrophin dependant. "Initial recruitment" refers to recruitment of primordial follicles, while "cyclic recruitment" refers to the recruitment and selection of the dominant follicle. The diagram is based on data presented in one reference (Gougeon, 1986).

Figure 2.2. Members of the superfamily of TGF-β predominantly produced by the theca cells, granulosa cells, and the oocyte. Paracrine effects are exerted between the theca and the granulosa cells as well as between the granulosa cells and the oocyte. Autocrine effects are also likely. The diagram is based on data presented in one reference (Knight and Glister, 2006).

of primordial follicles (May et al., 1990; Adashi, 1998; Knight and Glister, 2006). A group of such factors, members of the TGF-β superfamily, are shown in Figure 2.2. Another factor, produced particularly in primordial and primary follicles, is Wilms tumor suppressor gene (*WT1*) that may have a suppressive role in the expression of genes of various growth factors, maintaining thus the follicles at the resting stage (Hsu et al., 1995). Similarly, retinoblastoma protein (pRb) may also have a suppressive effect by inhibiting proliferation of granulosa cells even in humans (Bukovsky et al., 1995a, 1995b). A role in the transition from the primordial to the primary stage may be also played by the oncogene *myc* (Piontkewitz et al., 1997), the *steel* locus encoding the kit ligand (Huang et al., 1993), and the platelet-derived growth factor (Nilsson et al., 2006). Finally, neurotrophin molecules, such as nerve growth factor (NGF)

may also play a role in mice for early follicular development (Dissen et al., 2001).

During follicle growth, the oocyte undergoes functional changes in order to become fertilizable at ovulation. However, various factors derived from the oocyte seem to play a crucial role for preantral follicle development (Erickson and Shimasaki, 2001). For example, growth differentiation factor-9 (GDF-9), a member of TGF-β superfamily, is expressed by oocytes (McGrath et al., 1995) and stimulates granulosa cell proliferation and DNA synthesis in preantral and dominant follicles (Vitt et al., 2000). This factor also stimulates preantral follicle growth in vitro (Hayashi et al., 1999). It has been hypothesized that a concentration gradient of GDF-9 is established in the graafian follicle with the highest levels nearest the oocyte (Erickson and Shimasaki, 2000). This gradient in GDF-9 concentrations influences granulosa cell differentiation in response to FSH stimulation that leads to granulosa cell heterogeneity. For example, in the membrana cells, the expression of genes encoding LH receptors, P450 aromatase, P450 side chain cleavage, kit ligand, and urokinase-type plasminogen activator is facilitated by GDF-9, while in the cumulus cells, genes encoding IGF-1, hyaluronic acid synthase-2, and cycloxygenase-2 (COX-2) are expressed (Erickson and Shimasaki, 2000). Nevertheless, the effects of GDF-9 are different in preantral and dominant follicles.

Another protein that is also produced by the oocyte is bone morphogenetic protein-15 (BMP-15 or GDF-9B) (Dube et al., 1998). Similar to GDF-9, this protein stimulates granulosa cell mitosis in vitro (Otsuka et al., 2000). Furthermore, BMP-15 promotes early follicle growth but restrains the transition of follicles to the preovulatory stage, while it inhibits the expression of FSH receptors and prevents premature luteinization (Moore and Shimasaki, 2005). GDF-9 and BMP-15 are obligatory for normal folliculogenesis and female fertility. GDF-9 knockout mice remain infertile, with follicles being arrested at the primary stage (Carabatsos et al., 1998). Similarly, in sheep homozygous for point mutations of BMP-15 or GDF-9 genes or in animals immunized against these two factors, follicles fail to develop beyond the primary stage (McNatty et al., 2005). Finally, in women, a BMP-15 mutation causes ovarian dysgenesis with hypergonadotrophic ovarian failure (Di Pasquale et al., 2004). Apart from these two factors, other substances produced by the oocyte, such as BMP-6, fibroblast growth factor-8 (FGF-8), and TGF-β2, have been investigated to a lesser extent (Erickson and Shimasaki, 2000). Nevertheless, BMP-4 and BMP-7 produced by ovarian stroma and theca cells have been associated with the transition of follicles from the primordial to the primary stage (Knight and Glister, 2006).

GROWTH OF ANTRAL FOLLICLES: DOMINANT FOLLICLE

FSH Intercycle Rise

The growth of large antral follicles is depended on gonadotrophins. These hormones are obligatory for follicle maturation during the follicular phase of the cycle. Despite the apparently low FSH levels in the follicular and the luteal phase of the cycle (Messinis and Templeton, 1988a), important changes in the secretion of this hormone take place during the luteal-follicular transition. In particular, FSH levels increase in late luteal phase up to the onset of menstruation and the early follicular phase of the following cycle (Mais et al., 1987; Messinis et al., 1993).

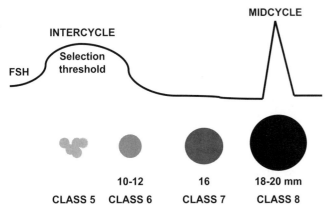

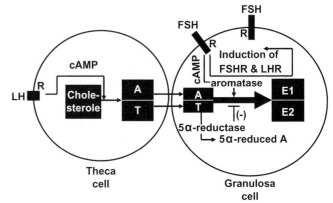

Figure 2.3. Intercycle rise of FSH during the luteal-follicular transition creating a selection threshold for the dominant follicle. Following selection, further growth of the follicle up to the preovulatory stage takes place despite the decreasing levels of FSH.

Figure 2.4. Two-cell two-gonadotrophin theory. Androgens are produced by the theca cells under the influence of LH. Aromatization of androgens in the granulosa cells takes place under the influence of FSH. 5α-reductase reduces androgens to 5α-reduced products and inhibits aromatase production. FSH overcomes the action of 5α-reductase by stimulating the production of aromatase.

The increase in FSH levels is the result of the decline in estradiol, progesterone, and inhibin A levels due to the demise of the corpus luteum (Groome et al., 1996; Messinis, 2006).

The "intercycle rise" of FSH, also named "FSH window," is the key factor for the selection of the dominant follicle during the normal menstrual cycle (Figure 2.3). Both the duration and the magnitude of FSH increase are important for stimulation of follicle maturation. An increase in FSH of 30–50 percent above the basal value is attained during that time, which is sufficient to induce follicle growth. Such an increase was recognized almost thirty years ago as a critical step during ovulation induction in anovulatory women with the use of exogenous FSH and is known as the "FSH threshold" concept (Brown et al., 1969).

Selection of the dominant follicle is a multifactorial process, although FSH is an absolute requirement (Zeleznik, 1981; Baird, 1983). The intercycle rise of FSH stimulates "cyclic recruitment" of a cohort of approximately four to six healthy antral follicles that usually belong to class 4 or class 5 according to the already discussed classification (Gougeon and Lefevre, 1983). These follicles accumulate FSH in their follicular fluid, which in the follicle destined to become dominant is concentrated at a critical threshold (McNatty et al., 1975). In that follicle, FSH stimulates the production of estradiol in excess of the production in the nondominant follicles, with the resultant increase of the concentrations of this steroid in its follicular microenvironment (McNatty et al., 1975; Van Dessel et al., 1996a). At the same time, proliferation of the granulosa cells at a fast rate and promotion of follicular fluid formation take place, so that a relationship between the number of granulosa cells and follicle diameter is established (McNatty et al., 1979a). Only in follicles with detectable levels of FSH in their follicular fluid, the concentrations of estradiol correlate significantly with the number of granulosa cells (McNatty and Baird, 1978). An increase in the rate of mitosis has been found in the cohort follicles as early as in late luteal phase in response to treatment with human menopausal gonadotrophin (Gougeon and Testart, 1990). It may be assumed that follicle selection takes place at that time of the cycle.

Steroids Production

Steroidogenesis is a critical process for follicle selection (Figure 2.4). It has been established that the theca cells are the site of androgen production, while granulosa cells produce estrogen only in the presence of androgen (Hillier et al., 1994). In vitro experiments have shown the expression of P450c17 enzyme, converting progesterone to androgens, in the theca layer and P450 aromatase enzyme in the granulosa cells of dominant follicles (Smyth et al., 1993; Hillier et al., 1994). Although FSH is important for follicle growth, steroidogenesis in the early follicular phase is the result of the cooperation of FSH and LH in the context of the two-cell two-gonadotrophin theory (Hillier et al., 1994). In particular, LH acts on the theca cells via specific receptors and stimulates changes in gene expression that are critical for the production of androgens (androstenedione and testosterone) (Erickson et al., 1985). Androgens produced under these conditions are transferred into the granulosa cells where they are used as aromatase substrate for the production of estrogens (estrone and estradiol, respectively) (McNatty et al., 1979b). P450 aromatase is produced under the influence of FSH (Whitelaw et al., 1992), which acts on the granulosa cells via specific receptors (Roy et al., 1987). At the same time, FSH upregulates its own receptors on the same cells (Dorrington and Armstrong, 1979). Only dominant follicles contain augmented aromatase activity and produce increased amounts of estrogens that are released in the circulation (McNatty et al., 1979c). The latter interfere with the ovarian negative feedback system and render the remaining cohort follicles devoid of FSH support, resulting thus in single-follicle selection (Fauser and Van Heusden, 1997).

The process of steroidogenesis is controlled by the paracrine/autocrine action of various factors produced locally in the follicle that modulate the effects of FSH and LH. Such factors are the system of inhibin/activin, the system of IGFs (IGF-1 and IGF-2) and their binding proteins (IGFBPs), androgens, and estrogens (Hillier, 2001).

Inhibin/Activin System

Inhibin is a member of the superfamily of TGF-β (de Kretser et al., 2002). Both inhibin and activin are produced by granulosa cells and exert intraovarian effects. Activin is produced by immature follicles in higher amounts as compared to inhibin, while inhibin predominates in progressively maturing follicles

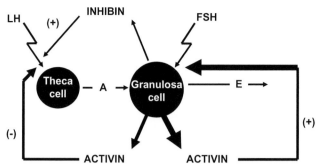

Figure 2.5. The role of inhibin and activin in the control of steroidogenesis in the early follicular phase during the selection of the dominant follicle. Inhibin enhances the action of LH on the theca cells and the production of androgens, while activin inhibits the action of inhibin. At the same time, activin facilitates the action of FSH on the granulosa cells and the aromatization of androgens to estrogens.

(Nakatani et al., 1991; Miro and Hiller, 1996). In vitro studies have suggested that inhibin and activin participate in the process of steroidogenesis at least in small antral follicles (Figure 2.5). Especially, inhibin enhances the action of LH on androgen production in theca cells, a process that is suppressed by activin (Hillier, 2001). As a result of a balance, relatively low amounts of androgens are produced at that stage of follicle development, which, however, are adequate for estrogen production in the granulosa cells. The latter is facilitated by activin, which enhances the actions of FSH, including FSH-induced mitosis and steroidogenesis (Hillier, 2001). Therefore, activin promotes rapid estrogenization of the follicular environment that is important for the expression of dominance. Recent in vitro data in bovine follicles have shown a marked increase in intrafollicular activin "tone" at the critical time of FSH-depended follicle selection (Glister et al., 2006).

IGFs/IGFBPs

In vitro data have suggested that the system of IGFs and the IGFBPs participates in folliculogenesis during the early follicular phase of the cycle. Receptors of IGF-1, activated by both IGF-1 and IGF-2, have been detected in the granulosa cells of dominant follicles, while receptors of IGF-2 have been found in theca and granulosa cells (Mazerbourg et al., 2003). The action of IGFs is locally regulated by the binding proteins. Five of the six known binding proteins are expressed in the human ovary (Wang and Chard, 1999). Of these, IGFBP-4 gains great interest since it inhibits in vitro FSH-induced production of estradiol by human granulosa cells (Mason et al., 1998). IGFBP-4 binds IGFs and neutralizes their biological activity. However, under the influence of the intercycle rise of FSH, the granulosa cells of the follicle that is destined to become dominant and, therefore, has the highest receptivity for FSH produce a protease that degrades IGFBP-4 and possibly IGFBP-5 and IGFBP-2, increasing thus the levels of free IGFs (Spicer, 2004).

Recent data have shown that pregnancy-associated plasma protein-A (PAPP-A), a metalloproteinase, contains activity of IGFBP-4ase (Lawrence et al., 1999). Since PAPP-A is present in the follicular fluid (Conover et al., 1999), while the gene encoding this protease is expressed in human ovaries (Hourvitz et al., 2000), it is possible that it plays a physiological role in the process of dominant follicle selection. It has been suggested

that PAPP-A is acquired by the future dominant follicle under the influence of FSH before it becomes larger than the remaining follicles of the recruited cohort (Rivera and Fortune, 2003). PAPP-A is expressed only in healthy follicles, while IGFBP-4 is expressed in atretic follicles (Hourvitz et al., 2000).

The proteolytic cleavage of IGFBP-4/5 results in bioavailable IGF-1 and IGF-2, which participate in the control of follicle maturation. The importance of IGF-1 in human folliculogenesis is less clear than that of IGF-2. IGF-1 is expressed in the granulosa cells of various species but not of women (El-Roeiy et al., 1993). In addition, clinical data in women with Laron-type dwarfism characterized by IGF-1 deficiency indicate that IGF-1 may not play an important role in folliculogenesis (Dor et al., 1992). Nevertheless, this factor is expressed in human theca cells (Mason et al., 1996) and is detectable in human follicular fluid (Eden et al., 1990), while its receptors have been found in antral follicles (Hernandez et al., 1988; Zhou and Bondy, 1993). In vitro studies have shown that IGF-1 stimulates the production of estradiol by human granulosa and granulosa-lutein cells in culture as well as proliferation and differentiation of granulosa cells (Bergh et al., 1991). It is assumed that at least in an animal model, IGF-1 produced by granulosa cells exerts paracrine actions on the theca cells, increasing the number of LH receptors and stimulating postreceptor events including steroidogenesis (Magoffin and Weitsman, 1994). IGF-1 also exerts autocrine effects, enhancing the responsiveness of the ovary to FSH by increasing the number of functional FSH receptors (Minegishi et al., 2000). The possibility of extragonadal IGF-1 synthesized in the liver under the influence of growth hormone to play a physiological endocrine role in the human ovary cannot be excluded.

In contrast to IGF-1, IGF-2 is produced both by the theca and the granulosa cells in women (El-Roeiy et al., 1993). This is evident not only in small antral follicles but also in the granulosa cells of preovulatory follicles (Geisthovel et al., 1989). IGF-2 is also detectable in human follicular fluid (Barreca et al., 1996; Van Dessel et al., 1996b), and its receptors are present in the theca and the granulosa cells (El-Roeiy et al., 1993). In vitro data have demonstrated that, similar to IGF-1, IGF-2 stimulates estradiol production as well as proliferation of the granulosa and granulosa-lutein cells (Kamada et al., 1992). It is possible that IGF-2 produced by the theca cells exerts autocrine effects, enhancing the action of LH and the production of androgen as well as paracrine effects on the granulosa cells facilitating the actions of FSH on the production of estrogen and cell proliferation (Di Blasio et al., 1994; Mason et al., 1994).

Follicle Rescue/Atresia

The described interrelationships between FSH and IGFs indicate that follicle development is a self-supported event via a functional loop, with various links involving different local factors. For instance, inhibin not only affects steroidogenesis by enhancing the action of LH on the theca cells but also augments in vitro the actions of IGF-1 and IGF-2 on thecal androgen production (Nahum et al., 1995). The effects of FSH on follicle maturation are also facilitated (Campbell, 1999). The end point of these events is the increase in the concentrations of estradiol in the follicular fluid of the dominant follicle. The follicles that do not contain adequate number of FSH receptors in their granulosa cells during the intercycle rise of FSH are able to aromatize androgens to estrogens only to a limited extent, and therefore, androgens are the predominant steroids in their follicular environment. The ability of granulosa cells to metabolize androgens to estrogens is demonstrated in vitro only in follicles larger than 8 mm in diameter, a process regulated by FSH (Mason et al., 1994). Healthy human antral follicles with a diameter greater than 8 mm contain an increased ratio of estrogens to androgens in their follicular fluid as compared to smaller follicles, which contain higher levels of androgens (van Dessel et al., 1996a). In large dominant follicles, follicle diameter correlates significantly with intrafollicular concentrations of estradiol and negatively with the concentrations of androstenedione (Westergaard et al., 1986; van Dessel et al., 1996a).

Follicles with an estrogenic environment are rescued for further growth, while follicles with an androgenic environment become atretic. Atresia is a process that takes place at all stages of human folliculogenesis. The underline mechanism is apoptotic cell death, although the signaling pathways are not clear. Although an androgen-rich environment may be the result rather than the cause of atresia, evidence has been provided that androgens themselves increase DNA fragmentation and, therefore, apoptosis, while estrogens decrease DNA fragmentation (Billig et al., 1993). Various genes are involved in this process, such as *p53, c-myc, c-fox, bax, bcl-x*, and others. The system of *Fas-Fas* ligand is also implicated, while various caspases are also involved (Hussein, 2005). Apoptosis is defective if genes are defective, such as for instance in mice with the lack of the proapoptotic protein *bax* (Perez et al., 1999). Antiapoptotic factors are FSH and LH as well as IGF-1, EGF, bFGF, TGF-α, interleukin-1β (IL-1β), bcl-2, bcl-x, insulin, and ovarian steroids (Hussein, 2005; Rolaki et al., 2005). Atretogenic factors include TGF-β, IL-6, androgens, reactive oxygen species, *bax, Fas* antigens, *p53*, tumor necrosis factor (TNF), and caspases (Hussein, 2005; Rolaki et al., 2005). The lack of FSH at the critical time of follicle selection leads to atresia of the recruited follicles. In these follicles, PAPP-A is absent and, therefore, IGFBP-4 is not degraded, while aromatase enzyme is limited (Mazerbourg et al., 2003). This means that androgens are not converted to estrogens, a situation that favors apoptosis.

Androgens

Despite the atretogenic effects of androgens, in vitro data in rats and primates have demonstrated that these steroids may play a positive role in folliculogenesis. Androgen receptors are present in the granulosa cells of early antral but not of preovulatory follicles (Tetsuka et al., 1995). It has been suggested that androgens, apart from serving as a substrate for the production of estrogens, sensitize granulosa cells to FSH simulation in early antral follicles. Especially, low amounts of androgens amplify FSH-induced protein kinase A signaling in rat granulosa cells in vitro (Tetsuka and Hillier, 1996). In more advanced stages of follicle development, such as during the late preovulatory period, the number of androgen receptors in the granulosa cells declines, and therefore, the sensitivity of the follicle to FSH is diminished, delaying any effects of gonadotrophins on terminal differentiation and luteinization of granulosa cells until the onset of the LH surge (Hillier and Tetsuka, 1997).

Estrogens

The role of estrogens in the process of follicle maturation is less clear. Estrogen receptors-α and -β are present in the ovaries (Pelletier and El-Alfy, 2000; Scobie et al., 2002), suggesting

a local action of estradiol. Nevertheless, although this steroid is important for follicle development in animals, its significance in women has not been clarified (Findlay et al., 2000). In rats, estradiol acts synergistically with FSH to promote granulosa cell proliferation and to increase the FSH receptors and the production of aromatase, thus preventing atresia (Wang and Greenwald, 1993; Fauser and Van Heusden, 1997).

In terms of estrogen receptors, the β-subtype appears to play in the ovary a more important role than the α-form. Estrogen receptor-β knockout female mice have an increased number of atretic follicles with no progression from early to large antral stage and show decreased production of estradiol and a reduced ovulation rate (Emmen et al., 2005). Also, in the same animals, in the absence of estrogen receptors-β, preovulatory follicles are able to aromatize androgens to estrogens to a limited extent and show inadequate response to FSH in terms of differentiation and induction of LH receptors and a reduced rate of follicle rupture (Couse et al., 2005).

In women with 17α-hydroxylase/17,20-lyase deficiency, administration of exogenous FSH after pituitary desensitization stimulated follicle maturation but the synthesis of estrogen was very low (Rabinovici et al., 1989). Also, women with the aromatase deficiency syndrome developed follicular cysts with high FSH and low estradiol levels (Mullis et al., 1997). Similarly, women with hypogonadotrophic hypogonadism, when treated with FSH without LH, developed multiple preovulatory follicles despite the low serum estradiol levels (Schoot et al., 1992). Follicle aspiration in these women confirmed the low intrafollicular concentrations of estradiol. It is evident from these data that follicles can mature from the antral to the preovulatory stage under stimulation with FSH in the absence of high estradiol concentrations, suggesting that this steroid is not required for follicle development in women. However, it remains to be elucidated whether the increase in follicle size in patients with low estrogen is accompanied by granulosa cell proliferation in a pattern similar to that in normal women.

Other Factors

Progesterone is an ovarian steroid, whose concentrations in serum during the follicular phase of the cycle are very low. It has been considered that the main source of circulating progesterone at that stage of the cycle is the adrenal glands (Judd et al., 1992), but clinical evidence has demonstrated that the ovaries also contribute (Alexandris et al., 1997). Although this steroid may have an endocrine role during the follicular phase (Dafopoulos et al., 2004), a role in follicle selection is rather unlikely since progesterone receptors are not present in the granulosa cells until the onset of the midcycle LH surge (Hild-Petito et al., 1988; Iwai et al., 1990). The role of glucocorticoids in the ovary is not clear. In vitro data have shown a protective effect, via bcl-2, of dexamethasone and hydrocortisone on apoptosis induced by TNF-α in preovulatory human granulosa cells (Sasson and Amsterdam, 2002).

Other factors that may play a role in follicle development include EGF, FGF, TGF-α, and TGF-β that modulate the action of FSH in vitro. The vascular endothelial growth factor (VEGF) may also play a role in folliculogenesis since in vitro data have shown that when angiogenesis was inhibited for a short period of time by an anti-VEGF-blocking antibody during the growth of the dominant follicle, the follicular phase was lengthened (Zimmermann et al., 2003).

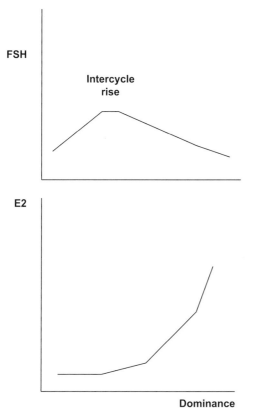

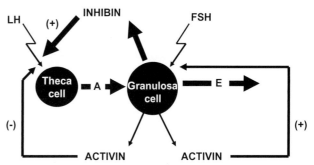

Figure 2.7. The role of inhibin and activin in the control of follicle maturation during the late follicular phase. Inhibin enhances the effect of LH on the production of androgens, leading to the production of high amounts of estrogens.

Figure 2.6. Selection of the dominant follicle is followed by increasing estradiol concentrations in the circulation that suppress FSH levels and terminate the intercycle rise of this hormone. This mechanism leads to single-follicle maturation during the normal menstrual cycle. The diagram is based on data presented in van Santbrink et al., 1995.

SINGLE-FOLLICLE SELECTION

Estrogens produced by the dominant follicle are released in the circulation and increase serum concentrations of estradiol (Figure 2.6). It has been suggested that increasing serum estradiol levels by suppressing, via a negative feedback mechanism, the secretion of FSH from the pituitary terminate the intercycle rise of this hormone (van Santbrink et al., 1995). That rising estradiol values can suppress serum FSH levels has been shown in experiments performed in women during the early and midfollicular phase of the cycle (Messinis and Templeton, 1990a; Messinis et al., 1994). In addition, an inverse relationship between the magnitude of FSH decrease and the estradiol rise has been found in the follicular phase of the natural cycle (van Santbrink et al., 1995). Therefore, under these conditions, the FSH window is narrowed, precluding follicles that are at a less advanced stage of development than the dominant follicle from selection and further growth. These follicles will not attain the appropriate threshold of FSH in their environment, although in the meantime they may have acquired the appropriate number of FSH receptors. Data in monkeys have shown that an earlier increase in serum estradiol values reduced FSH levels prematurely and this jeopardized the survival of the dominant follicle (Zeleznik, 1981). In the same animals, passive immunization against estradiol with the administration of an antibody prevented the decrease in FSH levels in mid- to late follicular

phase and resulted in multiple follicular development (Zeleznik et al., 1987). It is clear, therefore, that not only the magnitude but also the duration of the FSH window is important.

In vivo experiments in women have demonstrated that estradiol is not the only factor that terminates FSH intercycle rise (Messinis, 2006). Administration of the antiestrogenic compound, clomiphene, to normal women in the early and midfollicular phase of the cycle prolonged the FSH rise, supporting thus the role of estrogen, but also provided a role for inhibin in the control of FSH intercycle rise (Messinis and Templeton, 1988b). Serum levels of inhibin B increase rapidly in the early follicular phase of the cycle and decline as FSH rise is terminated (Groome et al., 1996). It is possible, therefore, that inhibin B produced by the dominant follicle under the intercycle rise of FSH participates in the mechanism that "closes" the FSH window. Nevertheless, although experiments in rhesus monkeys have demonstrated that inhibin A can suppress FSH secretion from the pituitary (Molskeness et al., 1996), the role of these proteins in the secretion of FSH in women is rather unclear (Klein et al., 2004).

GROWTH OF THE DOMINANT FOLLICLE

Following termination of FSH intercycle rise, FSH values remain low for the rest of the follicular phase. Despite this, the selected dominant follicle continues to grow until the ovulatory stage (Figure 2.3). Although the mechanism of this process is not clear, it has been assumed that the dominant follicle becomes increasingly sensitive to FSH after the completion of the selection process (Zeleznik, 2004). This hypothesis has been tested in cynomolgous monkeys during the exogenous administration of highly purified FSH and LH following blockage of endogenous gonadotrophin secretion by a GnRH antagonist (Zeleznik and Kubik, 1986). It was found that from the time estradiol levels started to increase, the progressive reduction in FSH levels after lowering the FSH dose did not affect follicle growth.

There are two possible explanations for the increased sensitivity of the growing follicle to FSH. First, various intrafollicular regulators may play a role within the follicle, and second, from midfollicular phase onward, the follicle becomes dependent on LH. Of the intrafollicular regulators an important role is played by inhibin/activin (Figure 2.7). In contrast to early follicular phase, in late stages of follicle development, high amounts of androgens are required for the synthesis of estrogens. At these stages, the stimulating effect of inhibin on LH-induced steroidogenesis in the theca cells overcomes the inhibiting effect of activin. The latter, however, enhances the action of FSH on the granulosa cells, facilitating aromatization of androgens to estrogens (Hillier, 2001). The role of follistatin is less clear. This substance binds activin and neutralizes its bioactivity and possibly the activity of BMPs, facilitating thus luteinization and/or atresia (Knight and Glister, 2003).

Apart from the system of inhibin/activin, growth factors, such as EGF, TGF-α, FGF, VEGF, NGF, and TNF-α may also play a role. The superfamily of TGF-β is also important (Figure 2.2). For example, BMP-2, BMP-5, and BMP-6 derived from the granulosa cells; BMP-4 and BMP-7 derived from the theca cells; and BMP-6 derived from the oocyte promote granulosa cell proliferation and facilitate the secretion of estradiol and inhibin, while suppressing progesterone production by bovine granulosa cells in vitro, protecting thus the follicle from atresia and early luteinization (Knight and Glister, 2003, 2006). In terms of the action of estradiol, it has been generally accepted that this steroid exerts an autocrine effect that facilitates the action of FSH (Adashi and Hseuh, 1982; Reilly et al., 1996).

As it was mentioned previously, LH receptors are present only in the theca cells of growing antral follicles, while granulosa cells possess FSH receptors. However, following the selection of the dominant follicle, LH receptors are also acquired by the granulosa cells under the influence of FSH (Piquette et al., 1991). Aromatase is functionally coupled with these receptors, so that estrogen synthesis is directly regulated by LH (Zeleznik and Hillier, 1984; Zeleznik 2001). In vitro data have demonstrated that human granulosa cells become responsive to LH and produce estradiol and progesterone if they are obtained from follicles 10 mm or greater (Willis et al., 1998). Also, data in women have shown the ability of recombinant LH alone to maintain the growth of a follicle from the stage of ≈14 mm following recruitment-selection by recombinant FSH (Sullivan et al., 1999). It is evident, therefore, that the dominant follicle in late follicular phase becomes less depended on FSH partly because it acquires responsiveness to LH that facilitates its growth to the preovulatory stage despite the low concentrations of FSH in the circulation. Although the action of LH on follicle growth in humans is restricted to the advanced stages of this process, animal data have demonstrated that, to a lesser extent than FSH, LH can support the survival of preantral follicles and induce the formation of an antrum-like cavity in vitro (Cortvrindt et al., 1998).

Over the past few years, in an effort to explain follicle selection, research has been also focused on interactions between neighbor cells and follicles in the context of "inductive signaling" and "lateral specification" (Baker and Spears, 1999). It is believed that apart from endocrine factors, these interactions possibly play roles at the early stages of follicle development as well as at the stage of "cyclic" recruitment and selection. Possible factors, such as granulosa cell inhibitory factor (GCIF), produced by a certain follicle may inhibit proliferation of small- and medium-sized follicles.

At the end of the selection process, the dominant follicle is about 10–12 mm in diameter (van Santbrink et al., 1995). This coincides with the time of the first significant rise in serum estradiol concentrations. The dominant follicle of that size becomes easily visible by transvaginal ultrasound. The growth to the preovulatory stage is almost linear, with a rate of growth of about 1.5–2.0 mm/day (Templeton et al., 1986). A significant correlation has been found between follicle diameter calculated by ultrasound and that calculated from follicle aspirates at laparoscopy (Messinis and Templeton, 1986). The growth of the dominant follicle is due not only to the expansion in follicular fluid volume but also to the proliferation of the granulosa cells, the number of which increases exponentially (McNatty et al., 1979a).

During the developmental process, marked changes occur in the granulosa cells including proliferation and differentiation. In primordial follicles, only a layer of flattened pregranulosa cells exists surrounding the oocyte. As the follicle leaves the resting pool, the granulosa cells proliferate and become cuboidal. At the stage of approximately 2,000 cells, formation of the antrum takes place and the granulosa cells differentiate to form three major populations (Gosden et al., 1993). Depending on their location, the membrana or mural granulosa cells in the outer part, the cumulus granulosa cells in the inner part close to the oocyte, and the intermediate or periantral granulosa cells have been demonstrated by quantitative cytochemistry (Zoller and Weisz, 1979). However, with respect to the method used, further differentiation has been demonstrated. For instance, flow cytometry of human follicular aspirates following the administration of hCG has demonstrated two distinct luteinized cell populations (Whitman et al., 1991). Certainly, the situation may be different in women undergoing superovulation induction for IVF as a high percentage of aneuploid granulosa-lutein cells has been found by flow cytometry (Grunwald et al., 1998).

This heterogeneity in granulosa cell population reflects morphological as well as functional differences between the cells as assessed by differences in size, protein expression, lectin binding, enzymes, FSH receptors, etc. (Kerketze et al., 1996; Marrone and Crissman, 1988). The mechanism of this heterogeneity is not clear; however, oocyte-derived morphogens, such as GDF-9 and BMP-15, by establishing a concentration gradient, may direct selective physiological responses to FSH in the different cell populations (Erickson and Shimasaki, 2000). In brief, cumulus cells show a high mitotic index with continuous proliferation, while membrana granulosa cells express LH receptors and steroidogenic enzymes.

MULTIPLE FOLLICULAR DEVELOPMENT

Following the delivery of the first IVF baby in 1978 and in an effort to maximize the success rate of the treatment, superovulation induction was adopted as the principal way of obtaining more than one oocyte. This is achieved with the injection of exogenous FSH or the stimulation of increased secretion of endogenous FSH from the pituitary that widen the FSH window and, therefore, the process of single-follicle selection is overridden (Messinis, 1989; Salha and Balen, 2000). Nevertheless, under these conditions, follicle development is always asynchronous. Despite this, the process of multiple follicular development has provided important information for the understanding of the physiology of human folliculogenesis. In contrast, knowledge of the physiological process of follicle maturation provides the basis for the development of protocols that might increase the standard of success in assisted reproduction. When multiple follicular development is induced, marked changes in the relationship between the ovaries and the hypothalamic-pituitary system take place (Messinis, 2006). For instance, circulating estradiol levels become supraphysiological and inhibin levels increase, while the activity of substances such as gonadotrophin surge–attenuating factor

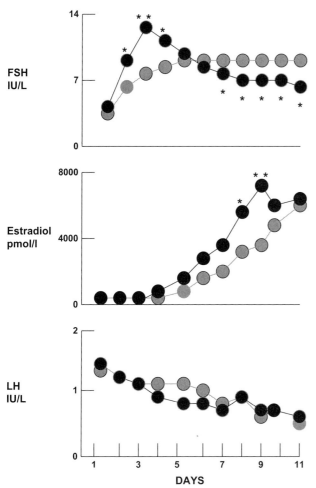

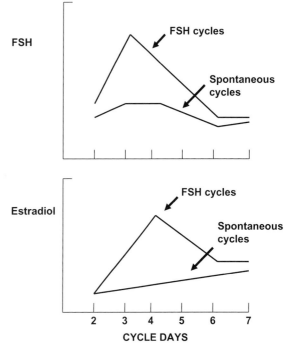

Figure 2.9. Changes in FSH and estradiol concentrations following the injection of a single dose of 450 IU FSH to normal women on cycle day 2. Comparison with spontaneous cycles of the same women. The diagram is based on data presented in Messinis et al., 1994.

Figure 2.8. Mean values of FSH, estradiol, and LH during stimulation with exogenous FSH. Comparison between two protocols, the step-up and the step-down. Forty-five normally cycling women were treated with the two protocols in two different cycles. In the step-up protocol, the starting dose of FSH was 150 IU increasing after five days if necessary according to the ovarian response. In the step-down protocol, the starting dose of FSH was 300 IU for the first two days followed by 150 IU for the rest of the treatment period. The diagram is based on unpublished data.

(GnSAF) that affect the onset and the amplitude of the endogenous LH surge becomes evident.

FSH Thresholds

Two main protocols of ovarian stimulation with FSH are in use now, the step-up and the step-down (Fauser and Van Heusden, 1997). With the step-up protocol, FSH dose increases gradually depending on the ovarian response, while with the step-down, which is closer to the physiological process of follicle selection, a higher dose is given initially that leads to a rapid increase in FSH concentrations and the dose is decreased thereafter, resulting in a gradual decline in FSH levels.

Which of the two protocols is better in clinical terms has not been evaluated. However, based on a recent study (unpublished data), the profile of circulating ovarian hormones differs greatly between the two protocols, reflecting differences in the time at which specific events of folliculogenesis take place. In

particular, with the step-down protocol, estradiol concentrations increased earlier than with the step-up but eventually similar levels were attained toward the end of the treatment (Figure 2.8). Since, in the context of these schedules, eventually a similar number of preovulatory follicles developed, it is suggested that due to the rapid increase in serum FSH levels, follicles were recruited earlier with the step-down than with the step-up protocol. However, not all of them were selected for further growth to the preovulatory stage probably by losing FSH support during the declining part of the levels of this hormone. These results demonstrate that the FSH dose given during the mid- and late follicular phase in the step-down protocol was not adequate to support the growth of all recruited follicles. It is suggested that follicles recruited with the exogenous administration of FSH require certain levels of this hormone during the rest of the follicular phase for further growth.

Similar information has been also obtained from a previous study in which a single high dose of FSH (450 IU) was given to normal women on day 2 of a spontaneous cycle (Messinis et al., 1994). In comparison with an untreated spontaneous cycle of the same women, the FSH injection resulted in a temporal but significant increase of serum FSH levels, which was accompanied by a significant and similar duration increase in serum estradiol concentrations (Figure 2.9). Following this and up to midcycle, the levels of FSH and estradiol were similar to those in the spontaneous cycles and therefore compatible with single-follicle development. These results indicate that the temporal increase in estradiol values after the single dose of FSH was due to the recruitment of multiple follicles, which, however, were unable to achieve further maturation. This means that serum levels of FSH in mid- and late follicular phase that

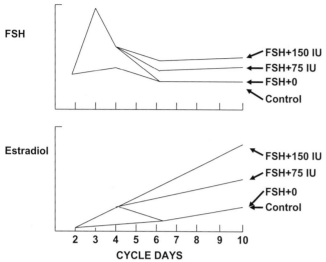

Figure 2.10. FSH and estradiol concentrations during treatment of normal women with FSH. Initially a single dose of 450 IU FSH was given on cycle day 2. Then, from cycle day 4, the women received either no treatment (FSH plus 0) or FSH at the dose of one ampoule (FSH plus 75 IU) or two ampoules (FSH plus 150 IU). Comparison with spontaneous cycles of the same women (control). The estradiol concentrations increased in proportion to the increase in FSH concentrations. The diagram is based on data presented in Lolis et al., 1995.

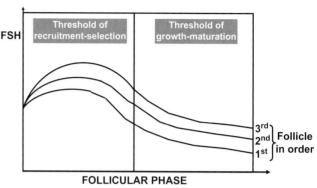

Figure 2.11. A theoretic approach to the FSH thresholds during folliculogenesis in humans. Each follicle has a threshold of recruitment-selection and a threshold of further growth-maturation.

were adequate to stimulate the growth of a dominant follicle were inadequate to support further growth of follicles recruited under the temporal increase of FSH. A hypothesis is supported from these results that follicles recruited with the exogenous administration of FSH require higher FSH levels for further growth than those needed for the growth of the dominant follicle in the natural cycle.

This hypothesis was tested in a subsequent study in which the injection of a single dose of 450 IU FSH on day 2 of the cycle was followed by additional FSH given from day 4 onward at different daily doses (Lolis et al., 1995). It was found that the concentrations of estradiol and the number of follicles that reached the preovulatory stage were increased in proportion to the extra dose of FSH given in mid- and late follicular phase (Figure 2.10). Although the growth rate of the first in order follicle was not affected by the administration of additional FSH, the growth rate of the second and the third in order follicle was increased in proportion to the increasing FSH levels. It is suggested that, although supraphysiological concentrations of FSH are required to induce multiple follicular development in the early follicular phase, the key factor that determines the final number of preovulatory follicles is the FSH levels during the rest of the follicular phase. These data were confirmed in a more recent study that showed that when FSH levels increased above the threshold in the early follicular phase after the exogenous administration of this hormone, the development of the dominant follicle was not affected, although the number of small antral follicles increased (Schipper et al., 1998). However, multiple follicular development occurred only when FSH levels remained high also in mid- and late follicular phase.

It is clear from these data that during superovulation induction, each follicle has its own thresholds, one for recruitment-selection and one for further maturation (Figure 2.11). The first in order follicle has thresholds that are similar to those of the dominant follicle in the spontaneous cycle, or in other words, superovulation induction in normally cycling women does not affect recruitment-selection and further growth of the dominant follicle. The FSH thresholds of the second in order follicle are higher than those of the first follicle, and those of the third follicle are higher than those of the second follicle etc. However, in all follicles, the threshold of recruitment and selection is always higher than the threshold of further maturation.

Follicle recruitment is a timeless process that can happen whenever the FSH threshold of a particular follicle is exceeded. In cycles in which a high dose of FSH is given every day throughout the whole follicular phase, new follicles are recruited continuously, leading to asynchronous follicle maturation. In two recent studies (Hohmann et al., 2001, 2005) in which women with normal cycles were treated with a low-dose regimen of FSH (75 IU/day), multiple follicles developed and estradiol levels increased regardless of the time of onset of FSH administration (cycle days 3, 5, or 7). Administration of FSH on cycle day 5 or 7 interfered with the declining pattern of FSH that was a prerequisite for single-follicle development. Therefore, not only the increase in the levels but also the extension of the FSH intercycle rise by the exogenous administration of this hormone can override the process of single-follicle selection.

The FSH increase in the early follicular phase of the cycle is important both for recruiting multiple follicles and for determining the duration of the follicular phase (Figure 2.12). In a study in which increased FSH levels of different magnitude were achieved on day 4 or 6 of the cycle with the use of different treatment regimens, an inverse relationship was found between these levels and the duration of the follicular phase (Messinis and Templeton, 1990b). Since the length of the follicular phase did not correlate with the levels of FSH in mid- and late follicular phases, it is suggested that in these cycles, increasing levels of FSH early in the cycle advanced follicle selection. The physiological importance of this finding is not clear; however, variability in the magnitude of FSH increase during the intercycle period could explain the varying duration of the follicular phase seen in otherwise normally cycling women.

It is clear from the above discussion that synchronizing multiple follicular development with exogenous FSH is rather unlikely. This is due to the fact that at the time of the FSH rise, there is always at least one follicle that is in a more advanced

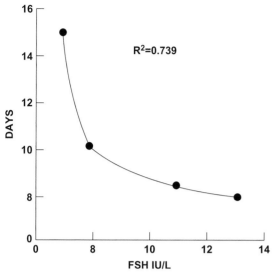

Figure 2.12. Correlation between early follicular phase serum FSH values and the duration of the follicular phase during ovarian stimulation for multiple follicular development. The duration of the follicular phase decreased in proportion to the increase in FSH values but could not be shorter than eight days. The diagram is based on data presented in Messinis and Templeton, 1990b.

stage of development in terms of FSH receptors and increased sensitivity to this hormone than the other follicles of the same cohort. The use of different FSH isoforms might be useful (Wide, 1982; Baird, 2001), however, such isoforms are not available. The only FSH isoform that has been used in clinical practice so far is FSH-CTP, which is a long-acting substance (Duijkers et al., 2002). A single injection of this isoform induces high FSH levels for about one week, creating a long-lasting FSH window (Beckers et al., 2003). Although under the circumstances multiple follicles are selected, folliculogenesis is asynchronous. Therefore, such a substance does not appear to be suitable for optimizing the process of ovarian stimulation.

LH Thresholds

It has been established that besides FSH, LH is also important for follicle maturation in women. Apart from the action on the theca cells, LH acts also via specific receptors that appear on the granulosa cells of the dominant follicle during the second half of the follicular phase of the cycle, that is, after the selection process is completed. It has been found that an LH threshold level is required for normal folliculogenesis, and if serum LH is below it, follicles will not grow further. Administration of a GnRH antagonist to normal women in the second half of the follicular phase resulted in a marked suppression of LH concentrations, while the growth of the dominant follicle was arrested (Leroy et al., 1994).

In vitro and in vivo experiments have shown that an upper limit of LH levels is also important. The concept of LH "ceiling" denotes that when LH exceeds a certain level, it becomes detrimental for follicle maturation (Hillier, 1994). When granulosa cells were treated in vitro with "low-dose" LH, cell proliferation, steroidogenesis, and DNA synthesis were augmented, while with "high-dose" LH, progesterone production was increased, aromatase activity was suppressed, and granulosa cell

growth was inhibited (Yong et al., 1992). Similarly, studies in anovulatory women treated with recombinant FSH have demonstrated that the dose of recombinant LH given during the second half of the follicular phase can control the number of preovulatory follicles (Loumaye et al., 2003; Hugues et al., 2005). Such a dual action of LH might have a potential application in IVF programs to control the number of follicles that develop during the exogenous administration of FSH, particularly in patients prone to excessive response of the ovaries, such as in polycystic ovary syndrome.

MIDCYCLE ENDOGENOUS LH SURGE

The selected dominant follicle that becomes preovulatory secretes in the circulation during the late follicular phase of the cycle high amounts of estradiol that exert a positive feedback effect on the hypothalamic-pituitary system (Rizk, 2008). As a result, the endogenous gonadotrophin surge occurs. With the onset of the LH surge, the granulosa cells begin to undergo terminal differentiation and express a luteal-specific pattern of genes (Richards, 1994). The onset of the luteinization process means a shift in steroidogenesis within the follicle with a dramatic decrease in estradiol concentrations and a gradual increase in serum progesterone values (McNatty et al., 1979a, 1979c). Luteinization is a vital process for the transition of the granulosa and theca cells to the luteal phenotype.

It has become clear that following the onset of the LH surge, the granulosa cells cease to divide as a result of the rapid loss of cell cycle activators including cycling D2 and cycling E and a corresponding increase of cell cycle inhibitors, such as p21cip1 and p27kip1 (Richards, 1994; Richards et al., 1998). The process of cessation of cell division and the process of luteinization are interrelated because normal luteinization fails in mice deficient in p27kip1 (Richards et al., 1998). Oocyte-derived factors, such as GDF-9 and BMP-15, may play a role in luteinization by reducing estradiol production from the surrounding granulosa cells and by promoting the secretion of progesterone (Knight and Glister, 2003). In spite of the fact that following the onset of the LH surge granulosa cells cease to divide, clinical data have demonstrated that follicle diameter continues to increase during the LH surge. The rate of follicle growth during the endogenous LH surge is similar to that during the days preceding the onset of the LH surge, both in spontaneous and FSH superovulated cycles (Messinis and Templeton, 1987). Whether this increase in follicle size is due only to the increase in the follicular fluid volume is not known.

Following the onset of the LH surge, a series of events take place that lead to the rupture of the follicle (Richards et al., 1998). The LH surge induces the expression of progesterone receptors (PR) and prostaglandin endoperoxide synthase-2 (PGS-2) or COX-2 in the granulosa cells. Various proteases are also synthesized to change the integrity of the extracellular matrix, a process that is controlled by PR and PGS-2. The PR may also regulate the response of ovarian cells to prostaglandins. Other pathways include the modification by the PR and PGS-2 of the function of fibroplasts and chemokines, while other growth factors, such as VEGF that is responsible for initiation of angiogenesis, are also important. The ovarian surface epithelium is degraded by the various proteases (metalloproteinases) that are activated by the PR and PGS-2, leading to ovulation.

The process of follicle rupture leads to serial injury and repair of ovarian surface epithelium. In this process, which is an inflammatory event, a compensatory anti-inflammatory mechanism is involved in which cortisol plays a pivotal role (Rae and Hillier, 2005). Inflammatory cytokines such as IL-1α increase the expression of 11β-hydroxysteroid dehydrogenase that reduces cortisone to cortisol, which in turn suppresses IL-1α–induced increase in COX-2 levels in vitro (Rae and Hillier, 2005). This interaction between inflammatory and anti-inflammatory signaling provides possibly the natural mechanism of the healing process after ovulation.

REFERENCES

Adashi E.Y. (1998) The IGF family and folliculogenesis. *J. Reprod. Immunol.* 39, 13–19.

Adashi E.Y. and Hsueh A.J. (1982) Estrogens augment the stimulation of ovarian aromatase activity by follicle-stimulating hormone in cultured rat granulosa cells. *J. Biol. Chem.* 257, 6077–83.

Alexandris E., Milingos S., Kollios G., Seferiadis K., Lolis D. and Messinis I.E. (1997) Changes in gonadotrophin response to gonadotrophin releasing hormone in normal women following bilateral ovariectomy. *Clin. Endocrinol. (Oxf.)* 47, 721–6.

Baird D.T. (1983) Factors regulating the growth of the preovulatory follicle in the sheep and human. *J. Reprod. Fertil.* 69, 343–52.

Baird D.T. (2001) Is there a place for different isoforms of FSH in clinical medicine? IV. The clinician's point of view. *Hum. Reprod.* 16, 1316–18.

Baker S.J. and Spears N. (1999) The role of intra-ovarian interactions in the regulation of follicle dominance. *Hum. Reprod. Update* 5, 153–65.

Barreca A., Del Monte P., Ponzani P., Artini P.G., Genazzani A.R. and Minuto F. (1996) Intrafollicular insulin-like growth factor-II levels in normally ovulating women and in patients with polycystic ovary syndrome. *Fertil. Steril.* 65, 739–45.

Beckers N.G., Macklon N.S., Devroey P., Platteau P., Boerrigter P.J. and Fauser B.C. (2003) First live birth after ovarian stimulation using a chimeric long-acting human recombinant follicle-stimulating hormone (FSH) agonist (recFSH-CTP) for in vitro fertilization. *Fertil. Steril.* 79, 621–3.

Bergh C., Olsson J.H. and Hillensjo T. (1991) Effect of insulin-like growth factor I on steroidogenesis in cultured human granulosa cells. *Acta. Endocrinol. (Copenh).* 125, 177–85.

Billig H., Furuta I. and Hsueh A.J. (1993) Estrogens inhibit and androgens enhance ovarian granulosa cell apoptosis. *Endocrinology* 133, 2204–12.

Brown J.B., Evans J.H., Adey F.D. and Taft H.P. (1969) Factors involved in the induction of fertile ovulation with human gonadotrophins. *J. Obstet. Gynaecol. Br. Commonw.* 76, 289–307.

Bukovsky A., Caudle M.R., Keenan J.A., Wimalasena J., Foster J.S. and Van Meter S.E. (1995a) Quantitative evaluation of the cell cycle-related retinoblastoma protein and localization of Thy-1 differentiation protein and macrophages during follicular development and atresia, and in human corpora lutea. *Biol. Reprod.* 52, 776–92.

Bukovsky A., Caudle M.R., Keenan J.A., Wimalasena J., Foster J.S., Upadhyaya N.B. and van Meter S.E. (1995b) Expression of cell cycle regulatory proteins (p53, pRb) in the human female genital tract. *J. Assist. Reprod. Genet.* 12, 123–31.

Campbell B.K. (1999) The modulation of gonadotrophic hormone action on the ovary by paracrine and autocrine factors. *Anat. Histol. Embryol.* 28, 247–51.

Carabatsos M.J., Elvin J., Matzuk M.M. and Albertini D.F. (1998) Characterization of oocyte and follicle development in growth differentiation factor-9-deficient mice. *Dev. Biol.* 204, 373–84.

Carlsson I.B., Scott J.E., Visser J.A., Ritvos O., Themmen A.P. and Hovatta O. (2006) Anti-Mullerian hormone inhibits initiation of growth of human primordial ovarian follicles in vitro. *Hum. Reprod.* 21, 2223–7.

Conover C.A., Oxvig C., Overgaard M.T., Christiansen M. and Giudice L.C. (1999) Evidence that the insulin-like growth factor binding protein-4 protease in human ovarian follicular fluid is pregnancy associated plasma protein-A. *J. Clin. Endocrinol. Metab.* 84, 4742–5.

Cortvrindt R., Hu Y. and Smitz J. (1998) Recombinant luteinizing hormone as a survival and differentiation factor increases oocyte maturation in recombinant follicle stimulating hormone-supplemented mouse preantral follicle culture. *Hum. Reprod.* 13, 1292–302.

Couse J.F., Yates M.M., Deroo B.J. and Korach K.S. (2005) Estrogen receptor-beta is critical to granulosa cell differentiation and the ovulatory response to gonadotropins. *Endocrinology* 146, 3247–62.

Dafopoulos K.C., Kotsovassilis C.P., Milingos S.D., Kallitsaris A.T., Georgadakis G.S., Sotiros P.G. and Messinis I.E. (2004) Changes in pituitary sensitivity to GnRH in estrogen-treated postmenopausal women: evidence that gonadotrophin surge attenuating factor plays a physiological role. *Hum. Reprod.* 19, 1985–92.

de Kretser D.M., Hedger M.P., Loveland K.L. and Phillips D.J. (2002) Inhibins, activins and follistatin in reproduction. *Hum. Reprod. Update* 8, 529–41.

Di Blasio A.M., Vigano P. and Ferrari A. (1994) Insulin-like growth factor-II stimulates human granulosa-luteal cell proliferation in vitro. *Fertil. Steril.* 61, 483–7.

Di Pasquale E., Beck-Peccoz P. and Persani L. (2004) Hypergonadotropic ovarian failure associated with an inherited mutation of human bone morphogenetic protein-15 (BMP15) gene. *Am. J. Hum. Genet.* 75, 106–11.

Dissen G.A., Romero C., Hirshfield A.N. and Ojeda S.R. (2001) Nerve growth factor is required for early follicular development in the mammalian ovary. *Endocrinology* 142, 2078–86.

Dor J., Ben-Shlomo I., Lunenfeld B., Pariente C., Levran D., Karasik A., Seppala M. and Mashiach S. (1992) Insulin-like growth factor-I (IGF-I) may not be essential for ovarian follicular development: evidence from IGF-I deficiency. *J. Clin. Endocrinol. Metab.* 74, 539–42.

Dorrington J.H. and Armstrong D.T. (1979) Effects of FSH on gonadal functions. *Recent Prog. Horm. Res.* 35, 301–42.

Dube J.L., Wang P., Elvin J., Lyons K.M., Celeste A.J. and Matzuk M.M. (1998) The bone morphogenetic protein 15 gene is X-linked and expressed in oocytes. *Mol. Endocrinol.* 12, 1809–17.

Duijkers I.J., Klipping C., Boerrigter P.J., Machielsen C.S., De Bie J.J., and Voortman G. (2002) Single dose pharmacokinetics and effects on follicular growth and serum hormones of a long-acting recombinant FSH preparation (FSH-CTP) in healthy pituitary-suppressed females. *Hum. Reprod.* 17, 1987–93.

Eden J.A., Jones J., Carter G.D. and Alaghband-Zadeh J. (1990) Follicular fluid concentrations of insulin-like growth factor 1, epidermal growth factor, transforming growth factor-alpha and sex-steroids in volume matched normal and polycystic human follicles. *Clin. Endocrinol. (Oxf).* 32, 395–405.

El-Roeiy A., Chen X., Roberts V.J., LeRoith D., Roberts C.T., Jr. and Yen S.S. (1993) Expression of insulin-like growth factor-I (IGF-I) and IGF-II and the IGF-I, IGF-II, and insulin receptor genes and localization of the gene products in the human ovary. *J. Clin. Endocrinol. Metab.* 77, 1411–18.

Emmen J.M., Couse J.F., Elmore S.A., Yates M.M., Kissling G.E. and Korach K.S. (2005) In vitro growth and ovulation of follicles from ovaries of estrogen receptor (ER){alpha} and ER{beta} null mice indicate a role for ER{beta} in follicular maturation. *Endocrinology* 146, 2817–26.

Erickson G.F. and Shimasaki S. (2000) The role of the oocyte in folliculogenesis. *Trends Endocrinol. Metab.* 11, 193–8.

Erickson G.F. and Shimasaki S. (2001) The physiology of folliculogenesis: the role of novel growth factors. *Fertil. Steril.* 76, 943–9.

Erickson G.F., Magoffin D.A., Dyer C.A. and Hofeditz C. (1985) The ovarian androgen producing cells: a review of structure/function relationships. *Endocr. Rev.* 6, 371–99.

Fauser B.C. and Van Heusden A.M. (1997) Manipulation of human ovarian function: physiological concepts and clinical consequences. *Endocr. Rev.* 18, 71–106.

Findlay J.K., Drummond A.E., Britt K.L., Dyson M., Wreford N.G., Robertson D.M., Groome N.P., Jones M.E. and Simpson E.R. (2000) The roles of activins, inhibins and estrogen in early committed follicles. *Mol. Cell. Endocrinol.* 163, 81–7.

Geisthovel F., Moretti-Rojas I., Asch R.H. and Rojas F.J. (1989) Expression of insulin-like growth factor-II (IGF-II) messenger ribonucleic acid (mRNA), but not IGF-I mRNA, in human preovulatory granulosa cells. *Hum. Reprod.* 4, 899–902.

Glister C., Groome N.P. and Knight P.G. (2006) Bovine follicle development is associated with divergent changes in activin-A, inhibin-A and follistatin and the relative abundance of different follistatin isoforms in follicular fluid. *J. Endocrinol.* 188, 215–25.

Gosden R.G., Huntley J.F., Douglas A., Inglis L. and Miller H.R. (1993) Quantitative and cytochemical studies of mast cell proteases in rat ovaries and uteri in various reproductive states. *J. Reprod. Fertil.* 98, 577–82.

Gougeon A. (1986) Dynamics of follicular growth in the human: a model from preliminary results. *Hum. Reprod.* 1, 81–7.

Gougeon A. and Lefevre B. (1983) Evolution of the diameters of the largest healthy and atretic follicles during the human menstrual cycle. *J. Reprod. Fertil.* 69, 497–502.

Gougeon A. and Testart J. (1990) Influence of human menopausal gonadotropin on the recruitment of human ovarian follicles. *Fertil. Steril.* 54, 848–52.

Groome N.P., Illingworth P.J., O'Brien M., Pai R., Rodger F.E., Mather J.P. and McNeilly A.S. (1996) Measurement of dimeric inhibin B throughout the human menstrual cycle. *J. Clin. Endocrinol. Metab.* 81, 1401–5.

Grunwald K., Feldmann K., Melsheimer P., Rabe T., Neulen J. and Runnebaum B. (1998) Aneuploidy in human granulosa lutein cells obtained from gonadotrophin-stimulated follicles and its relation to intrafollicular hormone concentrations. *Hum. Reprod.* 13, 2679–87.

Hayashi M., McGee E.A., Min G., Klein C., Rose U.M., van Duin M. and Hsueh A.J. (1999) Recombinant growth differentiation factor-9 (GDF-9) enhances growth and differentiation of cultured early ovarian follicles. *Endocrinology* 140, 1236–44.

Hernandez E.R., Resnick C.E., Svoboda M.E., Van Wyk J.J., Payne D.W. and Adashi E.Y. (1988) Somatomedin-C/insulin-like growth factor I as an enhancer of androgen biosynthesis by cultured rat ovarian cells. *Endocrinology* 122, 1603–12.

Hild-Petito S., Stouffer R.L. and Brenner R.M. (1988) Immunocytochemical localization of estradiol and progesterone receptors in the monkey ovary throughout the menstrual cycle. *Endocrinology* 123, 2896–905.

Hillier S.G. (1994) Current concepts of the roles of follicle stimulating hormone and luteinizing hormone in folliculogenesis. *Hum. Reprod.* 9, 188–91.

Hillier S.G. (2001) Gonadotropic control of ovarian follicular growth and development. *Mol. Cell. Endocrinol.* 179, 39–46.

Hillier S.G. and Tetsuka M. (1997) Role of androgens in follicle maturation and atresia. *Baillieres Clin. Obstet. Gynaecol.* 11, 249–60.

Hillier S.G., Whitelaw P.F. and Smyth C.D. (1994) Follicular oestrogen synthesis: the 'two-cell, two-gonadotrophin' model revisited. *Mol. Cell. Endocrinol.* 100, 51–4.

Hirshfield A.N. (1991) Development of follicles in the mammalian ovary. *Int. Rev. Cytol.* 124, 43–101.

Hohmann F.P., Laven J.S., de Jong F.H., Eijkemans M.J. and Fauser B.C. (2001) Low-dose exogenous FSH initiated during the early, mid or late follicular phase can induce multiple dominant follicle development. *Hum. Reprod.* 16, 846–54.

Hohmann F.P., Laven J.S., de Jong F.H. and Fauser B.C. (2005) Relationship between inhibin A and B, estradiol and follicle growth dynamics during ovarian stimulation in normo-ovulatory women. *Eur. J. Endocrinol.* 152, 395–401.

Hourvitz A., Widger A.E., Filho F.L., Chang R.J., Adashi E.Y. and Erickson G.F. (2000) Pregnancy-associated plasma protein-A gene expression in human ovaries is restricted to healthy follicles and corpora lutea. *J. Clin. Endocrinol. Metab.* 85, 4916–20.

Hsu S.Y., Kubo M., Chun S.Y., Haluska F.G., Housman D.E. and Hsueh A.J. (1995) Wilms' tumor protein WT1 as an ovarian transcription factor: decreases in expression during follicle development and repression of inhibin-alpha gene promoter. *Mol. Endocrinol.* 9, 1356–66.

Huang E.J., Manova K., Packer A.I., Sanchez S., Bachvarova R.F. and Besmer P. (1993) The murine steel panda mutation affects kit ligand expression and growth of early ovarian follicles. *Dev. Biol.* 157, 100–9.

Hugues J.N., Soussis J., Calderon I., Balasch J., Anderson R.A. and Romeu A. (2005) Recombinant LH Study Group. Does the addition of recombinant LH in WHO group II anovulatory women over-responding to FSH treatment reduce the number of developing follicles? A dose-finding study. *Hum. Reprod.* 20, 629–35.

Hussein M.R. (2005) Apoptosis in the ovary: molecular mechanisms. *Hum. Reprod. Update* 11, 162–77.

Iwai T., Nanbu Y., Iwai M., Taii S., Fujii S. and Mori T. (1990) Immunohistochemical localization of oestrogen receptors and progesterone receptors in the human ovary throughout the menstrual cycle. *Virchows Arch A. Pathol. Anat. Histopathol.* 417, 369–75.

Judd S., Terry A., Petrucco M. and White G. (1992) The source of pulsatile secretion of progesterone during the human follicular phase. *J. Clin. Endocrinol. Metab.* 74, 299–305.

Kamada S., Kubota T., Taguchi M., Ho W.R., Sakamoto S. and Aso T. (1992) Effects of insulin-like growth factor-II on proliferation and differentiation of ovarian granulosa cells. *Horm. Res.* 37, 141–9.

Kerketze K., Blaschuk O.W. and Farookhi R. (1996) Cellular heterogeneity in the membrana granulosa of developing rat follicles: assessment by flow cytometry and lectin binding. *Endocrinology* 137, 3089–100.

Klein N.A., Houmard B.S., Hansen K.R., Woodruff T.K., Sluss P.M., Bremner W.J. and Soules M.R. (2004) Age-related analysis of inhibin A, inhibin B, and activin A relative to the intercycle monotropic follicle-stimulating hormone rise in normal ovulatory women. *J. Clin. Endocrinol. Metab.* 89, 2977–81.

Knight P.G. and Glister C. (2003) Local roles of TGF-beta superfamily members in the control of ovarian follicle development. *Anim. Reprod. Sci.* 78, 165–83.

Knight P.G. and Glister C. (2006) TGF-beta superfamily members and ovarian follicle development. *Reproduction* 32, 191–206.

Lawrence J.B., Oxvig C., Overgaard M.T., Sottrup-Jensen L., Gleich G.J., Hays L.G., Yates J.R., 3rd and Conover C.A. (1999) The insulin-like growth factor (IGF)-dependent IGF binding protein-4 protease secreted by human fibroblasts is pregnancy-associated plasma protein-A. *Proc. Natl. Acad. Sci. U. S. A.* 96, 3149–53.

Leroy I., d'Acremont M., Brailly-Tabard S., Frydman R., de Mouzon J. and Bouchard P. (1994) A single injection of a gonadotropin-releasing hormone (GnRH) antagonist (Cetrorelix) postpones the luteinizing hormone (LH) surge: further evidence for the role of GnRH during the LH surge. *Fertil. Steril.* 62, 461–7.

Lolis D.E., Tsolas O. and Messinis I.E. (1995) The follicle-stimulating hormone threshold level for follicle maturation in superovulated cycles. *Fertil. Steril.* 63, 1272–7.

Loumaye E., Engrand P., Shoham Z., Hillier S.G. and Baird D.T. (2003) Clinical evidence for an LH 'ceiling' effect induced by administration of recombinant human LH during the late follicular phase of stimulated cycles in World Health Organization type I and type II anovulation. *Hum. Reprod.* 18, 314–22.

MacNatty K.P., Hunter W.M., MacNeilly A.S. and Sawers R.S. (1975) Changes in the concentration of pituitary and steroid hormones in the follicular fluid of human graafian follicles throughout the menstrual cycle. *J. Endocrinol.* 64, 555–71.

Magoffin D.A. and Weitsman S.R. (1994) Insulin-like growth factor-I regulation of luteinizing hormone (LH) receptor messenger ribonucleic acid expression and LH-stimulated signal transduction in rat ovarian theca-interstitial cells. *Biol. Reprod.* 51, 766–75.

Mais V., Cetel N.S., Muse K.N., Quigley M.E., Reid R.L. and Yen S.S. (1987) Hormonal dynamics during luteal-follicular transition. *J. Clin. Endocrinol. Metab.* 64, 1109–14.

Marrone B.L. and Crissman H.A. (1988) Characterization of granulosa cell subpopulations from avian preovulatory follicles by multiparameter flow cytometry. *Endocrinology* 122, 651–8.

Mason H.D., Willis D.S., Holly J.M. and Franks S. (1994) Insulin preincubation enhances insulin-like growth factor-II (IGF-II) action on steroidogenesis in human granulosa cells. *J. Clin. Endocrinol. Metab.* 78, 1265–7.

Mason H.D., Cwyfan-Hughes S.C., Heinrich G., Franks S. and Holly J.M. (1996) Insulin-like growth factor (IGF) I and II, IGF-binding proteins, and IGF-binding protein proteases are produced by theca and stroma of normal and polycystic human ovaries. *J. Clin. Endocrinol. Metab.* 81, 276–84.

Mason H.D., Cwyfan-Hughes S., Holly J.M. and Franks S. (1998) Potent inhibition of human ovarian steroidogenesis by insulin-like growth factor binding protein-4 (IGFBP-4). *J. Clin. Endocrinol. Metab.* 83, 284–7.

Matthews C.H., Borgato S., Beck-Peccoz P., Adams M., Tone Y., Gambino G., Casagrande S., Tedeschini G., Benedetti A. and Chatterjee V.K. (1993) Primary amenorrhoea and infertility due to a mutation in the beta-subunit of follicle-stimulating hormone. *Nat. Genet.* 5, 83–6.

May J.V., Frost J.P. and Bridge A.J. (1990) Regulation of granulosa cell proliferation: facilitative roles of platelet-derived growth factor and low density lipoprotein. *Endocrinology* 126, 2896–905.

Mazerbourg S., Bondy C.A., Zhou J. and Monget P. (2003) The insulin-like growth factor system: a key determinant role in the growth and selection of ovarian follicles? A comparative species study. *Reprod. Domest. Anim.* 38, 247–58.

McGee E.A. and Hsueh A.J. (2000) Initial and cyclic recruitment of ovarian follicles. *Endocr. Rev.* 21, 200–14.

McGee E., Spears N., Minami S., Hsu S.Y., Chun S.Y., Billig H. and Hsueh A.J. (1997) Preantral ovarian follicles in serum-free culture: suppression of apoptosis after activation of the cyclic guanosine 3',5'-monophosphate pathway and stimulation of growth and differentiation by follicle-stimulating hormone. *Endocrinology* 138, 2417–24.

McGee E.A., Smith R., Spears N., Nachtigal M.W., Ingraham H. and Hsueh A.J. (2001) Mullerian inhibitory substance induces growth of rat preantral ovarian follicles. *Biol. Reprod.* 64, 293–8.

McGrath S.A., Esquela A.F. and Lee S.J. (1995) Oocyte-specific expression of growth/differentiation factor-9. *Mol. Endocrinol.* 9, 131–6.

McNatty K.P. and Baird D.T. (1978) Relationship between follicle-stimulating hormone, androstenedione and oestradiol in human follicular fluid. *J. Endocrinol.* 76, 527–31.

McNatty K.P., Smith D.M., Makris A., Osathanondh R. and Ryan K.J. (1979a) The microenvironment of the human antral follicle: interrelationships among the steroid levels in antral fluid, the population of granulosa cells, and the status of the oocyte in vivo and in vitro. *J. Clin. Endocrinol. Metab.* 49, 851–60.

McNatty K.P., Makris A., Reinhold V.N., De Grazia C., Osathanondh R. and Ryan K.J. (1979b) Metabolism of androstenedione by human ovarian tissues in vitro with particular reference to reductase and aromatase activity. *Steroids* 34, 429–43.

McNatty K.P., Makris A., DeGrazia C., Osathanondh R. and Ryan K.J. (1979c) The production of progesterone, androgens, and estrogens by granulosa cells, thecal tissue, and stromal tissue from human ovaries in vitro. *J. Clin. Endocrinol. Metab.* 49, 687–99.

McNatty K.P., Juengel J.L., Reader K.L., Lun S., Myllymaa S., Lawrence S.B., Western A., Meerasahib M.F., Mottershead D.G., Groome N.P., Ritvos O. and Laitinen M.P.E. (2005) Bone morphogenetic protein 15 and growth differentiation factor 9 co-operate to regulate granulosa cell function. *Reproduction* 129, 473–80.

Messinis I.E. (1989) Drugs used in in vitro fertilisation procedures. *Drugs* 38, 148–59.

Messinis I.E. (2006) Ovarian feedback, mechanism of action and possible clinical implications. *Hum. Reprod. Update* 12, 557–71.

Messinis I.E. and Templeton A. (1986) Urinary oestrogen levels and follicle ultrasound measurements in clomiphene induced cycles with an endogenous luteinizing hormone surge. *Br. J. Obstet. Gynaecol.* 93, 43–9.

Messinis I.E. and Templeton A.A. (1987) Endocrine and follicle characteristics of cycles with and without endogenous luteinizing hormone surges during superovulation induction with pulsatile follicle-stimulating hormone. *Hum. Reprod.* 2, 11–16.

Messinis I.E. and Templeton A.A. (1988a) The endocrine consequences of multiple folliculogenesis. *J. Reprod. Fertil. Suppl.* 36, 27–37.

Messinis I.E. and Templeton A. (1988b) Blockage of the positive feedback effect of oestradiol during prolonged administration of clomiphene citrate to normal women. *Clin. Endocrinol. (Oxf).* 29, 509–16.

Messinis I.E. and Templeton A.A. (1990a) Effects of supraphysiological concentrations of progesterone on the characteristics of the oestradiol-induced gonadotrophin surge in women. *J. Reprod. Fertil.* 88, 513–19.

Messinis I.E. and Templeton A.A. (1990b) The importance of follicle-stimulating hormone increase for folliculogenesis. *Hum. Reprod.* 5, 153–6.

Messinis I.E., Koutsoyiannis D., Milingos S., Tsahalina E., Seferiadis K., Lolis D. and Templeton A.A. (1993) Changes in pituitary response to GnRH during the luteal-follicular transition of the human menstrual cycle. *Clin. Endocrinol. (Oxf).* 38, 159–63.

Messinis I.E., Lolis D., Zikopoulos K., Tsahalina E., Seferiadis K. and Templeton A.A. (1994) Effect of an increase in FSH on the production of gonadotrophin-surge-attenuating factor in women. *J. Reprod. Fertil.* 101, 689–95.

Minegishi T., Hirakawa T., Kishi H., Abe K., Abe Y., Mizutani T. and Miyamoto K. (2000) A role of insulin-like growth factor I for follicle-stimulating hormone receptor expression in rat granulosa cells. *Biol. Reprod.* 62, 325–33.

Miro F. and Hillier S.G. (1996) Modulation of granulosa cell deoxyribonucleic acid synthesis and differentiation by activin. *Endocrinology* 137, 464–8.

Molskness T.A., Woodruff T.K., Hess D.L., Dahl K.D. and Stouffer R.L. (1996) Recombinant human inhibin-A administered early in the menstrual cycle alters concurrent pituitary and follicular, plus subsequent luteal, function in rhesus monkeys. *J. Clin. Endocrinol. Metab.* 81, 4002–6.

Moore R.K. and Shimasaki S. (2005) Molecular biology and physiological role of the oocyte factor, BMP-15. *Mol. Cell. Endocrinol.* 234, 67–73.

Mullis P.E., Yoshimura N., Kuhlmann B., Lippuner K., Jaeger P. and Harada H. (1997) Aromatase deficiency in a female who is compound heterozygote for two new point mutations in the P450arom gene: impact of estrogens on hypergonadotropic hypogonadism, multicystic ovaries, and bone densitometry in childhood. *J. Clin. Endocrinol. Metab.* 82, 1739–45.

Nahum R., Thong K.J. and Hillier S.G. (1995) Metabolic regulation of androgen production by human thecal cells in vitro. *Hum. Reprod.* 10, 75–81.

Nakatani A., Shimasaki S., Depaolo L.V., Erickson G.F. and Ling N. (1991) Cyclic changes in follistatin messenger ribonucleic acid and its protein in the rat ovary during the estrous cycle. *Endocrinology* 129, 603–11.

Nilsson E.E., Detzel C. and Skinner M.K. (2006) Platelet-derived growth factor modulates the primordial to primary follicle transition. *Reproduction* 31, 1007–15.

Otsuka F., Yao Z., Lee T., Yamamoto S., Erickson G.F. and Shimasaki S. (2000) Bone morphogenetic protein-15. Identification of target cells and biological functions. *J. Biol. Chem.* 275, 39523–8.

Pelletier G. and El-Alfy M. (2000) Immunocytochemical localization of estrogen receptors alpha and beta in the human reproductive organs. *J. Clin. Endocrinol. Metab.* 85, 4835–40.

Perez G.I., Robles R., Knudson C.M., Flaws J.A., Korsmeyer S.J. and Tilly J.L. (1999) Prolongation of ovarian lifespan into advanced chronological age by Bax-deficiency. *Nat. Genet.* 21, 200–3.

Peters H., Byskov A.G. and Grinsted J. (1978) Follicular growth in fetal and prepubertal ovaries of humans and other primates. *J. Clin. Endocrinol. Metab.* 7, 469–85.

Piontkewitz Y., Sundfeldt K. and Hedin L. (1997) The expression of c-myc during follicular growth and luteal formation in the rat ovary in vivo. *J. Endocrinol.* 152, 395–406.

Piquette G.N., LaPolt P.S., Oikawa M. and Hsueh A.J. (1991) Regulation of luteinizing hormone receptor messenger ribonucleic acid levels by gonadotropins, growth factors, and gonadotropin-releasing hormone in cultured rat granulosa cells. *Endocrinology* 128, 2449–56.

Rabin D., Spitz I., Bercovici B., Bell J., Laufer A., Benveniste R. and Polishuk W. (1972) Isolated deficiency of follicle-stimulating hormone. Clinical and laboratory features. *N. Engl. J. Med.* 287, 1313–17.

Rabinovici J., Blankstein J., Goldman B., Rudak E., Dor Y., Pariente C., Geier A., Lunenfeld B. and Mashiach S. (1989) In vitro fertilization and primary embryonic cleavage are possible in 17 alpha-hydroxylase deficiency despite extremely low intrafollicular 17 beta-estradiol. *J. Clin. Endocrinol. Metab.* 68, 693–7.

Rae M.T. and Hillier S.G. (2005) Steroid signalling in the ovarian surface epithelium. *Trends Endocrinol. Metab.* 16, 327–33.

Reilly C.M., Cannady W.E., Mahesh V.B., Stopper V.S., De Sevilla L.M. and Mills T.M. (1996) Duration of estrogen exposure prior to follicle-stimulating hormone stimulation is critical to granulosa cell growth and differentiation in rats. *Biol. Reprod.* 54, 1336–42.

Richards J.S. (1994) Hormonal control of gene expression in the ovary. *Endocr. Rev.* 15, 725–51.

Richards J.S., Russell D.L., Robker L., Dajee M. and Alliston T.N. (1998) Molecular mechanisms of ovulation and luteinization. *Mol. Cell. Endocrinol.* 145, 47–54.

Rivera G.M. and Fortune J.E. (2003) Proteolysis of insulin-like growth factor binding proteins -4 and -5 in bovine follicular fluid: implications for ovarian follicular selection and dominance. *Endocrinology* 144, 2977–87.

Rizk B. (Ed.). 2008 Ultrasonography in reproductive medicine and infertility. Cambridge: United Kingdom, Cambridge University Press (in press).

Rolaki A., Drakakis P., Millingos S., Loutradis D. and Makrigiannakis A. (2005) Novel trends in follicular development, atresia and corpus luteum regression: a role for apoptosis. *Reprod. Biomed. Online* 11, 93–103.

Roy S.K., Wang S.C. and Greenwald G.S. (1987) Radioreceptor and autoradiographic analysis of FSH, hCG and prolactin binding sites in primary to antral hamster follicles during the periovulatory period. *J. Reprod. Fertil.* 79, 307–13.

Salha O. and Balen A.H. (2000) New concepts in superovulation strategies for assisted conception treatments. *Curr. Opin. Obstet. Gynecol.* 12, 201–6.

Sasson R. and Amsterdam A. (2002) Stimulation of apoptosis in human granulosa cells from in vitro fertilization patients and its prevention by dexamethasone: involvement of cell contact and bcl-2 expression. *J. Clin. Endocrinol. Metab.* 87, 3441–51.

Schipper I., Hop W.C. and Fauser B.C. (1998) The follicle-stimulating hormone (FSH) threshold/window concept examined by different interventions with exogenous FSH during the follicular phase of the normal menstrual cycle: duration, rather than magnitude, of FSH increase affects follicle development. *J. Clin. Endocrinol. Metab.* 83, 1292–8.

Schoot D.C., Coelingh Bennink H.J., Mannaerts B.M., Lamberts S.W., Bouchard P. and Fauser B.C. (1992) Human recombinant follicle-stimulating hormone induces growth of preovulatory follicles without concomitant increase in androgen and estrogen biosynthesis in a woman with isolated gonadotropin deficiency. *J. Clin. Endocrinol. Metab.* 74, 1471–3.

Scobie G.A., Macpherson S., Millar M.R., Groome N.P., Romana P.G. and Saunders P.T. (2002) Human oestrogen receptors: differential expression of ER alpha and beta and the identification of ER beta variants. *Steroids* 67, 985–92.

Smyth C.D., Miro F., Whitelaw P.F., Howles C.M. and Hillier S.G. (1993) Ovarian thecal/interstitial androgen synthesis is enhanced by a follicle-stimulating hormone-stimulated paracrine mechanism. *Endocrinology* 133, 1532–8.

Spicer L.J. (2004) Proteolytic degradation of insulin-like growth factor binding proteins by ovarian follicles: a control mechanism for selection of dominant follicles. *Biol. Reprod.* 70, 1223–30.

Sullivan M.W., Stewart-Akers A., Krasnow J.S., Berga S.L. and Zeleznik A.J. (1999) Ovarian responses in women to recombinant follicle-stimulating hormone and luteinizing hormone (LH): a role for LH in the final stages of follicular maturation. *J. Clin. Endocrinol. Metab.* 84, 228–32.

Templeton A., Messinis I.E. and Baird D.T. (1986) Characteristics of ovarian follicles in spontaneous and stimulated cycles in which there was an endogenous luteinizing hormone surge. *Fertil. Steril.* 46, 1113–17.

Tetsuka M. and Hillier S.G. (1996) Androgen receptor gene expression in rat granulosa cells: the role of follicle-stimulating hormone and steroid hormones. *Endocrinology* 137, 4392–7.

Tetsuka M., Whitelaw P.F., Bremner W.J., Millar M.R., Smyth C.D. and Hillier S.G. (1995) Developmental regulation of androgen receptor in rat ovary. *J. Endocrinol.* 145, 535–43.

Touraine P., Beau I., Gougeon A., Meduri G., Desroches A., Pichard C., Detoeuf M., Paniel B., Prieur M., Zorn J.R., Milgrom E., Kuttenn F. and Misrahi M. (1999) New natural inactivating mutations of the follicle-stimulating hormone receptor: correlations between receptor function and phenotype. *Mol. Endocrinol.* 13, 1844–54.

van Dessel H.J., Schipper I., Pache T.D., van Geldorp H., de Jong F.H. and Fauser B.C. (1996a) Normal human follicle development: an evaluation of correlations with oestradiol, androstenedione and progesterone levels in individual follicles. *Clin. Endocrinol. (Oxf).* 44, 191–8.

van Dessel H.J., Chandrasekher Y., Yap O.W., Lee P.D., Hintz R.L., Faessen G.H., Braat D.D., Fauser B.C. and Giudice L.C. (1996b) Serum and follicular fluid levels of insulin-like growth factor I (IGF-I), IGF-II, and IGF-binding protein-1 and -3 during the normal menstrual cycle. *J. Clin. Endocrinol. Metab.* 81, 1224–31.

van Santbrink E.J., Hop W.C., van Dessel T.J., de Jong F.H. and Fauser B.C. (1995) Decremental follicle-stimulating hormone and dominant follicle development during the normal menstrual cycle. *Fertil. Steril.* 64, 37–43.

van Wezel I.L. and Rodgers R.J. (1996) Morphological characterization of bovine primordial follicles and their environment in vivo. *Biol. Reprod.* 55, 1003–11.

Visser J.A. and Themmen A.P. (2005) Anti-Mullerian hormone and folliculogenesis. *Mol. Cell. Endocrinol.* 234, 81–6.

Vitt U.A., Hayashi M., Klein C. and Hsueh A.J. (2000) Growth differentiation factor-9 stimulates proliferation but suppresses the follicle-stimulating hormone-induced differentiation of cultured granulosa cells from small antral and preovulatory rat follicles. *Biol. Reprod.* 62, 370–7.

Wang H.S. and Chard T. (1999) IGFs and IGF-binding proteins in the regulation of human ovarian and endometrial function. *J. Endocrinol.* 161, 1–13.

Wang X.N. and Greenwald G.S. (1993) Synergistic effects of steroids with FSH on folliculogenesis, steroidogenesis and FSH- and hCG-receptors in hypophysectomized mice. *J. Reprod. Fertil.* 99, 403–13.

Westergaard L., McNatty K.P. and Christensen I.J. (1985) Steroid concentrations in fluid from human ovarian antral follicles during pregnancy. *J. Endocrinol.* 107, 133–6.

Westergaard L., Christensen I.J. and McNatty K.P. (1986) Steroid levels in ovarian follicular fluid related to follicle size and health status during the normal menstrual cycle in women. *Hum. Reprod.* 1, 227–32.

Whitelaw P.F., Smyth C.D., Howles C.M. and Hillier S.G. (1992) Cell-specific expression of aromatase and LH receptor mRNAs in rat ovary. *J. Mol. Endocrinol.* 9, 309–12.

Whitman G.F., Boldt J.P., Martinez J.E. and Pantazis C.G. (1991) Flow cytometric analysis of induced human graafian follicles. I. Demonstration and sorting of two luteinized cell populations. *Fertil. Steril.* 56, 259–64.

Wide L. (1982) Male and female forms of human follicle-stimulating hormone in serum. *J. Clin. Endocrinol. Metab.* 55, 682–8.

Willis D.S., Watson H., Mason H.D., Galea R., Brincat M. and Franks S. (1998) Premature response to luteinizing hormone of granulosa cells from anovulatory women with polycystic ovary syndrome: relevance to mechanism of anovulation. *J. Clin. Endocrinol. Metab.* 83, 3984–91.

Yong E.L., Baird D.T., Yates R., Reichert L.E. Jr. and Hillier S.G. (1992) Hormonal regulation of the growth and steroidogenic function of human granulosa cells. *J. Clin. Endocrinol. Metab.* 74, 842–9.

Zeleznik A.J. (1981) Premature elevation of systemic estradiol reduces serum levels of follicle-stimulating hormone and lengthens the follicular phase of the menstrual cycle in rhesus monkeys. *Endocrinology* 109, 352–5.

Zeleznik A.J. (2001) Follicle selection in primates: "many are called but few are chosen". *Biol. Reprod.* 65, 655–9.

Zeleznik A.J. (2004) The physiology of follicle selection. *Reprod. Biol. Endocrinol.* 2, 31.

Zeleznik A.J. and Hillier S.G. (1984) The role of gonadotropins in the selection of the preovulatory follicle. *Clin. Obstet. Gynecol.* 27, 927–40.

Zeleznik A.J. and Kubik C.J. (1986) Ovarian responses in macaques to pulsatile infusion of follicle-stimulating hormone (FSH) and luteinizing hormone: increased sensitivity of the maturing follicle to FSH. *Endocrinology* 119, 2025–32.

Zeleznik A.J., Hutchinson J.S. and Schuler H.M. (1987) Passive immunization with anti-oestradiol antibodies during the luteal phase of the menstrual cycle potentiates the perimenstrual rise in serum gonadotrophin concentrations and stimulates follicular growth in the cynomolgus monkey (Macaca fascicularis). *J. Reprod. Fertil.* 80, 403–10.

Zhou J. and Bondy C. (1993) Anatomy of the human ovarian insulin-like growth factor system. *Biol. Reprod.* 48, 467–82.

Zimmermann R.C., Hartman T., Kavic S., Pauli S.A., Bohlen P., Sauer M.V. and Kitajewski J. (2003) Vascular endothelial growth factor receptor 2-mediated angiogenesis is essential for gonadotropin-dependent follicle development. *J. Clin. Invest.* 112, 659–69.

Zoller L.C. and Weisz J. (1979) A quantitative cytochemical study of glucose-6-phosphate dehydrogenase and delta 5-3 beta-hydroxysteroid dehydrogenase activity in the membrana granulosa of the ovulable type of follicle of the rat. *Histochemistry* 62, 125–35.

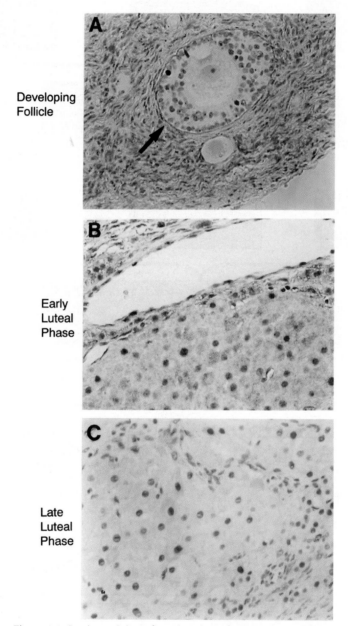

Developing
Follicle

Early
Luteal
Phase

Late
Luteal
Phase

Figure 1.1. In situ staining of ovarian tissue for expression of Flt-1.
Ovarian tissue was stained with antibodies against Flt-1 to determine
its expression in developing follicles and during CL formation and
regression. Flt-1 was not detected in developing follicles (A, arrows)
but was present on the GCs of early luteal phase (B), expression that
was not evident during the late luteal phase (C). (magnification: ×400).

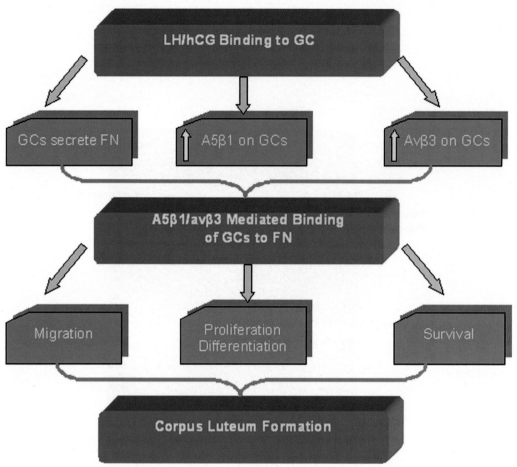

Figure 1.2. Proposed mechanism for the involvement of fibronectin and two of its integrin ligands in CL formation and their regulation by hCG through VEGF in this process.

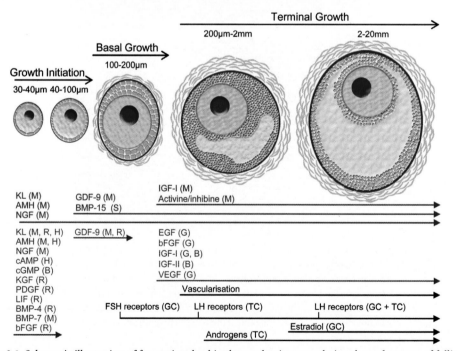

Figure 3.1. Schematic illustration of factors involved in the mechanisms regulating the early stages of follicular development: data from in vivo (green) and in vitro (blue) experiments. AMH, anti-Mullerian hormone; bFGF, basic fibroblast growth factor; BMP, bone morphogenetic protein; cAMP, cyclic adenosine mono phosphate, cGMP, cyclic guanosine monophosphate; EGF, epidermal growth factor; FSH, follicle-stimulating hormone; GDF-9, growth differentiation factor 9; IGF, insulin-like growth factor; KL, kit ligand; KGF, ker-atinocyte growth factor; LIF, leukemia inhibitory factor; LH, luteinizing hormone; NGF, nerve growth factor; PDGF, platelet-derived growth factor; VEGF, vascular endothelial growth factor; GC, granulosa cells; TC, theca cells; H, humans; B, bovine; G, goat; M, mouse; R, rat; S, sheep.

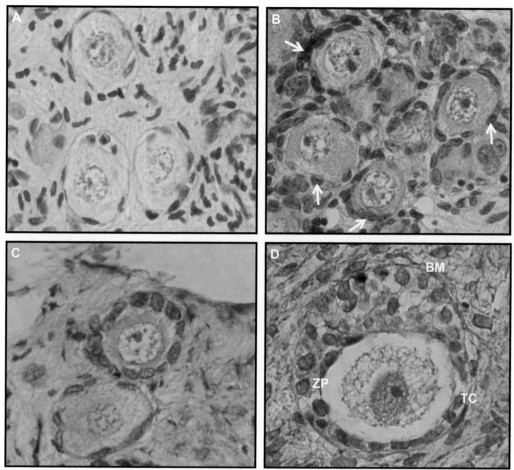

Figure 3.2. Early follicular development in the human ovarian cortex. (A) Histology of primordial follicles surrounded with flattened granulosa cells after cryopreservation/thawing. (B) Individual granulosa cells become cuboidal after primordial follicle activation in culture. (C) Further development in vitro involved differentiation of granulosa cells and formation of primary follicles with one layer of granulosa cells. (D) Granulosa cells divide to produce secondary follicles. Oocyte growth is associated with deposition of zona pellucida (ZP), recruitment of theca cells (TC), and formation of a basal membrane (BM). Original magnification (A–C) ×200; (D) ×400.

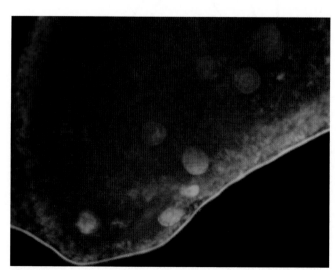

Figure 3.4. Localization of early-stage follicles in the human ovarian cortex after cryopreservation/thawing. Viable follicles are stained with calcein AM (green fluorescence) and dead cells with ethidium homo-dimer (red fluorescence).

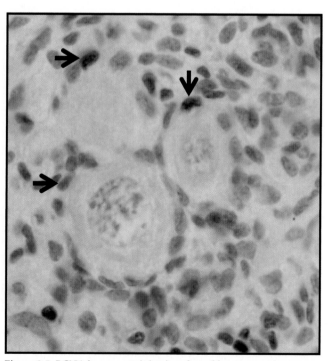

Figure 3.5. PCNA immunostaining in cultured human ovarian cortex. Cuboidal granulosa cells display positive PCNA staining (arrows), indication of granulosa cell division upon activation for growth initiation in culture. Original magnification ×200.

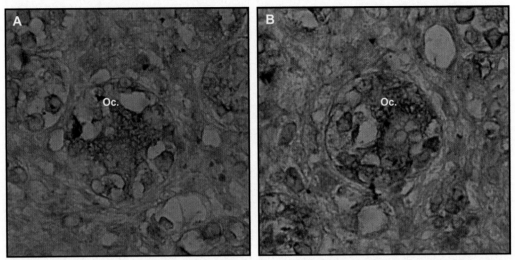

Figure 3.6. Immunohistochemical detection of GDF-9 in cultured human ovarian follicles. Positive GDF-9 immunostaining is localized to the oocytes (Oc.) of primary follicles grown in culture. Original magnification ×400.

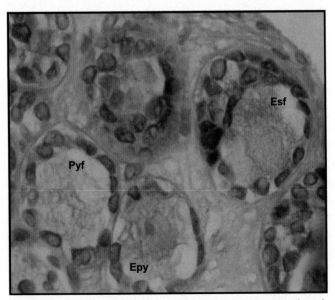

Figure 3.7. Immunohistochemical detection of AMH in cultured human ovarian follicles. Positive AMH immunostaining is localized to granulosa cells of growing early primary (Epy), primary (Pyf), and early secondary (Esf) follicle. Original magnification ×400.

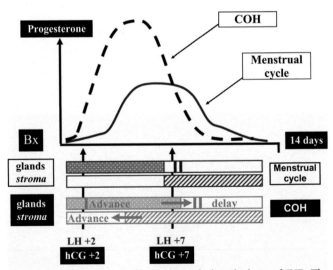

Figure 4.1. Hormonal profile in the early luteal phase of IVF. The diagram depicts the patterns of progesterone levels encountered in the menstrual cycle and in COH. In COH, plasma progesterone peaks earlier and reaches higher levels. Concomitantly, analyses of endometrial histology show a delay in the secretory transformation of glands (after a transitory slight advance within two days of hCG administration), whereas predecidualization of endometrial stroma is characteristically advanced.

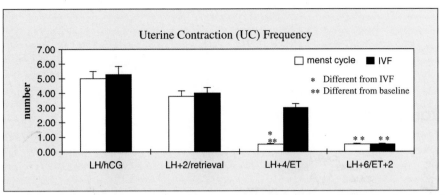

Figure 4.3. Uterine contractility in the menstrual cycle and IVF. Uterine contractility during the luteal phase of the menstrual cycle and in IVF. In the menstrual cycle, a profound decrease of uterine contractility is observed on the fourth day after LH surge. When the same patients underwent IVF, a characteristic delay in the response to the uteroquiescent properties of progesterone was observed (from: Ayoubi et al.; 58).

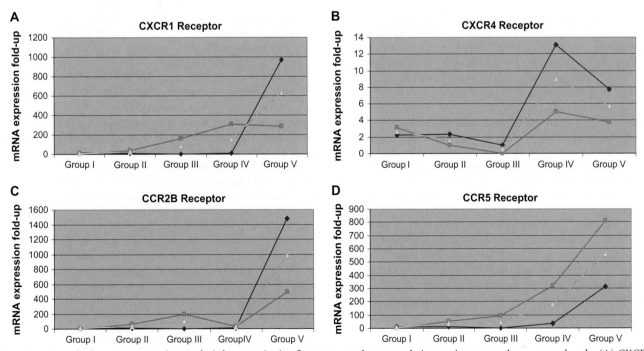

Figure 5.1. Quantitative gene expression analysis by quantitative fluorescent polymerase chain reaction across the menstrual cycle. (A) CXCR1 receptor expression. (B) CXCR4 receptor. (C) CCR2B receptor. (D) CCR5 receptor. Endometrial biopsies were distributed in five groups: group I, early to mid-proliferative (days 1–8); group II, late proliferate phase (days 9–14); group III, early secretory (days 15–18); group IV, mid-secretory (days 19–22); and group V, late secretory phase (days 23–28). Squares: set one; rhombus: set two; triangles: media.

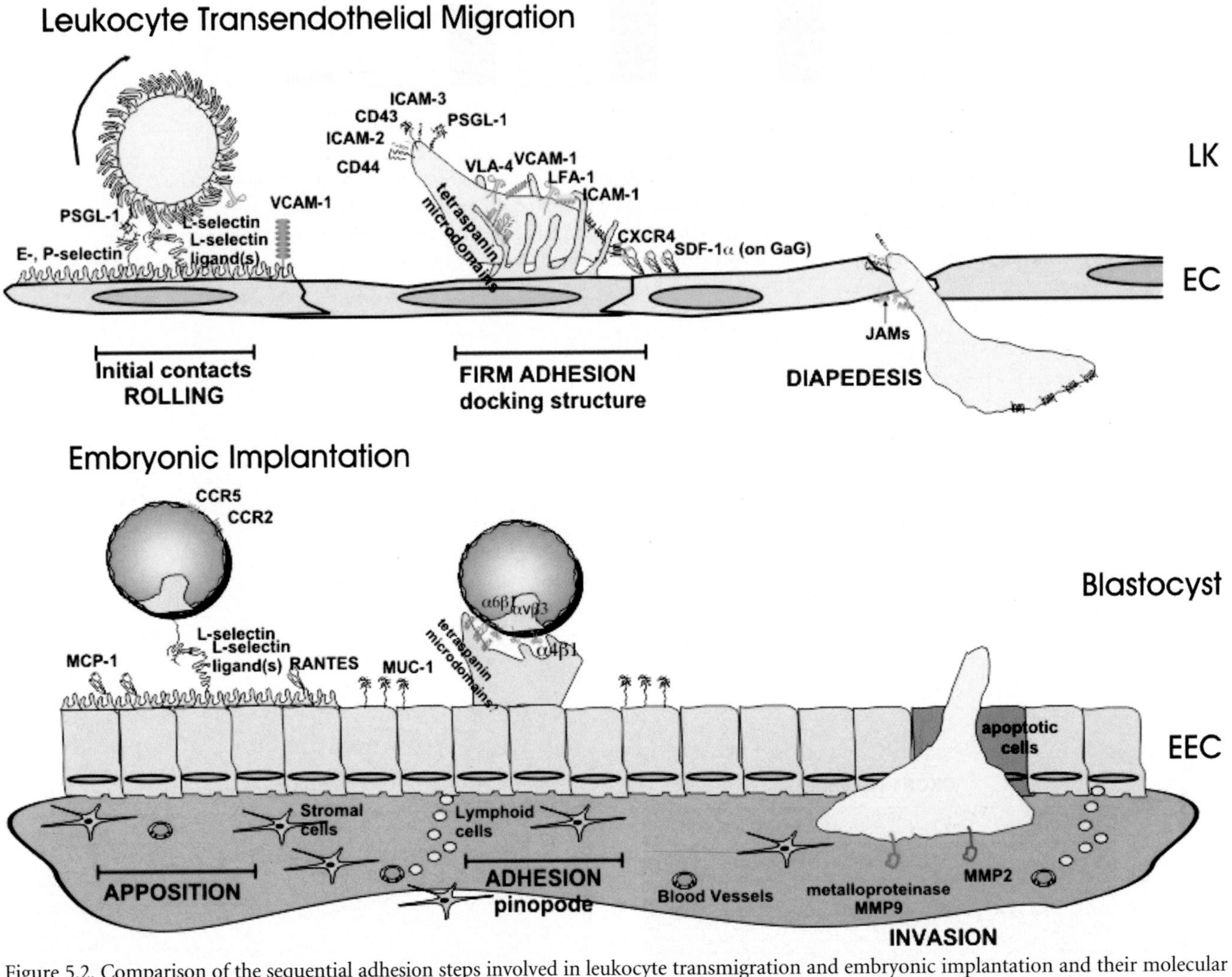

Figure 5.2. Comparison of the sequential adhesion steps involved in leukocyte transmigration and embryonic implantation and their molecular players. Leukocyte *rolling*, via the interaction of selectins with their carbohydrate ligands, slows down the leukocyte and facilitates the binding of chemokines to their GPCR receptors. Chemokines induce the high-affinity conformation of leukocyte integrins, which bind to ICAM-1 and VCAM-1, included into tetraspanin microdomains and anchored to the cortical actin cytoskeleton on the apical surface of endothelial cells. Upon leukocyte *adhesion*, endothelial cells develop a three-dimensional *docking structure* that prevents the detachment of the adhered leukocyte, allowing it to proceed to diapedesis. During *diapedesis* leukocyte integrins interact with endothelial JAM adhesion molecules that reseal the junction by homophilic interactions once the leukocyte has traversed the monolayer. In embryonic implantation, chemokines are implicated in embryonic *apposition*. Blastocyst presents CCR5 and CCR2 receptors on its surface, whereas chemokine ligands adhere to glycosaminoglycans in the endometrial epithelium. L-Selectin/L-selectin ligands' initial contacts are also important in this first phase. Adhesion and anti-adhesion molecules such as integrin subunits on *pinopode* structures and MUC-1 on the endometrial surface facilitates/prevents the embryo *adhesion*. The role of tetraspanin microdomains is still unknown in blastocyst attachment. In the final *invasion* phase, the blastocyst breaches the epithelial barrier, increasing the number of apoptotic cells beneath it and then the trophoblast advances through the stroma, expressing different metalloproteinases like MMP-2 and -9.

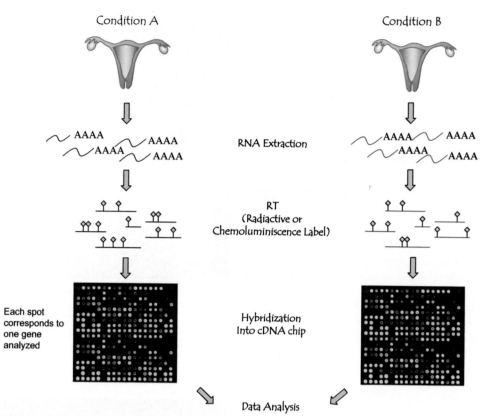

Condition A

Condition B

RNA Extraction

RT
(Radiactive or
Chemoluminiscence Label)

Each spot
corresponds to
one gene
analyzed

Hybridization
Into cDNA chip

Data Analysis

Figure 5.3. Diagram of the process of an array experiment. We can study the gene expression profile of two different conditions extracting RNA from conditions A and B and transforming the RNA into cDNA (labeled with radiactive or chemoluminiscence signal). These probes are hybridized into arrays/chips of thousands of genes. Differential data profiles obtained from these comparison studies should be processed by powerful software in order to obtain confident data.

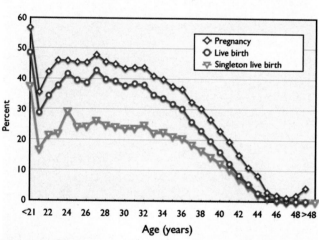

Figure 6.2. Pregnancy rates, live birth rates, and singleton live birth rates for ART cycles using fresh nondonor eggs or embryos, by age of woman, 2005. (adapted from Centers for Disease Control and Prevention, American Society for Reproductive Medicine, Society for Assisted Reproductive Technology. 2005 Assisted reproductive technology success rates: national summary and fertility clinic reports. Atlanta, GA: Centers for Disease Control and Prevention; 2007).

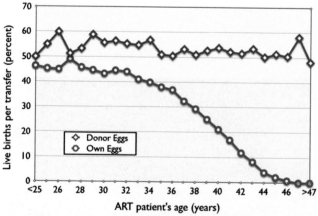

Figure 6.3. Live births per transfer for ART cycles using fresh embryos from own and donor eggs, by ART patient's age, 2005. The average live birth per transfer rate using donor eggs is 51 percent. In contrast, the live birth rates for cycles using embryos from women's own eggs decline steadily as women get older (adapted from Centers for Disease Control and Prevention, American Society for Reproductive Medicine, Society for Assisted Reproductive Technology. 2005 Assisted reproductive technology success rates: national summary and fertility clinic reports. Atlanta, GA: Centers for Disease Control and Prevention; 2007).

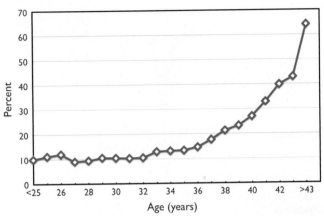

Figure 6.4. Miscarriage rates among women who had ART cycles using fresh nondonor eggs or embryos, by age of woman, 2005. A woman's age not only affects the chance for pregnancy when her own eggs are used but also affects her risk for miscarriage (adapted from Centers for Disease Control and Prevention, American Society for Reproductive Medicine, Society for Assisted Reproductive Technology. 2005 Assisted reproductive technology success rates: national summary and fertility clinic reports. Atlanta, GA: Centers for Disease Control and Prevention; 2007).

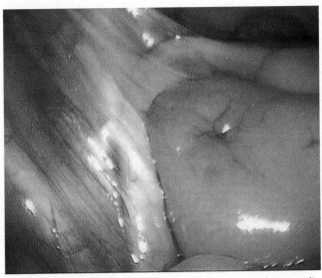

Figure 6.7. Laparoscopic image showing adhesions around the appendix.

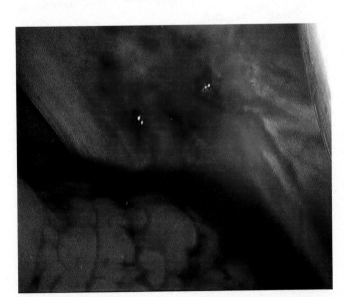

Figure 6.6. Laparoscopic view of pelvic endometriosis stage III.

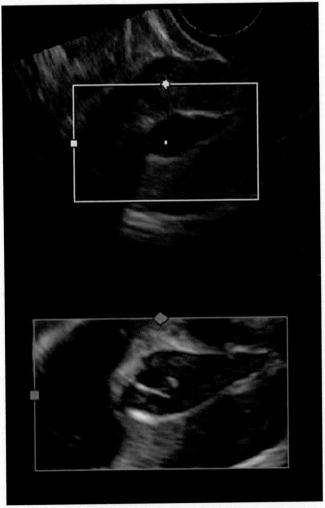

Figure 6.10. Sonohysterography showing intrauterine synechae.

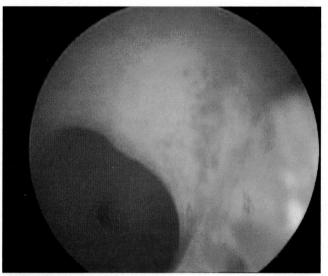

Figure 6.11. Hysteroscopy of a patient with a uterine septum.

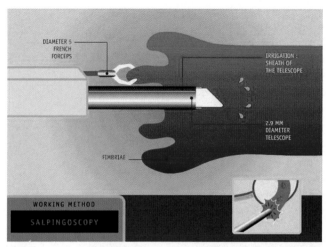

Figure 7.3. Salpingoscopy.

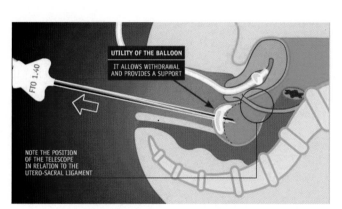

Figure 7.1. Principle of fertiloscopy.

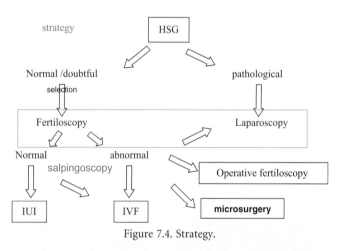

Figure 7.4. Strategy.

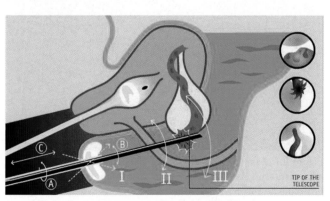

Figure 7.2. Optics movements during hydropelviscopy.

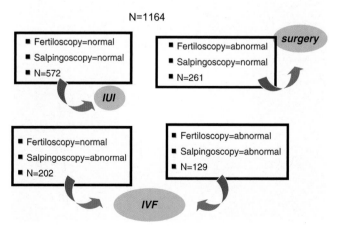

Figure 7.5. The four groups of patients according to tubal mucosa status.

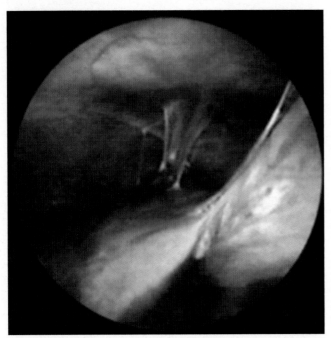

Figure 8.1. Fitz-Hugh Curtis syndrome. In Almeida O (ed.), Micro-laparoscopy. Wiley-Liss, Inc.; New York 2000.

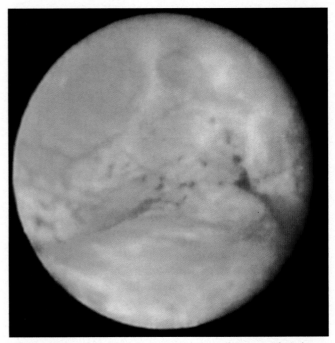

Figure 8.3. A typical red endometriotic lesions (hypervascularity) over the bladder peritoneum. Atlas. In Almeida O (ed.), Microlaparoscopy. Wiley-Liss, Inc.; New York 2000.

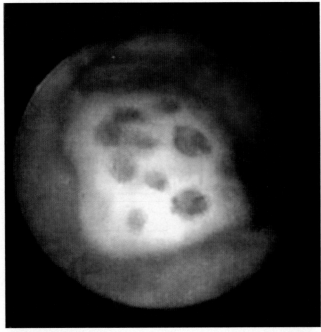

Figure 8.2. Microlaparoscopic ovarian drilling. Atlas. In Almeida O (ed.), Microlaparoscopy. Wiley-Liss, Inc; New York.

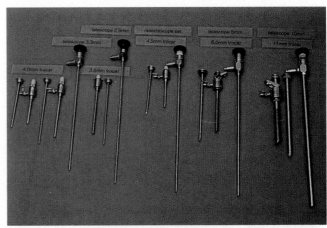

Figure 9.1. Laparoscopes of varying sizes for use in pediatric and adolescent surgery. Reprinted from Atlas of Pelvic Anatomy and Gynecologic Surgery, Baggish and Karram, Page No. 677, 2001, with permission from Elsevier.

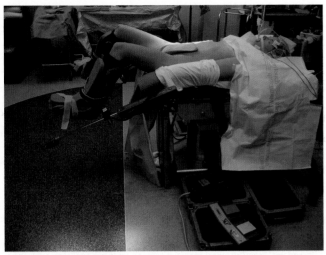

Figure 9.2. Proper patient positioning with legs secured in Allen stirrups and arms tucked at the side.

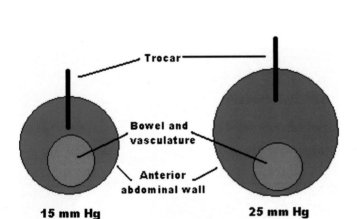

Figure 9.3. Transiently increasing the insufflation pressure to 25 mmHg prior to primary trocar insertion increases the distance between the trocar tip and the underlying bowel and vasculature.

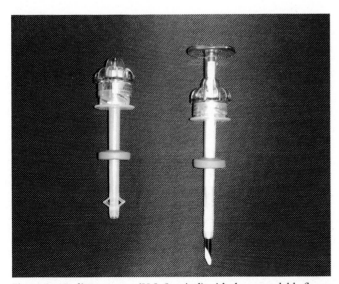

Figure 9.4. Pediport trocar (U.S. Surgical) with the expandable flange deployed (left) and retracted (right).

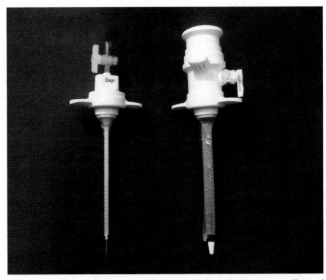

Figure 9.5. Versa-step trocar (U.S. Surgical) with Veress needle and unexpanded sheath (left) and dilating blunt trocar and expanded sheath (right).

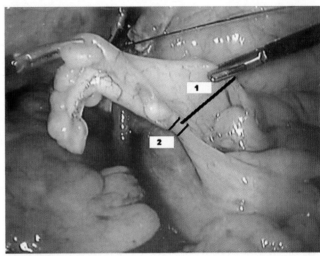

Figure 9.6. Normal appendix. 1. Level at which the mesoappendix and appendiceal artery should be controlled. 2. Level at which the appendix should be transected.

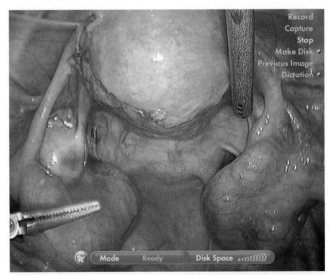

Figure 9.7. Sequela of PID. This patient has bilateral hydrosalpinges, tubal occlusion, and pelvic pain.

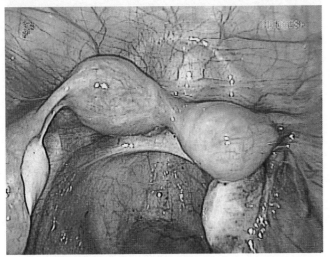

Figure 9.8. Uterus didelphys that presented as an adnexal mass.

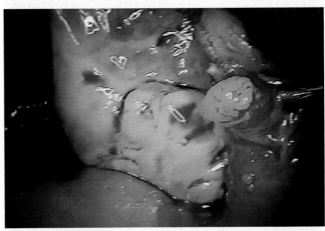

Figure 10.2. Healthy tubal mucosa after the edges have been refreshed.

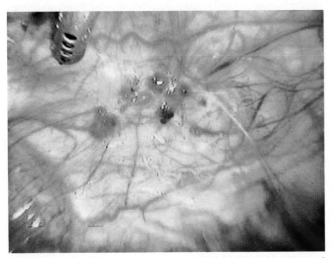

Figure 9.9. Endometriotic lesion in a young girl. The lesion was red and vesicular.

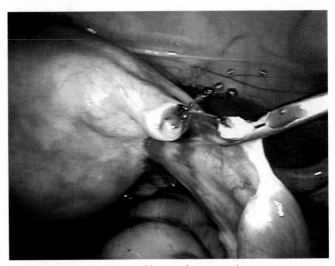

Figure 10.3. Proximal lumen demonstrating patency.

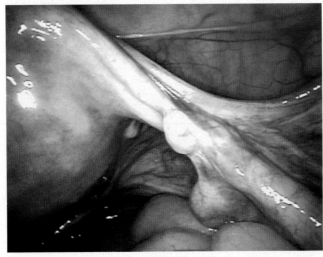

Figure 10.1. Falope ring in place prior to resection.

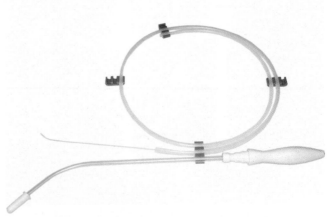

Figure 10.4. Tubal cannulator with accompanying 3F stent.

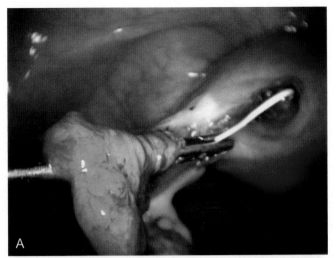

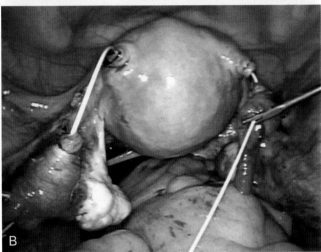

Figure 10.5. A) Demonstration of distal segment patency, preparing to pull stent through. B) Cannulation completed.

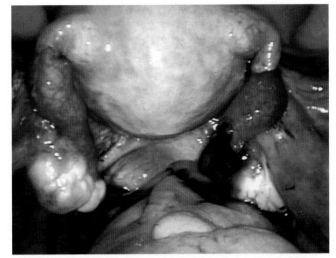

Figure 10.7. Inspection of completed bilateral anastomosis after removal of stents. Note good filling of distal segments and free flow of indigo-carmine dye through fimbriated ends.

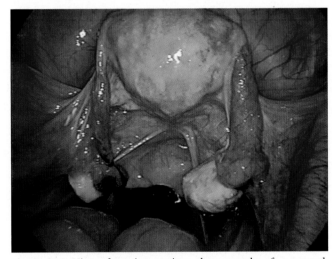

Figure 10.8. View of previous patient, three months after reversal, during a laparoscopic cholecystectomy.

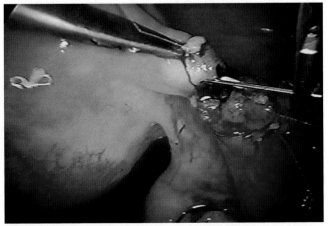

Figure 10.6. Placement of suture (7–0) in the thick muscular layer of the isthmic portion, with a clear view of the tubal lumen.

Outcome Rates for All 127 Pregnancies by Anastomosis by Age

Figure 10.9. Summary of pregnancy outcomes based upon anastomosis and age.

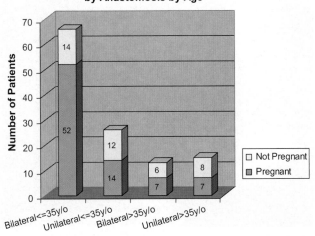

Number of Patients Who Became Pregnant by Anastomosis by Age

Figure 10.10. Pregnancy summary based upon anastomosis and age.

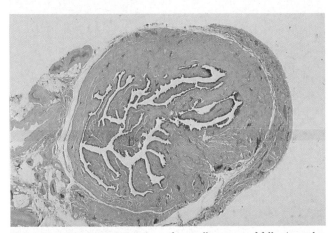

Figure 11.1. Microscopic section of ampullary part of fallopian tube. Normal rugae of mucosa.

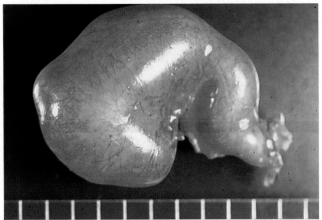

Figure 11.2. Gross picture of hydrosalpinx – marked distension of the fallopian tube, with absent fimbria and complete obstruction of distal end.

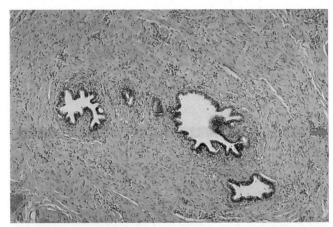

Figure 11.3. Microscopic section of the isthmus of the fallopian tube showing endosalpingiosis (salpingitis isthmica nodosa).

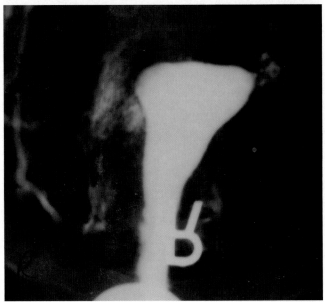

Figure 11.4. Hysterosalpingogram showing salpingitis. Isthmica nodesa (honeycomb appearance).

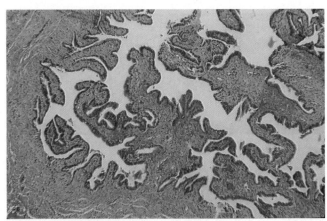

Figure 11.5. Microscopic section of fallopian tube stump removed during tubal anastomosis after Pomeroy sterilization. Note the normal mucosa with normal rugae.

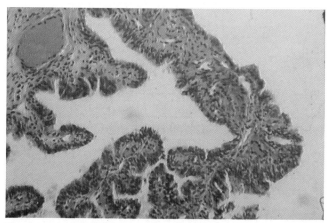

Figure 11.6. Microscopic section of fallopian tube stump removed during anastomosis, after tubal sterilization using falopi ring. Note the healthy tubal mucosa. Hysterosalpingogram showing marked dilatation of the fallopian tube (hydrosalpinx) in an infertile patient.

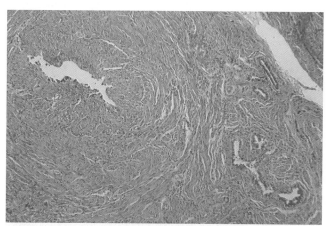

Figure 11.9. Microscopic section of the fallopian tube with ectopic endometrium representing endometriosis.

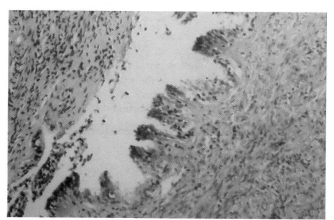

Figure 11.7. Microscopic section of fallopian tube stump removed during tubal anastomosis following unipolar coagulation for sterilization. Note the absence of tubal mucosa in part of the lumen and fimbriotic changes in tubal wall.

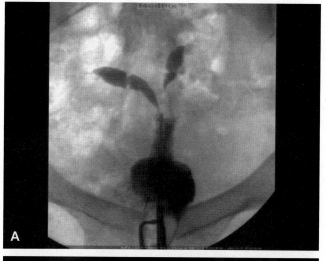

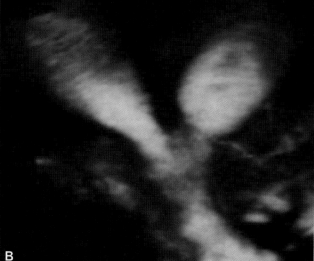

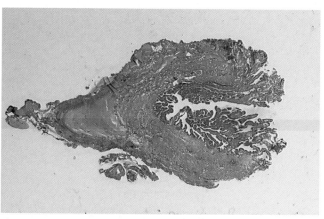

Figure 11.8. Microscopic section of fallopian tube stump removed during anastomosis after tubal sterilization using bipolar cautery. Note the healthy tubal mucosa.

Figure 13.3. The figure shows two hysterosalpingograms of complete uterine septum (A) and bicornuate uterus (B). Notice the wider angle between the two sides of the uterine cavity in the hysterosalpingogram picture of the uterine septum. Such an angle is much smaller in case of the bicornuate uterus.

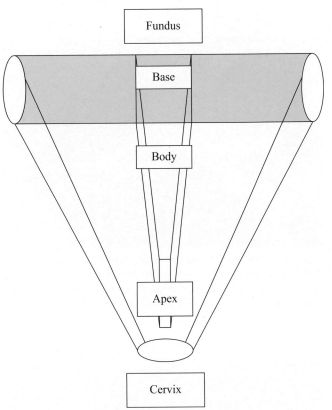

Drawing 13.1. Shows the different parts of the uterine septum in relation to the uterine walls: base of the septum where it meets the fundus, body of the septum that extends down dividing the uterine cavity into two sides, and apex of the septum that is the lower most part of the septum.

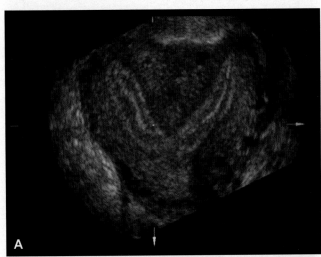

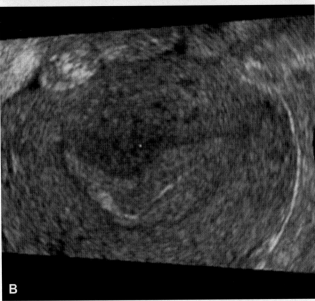

Figure 13.5. Three-dimensional transvaginal ultrasonography showing incomplete uterine septum (A), and the subtype of the incomplete uterine septum that we call as asymmetrical, incomplete uterine septum (B). Notice the advantages of this ultrasound technique in visualizing the dimensions of the septum, relationship to different parts of the uterine cavity, as well as the external contour of the uterus.

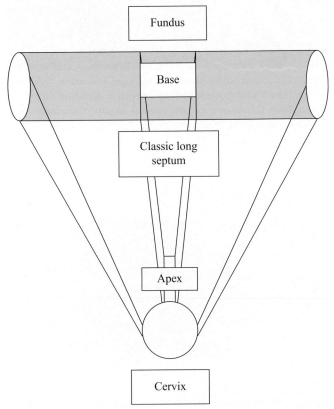

Drawing 13.2. Shows the complete or long septum type (septate uterus). In this type of the uterine septum, the body of the septum extends all the way down from the fundus to the cervix, completely separating the uterine cavity into two sides.

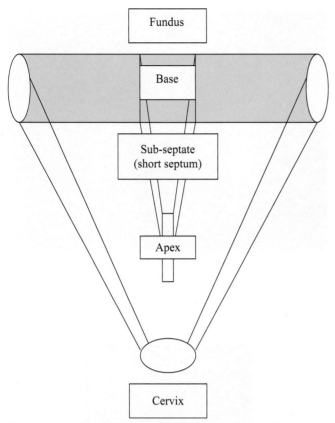

Drawing 13.3. Shows the incomplete short type of the uterine septum (subseptate uterus). In this type, the apex of the septum stops somewhere below the fundus before reaching the cervix.

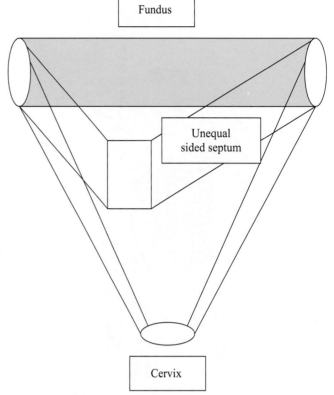

Drawing 13.5. Shows another subtype of the short septum (asymmetrical). In this type, the two sides of the uterine cavity are unequal. The apex of the septum is deviated more toward one side.

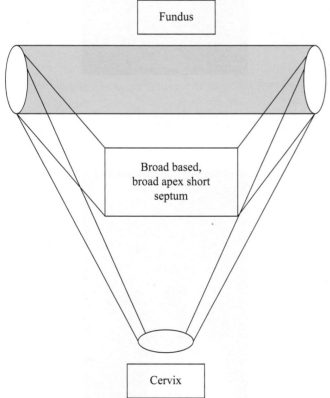

Drawing 13.4. Shows a subtype of the short septum. We call it broad-based short septum. In this type, the base of the septum is very broad, extending between almost the whole distance between the two tubal ostia. The base in this subtype is usually broad.

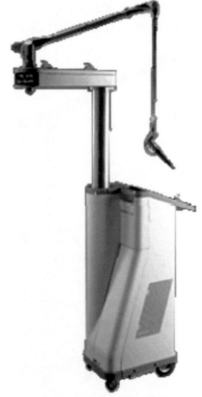

Figure 14.2. CO_2 Laser.

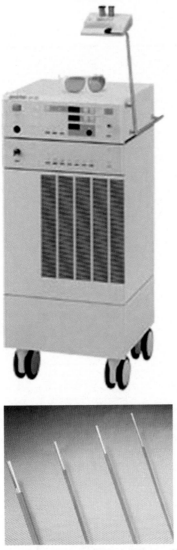

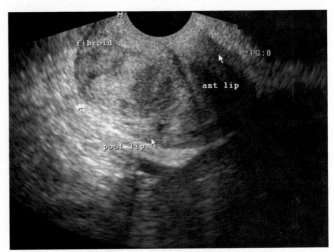

Figure 16.6. Cervical fibroid.

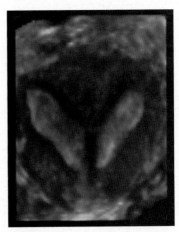

Figure 14.3. NdYAG Laser and different fibres.

Figure 16.7. Mullerian anomaly, 3D image of uterus didelphys.

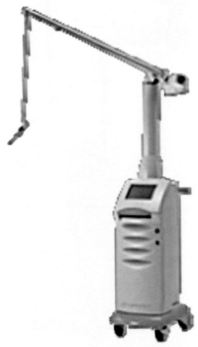

Figure 14.4. Ultrapulse Laser.

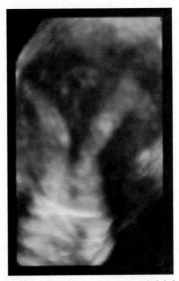

Figure 16.8. 3D image of uterus didelphys.

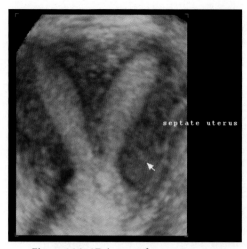

Figure 16.9. 3D image of septate uterus.

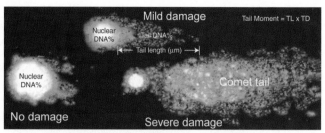

Single Cell Gel electrophoresis (Comet assay)

Figure 19.2. COMET assay uses the electro gel electrophoresis principle to assess the DNA damage. After DNA extraction and gel electrophoresis, damaged DNA looks like a "comet." The level of DNA fragmentation is measured using special software after transferring a live video image of the microscopic field into the computer. One of the indices used is "tail moment," which is a relation between the size and density (DNA percent) of the comet head and tail [= TL (tail length) × TD (tail density)]. The tail moment lies in one of three levels: mild, moderate, and severe, and their percentage in the sample are given.

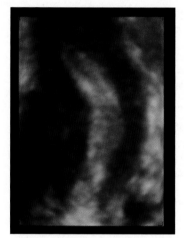

Figure 16.10. 3D image of unicornuate uterus.

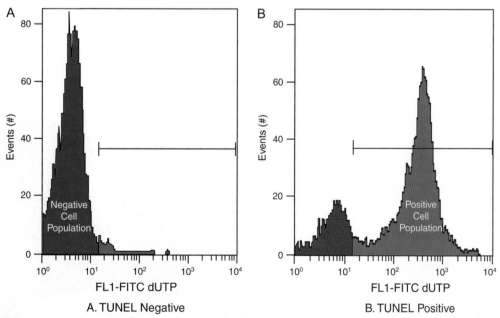

Figure 19.1. TUNEL assay fluorescent activated cell sorting (FACS) histograms with markers (|———|) for detection of fluorescence set at 650 nm. (A) A semen sample with low percentage of sperm DNA fragmentation; (B) a semen sample with high percentage of sperm DNA fragmentation.

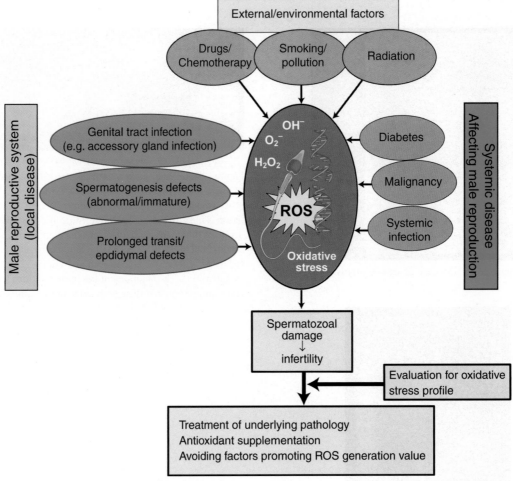

Figure 19.3. Etiology and management of oxidative stress. Many factors, including primary pathological condition of male reproductive system, systemic disorders, and environmental factors, increase oxidative stress status, which causes spermatozoa dysfunction leading to infertility.

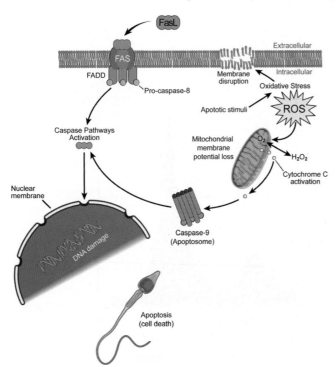

Figure 19.4. ROS-induced apoptosis. ROS (apoptotic stimulus) trigger mitochondria to release cytochrome *c*, initiating a caspase cascade. Interaction between Fas and Fas ligand is also necessary in apoptotic mechanism. DNA fragmentation occurs as a result of activation of effector caspases (caspases 3, 6, and 9), eventually causing apoptosis.

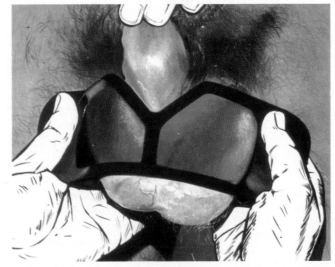

Figure 20.1. Varicoscreen application for contact thermography.

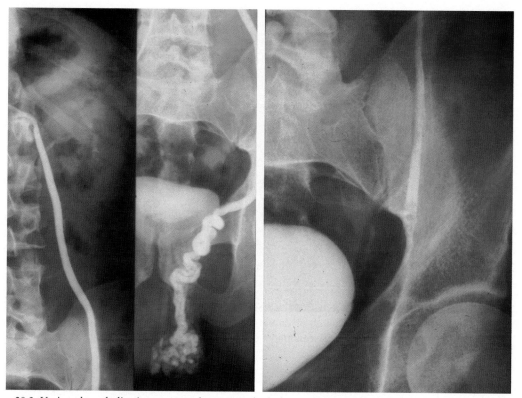

Figure 20.2. Varicocele embolization; retrograde venography before and after embolization (courtesy Dr. Jan Kunnen).

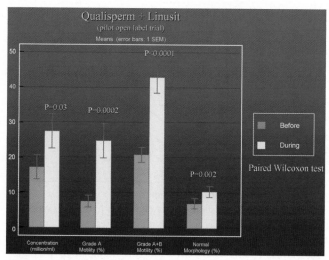

Figure 20.3. Histogram of sperm characteristics before and after three months of complementary intake of Qualisperm® plus linseed oil in patients treated for male infertility.

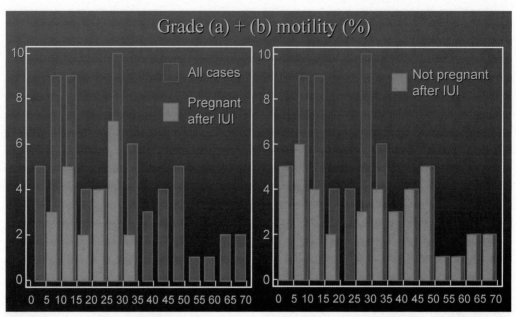

Figure 20.4. Proportion of couples that do or do not attain pregnancy by means of IUI in relation to the percentage of spermatozoa with progressive motility (grade "a" and "b" added) in the native semen (52).

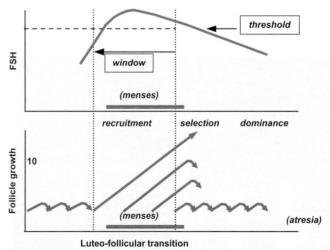

Figure 22.2. The FSH threshold/window concept. In the physiological situation (left panel), early follicular phase increase in serum FSH concentration above the FSH threshold induces follicular growth; when followed by FSH decrease (narrow FSH window), this prevents selection of multiple follicles (left panel). In ovarian hyperstimulation, intentional multiple follicle development results from absence of FSH decrease (upper line, right panel).

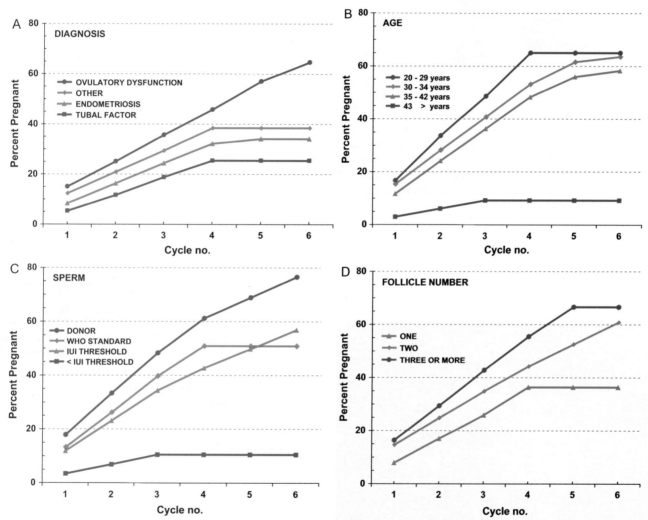

Figure 23.7. Cumulative pregnancy rate. (A) Diagnosis: ovulatory dysfunction = anovulatory, PCO, or luteal insuffiency; endometriosis = with or without tubal involvement; tubal factor = unilateral tubal obstruction or tubal adhesions without endometriosis; other = cervical factor, male factor, or unexplained infertility and normal cycles without endometriosis or tubal factor. Patient's age greater than or equal to forty-three and cycles with total initial motile sperm count less than five million or motility <30 percent excluded. (B) Age, patients with endometriosis, tubal impairment, and cycles with total initial motile sperm count less than five million or motility <30 percent excluded. (C) Sperm, WHO: initial sperm quality greater than or equal to World Health Organization (1(4)1992) criteria of twenty million concentration, forty million total count, 50 percent progressive motility, 30 percent normal forms. IUI threshold; initial sperm quality less than WHO criteria but greater than or equal to five million total motile sperm and ≥ 30 percent initial motility. Sub-IUI threshold: initial motile sperm count less than five million or motility <30 percent. Patient's age greater than or equal to forty-three, and patients with endometriosis and tubal factor excluded. (D) Follicle number, patient's age greater than or equal to forty-three, and patients with endometriosis and tubal factor, and cycles with total initial motile sperm count less than five million or motility <30 percent excluded. Adapted from Dickey et al. ((27)2002). Reproduced with permission of the publishers.

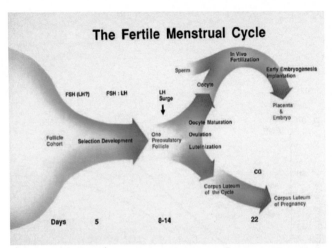

Figure 25.1. Diagram of the events occurring in the ovary and reproductive tract during the initial three weeks of the fertile menstrual cycle leading to natural reproduction in primates. From: Stouffer and Zelinski-Wooten: *Reproductive Biology and Endocrinology* 2: 32, 2004. http://www.rbej.com/content/2/1/32.

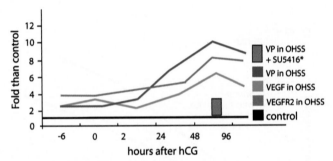

Figure 27.1. VP, VEGF, and VEGFR-2 mRNA expression over time in hyperstimulated rats. The profound effect of a specific VEGFR-2 blocker (SU5416) on VP is also showed in a brown barr. (Adapted from reference 39.)

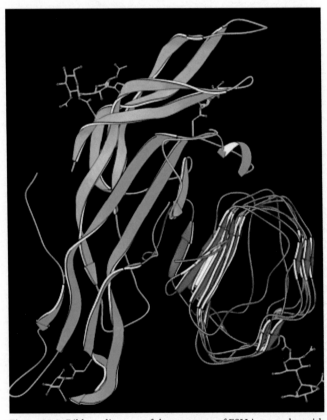

Figure 25.3. Ribbon diagram of the structure of FSH in complex with the FSHR. FSH α-chains are in green. FSH β-chains are in blue. FSHR is in red. N-linked glycosylation sites (of both the FSH molecule and the FSHR) are in yellow. From: Fan and Hendrickson: *Nature* 433: 269–277, 2005. Macmillan Publishers Ltd.

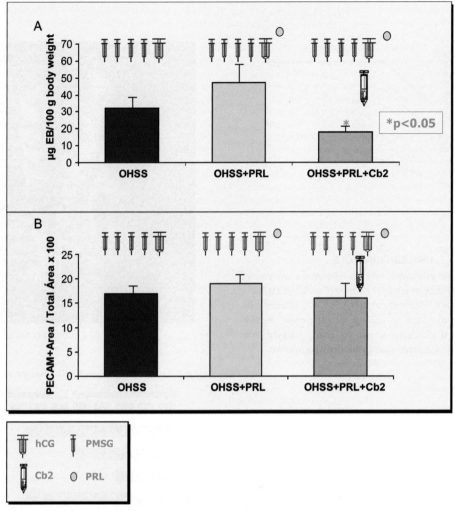

Figure 27.4. The effects of low-dose Cb2 in the treatment of increased VP in prolactin-supplemented OHSS rats. The state of increased vascular permeability (A) (as micrograms of extravasated EB dye per 100 g animal weight) was significantly reversed after Cb2 administration in prolactin-supplemented OHSS rats. These changes in VP in the experimental group were not mediated by luteolytic effects since luteal vascular density (B) (as the percentage of PECAM, a specific endothelial cell marker) was not affected. (Adapted from reference 121.)

UNITED STATES TOTAL TWIN AND TRIPLET BIRTHS

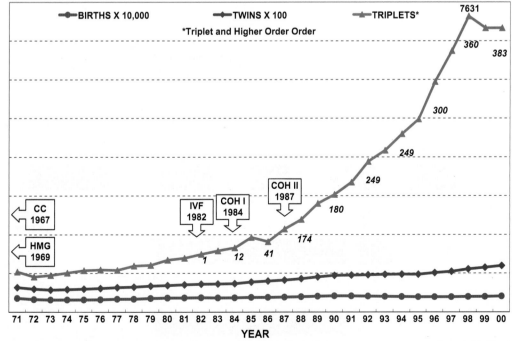

Figure 28.2. Total, twin, and triplet or higher order births, United States 1971–2000. Data show individual births. Italic numbers indicate number of IVF clinics. Adapted from Dickey and Sartor ((9)2005). Reprinted with publisher's permission.

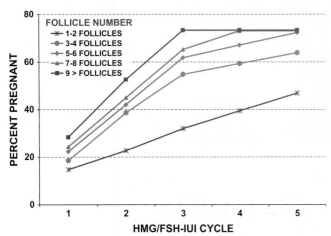

Figure 28.3. Cumulative pregnancy rate in relation to number of preovulatory follicles 10 mm or larger for first five cycles of HMG or FSH–IUI; for patients age <38, without tubal factor, endometriosis, total initial motile sperm count <5 million, or progressive motility <30 percent. Number of follicles as shown on chart. Adapted from Dickey et al. ((21)2005). Reprinted with publisher's permission.

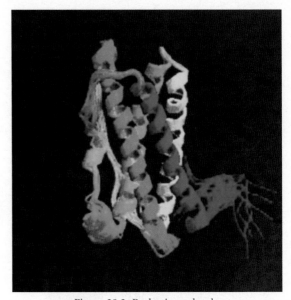

Figure 29.2. Prolactin molecule.

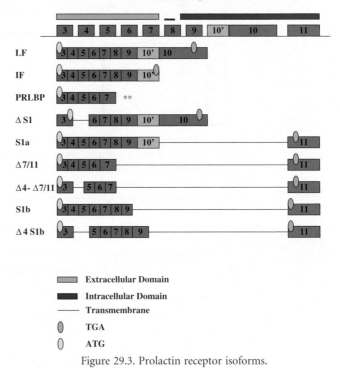

Figure 29.3. Prolactin receptor isoforms.

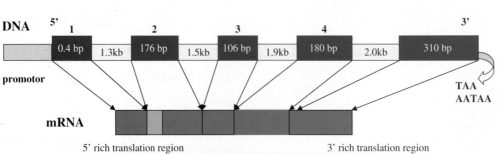

Figure 29.1. Prolactin gene transcription.

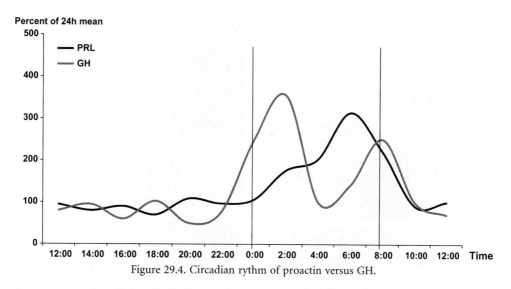

Figure 29.4. Circadian rythm of proactin versus GH.

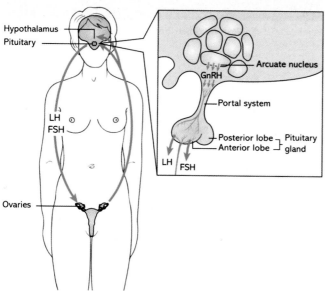

Figure 33.1. Pulsatile secretion of GnRH and stimulation of FSH and LH from the ovary. Reproduced with permission from Rizk and Abdalla (1) and Health Press, Oxford, UK.

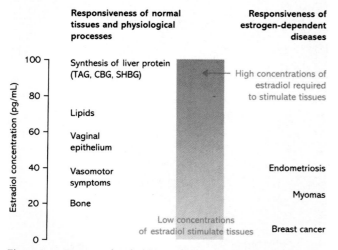

Figure 33.2. Estrogen threshold hypothesis. Reproduced with permission from Barbieri (31).

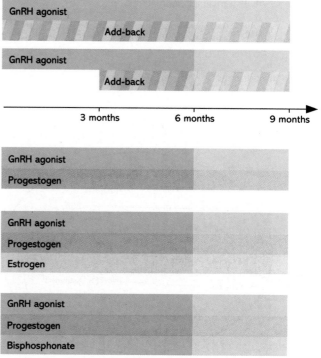

Figure 33.3. Add-back therapy for bone protection for conventional bone loss during GnRh treatment. Reproduced with permission from Rizk and Abdalla (1) and Health Press, Oxford, UK.

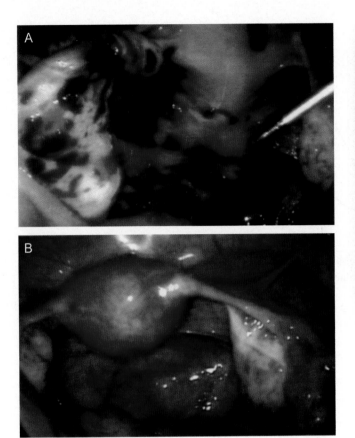

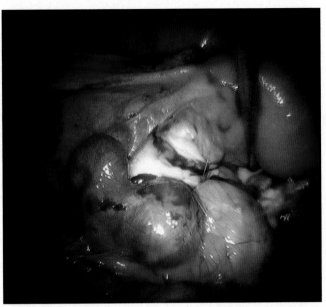

Figure 34.2. Severe endometriosis with adnexal and cul-de-sac adhesions.

Figure 33.4. Pelvic endometriosis before and after treatment with GnRH antagonist. Reproduced with permission from Kupker (40).

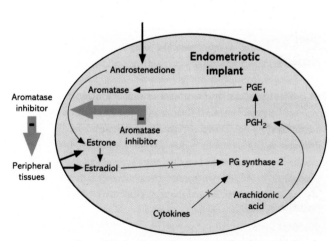

Figure 33.5. The molecular basis of treatment of endometriosis using an aromatase inhibitor. Reproduced with permission from Rizk and Abdalla (1) and Health Press, Oxford, UK.

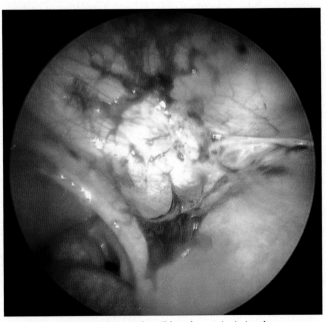

Figure 34.3. Pelvis with mild endometriosis implants.

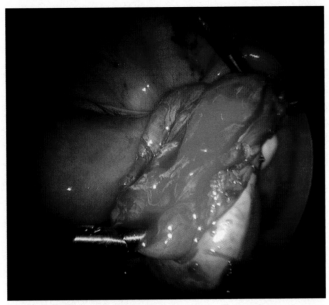

Figure 34.4. Endometrioma cyst wall resection.

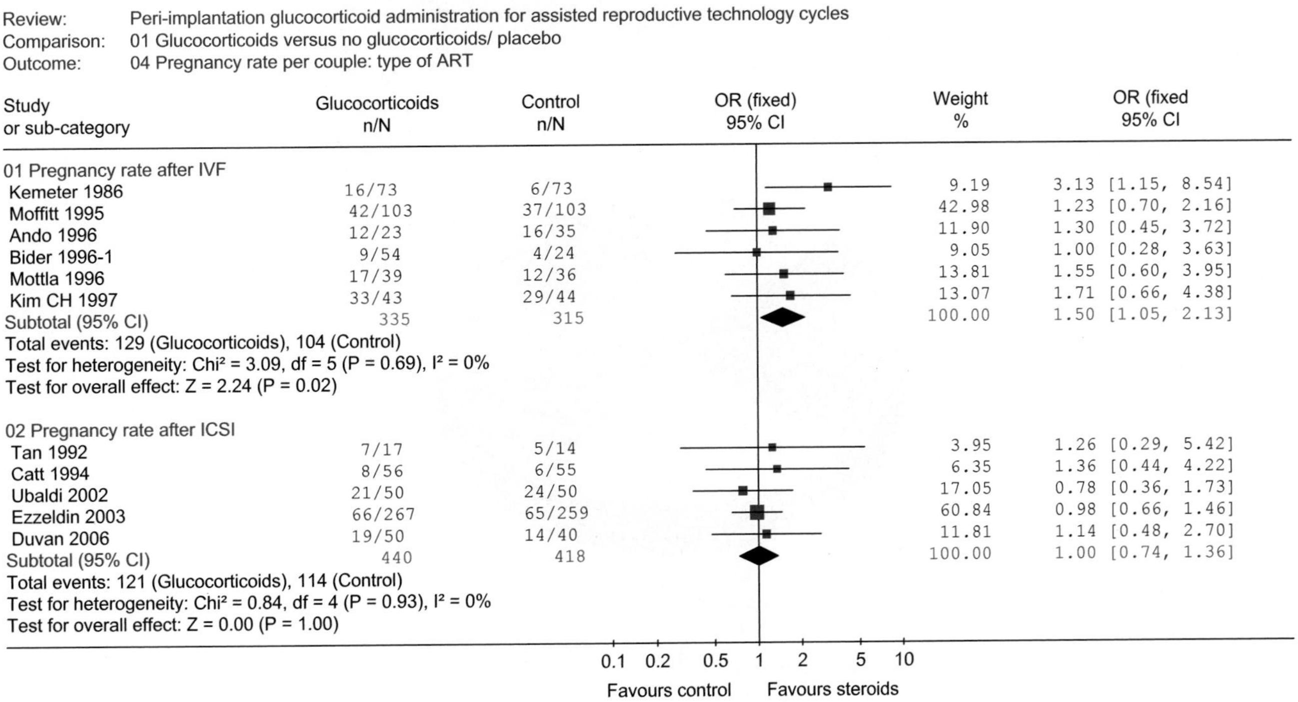

Review: Peri-implantation glucocorticoid administration for assisted reproductive technology cycles
Comparison: 01 Glucocorticoids versus no glucocorticoids/ placebo
Outcome: 04 Pregnancy rate per couple: type of ART

Study or sub-category	Glucocorticoids n/N	Control n/N	OR (fixed) 95% CI	Weight %	OR (fixed) 95% CI
01 Pregnancy rate after IVF					
Kemeter 1986	16/73	6/73		9.19	3.13 [1.15, 8.54]
Moffitt 1995	42/103	37/103		42.98	1.23 [0.70, 2.16]
Ando 1996	12/23	16/35		11.90	1.30 [0.45, 3.72]
Bider 1996-1	9/54	4/24		9.05	1.00 [0.28, 3.63]
Mottla 1996	17/39	12/36		13.81	1.55 [0.60, 3.95]
Kim CH 1997	33/43	29/44		13.07	1.71 [0.66, 4.38]
Subtotal (95% CI)	335	315		100.00	1.50 [1.05, 2.13]
Total events: 129 (Glucocorticoids), 104 (Control)					
Test for heterogeneity: Chi² = 3.09, df = 5 (P = 0.69), I² = 0%					
Test for overall effect: Z = 2.24 (P = 0.02)					
02 Pregnancy rate after ICSI					
Tan 1992	7/17	5/14		3.95	1.26 [0.29, 5.42]
Catt 1994	8/56	6/55		6.35	1.36 [0.44, 4.22]
Ubaldi 2002	21/50	24/50		17.05	0.78 [0.36, 1.73]
Ezzeldin 2003	66/267	65/259		60.84	0.98 [0.66, 1.46]
Duvan 2006	19/50	14/40		11.81	1.14 [0.48, 2.70]
Subtotal (95% CI)	440	418		100.00	1.00 [0.74, 1.36]
Total events: 121 (Glucocorticoids), 114 (Control)					
Test for heterogeneity: Chi² = 0.84, df = 4 (P = 0.93), I² = 0%					
Test for overall effect: Z = 0.00 (P = 1.00)					

0.1 0.2   0.5   1   2   5   10

Favours control   Favours steroids

Figure 38.2. Adjuvant glucocorticoid administration and pregnancy outcome in IVF and ICSI. From Boomsma et al. (in press).

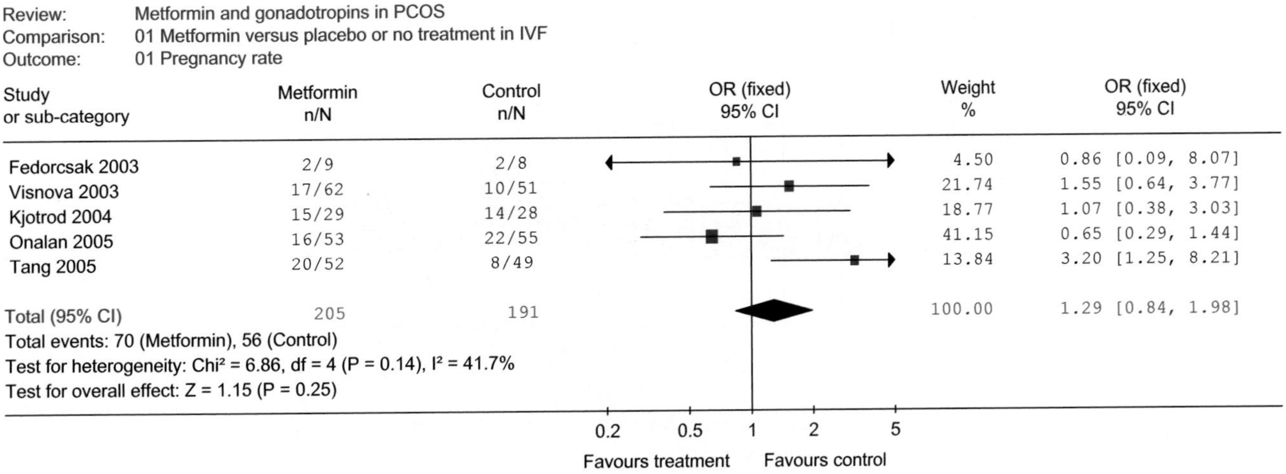

Review: Metformin and gonadotropins in PCOS
Comparison: 01 Metformin versus placebo or no treatment in IVF
Outcome: 01 Pregnancy rate

Study or sub-category	Metformin n/N	Control n/N	OR (fixed) 95% CI	Weight %	OR (fixed) 95% CI
Fedorcsak 2003	2/9	2/8		4.50	0.86 [0.09, 8.07]
Visnova 2003	17/62	10/51		21.74	1.55 [0.64, 3.77]
Kjotrod 2004	15/29	14/28		18.77	1.07 [0.38, 3.03]
Onalan 2005	16/53	22/55		41.15	0.65 [0.29, 1.44]
Tang 2005	20/52	8/49		13.84	3.20 [1.25, 8.21]
Total (95% CI)	205	191		100.00	1.29 [0.84, 1.98]
Total events: 70 (Metformin), 56 (Control)					
Test for heterogeneity: Chi² = 6.86, df = 4 (P = 0.14), I² = 41.7%					
Test for overall effect: Z = 1.15 (P = 0.25)					

0.2   0.5   1   2   5

Favours treatment   Favours control

Figure 38.3. Effect of metformin versus placebo/no treatment in IVF on pregnancy rates. Adapted from Costello et al. ((22)2006). ©European Society of Human Reproduction and Embryology. Reproduced by permission of Oxford University Press/Human Reproduction.

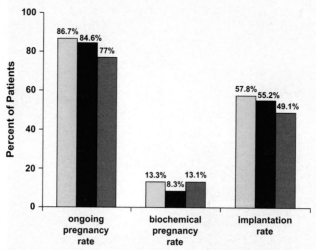

Figure 39.1. Cycle outcomes of patients undergoing oocyte donation (Surrey et al., 82). Reprinted with permission from the American Society for Reproductive Medicine. (☐) Group A: hysteroscopic myomectomy; (■) Group B: myomectomy at laparotomy; (■) Group C: recipient controls.

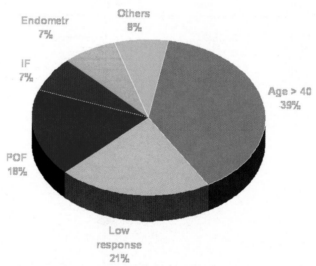

Figure 48.1. Oocyte donation indications in IVI.

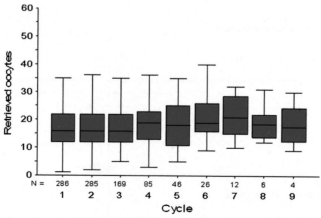

Figure 48.2. Oocyte recovery after successive ovarian stimulation cycles in oocyte donors.

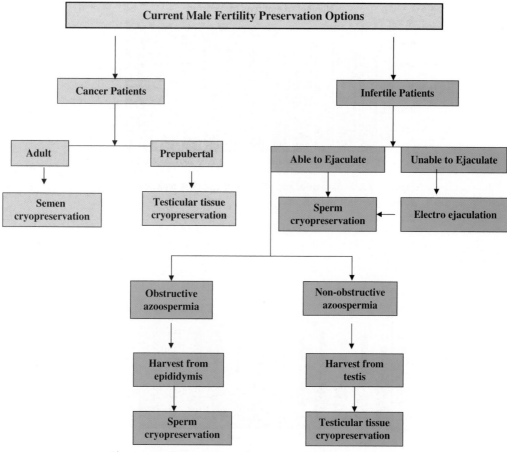

Figure 51.1. Current approaches to male fertility preservation.

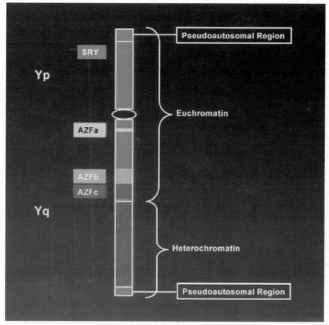

Figure 52.1. Diagram of the Y chromosome depicting the location of AZF regions a, b, and c. SRY, sex-determining region of the Y chromosome. From Choi et al. (2002).

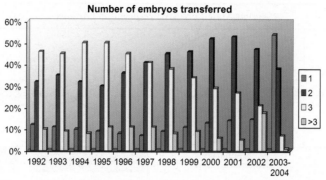

Figure. 55.3. Evolution of the number of embryos replaced over the years 1992–2004 in Belgium.

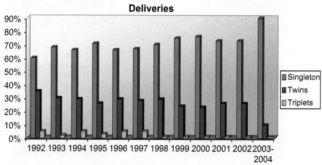

Figure. 55.4. Evolution of the number of singleton, twin, and triplet deliveries over the years 1992–2004 in Belgium.

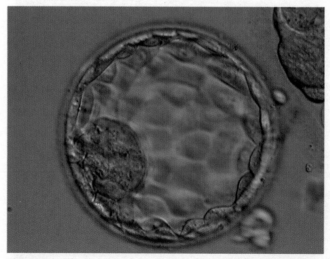

Figure 56.2. Photomicrograph of a day 5 human blastocyst. The embryo in the figure was cultured for four days from the pronucleate oocyte stage: forty-eight hours in medium G1, followed by forty-eight hours in medium G2. The gas phase was 6 percent carbon dioxide and 5 percent oxygen, the remaining 89 percent of the gas being nitrogen. The blastocyst was graded as 4AA.

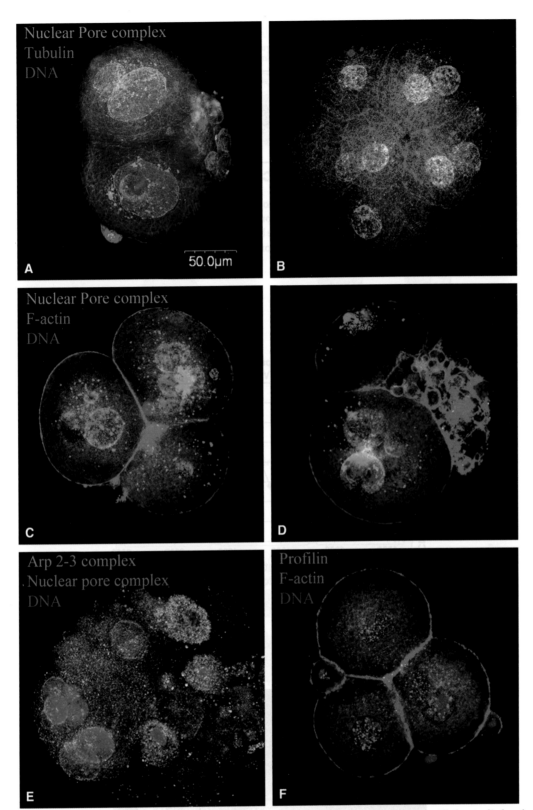

Figure 57.2. Confocal microscopy of different cytoskeletal components of multinucleated human embryos. All the studied embryos developed from normally fertilized eggs and showed at least one blastomere with more than two nuclei on day 2. (A) Microtubules (red) are uniformly distributed throughout the cytoplasm and concentrated in different fragments. Note that this embryo has asymmetric binucleated blastomeres (two uneven-sized interphase nuclei) with disorganized nuclear envelopes (green). (B) This binucleated embryo has microtubules (red) uniformly distributed throughout the cytoplasm. No abnormal patterns can be seen. In this case, smooth and organized nuclear envelopes are visualized in each even-sized nuclei. (C) F-actin is distributed in the cytoplasm and enriched at the cortex of a three-cell multinucleated embryo. As seen in A, nuclear envelopes are disorganized resembling the features of an apoptotic cell. (D) Two-cell embryo with abnormal distribution and absence of homogenous actin filaments (red). The upper blastomere has just a very small amount of spread DNA surrounded by disorganized nuclear envelopes. The presence of four nuclei can be seen in the lower blastomere. Anucleate fragments enriched with actin are also visualized. (E) Arp 2/3 complex (green) is present in the cytoplasm and inside each nuclei taking part of "the nucleoskeleton." Variable intense fluorescence signal can be observed in each blastomere. (F) Profilin (green) is dispersed in the cytoplasm and is present inside each nuclei in a punctuated pattern. This pattern resembles what has been observed in normal bovine embryos (20). Actin filaments seem to be normally distributed. Embryos were examined under a spectral confocal microscope (Olympus), using laser lines at 488, 568, and 633 nm wavelengths (University of Buenos Aires, Faculty of Exact and Natural Sciences). Images were edited using Adobe Photoshop 7.0.

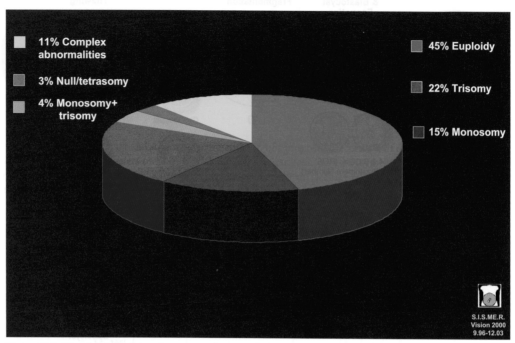

Figure 65.1. Distribution of the chromosomal status of 3,937 oocytes tested by FISH analysis of the first polar body.

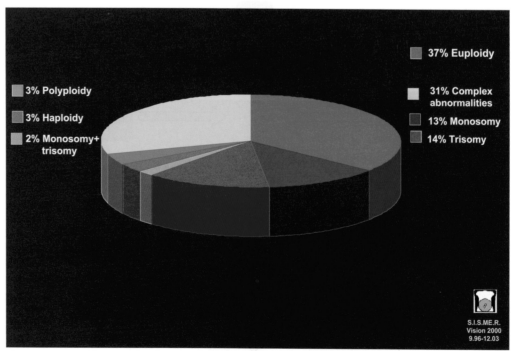

Figure 65.2. Distribution of the chromosomal status of 5,217 in vitro generated embryos tested by FISH analysis of one blastomere.

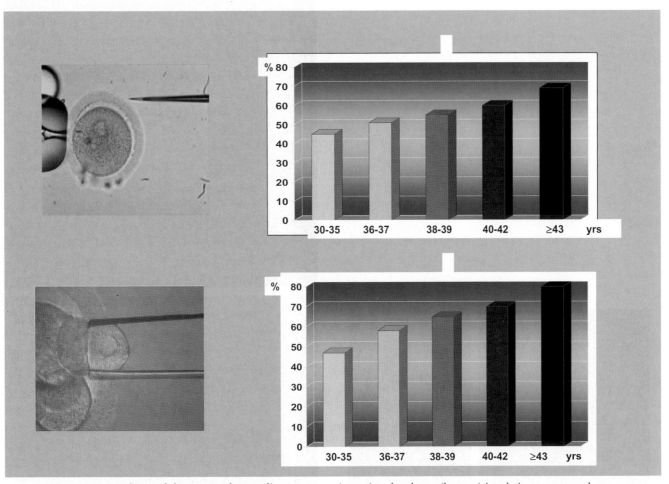

Figure 65.3. Incidence of chromosomal anomalies on oocytes (upper) and embryos (bottom) in relation to maternal age.

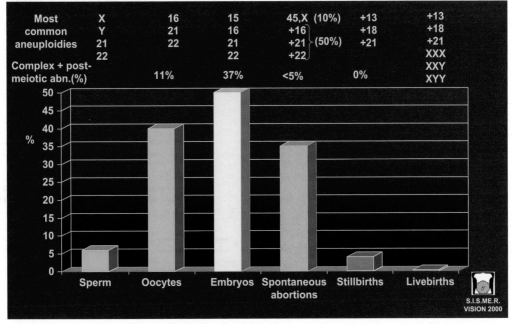

Most common aneuploidies	X Y 21 22	16 21 22	15 16 21 22	45,X (10%) +16 +21 } (50%) +22	+13 +18 +21	+13 +18 +21 XXX XXY XYY
Complex + post-meiotic abn.(%)		11%	37%	<5%	0%	

S.I.S.ME.R.
VISION 2000

Figure 65.7. Frequency of chromosomal anomalies in different stages of the human reproductive process.

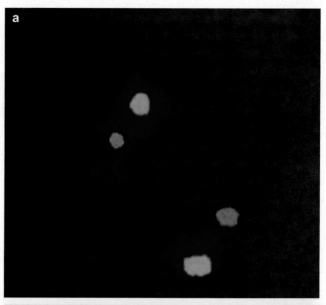

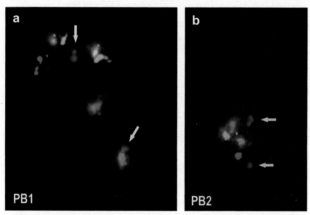

Figure 66.2. PGD of X-linked disorders using FISH. Two nuclei that have been hybridized with probes that are complementary to sequences on chromosomes X (green), Y (red), and 18 (blue). (a) A nucleus from the blastomere of a normal female embryo has two green and two blue signals, whereas (b) a nucleus from a normal male has one red, one green, and two blue signals. [Yacoub Khalaf (2007). Preimplantation genetic diagnosis. *Obstetrics, Gynecology and Reproductive Medicine* 17:1.]

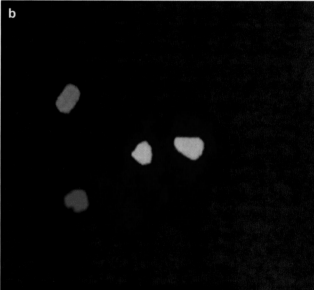

Figure 66.3. Polar body biopsy showing meiosis II error leading to monosomy 13. In PB1, there are two red signals for chromosome 13 (one of them is split). In PB2, there are two signals for chromosome 13 indicating monosomy in the oocyte. (Verlinsky Y and Anver Kuliev. Preimplantation diagnosis for aneuploidies. In Verlinsky Y and Anver Kuliev, eds. Atlas of preimplantation genetic diagnosis. Taylor and Francis, Abingdon, UK, 2005; pp. 156).

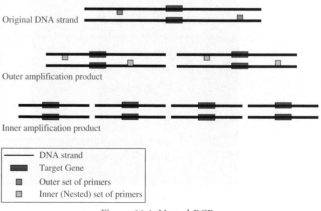

Figure 66.4. Nested PCR.

G₂ Ph
Specia
and RN

S Pha:
DNA sy

Figure 70
gonadoto
peutic age
lotoxins a
paclitaxel;
bleomycin
antipurine
abine, flu
urea, proca
as carmust
diglycoalde
alkylating
mechloreth
rubicin, da
neous: DTI
acts in G0.

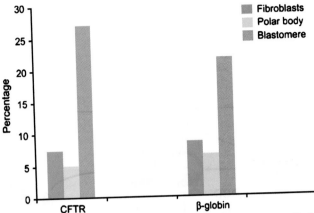

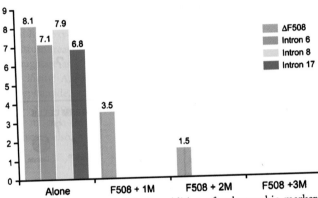

Figure 66.5. Allele dropout in different types of single cells. (Verlinsky Y and Anver Kuliev. Preimplantation diagnosis for single-gene disorders. In Verlinsky Y and Anver Kuliev, eds. Atlas of preimplantation genetic diagnosis. Taylor and Francis, Abingdon, UK, 2005; pp. 233).

Figure 66.6. ADO rate with the addition of polymorphic markers. Simultaneous analysis of two linked loci decrease the rate of ADO to 3.5 percent, while simultaneous analysis of three loci decrease that rate to 1.5 percent. (Verlinsky Y and Anver Kuliev. Preimplantation diagnosis for single-gene disorders. In Verlinsky Y and Anver Kuliev, eds. Atlas of preimplantation genetic diagnosis. Taylor and Francis, Abingdon, UK, 2005; pp. 233).

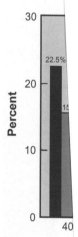

Pregnancy
Figure 72.1. Pre
rates for ART
women aged for

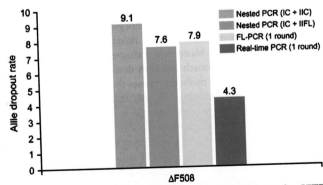

Figure 66.7. ADO rates in the analysis of F508 mutation in the CFTR gene following different types of PCR. The red bar indicates nested conventional PCR, the blue bar nested combined PCR (first round is conventional and the second round fluorescent), the yellow bar fluorescent PCR, and the green bar real-time PCR, which is the most sensitive. (Verlinsky Y and Anver Kuliev. Preimplantation diagnosis for single-gene disorders. In Verlinsky Y and Anver Kuliev, eds. Atlas of preimplantation genetic diagnosis. Taylor and Francis, Abingdon, UK, 2005; pp. 234).

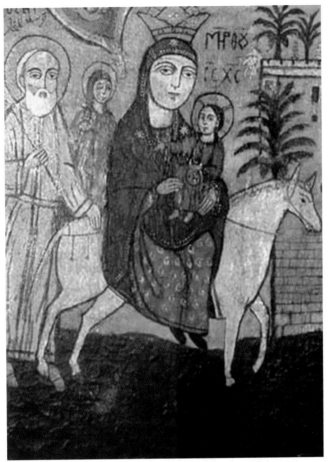

Figure 73.2. The Holy Family's flight to Egypt.

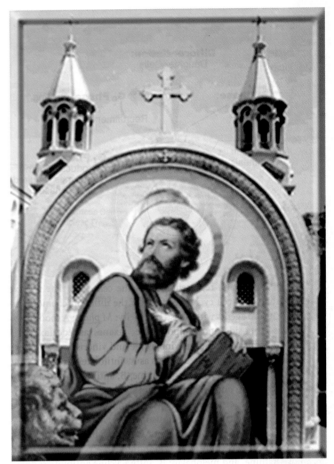

Figure 73.4. St. Mark, the founder of Christianity in Egypt and his Cathedral in Alexandria.

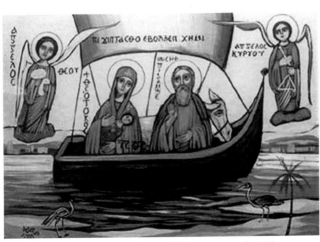

Figure 73.3. The Holy Family's journey on the Nile.

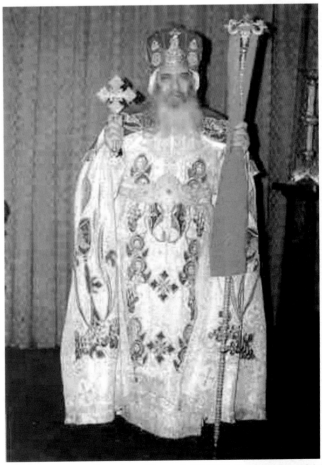

Figure 73.5. His Holiness Pope Shenouda III 117th Pope of Alexandria and Patriarch of the See of St. Mark.

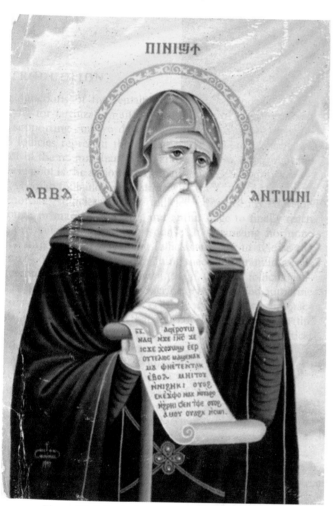

Figure 73.6. St. Anthony, founder of Monasticism.

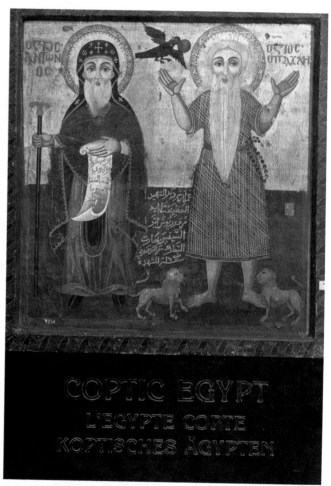

Figure 73.7. St. Anthony and St. Paul depiction of their historic meeting.

57. Hirao Y, Nagai T, Kubo M, Miyano T, Miyake M, Kato S. (1994). In vitro growth and maturation of pig oocytes. *J Reprod Fertil*;**100**:333–9.

58. Mao J, Wu G, Smith MF, McCauley TC, Cantley TC, Prather RS, et al. (2002). Effects of culture medium, serum type, and various concentrations of follicle-stimulating hormone on porcine preantral follicular development and antrum formation in vitro. *Biol Reprod*;**67**:1197–203.

59. Wu J, Emery BR, Carrell DT. (2001). In vitro growth, maturation, fertilization, and embryonic development of oocytes from porcine preantral follicles. *Biol Reprod*;**64**:375–81.

60. Yang MY, Fortune JE. (2007). Vascular endothelial growth factor stimulates the primary to secondary follicle transition in bovine follicles in vitro. *Mol Reprod Dev*;**74**:1095–104.

61. Nugent DNH, Gosden RG, Rutherford AJ. (1998). Investigation of follicle survival after human heterotopic autografting. *Hum Reprod*;**13**:22–3 (O-046).

62. Van Den Broecke R, Van Der Elst J, Liu J, Hovatta O, Dhont M. (2001). The female-to-male transsexual patient: a source of human ovarian cortical tissue for experimental use. *Hum Reprod*;**16**:145–7.

63. Abir R, Fisch B, Nitke S, Okon E, Raz A, Ben Rafael Z. (2001). Morphological study of fully and partially isolated early human follicles. *Fertil Steril*;**75**:141–6.

64. Roy SK, Terada DM. (1999). Activities of glucose metabolic enzymes in human preantral follicles: in vitro modulation by follicle-stimulating hormone, luteinizing hormone, epidermal growth factor, insulin-like growth factor I, and transforming growth factor beta1. *Biol Reprod*;**60**:763–8.

65. Dolmans MM, Michaux N, Camboni A, Martinez-Madrid B, Van Langendonckt A, Nottola SA, et al. (2006). Evaluation of liberase, a purified enzyme blend, for the isolation of human primordial and primary ovarian follicles. *Hum Reprod*;**21**:413–20.

66. Eppig JJ, O'Brien MJ. (1996). Development in vitro of mouse oocytes from primordial follicles. *Biol Reprod*;**54**:197–207.

67. Cortvrindt R, Smitz J, Van Steirteghem AC. (1996). In-vitro maturation, fertilization and embryo development of immature oocytes from early preantral follicles from prepuberal mice in a simplified culture system. *Hum Reprod*;**11**:2656–66.

68. O'Brien MJ, Pendola JK, Eppig JJ. (2003). A revised protocol for in vitro development of mouse oocytes from primordial follicles dramatically improves their developmental competence. *Biol Reprod*;**68**:1682–6.

69. Isachenko E, Isachenko V, Rahimi G, Nawroth F. (2003). Cryopreservation of human ovarian tissue by direct plunging into liquid nitrogen. *Eur J Obstet Gynecol Reprod Biol*; **108**:186–93.

70. Isachenko V, Montag M, Isachenko E, van der Ven K, Dorn C, Roesing B, Braun F, Sadek F, van der Ven H. (2006). Effective method for in-vitro culture of cryopreserved human ovarian tissue. *Reprod Biomed Online*;**13**:228–34.

71. Isachenko V, Isachenko E, Reinsberg J, Montag M, van der Ven K, Dorn C, Roesing B, van der Ven H. (2007). Cryopreservation of human ovarian tissue: comparison of rapid and conventional freezing. *Cryobiology*;**55**:261–8.

72. Scott JE, Carlsson IB, Bavister BD, Hovatta O. (2004). Human ovarian tissue cultures: extracellular matrix composition, coating density and tissue dimensions. *Reprod Biomed Online*;**9**: 287–93.

73. Telfer E, Torrance C, Gosden RG. (1990). Morphological study of cultured preantral ovarian follicles of mice after transplantation under the kidney capsule. *J Reprod Fertil*;**89**:565–71.

74. Kreeger PK, Deck JW, Woodruff TK, Shea LD. (2006). The in vitro regulation of ovarian follicle development using alginate-extracellular matrix gels. *Biomaterials*;**27**:714–23.

75. Nayudu PL, Osborn SM. (1992). Factors influencing the rate of preantral and antral growth of mouse ovarian follicles in vitro. *J Reprod Fertil*;**95**:349–62.

76. Roy SK, Greenwald GS. (1989). Hormonal requirements for the growth and differentiation of hamster preantral follicles in long-term culture. *J Reprod Fertil*;**87**:103–14.

77. Roy SK, Greenwald GS. (1996). Methods of separation and in-vitro culture of pre-antral follicles from mammalian ovaries. *Hum Reprod Update*;**2**:236–45.

78. Spears N, Boland NI, Murray AA, Gosden RG. (1994). Mouse oocytes derived from in vitro grown primary ovarian follicles are fertile. *Hum Reprod*;**9**:527–32.

79. Lenie S, Cortvrindt R, Adriaenssens T, Smitz J. (2004). A reproducible two-step culture system for isolated primary mouse ovarian follicles as single functional units. *Biol Reprod*;**71**: 1730–8.

80. Eppig JJ, Schroeder AC. (1989). Capacity of mouse oocytes from preantral follicles to undergo embryogenesis and development to live young after growth, maturation, and fertilization in vitro. *Biol Reprod*;**41**:268–76.

81. Tilly JL. (2003). Ovarian follicle counts—not as simple as 1, 2, 3. *Reprod Biol Endocrinol*;**1**:11.

82. Cortvrindt RG, Smitz JE. (2001). Fluorescent probes allow rapid and precise recording of follicle density and staging in human ovarian cortical biopsy samples. *Fertil Steril*;**75**:588–93.

83. Schotanus K, Hage WJ, Vanderstichele H, van den Hurk R. (1997). Effects of conditioned media from murine granulosa cell lines on the growth of isolated bovine preantral follicles. *Theriogenology*;**48**:471–83.

84. Reynaud K, Nogueira D, Cortvrindt R, Kurzawa R, Smitz J. (2001). Confocal microscopy: principles and applications to the field of reproductive biology. *Folia Histochem Cytobiol*;**39**:75–85.

85. Cortvrindt RG, Hu Y, Liu J, Smitz JE. (1998). Timed analysis of the nuclear maturation of oocytes in early preantral mouse follicle culture supplemented with recombinant gonadotropin. *Fertil Steril*;**70**:1114–25.

86. Gougeon A. (1996). Regulation of ovarian follicular development in primates: facts and hypotheses. *Endocr Rev*;**17**: 121–55.

87. Cortvrindt R, Liu J, Smitz J. (1998). Validation of a simplified culture system for primary mouse follicles by birth of live young. In: Ares Serono Symposia; 1998; XI International Workshop on Development and Function of the Reproductive Organ; Artis Zoo, Amsterdam, The Netherlands.

88. Cecconi S, Barboni B, Coccia M, Mattioli M. (1999). In vitro development of sheep preantral follicles. *Biol Reprod*;**60**: 594–601.

89. Kezele PR, Nilsson EE, Skinner MK (2002). Insulin but not insulin-like growth factor-1 promotes the primordial to primary follicle transition. *Mol Cell Endocrinol*;**192**:37–43.

90. Nilsson EE, Detzel C, Skinner MK. Platelet-derived growth factor modulates the primordial to primary follicle transition. (2006). *Reproduction*;**131**:1007–15.

91. Silva JR, van den Hurk R, van Tol HT, Roelen BA, Figueiredo JR. (2006). The Kit ligand/c-Kit receptor system in goat ovaries: gene expression and protein localization. *Zygote*;**14**:317–28.

92. Abir R, Roizman P, Fisch B, Nitke S, Okon E, Orvieto R, Ben Rafael Z. (1999). Pilot study of isolated early human follicles cultured in collagen gels for 24 hours. *Hum Reprod*;**14**:1299–301.

93. Hulshof SC, Figueiredo JR, Beckers JF, Bevers MM, van den Hurk R. (1994). Isolation and characterization of preantral follicles from foetal bovine ovaries. *Vet Q*;**16**:78–80.

94. Thomas FH, Leask R, Srsen V, Riley SC, Spears N, Telfer EE. (2001). Effect of ascorbic acid on health and morphology of bovine preantral follicles during long-term culture. *Reproduction*;**122**:487–95.

95. Wandji SA, Eppig JJ, Fortune JE. (1996). FSH and growth factors affect the growth and endocrine function in vitro of granulosa cells of bovine preantral follicles. *Theriogenology*;**45**:817–32.

96. Santos RR, van den Hurk R, Rodrigues AP, Costa SH, Martins FS, Matos MH, Celestino JJ, Figueiredo JR. (2007). Effect of cryopreservation on viability, activation and growth of in situ and isolated ovine early-stage follicles. *Anim Reprod Sci*;**99**:53–64.

97. Kreeger PK, Fernandes NN, Woodruff TK, Shea LD. (2005). Regulation of mouse follicle development by follicle-stimulating hormone in a three-dimensional in vitro culture system is dependent on follicle stage and dose. *Biol Reprod*;**73**:942–50.

4

ENDOMETRIAL RECEPTIVITY

Dominique de Ziegler, Timothee Fraisse, Charles Chapron

INTRODUCTION

Twenty-five years into the history of in vitro fertilization (IVF), endometrial receptivity remains both puzzling and challenging. The challenge comes from the fact that embryo implantation rates, however markedly improved in the later years, remain the bottleneck of assisted reproduction treatments (ART). In contrast to all the steps that take place earlier in the chain of ART measures such as notably multiple follicular stimulation, oocyte retrieval, fertilization, and cleavage rates, which have an efficacy largely more than 50 percent, embryo implantation rates continue to lag behind.

The puzzling fact about endometrial receptivity is that the simplest way of priming it is with the sole use of exogenous E2 and progesterone, as it was conceived for women whose ovaries have prematurely failed over twenty years ago. Indeed, implantations rates achieved in hormonal regimens developed for recipients of donor egg IVF remain remarkable even by today's standards, being at best equaled but to this date never surpassed, either in natural cycles or in any type of ART.

The lasting lesson that donor egg IVF has been teaching us is that E2 and progesterone suffice for triggering an optimal endometrial receptivity. This implies that other factors produced by the ovary such as notably androgens are at best unnecessary but often capable of harming. In controlled ovarian hyperstimulation (COH), as performed in ART, the ovaries are stimulated with supraphysiological levels of gonadotropins. This not only increases the production of E2 and after ovulation that of progesterone but also stimulates a host of other factors that are also sensitive to gonadotropins. As we will see, some of these latter products are susceptible of harming endometrial receptivity. This hypothesis put forth for explaining the deleterious effects of COH on the endometrium will be addressed in the section of this chapter entitled the *Third Factor Theory*.

THE MENSTRUAL CYCLE: A SEQUENCE OF ENDOMETRIAL CHANGES LEADING TO RECEPTIVITY

The Two Endometrial Constituents: The Glands and Stroma

In the menstrual cycle, exposure to E2 takes place during the follicular phase. It has been amply documented that this represents a necessary priming step during which the endometrium acquires receptors to E2 (ER) and progesterone (PR)

(1, 2). We know today that the follicular phase is of variable length in part because of the uncertainty about when its functional onset, the intercycle FSH elevation, truly takes place (3). Yet, this variability in the length of the follicular phase appears to not affect the quality of endometrial priming and has no practical consequences on endometrial responsiveness during the ensuing luteal phase (4–6).

The endometrial changes that take place during the luteal phase of the menstrual cycle have been described in detail by Noyes et al. (7). Amazingly, the original description made by Noyes and Haman remains valid today, over fifty years after it was originally published. Yet, these authors did not mention in their description a fairly important consideration that is crucial for our understanding of the changes in endometrial morphology taking place in COH: the parameters retained for describing the sequence of changes seen in the endometrium during the luteal phase occur first in the endometrial glands and later in the stroma for the first and second half of the luteal phase, respectively.

Work done in the donor egg model in order to elucidate the so-called glandular-stromal dyssynchrony led to postulate and ultimately demonstrate that endometrial glands and stroma have different sensitivities to progesterone (8–12). While glands are more sensitive to the action of progesterone, the endometrial stroma tends to be advanced as compared to findings made in the menstrual cycle in case of strong response to COH (13). In COH, therefore, it is possible to see at the theoretical time of implantation the combination of a glandular delay and stromal advance, a finding from which came the concept glandular-stromal dyssynchrony. The former (glandular delay) is believed to result from the suppression of late – follicular phase progesterone elevation in COH by GnRH-a (contrary to the menstrual cycle). Conversely, the latter (stromal advance) reflects the higher levels of progesterone early after multiple ovulation than normally seen in the menstrual cycle (Figure 4.1).

Endometrial Markers of Receptivity: From Integrins to Pinopodes

Integrins are molecules involved in cell-to-cell adhesion that are present at the surface of essentially all human cells. Based on immunoperoxidase staining, different forms of integrins are expressed in the endometrium at different times throughout the cycle. Of particular interest is the fact that immunostaining for the β3-subunit appears abruptly, precisely on day 20 of the menstrual cycle. This corresponds with the short interval of endometrial receptivity to embryo implantation or *window of*

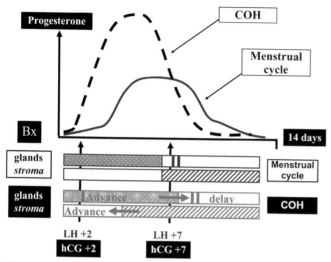

Figure 4.1. Hormonal profile in the early luteal phase of IVF. The diagram depicts the patterns of progesterone levels encountered in the menstrual cycle and in COH. In COH, plasma progesterone peaks earlier and reaches higher levels. Concomitantly, analyses of endometrial histology show a delay in the secretory transformation of glands (after a transitory slight advance within two days of hCG administration), whereas predecidualization of endometrial stroma is characteristically advanced.

implantation (14). Conversely, out of phase endometrial biopsies from infertile patients have been associated with delayed and/or absent expression of β3-integrins, a finding that has been proposed to reflect impaired fertility due to implantation problems (15). As discussed in later sections of this chapter, aberrant expression of β3-integrins has been described in two situations, endometriosis (16) and E2 and progesterone cycles prepared for recipients of donor egg IVF (17). The former situation is associated with diminished receptivity, while the latter is not.

Great hopes of holding an assessable marker of endometrial receptivity came from the early reports that related the development of specific surface structures known as pinopodes at the time of endometrial receptivity (18). Interest for pinopodes was bolstered by observations that pinopodes expression was altered in IVF, possibly offering a reflection of the decreased endometrial receptivity that characterizes these cycles (19, 20). Dyssynchronous expression of pinopodes in women receiving E2 and progesterone, as designed for donor egg IVF (18), seriously threw into question the postulate that synchronous expression of pinopodes is a prerequisite for endometrial receptivity. Rather, it became apparent that the forward shift in pinopode expression (or delay) observed in E2 and progesterone cycles paralleled the changes in β3 integrin and histological changes in glands and stroma. Yet this dyssynchrony had no impact on endometrial receptivity in the donor egg model, as receptivity is there as good as it gets in E2 and progesterone substitution cycles.

More recently, the role of the homeobox (HOX) genes has been proposed as possible mediator if not organizer of hormonal effects on the endometrium. HOX genes are evolutionary conserved structures responsible for body axis patterning during embryogenesis (21). While primarily active during embryogenesis, HOX genes are also involved in the adult in certain tissues that undergo rapid developmental changes such as notably the hematopoietic system and endometrium. In the

endometrium, cyclical activation of the HOX gene coding for the endometrium, HOXA-10, takes place during the follicular and luteal phases of each menstrual cycle, as if the endometrium was reborn every month. Expression of HOXA-10 is stimulated by E2 and further so by the association of E2 and progesterone (22, 23). Hence, rather than opposing the effects of E2 as for endometrial proliferation, progesterone amplifies the action of E2 on HOXA-10 expression, an action that is only surpassed by the further hormonal enhancement encountered in case of pregnancy. Conversely, HOXA-10 expression is inhibited by certain (testosterone, dihydrotestosterone or DHT) but not all androgens (Δ4 androstenedione), as illustrated in Figure 4.2 (22, 23). Similarly, HOXA-10 expression is hampered in case of hydrosalpinx (24), a condition known to be associated with diminished endometrial receptivity. As discussed later in this chapter, HOXA-10 expression is also decreased in other conditions also associated with decreased endometrial receptivity such as, notably, endometriosis.

DONOR EGG IVF: A REFERENCE FOR ENDOMETRIAL RECEPTIVITY AND A STUDY MODEL

The advent of IVF opened the possibility to revert to donated oocytes for cases of infertility linked to premature ovarian failure (POF). For being effective, however, donor egg IVF required that the endometrium was rendered receptive with the sole use of the exogenous hormones E2 and progesterone. At first, this appeared heroic to the early players who attempted to render the endometrium receptive by duplicating the hormonal profile seen in the menstrual cycle with the sole use of exogenous hormones. Following the first reports of success with donor egg IVF (25, 26), it soon became apparent that pregnancy rates achieved in recipient of donated oocytes exceeded those commonly encountered in regular IVF (27). Today, twenty years into the history of donor egg IVF, it remains true that embryo implantation rates are exceptionally high, being at best equaled but never exceeded in any other form of treatment or even in the menstrual cycle.

The first lesson learned from the donor egg model was that all that is needed for an optimal endometrium is an E2 priming of sufficient duration followed by exposure to progesterone with proper respect of the respective endometrial and embryo exposures to progesterone. Donor egg IVF also allowed to precisely determine the timing of endometrial receptivity (28). Comparing embryo implantation rates to the timing of embryo transfers in relation to the onset of progesterone administration established the bases of our knowledge of the period of optimal results or window of transfers. From the early reports, we know that optimal results for two to eight cell embryos are obtained when transfers are programmed between the third and fourth days of exposure to exogenous progesterone (29, 30). While some pregnancies have been seen with early transfers (as early as on the last day of E2 only), none took place beyond the fifth day of exposure to progesterone, leading to delineate the limits of the window of transfer.

Early works also compared the efficacy of the different routes available for hormone administration. This allowed to establish that transdermal and oral E2 are equally effective at priming endometrial receptivity in spite of different hormonal profiles of estrone (E1) and E2 ratios (31). Similarly, vaginal and IM progesterone preparations have been found equally

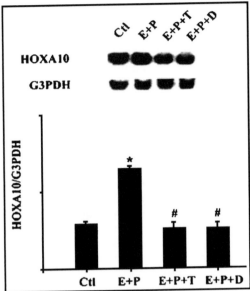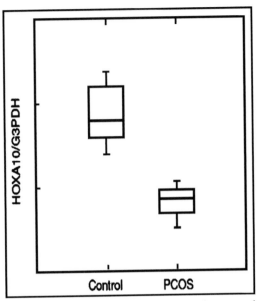

Figure 4.2. HOXA-10 expression in response to sex steroids. HOXA-10 expression in the presence of E2, E2 and progesterone, and E2 and progesterone plus testosterone (T) or dihydrotestosterone (DHT). E2 and progesterone induce a more important expression of HOXA-10 than E2 alone. On the contrary, the addition of T or DHT profoundly hampers the effect of E2 and progesterone on HOXA-10. In POCS, endogenous production of T also interferes with HOXA-10 expression (from: Daftary and Taylor; 21).

effective, a finding that has not been disputed in spite of the large number of trials that looked into this issue (32).

The remarkable efficacy of E2 and progesterone cycles at priming endometrial receptivity in donor egg IVF has led several investigators to use these cycles as study models for delineating the respective roles played by each hormonal constituent. In the early days of IVF, one of the prevailing concerns regarding endometrial receptivity in IVF was that the high E2 levels induced by COH altered endometrial receptivity (33) by creating an imbalance of theoretically normal E2 to progesterone ratio (34–37). Yet, in this quest toward an ideal E2 to progesterone ratio, it became apparent to us that the effects of one of the terms of the E2 to progesterone ratio, luteal E2 produced by the corpus luteum after ovulation, were unknown. In a prospective trial, we compared the effects of progesterone on endometrial glands (day 20) and stroma (day 24) in women who either received a physiological E2 and progesterone replacement paradigm or in whom E2 supplementation was stopped as soon as progesterone was initiated on cycle day 15 (38). In this latter group, therefore, women received E2 priming that mimicked the follicular phase of the menstrual cycle while progesterone was administered without concomitant administration of E2. This therefore constituted a no-luteal E2 model. To our surprise, endometrial changes were unaltered in the no-luteal E2 group, either on day 20 or on day 24 biopsies. This, thereby, indicated that luteal E2 bears no effect on endometrial morphology (38), a findings subsequently confirmed by others (40). We subsequently performed the opposite hormonal manipulation, which consisted in administrating pharmacological amounts of E2 together with progesterone supplementation. In this group too, endometrial changes observed in endometrial glands and stroma after six and ten days of exposure to progesterone (days 20 and 24, respectively) were unaltered as compared to findings made in the menstrual cycle and in women receiving physiological E2 and progesterone replacement (40).

In further manipulations of E2 and progesterone cycles, Navot et al. (4) indicated that the duration of the E2-only phase of the treatment could be shortened to six days only. Subsequently, Simon's group in Spain determined that the E2 priming phase can be lengthened to up to hundred days without deleterious consequences (41).

IN COH: BASES FOR THE *THIRD FACTOR THEORY* AND RATIONALE FOR MINIMAL STIMULATION

In spite of the lack of proven effects of high E2 levels on endometrial morphology, numerous reports have documented that strong responses to COH with high E2 levels adversely affect endometrial morphology (13) and IVF outcome (42). We fully believe the clinical relevance of each of these findings but question, however, the interpretation that has been made postulating that endometrial alterations (13) and a poor IVF outcome (42) truly result from an effect of the high E2 levels.

Opposing the commonly stated axiom postulating that it is the high E2 levels encountered in certain COH protocols that adversely affect endometrial morphology and receptivity, we offered an alternate hypothesis. This alternate paradigm postulates that the high levels of gonadotropins achieved in COH stimulate other ovarian factors beyond just E2 and luteal progesterone (hence, the *third factor hypothesis* concept) that are susceptible of altering endometrial receptivity. First on the list of candidates for playing the role of the hypothetical *third factor* responsible for altering endometrial receptivity in COH are ovarian androgens. These are increased by gonadotropins (43–45) to various degrees according to individual characteristics and are susceptible of altering endometrial quality, notably by interfering with HOX-A10 expression (46).

Awareness of the possibility that COH may harm the endometrium through ovarian factors other than E2 and progesterone and thus not commonly monitored led us to avoid excessive FSH/hMG exposure in the later stages of COH. This precautionary move is accomplished by reducing FSH/hMG doses (47) or opting to LH dominance in the later stages of COH (48).

Uterine Contractility and Receptivity

Originally, it was solely the effects that hormones exerted on the endometrium that were taken into account when studying uterine receptivity to embryo implantation. It became later obvious that myometrial factors were also susceptible of affecting embryo implantation by their effects on contractility, which could alter the outcome of embryo transfers (ET). In this review, it is therefore necessary to summarize the endocrine control of myometrial contractility and survey the possible alterations that are susceptible of altering uterine receptivity to embryo implantation.

Characteristically, there are three patterns of contractility that have been recognized in the menstrual cycle. These are encountered during the intercycle interval, the late follicular phase, and during the luteal phase. During the intercycle interval, uterine contractions (UC) present a marked increase in amplitude and duration, whereas UC frequency is only moderately increased (49, 50). Moreover, resting intrauterine pressure is elevated during the intercycle interval (50, 51). At this stage of the menstrual cycle, UC involve all the layers of the myometrium and may be perceived by women. In the physiological sense, UC encountered during the intercycle interval constitute a mini replica of the pattern of contractions that take place during labor (52). In a variant of this pattern, all the parameters of UC are further increased and the perception of UC is described as frankly painful by women in a condition known as dysmenorrhea (53, 54). A long-lasting history of dysmenorrhea is classically found in women diagnosed with endometriosis, a condition that is associated with a possible decrease in endometrial receptivity (55, 56). Yet, dysmenorrhea per se is not known to be associated with decreased fertility and/or receptivity to embryo implantation.

Finally, in the late follicular phase, there is a progressive increase in UC frequency under the influence of rising E2 levels (57). These contractions only affect the subendometrial layers of the myometrium and, remarkably, are not perceived by women.

UC frequency is high however, reaching approximately five per minute just prior to ovulation, which constitutes the highest value encountered at any time during the menstrual cycle. A wealth of evidences that indicate a predominance of retrograde contraction in the late follicular phase has been accumulated (52). Using labeled macroalbumin aggregates, Leyendecker's team has documented that retrograde cervix to fundus transport predominates during the late follicular phase, with a preference of transport toward the side bearing the developing follicle (52). Taken together, these pieces of information have led to conclude that the primary function of UC in the late follicular phase is to facilitate sperm transport toward the tubes and ultimately the distal end of it where fertilization takes place.

The luteal phase is characterized by a state of uterine quiescence that is brought by progesterone secreted by the corpus luteum after ovulation. In the natural cycle, a profound decrease in UC frequency takes place within two to four days of ovulation (49, 50). In women prematurely deprived of ovarian function and primed with exogenous E2, progesterone administered vaginally induced a similar decrease in UC frequency that followed a similar time course (58). In contrast with these findings, however, UC remains elevated at the time of ET in IVF, in spite of ET taking place four days or later after ovulation, a time when the uterus is quiescent in the menstrual cycle (59). In our trial conducted in women who all had three good looking embryos available for transfer, we observed that pregnancy rates were markedly decreased in women whose UC frequency remained elevated at the time of ET (59).

In a prospective trial, we compared UC frequency in women undergoing IVF and in the menstrual cycle that immediately preceded IVF (60). For this, women were studied and UC frequency assessed on the day of LH surge (menstrual cycle) or hCG administration (IVF) and every two days thereafter until the sixth day after LH surge or hCG administration. Results are illustrated in Figure 4.3. On the day of hCG administration, UC frequency was comparable at five per minute to findings made in the same women on the day of LH surge (60). It can be concluded that the higher E2 levels encountered in IVF did not result in higher UC frequency in the IVF cycle, suggesting that the E2 levels achieved in the menstrual cycle already achieved maximal stimulation on uterine contractility. On the fourth day after LH surge and hCG administration, UC frequency differed markedly between the menstrual and IVF

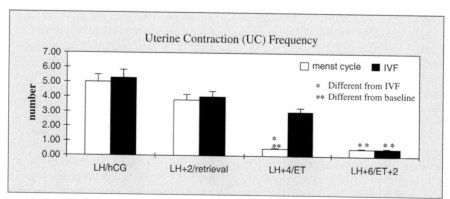

Figure 4.3. Uterine contractility in the menstrual cycle and IVF. Uterine contractility during the luteal phase of the menstrual cycle and in IVF. In the menstrual cycle, a profound decrease of uterine contractility is observed on the fourth day after LH surge. When the same patients underwent IVF, a characteristic delay in the response to the uteroquiescent properties of progesterone was observed (from: Ayoubi et al.; 58).

cycle. In the former, UC frequency was markedly reduced as previously reported by other authors (49) and seen after exogenous progesterone administration, thereby reflecting the state of uteroquiescence that characterizes the luteal phase (58). When the same women underwent IVF, UC frequency remained elevated on the fourth day after hCG administration at values nearing those seen in the late follicular phase. On the sixth day after hCG, however, UC frequency had finely decreased as seen in the luteal phase. We conclude from these results that the high E2 levels of IVF do not further stimulate UC frequency above the finding seen in the follicular phase of the menstrual cycle but induce a state of relative resistance to the uterorelaxing effects of progesterone.

In a prospective trial, Fanchin et al. (61) showed that an earlier start of luteal support with vaginal progesterone on the day of oocyte retrieval resulted in decreased UC frequency two days later at the time of ET as compared to controls in whom luteal support had not been started yet. From these sets of studies, we decided to initiate luteal support immediately after conducting the oocyte retrieval, using in our hands soft gelatin capsules of progesterone administered vaginally (300 mg/day). All attempts that we have been aware of to further decrease UC prior to ET in IVF with beta mimetics or NO donors did not improve embryo implantation rates (62). An alternate option when UC frequency remains too elevated two to three days after oocyte retrieval is to delay ETs until the blastocyst stage, five days after oocyte retrieval (63).

One practical conclusion drawn from this review of the hormonal effects on uterine contractility is that one should not limit analyses to the endometrium when assessing issues pertinent to uterine receptivity to embryo implantation. It is likely that part of the benefit of luteal support with exogenous progesterone is mediated by an effect on the myometrium. The impact of uterine contractility on IVF outcome also stresses the role of precautions that need to accompany ET in an attempt to minimize the impact the measures themselves have on UC (64).

CONDITIONS WITH DECREASED ENDOMETRIAL RECEPTIVITY: ENDOMETRIOSIS AND ENDOMETRITIS

Endometriosis and Decreased Receptivity

Several conditions have been claimed to impact on the endometrium's ability to accept embryo implantation (65). One of these is endometriosis. Unquestionably, the primary impact of endometriosis is on the peritoneal stage of reproduction with a characteristically impaired sperm oocyte interaction. Yet, a host of data have accumulated that also lend credence to the hypothesis that endometriosis hampers endometrial receptivity to embryo implantation. The suspicion that endometriosis hampers endometrial receptivity is rooted in various sorts of evidences.

On the one side, reports abound that describe decreased implantation rates in case of endometriosis (66). Yet to this date, it is still difficult to definitively single out the mechanism(s) at play in the harm created by endometriosis on pregnancy and implantation rates in ART. Does this result from impaired oocyte quality itself caused by the impact of endometriosis on ovarian function or is this the direct result of an impact of the disease on the endometrium?

On the other side, a host of studies have focused on altered, let alone absent, biomarkers of uterine receptivity in case of endometriosis (67). In studies that are now classical, Lessey et al. documented reduced expression of the cell adhesion molecule β-integrin at the theoretical time of implantation (16). Questions arose about the clinical meaningfulness of this finding when it was reported that the expression of β-integrin was delayed in E2 and progesterone substitution cycles designed for donor-egg recipients (17). Yet, the recent report indicating that aberrant absence of β-integrin expression results from an abnormal persistence and inappropriate overexpression of ERa during the midsecretory phase (68) is shedding new lights on the possible mechanism(s) at play. According to this hypothesis, an intrinsic disorder of ERα regulation in the endometrium might exist in endometriosis as a result of local production of E2 through activation of the aromatase gene (69–71), possibly through an increased production of PG-E2 (72). Recent data indicate that altered aromatase expression might represent a generalized and ubiquitous manifestation of inflammation not specific to endometriosis (73–75).

Recently, converging reports have stressed the possible therapeutic role of aromatase inhibitors in the medical treatment of endometriosis (76, 77). The reader is urged to follow the literature for reports on the possible value of using combined oral contraceptive pill and aromatase inhibitors for restoring optimal endometrial receptivity in women suffering from endometriosis.

Arguments fueling credit to the concept that endometrial receptivity is impaired in endometriosis came from the observation that ovarian suppression with GnRH agonists (GnRH-a) prior to IVF significantly improved the outcome. In a prospective trial, Surrey et al. (78) showed that women diagnosed with endometriosis in the past sixty months had better IVF outcome if they received three months of treatment with GnRH-a prior to IVF. Interestingly, in this trial, women were attributed FSH/hMG doses prior to their randomization into the GnRH-a or control direct IVF arm. Hence, it can be reasonably ascertained that the three-month treatment with GnRH-a did not hamper ovarian response in spite of the suspicions that exist. Instrumental in the lack of excessive suppression encountered in the GnRH-a arm was the fact that COH for IVF was started forty-five days after the last twenty-eight days following long-acting GnRH-a injection, a measure that may prove to have been well inspired.

Contrasting with this host of studies that speak for an impairment of endometrial receptivity in case of endometriosis, a prospective trial stands alone in claiming a lack of alteration of endometrial receptivity in women affected by endometriosis (79). In their study, Diaz et al. compared implantation rates of embryo obtained from donated oocytes following their transfers in recipients who suffered from severe endometriosis or not. In their hands, embryo implantation rates were similar in women who had severe endometriosis and in unaffected controls. It is noteworthy to underscore, however, that the number of embryos transferred in this trial was relatively limited. Moreover, this trial stood aside of the commonly encountered circumstances in that women suffering from endometriosis had their ovaries suppressed by the E2 and progesterone replacement regimen received for priming embryo transfers. Hence, any putative ovarian factor susceptible of harming receptivity is likely to not have been expressed in this study paradigm contrary to what would be encountered in women affected by endometriosis undergoing regular IVF.

Endometritis: An Elusive Diagnosis

Endometritis is a condition in which there is an inflammation and/or infection of the endometrium. Acute forms of endometritis commonly either are associated with other facets of pelvic infection as part of pelvic inflammatory disease or constitute a complication of deliveries, dilatation, and curettage and/or other instrumentations of the uterus. Acute endometritis found in the follow up of therapeutic abortions are most often associated with retained product of conception and rarely constitute an issue in infertility cases unless for possible squealae in the form of Asherman syndrome.

More recently, however, the attention of infertility specialists has been drawn to the concept of low-grade chronic endometritis (CE) as possible cause of otherwise unexplained infertility (80). Histologically, the diagnosis of CE is generally based on finding an excessive number of neutrophils and plasma cell infiltrates in endometrial biopsies (81, 82). In support of this emerging new concept, there are a slew of publications describing a chronically inflamed endometrium in a sizable fraction of women undergoing diagnostic hysteroscopy as part of infertility work up. In the descriptions made, the uterine cavity is covered by one or several spots where the mucosa appears thickened. Often endometritis appear as sets of white dots laid over these reddish areas that justify their description as strawberry-like patches (80).

A recent finding bears common interest for treating the possible harmful consequences of these two conditions, endometriosis and endometritis, on the endometrium. It has recently been identified that aromatase, the enzyme controlling the last step in the synthesis of estrogen, may be activated in various sorts of tissues. While originally believed to be the exclusive attribute of steroid-synthesizing organs (ovaries, testicles, and adrenals) and adipose tissue, it has been documented that activation of the aromatize gene is an ubiquitous reaction linked to inflammation (74). Depending on the organ involved, the local production of estrogen may play a specific role in the disease itself. In the case in endometriosis, the local activation of aromatase (70) leads to the local production of E2, which further enhances the symptoms and aggravates a condition that is likely to further hamper endometrial receptivity to embryo implantation.

KEY POINTS

■ Endometrial receptivity to embryo implantation has been an enduring bottleneck of the reproductive system in humans. In assisted reproduction, oocyte retrieval, fertilization rates, and embryo cleavage rates all yield results in the 60–90 percent rates. On the contrary, embryo implantation rates continue to lag behind in spite of recent progress made in the IVF overall success rates. The possibility that hormonal imbalances resulting from hormonal regimens prescribed for inducing multiple ovulation has been a clinical preoccupation since day 1 of IVF. First among the set of data that fueled this hypothesis has been the repeated observation that pregnancy and embryo implantation rates tend to be higher in donor egg IVF than in regular IVF in programs offering both services.

■ While high E2 levels have been blamed for the possible harm caused by COH prescribed in IVF, we contend that other ovarian factors also increased in COH may actually be the primary culprits. This third factor hypothesis is based on high E2 levels, having no deleterious effects in the donor egg exogenous E2 and progesterone model. Conversely, COH may increase other ovarian factors such as androgens that possibly harm endometrial receptivity. The recent uncovering of the role played by HOX genes in endometrial development throughout the menstrual cycle offers support for a deleterious role of androgens on the endometrium. While E2 and progesterone leads to full expression of the HOX system, this is hampered by exogenous or endogenous androgens. In daily clinical practice, our current understanding of hormonal effects on the endometrium call for minimizing gonadotropin stimulation notably, FSH doses, toward the end stages of COH. Minimizing ovarian stimulation may be facilitated by step-down regimens, calling for slightly higher initial doses of gonadotropins in COH.

REFERENCES

1. Garcia E, Bouchard P, De Brux J, Berdah J, Frydman R, Schaison G, Milgrom E, Perrot-Applanat M. Use of immunocytochemistry of progesterone and estrogen receptors for endometrial dating. *J Clin Endocrinol Metab.* 1988;67:80–7.

2. Bergeron C, Ferenczy A, Toft DO, Schneider W, Shyamala G. Immunocytochemical study of progesterone receptors in the human endometrium during the menstrual cycle. *Lab Invest.* 1988;59:862–9.

3. le Nestour E, Marraoui J, Lahlou N, Roger M, de Ziegler D, Bouchard P. Role of estradiol in the rise in follicle-stimulating hormone levels during the luteal-follicular transition. *J Clin Endocrinol Metab.* 1993;77:439–42.

4. Navot D, Bergh PA, Williams M, Garrisi GJ, Guzman I, Sandler B, Fox J, Schreiner-Engel P, Hofmann GE, Grunfeld L. An insight into early reproductive processes through the in vivo model of ovum donation. *J Clin Endocrinol Metab.* 1991;72:408–14.

5. Navot D, Bergh P. Preparation of the human endometrium for implantation. *Ann N Y Acad Sci.* 1991;622:212–9. Review. No abstract available.

6. Navot D, Anderson TL, Droesch K, Scott RT, Kreiner D, Rosenwaks Z. Hormonal manipulation of endometrial maturation. *J Clin Endocrinol Metab.* 1989;68:801–7.

7. Noyes RW, Haman JO. Accuracy of endometrial dating; correlation of endometrial dating with basal body temperature and menses. *Fertil Steril.* 1953;4:504–17.

8. Navot D, Anderson TL, Droesch K, Scott RT, Kreiner D, Rosenwaks Z. Hormonal manipulation of endometrial maturation. *J Clin Endocrinol Metab.* 1989;68:801–7.

9. Navot D, Scott RT, Droesch K, Veeck LL, Liu HC, Rosenwaks Z. The window of embryo transfer and the efficiency of human conception in vitro. *Fertil Steril.* 1991;55:114–8.

10. Bergh PA, Navot D. The impact of embryonic development and endometrial maturity on the timing of implantation. *Fertil Steril.* 1992;58:537–42.

11. de Ziegler D. Hormonal control of endometrial receptivity. *Hum Reprod.* 1995;10:4–7.

12. de Ziegler D, Bouchard P. Understanding endometrial physiology and menstrual disorders in the 1990s. *Curr Opin Obstet Gynecol.* 1993;5:378–88.

13. Basir GS, O WS, Ng EH, Ho PC. Morphometric analysis of peri-implantation endometrium in patients having excessively high oestradiol concentrations after ovarian stimulation. *Hum Reprod.* 2001;16:435–40.

14. Lessey BA, Damjanovich L, Coutifaris C, Castelbaum A, Albelda SM, Buck CA. Integrin adhesion molecules in the human endometrium. Correlation with the normal and abnormal menstrual cycle. *J Clin Invest.* 1992;90:188–95.

15. Lessey BA. The use of integrins for the assessment of uterine receptivity. *Fertil Steril.* 1994;61:812–4.

16. Lessey BA, Castelbaum AJ, Sawin SW, Buck CA, Schinnar R, Bilker W, Strom BL. Aberrant integrin expression in the endometrium of women with endometriosis. *J Clin Endocrinol Metab.* 1994;79:643–9.

17. Damario MA, Lesnick TG, Lessey BA, Kowalik A, Mandelin E, Seppala M, Rosenwaks Z. Endometrial markers of uterine receptivity utilizing the donor oocyte model. *Hum Reprod.* 2001; 16:1893–9.

18. Nikas G, Drakakis P, Loutradis D, Mara-Skoufari C, Koumantakis E, Michalas S, Psychoyos A. Uterine pinopodes as markers of the 'nidation window' in cycling women receiving exogenous oestradiol and progesterone. *Hum Reprod.* 1995;10:1208–13.

19. Nikas G, Develioglu OH, Toner JP, Jones HW Jr. Endometrial pinopodes indicate a shift in the window of receptivity in IVF cycles. *Hum Reprod.* 1999;14:787–92.

20. Bentin-Ley U, Sjogren A, Nilsson L, Hamberger L, Larsen JF, Horn T. Presence of uterine pinopodes at the embryo-endometrial interface during human implantation in vitro. *Hum Reprod.* 1999; 14:515–20.

21. Daftary GS, Taylor HS. Endocrine regulation of HOX genes. *Endocr Rev.* 2006;27:331–55.

22. Taylor HS, Arici A, Olive D, Igarashi P. HOXA10 is expressed in response to sex steroids at the time of implantation in the human endometrium. *J Clin Invest.* 1998;101:1379–84.

23. Taylor HS. Transcriptional regulation of implantation by HOX genes. *Rev Endocr Metab Disord.* 2002;3:127–32.

24. Daftary GS, Taylor HS. Hydrosalpinx fluid diminishes endometrial cell HOXA10 expression. *Fertil Steril.* 2002;78:577–80.

25. Lutjen PJ, Leeton JF, Findlay JK. Oocyte and embryo donation in IVF programmes. *Clin Obstet Gynaecol.* 1985;12:799–813.

26. Navot D, Laufer N, Kopolovic J, Rabinowitz R, Birkenfeld A, Lewin A, Granat M, Margalioth EJ, Schenker JG. Artificially induced endometrial cycles and establishment of pregnancies in the absence of ovaries. *N Engl J Med.* 1986;314:806–11.

27. Rosenwaks Z, Veeck LL, Liu HC. Pregnancy following transfer of in vitro fertilized donated oocytes. *Fertil Steril.* 1986;45:417–20.

28. Rosenwaks Z, Garcia-Velasco JA, Isaza V, Caligara C, Pellicer A, Remohi J, Simon C. Factors that determine discordant outcome from shared oocytes. *Fertil Steril.* 2003;80:54–60.

29. Rosenwaks Leeton J, Chan LK, Trounson A, Harman J. Pregnancy established in an infertile patient after transfer of an embryo fertilized in vitro where the oocyte was donated by the sister of the recipient. *J In Vitro Fert Embryo Transf.* 1986;3:379–82.

30. Sauer MV, Paulson RJ, Lobo RA. Simultaneous establishment of pregnancies in two ovarian failure patients using one oocyte donor. *Fertil Steril.* 1989;52:1072–3.

31. Smitz J, Devroey P, Faguer B, Bourgain C, Camus M, Van Steirteghem AC. A prospective randomized comparison of intramuscular or intravaginal natural progesterone as a luteal phase and early pregnancy supplement. *Hum Reprod.* 1992;7:168–75.

32. Steingold KA, Matt DW, de Ziegler D, Sealey JE, Fratkin M, Reznikov S. Comparison of transdermal to oral estradiol administration on hormonal and hepatic parameters in women with premature ovarian failure. *J Clin Endocrinol Metab.* 1991;73:275–80.

33. Forman R, Fries N, Testart J, Belaisch-Allart J, Hazout A, Frydman R. Evidence for an adverse effect of elevated serum estradiol concentrations on embryo implantation. *Fertil Steril.* 1988;49:118–22.

34. Mahadevan MM, Fleetham J, Taylor PJ. Effects of progesterone on luteinizing hormone release and estradiol/progesterone ratio in the luteal phase of women superovulated for in vitro fertilization and embryo transfer. *Fertil Steril.* 1988;50:935–7.

35. Maclin VM, Radwanska E, Binor Z, Dmowski WP. Progesterone: estradiol ratios at implantation in ongoing pregnancies, abortions, and nonconception cycles resulting from ovulation induction. *Fertil Steril.* 1990;54:238–44.

36. Gorkemli H, Ak D, Akyurek C, Aktan M, Duman S. Comparison of pregnancy outcomes of progesterone or progesterone + estradiol for luteal phase support in ICSI-ET cycles. *Gynecol Obstet Invest.* 2004;58:140–4.

37. Gelety TJ, Buyalos RP. The influence of supraphysiologic estradiol levels on human nidation. *J Assist Reprod Genet.* 1995;12: 406–12.

38. de Ziegler D, Bergeron C, Cornel C, Medalie DA, Massai MR, Milgrom E, Frydman R, Bouchard P. Effects of luteal estradiol on the secretory transformation of human endometrium and plasma gonadotropins. *J Clin Endocrinol Metab.* 1992;74:322–31.

39. Younis JS, Ezra Y, Sherman Y, Simon A, Schenker JG, Laufer N. The effect of estradiol depletion during the luteal phase on endometrial development. *Fertil Steril.* 1994;62:103–7.

40. de Ziegler D, Fanchin R, de Moustier B, Bulletti C. The hormonal control of endometrial receptivity: estrogen (E2) and progesterone. *J Reprod Immunol.* 1998;39:149–66.

41. Remohi J, Gutierrez A, Cano F, Ruiz A, Simon C, Pellicer A. Long oestradiol replacement in an oocyte donation programme. *Hum Reprod.* 1995;10:1387–91.

42. Simon C, Garcia Velasco JJ, Valbuena D, Peinado JA, Moreno C, Remohi J, Pellicer A. Increasing uterine receptivity by decreasing estradiol levels during the preimplantation period in high responders with the use of a follicle-stimulating hormone step-down regimen. *Fertil Steril.* 1998;70:234–9.

43. Fanchin R, de Ziegler D, Castracane VD, Taieb J, Olivennes F, Frydman R. Physiopathology of premature progesterone elevation. *Fertil Steril.* 1995;64:796–801.

44. Fanchin R, Righini C, Olivennes F, Taieb J, de Ziegler D, Frydman R. Premature plasma progesterone and androgen elevation are not prevented by adrenal suppression in in vitro fertilization. *Fertil Steril.* 1997;67:115–9.

45. Fanchin R, de Ziegler D, Taieb J, Olivennes F, Castracane VD, Frydman R. Human chorionic gonadotropin administration does not increase plasma androgen levels in patients undergoing controlled ovarian hyperstimulation. *Fertil Steril.* 2000;73:275–9.

46. Daftary GS, Taylor HS. Endocrine regulation of HOX genes. *Endocr Rev.* 2006;27:331–55.

47. de Ziegler D, Fanchin R, Freitas S, Bouchard P. The hormonal control of endometrial receptivity in egg donation and IVF: from a two to a multi-player scenario. *Acta Eur Fertil.* 1993;24: 147–53.

48. de Ziegler D, Mattenberger C, Schwarz C, Ibecheole V, Fournet N, Bianchi-Demicheli F. New tools for optimizing endometrial receptivity in controlled ovarian hyperstimulation: aromatase inhibitors and LH/(mini)hCG. *Ann N Y Acad Sci.* 2004;1034: 262–77.

49. Bulletti C, de Ziegler D, Polli V, Diotallevi L, Del Ferro E, Flamigni C. Uterine contractility during the menstrual cycle. *Hum Reprod.* 2000;15:81–9.

50. Martinez-Gaudio M, Yoshida T, Bengtsson LP. Propagated and nonpropagated myometrial contractions in normal menstrual cycles. *Am J Obstet Gynecol.* 1973;115:107–11.

51. Bulletti C, Rossi S, Albonetti A, Polli VV, de Ziegler D, Massoneau M, Flamigni C. Uterine contractility in patients with endometriosis. *J Am Assoc Gynecol Laparosc.* 1996;34:S5.

52. Kunz G, Leyendecker G. Uterine peristaltic activity during the menstrual cycle: characterization, regulation, function and dysfunction. *Reprod Biomed Online.* 2002;4:5–9.

53. Leyendecker G, Kunz G, Herbertz M, Beil D, Huppert P, Mall G, Kissler S, Noe M, Wildt L. Uterine peristaltic activity and the development of endometriosis. *Ann N Y Acad Sci.* 2004;1034: 338–55.

54. Lumsden MA, Baird DT. Intra-uterine pressure in dysmenorrhea. *Acta Obstet Gynecol Scand.* 1985;64:183–6.

55. Fauconnier A, Chapron C. Endometriosis and pelvic pain: epidemiological evidence of the relationship and implications. *Hum Reprod Update.* 2005;11:595–606.

56. Milingos S, Protopapas A, Kallipolitis G, Drakakis P, Makrigiannakis A, Liapi A, Milingos D, Antsaklis A, Michalas S. Laparoscopic evaluation of infertile patients with chronic pelvic pain. *Reprod Biomed Online.* 2006;12:347–53.

57. de Ziegler D, Bulletti C, Fanchin R, Epiney M, Brioschi PA. Contractility of the non-pregnant uterus: the follicular phase. *Ann N Y Acad Sci.* 2001;943:172–84.

58. Ayoubi JM, Fanchin R, Kaddouz D, Frydman R, de Ziegler D. Uterorelaxing effects of vaginal progesterone: comparison of two methodologies for assessing uterine contraction frequency on ultrasound scans. *Fertil Steril.* 2001;76:736–40.

59. Fanchin R, Righini C, Olivennes F, Taylor S, de Ziegler D, Frydman R. Uterine contractions at the time of embryo transfer alter pregnancy rates after in-vitro fertilization. *Hum Reprod.* 1998;13:1968–74.

60. Ayoubi JM, Epiney M, Brioschi PA, Fanchin R, Chardonnens D, de Ziegler D. Comparison of changes in uterine contraction frequency after ovulation in the menstrual cycle and in in vitro fertilization cycles. *Fertil Steril.* 2003;79:1101–5.

61. Fanchin R, Righini C, de Ziegler D, Olivennes F, Ledee N, Frydman R. Effects of vaginal progesterone administration on uterine contractility at the time of embryo transfer. *Fertil Steril.* 2001;75:1136–40.

62. Schoolcraft WB, Surrey ES, Gardner DK. Embryo transfer: techniques and variables affecting success. *Fertil Steril.* 2001;76: 863–70.

63. Fanchin R, Ayoubi JM, Righini C, Olivennes F, Schonauer LM, Frydman R. Uterine contractility decreases at the time of blastocyst transfers. *Hum Reprod.* 2001;16:1115–19.

64. Mansour R. Minimizing embryo expulsion after embryo transfer: a randomized controlled study. Hum Reprod. 2005 Jan; 20(1):170–4. Epub 2004 Nov 26. *Erratum in: Hum Reprod.* 2005;20:1118.

65. Selam B, Arici A. Implantation defect in endometriosis: endometrium or peritoneal fluid. *J Reprod Fertil* Suppl. 2000;55: 121–8.

66. Garcia-Velasco JA, Arici A. Is the endometrium or oocyte/embryo affected in endometriosis? *Hum Reprod.* 1999;14:77–89.

67. Garrido N, Navarro J, Garcia-Velasco J, Remoh J, Pellice A, Simon C. The endometrium versus embryonic quality in endometriosis-related infertility. *Hum Reprod Update.* 2002;8:95–103.

68. Lessey BA, Palomino WA, Apparao K, Young SL, Lininger RA. Estrogen receptor-alpha (ER-alpha) and defects in uterine receptivity in women. *Reprod Biol Endocrinol.* 2006;4:S9.

69. Noble LS, Simpson ER, Johns A, Bulun SE. Aromatase expression in endometriosis. *J Clin Endocrinol Metab.* 1996;81:174–9.

70. Fazleabas AT, Brudney A, Chai D, Langoi D, Bulun SE. Steroid receptor and aromatase expression in baboon endometriotic lesions. *Fertil Steril.* 2003;80:820–7.

71. Attar E, Bulun SE. Aromatase and other steroidogenic genes in endometriosis: translational aspects. *Hum Reprod Update.* 2006; 12:49–56.

72. Noble LS, Takayama K, Zeitoun KM, Putman JM, Johns DA, Hinshelwood MM, Agarwal VR, Zhao Y, Carr BR, Bulun SE. Prostaglandin E2 stimulates aromatase expression in endometriosis-derived stromal cells. *J Clin Endocrinol Metab.* 1997;82: 600–6.

73. Jakob F, Homann D, Seufert J, Schneider D, Kohrle J. Expression and regulation of aromatase cytochrome P450 in THP 1 human myeloid leukaemia cells. *Mol Cell Endocrinol.* 1995;110:27–33.

74. Schmidt M, Weidler C, Naumann H, Anders S, Scholmerich J, Straub RH. Androgen conversion in osteoarthritis and rheumatoid arthritis synoviocytes—androstenedione and testosterone inhibit estrogen formation and favor production of more potent 5alpha-reduced androgens. *Arthritis Res Ther.* 2005;7:R938–48.

75. Schmidt M, Naumann H, Weidler C, Schellenberg M, Anders S, Straub RH. Inflammation and sex hormone metabolism. *Ann N Y Acad Sci.* 2006;1069:236–46.

76. Attar E, Bulun SE. Aromatase inhibitors: the next generation of therapeutics for endometriosis? *Fertil Steril.* 2006;85:1307–18.

77. Amsterdam LL, Gentry W, Jobanputra S, Wolf M, Rubin SD, Bulun SE. Anastrazole and oral contraceptives: a novel treatment for endometriosis. *Fertil Steril.* 2005;84:300–4.

78. Surrey ES, Silverberg KM, Surrey MW, Schoolcraft WB. Effect of prolonged gonadotropin-releasing hormone agonist therapy on the outcome of in vitro fertilization-embryo transfer in patients with endometriosis. *Fertil Steril.* 2002;78:699–704.

79. Diaz I, Navarro J, Blasco L, Simon C, Pellicer A, Remohi J. Impact of stage III-IV endometriosis on recipients of sibling oocytes: matched case-control study. *Fertil Steril.* 2000;74:31–4.

80. Cicinelli E, de Ziegler D, Nicoletti R, et al. Chronic endometritis: correlation among hysteroscopic, histologic and bacteriologic findings in a prospective trial with 2190 consecutive office hysteroscopies. *Fertil Steril.* 2008;89(3):677–84.

81. Kiviat NB, Wolner-Hanssen P, Eschenbach DA, Wasserheit JN, Paavonen JA, Bell TA, et al. Endometrial histopathology in patients with culture-proved upper genital tract infection and laparoscopically diagnosed acute salpingitis. *Am J Surg Pathol.* 1990;14:167–75.

82. Greenwood SM, Moran JJ. Chronic endometritis: morphologic and clinical observations. *Obstet Gynecol* 1981;58:176–84.

5

MOLECULAR MECHANISMS OF IMPLANTATION

F. Domínguez, Carlos Simón, Juan A. Garcia-Velasco

INTRODUCTION

Successful implantation requires a functionally normal embryo at the blastocyst stage and a receptive endometrium, while a communication link between them is also vital. This process is a highly regulated mechanism with the involvement of many systems at the paracrine-autocrine levels. Not only human implantation needs this kind of dialogue, but also in other species, like mouse or primates, this cross-communication has been described before (1,2).

During apposition, human blastocysts find a location to implant, in a specific area of the maternal endometrium. In the adhesion phase, which occurs six to seven days after ovulation, within the "implantation window," direct contact occurs between the endometrial epithelium (EE) and the trophoectoderm (TE). Finally, in the invasion phase, the embryonic trophoblast breaches the basement membrane, invading the endometrial stroma and reaching the uterine vessels.

The EE is a monolayer of cuboidal cells that covers the interior of the uterus. As a reproductive tract mucosal barrier, EE must provide continuous protection against pathogens that gain access to the uterine cavity, while allowing embryonic implantation, a unique event crucial for the continuation of the species in mammals. Initial adhesion of the TE of the embryo to the EE plasma membrane is the prerequisite for implantation and placental development. EE is a specialized hormonally regulated cell population that must undergo cyclical morphological and biochemical changes to maintain an environment suitable for pre-implantation embryonic development. Acting as a modulator, it translates and controls the impact of the embryo on the stromal and vascular compartment and converts hormonal signals into embryonic signals.

Scientific knowledge of the endometrial receptivity process has been fundamental for the understanding of human reproduction, but so far, none of the proposed biochemical markers for endometrial receptivity has been proven to be clinically or functionally useful.

In this chapter, we will summarize the information concerning the systems implicated in the regulation of implantation and endometrial receptivity in humans. We will focus on the chemokine system and the comparison of two similar processes, human implantation and leukocyte transendothelial migration. We will also present new strategies based on array technology that aim to clarify the fragmented information existing in the field.

CHEMOKINES IN IMPLANTATION

Chemokines (short for chemoattractant cytokines), a family of small polypeptides with molecular weight in the range of 8–12 kD, attract specific leukocyte subsets by binding to cell surface receptors. Two main subfamilies are distinguished by the arrangement of the first two of four (second and fourth) conserved cysteine residues near the amino terminus. CXC chemokines attract neutrophils and CC chemokines act upon monocytes, eosinohils, T lymphocytes, and natural killer cells. The other two subfamilies are CX3C (fractalkine or neurotactin) with three amino acids between the two cysteines and the C subfamily also named lymphotactins (3), with only a single cysteine near the N-terminal domain eliciting potent lymphocyte chemoattractant capacity but no action on monocytes. Chemokines act through cell surface G-protein–coupled receptors (GPCRs) (4). One receptor might bind one or more chemokines from the same subfamily, and chemokines can bind several different receptors (5). Consequently, the activity of chemokines is the outcome of a complex cascade that depends on the cell type, the ligand, the structure and configuration of the receptor, and the activation enzymes.

In reproductive biology, these molecules have been implicated in crucial processes such as ovulation, menstruation, embryo implantation, and parturition and in pathological processes such as preterm delivery, HIV infection, endometriosis, and ovarian hyperstimulation syndrome (6,7). Chemokines produced and incorporated by the endometrial epithelium and the human blastocyst are implicated in this molecular network. We know that different subsets of leukocytes are recruited into the endometrium during implantation. The regulation of the uterine tissue during this process is thought to be orchestrated by uterine epithelial cells, which release an array of chemokines in a precise temporal pattern driven mainly by ovarian steroids (8). Chemokines act on a range of leukocyte subsets, which in turn release a number of proteases and other mediators that facilitate embryo invasion (9).

Chemokine receptors belong to the superfamily of GPCRs. These receptors display seven sequences of twenty to twenty-five hydrophobic residues that form an α-helix and span the plasma membrane, an extracellular N-terminus, three extracellular loops, three intracellular domains, and an intracellular C-terminal tail. These receptors transmit information to the cell about the presence of chemokine gradients in the extracellular environment. They are named depending on the structure of their ligand (CXC or CC).

Chemokine expression has been found in EE cells, including regulated and normal T cells expressed and secreted (RANTES), macrophage inflammatory protein (MIP-1α and MIP-1β), and macrophage chemotactic protein (MCP-1) and others.

Interleukin-8 (IL-8), a CXC chemokine with neutrophil chemotactic/activating and T-cell chemotactic activity, is produced by human endometrial stromal and glandular cells in culture. IL-8 is found in both the surface epithelium and the glands throughout the menstrual cycle. It has been suggested that it might be implicated in the recruitment of neutrophils and lymphocytes into the endometrium (10). After ovulation, the number of large granular lymphocytes increases in the uterus (11), and this effect might be mediated by endometrial epithelial chemokines. There is a synergism between prostaglandin E (PGE) and IL-8 in the infiltration of neutrophils from the peripheral circulation (12). Cyclooxygenase 2 (COX-2), IL-8, and MCP-1 also have similar modulators; IL-1β upregulates MCP-1, IL-8, and COX-2 production, and this induction can be inhibited by dexamethasone and progesterone (P), and endometrial explants in culture produce IL-8, which is inhibited by P (13). Estrogen (E2) has also been implicated in the control of endometrial leukocyte migration by regulating the production of granulocyte-macrophage colony-stimulating factor (GM-CSF) by endometrial epithelial cells (14). In summary, P and E2 withdrawal initiates a cascade of events involving EE chemokine production (IL-8, MCP-1, and GM-CSF), which plays a role in inducing the premenstrual influx of leukocytes.

In rodents, on day 1 of pregnancy, there is a high density of leukocytes in the luminal epithelium, macrophages being the most predominant cell type. Granulocytes crawl across the epithelium into the lumen to phagocytose sperm debris, suggesting that semen may contain granulocyte-specific chemokines.

On day 3 (when apposition occurs), macrophages decrease and are evenly distributed through the uterine tissue (15). On day 5 (when adhesion occurs), they become more closely associated with the epithelium. All these findings suggest that there is a preimplantation surge of chemokines including RANTES, MCP-1, and GM-CSF produced by the EE in response to ovarian steroids that may contribute to the initiation of implantation. Endometrial epithelial chemokines can be regulated also by the embryo. Examination of the embryonic regulation of IL-8 mRNA (16) and production and secretion in human endometrial epithelial cells demonstrates no effect of the human blastocyst on EE IL-8 production and secretion. However, four to eight cell embryos inhibit IL-8 secretion by EEC, suggesting that endometrial IL-8 might be relevant for migration of the early preimplantation embryo. Interestingly, there is an upregulation of IL-8 mRNA expression on EEC cocultures with embryos compared to those without embryos (16).

Our group has analyzed the mRNA expression of four chemokine receptors (CXCR4, CXCR1, CCR5, and CCR2) throughout the natural cycle using fluorescence quantitative PCR. CXCR1 and CCR5 receptors showed a progesterone-dependent pattern in the early secretory phase that continued into the mid-secretory phase and was maximal in the late secretory phase (Figure 5.1). CXCR4 (SDF-1 receptor) presented a more pronounced upregulation in the mid-luteal phase than in the early and late luteal phases (an increase of ninefold versus increases of 0.5-fold and 5.7-fold, respectively). Therefore, this receptor, which is located in the endometrial epithelium, is specifically upregulated during the implantation window (17).

To study the "in vivo" hormonal regulation of the four chemokine receptors, endometrial biopsies were analyzed by

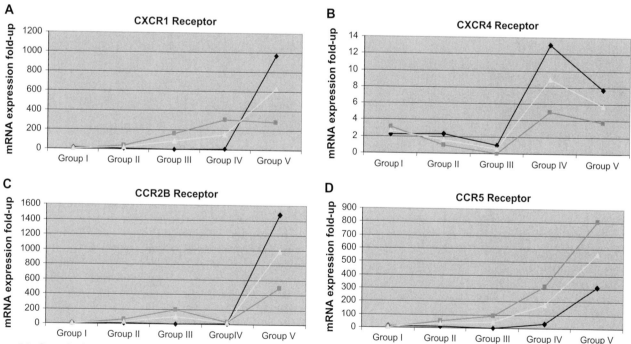

Figure 5.1. Quantitative gene expression analysis by quantitative fluorescent polymerase chain reaction across the menstrual cycle. (A) CXCR1 receptor expression. (B) CXCR4 receptor. (C) CCR2B receptor. (D) CCR5 receptor. Endometrial biopsies were distributed in five groups: group I, early to mid-proliferative (days 1–8); group II, late proliferate phase (days 9–14); group III, early secretory (days 15–18); group IV, mid-secretory (days 19–22); and group V, late secretory phase (days 23–28). Squares: set one; rhombus: set two; triangles: media.

immunohistochemistry. On day 13, when patients were treated solely with estradiol, a very weak staining for CCR2B, CCR5, and CXCR4 was localized in the luminal and glandular epithelium and endothelial cells. During the prereceptive and receptive periods (days 18 and 21, respectively), an increase of staining intensity for CXCR1 receptor was noted in the glandular compartment. CCR5 receptor was also immunolocalized, mainly at the luminal epithelium but also in the stromal and perivascular cells, showing a slight increase compared to the nonreceptive phase. CCR2B receptor showed a moderate increase of staining on days 18 and 21 in the luminal epithelium, while no staining was observed in endothelial cells or stroma. CXCR4 receptor showed the same staining as CCR5, mainly expressed in the epithelium on days 18 and 21. Endothelial and stromal cells were also positive (17).

The embryonic impact on immunolocalization and polarization of chemokine receptors CXCR1, CXCR4, CCR5, and CCR2B in cultured EEC was investigated using our apposition model for human implantation. This model consists in culture human blastocysts with a monolayer of EEC cells. When the blastocyst was absent, chemokine receptors CXCR1, CXCR4, and CCR5 are barely detectable in few cells at the EEC monolayer. However, when a human blastocyst was present, there was an increase in the number of stained cells for CXCR1, CXCR4, and CCR5 and polarization of these receptors in one of the cell poles of the endometrial epithelium was observed. Immunolocalization and polarization changes in CCR2B receptor were not present in the EEC monolayer, and this receptor was not upregulated by the presence of the human blastocyst.

Finally, we have detected immunoreactive CCR2B and CCR5 receptors in the human blastocyst. CCR2B staining was localized mainly at the inner cell mass, whereas CCR5 staining can be visualized across the TE. In all cases ($n = 3$), CCR5 staining was more intense than that of CCR2B receptor, while the pellucide zone was not stained in any case. Immunoreactive CXCR4 and CXCR1 were not detected in human blastocysts.

Other clues about the relevance of the chemokines in the process of implantation come from the chemokine interferon-inducible protein 10 kDa (IP-10). IP-10 has been involved in the regulation of blastocyst migration, apposition, and initial adhesion in ruminants (18). More indirect evidence on the implication of chemokines in the attraction of the blastocyst comes from clinical trials, demonstrating that scar tissue from previous cesarean section or endometrial surgery (that is a persistent inflammatory focus) became an attractive implantation site (19).

HUMAN IMPLANTATION VERSUS TRANSENDOTHELIAL MIGRATION

A parallelism between the different steps in human embryo-endometrial apposition/adhesion/invasion and leukocyte-endothelium rolling/adhesion/extravasation has been established in the recent years (20–22). Cascades of multiple events that take place during both processes show similarities although some details with respect to time scale, size of cells, identity of involved molecules, and others are obviously different.

For example, during the apposition phase in implantation and leukocyte adhesion, the blastocyst/endometrium and leukocyte/endothelium dialogue relies on a first wave of soluble mediators, such as cytokines, chemokines, and other factors,

produced and acting in a bidirectional fashion (23,24). These molecules regulate the expression and functional activity of adhesion molecules such as L-selectin and integrins that mediate both processes.

The first step into the extravasation sequence in leukocytes corresponds to the interaction of selectins with their carbohydrate-based ligands (25). This interaction, named as tethering, allows the leukocyte to roll on the endothelial cell wall. These selectin interactions are highly dynamic and quick, so they are able to slow down the leukocyte through transient contacts with the endothelial monolayer facilitating their firm adhesion (Figure 5.2). Leukocytes express L-selectin, which is shed from their surface to allow the transmigration process to proceed.

The L-selectin system is also critically involved in the embryonic apposition phase (21). Carbohydrate ligands that bind L-selectin are localized on the luminal epithelium at the time of implantation, while the TE expresses L-selectin strongly after hatching. Trophoblast lineages use L-selectin to bind to uterine epithelial oligosaccharide ligands, and when L-selectin is blocked with specific antibodies, adhesion to the epithelium is impaired (21).

Also exposed in the glycocalix of human endometrial epithelial cells (EEC) are mucins such as MUC1, which increases its expression from the proliferative to secretory phase in endometrial tissue (26) and is also induced by the human blastocyst (27). The possible substrate candidates for MUC1 binding include L-selectins (26), or intercellular adhesion molecules; however, its function as adhesion or anti-adhesion molecule is still controversial.

During the leukocyte rolling, chemokines induce the activation in situ of leukocyte integrins (28) and, in cooperation with integrin-dependent signals, the polarization of the cell (29,30). Many papers have studied the integrins in the human implantation. A subset of epithelial endometrial integrin subunits may be relevant to the process of implantation based on spatiotemporal considerations. The β3 subunit has a striking apical distribution on both glandular and luminal epithelium (31). The α1 subunit is present during the luteal phase (days 15–28 of the menstrual cycle). It has been proposed that the appearance of β3 opens the implantation window (days 20–24), while disappearance of α4 could close it (days 14–24). The appearance of epithelial β3 integrin is correlated with the clearance of progesterone receptors from the glandular epithelium (32). Indeed, the human blastocyst is able to selectively upregulate EE β3 integrin through the embryonic IL-1 system (33). Therefore, the embryo could induce a favorable epithelial integrin pattern for its implantation. Integrin knockout studies reveal that in β1−/− mice, embryos develop normally to the blastocyst stage but fail to implant (34). However, no implantation-related phenotypes have been observed in other integrins knockouts.

In the diapedesis step, leukocytes have to squeeze into the endothelial cell-to-cell junctions. During this process, the permeability of the endothelial monolayer is not usually compromised. Leukocyte integrins interact with tight junction molecules such as junctional adhesion molecules (JAMs), establishing heterotypic connections that are replaced by JAM-JAM homotypic interactions once the leukocyte has traversed the monolayer, thus restoring the initial situation (35,36).

In the invasion of the blastocyst, the size of the blastocyst prevents the migration between EEC; therefore, another strategy is needed. In humans and mice, when the blastocyst adheres

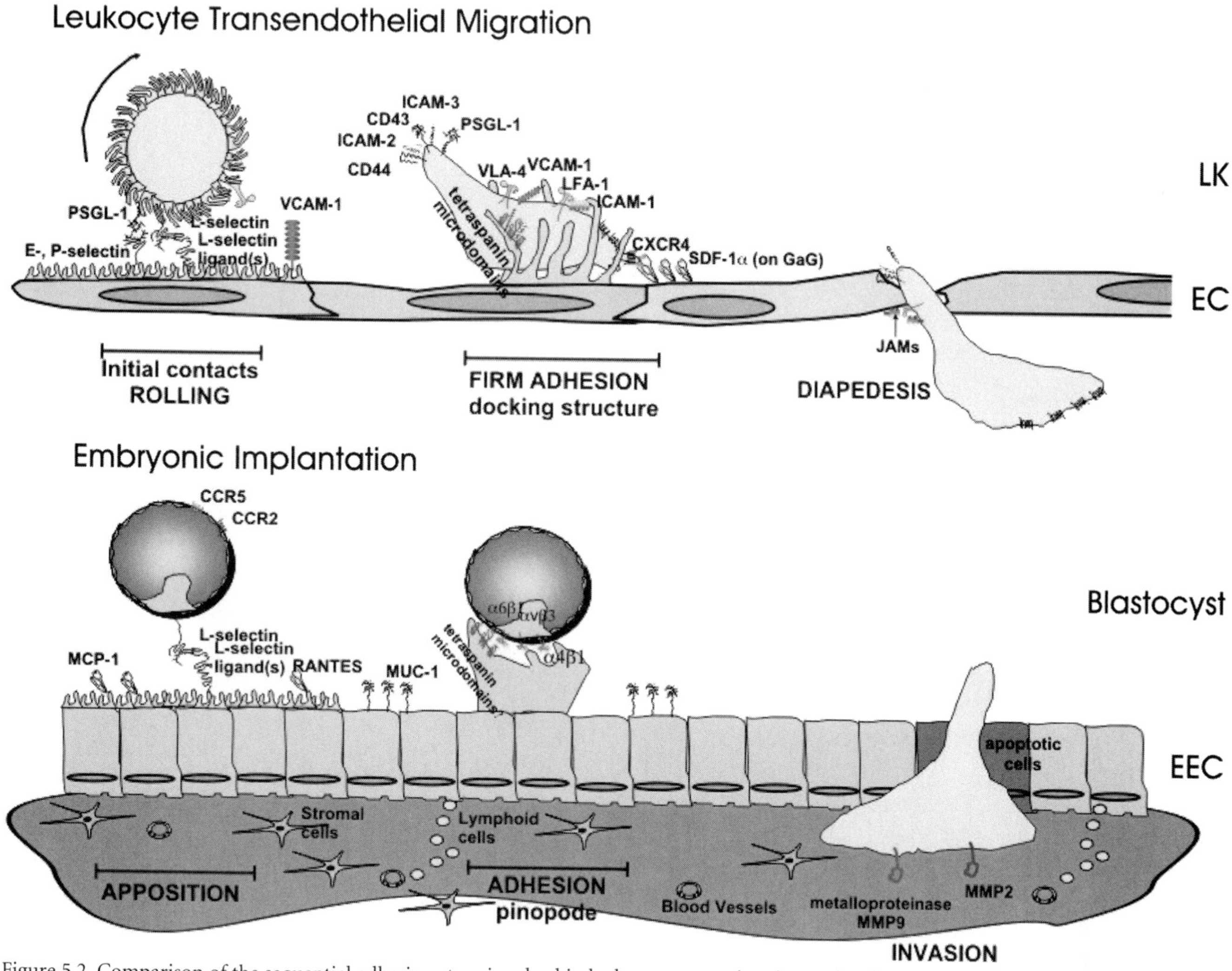

Leukocyte Transendothelial Migration

Embryonic Implantation

Figure 5.2. Comparison of the sequential adhesion steps involved in leukocyte transmigration and embryonic implantation and their molecular players. Leukocyte *rolling*, via the interaction of selectins with their carbohydrate ligands, slows down the leukocyte and facilitates the binding of chemokines to their GPCR receptors. Chemokines induce the high-affinity conformation of leukocyte integrins, which bind to ICAM-1 and VCAM-1, included into tetraspanin microdomains and anchored to the cortical actin cytoskeleton on the apical surface of endothelial cells. Upon leukocyte *adhesion*, endothelial cells develop a three-dimensional *docking structure* that prevents the detachment of the adhered leukocyte, allowing it to proceed to diapedesis. During *diapedesis* leukocyte integrins interact with endothelial JAM adhesion molecules that reseal the junction by homophilic interactions once the leukocyte has traversed the monolayer. In embryonic implantation, chemokines are implicated in embryonic *apposition*. Blastocyst presents CCR5 and CCR2 receptors on its surface, whereas chemokine ligands adhere to glycosaminoglycans in the endometrial epithelium. L-Selectin/L-selectin ligands' initial contacts are also important in this first phase. Adhesion and anti-adhesion molecules such as integrin subunits on *pinopode* structures and MUC-1 on the endometrial surface facilitates/prevents the embryo *adhesion*. The role of tetraspanin microdomains is still unknown in blastocyst attachment. In the final *invasion* phase, the blastocyst breaches the epithelial barrier, increasing the number of apoptotic cells beneath it and then the trophoblast advances through the stroma, expressing different metalloproteinases like MMP-2 and -9.

to the EEC monolayer, a paracrine apoptotic reaction is induced (37,38). This embryo-induced apoptotic mechanism is triggered by direct contact between the blastocyst and EEC and is mediated at least in part by the Fas-Fas ligand system. To achieve successful invasion, trophoblasts must induce a repertoire of genes involved in the degradation of the extracellular matrix. MMP-9 is closely associated with the invasive phenotype of trophoblasts (39).

Hence, the comparison of these two unrelated processes points to several aspects of similarity and divergence that open new fields of research for both immunologists and reproductive biologists.

GENE REGULATION IN THE MATERNAL INTERFACE

DNA microarrays technology is, at this moment, one of the most widely used and potentially revolutionary research tools derived from the human genome project. This technique has been developed within the past decade and allows analyzing the

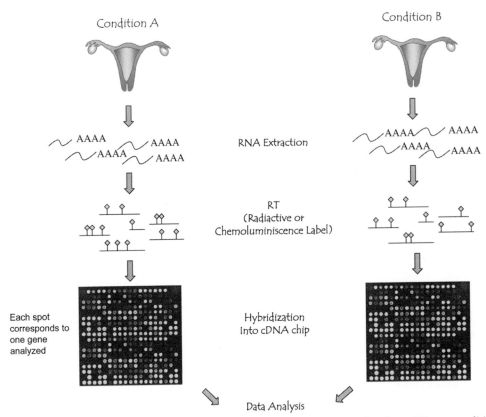

Figure 5.3. Diagram of the process of an array experiment. We can study the gene expression profile of two different conditions extracting RNA from conditions A and B and transforming the RNA into cDNA (labeled with radiactive or chemoluminiscence signal). These probes are hybridized into arrays/chips of thousands of genes. Differential data profiles obtained from these comparison studies should be processed by powerful software in order to obtain confident data.

practically total gene expression profile on one biological sample in a single experiment (40) (Figure 5.3). This capacity has produced a new way of understanding the biological investigation and has generated a large amount of options and applications in biology (41). It is important to have in mind that the gene expression profile of a tissue or a group of cells indicates how the genomic machinery is transcribing the genes into RNA. Transcriptional and posttranscriptional levels of regulation are an integral part of gene expression, and it is necessary to take them into account (42).

The action of progesterone on an estrogen-primed endometrium results in a particular gene expression profile, which renders the endometrium receptive (43,44). Several studies have analyzed, in a global way, the gene expression profile of the endometrium during the window of implantation (WOI) in comparison to other phases of the menstrual cycle (45–48). These analyses have produced long lists of genes that are up- or downregulated during this short period in which the endometrium is receptive. Some of the identified genes have known roles in human endometrial receptivity such as PP-14 (49) (glycodelin), osteopontin (50), or IGFBP-3 (51), but other genes were not previously known to be involved in endometrial receptivity. However, it is not clear from these studies which of the many genes altered during the WOI are functionally important for implantation. It is, therefore, important to analyze the gene expression profile of the endometrium in nonfertile or subfertile conditions. Several groups

have addressed this question by investigating mRNA expression in endometrium from women with endometriosis (45), or treated with RU486 (52), or under IVF protocols (53–54). These approaches have generated indirect evidence of the regulation or dysregulation of the WOI genes in those nonphysiological situations that produce a decrease in the embryonic implantation rate.

Although many significant results have been derived from microarray studies in the past decade, one of the most important limitations has been the lack of standards for presenting and exchanging such data. Some researchers have elaborated an interesting initiative, the Minimum Information About a Microarray Experiment, which describes the minimum information required to ensure that microarray data can be easily interpreted and that results derived from its analysis can be independently verified (55). The ultimate goal of this initiative is to establish a standard for recording and reporting microarray-based gene expression data, which will in turn facilitate the establishment of databases and public repositories and enable the development of data analysis tools.

CONCLUSIONS

The endometrium is a hormonally regulated tissue that responds through paracrine pathways to the presence of the blastocyst. The genomic and biochemical changes are thought to be crucial for the acquisition of receptivity, for example, chemokines produced locally by the epithelium may act to recruit leukocytes and further induce a second wave of cytokines that, through binding to their specific receptors, regulate the expression of adhesion molecules essential for the adhesion of the blastocyst. Furthermore, the development of new techniques of molecular biology such as microarray studies could shed light to decipher the genes and molecules implicated in this complex phenomenon.

KEY NOTES

■ Successful implantation requires a functional healthy embryo at the blastocyst stage, a receptive endometrium, and a communication link between them.

■ The EE is a key element where the initial adhesion of the TE's embryo occurs.

■ Chemokines have been implicated in crucial processes such as ovulation, menstruation, embryo implantation, and parturition and in pathological processes such as preterm delivery, HIV infection, endometriosis, and ovarian hyperstimulation syndrome.

■ Chemokines are produced and incorporated by the endometrial epithelium and are crucial mediators of the dialogue between the human blastocyst and the maternal endometrium.

■ Chemokine receptors are present on the surface of the human blastocyst and can transduce signals into the inner cells.

■ A clear parallelism between the different steps in human embryo-endometrial apposition/adhesion/invasion and leukocyte-endothelium rolling/adhesion/extravasation has been established in the recent years.

■ The comparison of these two unrelated processes point to several aspects of similarity and divergence that open new fields of research for both immunologists and reproductive biologists.

■ Using DNA microarray technology, we know the differential gene expression patterns between receptive and nonreceptive endometrium.

■ Using this technology, several groups have investigated the endometrium gene expression profiles in women with endometriosis, treated with RU486, or even under IVF protocols.

■ The ultimate goal of microarray-based gene expression data is to establish a standard for recording and reporting, which will in turn facilitate the establishment of databases and public repositories and enable the development of data analysis tools.

REFERENCES

1. Paria BC, Song H, Dey SK. Implantation: molecular basis of embryo-uterine dialogue. *Int J Dev Biol* 2001;45(3):597–605.
2. Cameo P, Srisuparp S, Strakova Z, et al. Chorionic gonadotropin and uterine dialogue in the primate. *Reprod Biol Endocrin* 2004;2:50.
3. Kelner GS, Kennedy J, Bacon KB, et al. Lymphotactin: a novel cytokine which represents a new class of chemokine. *Science* 1994;266:1395–9.
4. Vaddi K, Keller M, Newton RC. The chemokine fact book. London: Academic Press, 1997.
5. Horuk R, Peiper SC. Chemokines: molecular double agents. *Curr Biol* 1996;6:1581–2.
6. Cocchi F, DeVico AL, Garzino-Demo A, et al. Identification of RANTES, MIP-1 alpha, and MIP-1 beta as the major HIV-suppressive factors produced by CD8+ T cells. *Science* 1995;270: 1811–15.
7. Simón C, Caballero-Campo P, García-Velasco JA, et al. Potential implications of chemokines in the reproductive function: an attractive idea. *J Reprod Immunol* 1998;38:169–93.
8. Robertson SA, Mayrhofer G, Seamark RF. Ovarian steroid hormones regulate granulocyte-macrophage colony-stimulating factor synthesis by uterine epithelial cells in the mouse. *Biol Reprod* 1996;54:265–77.
9. Dudley DJ, Trantman MS, Mitchel MD. Inflammatory mediators regulate interleukin-8 production by cultured gestational tissues: evidence for a cytokine network at the chorio-decidual interface. *J Clin Endocrinol Metab* 1993;76:404–10.
10. Arici A, Seli E, Senturk LM, et al. Interleukin-8 in the human endometrium. *J Clin Endocrinol Metab* 1998;83:1783–7.
11. King A, Loke Y. Uterine large granular lymphocytes: a possible role in embryonic implantation. *Am J Obstet Gynecol* 1990;162: 308–10.
12. Colditz LG. Effects of exogenous prostaglandins E2 and actinomycin D on plasma leakage induced by neutrophil activating peptidel-interleukin-8. *Immunol Cell Biol* 1990;68:397–403.
13. Kelly RW, Illingworth P, Baldie G, et al. Progesterone control of IL-8 production in endometrium and chorio-decidual cells underlines the role of the neutrophil in menstruation and parturition. *Hum Reprod* 1994;9:253–8.
14. Robertson SA, Mau VJ, Tremellen KP, et al. Role of high molecular weight seminal vesicle proteins in eliciting the uterine inflammatory response to semen in mice. *J Reprod Fertil* 1996; 107:265–77.
15. De Choudhuri R, Wood GW. Determination of the number and distribution of macrophages, lymphocytes and granulocytes in the mouse uterus from mating through implantation. *J Leukoc Biol* 1991;50:252–62.
16. Caballero-Campo P, Dominguez F, Coloma J, et al. Hormonal and embryonic regulation of chemokines IL-8, MCP-1 and RANTES in the human endometrium during the window of implantation. *Mol Hum Reprod* 2002;8(4):375–84.
17. Dominguez F, Galan A, Martin JJ, et al. Hormonal and embryonic regulation of chemokine receptors CXCR1, CXCR4, CCR5 and CCR2B in the human endometrium and the human blastocyst. *Mol Hum Reprod* 2003;9:189–98.
18. Nagaoka K, Nojima H, Watanabe F, et al. Regulation of blastocyst migration, apposition, and initial adhesion by a chemokine, interferon gamma-inducible protein 10 kDa (IP-10), during early gestation. *J Biol Chem* 2003;278:29048–56.
19. Shufaro Y, Nadjari M. Implantation of a gestational sac in a cesarean section scar. *Fertil Steril* 2001;75:1217.
20. Dominguez F, Yanez-Mo M, Sanchez-Madrid F, et al. Embryonic implantation and leukocyte transendothelial migration: different processes with similar players? *FASEB J* 2005;19(9):1056–60.
21. Genbacev OD, Prakobphol A, Foulk RA, et al. Trophoblast L-selectin-mediated adhesion at the maternal-fetal interface. *Science* 2003;299:405–8.
22. Thie M, Denker HW, et al. In vitro studies on endometrial adhesiveness for trophoblast: cellular dynamics in uterine epithelial cells. *Cells Tiss Organs* 2002;172(3):237–52.
23. Paria BC, Reese J, Das SK, Dey SK. Deciphering the cross-talk of implantation: advances and challenges. *Science* 2002;296: 2185–8.
24. Moser B, Loetscher P. Lymphocyte traffic control by chemokines. *Nat Immunol* 2001;2:123–8.
25. Ley K, Kansas GS. Selectins in T-cell recruitment to non-lymphoid tissues and sites of inflammation. *Nat Rev Immunol* 2004;4:1–11.

26. Hey NA, Graham RA, Seif MW, et al. The polymorphic epithelial mucin MUC1 in human endometrium is regulated with maximal expression in the implantation phase. *J Clin Endocrinol Metab* 1994;78:337–42.

27. Meseguer M, Aplin JD, Caballero-Campo P, et al. Human endometrial mucin MUC1 is up-regulated by progesterone and down-regulated in vitro by the human blastocyst. *Biol Reprod* 2001;64:590–601.

28. Vicente-Manzanares M, Sánchez-Madrid F. Role of the cytoskeleton during leukocyte responses. *Nat Rev Immunol* 2004;4:110–22.

29. Vicente-Manzanares M, Sancho D, Yáñez-Mó M, et al. The leukocyte cytoskeleton in cell migration and immune interactions. *Int Rev Cytol* 2002;216:233–89.

30. Sanchez-Madrid F, del Pozo MA. Leukocyte polarization in cell migration and immune interactions. *EMBO J* 1999;18:501–11.

31. Aplin JD. Adhesion molecules in implantation. *Rev Reprod* 1997;2:84–93.

32. Lessey BA, Yeh Castelbaum AJ, et al. Endometrial progesterone receptors and markers of uterine receptivity in the window of implantation. *Fertil Steril* 1996;65:477–83.

33. Simón C, Gimeno MJ, Mercader A, et al. Cytokines-adhesion molecules-invasive proteinases. The missing paracrine/autocrine link in embryonic implantation? *Mol Hum Reprod* 1996;2:405–24.

34. Fássler R, Meyer M. Consequences of lack of β1 integrin gene expression in mice. *Genes Dev* 1995;9:1876–908.

35. Luscinskas FW, Ma S, Nusrat A, et al. The role of endothelial cell lateral junctions during leukocyte trafficking. *Immunol Rev* 2002;186:57–67.

36. Vestweber D. Regulation of endothelial cell contacts during leukocyte extravasation. *Curr Opin Cell Biol* 2002;14:587–93.

37. Galan A, Herrer R, Remohi J, et al. Embryonic regulation of endometrial epithelial apoptosis during human implantation. *Hum Reprod* 2000;15 (Suppl. 6):74–80.

38. Kamijo T, Rajabi MR, Mizunuma H, et al. Biochemical evidence for autocrine/paracrine regulation of apoptosis in cultured uterine epithelial cells during mouse embryo implantation in vitro. *Mol Hum Reprod* 1998;4:990–8.

39. Bischof P, Meisser A, Campana A. Control of MMP-9 expression at the maternal-fetal interface. *J Reprod Immunol* 2002;55:3–10.

40. Schena M., Shalon D, Davis RW, et al. Quantitative monitoring of gene expression patterns with a complementary DNA microarray. *Science* 1995;270:467–70.

41. Stoughton RB. Applications of DNA microarrays in biology. *Ann Rev Biochem* 2005;74:53–82.

42. Mata J, Marguerat S, Bahler J. Post-transcriptional control of gene expression: a genome-wide perspective. *Trend Biochem Sci* 2005;30:506–14.

43. Giudice LC. Elucidating endometrial function in the postgenomic era. *Hum Reprod Update* 2003;9:223–35.

44. Salamonsen LA, Nie G, Findlay JK. Newly identified endometrial genes of importance for implantation. *J Reprod Immunol* 2002;53(1–2):215–25.

45. Kao LC, Germeyer A, Tulac S, et al. Expression profiling of endometrium from women with endometriosis reveals candidate genes for disease-based implantation failure and infertility. *Endocrinology* 2003;144:2870–81.

46. Carson D, Lagow E, Thathiah A, et al. Changes in gene expression during the early to mid-luteal (receptive phase) transition in human endometrium detected by high-density microarray screening. *Mol Hum Reprod* 2002;8: 971–879.

47. Borthwick J, Charnock-Jones S, Tom B, et al. Determination of the transcript profile of human endometrium. *Mol Hum Reprod* 2003;9:19–33.

48. Riesewijk A, Martin J, Horcajadas JA, et al. Gene expression profiling of human endometrial receptivity on days LH+2 versus LH+7 by microarray technology. *Mol Hum Reprod* 2003;9: 253–64.

49. Julkunen M, Koistenen R, Sjoberg J, et al. Secretory endometrium synthesizes placental protein 14. *Endocrinology* 1986;118:1782–6.

50. Apparao KB, Murray MJ, Fritz MA, et al. Osteopontin and its receptor alpha (v) beta (3) integrin are coexpressed in the human endometrium during the menstrual cycle but regulated differentially. *J Clin Endocrinol Metab* 2001;86:4991–5000.

51. Zhou J, Dsupin BA, Giudice L, et al. Insulin-like growth factor system gene expression in human endometrium during the menstrual cycle. *J Clin Endocrinol Metab* 1994;79:1723–34.

52. Catalano RD, Yanaihara A, Evans AL, et al. The effect of RU486 on the gene expression profile in an endometrial explant model. *Mol Hum Reprod* 2003;9:465–73.

53. Horcajadas JA, Riesewijk A, Polman J, et al. Effect of controlled ovarian hyperstimulation in IVF on endometrial gene expression profiles. *Mol Human Reprod* 2005;11:195–205.

54. Simon C, Oberye J, Bellver J, et al. Similar endometrial development in oocyte donors treated with either high- or standard-dose GnRH antagonist compared to treatment with a GnRH agonist or in natural cycles. *Hum Reprod* 2005;20(12):3318–27.

55. Parkinson H, Sarkans U, Shojatalab MA, et al. ArrayExpress—a public repository for microarray gene expression data at the EBI. *Nucleic Acids Res* 2005;33(Database issue):D553–5.

PART II

INFERTILITY: EVALUATION AND MANAGEMENT

6

EVALUATION OF THE INFERTILE
FEMALE

Timothy N. Hickman, Rafael A. Cabrera, Laurie J. McKenzie, Hany F. Moustafa, Botros R. M. B. Rizk

INTRODUCTION

Infertility is defined as the inability to conceive after at least one year of unprotected intercourse. Using this definition, 7.4 percent of married women aged 15–44, or about 2.1 million women, were infertile in 2002 (1). The same survey showed that about 12 percent of women had "impaired fecundity" (that is difficulty in getting pregnant or carrying a baby to term), or 7.3 million women aged 15–44. The incidence of infertility clearly increases with age: In 2002, 11 percent of childless married women aged 15–29 had infertility, compared with 17 percent of those aged 30–34, 23 percent of those aged 35–39, and 27 percent of those aged 40–44.

Contrary to the public perception, rates of infertility and impaired fecundity have not changed significantly since 1965, but because of delayed childbearing and changes in population demographics, the number of older childless women increased substantially (2). In addition, the introduction of a variety of new fertility drugs and techniques received widespread news coverage and spurred public discussion about infertility. The greater range of treatment alternatives now available together with the increasing number of clinics and physicians specializing in infertility has resulted in a rise in the number of medical visits for infertility and in the amount of money spent to treat infertility.

EPIDEMIOLOGY OF INFERTILITY IN THE UNITED STATES

The first United States census was in 1790. At that time, the birth rate was 55 per 1,000 population; 200-plus years later, in 2005 it was 14.0 per 1,000 population, a decrease from 8 births per woman to 1.2 (3). Several speculative explanations have been offered for the decline in the US birth rate. They include greater interest in advanced education and career among women, postponement of marriage, delayed age of childbearing, increasing use of contraception and access to family planning services, concern over the environment, and decreased family size.

After World War II, the US total fertility rate reached a modern high of 3.8 births per woman in 1957 (4). The female offspring of this post-war "baby boom" generation, those born between 1946 and 1964, were the first to be afforded the means to safely and effectively control their fertility. This has resulted in reducing the number of unplanned pregnancies and births and helping women to avoid pregnancy until their education and career goals have been met and marriage and family have become a priority. The net result of these social changes has been a trend to delay childbearing among American women.

NORMAL REPRODUCTIVE EFFICIENCY

Human reproduction is not efficient. In presumably fertile couples, a maximal monthly fecundity rate of 20–30 percent is demonstrated (5–7). Likewise, pregnancy loss is common. This has been demonstrated as early as 1949, when Hertig and Rock reported in their now classic studies in which early embryos were recovered from 107 women who had intercourse at the estimated time of ovulation, prior to undergoing hysterectomy (8). One-third of the embryos was deemed to be abnormal; however, this was limited to the morphologic assessment of the embryos. Forty to sixty percent of conceptuses (as defined by a positive HCG value) fail to achieve twelve weeks of gestation, with the majority of losses occurring prior to the recognition of pregnancy by the mother (5–7). Miscarriage rates appear to be affected most by maternal age, with natural conception cycles resulting in losses for 7–15 percent of women less than thirty years, 8–21 percent for ages thirty to thirty-four, 17–28 percent for ages thirty-five to thirty-nine, and 34–52 percent for ages forty and above (9–11).

Age Effects

Female fertility begins to decline many years before menopause, despite continued regular ovulatory cycles. Decreased fecundity with increasing female age has long been recognized in demographic and epidemiological studies. A classic report that best reveals the effect of aging on female fertility and highlights the profound decline in fecundity after the age of forty years is that of the Hutterites in North America (12). This sect migrated to the United States from Switzerland in the 1870s and now lives in the Dakotas, Montana, and parts of Canada. The Hutterites promote large families and condemn the use of any form of contraception. As a result, the birth rate of the Hutterites is one of the highest on record, with an average of 11 live births per married woman. Only 5 of 209 women studied had no children, for an infertility rate of 2.4 percent. There was a definite decrease in fertility with advancing age; 11 percent of women bore no children after the age of 34, 33 percent of women had no children after the age of 40, and 87 percent of women were

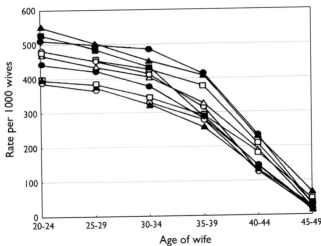

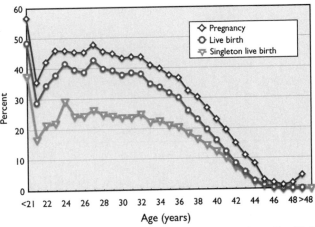

Figure 6.1. Marital fertility rates by five-year age groups (5). The ten populations (in descending order at ages twenty to twenty-four) are Hutterites, marriages 1921–30 (▲); Geneva bourgeoisie, husbands born 1600–49 (■); Canada, marriages 1700–30 (●); Normandy, marriages 1760–90 (○); Hutterites, marriages before 1921 (□); Tunis, marriages of Europeans 1840–59 (△); Normandy, marriages 1674–1742 (●); Norway, marriages 1874–76 (□); Iran, village marriages, 1940–50 (▲); Geneva bourgeoisie, husbands born before 1600 (○).

Figure 6.2. Pregnancy rates, live birth rates, and singleton live birth rates for ART cycles using fresh nondonor eggs or embryos, by age of woman, 2005. (adapted from Centers for Disease Control and Prevention, American Society for Reproductive Medicine, Society for Assisted Reproductive Technology. 2005 Assisted reproductive technology success rates: national summary and fertility clinic reports. Atlanta, GA: Centers for Disease Control and Prevention; 2007).

infertile by the age of 45. The average age of the last pregnancy was 40.9 years.

The Hutterite data along with the other population studies show a clear decline in fertility with increasing age, as seen in Figure 6.1. Fertility peaks when a woman is in her late teens and early twenties and begins to decline at age thirty, dropping more rapidly after age 35 years (13). Fertility plummets after age 40 and pregnancy after age 45 is rare (12, 14).

An analysis of historical date from population studies showed that the percentage of women not using contraception that remain childless rose steadily according to their age at marriage: 6 percent at age twenty to twenty-four, 9 percent at age twenty-five to twenty-nine, 15 percent at age thirty to thirty-four, 30 percent at age thirty-five to thirty-nine, and 64 percent at age forty to forty-four (14).

The biological basis of this decline in fecundity with increasing women age appears to involve several factors. Germ cells in the female are not replenished during life, the number of oocytes and follicles is determined in utero and declines following an exponential curve from the second trimester to menopause, the quality of remaining oocytes diminishes with age, and the frequency of sexual intercourse often declines with age.

Although there is an apparent decrease in the frequency of sexual intercourse with advancing age, this does not fully account for the decline in female fertility. Another factor frequently unaddressed is the males age. Increased male age is associated with a decline in semen volume, sperm motility, and sperm morphology but not with sperm concentration (15). There appears to be some decline in male fertility with age, particularly over the age of 50, but the data is confounded by the age of the female partners. There is no absolute age at which men cannot father a child. Thus, fertility is more dependent on the age of the female than the male.

A French study controlled for male factors (including age of male) and coital frequency by looking at women with azoo-

spermic husbands who were artificially inseminated (13). The cumulative pregnancy rate for women under the age of thirty was 73 percent after twelve insemination cycles. In women between the ages of thirty-one and thirty-five, the cumulative pregnancy rate fell to 62 and in women aged thirty-six to forty to only 54 percent. This decline in female fecundity is independent of frequency of sexual intercourse and is most dependent on maternal age.

Success rates achieved with ART also decline as the age of the women increases (Figure 6.2). A woman's age is the most important factor affecting the chances of a live birth when her own eggs are used. Among women in their 20s, pregnancy rates, live birth rates, and singleton live birth rates were relatively stable; however, success rates declined steadily from the mid-30s onward. According to the 2005 Assisted Reproductive Technology Success Rates, live birth rates per cycle were 37 percent in women under thirty-five, 30 percent in women aged thirty-five to thirty-seven, 20 percent in women aged thirty-eight to forty, 11 percent in women aged forty-one to forty-two, and approximately 4 percent in women aged 43 and older (16).

The effect of advancing maternal age on fertility is secondary to a larger proportion of abnormal embryos. Data from in vitro fertilization in which normal appearing embryos were examined with fluorescent in situ hybridization (FISH) revealed 39 percent abnormal embryos from women who are forty years of age or older compared to 5 percent from women who are twenty to thirty-four years of age (17). Live birth data from donor oocyte IVF also suggest that the age of the carrier of the pregnancy has little influence on the birth rate as seen in Figure 6.3.

Miscarriages are also more frequent as maternal age rises. The age-associated decline in female fecundity and increased rate of early pregnancy loss are largely attributed to abnormalities in the oocyte. The available data suggest that the regulatory mechanisms responsible for assembly of the meiotic spindle are significantly altered in older women, leading to the high prevalence of aneuploidy (18). A higher rate of aneuploidy is

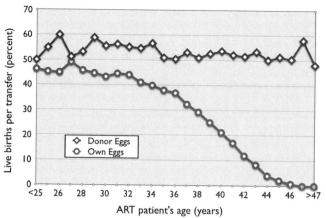

Figure 6.3. Live births per transfer for ART cycles using fresh embryos from own and donor eggs, by ART patient's age, 2005. The average live birth per transfer rate using donor eggs is 51 percent. In contrast, the live birth rates for cycles using embryos from women's own eggs decline steadily as women get older (adapted from Centers for Disease Control and Prevention, American Society for Reproductive Medicine, Society for Assisted Reproductive Technology. 2005 Assisted reproductive technology success rates: national summary and fertility clinic reports. Atlanta, GA: Centers for Disease Control and Prevention; 2007).

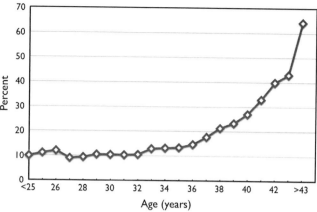

Figure 6.4. Miscarriage rates among women who had ART cycles using fresh nondonor eggs or embryos, by age of woman, 2005. A woman's age not only affects the chance for pregnancy when her own eggs are used but also affects her risk for miscarriage (adapted from Centers for Disease Control and Prevention, American Society for Reproductive Medicine, Society for Assisted Reproductive Technology. 2005 Assisted reproductive technology success rates: national summary and fertility clinic reports. Atlanta, GA: Centers for Disease Control and Prevention; 2007).

observed in the eggs and embryos of older women (19,20), and it is a major cause of increased spontaneous abortions and decreased live birth rates in women of advanced reproductive age. One of the best available estimates demonstrates that the prevalence of aneuploid oocytes is relatively low (<10 percent) before the age of thirty-five, reaches close to 30 percent by age forty, 50 percent by age forty-two, and 100 percent by age forty-five (21).

A large population based study based Danish health registries showed that 13.5% of the pregnancies intended to be carried to term ended with fetal loss. At age 42 years, more than half of such pregnancies resulted in fetal loss. The risk of a spontaneous abortion was 8.9% in women aged 20–24 years and increased to 74.7% in those aged 45 years or more (22).

The same pattern of increasing rate of miscarriage with increasing gestational age is observed in pregnancies resulting from ART (Figure 6.4). Figure 6.4 shows miscarriage rates for women of different ages who became pregnant using ART procedures in 2005. Miscarriage rates were below 13 percent among women younger than thirty-three. The rates began to increase among women in their mid- to late thirties and continued to increase with age, reaching 27 percent at age forty and 64 percent among women older than forty-three.

INDICATIONS FOR EVALUATION

Formal evaluation of infertility is generally indicated in women attempting pregnancy who fail to conceive after a year or more of regular, unprotected intercourse as 85 percent of couples will achieve pregnancy without assistance within this interval of time. Earlier evaluation and treatment is indicated in women with 1) age over 35 years, 2) history of oligomenorrhea/amenorrhea, 3) known or suspected uterine/tubal disease, endometriosis, or diminished ovarian reserve, or 4) a partner known to be or suspected to be subfertile. The pace and extent of evaluation should take into account the couple's wishes, patient age, the duration of infertility, and unique features of the medical history and physical examination.

Evaluation

The couple must be considered as a single unit as each partner contributes a share to the infertility potential of the couple. Initial consultation with the infertile couple should include a complete medical and menstrual history including a review of lifestyle and social habits, physical examination, and preconception counseling. The evaluation of female infertility assesses each component of reproductive physiology to identify an abnormality: the cervix, the uterus, the endometrium, the ovarian function, the fallopian tubes, and the peritoneum. The initial screening evaluation of the male partner should include, at a minimum, a reproductive history and two properly performed semen analyses. A careful history and physical examination of each partner can suggest a single or multifactorial etiology and can direct further investigation. Evaluation of both partners should be initiated simultaneously as it is imperative that infertility is approached as a "couple's disorder."

History

Couples attending their first visit to the reproductive center are asked to complete an extensive self-assessment questionnaire prior to their visit. The importance of this questionnaire is to ascertain relevant medical and surgical history. In the female partner, the woman's menstrual history, outcome of previous pregnancies, length of infertility, sexually transmitted diseases, outcome of previous surgeries, as well as prior fertility investigation and treatment are critical issues. Specifically, it is necessary to carefully review any prior treatment attempts, including evidence of ovulation with clomid, number of follicles developed in response to gonadotropin therapy, amount of drug utilized, peak estradiol levels, number of oocytes produced with ART, and embryo progression.

It is important to provide some privacy during history taking to allow the patient and her partner to disclose any relevant information that he or she may be reluctant to discuss in front of his or her partner. Such sensitive issues could include a history of sexually transmitted infections, coital difficulties, prior pregnancies and/or elective terminations, and so on. The regularity, length, and frequency of the woman's menstrual cycle, as well as associated symptoms such as pain, should be documented. A history of oligomenorrhea or amenorrhea and signs of androgen excess may be suggestive of polycystic ovary syndrome. Irregular vaginal bleeding may point to abnormalities within the uterus such as endometrial polyps or submucosal myomas. In addition, abnormally light menses or amenorrhea occurring after curettage may point toward Asherman's syndrome. Complains of chronic pelvic pain, dysmenorrhea, or dyspareunia may suggest the presence of endometriosis. Episodes of sexually transmitted disease, a history of prior pelvic/abdominal surgery, or a ruptured appendix may indicate significant pelvic adhesions tubal damage or obstruction. The history of previous abnormal pap smears and any subsequent treatment should be elicited. Cervical factors account for a very small percent (3–5 percent) of all infertility cases and may be present in patients with a history of multiple D&C, cone biopsy, cryosurgery, or LEEP. Prior surgical procedures of the cervix may also result in decreased cervical mucus production and cervical stenosis.

It is also important to obtain a detailed sexual history in terms methods of contraception, of the frequency and timing of intercourse, ability to reach orgasm, and incidents of separation. The couple should be questioned about the use of coital lubricants and postcoital douching because both are potentially spermicidal.

Other relevant aspect of the medical history includes: current medications and allergies; occupation and use of tobacco, alcohol and other drugs; family history of birth defects, premature ovarian failure, mental retardation or reproductive failure; symptoms of thyroid dysfunction, galactorrhea, hirsutism, pelvic pain, and dyspareunia.

Nutritional status, marked weight gain or loss, or intensive physical activity may signal ovulatory dysfunction. Often overlooked while eliciting a history are the social and lifestyle factors that can negatively impact fertility. These modifiable factors need to be addressed as part of a thorough assessment.

Elucidation of Lifestyle and Environmental Factors

Modifiable factors may have a significant impact on a couple's fertility. While obtaining a reproductive history, it is important not to overlook lifestyle and environmental influences, such as recent weight gain, tobacco use, toxin exposures, and over the counter preparations. NSAIDS are among the most widely used drugs in the developed world (23–25), although recent data suggests that prostaglandin inhibitors may have an adverse effect on reproductive outcomes. NSAID use particularly around the time of ovulation or use for duration greater than one week has been associated with an increased risk for miscarriage (hazard ratio 5.6, 95 percent confidence interval 2.3–13.7 and hazard ratio 8.1, 95 percent confidence interval 2.8–23.4, respectively) (26). Ovulation is a prostaglandin-mediated event as PGE2 increases markedly in human preovulatory follicular fluid, reaching maximal concentrations at ovulation (27), while prostaglandin inhibitors, such as indomethacin, inhibit rupture of the follicular wall (28). The enzymes that catalyze the rate-limiting step in prostaglandin synthesis, cyclooxygenase (COX) 1 and 2 (29), are present in the mammalian ovary (30) and rise dramatically in response to the ovulatory gonadotropin surge (31). Deletion of COX-2 in knockout mice decreases the number of ovulatory sites per ovary (32). Prostaglandins also mediate successful implantation (33). Until subsequent data further define the impact of NSAID use on reproduction, it may be prudent to avoid use of prostaglandin inhibitors around time of ovulation or during early pregnancy.

Employment has not been associated with infertility or reproductive loss (34), and this applies to even those hours accrued during medical residency training (35). An exception to this is worksite toxicant exposures. Antineoplastic drug exposure (36), tetrachloroethylene, a chemical constituent of the dry cleaning process (37), toluene, utilized for print manufacturing (38), and nitrous oxide, if inadequate scavenging equipment is lacking (39), may all increase risk of infertility and/or reproductive losses.

Smoking adversely affects the fertility of both men and women, with an odds ratio for the risk of infertility in female smokers versus nonsmokers of 1.6 (95 percent confidence interval, 1.34–1.91) (40). Smoking also negatively impacts success of ART. Female smokers have higher cycle cancellation rates, fewer oocytes recovered, higher gonadotropin requirements, lower fertilization rates, and lower clinical pregnancy rates than nonsmokers (41, 42). The data with male smokers is less compelling although tobacco use may decrease semen volumes by nearly 57 percent (43).

Alcohol use in pregnancy should be minimized or avoided for many reasons, particularly its association with a spectrum of characteristic abnormalities known as fetal alcohol spectrum disorders (FASD). Features of FASD include growth deficiency, structural defects, and problems with intellectual performance and behavior. Despite the established affect of alcohol on the developing fetal brain, it is not entirely clear how much alcohol must be consumed to affect reproductive capacity. A European study of greater than 4,000 couples determined that the waiting time to pregnancy was similar for all alcohol intake groups (44). A modest effect was demonstrated at high levels of consumption (more than eight drinks per week) (odds ratio 1.7, 95 percent confidence interval 1.3–2.4) compared to nondrinkers. In contrast, a subsequent study of 430 couples in Denmark trying to conceive for the first time observed that the odds ratio for a clinical pregnancy decreased with increased alcohol intake from 0.61 among women consuming between one and five drinks per week (95 percent confidence interval: 0.4–0.9) to 0.34 (95 percent confidence interval: 0.22–0.52) among women consuming more than ten drinks per week, demonstrating essentially 50 percent or more reduction in fecundity in women with any alcohol intake compared with nondrinkers (45). These results, however, were based upon a small study with highly selected participants. Reduced female fecundity with low weekly alcohol consumption (less than five drinks per week) had not been previously reported. Subsequent to the above study, 39,612 pregnant women recruited to the Danish National Birth Cohort reported their alcohol intake and waiting time to pregnancy (zero to two, three to five, six to twelve, and more than twelve months) (46). For nulliparous women, neither moderate nor high alcohol intake was related with longer waiting time to pregnancy compared with a low intake. For parous women, a modest association was seen only among those with an intake of more than fourteen drinks per week (subfecundity OR 1.3; 95 percent confidence interval 1.0–1.7).

Interestingly, women who reported no alcohol intake had a slightly longer waiting time (subfecundity OR 1.2; 95 percent confidence interval 1.1–1.3) than women with a moderate intake of alcohol. Despite these studies demonstrating the relative safety of modest alcohol consumption on fertility, women often continue their usual pattern of alcohol consumption into the early weeks of an unplanned pregnancy, a period during which the fetus is particularly vulnerable to alcohol exposure (47). The US Surgeon General has reiterated his recommendations regarding abstinence of alcohol consumption while pregnant and expanded that recommendation to apply to the preconception period as well (48).

A possible association between hair dyes and menstrual disorders and spontaneous abortions was raised with early epidemiologic studies that focused on hairdressers. Subsequent studies showed inconsistent results, probably due to methodological shortcomings (misclassification of exposure and small sample sizes). Time to conception, however, may be modestly affected by the chemical exposure. Self-administered questionnaires were sent to 5,289 Swedish hairdressers (response rate, 50 percent) and to 5,299 age-matched women from the general Swedish population (response rate, 54 percent) (49). Information was collected on time to pregnancy or trying time for women who had tried, but failed, to conceive at the time of the study. The hairdressers were less successful than the reference cohort in conceiving (fecundability ratio 0.91, 95 percent confidence interval 0.83–0.99). A recent population-based cohort study was conducted of 550 hairdressers and 3,216 shop assistants (reference group) by using data from the Danish National Birth Cohort between 1997 and 2003 (50). There were no significant differences in fetal loss, multiple births, gender ratio, preterm birth, small-for-gestational age, congenital malformations, or achievement of developmental milestones among the children of hairdressers and shop assistants. It is concluded that there is little evidence for reproductive disorders among hairdressers to date (51), and hair dye exposure during conception attempts or pregnancy is unlikely to be detrimental.

The prevalence of obesity in women of reproductive age continues to increase, and its impact on reproductive outcome has been the subject of debate. A study of 1,880 infertile women and 4,023 controls demonstrated that anovulatory infertility was three times more common in those with a BMI of >27 kg/m^2 (52). Furthermore, being overweight also adversely affects the reproductive outcome of ovulation induction. In a cohort of 270 women with polycystic ovary syndrome (PCOS) who received either clomiphene citrate or gonadotropins for ovulation induction, nearly 80 percent with a BMI of 18–24 kg/m^2 ovulated at six months compared with only 12 percent of women with a BMI >35 kg/m^2 (53). Overweight women also require higher doses of clomiphene and gonadotropins (54), and there is evidence that women who are extremely overweight have lower pregnancy rates with assisted reproduction technique cycles (55, 56). The chance of a live birth is also decreased due to an increased risk of miscarriage (57–60), although this has recently been contested (61). Lastly, pregnancy outcome is compromised by obesity-related complications of pregnancy. The long-term implications of obesity on fetal development have been well documented, including hypertension, gestational diabetes, preeclampsia, and macroso-

mia (62). The impact of obesity on reproductive outcome and the benefit of weight loss on the ability to conceive are yet other reasons to encourage obese patients to lose weight. Modest weight losses of ~10 percent in obese women have been demonstrated to be effective in improving hormonal profiles and menstrual regularity, ovulation, and pregnancy rates (63–68).

Modest caffeine consumption is controversial in regards to its reproductive effects. Most studies are retrospective and subject to participant recall in terms of daily consumption. In a retrospective study of 3,187 couples, caffeine consumption of more than 500 mg daily (approximately five cups of coffee) by the female partner was associated with a delay in time to conception as defined by the number of couples taking more than 9.5 months to conceive (odds ratio, 1.45; 95 percent CI, 1.03–2.04). In couples in which the woman drank no coffee, 16 percent of the couples had not conceived after 9.5 months. In couples in which the female partner drank five or more cups of coffee daily, 23 percent of the couples had not conceived by 9.5 months (69). An earlier study demonstrated a higher incidence of infertility when daily caffeine consumption exceeded 300 mg caffeine daily (OR of 2.65, 95 percent confidence interval: 1.38–5.07), with no increased risk with less than 300 mg daily (70). A recent small prospective study found caffeine consumption did not independently affect the probability of conception but may enhance alcohol's negative effects (71). Substantial caffeine consumption has been linked not only to infertility but also increased risk for pregnancy loss. When measuring serum paraxanthine levels, a metabolite of caffeine, there appeared to be nearly twice the risk for miscarriage when caffeine consumption exceeded the equivalent of six cups of coffee (1.9 OR, 95 percent confidence interval 1.2–1.8 for above 1,845 versus <50), with no increased risk at less. An exception may exist in individuals with alterations in caffeine metabolism. CYP1A2 is an enzyme primarily responsible for caffeine metabolism, and individuals with high CYP1A2 (homozygous *CYP1A2*1F* (A/A) genotype) activity and significant caffeine intake may have increased risks of recurrent pregnancy loss, even at lower levels of consumption (72–74).

Physical Examination

A thorough physical examination along with pelvic examination should be undertaken and focused on the issues that could be relevant to fertility. Absence of secondary sex characteristics should be noted, and stages of pubertal development could be relevant in some patients by using Tanner's scale. Scanty axillary and pubic hair may suggest testicular feminization syndrome, which is due to androgen resistance. Such patients are genetically males and phenotypically females. The absence of axillary and pubic hair accompanied by anosmia should raise suspicion to Kallmann's syndrome, which is due to congenital absence of the GnRH. Increased facial or midline hair may be indicative of androgen excess and highlight the possibility of polycystic ovarian syndrome or other relevant adrenal or ovarian disorders. It is important to realize that mild forms of late onset of adrenal hyperplasia due to 21-β-hydroxylase deficiency could be clinically indistinguishable from PCOS. This is due to the fact that partial enzyme deficiency is usually associated with normal cortisol and mineralocorticoid levels unlike the classical infantile type, which is characterized by decreased cortisol levels and high mineralocorticoid activity. The presence of acanthosis nigricans is a sign of insulin resistance and may be associated with PCOS, diabetes mellitus of thyroid dysfunction. Central obesity, buffalo neck, and moon faces may suggest Cushing's syndrome, which could be associated with abdominal striae and other pathognomonic features. Turner's syndrome is characterized by short stature, webbed neck, shield chest, undeveloped breasts, and cubitus valgus. The thyroid gland should be evaluated and palpated and features of multinodular goiter should be observed. Other features of thyroid disease should be noted (thin hair, myxedema, skin texture, bradycardia or tachycardia, tremors, diarrhea, weight loss, and exophthalmos). Both hypothyrodism and hyperthyroidism are associated with infertility. The former when present tends to be associated with some degree of hyperprolactinemia.

Breast examination for any evidence of galactorrhea should not be missed during the general examination. However, 50 percent of women reporting galactorrhea have normal prolactin levels. Other signs of prolactinomas should be assessed (headaches, anorexia, vomiting, and visual field defects).

Body mass index should be calculated if the patient is noted to be over or underweight. The body mass index (BMI) is calculated by dividing the weight in kilograms with the height in meters squared, with the normal range falling between 18.5 and 24.9 kg/m^2. The association between obesity and ovulatory dysfunction is well documented. Women with increased BMI are encouraged to reduce weight, which may help in the resumption of ovulation spontaneously and increase responsiveness to fertility therapy. On the contrary, severely underweight women should be encouraged to increase their weight to within the normal range prior to ovulation induction to decrease the risk of a low–birth weight baby.

The importance of pelvic examination can never be overemphasized and should be performed at the initial visit. Unfortunately, with the increasing use of ultrasound, many practitioners are reluctant in performing complete pelvic examination, which should not be the case. Congenital malformations of the vaginal tract should be screened for such as double cervices and vaginal septum. Congenital absence of the vagina (Mayer-Rokitansky-Küster-Hauser syndrome) remains to be the most frequent cause of primary amenorrhea.

Speculum examination and thorough evaluation of the cervix should be performed. Cervical smear and Chlamydia screening should be performed if not already done. Chlamydia infection is central in the pathogenesis of pelvic infection that may result in the development of tubal infertility, pelvic pain, and ectopic pregnancy.

Bimanual examination is helpful in determining the size, shape, and mobility of the uterus. The adnexa are examined for the presence of ovarian endometriomas or cysts. Nodularity in the uterosacral ligaments on rectovaginal examination suggests the presence of pelvic endometriosis.

In summary, as outlined in the ASRM 2006 Practice Committee Opinion, the history of the patient should include 1) gravidity, parity, pregnancy outcome, and associated complications, 2) age at menarche, cycle length and characteristics, and onset/severity of dysmenorrhea, 3) methods of contraception and coital frequency, 4) duration of infertility and results of any previous evaluation and treatment, 5) past surgery, its indications and outcome, previous hospitalizations, serious illnesses or injuries, pelvic inflammatory disease or exposure to sexually transmitted diseases, and unusual childhood disorders, 6) previous abnormal pap smears and any subsequent treatment, 7) current medications and allergies, 8) occupation and use of tobacco, alcohol, and other drugs, 9) family history of birth defects, mental retardation, or reproductive failure, and 10) symptoms of thyroid disease, pelvic or abdominal pain, galactorrhea, hirsutism, and dyspareunia. The physical examination should note the patient's weight and body mass index and identify any 1) thyroid enlargement, nodule, or tenderness, 2) breast secretions and their character, 3) signs of androgen excess, 4) pelvic or abdominal tenderness, organ enlargement, or mass, 5) vaginal or cervical abnormality, secretions, or discharge, 6) uterine size, shape, position, and mobility, 7) adnexal mass or tenderness, and 8) cul-de-sac mass, tenderness, or nodularity (75).

TESTING

It is important to realize that the approach to infertile couples may vary among infertility specialists, especially recently more than ever after the recent advances in assisted reproductive technology. There is a considerable debate on how far the female partner should be investigated prior to the commencement of fertility treatment, although there is a current shift from the classic diagnostic work-up of infertility towards a prognostic oriented approach, mostly due to the decrease in costs and increased success of ART. Still many authors advocate that infertile patients should be properly investigated before being offered any form of ART. On the other hand, care must be taken to avoid unnecessary expensive tests or procedures specially those with debatable diagnostic yields. The best diagnostic tools are those with high diagnostic accuracy and reliability, low cost, and minimal invasiveness. For women with advanced age (more than thirty-five years), the approach is somehow different than in younger patients. These patients have already lost a significant part of their fertility potential due to diminished ovarian reserve. Intense diagnostic effort is not warranted in these patients, and rapid movement towards ART treatment is always encouraged to insure better outcome without wasting more valuable time.

The first basic and simple investigation of the infertile couple is semen analysis, which is usually abnormal in almost 50 percent of the infertile patients. This is then simultaneously with investigations of the female partner.

Traditionally, the evaluation of the infertile female has consisted of: 1) ovulation assessment (ovulatory factors), 2) evaluation of the uterine morphology (uterine factors) and tubal patency (tubal factors), 3) assessment of the presence of pelvic pathology (by laparoscopy)(peritoneal factors), and 4) postcoital test (cervical factors), although the role of laparoscopy in the evaluation of infertility is controversial and the reliability and prognostic value of the postcoital test has been debated extensively. To this we have to add screening for ovarian reserve as it may provide important prognostic information that may have significant influence on treatment recommendations.

Ovulation Assessment

Disorders of ovulation account for approximately 15 percent of the problems identified in infertile couples and for up to 40 percent of the problems identified in infertile women (76). Detection of ovulation is an important component in the investigation and treatment of infertile couples. Several methods have been developed that can be used to predict or to confirm ovulation. Any method can be used in the investigation of infertility. The methods that predict ovulation are useful in order to time intercourse during the most fertile period in those

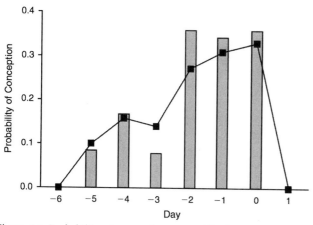

Figure 6.5. Probability of conception on specific days near the day of ovulation. The bars represent probabilities calculated from data on 129 menstrual cycles in which sexual intercourse was recorded to have occurred on only a single day during the six-day interval, ending on the day of ovulation (day 0). The solid line shows daily probabilities based on all 625 cycles. (from: Timing of sexual intercourse in relation to ovulation. Effects on the probability of conception, survival of the pregnancy, and sex of the baby. N Engl J Med 1995; 333; 1517–21.)

trying to get pregnant (Figure 6.5) (77) and for timed intrauterine inseminations in the treatment of infertility.

With the exception of serial transvaginal ultrasonography, as will be discussed below, all the methods depend on measuring the hormones that characterize the normal menstrual cycle or their biological effects. None of the test described here can prove that ovulation has actually occurred, and the occurrence of pregnancy is the only positive proof of ovulation.

Menstrual History

Menstrual history alone may be sufficient to determine whether the cycles are ovulatory or anovulatory. Women who have monthly menses (cycle lengths of twenty-two to thirty-five days) and report mittelschmerz and moliminal symptoms (such as bloating, headaches, and breast tenderness) are typically ovulatory. Patients with well-documented history of dysfunctional uterine bleeding, oligomenorrhea (cycle lengths greater than thirty-five days), or amenorrhea are typically anovulatory or oligoovulatory and do not require sophisticate diagnostic evaluation.

Serial Transvaginal Ultrasound

Transvaginal examination of the ovary can be used to demonstrate the growth of a dominant follicle and can provide presumptive evidence of ovulation and luteinization by observing collapse of the ovulatory follicle, the appearance of fluid in the pouch of Douglas, and a loss of clearly defined follicular margins and the appearance of internal echoes (78, 79). This method is expensive and is usually reserved for patients in whom other tests fail to provide evidence of ovulation or for the detection of luteinized unruptured follicle syndrome (LUF).

LUF occurs when, in spite of an LH surge and luteinization of the granulosa cells, the follicle wall does not rupture and the oocyte remains trapped within the follicle. Because the granulose cells are luteinized, there is minor or no disruption of the luteal phase with normal levels of progesterone. Serial ultrasound measurements demonstrate failure of the follicle to collapse, which persists as a cystic structure into the luteal phase.

LUF is a form of anovulation and is considered a subtle cause of female infertility.

LUF is seen in about 10 percent of menstrual cycles of normal fertile women (80). A higher incidence has been reported in infertile women (81, 82). LUF has been demonstrated in both spontaneous and stimulated cycles (83). The occurrence of LUF has been linked to unexplained infertility and the use of nonsteroidal anti-inflammatory drugs (NSAIDs) such as indomethacin, which inhibit the synthesis of prostaglandins (81, 84).

Systemic administration of COX inhibitors, including indomethacin and others, demonstrated that these drugs can cause delayed ovulation (85), failure of the follicle to rupture (80), and infertility (86).

Body Basal Temperature (BBT)

BBT charting is a simple and inexpensive means of documenting that ovulation has occurred and is dependent on the biological effect of progesterone on basal temperature. Recordings of BBT as a test of ovulation is based on the thermogenic properties of progesterone produced by the ovary as it appears to raise the hypothalamic set point for BBT by approximately 0.4–0.8°F. BBT is measured each morning, on awakening and before rising. In ovulatory cycles, the BBT often and gradually increases from 97°F to 98°F during the follicular phase, to greater than 98°F as the women's menstrual cycle progresses to the luteal phase. The BBT falls again to baseline levels in nonpregnancy cycles immediately before or after the onset of menses. A short luteal phase temperature elevation (less than eleven days) may indicate functional deficiency of the corpus luteum.

BBT is often imprecise and not a very reliable method to evaluate ovulation. Whereas a biphasic pattern is almost always associated with ovulation, some ovulatory women may exhibit monophasic BBT and the method cannot reliably define the time of ovulation (87, 88). The shift in BBT occurs when the serum progesterone levels reach a concentration of 5 ng/ml or more, and this can be one to five days after the midcycle LH surge, and from one day prior to 4 days after ovulation (89).

Serum Progesterone

Measurement of serum progesterone is another indirect method of confirming that ovulation has occurred. The concentration of progesterone in blood generally is below 1 ng/ml in the follicular phase, begins to rise within twelve hours of the start of the LH surge, and reaches its peak about seven to eight days after ovulation. A serum progesterone level of 3 ng/ml provides presumptive evidence of ovulation (90). The best time to measure ovulation is in the midluteal phase when it reaches its peak. Considering the normal range of cycle length (twenty-one to thirty-five days) with thirteen to sixteen day luteal phase, it is more practical to aim for approximately a week before the expected menses instead of the popular recommendation of performing the test on day 21 of the cycle.

In the mid- and late luteal phase, progesterone secretion is episodic and correlates with LH pulsatile release. Progesterone concentration fluctuates rapidly from levels as low as 2.3 to peaks of 40.1 ng/ml, often within the course of minutes (91). In spite of this, a single midluteal phase serum progesterone determinations has been used as a marker for adequacy of ovulation and corpus luteum function. In natural cycles, midluteal progesterone concentrations less than 10 ng/ml have been associated with a lower per-cycle pregnancy rate than progesterone levels above 10 ng/ml (92). In the same way, levels greater than 10 ng/ml have been shown to correlate well with normal "in phase" endometrial histology (93).

Urinary Luteinizing Hormone (LH)

As the midcycle approaches, the rise in estrogen originating from the dominant follicle initiates an LH surge. Ovulation typically occurs thirty-four to thirty-six hours after the onset of the serum LH surge and approximately ten to twelve hours after the LH peak. The onset of the LH surge is the most reliable indicator of impending ovulation, and the LH surge is relatively brief typically lasting forty-eight to fifty hours (94). The LH has a short half-life and is rapidly cleared in the urine.

The demonstration of an LH surge in the urine is also a presumptive evidence of ovulatory cycles. All the self-testing kits (generally known as "ovulation or LH prediction kits") are based on measurements of LH in the urine, which is easy to collect. Ovulation generally occurs within fourteen to twenty-six hours after detection of the urine LH surge and almost always within forty-eight hours (95). The day after the first positive is generally the best one day for timing intercourse or intrauterine insemination. In women with regular cycles, home LH testing may help to define the interval in which conception is more likely for future cycles: the five days prior to and the day of ovulation (Figure 6.5).

The accuracy, reliability, and ease of use vary among products. Home LH testing when performed under routine clinical conditions can lead to false-positive results in more than 7 percent of the times (96). Women scheduled to undergo procedures or testing related to ovulation may benefit from an alternative method to confirm their ovulatory status.

Endometrial Biopsy

An endometrial biopsy is an indirect method of confirming that ovulation has occurred that depends on the biological effect of progesterone. After ovulation, the progesterone secreted by the corpus luteum causes secretory transformation of the endometrium. In the absence of a recent exposure to exogenous progesterone or synthetic progestins, a secretory histology implies ovulation.

During the luteal phase, the morphological changes seen in the endometrium occur in a predictable pattern (97). Traditionally, a timed endometrial biopsy with histologic "dating" of the endometrium and the demonstration of a consistent maturation delay of more than two days was used for diagnosing a luteal phase defect (LPD).

However, controversies exist regarding the accuracy of these diagnostic criteria, the best timing for the biopsy, the prevalence of LPD, and its clinical relevance as a cause of infertility. The high prevalence of out-of-phase endometrial biopsies in fertile women makes histological dating of the endometrium of no use in the routine evaluation of infertility (98). An endometrial biopsy is an invasive procedure and should be reserved for when endometrial pathology (such as cancer, hyperplasia, or chronic endometritis) is suspected.

It has been suggested that defective luteal function or LPD may be a cause of infertility and early pregnancy loss. In clinical practice, LPD is best regarded as a real disorder that most likely represents a subtle form of ovulation dysfunction. It is characterized by a short luteal phase and/or inadequate secretion of progesterone. Histological dating of the endometrium is not a valid diagnostic method due to the high frequency of out-of-phase endometrium in the fertile women. In addition, the pul-

satile nature of progesterone secretion by the corpus luteum precludes the reliable interpretation of a single, well-timed serum progesterone level. The most objective and reliable test for LPD remains the demonstration of a short luteal phase (less than thirteen days), measured as the interval between the detection of the LH surge to the onset of menses.

Novel methods are being investigated, which are based on differential expression of endometrial proteins during the putative window of implantation. These may prove to be reliable measures of endometrial function and receptivity, and the endometrial biopsy may once again be considered a standard test in the evaluation of infertility in women.

Additional Evaluation

In women found to be anovulatory or to have ovulatory dysfunction, additional evaluation may help determine the underlying cause and define the most appropriate treatment. History, physical examination, and estimation of follicle stimulating hormone (FSH), TSH, and prolactin will identify the most common causes of amenorrhea. Although the list of potential causes of amenorrhea is extensive, the majority of cases are accounted for by four conditions: polycystic ovary syndrome (PCOS), hypothalamic amenorrhea, hyperprolactinemia, and ovarian failure. Checking serum thyroid – stimulating hormone (TSH) and prolactin will identify women with thyroid problems and/or hyperprolactinemia. Measurement of TSH is useful to rule out subclinical hypothyroidism, even in the absence of thyroid related symptoms. Thyroid abnormalities have also been associated with early pregnancy failure. A high FSH level indicates ovarian failure. Low or normal FSH levels are most common in patients with polycystic ovary syndrome (PCOS) and hypothalamic amenorrhea. Women with oligomenorrhea or amenorrhea and signs of androgen excess need to be evaluated for PCOS.

Evaluation of ovarian reserve with cycle day 3 FSH or clomiphene citrate challenge test may provide important prognostic information (that may have significant influence on treatment recommendations) in women with age over thirty-five, single ovary or history of ovarian surgery, poor response to exogenous gonadotropins, exposure to chemotherapeutic agents or ionizing radiation, and unexplained infertility. Obtaining an antral follicle count via transvaginal ultrasonography can be useful in evaluating ovarian reserve. The number of small antral follicles visible on transvaginal ultrasound appears to correlate directly with ovarian response to gonadotropins (99, 100), which is useful when considering treatment options. Serum inhibin B levels is not recommended for the routine use in the assessment of ovarian reserve due to limited availability of reliable assays and conflicting data regarding its prognostic value (101). An emerging diagnostic marker of ovarian function is mullerian inhibiting substance (MIS), also known as antimullerian hormone (AMH). Unlike other early follicular phase markers such as serum FSH, inhibin B, and estradiol, MIS/AMH serum levels offer potential advantages: 1) MIS is the earliest marker to change with age; 2) it has the least intercycle variability; 3) it has the least intracycle variability; and 4) it may be informative if randomly obtained during the cycle (102). The findings of the initial studies are promising, and widespread clinical use of MIS for evaluation of the ovarian reserve may be possible once international standards and reliable assays for MIS become available.

Women with diminished ovarian reserve have uniformly poor prognosis, regardless of age, other identified causes of infertility, or type of treatment. When ovarian reserve testing is normal age remains an important prognostic factor. When the ovarian reserve is abnormal, the best course of action is compassionate honest counseling. Ovarian reserve tests are generally reliable but certainly not infallible. An abnormal test does not preclude the possibility of pregnancy. Except perhaps when grossly abnormal, test results should not be used to deny treatment but only to obtain prognostic information that can help guide the choice of treatment and best use of available resources.

ASSESSMENT OF ANATOMICAL FACTORS

Cervical Factors

At coitus, human sperm are deposited into the anterior vagina, where they rapidly contact cervical mucus. Cervical mucus then filters out sperm with poor morphology and motility and as such only a minority of ejaculated sperm actually enter the cervix (103). The postcoital test (also known as Sims-Hauser test) has been used in many clinics as a fundamental part of the study of the infertile couple. The postcoital test was proposed to determine the adequacy of sperm, and the receptivity of cervical mucus, however, has been the subject of debate over the last ten years. In a randomized 24-month study, female patients with abnormal postcoital tests were compared to those with normal tests (104). There was no difference in pregnancy rates between the two groups. In a literature review assessing use of the postcoital test, the sensitivity of the test ranged from 0.09 to 0.71, specificity from 0.62 to 1.00, predictive value of abnormal from 0.56 to 1.00, and predictive value of normal from 0.25 to 0.75 (105). In addition to the problem of poor validity, the test suffers from a lack of standard methodology, lack of a uniform definition of normal, and unknown reproducibility. Results are subjective and exhibit high intra- and inter-observer variability. Its use is also limited by the fact that current treatments for otherwise unexplained infertility (superovulation with intrauterine insemination, and in vitro fertilization) effectively negate any unrecognized cervical factor.

Tubal Factors

Tuboperitoneal factors (postinfection tubal damage, tubal obstruction, and pelvic adhesions) are the most common identifiable cause of infertility. It is the primary diagnosis in approximately 30–40 percent of infertility couples. The factors responsible for tubal disease are diverse and include infection, pelvic surgery, and endometriosis, but, in some cases, the specific cause is undetermined.

Pelvic inflammatory disease is the major cause of tubal damage. The majority of cases of PID are caused by Chlamydia trachomatis, Neisseria gonorrhoea, or both. Studies on the prevalence of C. trachomatis in patients with proven PID have shown that more than half of PID cases are caused by C. trachomatis (106).

Hysterosalpingography (HSG)

HSG is the traditional and standard method for evaluating tubal patency. It also yields information about the uterine cavity. HSG does involve exposure to ionizing radiation and iodized contrast material. It is also uncomfortable and often

painful. Pretreatment with NSAID thirty to sixty minutes before is helpful is reducing the discomfort.

Complications are rare but can be serious when they happen. Infections have been reported in up to 1–4 percent of women, and the risk is increased when there is distal tubal occlusion (approximately 10 percent) (107, 108). The use of prophylactic antibiotics (such as doxycycline 100 mg twice a day for five days, starting two days before the procedure) can prevent infections following instrumentation of the uterus. If not done universally, antibiotic prophylaxis is indicated when the HSG shows dilated or distally occluded tubes.

HSG can document proximal and distal tubal obstruction and help determine the magnitude of the disease process as well as provide information of the tubal mucosa. It can also demonstrate salpingitis isthmica nodosa and suggest the presence of fimbrial phimosis or peritubal adhesions when there is delayed spillage or loculation of the contrast. Findings suggesting proximal tubal occlusion require further investigation to exclude the possibility of "tubal spasm." False-positive results can also occur if the test is stopped too soon in patients with large hydrosalpinges. In these cases, dilution of the contrast with the fluid within the tube can be misinterpreted as evidence of tubal patency.

A recent meta-analysis of all studies comparing HSG with diagnostic laparoscopy (considered the gold standard in the evaluation of tubal patency) with respect to the detection of tubal pathology showed that the sensitivity of HSG in the diagnosis of tubal obstruction was 65 percent, with a specificity of 83 percent in a typical infertility population (109). The predictive value of an abnormal test (i.e., blocked tubes if HSG is abnormal) was 38 percent, and the predictive value of a normal test (i.e., open tubes if HSG is normal) was 94 percent (110). This has important clinical implications. It indicates that, in the typical infertility population, if HSG suggests blocked tubes, tubal blockage is not confirmed at laparoscopy (tubes are open) in as many as 62 percent of patients. If, however, HSG suggests patent tubes, tubal blockage is highly unlikely (6 percent) (109, 110).

Fluoroscopic or hysteroscopic selective tubal cannulation can confirm or exclude any proximal tubal occlusion seen on HSG. It also provides the means for possible recanalization of the tube using specialized catheters (111, 112).

Laparoscopy

The role of laparoscopy in the evaluation of infertility is controversial. Laparoscopy is invasive and expensive and does not usually alter the treatment of the infertile couple, particularly in couples in whom the HSG is normal. Laparoscopy with "chromotubation" with a diluted solution of indigo carmine or methylene blue is considered the best available test for demonstrating tubal patency or demonstrating tubal obstruction, and it is the accepted reference test in the evaluation of the diagnostic performance of other.

Compared to the HSG, it provides additional information about the pelvis including pelvic/peritubal adhesions, endometriosis, and tubal pathology (Figures 6.6 and 6.7). It also affords the opportunity to treat any existing pathology. Contrary to the HSG, it does not provide information about the uterine cavity or the internal architecture of the tubal lumen. Laparoscopy is generally indicated in women with symptomatic endometriosis and in those whose HSG suggests tubal disease that may be amenable to repair, especially if IVF is not a valid alternative.

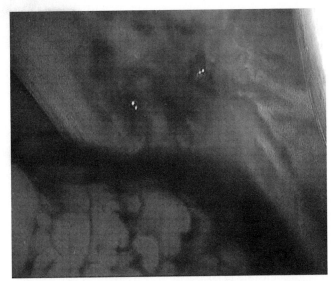

Figure 6.6. Laparoscopic view of pelvic endometriosis stage III.

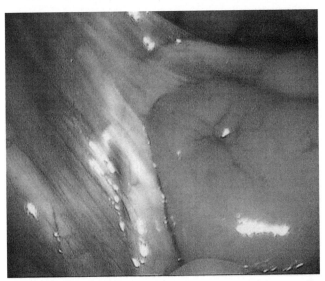

Figure 6.7. Laparoscopic image showing adhesions around the appendix.

It has an additional benefit for the patient in being a combined pelvic ultrasound assessment and tubal patency test (115, 116).

Chlamydia Antibody Testing

In women, the majority of tubal pathology is due to Chlamydia infections, and Chlamydia antibody testing (CAT) in serum was introduced as a screening method for tubal infertility (117). The aim was to use an inexpensive and noninvasive screening test that could serve to select patients that would benefit most from a laparoscopy.

Chlamydia antibody testing is a simple and cheap screening test for the likelihood of tubal infertility. The predictive value of testing will depend on the cut-off level of the immunoglobulin G titer chosen and the criteria applied for tubal factor infertility (CAT is more accurate in predicting distal tubal pathology). The role of CAT in infertility evaluation is still not very well defined. A positive screening should alert the physician to the possibility of tubal pathology but does not justify the universal use of laparoscopy based on positive testing.

Uterine Factors

Hysterosalpingography (HSG)

HSG defines the size and shape of the uterine cavity. It provides adequate images of most uterine developmental anomalies (although HSG alone cannot reliably distinguish between a uterine septum or bicornuate uterus) and most acquired abnormalities (submucosal myomas, endometrial polyps, and intrauterine adhesions) with potential effects on fertility (118) (Figure 6.8). Abnormalities found on HSG generally require further evaluation by laparoscopy, hysteroscopy, or other imaging modalities (ultrasonography or magnetic resonance imaging).

Sonohysterography

Sonohysterography involving transvaginal ultrasound after introduction of sterile water or saline will also document the size and shape of the uterine cavity and is a highly sensitive method for diagnosis of polyps, submucous myomas, and synechiae (119). (Figures 6.9 and 6.10) Compared with HSG the diagnostic accuracy of the sonohysterogram exceeds that of the HSG. It has an additional benefit for the patient in that it provides an ultrasound assessment of pelvic pathology such

Hystero-Salpingo Contrast Sonography (HyCoSy)

The development of HyCoSy offers an alternative to the above mentioned modes of investigation. HyCoSy is an ultrasound contrast technique that uses fluid for contrast injected into the Fallopian tubes via the uterine cavity. This is a simple, inexpensive, fast, and well tolerated procedure that can be performed in an office outpatient setting. The use of echo-enhancing agents such as Echovist® allows more consistent visualization of the Fallopian tubes using transvaginal ultrasound. Echovist® consists of a suspension of galactose microparticles in a 20% galactose solution which, when agitated, produces a suspension of microscopic air bubbles. The flow of the contrast solution through the Fallopian tubes is then visible by ultrasound and is indicative of tubal patency. Several groups have compared HyCoSy screening with either HSG or laparoscopy. In comparison with HSG it appears to provide similar information with respect to both the uterine cavity and tubal patency (113–115).

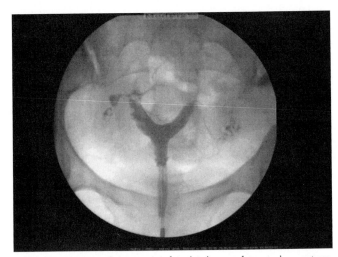

Figure 6.8. Hysterosalpingogram showing incomplete uterine septum.

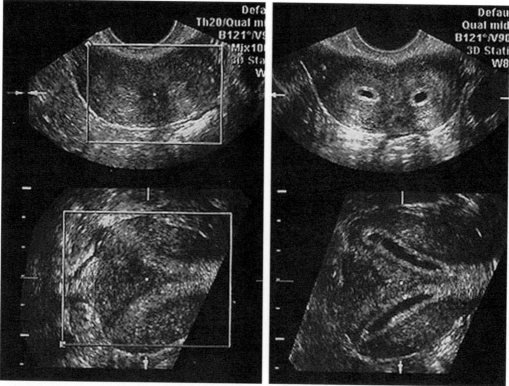

Figure 6.9. Three-D ultrasound of a complete uterine septum before and after infusion of saline during a sonohysterogram. (Courtesy of Dr. Frederick Larsen, Walter Reed Army Medical Center).

as adnexal masses, uterine fibroids, adenomyomas, and hydrosalpinges. When combined with 3-D ultrasonography it has diagnostic accuracy compared to MRI for the diagnosis of uterine developmental anomalies (120).

Hysteroscopy

Hysteroscopy is the definitive method for evaluation of the uterine cavity and diagnosis of associated abnormalities (Figure 6.11). As hysteroscopy in the operating room is also the most costly and invasive method, it is generally reserved for further evaluation and treatment of abnormalities defined by less invasive methods (HSG, sonohysterography). However, office hysteroscopy utilizing small (<3.4 mm) diameter flexible hysteroscopes with either saline or CO2 distention are now available and make definitive evaluation of the uterus quick, efficient, and well tolerated by patients.

Magnetic Resonance Imaging (MRI)

Ultrasound is the screening method of choice for evaluation of pelvic anatomy. However, there are times when the sonographic diagnosis is nonspecific, and MRI is helpful in clarifying abnormalities. MRI provides a detailed view of anatomy in three dimensions, and has the ability to characterize tissues. MRI allows for the assessment of mullerian anomalies and in most cases for the distinction between adenomyomas and fibroids (Figure 6.12).

KEY POINTS

- Infertility rates have not changed significantly since 1965. However, due to delayed childbearing and changes in population demographics, the number of older childless women increased substantially.
- Age is the most important factor affecting the female fertility. Fertility in women begins to decline many years before menopause, despite continued regular ovulatory cycles.
- During infertility evaluation, the couple must be considered as a single unit as each partner contributes a share to the infertility problem.
- Privacy during history taking is important to allow the patient and her partner to disclose any relevant information that he or she may be reluctant to discuss in front of his or her partner.
- Evaluation of the infertile female focuses on the assessment of each component of the reproductive physiology to identify any abnormality involving the cervix, the uterus, the endometrium, the ovarian function, the fallopian tubes or the peritoneum.
- Smoking adversely affects the fertility of both men and women, with an odds ratio for the risk of infertility in female smokers versus nonsmokers of 1.6.
- Alcohol use in pregnancy should be minimized or avoided for many reasons, particularly its association with a spectrum of characteristic abnormalities known as fetal alcohol spectrum disorders (FASD).
- The first basic and simple investigation of the infertile couple is semen analysis, which is usually abnormal in almost 50 percent of the infertile patients.
- Disorders of ovulation account for approximately 15 percent of the problems identified in infertile couples and for up to 40 percent of the problems identified in infertile women.

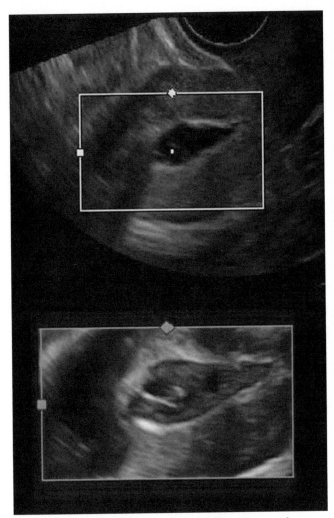

Figure 6.10. Sonohysterography showing intrauterine synechae.

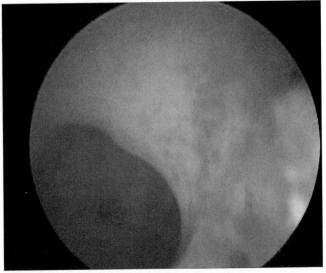

Figure 6.11. Hysteroscopy of a patient with a uterine septum.

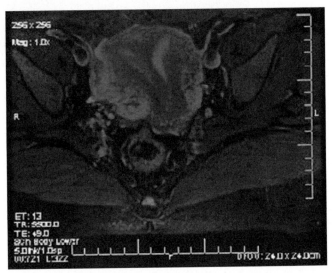

Figure 6.12. MRI showing a complete uterine septum.

- Currently, the best method to monitor ovulation is transvaginal ultrasound can be used to demonstrate the growth of a dominant follicle and provide presumptive evidence of ovulation and luteinization by observing collapse of the ovulatory follicle, the appearance of fluid in the pouch of Douglas, and a loss of clearly defined follicular margins and the appearance of internal echoes.
- Tuboperitoneal factors are the most common identifiable cause of female infertility affecting approximately 30–40 percent of infertility couples.
- Hysterosalpingogram is the traditional and standard method for evaluating tubal patency. It also yields information about the uterine cavity.
- Sonohysterography allows proper assessment of the uterine cavity with high sensitivity for detecting endometrial polyps, submucous fibroids and synechiae.
- Hysteroscopy remains the definitive method for evaluation of the uterine cavity and diagnosis of associated abnormalities.
- The role of laparoscopy as a first-line investigation tool for infertility is changing. It is now accepted that ovulation induction should be offered to selected couples who otherwise have a normal infertility work-up and normal

hysterosalpingogram (HSG), for at least three months before the need of having endoscopic evaluation.

REFERENCES

1. Chandra A, Martinez GM, Mosher WD, Abma JC, Jones J. Fertility, family planning, and reproductive health of U.S. women: data from the 2002 National Survey of Family Growth. Vital Health Stat 23 2005;(25):1–160.
2. Mosher WD, Bachrach CA. Understanding U.S. fertility: continuity and change in the National Survey of Family Growth, 1988–1995. *Fam Plann Perspect* 1996;28:4–12.
3. Hamilton BE, Miniño AM, Martin JA, Kochanek KD, Strobino DM, Guyer B. Annual summary of vital statistics: 2005. *Pediatrics* 2007;119:345–60.
4. National Center for Health Statistics. Vital statistics of the United States, 1968, vol. I natality. U.S. Department of Health, Education, and Welfare. Public Health Service. Rockville, MD.

1970. Available from: http://www.cdc.gov/nchs/data/vsus/vsus_1968_1.pdf.

5. Wilcox AJ, Weinberg CR, O'Connor JF, Baird DD, Schlatterer JP, Canfield RE, Armstrong EG, Nisula BC. Incidence of early loss of pregnancy. *N Engl J Med* 1988;319:189–94.

6. Zinaman MJ, Clegg ED, Brown CC, O'Connor J, Selevan SG. Estimates of human fertility and pregnancy loss. *Fertil Steril* 1996;65:503–9.

7. Edmonds DK, Lindsay KS, Miller JF, Williamson E, Wood PJ. Early embryonic mortality in women. *Fertil Steril* 1982;38:447–53.

8. Hertig AT, Rock J. Series of potentially abortive ova recovered from fertile women prior to the first missed menstrual period. *Am J Obstet Gynecol* 1949;58:968–93.

9. Stein ZA. A woman's age: childbearing and child rearing. *Am J Epidemiol* 1985;121:327–42.

10. Hassold T, Chiu D. Maternal age-specific rates of numerical chromosome abnormalities with special reference to trisomy. *Hum Genet* 1985;70:11–17.

11. Warburton D, Kline J, Stein Z, Strobino B. Cytogeneic abnormalities in spontaneous abortions of recognized conceptions. In: Porter IH, ed. *Perinatal Genetics: Diagnosis and Treatment*, Academic Press, New York, 1986. 133 pp.

12. Tietze C. Reproductive span and rate of reproduction among Hutterite women. *Fertil Steril* 1957;8:89–97.

13. Schwartz D, Mayaux MJ. Female fecundity as a function of age: results of artificial insemination in 2193 nulliparous women with azoospermic husbands. Federation CECOS. *N Engl J Med* 1982;306:404–10.

14. Menken J, Trussell J, Larsen U. Age and infertility. *Science.* 1986;233:1389–94.

15. Kidd SA, Eskenazi B, Wyrobek AJ. Effects of male age on semen quality and fertility: a review of the literature. *Fertil Steril* 2001;75:237–48.

16. Centers for Disease Control and Prevention, American Society for Reproductive Medicine, Society for Assisted Reproductive Technology. 2005 Assisted Reproductive Technology Success Rates: National Summary and Fertility Clinic Reports, Atlanta: Centers for Disease Control and Prevention; 2007.

17. Munné S, Alikani M, Tomkin G, Grifo J, Cohen J. Embryo morphology, developmental rates, and maternal age are correlated with chromosome abnormalities. *Fertil Steril* 1995;64:382–91.

18. Battaglia DE, Goodwin P, Klein NA, Soules MR. Influence of maternal age on meiotic spindle assembly in oocytes from naturally cycling women. *Hum Reprod* 1996;11:2217–22.

19. Platteau P, Staessen C, Michiels A, Van Steirteghem A, Liebaers I, Devroey P. Preimplantation genetic diagnosis for aneuploidy screening in women older than 37 years. *Fertil Steril* 2005;84:319–24.

20. Benadiva CA, Kligman I, Munné S. Aneuploidy 16 in human embryos increases significantly with maternal age. *Fertil Steril* 1996;66:248–55.

21. Pellestor F, Andréo B, Arnal F, Humeau C, Demaille J. Maternal aging and chromosomal abnormalities: new data drawn from in vitro unfertilized human oocytes. *Hum Genet* 2003;112:195–203.

22. Nybo Andersen AM, Wohlfahrt J, Christens P, Olsen J, Melbye M. Maternal age and fetal loss: population based register linkage study. *BMJ* 2000;320:1708–12.

23. Setter SM, Corbett C, Gates BJ, Terriff C, Johns CA, Sclar DA, et al. Nonsteroidal anti-inflammatory drugs: The need for assessment and education. *Home Care Provid* 2001;6:100–5.

24. Brooks P. Use and benefits of nonsteroidal anti-inflammatory drugs. *Am J Med* 1998;104:9–13S.

25. Hernandez-Diaz S, Garcia-Rodriguez LA. Epidemiologic assessment of the safety of conventional nonsteroidal anti-inflammatory drugs. *Am J Med* 2001;110(Suppl. 3A):20–7S.

26. Li DK, Liu L, Odouli R. Exposure to non-steroidal anti-inflammatory drugs during pregnancy and risk of miscarriage: population based cohort study. *BMJ* 2003;327:368.

27. LeMaire W, Linder R, Marsh J. Pre and postovulatory changes of prostaglandins in rat Graffian follicles. *Prostaglandins* 1975;9:221–9.

28. Armstrong D, Grinwich D. Blockade of spontaneous LH-induced ovulation in rats by indomethacin, an inhibitor of prostaglandin synthesis. *Prostaglandins* 1972;1:21–8.

29. Duffy DM, Stouffer RL. Progesterone receptor messenger ribonucleic acid in the primate corpus luteum during the menstrual cycle: possible regulation by progesterone. *Endocrinology* 1995;136:1869–76.

30. Vane JR, Bakhle YS, Botting RM. Cyclooxygenases 1 and 2. *Annu Rev Pharmacol Toxicol* 1998;38:97–120.

31. Wong WYL, Richards JS. Evidence for two antigenically distinct molecular weight variants of prostaglandin H synthase in the rat ovary. *Mol Endocrinol* 1991;5:1269–79.

32. Lim H, Paria BC, Das SK, et al. Multiple female reproductive failures in cyclooxygenase 2-deficient mice. *Cell* 1997;91:197–208.

33. Dawood MY. Nonsteroidal antiinflammatory drugs and reproduction. *Am J Obstet Gynecol* 1993;169:1255–65.

34. Ahlborg G, Hogstedt C, Bodin L, Bárány S. Pregnancy outcome among working women. *Scand J Work Environ Health* 1989;15:227–33.

35. Klebanoff MA, Shiono PH, Rhoads GG. Outcomes of pregnancy in a national sample of resident physicians. *N Engl J Med* 1990;323:1040–5.

36. Stücker I, Caillard JF, Collin R, Gout M, Poyen D, Hemon D. Risk of spontaneous abortion among nurses handling antineoplastic drugs. *Scand J Work Environ Health* 1990;16:102–7.

37. Kyyronen P, Taskinen H, Lindbohm M-L, Hemminki K, Heinonen OP. Spontaneous abortions and congenital malformations among women exposed to tetrachloroethylene in dry cleaning. *J Epidemiol Comm Health* 1989;43:346–51.

38. Plenge-Bomig A, Karmaus W. Exposure to toluene in the printing industry is associated with subfecundity in women but not in men. *Occup Environ Med* 1999;56:443–8.

39. Rowland AS, Baird D, Shore D, Weinburg C, Savitz D, Wilcox A. Nitrous oxide and spontaneous abortion in female dental assistants. *Am J Epidemiol* 1995;141:531–8.

40. Augood C, Duckitt K, Templeton AA. Smoking and female infertility: systematic review and meta-analysis. *Hum Reprod* 1998;13:1532–9.

41. El-Nemr A, Al-Shawaf T, Sabatini L, Wilson C, Lower AM, Grudzinskas JG. Effect of smoking on ovarian reserve and ovarian stimulation in in-vitro fertilization and embryo transfer. *Hum Reprod* 1998;13:2192–8.

42. Bolumar F, Olsen I, Boldsen J. Smoking reduces fecundity: a European multicenter study on infertility and subfecundity. The European Study Group on Infertility and Subfecundity. *Am J Epidemiol* 1996;143:578–87.

43. Chia SE, Tay SK, Lim ST. What constitutes a normal semen analysis? Semen parameters of 243 fertile men. *Hum Reprod* 1998;13:3394–8.

44. Olsen J, Bolumar F, Boldsen J, Bisanti L. Does moderate alcohol intake reduce fecundability? A European multicenter study on infertility and subfecundity. European Study Group on Infertility and Subfecundity. *Alcohol Clin Exp Res* 1997;21:206–12.

45. Jensen TK, Hjollund NH, Henriksen TB, Scheike T, Kolstad H, Giwercman A, Ernst E, Bonde JP, Skakkebaek NE, Olsen J. Does

moderate alcohol consumption affect fertility? Follow up study among couples planning first pregnancy. *Br Med J* 1998;317:505–10.

46. Juhl M, Andersen A, Grønbaek M, Olsen J. Moderate alcohol consumption and waiting time to pregnancy. *Hum Reprod* 2001;12:2705–09.

47. Jones KL, Chambers CD, Hill LL, Hull AD, Riley EP. Alcohol use in pregnancy: inadequate recommendations for an increasing problem. *BJOG* 2006;113:967–8.

48. US Surgeon General. Urges women who are pregnant or who may become pregnant to abstain from alcohol. (www.surgeongeneral.gov/pressreleases/sg02222005.html) Press release Feb 21, 2005.

49. Axmon A, Rylander L, Lillienberg L, Albin M, Hagmar L. Fertility among female hairdressers. *Scand J Work Environ Health* 2006;32:51–60.

50. Zhu JL, Vestergaard M, Hjollund NH, Olsen J. Pregnancy outcomes among female hairdressers who participated in the Danish National Birth Cohort. *Scand J Work Environ Health* 2006;32:61–6.

51. Kersemaekers WM, Roelevend N, Zielhuis GA. Reproductive disorders due to chemical exposures among hairdressers. *Scand J Work Environ Health* 1995;27:699–713.

52. Grodstein F, Goldman MB, Cramer DW. Body mass index and ovulatory infertility. *Epidemiology* 1994;5:247–50.

53. Al-Azemi M, Omu FE, Omu AE. The effect of obesity on the outcome of infertility management in women with polycystic ovary syndrome. *Arch Gynecol Obstet* 2004;270:205–10.

54. Norman RJ, Noakes M, Wu R, Davies MJ, Moran L, Wang JX. Improving reproductive performance in overweight/obese women with effective weight management. *Hum Reprod Update* 2004;10:267–80.

55. Koloszar S, Daru J, Kereszturi A, Zavaczki Z, Szollosi J, Pal A. Effect of female body weight on efficiency of donor AI. *Arch Androl* 2002;48:323–7.

56. Lintsen AM, Pasker-de Jong PC, de Boer EJ, Burger CW, Jansen CA, Braat DD, et al. Effects of subfertility cause, smoking and body weight on the success rate of IVF. *Hum Reprod* 2005;20:1867–75.

57. Wang JX, Davies MJ, Norman RJ. Obesity increases the risk of spontaneous abortion during infertility treatment. *Obes Res* 2002;10:551–4.

58. Lashen H, Fear H, Sturdee D. Obesity is associated with increased risk of first trimester and recurrent miscarriage: matched case control study. *Hum Reprod* 2004;19:1644–6.

59. Bellver J, Rossal LP, Bosch E, Zúñiga A, Corona JT, Meléndez F, Gómez E, Simón C, Remohí J, Pellicer A. Obesity and the risk of spontaneous abortion after oocyte donation. *Fertil Steril* 2003;79:1136–40.

60. Bellver J, Melo MB, Bosch E, Serra V, Remohi J, Pellicer A. Obesity and poor reproductive outcome: the potential role of endometrium. *Fertil Steril* 2007;88:446–451.

61. Styne-Gross A, Elkind-Hirsch K, Scott Jr RT. Obesity does not impact implantation rates or pregnancy outcome in women attempting conception through oocyte donation. *Fertil Steril* 2005;83:1629–34.

62. Hall LF, Neubert AG. Obesity and pregnancy. *Obstet Gynecol Surv* 2005;60:253–60.

63. Falsetti L, Pasinetti E, Mazzani MD, Gastaldi A. Weight loss and menstrual cycle: clinical and endocrinological evaluation. *Gynecol Endocrinol* 1992;6:49–56.

64. Kumar A, Mittal S, Buckshee K, Farooq A. Reproductive functions in obese women. *Prog Food Nutr Sci* 1993;17:89–98.

65. Clark AM, Ledger W, Galletly C, Tomlinson L, Blaney F, Wang X, Norman RJ. Weight loss results in significant improvement in pregnancy and ovulation rates in anovulatory obese women. *Hum Reprod* 1995;10:2705–12.

66. Galletly C, Clark A, Tomlinson L, Blaney F. Improved pregnancy rates for obese, infertile women following a group treatment program. An open pilot study. *Gen Hosp Psychiat* 1996;18:192–5.

67. Hollmann M, Runnebaum B, Gerhard I. Effects of weight loss on the hormonal profile in obese, infertile women. *Hum Reprod* 1996;11:1884–91.

68. Norman RJ, Clark AM. Obesity and reproductive disorders: a review. *Reprod Fertil Dev* 1998;10:55–63.

69. Bolumar F, Olsen J, Rebagliato M, Bisanti L. Caffeine intake and delayed conception: a European multicenter study on infertility and subfecundity. *Am J Epidemiol* 1997;145:324–34.

70. Stanton CK, Gray RH. Effects of caffeine consumption on delayed conception. *Am J Epidemiol* 1995;142:1322–9.

71. Hakim RB, Gray RH, Zacur H. Alcohol and caffeine consumption and decreased fertility. *Fertil Steril* 1998;70:632–7.

72. Sachse C, Brockmoller J, Bauer S, Roots I. Functional significance of a C→A polymorphism in intron 1 of the cytochrome P450 CYP1A2 gene tested with caffeine. *Br J Clin Pharmacol* 1999;47:445–9.

73. Signorello LB, Nordmark A, Granath F, Blotm WJ, McLaughlin JK, Anneren G, Lundgren S, Ekbom A, Rane A, Cnattingius S. Caffeine metabolism and the risk of spontaneous abortion of normal karyotype fetuses. *Obstet Gynecol* 2001;98:1059–66.

74. Sata F, Yamada H, Suzuki K, Saijo Y, Kato EH, Morikawa M, Minakami H, Caffeine intake, Kishi R. CYP1A2 polymorphism and the risk of recurrent pregnancy loss. *Mol Hum Reprod* 2005;11:357–60.

75. American Society for Reproductive Medicine Practice Committee Opinion. Optimal evaluation of the infertile female. *Fertil Steril* 2006;86(Suppl. 4):S264–7.

76. Mosher WD, Pratt WF. Fecundity and infertility in the United States: incidence and trends. *Fertil Steril* 1991;56:192–3.

77. Wilcox AJ, Weinberg CR, Baird DD. Timing of sexual intercourse in relation to ovulation. Effects on the probability of conception, survival of the pregnancy, and sex of the baby. *N Engl J Med* 1995;333:1517–21.

78. de Crespigny LC, O'Herlihy C, Robinson HP. Ultrasonic observation of the mechanism of human ovulation. *Am J Obstet Gynecol* 1981;139:636–9.

79. Ecochard R, Marret H, Rabilloud M, Bradaï R, Boehringer H, Girotto S, Barbato M. Sensitivity and specificity of ultrasound indices of ovulation in spontaneous cycles. *Eur J Obstet Gynecol Reprod Biol* 2000;91:59–64.

80. Killick S, Elstein M. Pharmacologic production of luteinized unruptured follicles by prostaglandin synthetase inhibitors. *Fertil Steril* 1987;47:773–7.

81. Marik J, Hulka J. Luteinized unruptured follicle syndrome: a subtle cause of infertility. *Fertil Steril* 1978;29:270–4.

82. Smith G, Roberts R, Hall C, Nuki G. Reversible ovulatory failure associated with the development of luteinized unruptured follicles in women with inflammatory arthritis taking non-steroidal anti-inflammatory drugs. *Br J Rheumatol* 1996;35:458–62.

83. Qublan H, Amarin Z, Nawasreh M, Diab F, Malkawi S, Al-Ahmad N, Balawneh M. Luteinized unruptured follicle syndrome: incidence and recurrence rate in infertile women with unexplained infertility undergoing intrauterine insemination. *Hum Reprod* 2006;21:2110–3.

84. Katz E. The luteinized unruptured follicle and other ovulatory dysfunctions. *Fertil Steril* 1988;50:839–50.

85. Pall M, Fridén BE, Brännström M. Induction of delayed follicular rupture in the human by the selective COX-2 inhibitor rofecoxib: a randomized double-blind study. *Hum Reprod* 2001;16:1323–8.

86. Mendonça LL, Khamashta MA, Nelson-Piercy C, Hunt BJ, Hughes GR. Non-steroidal anti-inflammatory drugs as a possible cause for reversible infertility. *Rheumatology* 2000;39:880–2.

87. Luciano AA, Peluso J, Koch EI, Maier D, Kuslis S, Davison E. Temporal relationship and reliability of the clinical, hormonal, and ultrasonographic indices of ovulation in infertile women. *Obstet Gynecol* 1990;75:412–16.

88. Guermandi E, Vegetti W, Bianchi MM, Uglietti A, Ragni G, Crosignani P. Reliability of ovulation tests in infertile women. *Obstet Gynecol* 2001;97:92–6.

89. Andersen AG, Als-Nielsen B, Hornnes PJ, Franch Andersen L. Time interval from human chorionic gonadotrophin (HCG) injection to follicular rupture. *Hum Reprod* 1995;10:3202–5.

90. Wathen NC, Perry L, Lilford RJ, Chard T. Interpretation of single progesterone measurement in diagnosis of anovulation and defective luteal phase: observations on analysis of the normal range. *Br Med J* 1984;288:7–9.

91. Filicori M, Butler JP, Crowley WF Jr. Neuroendocrine regulation of the corpus luteum in the human. Evidence for pulsatile progesterone secretion. *J Clin Invest* 1984;73:1638–47.

92. Hull MG, Savage PE, Bromham DR, Ismail AA, Morris AF. The value of a single serum progesterone measurement in the mid-luteal phase as a criterion of a potentially fertile cycle ("ovulation") derived form treated and untreated conception cycles. *Fertil Steril* 1982;37:355–60.

93. Jordan J, Craig K, Clifton DK, Soules MR. Luteal phase defect: the sensitivity and specificity of diagnostic methods in common clinical use. *Fertil Steril* 1994;62:54–62.

94. Hoff JD, Quigley ME, Yen SS. Hormonal dynamics at midcycle: a reevaluation. *J Clin Endocrinol Metab* 1983;57:792–6.

95. Miller PB, Soules MR. The usefulness of a urinary LH kit for ovulation prediction during menstrual cycles of normal women. *Obstet Gynecol* 1996;87:13–17.

96. McGovern PG, Myers ER, Silva S, Coutifaris C, Carson SA, Legro RS, Schlaff WD, Carr BR, Steinkampf MP, Giudice LC, Leppert PC, Diamond MP; NICHD National Cooperative Reproductive Medicine Network. Absence of secretory endometrium after false-positive home urine luteinizing hormone testing. *Fertil Steril* 2004;82:1273–7.

97. Noyes RW, Hertig AW, Rock J. Dating the endometrial biopsy. *Fertil Steril* 1950;1:3.

98. Coutifaris C, Myers ER, Guzick DS, Diamond MP, Carson SA, Legro RS, McGovern PG, Schlaff WD, Carr BR, Steinkampf MP, Silva S, Vogel DL, Leppert PC; NICHD National Cooperative Reproductive Medicine Network. Histological dating of timed endometrial biopsy tissue is not related to fertility status. *Fertil Steril* 2004;82:1264–72.

99. Chang MY, Chiang CH, Hsieh TT, Soong YK, Hsu KH. Use of antral follicle count to predict the outcome of assisted reproductive technologies. *Fertil Steril* 1998;69:505–10.

100. Frattarelli JL, Lauria-Costab DF, Miller BT, Bergh PA, Scott RT. Basal antral follicle number and mean ovarian diameter predict cycle cancellation and ovarian responsiveness in assisted reproductive technology cycles. *Fertil Steril* 2000;74:512–17.

101. Corson SL, Gutmann J, Batzer FR, Wallace H, Klein N, Soules MR. Inhibin-B as a test of ovarian reserve for infertile women. *Hum Reprod* 1999;14:2818–21.

102. Seifer DB, Maclaughlin DT. Mullerian inhibiting substance is an ovarian growth factor of emerging clinical significance. *Fertil Steril* 2007;88:539–46.

103. Suarez SS, Pacey AA. Sperm transport in the female reproductive tract. *Hum Reprod Update* 2006;12:23–37.

104. Oei SG, Helmerhorst FM, Bloemenkamp KW, Hollants FA, Meerpoel DE, Keirse MJ. Effectiveness of the postcoital test: randomised controlled trial. *BMJ* 1998;317:502–5.

105. Griffith CS, Grimes DA. The validity of the postcoital test. *Am J Obstet Gynecol* 1990;162:615–20.

106. Paavonen J, Lehtinen M. Chlamydial pelvic inflammatory disease. *Hum Reprod Update* 1996;2:519–29.

107. Forsey JP, Caul EO, Paul ID, Hull MG. Chlamydia trachomatis, tubal disease and the incidence of symptomatic and asymptomatic infection following hysterosalpingography. *Hum Reprod* 1990;5:444–7.

108. Pittaway DE, Winfield AC, Maxson W, Daniell J, Herbert C, Wentz AC. Prevention of acute pelvic inflammatory disease after hysterosalpingography: efficacy of doxycycline prophylaxis. *Am J Obstet Gynecol* 1983;147:623–6.

109. Swart P, Mol BW, van der Veen F, van Beurden M, Redekop WK, Bossuyt PM. The accuracy of hysterosalpingography in the diagnosis of tubal pathology: a meta-analysis. *Fertil Steril* 1995;64:486–91.

110. Evers JL, Land JA, Mol BW. Evidence-based medicine for diagnostic questions. *Semin Reprod Med.* 2003;21:9–15.

111. Thumond AS. Selective salpingography and fallopian tube recanalization. *Am J Roentgenol* 1991;56:33–8.

112. Osada H, Kiyoshi Fujii T, Tsunoda I, Tsubata K, Satoh K, Palter SF. Outpatient evaluation and treatment of tubal obstruction with selective salpingography and balloon tuboplasty. *Fertil Steril* 2000;73:1032–6.

113. Campbell S, Bourne TH, Tan SL, Collins WP. Hysterosalpingo contrast sonography (HyCoSy) and its future role within the investigation of infertility in Europe. *Ultrasound Obstet Gynecol.* 1994;4:245–53.

114. Exacoustos C, Zupi E, Carusotti C, Lanzi G, Marconi D and Arduini D. Hysterosalpingo-contrast sonography compared with hysterosalpingography and laparoscopic dye pertubation to evaluate tubal patency. *J Am Assoc Gynecol Laparosc* 2003;10:367–72.

115. Strandell A, Bourne T, Bergh C, Granberg S, Thorburn J, Hamberger L. A simplified ultrasound based infertility investigation protocol and its implications for patient management. *J Assist Reprod Genet* 2000;17:87–92.

116. Strandell A, Bourne T, Bergh C, Granberg S, Asztely M, Thorburn J. The assessment of endometrial pathology and tubal patency: a comparison between the use of ultrasonography and X-ray hysterosalpingography for the investigation of infertility patients. *Ultrasound Obstet Gynecol.* 1999;14:200–4.

117. Land JA, Evers JL, Goossens VJ. How to use Chlamydia antibody testing in subfertility patients. *Hum Reprod* 1998;13:1094–8.

118. Badawy S. Hysterosalpingography. In Rizk B (ed) *Ultrasonography in reproductive medicine and infertility.* Cambridge; United Kingdom. Cambridge University Press 2008, (in press).

119. Brown W and Shwayder J. Sonohysterography. In Rizk B (ed) *Ultrasonography in reproductive medicine and infertility.* Cambridge; United Kingdom. Cambridge University Press 2008, (in press).

120. Garcia Velasco JA. Ultrasonography of endometriosis. In Rizk B (ed) *Ultrasonography in reproductive medicine and infertility.* Cambridge; United Kingdom. Cambridge University Press 2008, (in press).

7

FERTILOSCOPY

A. Watrelot

Reproductive medicine is now mainly in the hands of nonsurgical doctors. Several reasons may explain this fact: first of all, the success of IVF and therefore the decreasing of surgical indications especially in tubal surgery and then the fact that, since 1986, egg collection is performed through ultrasonography and so requires no surgical skill.

Indeed, it is was a major progress to be able to perform IVF procedure without the need of laparoscopy, but as a consequence, reproductive surgery was progressively abandoned even at the stage of diagnosis. Therefore, today, very frequently, only noninvasive methods like hysterosalpingography (HSG) or ultrasonography are used to assess the normality of the genitalia.

Using only nonsurgical method of diagnosis leads to a false-negative rate between 20 and 40 percent, according to the works published. Swart et al. (1) in a meta-analysis found for HSG a point estimate of 0.65 for sensitivity and of 0.83 for specificity and underline the fact that HSG was not suitable for the evaluation of periadnexal adhesions.

In contrast, laparoscopy is considered as the gold standard to explore tuboperitoneal infertility. Nevertheless, laparoscopy is often performed without discovering any significant pathology.

Unfortunately, laparoscopy presents some risks that can be very serious, as recently shown in the French register of laparoscopic accidents, where six major injuries occurred in diagnostic laparoscopies (2). The results are either a delay carrying out laparoscopy, which can be prejudicial to the patient, for instance, if an IVF procedure is decided on the basis of a wrong diagnosis, or the conducting of a great number of normal laparoscopies, with the potential risks that accompany such procedures.

Other diagnostic procedures such as hysterosonography or falloposcopy are not sufficiently accurate to support a therapeutic strategy. Culdoscopy could have been an alternative method but was abandoned in the 1970s in its classical version for laparoscopy.

More recent improvements have been suggested such as the use of dorsal decubitus (3), the use of hydroflotation (4), and transvaginal hydrolaparoscopy, which provides a very good imaging of the pelvis (Gordts and co-workers (5, 6)).

Following this initial work, we have defined the concept of *fertiloscopy* (Watrelot et al. 1997–1999 (7–9)) as the combination at the same time of a *transvaginal hydropelviscopy*, a *dye test*, a *salpingoscopy*, a *microsalpingoscopy*, and lastly a *hystéroscopy* performed under strict local anesthesia.

TECHNIQUE

Prior to the procedure, a careful vaginal examination is performed. This examination allows detecting pathology of the Douglas cul-de-sac, as nodule of the recto vaginal septum or fixed retroverted uterus. These situations represent the true contraindications of fertiloscopy.

When there is posterior endometriosis, the rectum is attracted close to the posterior vaginal vault and the risk of rectum injury is high when inserting the trocar. In case of fixed retroverted uterus, there is no space to penetrate the pouch of Douglas.

Anesthesia is either strictly local, or a general sedation is used.

Strict local anesthesia is very useful in the countries where office procedure is allowed. In the other cases, general sedation is proposed.

Sometimes, it is the choice of patients. Another advantage of general sedation is the possibility to practice operative fertiloscopy in the same time when pathology is found.

Strict local anesthesia consists of inserting first an anesthetic swab (Emla gel) for ten minutes; then, a classical paracervical block is performed using lignocaine.

General sedation is of the same kind of the one used for egg collection during IVF.

In all cases, fertiloscopy is performed as an ambulatory technique.

As already mentioned, there are five steps in the procedure:

1. Hydropelviscopy
2. Dye test
3. Salpingoscopy
4. Microsalpingoscopy
5. Hysteroscopy

1. Hydropelviscopy (Figure 7.1) is performed by inserting first a Veres needle in the pouch of Douglas. This needle is inserted 1 cm below the cervix; then, saline solution is instilled trough a perfusion line using no other pressure than gravity. When 150–200 cc have been instilled, Veres needle is removed and replaced by the fertiloscope (FTO 1-40-Gyneo, France). The sharp end of the fertiloscope allows a direct insertion without any incision. Also, fertiloscope is fitted at its extremity with a balloon, which prevents it from being inadvertently pulled out of the peritoneal cavity (Figure 7.1). Optic is then introduced in the fertiloscope. It is important to use a 30° telescope less than 4 mm of outer

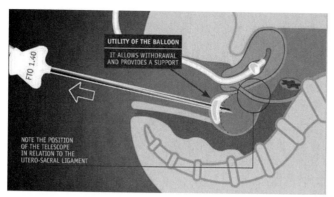

Figure 7.1. Principle of fertiloscopy.

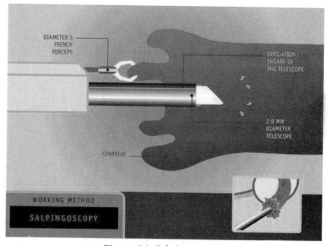

Figure 7.3. Salpingoscopy.

diameter. Observation may start (Figure 7.2). It is disorientating at the beginning because view is inverted. After a short learning curve, it becomes easy to see all the genital structures. It is important to have a systematic view of both ovaries, tubes, fossae ovaricae, posterior part of the uterus, uterosacral ligament, and pelvic peritoneum.

2. When anatomy has been assessed, a dye test is performed through the uterine fertiloscope (FH 1-29-Gyneo, France). Tubal patency is thus established.

3. Evaluation of the tubal mucosa is widely recognized as a major importance; therefore, salpingoscopy is systematically performed (Figure 7.3). It is rather easy to go in the tubal ampulla using the same scope. So salpingoscopy may be practiced as a routine evaluation that is not usually the case during laparoscopy where a second optic, a second cold light supply, and a separate irrigation are needed. Salpingoscopy is able to detect intratubal pathology such as intra-ampullary adhesions or flattened mucosal folds. These lesions are very important to be detected because the only valid therapeutic option in these cases is IVF.

4. Microsalpingoscopy is a further step. The concept was described by Marconi (10) who clearly demonstrated that after the dye test, the more the nuclei are dye stained by the methylene blue, the more pathological the tube is. Every dye-stained nucleus is a damaged cell (either inflammatory or in apoptosis). To perform microsalpingoscopy, a special optic is used (Hamou II- K. Storz, Germany), which allows to magnify the mucosa up to one hundred times, thus realizing a real "in vivo" histology. Findings are either normal (number of nuclei dye stained is few) or pathological when many nuclei are dye stained.

5. A standard hysteroscopy (through the same optic) is then practiced in order to have a complete evaluation of the genitalia.

At the end of the procedure, it is not necessary to close the vaginal puncture site and we do not give any antibiotics.

OPERATIVE FERTILOSCOPY

At the beginning, fertiloscopy was purely diagnostic. But rapidly and thanks to the operative channel provided on the fertiloscope, several attempts of treatment have been performed.

Now, we can routinely practice adhesiolysis, treatment of endometriosis, and ovarian drilling.

One of the prerequisite of operative fertiloscopy was to be as effective as the same procedure practiced during laparoscopy. Therefore, this obligation gives the limits of what we are able to perform.

The operative channel is unique and small (5 Fg), and only relatively limited adhesiolysis can be performed (especially when adhesions are found between distal part of the tubes, ovaries, and fossa ovarica) as well as endometriotic lesions can be treated only when minimal or moderate.

Another obligation is to avoid any bleeding during operative fertiloscopy since only few drops of blood will darken the visions. This is why a very careful hemostasis is compulsory. For that purpose, it was necessary to use a bipolar probe to be able to work in liquid environment. Several exist, and we mostly use the disposable Versapoint (Gynecare, USA). We have also developed the Ovadrill, which is reusable.

The use of 5-Fg (1.5 mm in diameter) bipolar probe gave the idea to Fernandez (11) to propose ovarian drilling through fertiloscopy.

Since then, a great number of fertiloscopic ovarian drilling has been made in polycystic ovarian syndrome (PCOS) patients. Pregnancy rate obtained is similar as the results observed after laparoscopic ovarian drilling.

The technique is simple: it requires after a careful exploration of the pelvis to visualize the landmark represented by the ovarian ligament and then the drilling itself is performed on both ovaries through a bipolar probe, six to eight holes being practiced on each side.

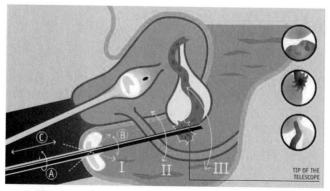

Figure 7.2. Optics movements during hydropelviscopy.

COMPLICATIONS

As for every surgical technique, some risks are involved in fertiloscopy.

They are never serious in diagnostic fertiloscopy. Nevertheless, all have to be made to avoid this situation.

The only real risk is the rectal injury for insertion of Veres needle and fertiloscope are made between the cervix and the rectum. In a normal situation, there is plenty of space. But if a pathology occurs in the pouch of Douglas, then the rectum is at risk to be injured.

It can be the case in endometriosis of the rectovaginal septum, which attracts the rectum close to the cervix. It is easy to diagnose this situation by a careful vaginal examination; if any pathology is detected, fertiloscopy is contraindicated.

Also we avoid proposing fertiloscopy in fixed retroverted uterus due to the risk of uterine injury.

We have demonstrated that rectal injury is a beginner complication and mostly occurs in the first fifty cases. After that initial period, the rate of injury is very low and less than 0.5 percent.

A major point is the management of such injuries.

We have already demonstrated that in case of rectal injury, the site of perforation is located where rectum is under the peritoneum. Therefore, the only treatment to do is to give antibiotics and to survey the patients. It is not necessary to perform a complementary laparoscopy that has no utility and that is unable to show the perforation due to its localization. In about twenty rectal injuries reported in several cases, temperature around 38°C was observed, which lasted no more than forty-eight hours (12).

The only one major complication is the inadvertent perforation of the bowel during an ovarian drilling. This very serious complication has been reported in two cases, leading to a laparotomy in order to treat the injured bowel (13). This complication is very easily avoided if ovarian drilling is performed only when *the utero-ovarian ligament* is in plain sight. If one is unable to see it correctly, the procedure has to be canceled.

RATIONALE OF FERTILOSCOPY

Fertiloscopy was first designed to avoid diagnostic laparoscopy. Operative possibilities were developed later.

So the fundamental question was to know if fertiloscopy was as accurate as laparoscopy, considered at that time as the "gold standard" in infertility investigation.

To be able to answer, we designed a special study: the FLY study (acronym for Fertiloscopy versus LaparoscopY) (14).

It was a multicentric prospective randomized study in which fertiloscopy and then laparoscopy were performed on the same infertile patient by two surgeons A and B, randomized for the procedure. Every procedure was video recorded, the files being seen by two independent reviewers. This trial was approved by the French ethic committee under the Huriet law.

Fourteen teaching hospital centers were enrolled (twelve in France, one in Belgium, and one in Tunisia).

Calculation of sensitivity and specificity was performed and concordance test using kappa score was established on six sites (both ovaries, tubes, peritoneum, and ovaries). Since ninety-two patients have been included, it was 552 sites that were compared. The kappa score was situated between 0.75 and 0.91, depending on the sites studied. A correlation between

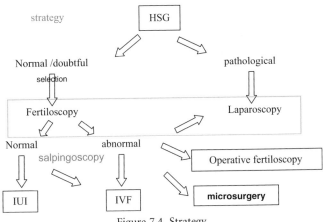

Figure 7.4. Strategy.

two diagnostic tools is considered as excellent when kappa score reaches 0.75 or more.

So the conclusion of FLY study was that fertiloscopy should replace laparoscopy in infertile women with no obvious pathology.

We, therefore, validated the following strategy in our unit.

STRATEGY FOR FERTILOSCOPY (FIGURE 7.4)

In our team, we consider that HSG is still the first-line examination. If HSG is evidently abnormal (for instance, in presence of big hydrosalpinx), there is no place for fertiloscopy and an operative laparoscopy is directly proposed.

In all other cases, when HSG is normal or doubtful and after at least one year of infertility, we propose to perform a fertiloscopy.

If the macroscopic findings are normal, then we consider the value of tubal mucosa (thanks to salpingoscopy and microsalpingoscopy). If tubal mucosa is abnormal, the patient is directly referred to IVF. If tubal mucosa appears to be normal, intrauterine insemination (IUI) is the preferred option.

When macroscopic findings are abnormal, we treat them according to the tubal mucosa status and the severity of lesions: mild and moderate lesions with normal mucosa will be treated by fertiloscopy, more severe cases by laparoscopy, and selected cases by microsurgery (in case of proximal obstruction); whatever the severity of lesions, if tubal mucosa is not normal, then the patient is also referred directly to IVF (15,16).

RESULTS

Global Results

From June 1997 to December 2005, we have proposed fertiloscopy in 1,802 infertile patients.

Some cases have to be excluded due to the lack of follow-up: it is the case for the 101 fertiloscopies practiced during live demonstrations in eighteen different countries. Obviously, we have very little record on what followed the procedure. Therefore, they were not taken in account in this series.

Also the 112 cases of fertiloscopic ovarian drilling were considered separately.

So 1,589 patients were enrolled in the study. Ninety-one patients (5.7 percent) were excluded during the selection process due to abnormalities discovered during the preoperative clinical examination. It was mainly endometriosis of the rectovaginal space or fixed retroverted uterus. These cases, being a contraindication to the technique, were referred to operative laparoscopy. Thus, 1,498 patients underwent fertiloscopy procedure.

Population characteristics were the following: mean age, thirty-two (twenty-two to forty-one); mean duration of infertility: 3.2 years (1–9); and 1,018 (67.9 percent) patients had primary infertility.

In 1,490 patients (99.5 percent), fertiloscopy was performed as an ambulatory procedure.

Fertiloscopy was performed under strict local anesthesia in 288 cases (19.2 percent).

In 1,210 (80.3 percent) others, fertiloscopy was done under general sedation, thus allowing to carry out operative fertiloscopy at the same time when necessary.

Global results were the following: in 1,006 (73.3 percent) patients, macroscopic findings appeared to be normal. We included in this category, patients with subtle lesions as paratubal cyst, nonconnective adhesions, very minimally endometriotic lesions, and minor tubal alterations like sacculation or accessory tube.

In the others (482, 26.7 percent), pathology was found. In 112 patients, endometriosis was found (7.4 percent), in seventy-nine (5.2 percent) cases, endometriosis was considered as mild, and in thirty-three cases (2.2 percent), endometriosis was severe. The frequency of endometriosis thus appears quite low. It is first due to the cancellation policy in the patient with endometriosis of the rectovaginal septum and second due to the patient with minimal endometriosis considered as subtle lesions and classified as normal or having very few impact on fertility. Therefore, we should add seventy-two cases of rectovaginal endometriosis and 139 cases of minimal endometriosis. So 323 (21.5 percent) patients presented endometriosis at various stage or location, which is consistent in an infertile population.

Pelvic adhesions and tubal pathology were the second main pathology encountered. Three hundred and seventy (25.6 percent) patients were found in this group.

We distinguished minimal adhesion situation with normal tubes in 104 (6.9 percent) patients, 208 (13.8 percent) patients with mild adhesions associated either to a phimosis or hydrosalpinx, and 58 (3.8 percent) patients having a severe adhesion status associated with tubal lesions (phimosis, hydrosalpinx, or proximal tubal blockage). The group of patients with severe adhesions is rather small because very often lesions were seen on HSG, and in these cases, patients were directly referred to operative laparoscopy as mentioned above.

At the beginning, fertiloscopy was exclusively diagnostic; then in 1999, we have included the routine practice of microsalpingoscopy, following the work of Marconi.

Two hundred and sixty-six fertiloscopies were performed in the first period (prior to January 1999) and 1,232 from that time.

We have shown that salpingoscopy and microsalpingoscopy are feasible routinely in a great number of cases. In our series, it was possible to achieve both techniques in at least one tube in 1,164 cases (94.3 percent).

From that time, the results of microsalpingoscopy were taken into account, allowing to distinguish four kinds of situation according to the value of tubal mucosa (Figure 7.5).

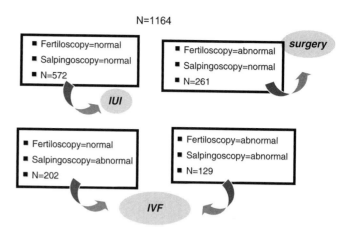

Figure 7.5. The four groups of patients according to tubal mucosa status.

The four groups were the following: Group 1, normal fertiloscopic findings and normal tubal mucosa; Group 2, normal fertiloscopic findings but abnormal tubal mucosa; Group 3, abnormal fertiloscopic findings but with normal tubal mucosa; and Group 4, abnormal fertiloscopic findings and abnormal tubal mucosa.

We had 572 patients in Group 1, 202 in Group 2, 261 in Group 3, and 129 in Group 4.

Patients of Groups 2 and 4 (i.e., with abnormal tubal mucosa were directly referred to IVF).

Patients of Group 1 were considered eligible for IUI, and lastly, patients of Group 3 have had subsequent surgical treatment.

So, respectively, 331 patients were referred for IVF (28.4 percent), 572 referred to IUI (49.1 percent), and 261 for surgery (22.4 percent).

Of 261 patients for whom surgery was decided, in 139 (53.2 percent) patients, treatment was achieved through operative laparoscopy; 105 (40.2 percent) were treated by operative fertiloscopy; and only 17 (6.5 percent) were treated by microsurgical proximal anastomosis.

When operative fertiloscopy was performed, it consisted in distal ovarosalpingolysis in seventy-eight cases and treatment of ovarian superficial lesions in twenty-seven cases.

We were able to have a complete follow-up for only six months due to various geographic origins of patients, thus preventing to have a longer follow-up.

Among the 572 patients referred to IUI, 118 (20.6 percent) became pregnant in the following six months and after one to three IUI attempts.

Among the 331 patients referred to IVF, 121 (35.2 percent) become pregnant after one to two attempts.

Among the 261 patients treated surgically, we obtained 121 (35.7 percent) pregnancies.

There is no significant difference between patients who have had IVF and patients who have undergone a surgical approach.

In all, 116 (28.4 percent) patients out of 331 became pregnant in the following six months.

Like in all surgical procedures, complications may occur.

Fortunately, they are not serious in fertiloscopy.

We have had three rectal injuries, all treated conservatively (i.e., antibiotics for five days without any further surgery).

Only one infection (0.01 percent) occurred despite the fact that no antibiotics are routinely given.

We also had two (0.02 percent) abnormal vaginal bleedings in which case a stitch on the vaginal wall was required, which is not commonly done.

Lastly, we have had eleven (0.07 percent) false route (i.e., when the fertiloscope is inserted between the peritoneum and the vaginal wall). This complication is the result of a bad technique typically linked with slow insertion of the needle in the pouch of Douglas. Instead, the insertion should be done with a firm movement.

We had no complications in patients having had operative fertiloscopy.

Results of Ovarian Drilling

In cases of patients having a PCOS, ovarian drilling per fertiloscopy was an alternative proposed when they were resistant to clomiphene citrate given during three to six months (17).

Criteria of Rotterdam (i.e., two criteria required among clinical hyperandrogenia, biological hyperandrogenia, and typical ultrasonographic aspect) were compulsory to be eligible for the ovarian drilling.

We performed 112 fertiloscopic ovarian drilling. Mean time of the procedure was fourteen minutes (range 9–18).

Ovulation was recovered in eighty-eight patients (78.5 percent), spontaneously in forty-seven cases and with the help of ovulation inductor in the remaining cases.

Cumulative pregnancy rate, of fifty-two patients, after six months was 6 percent (59/112) and the mean time to obtain a pregnancy was short: 3.9 months (range 1–11.8).

Among the fifty-nine pregnancies, there were nine miscarriages (15.2 percent), no ectopic pregnancy, and no multiple pregnancies.

We had no complication in this series.

DISCUSSION

This rather extensive series demonstrates that fertiloscopy may be practiced in a routine manner in any infertility center.

Learning curve is short, and we have estimated that ten fertiloscopies are sufficient for a laparoscopist to have the sufficient skill to introduce fertiloscopy in his panel of surgical procedures. However, it is true to say that fertiloscopy at the beginning may be disturbing due to the inverted view obtained. Also vision is not panoramic like in laparoscopy; but after some cases, this disadvantage becomes an advantage because of the magnification that provides a very accurate view. Genital tract is also inspected in physiological position, and there is no need (like in laparoscopy) to mobilize the organs with the risk of perturbing the anatomy.

We described first fertiloscopy under strict local anesthesia. It is always possible, but it depends on the health system considered. In the health system like in France where office procedure is not possible, we perform generally fertiloscopy under general sedation, which allows in case of abnormal findings to perform the treatment at the same time (operative fertiloscopy or laparoscopy). In this case, we use general sedation identical to those used for egg collection during IVF in the UK or United States where office procedure is allowed, then strict local anesthesia is a very good alternative due to the reduction of the cost.

The complication rate is low, almost always avoidable if contraindications are strictly respected. Fertiloscopy is very mini-invasive compared to laparoscopy. The FLY study has clearly shown that fertiloscopy should be the preferred option in infertile patients with no obvious pathology.

Compared to laparoscopy, fertiloscopy has also some advantages like the facility to perform salpingoscopy and microsalpingoscopy. Even if salpingoscopy has been described during laparoscopy, it is very rarely performed on a routine basis for technical reasons: during a laparoscopy, it is necessary to dispose of a second video camera, second cold light supply, irrigation with a traumatic risk, and so on. On the contrary, during fertiloscopy, everything is performed through the same optic, the fimbria being very close to the tip of the optic.

The routine practice allows selecting the best therapeutic option according to one of the most important parameter: the tubal mucosa.

We have demonstrated that even with only six months of follow-up, this approach seems valid: when tubal mucosa is altered, then no time is lost, the patient being directly referred to IVF. When tubal mucosa is normal, then surgical option is effective and the pregnancy rate obtained is not significantly different from those obtained in IVF. Also results of IUI when tubal mucosa is normal are satisfactory.

So the main interest of fertiloscopy is to give the best therapeutic option, avoiding in all cases any loss of time, which is critical in patients with a long history of infertility.

Also fertiloscopy shows that a good number of IVF has to be delayed and proposed only if the other alternatives have failed.

The need for a careful evaluation of the genital tract is also psychologically beneficial for the patients. This is because the diagnosis of unexplained infertility in itself is very distressful and the great majority of women are very keen to have a thorough evaluation in order to find "something" that may explain their infertile condition.

Concerning operative fertiloscopy, it becomes a reality because 40 percent of patients, requiring surgical procedure after fertiloscopy, were treated through operative fertiloscopy.

Procedures are obviously limited due to the unique operative channel but thanks to the magnification provided adhesiolysis is very accurate, providing that no bleeding occurs.

Therefore, one cannot imagine to practice operative procedure without a bipolar probe, allowing a complete hemostasis. When this prerequisite is respected, then the results are similar to those obtained by laparoscopy for the same lesions.

Endometriosis may also be treated by operative fertiloscopy, when minimal or moderate. If the lesions are extensive or severe, then laparoscopy has to be the preferred option.

Ovarian drilling is very effective in patients who have not responded to clomiphene citrate.

Results are similar to those observed after laparoscopic ovarian drilling, and the main interest compared to medical alternatives is the absence of ovarian hyperstimulation syndrome (OHSS) and the lack of multiple pregnancy.

Also the time necessary to conceive after fertiloscopic ovarian drilling appears to be very short (three to four months being the time average to conceive in our series).

CONCLUSIONS

Fertiloscopy appears to be a very safe and reproducible technique. Acceptance by the patients is very good for several reasons: there is no scar and no postoperative pain. Also patients are very keen to have a complete and thorough evaluation of all their parameters in order to find the origin of their infertility. The procedure is performed as an office procedure or at least as an ambulatory technique in countries (like in France), where the health system requires that every procedure, even minimally invasive, should be practiced in hospital. When practiced as office procedure, strict local anesthesia or conscious sedation is used. When practiced in hospital, general sedation is generally preferred; this option allowing to perform operative fertiloscopy or subsequent operative laparoscopy if needed.

Accuracy of fertiloscopy has been proved thanks to the FLY study, and therefore, it is legitimate to use fertiloscopy as the first option, provided that the contraindications to fertiloscopy have been diagnosed (in approximately six percent of cases).

We have seen that fertiloscopy, through salpingoscopy, allows for the first time to take in account the value of tubal mucosa routinely.

Microsalpingoscopy seems very promising because it confirms the fact that tubal permeability is necessary but not sufficient to achieve pregnancy. Microalterations of the tubal mucosa in patients with good tubal patency lead to propose IVF without delays. In the future, more works will have to be carried on to give a better understanding of tubal alterations and their consequences on tubal function.

Operative fertiloscopy is now a reality and will also need to be more standardized in the future. Some techniques like fertiloscopic ovarian drilling in PCOS patients have already demonstrated its interest in the pregnancy rate obtained without the risks of OHSS. Fertiloscopic ovarian drilling should become more and more a robust alternative to medical treatment of PCOS patients.

Finally, the rate of pathological findings is a strong argument for performing fertiloscopy early in the infertile work up and at least before IVF. Therefore, fertiloscopy should have a great future in these situations of the so-called "unexplained" infertility, which are frequently no longer unexplained after proper endoscopic evaluation.

BIBLIOGRAPHY

1. Swart P., Mol B.W., Van Beurden M., et al. The accuracy of hysterosalpingography in the diagnosis of tubal pathology: a meta-analysis. *Fertil. Steril.* 1995, 64, 486–91.

2. Chapron C., Querleu D., Bruhat M.A., et al. Surgical complications of diagnostic and operative gynaecologic laparoscopy: a serie of 29966 cases. *Hum. Reprod.* 1999, 13, 867–72.

3. Mintz M. Actualisation de la culdoscopie transvaginale en décubitus dorsal. Un nouvel endoscope à vision directe muni d'une aiguille à ponction incorporée dans l'axe. *Contr. Fertil. Sex* 1987, 15, 401–4.

4. Odent M. Hydrocolpotomie et hydroculdoscopie. *Nouv. Press. Med.* 1973, 2, 187.

5. Gordts S., Campo R., Rombauts L., Brosens I. Transvaginal hydrolaparoscopy as an outpatient procedure for infertility investigation. *Hum. Reprod.* 1998, 13, 99–103.

6. Brosens I., Campo R., Gordts S. Office hydrolaparoscopy for the diagnosis of endometriosis and tubal infertility. *Curr. Opin. Obstet. Gynec.* 1999, 11, 371–7.

7. Watrelot A., Gordts S., Andine J.P., Brosens I. Une nouvelle approche diagnostique: La Fertiloscopie. *Endomag* 1997, 21, 7–8.

8. Watrelot A., Dreyfus J.M., Andine J.P. Fertiloscopy; first results (120 cases report). *Fertil. Steril.* 1998, 70 (Suppl.), S 42.

9. Watrelot A., Dreyfus J.M., Andine J.P. Evaluation of the performance of fertiloscopy in 160 consecutive infertile patients with no obvious pathology. *Hum. Reprod.* 1999, 14, 3, 707–11.

10. Marconi G., Quintana R. Methylene blue dyeing of cellular nuclei during salpingoscopy, a new in vivo method to evaluate vitality of tubal epithelium. *Hum. Reprod.* 1998, 13, 3414–17.

11. Fernandez H., Alby J.D. De la culdoscopie à la fertiloscopie opératoire. *Endomag* 1999, 21, 5–6.

12. Gordts S., Watrelot A., Campo R., Brosens I. Risk and outcome of bowel injury during transvaginal pelvic endoscopy. *Fertil. Steril.* 2001, 76, 1238–41.

13. Chiesa-Montadou S., Rongieres C., Garbin O., Nisand I. A propos de deux complications au cours du drilling ovarien par fertiloscopie. *Gynecol. Obstet. Fertil.* 2003, 31, 844–6.

14. Watrelot A., Nisolle M., Hocke C., Rongieres C., Racinet C. Is laparoscopy still the gold standard in infertility assessment? A comparison of fertiloscopy versus laparoscopy in infertility. *Hum. Reprod.* 2003, 18, 834–9.

15. Surrey E. Microendoscopy of the human fallopian tube. *J. Am. Assoc. Gynaec. Laparosc.* 1999, 6(4), 383–90.

16. Watrelot A., Dreyfus J.M. Explorations intra-tubaires au cours de la fertiloscopie. *Reprod. Hum. et Horm.* 2000, 12, 39–44.

17. Rizk B., Nawar M.G. Laparoscopic ovarian drilling for ovulation induction in polycystic ovarian syndrome. In Allahbadia G. (Ed.) Manual of Ovulation Induction. Mumbai: India, Rotunda Medical Technologies, 2001, chapter, 140–4.

8

MICROLAPAROSCOPY

Botros R. M. B. Rizk, Hany F. Moustafa, Mary George Nawar, Christopher B. Rizk, Christine B. Rizk, David B. Rizk, Nicole Brooks, Craig Sherman, Stephen Varner

INTRODUCTION

The history of endoscopies goes back to 1805 when Bozzani managed to visualize the urethra using a very primitive tool known as Lichtleiter that depended on a candle as a light source (1).

It was not until 1910, when the term laparoscopy was designated by Jacobaeus (2), who reported the first human laparoscopy using a Nitze cystoscope (3) to visualize different body cavities, although he did not employ pneumoperitoneum at that time. Fevers (4) was the first to report operative laparoscopy in 1933, when he performed the lysis of some adhesions and obtained a number of biopsies.

In the 1940s, extensive laparoscopic research was done by Palmer (5) who advocated the use of Trendelenburg position for improved visualization during laparoscopy and later was the first to report human oocyte retrieval in 1961 (6).

Further technological advancements in the field of fiber optics along with the introduction of automatic CO_2 insufflators in the 1970s dramatically improved laparoscopic procedures (7).

The introduction of laparoscopy in the field of gynecology was a historic landmark as it gradually replaced the traditional laparotomy. Currently, most of the gynecologic surgeries are performed laparoscopically, which undoubtedly decreased the rate of morbidity and complications along with hastening the patient recovery.

In order to decrease the surgical trauma during endoscopic procedures, miniatures of traditional laparoscopies utilizing instruments 2–5 mm in diameter were developed (8, 9) and were known as minilaparoscopy or microlaparoscopy. Many researchers pioneered these techniques during the early 1990s and managed to perform increasingly advanced surgeries (9–13).

MICROLAPAROSCOPY

Microlaparoscopy refers to small-diameter laparoscopy (≤2 mm in diameter). Although these small endoscopes were available earlier and were utilized by orthopedics and otolaryngologists, they were not useful in the gynecologic field at that time due to the poor light sources that were employed, which made it difficult to visualize large dark areas in the abdomen and the pelvis.

Rapid evolution in the field of fiber optics and the introduction of diffused image bundle technology led to substantial improvement in visualization, which was the major draw back in small-diameter laparoscopies. The first generation microlaparoscopies had a 30,000-pixel fiber image bundle, while the currently used second generation microlaparoscopies have a 50,000-pixel fiber image bundle, which gives a 75 degree field of view with enhanced resolution.

Currently, microlaparoscopy is used for many diagnostic and operative gynecologic procedures with the same efficiency of traditional laparoscopies coupled with many other advantages, including the possibility of even performing it under conscious sedation without the need of general anesthesia (14).

WHY MICROLAPAROSCOPY?

Advances in the field of endoscopies have continuously aimed at creating the ultimate tool with the highest visualization potential and operative efficiency coupled with the lowest cost, morbidity, and minimal invasiveness. Unfortunately, such a tool does not exist yet, although the development of microlaparoscopy succeeded to meet many of these goals.

Microlaparoscopy offers the advantage of carrying out many diagnostic and operative gynecologic procedures in a rapid, minimally invasive approach (Tables 8.1 and 8.2). It can be carried out in an ambulatory surgical unit, both in emergent and nonemergent conditions (15).

General anesthesia has been associated with much of the morbidity and mortality during the laparoscopic procedures. Avoiding general anesthesia will also eliminate postoperative complaints due to intubation such as sore throat, nausea, and vomiting. The fact that with microlaparoscopy the procedure could be carried out under conscious sedation makes it very valuable in proper assessment of pelvic pain. This process is known as conscious pain mapping, where the patient provides the physician with feedback during his systematic probing during laparoscopy (16–19). The smaller instruments used during the procedure produce less surgical trauma than the traditional laparoscopic instruments, leading to less tissue damage and significant reduction in postoperative pain. Because of the smaller instrument size, it is safer than traditional laparoscopy in patients with previous multiple surgeries. It was also shown that microlaparoscopy could potentially decrease the operative costs, the scheduling days, and duration of hospital stay and allow fast recovery (14).

INSTRUMENTS

Full complete sets for diagnostic and operative microlaparoscopy are now widely available. Some of these instruments are

Table 8.1: Uses of Diagnostic Microlaparoscopy

Assessment of pelvic pain

Fertility assessment

Diagnosis of adenexial masses, hemorrhagic cysts, and adenexial torsion

Diagnosis of endometriosis

Diagnosis of pelvic adhesions

Diagnosis and monitoring of ectopic pregnancy

Assessment of the appendix when appendicitis is suspected

Table 8.2: Uses of Operative Microlaparoscopy

Tubal sterilization

Fulguration of endometriosis

Lysis of adhesions

Ovarian drilling

Laparoscopic uterosacral nerve ablation

Management of ectopic pregnancy

Management of hemorrhagic cysts and adenexial torsion

Appendectomy

In assisted reproduction (GIFT, ZIFT, and TET)

Laparoscopic assisted vaginal hysterectomy (LAVH)

meant for single use, while others are reusable. The choice of using either of them is personal, although the latter is more cost effective.

The primary trocars of microlaparoscopy interlock with a Verres needle, which averts the need of using two separate instruments. Once the pneumoperitoneum has been created, the Verres needle is removed.

Other instruments include forceps (serrated, atraumatic, and bipolar), suction irrigation cannulas, injection aspiration needles, endoloops, and scissors (cautery and noncautery, although all the available scissors are only the straight tip type to fit through the small trocars).

PATIENT SELECTION

Proper patient selection is very important for the success of the procedure. Marked obesity increases the likelihood of procedure failure. Patients with cardiac, pulmonary, and CNS diseases are not good candidates. Patients with a history of allergy to local anesthetics are not good candidates, unless there are some types of local anesthetics that they are not allergic to.

If the procedure is to be performed under conscious sedation, it is important to discuss with the patient the details of the procedures and the kind of discomfort she might experience, either due to insufflation or manipulation, in order to decrease unnecessary anxiety during the procedure.

All patients should receive routine preanesthetic assessment including medical, surgical, and anesthetic history, along with clinical and laboratory information about their cardiac, respiratory, renal, and hepatic functions.

All patients should be fasting for at least seven hours prior to the procedure and have a fleet enema the night before the surgery.

ANESTHESIA

Microlaparoscopy could be performed either with general anesthesia or with local anesthesia under conscious sedation, which is a state of depressed consciousness allowing communication with the patient during the procedure. Conscious sedation has the advantage of maintaining the protective respiratory reflexes and averts the need for artificial ventilation. It is generally preferred to do microlaparoscopy under general anesthesia except in patients with chronic pelvic pain, where conscious sedation is more valuable for pain mapping (20).

Conscious Sedation

There are many drugs that could be used for conscious sedation during microlaparoscopy; the aim is to maintain proper analgesia without excessive sedation. Ideally, the drugs used should have short duration of action, have minimal respiratory depressive effect, not induce histamine release, produce no or little dysphoric effect, and be easily reversible.

Before administering the anesthetic agents, atropine 0.2 mg is given to reduce the risk of vasovagal reaction. Also, an antiemetic should be given like ondansetron 4 mg, to prevent vomiting.

The most widely used combination is fentanyl with midazolam. Fentanyl is a synthetic narcotic analgesic with 100 times the potency of morphine. It has a rapid onset and a short duration of action with rapid recovery. Still, as with most other narcotics, it can cause respiratory depression and bradycardia. Reversal of these side effects could be achieved by the administration of naloxone. Although there are many other narcotics, their use is limited in conscious sedation. For example, morphine and meperidine are associated with marked sedation and histamine release. Alfentanil and sufentanil are very similar to fentanyl, except that they have a short duration of action and lower volume of distribution, which requires multiple dosing.

Midazolam is the anxiolytic agent of choice, as it has a rapid onset of action and a relatively short duration of action. Higher doses may cause respiratory depression, which can be reversed by the use of flumazenil. Diazepam is not preferred as it causes irritation at the injection site and has the tendency to crystallize in intravenous lines, not to mention that it has a long duration of action. Lorazipam is highly sedative and has a long duration of action as well.

Immediately before the procedure, the patient should be properly hydrated with IV fluids (i.e., lactated ringers solution), and oxygen via intranasal cannula or mask is provided. It is recommended to use a Foley catheter to evacuate the bladder to avoid bladder injury.

During the procedure, the patient should have continuous ECG monitoring, respiratory monitoring, and pulse oximetry. There is no need for the anesthesiologist to be present as long as a registered nurse with advanced cardiac life support training is present. Emergency resuscitative equipment and drugs should be available on site.

If the patient has decided to receive conscious sedation, she should be placed from the start in dorsolithotomy position since no general anesthesia is needed. The Trendelenburg position allows easy visualization of the pelvis. It is very important to ensure that the patient is positioned comfortably to avoid any anxiety during the procedure.

Once the patient is sedated, local anesthesia is injected at the primary trocar site at the umbilicus. This is achieved by the use of 10 ml of 1% lidocaine with epinephrine, 1:100,000 (to maintain local hemostasis and prolong the analgesic effect), buffered with sodium bicarbonate to decrease irritation. Marcaine may be used instead, but it has a slower onset and longer duration of action. The two drugs could be used together. All the abdominal wall layers down to the peritoneum should be infiltrated with the local anesthetic using a 17- to 22-gauge needle. Extra care should be taken in thin patients in order to avoid any injury to internal organs during infiltration and perhaps it is better to elevate the skin in these patients during injection.

THE PROCEDURE

An umbilical incision is made (a local anesthetic block is done first in a case of conscious sedation) through which the interlocking trocar with the Verres needle is introduced to the abdomen. After the patency of the Verres needle is checked, pneumoperitonium is created using either carbon dioxide or nitrous oxide. Both are inexpensive and are easily eliminated and absorbed. Although carbon dioxide is more widely used, it is preferred to use nitrous oxide in long procedures due to the lack of hemodynamic side effects seen with carbon dioxide (hypercarbia, respiratory acidosis, peritoneal irritation, tachycardia, and arrhythmia). Another advantage of nitrous oxide is that it has an anesthetic effect (21).

The volume of gas to be insufflated varies according to the type of anesthesia (general or local), the length of the procedure, and the patient habitus. It is important to realize that in patients who are not under general anesthesia, higher volumes of gas can cause significant distress and anxiety; accordingly, the gas volume and the operating time should be kept to the minimum. In most patients, insufflation of 1.5 L is very well tolerated. For long procedures, lower volumes are needed to decrease the patient's discomfort. In contrast, in obese patients, it is very difficult to obtain good visualization with such a small amount of gas and the volume could be increased up to 3 L. In general, the intra-abdominal pressure should be maintained at 10 mmHg.

Once pneumoperitoneum is created, the Verres needle is removed and the microlaparoscope is inserted through the primary trocar to visualize the abdomen and the entry site.

A secondary accessory trocar is then inserted in the suprapubic area (two fingers' breadth, cephalad to the symphysis pubis). Again, in case of conscious sedation, a local infiltration with anesthesia should be done first and the patient should be advised to perform Valsalva maneuver during the trocar insertion to avoid any possible internal organ injury, especially in the presence of such relatively low intra-abdominal pressure (21).

Depending on the nature of the procedure, other paraumbilical ancillary ports could be done. Occasionally, larger trocars may be needed especially during appendectomy, LAVH, or in some cases of tubal sterilization when clip applicators are used (22).

If there is any pain during the procedure in the consciously sedated patients due to instrument manipulation, reapplication of lidocaine at the trocar site will decrease the pain or discomfort. Lidocaine could be also applied directly to the peritoneum without the need for injection as it is readily absorbed. It is important to maintain communication with the patient during the procedure, not only to obtain feedback about any possible pain but also to decrease the patient's anxiety. Other factors that help to decrease the patient's anxiety include gentle handling of organs, limited manipulation, maintaining the lowest possible intra-abdominal pressure, and limiting the duration of the procedure to the minimum.

At the end of the procedures, the instruments are removed, and elimination of as much gas as possible should be done while the trocars are still in, to decrease postoperative discomfort.

There is no need for suturing the incision sites, but steri-strips are used to approximate the edges for better aesthetic outcome. Most of the patients can leave the office within one hour of the procedure.

MICROLAPAROSCOPY IN INFERTILITY AND ASSISTED REPRODUCTION

The role of microlaparoscopy in the field of infertility and assisted reproduction has grown exponentially over the past two decades. Microlaparoscopy is currently used for infertility assessment, surgical management of endometriosis, lysis of adhesions, ovarian drilling, gamete intrafallopian transfer, tubal embryo transfer, hydrosalpinx removal before IVF, and management of ectopic and heterotopic pregnancy.

Microlaparoscopy for Infertility Assessment

The role of laparoscopy as a first-line investigation tool for infertility has waxed and waned over the past few years. Until recently, infertility assessment was not considered complete until the female partner receives a laparoscopic assessment and was considered by all infertility algorithms to be the final diagnostic approach before the patient is given the diagnosis of unexplained infertility. Recently, the continuous need to simplify the fertility work up and the pressure to reduce its cost coupled with the rapid advances in ART have led to the recession of laparoscopic assessment as a first-line diagnostic tool in infertility. It is now accepted that ovulation induction should be offered to selected couples who otherwise have a normal infertility work up and normal hysterosalpingogram (HSG), for at least three months before the need of having endoscopic evaluation.

Some authors believe that it is very important not to proceed with ART without laparoscopic assessment as it is shown that laparoscopy can reveal abnormal findings in the pelvis in up to 68 percent in patients with normal HSG (23) and might lead to changes in ART treatment plans in up to 25 percent of cases (24) (see chapters 11,12).

Laparoscopic assessment is still considered the golden standard for the diagnosis of pelvic causes of infertility like peritubal adhesions, abnormal tubo-ovarian relationship, and endometriosis (25) (Figure 8.1). Diagnosis and treatment of these conditions is very important as it was evidently shown to have significant positive effect on the fertility outcome.

Lysis of Pelvic Adhesions

The presence of pelvic adhesions is an important cause of infertility. There is some evidence too that peritubal adhesions are associated with lower response to gonadotrophins during IVF treatment. Pelvic adhesions were also frequently claimed to

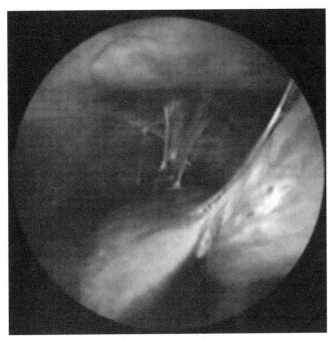

Figure 8.1. Fitz-Hugh Curtis syndrome. In Almeida O (ed.), Microlaparoscopy. Wiley-Liss, Inc.; New York 2000.

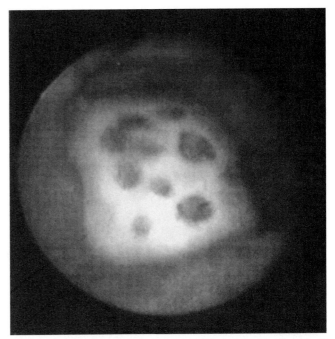

Figure 8.2. Microlaparoscopic ovarian drilling. Atlas. In Almeida O (ed.), Microlaparoscopy. Wiley-Liss, Inc; New York.

be a source of chronic pelvic pain, a fact that has been confirmed recently using conscious pain mapping.

Lysis of these adhesions could be effectively carried out using microlaparoscopy without general anesthesia. For thin filmy adhesions, there is no need for cautery; they could be simply cut by scissors after the local application of lidocain. For dense adhesions, they are better to be cut with the 2-mm monopolar coagulation scissors. Alternatively, they could be cauterized using the 2-mm bipolar forceps before excision. The use of Ringer's lactate during and after the procedure was shown to significantly decrease the rate of adhesions recurrence (26, 27).

Laparoscopic Removal of Hydrosalpinges

The presence of communicating hydrosalpinx was evidently shown to have a deleterious effect on fertility and IVF outcome. This is due to the fact that such embryo toxic fluid keeps seeping into the endometrial cavity, leading to reduced endometrial receptivity, diminished embryo survivability, improper implantation, and increased incidence of abortion (28, 29).

Many studies have demonstrated significant improvement in the implantation rate and live birth rate in IVF patients after the removal of hydrosalpinx (30, 31). According to the NICE guidelines and ASRM clinical practice committee, hydrosalpinx should be removed before the commencement of ART treatment to improve the implantation, pregnancy, and live birth rate (32, 33).

Although the presence of hydrosalpinx could be diagnosed with ultrasound and HSG, these tests have relatively low sensitivity and specificity when compared with laparoscopy with chromopertubation, which is considered the golden standard for diagnosis (34).

Laparoscopic Fulguration of Endometriosis

Endometriosis, regardless of its severity, has a negative impact on fertility, although the more severe is the disease, the more

negative is the impact. Patients with endometriosis were also shown to have 50 percent reduction in the chances of pregnancy after IVF.

Infertile patients with minimal to mild disease should be offered laparoscopic ablation with adhesiolysis, which is now proved to be more effective than ovarian suppression in improving infertility (35). Currently, there is no evidence to suggest that such surgical intervention enhances the pregnancy rate in patients with moderate to severe disease (36). Microlaparoscopy is very effective in surgical management of stage I and II endometriosis (Figure 8.2). For small superficial lesions less than 5 mm, local application of lidocain before their fulguration with 2-mm noncautery scissors in enough. Suctioning and reapplication of the local anesthetic several times ensures better local anesthesia. For deeper lesions, it might be necessary to inject lidocain before the lesion is excised. If the patient starts to develop discomfort during the procedure, more sedative hypnotic such as propofol could be used. It is not advised to manage advanced endometriosis with microlaparoscopy, specially without general anesthesia because of the greater chance of patient discomfort and potential complications.

Laparoscopic Ovarian Drilling (LOD)

Polycystic ovarian syndrome (PCOS) is the most common reproductive endocrinopathy in women, with estimated prevalence of 4–12 percent. Infertility is one of the main presenting symptoms of this syndrome for which there is a logistic stepwise management protocol. Weight loss is usually the first line of treatment, followed by ovulation induction with clomiphene citrate and insulin sensitizers such as metformin. Unfortunately, up to 25 percent of women with PCOS will show clomiphene citrate resistance and those patients could be managed either by LOD or by ovulation induction using gonadotrophins (37). A recent meta-analysis showed that both procedures are

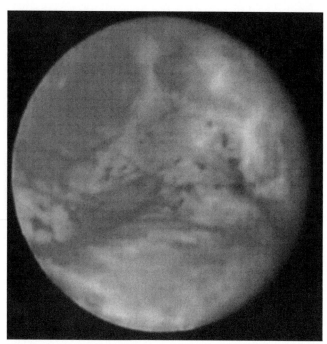

Figure 8.3. A typical red endometriotic lesions (hypervascularity) over the bladder peritoneum. Atlas. In Almeida O (ed.), Microlaparoscopy. Wiley-Liss, Inc.; New York 2000.

equally effective in terms of pregnancy rates (38). One of the advantages of LOD is the lower risk of complications such as ovarian hyperstimulation syndrome, which is more common in this subset of patients, and a lower risk of multiple pregnancies (39, 40). Another advantage of LOD is improved menstrual regularity and long-term reproductive performance. For further details about medical versus surgical management of PCOS, refer to Chapters 30 and 31.

The procedure can be done by microlaparoscopy under conscious sedation. After starting the standard anesthetic protocol detailed earlier, the patient should also receive a paracervical block before the placement of a uterine manipulator. The ovary is then stabilized by holding the utero-ovarian ligament, and local anesthesia is applied to the surface of the ovary. Using the 2-mm cautery scissors, ten to twelve punctures of 5-mm depth should be done for each ovary (Figure 8.3).

KEY POINTS

■ Microlaparoscopy refers to small-diameter laparoscopies (≤2 mm in diameter), which are less invasive than traditional laparoscopies.

■ Currently, microlaparoscopy is used for many diagnostic and operative gynecologic procedures with the same efficiency of traditional laparoscopies.

■ It has many advantages over the traditional laparoscopy, including less operative trauma and tissue damage, shorter hospital stay, faster recovery, and significant reduction of postoperative pain.

■ Microlaparoscopy could be performed either under general anesthesia or conscious sedation, which is a state of depressed consciousness.

■ The use of conscious sedation lowers the morbidity and mortality associated with general anesthesia and reduces many postoperative complaints due to intubation.

■ The use of conscious sedation was shown to be particularly useful during assessment of pelvic pain. This process is known as conscious pain mapping.

■ Proper patient selection is important for the success of the procedure. Marked obesity increases the likelihood of procedure failure.

■ Some of the current uses of microlaparoscopy include tubal sterilization, diagnosis and monitoring of ectopic pregnancy, infertility assessment, lysis of pelvic adhesions, LOD, fulguration of endometriosis, laparoscopic removal of hydrosalpinges, and laparoscopic uterosacral nerve ablation.

REFERENCES

1. Belt AE, Charnock DA. The history of the cystoscope. In Cabol H, ed., Modern Urology. Philadelphia: Lea and Febiger, 1936; pp. 15–50.
2. Jacobaeus HC. Uber die Moglichkeit die Zystoskopie bei Untersuchung seroser Hohlungen anzuwenden. *Munch Med Wochenschr* 1910;57:2090–2.
3. Nitze M. Uber eine neue Beleuchtungsmethode der Hohlen des menschlichen Korpers. *Wien Med Presse* 1879;20:851–8.
4. Fevers C. Die laparoskopie mit dem cystoskop: ein beitrag zur vereinfachng der technik und zur endoskopischen Strangdurtrennung in der Bauchhohle. *Med Klin* 1933;29:1042–5.
5. Palmer R. Instrumentation et technique de la coelioscopie gynecologique. *Gynecol Obstet* 1947;46:420–31.
6. Klein R, Palmer R. Technique de prelevement ovules humaines par ponction folliculaire sans coelioscopie. *C R Soc Biol (Paris)* 1961;155:1918–21.
7. Semm K. Atlas of gynecologic laparoscopy and hysteroscopy. Philidelphia: Saunders, 1977.
8. Palter SF. Microlaparoscopy under local anesthesia and conscious pain mapping for the diagnosis and management of pelvic pain. *Curr Opin Obstet Gynecol* 1999;11(4):387–93.
9. Dorsey JH, Tabb CR. Mini-laparoscopy and fiber-optic lasers. *Obstet Gynecol Clin North Am* 1991;18(3):613–17.
10. Palter SF. Office microlaparoscopy under local anesthesia. *Obstet Gynecol Clin North Am* 1999;26(1):109–20, vii.
11. Childers JM, Hatch KD, Surwit EA. Office laparoscopy and biopsy for evaluation of patients with intraperitoneal carcinomatosis using a new optical catheter. *Gynecol Oncol* 1992;47(3):337–42.
12. Risquez F, Pennehouat G, Fernandez R, Confino E, Rodriguez O. Microlaparoscopy: a preliminary report. *Hum Reprod* 1993;8(10):1701–2.
13. Bauer O, Devroey P, Wisanto A, Gerling W, Kaisi M, Diedrich K. Small diameter laparoscopy using a microlaparoscope. *Hum Reprod* 1995;10(6):1461–4.
14. Risquez F, Pennehoaut G, McCorvey R, Love B, Vazquez A, Partamian J, Rebon P, Lucena E, Audebert A, Confino E. Diagnostic and operative microlaparoscopy: a preliminary multicentre report. *Hum Reprod* 1997;12(8):1645–8.
15. Tulandi T. Modern surgical approaches to female reproductive tract. *Hum Reprod Update* 1996;2:419–27.
16. Almeida OD, Val-Gallas JM. Conscious pain mapping. *J Am Assoc Gynecol Laparosc* 1997;4(5):587–90.
17. Howard FM, El-Minawi AM, Sanchez RA. Conscious pain mapping by laparoscopy in women with chronic pelvic pain. *Obstet Gynecol* 2000;96(6):934–9.
18. Almeida OD, Val-Gallas JM. Office microlaparoscopy under local anesthesia in the diagnosis and treatment of chronic pelvic pain. *J Am Assoc Gynecol Laparosc* 1998;5(4):407–10.

19. Palter SF, Olive DL. Office microlaparoscopy under local anesthesia for chronic pelvic pain. *J Am Assoc Gynecol Laparosc* 1996;3(3):359–64.

20. Almeida OD, Val-Gallas JM, Browning JL. A protocol for conscious sedation in microlaparoscopy. *J Am Assoc Gynecol Laparosc* 1997;4(5):591–4.

21. Ikeda F, Abrão MS, Podgaec S, Nogueira AP, Neme RM, Pinotti JA. Microlaparoscopy in gynecology: analysis of 16 cases and review of literature. *Rev Hosp Clin Fac Med Sao Paulo* 2001; 56(4):115–18.

22. Almeida OD, Val-Gallas JM, Rizk B. Appendectomy under local anaesthesia following conscious pain mapping with microlaparoscopy. *Hum Reprod* 1998;13(3):588–90.

23. Corson SL, Cheng A, Gutmann JN. Laparoscopy in the "normal" infertile patient: a question revisited. *J Am Assoc Gynecol Laparosc* 2000;7(3):317–24.

24. Tanahatoe S, Hompes PG, Lambalk CB. Accuracy of diagnostic laparoscopy in the infertility work-up before intrauterine insemination. *Fertil Steril* 2003;79:361–6.

25. Surrey ES. Endoscopy in the evaluation of the woman experiencing infertility. *Clin Obstet Gynecol* 2000;43(4):889–96.

26. Tulandi T, Murray C, Guralnick M. Adhesion formations and reproductive outcome after myomectomy and second-look laparoscopy. *Obstet Gynecol* 1993;82:213–15.

27. Pagidas K, Tulandi T. Effects of Ringer's lactate, Interceed (TC&) and Gene-Tex surgical membrane or postsurgical adhesion formation. *Fertil Steril* 1992;57:199–201.

28. Zeyneloglu HB, Arici A, Olive DL. Adverse effects of hydrosalpinx on pregnancy rates after in vitro fertilization-embryo transfer. *Fertil Steril* 1998;70:492.

29. Spielvogel K, Shwayder J, Coddington CC. Surgical management of adhesions, endometriosis, and tubal pathology in the woman with infertility. *Clin Obstet Gynecol* 2000;43(4):916–28.

30. Shelton KE, Butler L, Toner JP, Oehninger S, Muasher SJ. Salpingectomy improves the pregnancy rate in in-vitro fertilization with hydrosalpinx. *Hum Reprod* 1996;11:523–5.

31. Johnson NP, Mak W, Sowter MC. Laparoscopic salpingectomy for women with hydrosalpinges enhances the success of IVF: a Cochrane review. *Hum Reprod* 2002;17:543.

32. Practice Committee of the American Society for Reproductive Medicine. Salpingectomy for hydrosalpinx prior to in vitro fertilization. Fertil Steril 2006;86 (Suppl. 5):S200–1.

33. National Institute of Clinical Excellence. Fertility: assessment and treatment of people with fertility problems, Clinical guidelines No. 11. London: Abba Litho Ltd UK, 2004.

34. Spielvogel K, Shwayder J, Coddington CC. Surgical management of adhesions, endometriosis, and tubal pathology in the woman with infertility. *Clin Obstet Gynecol* 2000;43(4): 916–28.

35. Nezhat C, Crowgey SR, Garrison CP. Surgical treatment of endometriosis via laser laparoscopy. *Fertil Steril* 1986;45(6): 778–83.

36. Kennedy S, Bergqvist A, Chapron C, D'Hooghe T, Dunselman G, Greb R, Hummelshoj L, Prentice A, Saridogan E; on behalf of the ESHRE Special Interest Group for Endometriosis and endometrium Guideline Development Group. ESHRE guideline for the diagnosis and treatment of endometriosis. *Hum Reprod* 2005; 20(10):2698–704.

37. Unlu C, Atabekoglu CS. Surgical treatment in polycystic ovary syndrome. *Curr Opin Obstet Gynecol* 2006;18(3):286–92.

38. Farquhar C, Lilford RJ, Marjoribanks J, Vandekerckhove P. Laparoscopic "drilling" by diathermy or laser for ovulation induction in anovulatory polycystic ovary syndrome. *Cochrane Database Syst Rev* 2005;(3):CD001122.

39. Rizk B, Nawar MG. Laparoscopic ovarian drilling for ovulation induction in polycystic ovarian syndrome. In Allahbadia G (Ed.) Manual of ovulation Induction. Mumbai: India, Rotunda Medical Technologies, 2001, chapter 18, 140–4.

40. Rizk B. Prevention of ovarian hyperstimulation syndrome. In Rizk B (Ed.) Ovarian hyperstimulation syndrome. Cambridge: United Kingdom, Cambridge University Press, 2006, chapter 7, 130–99.

PEDIATRIC AND ADOLESCENT GYNECOLOGIC LAPAROSCOPY

Suketu M. Mansuria, Joseph S. Sanfilippo

SYNOPSIS

The use of laparoscopy by gynecologists in treating pediatric and adolescent patients is a relatively new phenomenon. We present the specialized instrumentation prerequisite to operating on patients in the pediatric-adolescent age-group. Preoperative considerations and generalized techniques unique to this population are discussed. Though laparoscopy has a myriad of indications, the main focus will be on treatment and diagnosis of pelvic pain, adnexal masses, and pelvic inflammatory disease. A discussion of incidental appendectomy in these patients will also be presented.

INTRODUCTION

Endoscopic surgery dates back to the Babylonian Talmud (Niddah Treatise, Section 65b). A lead funnel with a bent mouthpiece was introduced into the vagina, enabling direct visualization of the cervix. The first true laparoscopic procedure is credited to Ott in 1901, when he inserted a speculum through a small incision and, using a head mirror to focus light through the incision, inspected the abdominal viscera. Since that time, advances in the field have allowed surgeons to perform ever more complicated and intricate procedures. Of all the fields of surgery to benefit from laparoscopy, pediatric surgery is considered the newcomer. It was not until the production of high-quality, miniaturized instrumentation that surgeons began to look for applications of laparoscopy in the pediatric patient population. Few procedures were performed laparoscopically in this age-group before 1970 mainly because attempts at making smaller scopes resulted in unacceptable poor visualization. With the advent of fiber optic light sources and the Hopkins rod-lens system, smaller scopes with superior visualization allowed surgeons to apply minimally invasive techniques in the treatment of pediatric and adolescent patients. Gans is credited with advancing the technique of laparoscopic surgery in this population in the early 1970s (Schropp, 1994). After his initial push, surgeons from different specialties began to assimilate his techniques within their own areas of interest.

INSTRUMENTATION

Without the rigid endoscope, laparoscopy would not be possible. The majority of procedures can be performed with 5- or 10-mm scopes, but 2-mm endoscopes are available for use in smaller patients (Figure 9.1). The most common lens configuration for gynecologic procedures is 0°, but angled scopes are available for when it is required to evaluate "around" an obstructing structure. The reason that the 0° lens is the most commonly used by gynecologists is that it provides the least amount of distortion and that the pelvic organs are situated in a straight "line of sight" from the umbilicus, the most common site of scope placement. Unless the surgeon plans on operating on young children or infants, the 5- and 10-mm scopes should suffice. Both should be available because sometimes it becomes necessary to transfer the scope to a 5-mm auxiliary port from a 10-mm umbilical port for improved visualization. Unless the surgeon is using an insufflator with the capability of providing warmed CO_2, fogging during the case can be an annoyance and a hazard. Fogging is due to condensation on the tip of the scope. Condensation occurs when the scope is cooler than the surrounding air and body. Antifog solutions are available, but often they are not effective. A cheap alternative is to keep a sterile thermos filled with warmed (37–50°C) water. When fogging occurs, the scope is inserted into the thermos. This will not only clean the scope lens but it will also raise the scope's temperature, which will prevent fogging.

After the rigid endoscope, the other essential pieces of equipment include the insufflator, light and video system, and trocars. We recommend an insufflation system capable of up to 20 L/min of flow. This allows immediate replacement of any gas that is taken up during aspiration with the suction irrigator. This is especially important in the pediatric and adolescent population as the total volume of insufflation in their abdomens during surgery is usually much less than adults; thus, aspiration with the suction irrigator in younger patients will reduce the intra-abdominal volume of gas to a relatively greater extent than in larger, older patients. The ability to insufflate the abdomen at greater rates of flow will prevent the collapse of the anterior abdominal wall due to the loss of pneumoperitoneum intraoperatively. Newer insufflators (e.g., Stryker, Kalamazoo, MI) are equipped with the ability to insufflate with warmed CO_2 to reduce fogging during the case and prevent hypothermia in the patient. The light and video system plays a crucial role in image quality. Even the most expensive scope will provide poor image quality if coupled to an inferior light and video system. The light cords are usually made from bundles of fiber optic strands. These strands transmit light from the (light) source to the scope. Unfortunately, these fiber optic strands

Laparoscopic Tubal Anastomosis

Carlos Rotman, Nasir Rana, Jonathan Y. Song, Edgardo Yordan, Carlos E. Sueldo

INTRODUCTION

Bilateral tubal ligation as a form of permanent sterilization has been carried out in females for more than a century (1). Patients who have completed their desired family size and are certain about the lack of interest in future pregnancies find this procedure to be cost effective, relatively simple, and generally free of complications. Patients find this permanent procedure convenient since they do not have to deal with the costs and potential complications of different types of ongoing contraceptive methods, such as birth control pills and intrauterine contraceptive devices.

The procedure can be accomplished effectively by different routes, including vaginal or abdominal approaches, either through a mini-laparotomy or by laparoscopy. The timing of the procedure is variable as it can be performed right after a vaginal delivery or at the time of a cesarean section. Also, it can be accomplished in a gynecologic patient (interval tubal ligation) during the preovulatory phase of the menstrual cycle, commonly by laparoscopy. As for the methods used, the fallopian tubes can be sectioned and a segment of the tube removed, or if a laparoscopic approach is used, bipolar cauterization of the tubes or application of silastic rings or clips are popular alternatives (2–4).

It is estimated that as many as 700,000 procedures are performed each year in the United States, roughly half after delivery or at the time of a cesarean section and half by laparoscopic (interval) tubal ligation (5).

A number of these patients, however, change their minds later in life, most commonly due to divorce followed by a new relationship, leading to a desire for a new pregnancy. A subsequent consultation with a reproductive surgeon takes place, discussing the possibility of having the tubal ligation reversed. It is estimated that approximately 1 percent of all patients will seek consultation for a tubal reversal within a few years after the procedure (6); prior to surgery, an appropriate evaluation of the couple is required to determine whether tubal reversal or perhaps in vitro fertilization–embryo transfer would be a better reproductive option.

Documenting the presence of ovulation and performing a complete semen analysis including a strict morphology assessment (Kruger) to rule out the presence of a male factor problem (7), even in those that have fathered children in the past, are required. Also, it is important to conduct some form of assessment of the uterine cavity, even in asymptomatic patients, in order to rule out significant intracavitary pathology (e.g., submucous fibroids, large polyps, or intrauterine adhesions)

prior to performing tubal surgery. An office hysteroscopy and/or a sonohysterogram should be performed during the preoperative work up.

Assessment of the type of tubal ligation performed is also important since it might determine whether or not a tubal reversal is indicated. For example, tubal cauterization, especially by unipolar energy, typically causes significant damage to the blood supply of the fallopian tube and is unlikely to result in a successful outcome if tubal anastomosis is performed, despite the results published recently by Yoon et al. (8). On the other hand, silastic rings, clips, as well as the Pomeroy-type of tubal ligation (commonly done for puerperal sterilization and also at the time of cesarean sections) typically result in limited damage to the fallopian tubes. Most often, a tubal anastomosis can be performed in those cases.

The success rate of tubal anastomosis, measured as the rate of intrauterine gestations after surgery, is generally quite high, especially if there is an appropriate patient selection and evaluation prior to surgery. Large series frequently quote intrauterine pregnancy rates in the 60–80 percent range (9).

As in other areas of reproductive medicine, the age of the female is an important factor in determining success, and evaluation of the ovarian reserve, either with an antral follicle count and/or with hormone evaluation on cycle day three in patients older than thirty-five years (10), may be a contributing factor in determining the best treatment approach. Also, as mentioned, the presence of other infertility factor(s), especially male factor infertility, may be enough reason to indicate assisted reproductive technology procedures instead of tubal surgery (11) since by using intracytoplasmic sperm injection for fertilization, the patient is more likely to get pregnant, as opposed to undergoing tubal surgery and subsequent sexual intercourse or intrauterine insemination.

Once the couple has made a decision about having a tubal anastomosis, the surgeon determines the best surgical approach to be used in order to accomplish a successful tubal reversal. The procedure can be accomplished by laparotomy or by laparoscopy; laparotomy is the more traditional method, and over the years, by using tubal microsurgical techniques, it has developed a proven record of good pregnancy rates (12). With improvements in laparoscopic equipment and the availability of experienced laparoscopic surgeons, more and more patients are being treated by laparoscopy, with equal degrees of success as those seen with laparotomy in the past.

The advantages of laparoscopy are the same as in other areas of gynecology: an ambulatory procedure, a more rapid recovery after surgery, less postoperative morbidity, and equal rates of pregnancy as those performed via laparotomy. There are many laparoscopic techniques described for tubal anastomosis: sutureless technique (13), application of titanium staples (14), robotically assisted laparoscopic tubal reversal (15), and the use of LASER (16).

Our group has vast experience with laparoscopic reconstructive surgery in the management of tubal conditions resulting from a myriad of pathological conditions. This presentation however, will be limited to the use of laparoscopy as a means to restore fertility in patients that have previously undergone tubal sterilization.

Our laparoscopic technique of tubal anastomosis was developed in 1998 after many years of performing mini-laparotomy and traditional microsurgery in several hundred cases. The laparoscopic approach is essentially identical to that of the open-abdomen technique except for the use of specialized instrumentation to facilitate its performance via laparoscopy. Most tubal anastomosis at our center are performed for sterilization reversal, but the same technique is applied to cases of tubal occlusion secondary to pathologic processes.

As our experience evolved, numerous changes were implemented to overcome technical challenges, enhancing the procedure to make it easier, faster, and hopefully more successful. These changes included selection of suture material, type of tubal closure (one vs. two layers), tubal stump preparations, tubal cannulation, and the type of electric current best suited for these cases. Last but not least, placement of interrupted sutures versus a continuous closure was also investigated.

Videotaping of the surgical procedure from beginning to end is crucial for evaluating the different steps. It also allows the surgeons to return later and review the surgery, providing the opportunity to think, study, and improve, enhancing the technique to make it better and more efficient.

PRELIMINARY WORK UP

Prior to surgery, the preliminary work up consists of the following: 1) a thorough review of all pertinent medical records if available; 2) a carefully obtained medical and surgical history and full examination; 3) a day 3 serum FSH and estradiol to ascertain ovarian reserve, a midluteal phase serum progesterone to document ovulation, and a complete semen analysis on the husband/partner, including a Kruger index of sperm morphology; and 4) a complete pelvic ultrasound and sonohysterogram.

We try to obtain previous medical records on all of our patients prior to surgery for review; however, in some circumstances, these records may not be available (international patients, records destroyed due to age, etc.). In certain cases, we have also found that the operative report was inconsistent with true surgical findings at the time of the operation. For example, according to some operative reports, a modified Pomeroy technique was performed for tubal sterilization; however, upon entering the abdomen, we discovered instead evidence of bilateral fimbriectomy. Other findings included multiple Hulka clip or Falope ring applications per tube (decreasing the actual length of repairable tube), when the operative report stated that a single clip or ring was placed on each tube.

We do not routinely perform a preoperative hysterosalpingogram (HSG). Not only does it not provide the length of the distal segment but it will also not accurately determine the length and quality of the proximal segment. Only after entering the abdomen are the surgeons able to ascertain pertinent information for the procedure. A pelvic ultrasound and sonohysterogram are performed in the office on all potential candidates. If we identify any intrauterine pathology (e.g., submuous fibroids, polyps, and intrauterine adhesions), they are either addressed at the time of our laparoscopic tubal surgery or beforehand, depending on the type and severity of the pathology.

During our preoperative counseling and work up, the patients are informed of our pregnancy, ectopic, and abortion rates as stated in the results section later in this chapter. Also, we discuss the main advantages and disadvantages of this procedure versus the use of in vitro fertilization–embryo transfer. After the preoperative work up is completed, the patient is scheduled for laparoscopic surgery.

SURGICAL TECHNIQUE

Prior to commencing, the entire surgical team gets together to review all pertinent information about the case. The patient is then reassured, and anesthesia is given.

Patient positioning is the responsibility of the primary surgeon. If this step is done by other team members, the surgeon should walk around the operating table to ensure that everything is in place prior to proceeding. We prefer a dorsolithotomy position with arms tucked in, shoulder stoppers placed to prevent intra-operative sliding, and legs slightly bent at the knees and hips. Well-cushioned, adjustable leggings are a must to prevent lower-limb nerve injury.

With the anesthesiologist's permission, a thorough pelvic examination is performed, and the patient is prepped and draped in the usual manner. A Foley catheter (connected to a bag) is placed in the bladder. After completion of any hysteroscopy or endometrial biopsy where warranted, a manipulator is introduced into the uterine cavity. A vaginal assistant, responsible for keeping the uterus properly positioned as per the surgeon's instructions during the procedure, is seated between the patient's legs, facing a slave monitor located overhead or at either side of the surgical table. A primary monitor is placed behind the vaginal assistant, directly facing the surgeons. We videotape all surgeries in both SVHS and miniDV formats. Beyond the significant educational value, videotaping will most often protect you and your facility in the event of litigation.

To gain access into the abdomen, we advocate the use of an open technique (17); but surgeons should choose the method with which they feel most comfortable.

Once the laparoscope is introduced into the abdomen, we proceed with a thorough evaluation of the pelvic and abdominal cavity; this is accomplished much better by laparoscopy than through an open abdomen. In all of our cases, a total of four ports are utilized: one 10 mm at the umbilicus for the laparoscope and three ancillary 5-mm ports, of which two are placed on each side of the abdomen in the lower quadrant, lateral to the inferior epigastric vessels, and one placed suprapubically anywhere between the umbilicus and the symphysis pubis, depending on the size of the uterus. The tubes are then evaluated for length, type, and location of the obstruction; associated pathology; and quality of the fimbriated ends (Figure 10.1).

The obstructed segments are resected using laparoscopic microbipolar cautery and scissors. It is very important to use the minimum amount of current needed to achieve adequate

Table 10.3: Summary and Cross-Match for All Groups

Age (years)	Anastomosis, rate (%)	Pregnancy, rate (%)	Abortion, rate (%)	Ectopic, rate (%)	Successful pregnancies, rate (%)
≤35	Bilateral	52/66 (79)	23/90 (26)	1/90 (1.1)	66/90 (73)
	Unilateral	14/26 (54)	5/19 (26)	0/19 (0)	14/19 (74)
	Overall	66/92 (72)	28/109 (26)	1/109 (0.9)	80/109 (73)
>35	Bilateral	7/13 (54)	4/9 (44)	0/9 (0)	5/9 (56)
	Unilateral	7/15 (47)	5/9 (56)	1/9 (11)	3/9 (33)
	Overall	14/28 (50)	9/18 (50)	1/18 (5.5)	8/18 (44)

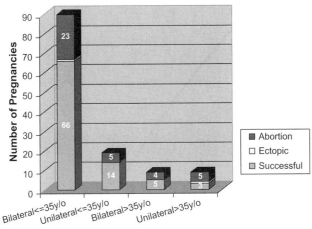

Figure 10.9. Summary of pregnancy outcomes based upon anastomosis and age.

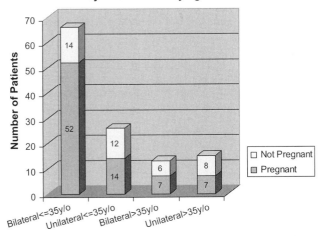

Figure 10.10. Pregnancy summary based upon anastomosis and age.

One must also realize that in interpreting the results of our data, our experience involved working with fertile patients. These patients underwent an elective procedure to render them sterile; therefore, the pregnancy rate in our patients may not be reflective of those who experience primary or secondary infertility due to tubal pathology and undergo a similar laparoscopic procedure.

Based on our experience, we would be cautious in recommending a laparoscopic tubal anastomosis to patients who are older than 35 years, unless they are willing to accept a much lower pregnancy rate and a higher miscarriage rate. The treatment alternative to tubal anastomosis in this age-group, IVF-ET, is also known for having a lower pregnancy rate as well as an increased abortion rate, mostly due to an increased incidence of chromosomal anomalies in the embryos that these patients generate.

That is why it is important during counseling to inform these couples about the success rates with both techniques. The older groups (C and D) in our study represented the lowest pregnancy rate at 50 percent (14/28), the highest spontaneous abortion rate at 50 percent (9/18), as well as the highest ectopic pregnancy rate at 5.5 percent (1/18). The fact that we were cautious in counseling older patients about undergoing laparoscopic tubal anastomosis reduced our sample size for this population, which affected our numerical analysis.

We have also found that in our hands, interstitial to isthmic, and ampullary to fimbria anastomosis with a less than 1-cm distance from the fimbria to the anastomotic site, yielded no pregnancies, regardless of the length of tube pre- or post reconstruction. Also as a rule, we do not attempt a laparoscopic tubal anastomosis if the pre-procedure length of the tube is less than 5 cm.

The intraoperative placement of tubal stents resulted in a much easier and faster operation and is now performed routinely in all of our laparoscopic tubal reversals. Contrary to our expectations, however, it did not significantly improve our pregnancy rate. Nevertheless, we do advocate its use, especially at the beginning of the learning curve of this technically challenging procedure.

In cases where the tubes are not repairable (e.g., a total pre-procedure tubal length less than 5 cm, unilateral hydrosalpinx, previous fimbriectomy, etc.), we recommend performing a salpingectomy to prevent possible ectopic pregnancies from occurring in the future, exercising the "use-it or lose-it" concept stated earlier in this chapter. If the salpingectomy is performed correctly, compromised ovarian blood supply should be of minimal concern.

Finally, we must also realize that in real time, the data we have presented thus far are constantly subject to change. Since information on new pregnancies is collected on an ongoing basis, and will continue for years to come, we must be very careful when interpreting favorable or negative results until enough time has passed and many more cases are performed by different groups in order to obtain meaningful and more definitive results.

CONCLUSIONS

The role and techniques of traditional microsurgery have paved the way for reproductive surgery and laid the conventional foundation for surgical principles pertaining to tubal reconstructive surgery. We have simply used this foundation as a platform to develop, build, and master laparoscopic applications for tubal surgery. When a meticulous technique is followed, the magnification and clarity of view afforded by laparoscopy, combined with performance of the procedure in a closed environment, makes the laparoscopic approach ideally suited for this kind of surgery. In an organized and well-trained surgical setting, and with proper patient selection based on past experience, laparoscopic tubal surgery has the potential to become the superior and preferred method over the traditional mini-laparotomy/microsurgery technique.

KEY POINTS

■ A proper preoperative evaluation of the ovarian reserve and male factor are important determinants as to whether the patient will be best served by having a laparoscopic tubal anastomosis or in vitro fertilization.

■ Age of the female patient at surgery is a major factor in the overall success of the procedure.

■ Proper preparation of both the proximal and distal tubal stumps is the most important part of the entire procedure, and the one that will ultimately determine the success or failure of the operation.

■ The innovative use of the stent easily placed transcervically greatly facilitates the performance of the tubal anastomosis.

■ For isthmic-to-isthmic anastomosis, use *interrupted* stitches placed at 6, 3, 9, and 12 o'clock positions, in that sequence without penetrating the tubal lumen, incorporating muscularis and serosa together.

■ For isthmic-to-ampullary or ampullary-to-ampullary anastomosis, use a *continuous* running suture. Great care should be applied to avoid placing the suture into the lumen on the isthmic portion, but through and through stitches in the ampullary section is fine since the muscularis layer is almost nonexistent, and penetration of the tubal lumen is inconsequential due to its large diameter.

■ Perform an HSG twelve weeks post-op to evaluate tubal patency.

REFERENCES

1. Lungren SS. A case of c-section twice successfully performed on the same patient: remarks on the time, indications and details of the operation. *Am J Obstet Gynecol* 1881;14:76.
2. Ryder RM, Vaughan MC. Laparoscopic tubal sterilization: methods, effectiveness and sequelae. *Obstet Gynecol Clin North Am* 1999;26(1)83–97.
3. Meyer JH. A five year experience with laparoscopic tubal ligation by falope ring application. *Int J Gynecol Obstet* 1982;20(3):183–7.
4. Dominik R, et al. Two randomized controlled trials comparing the Hulka and Filshie clips for tubal sterilization. *Contraception* 2000;62(4):169–75.
5. Mackay AP, Kieke BA, et al. Tubal sterilizations in the Unites States 1994–96. *Fam Plann Perspect* 2001;33(4):161–65.
6. Liskin KL, Rinehart W, et al. Minilaparotomy and laparoscopy: safe, effective and widely used. *Popul Rep* 1985;C9, C125–67.
7. Lundin K, Suderland B, et al. The relationship between sperm morphology and rates of fertilization, pregnancy and spontaneous abortion in an IVF-ICSI program. *Hum Reprod* 1997;12(12):2676–81.
8. Yoon TK, Sung HR, et al. Laparoscopic tubal anastomosis: fertility outcome in 202 cases. *Fertil Steril* 1999;72:1121–6.
9. Koh CH, Janick GM. Laparoscopic microsurgical tubal anastomosis. *Obstet Gynecol Clin North Am* 1999;26:189–200.
10. Hendriks DJ, Mol BW, et al. Antral follicle count in the prediction of poor ovarian reserve and pregnancy after in vitro fertilization: a meta-analysis and a comparison with basal FSH level. *Fertil Steril*, 2005;83(2):291–301.
11. Devroey P, Van Steirteghem A, et al. Ten years experience with ICSI. *Hum Reprod Update* 2004;10(1):19–28.
12. Gomel V. Microsurgical reversal of tubal sterilization: a reappraisal. *Fertil Steril* 1980;33:587–97.
13. Wiegereinck M, Roukema M, et al. Sutureless reanastomosis by laparoscopy vs. microsurgical reanastomosis by laparotomy for sterilization reversal: a matched cohort study. *Hum Reprod* 2005;20(8):2355–8.
14. Stadmauer L, Sauer M. Reversal of tubal sterilization using laparoscopically placed staples: preliminary experience. *Hum Reprod* 1997;12:647–9.
15. Margossian H, Garcia-Ruiz A, Falcone T, et al. Robotically assisted laparoscopic tubal anastomosis in a porcine model: a pilot study. *J Laparoendosc Adv Surg Tech* 1998;8:69–73.
16. Kao LW, Giles HR. Laser assisted tubal anastomosis. *J Reprod Med* 1995;40:585–9.
17. Hasson HM, Rotman C, Rana N, et al. Open laparoscopy: 29-year experience. *Obstet Gynecol*, 2000;96(5)P1:763–6.
18. Gelbaya TA, Nardo LG, Fitzgerald CT, et al. Ovarian response to gonadotropins after laparoscopic salpingectomy or the division of fallopian tubes for hydrosalpinges. *Fertil Steril* 2006;85(5):1464–8.
19. Moon HS, Joo BS, Park SJ, et al. Effective method and successful pregnancy in microsurgical tubal reanastomosis: a report of 715 cases. *Fertil Steril* 2000;74(3):S201.
20. Hanafi MM. Factors affecting the reproductive outcome after microsurgical tubal ligation reversal. *Fertil Steril* 2002;78(S1):S113.

11

Tubal Microsurgery versus Assisted Reproduction

Shawky Z. A. Badawy, Frances Shue, Jennifer Shinners

ANATOMY OF THE FALLOPIAN TUBE

The fallopian tube develops as part of the paramesonephric ducts. These ducts develop as invaginations of the celomic epithelium around the four to six weeks of embryonic life after fertilization. The proximal portion of the paramesonephric ducts will lead to the development of the fallopian tubes. The distal portions will lead to the development of the uterus, cervix, and upper part of the vagina (1).

The human fallopian tube varies in length between 7 and 14 cm, with an average of 10 cm. It has various segments that vary in length and lumen diameter. The interstitial portion of the fallopian tube is contained within the cornual portion of the uterus, and it is about 1 cm in length. This will lead to the isthmic portion of the fallopian tube, which is about 2–3 cm in length and a lumen about 1 mm in diameter. The isthmus then is connected to the ampulla of the fallopian tube, which is the longest portion of the tube about 5–7 cm. The lumen is about 1–2 mm in diameter. This will lead after that to the infundibulum, which is about 3 cm wide and leads to the fimbrial end of the fallopian tube. The fimbria embrace the ovary, and this is assisted with the longest fimbria known as fimbriaovarica especially around the time of ovulation, and this process is important in the ovum pickup phenomena (2–4).

The fallopian tube has a muscle wall and is lined with an epithelial layer. The muscle wall at the isthmus of the tube has three layers including an inner and outer longitudinal layers and a middle circular layer. As the muscle layer expands toward the distal end of the fallopian tube, it gets thinner. The lumen of the tube is lined with epithelial layer that has four types of cells: ciliary, secretory, intercalary, and peg cells. The intercalary and peg cells are nonfunctioning. The functions of the ciliary and secretory cells are essential for the embryo survival and its motion toward the uterine cavity (Figure 11.1).

The blood supply to the fallopian tube includes both arterial and venous blood. The arterial blood supply comes from branches of the ovarian artery and the uterine artery. These branches meet in the mesosalphinx, and tributaries from them supply the fallopian tube. The venous drainage follows the arterial blood supply. A part of it goes to the uterine vein, and part of it goes to the ovarian vein. The lymphatic drainage follows the course of the venous drainage.

The fallopian tube has both sympathetic and parasympathetic nerve supply. The sympathetic fibers are part of the sympathetic network originating at thoracic five to ten, and the parasympathetic fibers come from sacral two to four. This is part of the nerve supply to the rest of the paramesonephric duct system.

The function of the fallopian tube is to achieve the pickup of the oocyte around ovulation time and to facilitate the meeting of the oocyte with the sperm in the distal portion of the fallopian tube where fertilization happens (5). The oocyte remains in the fallopian tube, distal to the ampullary isthmus junction until fertilization happens. That takes about three days. Then, the early embryonic stage of the human development will proceed through the isthmic portion of the fallopian tube to reach the uterus about six days after ovulation. The biological phenomenon of the fallopian tube that helps this function is due to the changes that occur in the cellular lining of the tube as well as the muscle contractility that occurs at the same time. During the proliferative phase of the menstrual cycle, the estrogens will lead to an increase in the size of the secretory as well as ciliary cells. The secretions from the secretory cells are essential to help the survival of the oocyte, sperm, and the developing embryo. This fluid contains glycoproteins and various electrolytes, and that is the basis for developing culture media for in vitro fertilization to mimic the environment within the lumen of the fallopian tube (6). During the luteal phase and with the secretion of progesterone from the ovary, these cells become shorter and less active. In addition to the effect of ovarian steroids, the fallopian tube is also under the effect of various kinds of prostaglandins secreted by the ovary that will help both the ciliary motion as well as the contractility of the muscle wall of the fallopian tube, thus contributing the embryo toward the uterine cavity (7–9).

Both patency and normal anatomy of the fallopian tube are essential for the reproductive process. Disruption of the normal anatomy of the fallopian tube will lead to negative effects on reproduction, depending on the degree of damage.

Along the centuries, the fallopian tube received attention and recognition from scientist because of its significance to the process of reproduction. For example, Herophilus in the third century BC and Soranus 100 years AD described these tubes as structures that carry the female semen from the ovaries to the urinary bladder. However, Galen, 130–200 AD, described the tubes as leading from the ovaries to the uterus, but still he described them as carrying semen. The credit of describing the proper anatomy of the fallopian tube goes to Gabriel Fallopius in 1561. He named the fallopian tube as tuba uteri. Since Gabriel Fallopius till the present time, the fallopian tube has been the subject of many studies to understand the

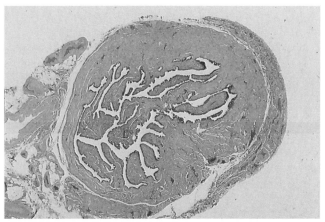

Figure 11.1. Microscopic section of ampullary part of fallopian tube. Normal rugae of mucosa.

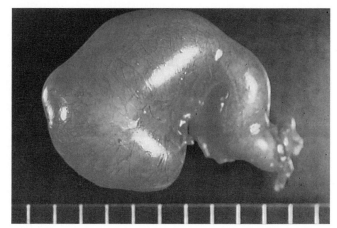

Figure 11.2. Gross picture of hydrosalpinx – marked distension of the fallopian tube, with absent fimbria and complete obstruction of distal end.

pathology that interferes with its proper anatomy and function. Certainly, there are many pathological conditions that affect the fallopian tube and consequently affect human reproduction. As a result, both medical and surgical interventions have been introduced to correct the normal pathology. During the past twenty-eight years, the introduction of in vitro fertilization helped many infertile couples to achieve successes, despite tubal pathology.

TUBAL PATHOLOGY AND EFFECT ON HUMAN REPRODUCTION

Acute and Chronic Salpingitis

Pelvic inflammatory disease results from infections due to *Neisseria gonorrhea*, *Chlamydia trachomatis*, and anerobic bacteria. These sexually transmitted diseases are on the rise. Failure of early diagnoses and treatment results in tubal obstruction and infertility. Ascending infection by the these microorganisms reaches the lumen of the fallopian tube and leads to inflammatory changes, leading to increased vascularity, exudation, and eventually destruction of the mucus membrane lining of the fallopian tube. Furthermore, the infection will spread through the wall of the tube into the peritoneal cavity, leading to pelvic inflammatory disease, and in severe cases, it will lead to tubo-ovarian abscess and cul-de-sac abscess.

Early diagnosis and treatment with antibiotics that cover both aerobic and anaerobic microorganisms may lead to cure of these cases and minimal damage to the fallopian tube. However, many of these infections, especially due to *Chlamydia*, are asymptomatic and the tubal damage might have occurred before these patients receive proper treatment. The end result will be destruction of the lining of the fallopian tubes; therefore, the ciliary cells will be absent from many parts of the lumen of the fallopian tube. The fimbriated end becomes agglutinated, and the secretions in the tube will lead to distention and thinning of the wall of the tube, resulting in the formation of hydrosalpinx (10, 11).

In addition, fibrinous exudates as a result of the infection will lead to the occurrence of peritubal and periovarian adhesions. These adhesions will prevent the proper mechanism of ovum capture around ovulation because of the mechanical

fixation of the tube and ovary to the lateral pelvic wall, posterior surface of the uterus, and cul-de-sac.

In order to prevent all these sequence of events of tubal infection, it is essential to reach an early diagnosis and to be aggressive in the management using intravenous antibiotic therapy. If there is doubt in the diagnosis or there is no response within twenty-four to forty-eight hours, these patients should be taken to the operating room for laparoscopic surgery. This will allow proper diagnosis, drainage of an abscess early enough, and lyses of early adhesions. This has been found to be effective in early cure of these cases and also preservation of fertility potential.

In some situations, the effect of the inflammatory process might be more pronounced on one fallopian tube more than the other. Sometimes, we find during the infertility evaluation using hysterosalpingogram the presence of hydrosalpinx on one side and the other tube is still patent. However, the patent tube may have some microscopic disease that is interfering with pregnancy. Recently, researchers focused on the effect of hydrosalpinx and especially the hydrosalpinx fluid on the fertility potential. The studies demonstrated that patients with hydrosalpinx have low pregnancy rates. Furthermore, in vitro fertilization in patients with hydrosalpinx has a lower implantation and pregnancy rate than in patients without hydrosalpinx (Figure 11.2).

The studies also have shown that the hydrosalpinx fluid affects implantation adversely by washing out the early embryos from the uterus. With the high contents of interleukins and prostaglandins, hydrosalpinx fluid is also toxic to the embryos. The subendometrial vascularity is also decreased in patients with hydrosalpinx. The integrins that are necessary for implantation also have been found to be decreased in the endometrium of patients with hydrosalpinx. Furthermore, recent studies documented the presence of inflammatory reaction and increase in interleukin-2 in the endometrium of patients with hydrosalpinx. This inhibits embryo implantation (12–14).

Hysterosalpingogram studies in patients with hydrosalpinx reveals characteristic picture in which the tube is obstructed distally and distended with the dye. It is very interesting to note that the normal rugae of tubal lumen that are present in a normal fallopian tube are completely absent, and this suggests a poor prognosis for the fallopian tube if neosalpingostomy is done to correct this type of tubal obstruction.

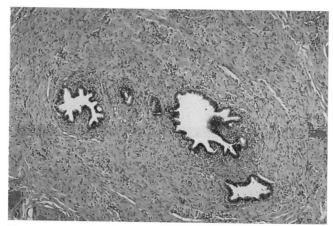

Figure 11.3. Microscopic section of the isthmus of the fallopian tube showing endosalpingiosis (salpingitis isthmica nodosa).

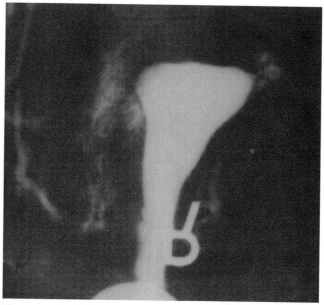

Figure 11.4. Hysterosalpingogram showing salpingitis. Isthmica nodesa (honeycomb appearance).

Salpingitis Isthmica Nodosa

This is a disease process that mostly affects the isthmus of the fallopian tube; however, other segments of the fallopian tube may also be affected (15). It was thought early that this is due to ascending infection from the uterus, and some studies related this process to the IUD use. However, there is no evidence to correlate this type of tubal disease with any infection or IUD use.

Salpingitis ishmica nordosa is now believed to be a proliferative process of the endosalpinx into the myosalpinx, leading to hypertropic process and fibrosis in the wall of the fallopian tube and the isthmus (Figure 11.3). In severe cases, this leads to complete obstruction of the isthmus, and in some cases, the isthmus may be open with a very narrow lumen. The hysterosalpingogram picture in these cases shows a honeycomb appearance, where the dye goes from the tubal lumen into the outgrowing pouches of the endosalpinx into the wall of the fallopian tube. Some investigators called this condition endosalpingiosis (16, 17) (Figure 11.4).

These patients are usually asymptomatic until they present with either infertility or ectopic pregnancy.

Tubal Sterilization

Tubal sterilization is performed for women who completed their family or who have a disease process that contraindicates pregnancy. Patients are usually counseled that this type of technology leads to permanent sterility. However, infertility specialists have been seeing women with history of tubal sterilization presenting for tubal reversal because either they have changed their mind, feeling regret for being sterilized, or getting remarried and wish to have a new family (18). It is essential to review the operative report before committing these patients for microsurgical reconstruction of the fallopian tubes.

Certain types of tubal sterilization are amenable for reversal while others are not. Patients who had salpingectomy, especially with the removal of the fimbriated end of the fallopian tube, are not candidates for the microsurgical tubal reconstruction. Also, patients who have partial salpingectomy with the removal of a large portion of the fallopian tube will not be a good candidate for reconstruction because the remaining tube is going to be short and will not lead to the proper function.

We have to have at least 5–6 cm of the fallopian tube left behind to be able to have a successful outcome. The pregnancy rate after tubal anastomosis improves with the increasing length of the fallopian tube that is left behind. Patients who had Pomeroy tubal sterilization, the use of the clip, or using the ring are all suitable cases for microsurgical tubal anastomosis (Figures 11.5 and 11.6). Laparoscopic tubal coagulation should be evaluated thoroughly because the length of the tubal segment that is coagulated could make a difference. If more than 3 cm of the tube is coagulated, then it will not be suitable for microsurgical tubal anastomosis. This is due to the fact that extension of the thermal damage could occur beyond the 3 cm margin and therefore leaves short healthy segments of the tube that are not amenable to anastomosis. This is especially the case when unipolar coagulation was used (Figure 11.7). The bipolar coagulation is the method of coagulation used these days and therefore

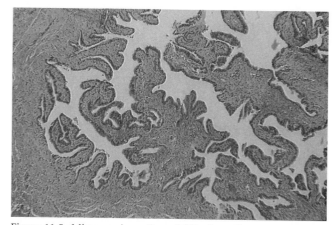

Figure 11.5. Microscopic section of fallopian tube stump removed during tubal anastomosis after Pomeroy sterilization. Note the normal mucosa with normal rugae.

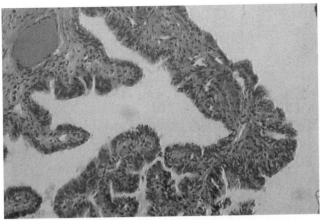

Figure 11.6. Microscopic section of fallopian tube stump removed during anastomosis, after tubal sterilization using falopi ring. Note the healthy tubal mucosa. Hysterosalpingogram showing marked dilatation of the fallopian tube (hydrosalpinx) in an infertile patient.

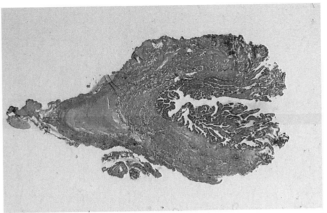

Figure 11.8. Microscopic section of fallopian tube stump removed during anastomosis after tubal sterilization using bipolar cautery. Note the healthy tubal mucosa.

the extent of damage is far less than the unipolar methods (Figure 11.8).

In cases of doubt about the remaining length of the fallopian tube, the surgeon should do laparoscopic evaluation before attempting to do the anastomosis so as to save time and unnecessary surgical intervention. Certainly, cases that are not suitable for microsurgical tubal anastomosis are good candidates for in vitro fertilization.

Endometriosis of the Fallopian Tube

The fallopian tube could be affected with endometriosis directly or indirectly. Endometriosis is a disease process that affects women during reproductive years. The incidence is about 30 percent in women during their reproductive years (19). However, the incidence is certainly higher in women presenting with infertility. Endometriosis affects various areas in the pelvic cavity including the fallopian tubes. The indirect effect of endometriosis on the fallopian tube could be related

to the presence of adhesions that could be filmy or fibrous, fixing the fallopian tube to the ovary or to the lateral pelvic wall. This is the result of a pelvic reaction for the presence of endometriosis. These adhesions will lead to interference with the ovum pickup phenomenon.

The presence of pelvic endometriosis has been shown to lead to activation of the immune system with increase in macrophages, T lymphocytes, and B lymphocytes. The activated macrophages secrete both cytokines and prostaglandins. The concentration of prostaglandin F_{2x} and prostaglandin E_2 has been found to be high in women with pelvic endometriosis compared to normal women. Increased concentration of these types of prostaglandins will lead to tubal dysfunction in the form of either increased motility or decreased motility, depending on the concentration of both these prostaglandins. It also will lead to dysfunction of the ciliary action in the endosalpinx. Because of all these phenomenon, either interference with the ovum pickup will occur or, if the ovum gains access to the fallopian tube, it might go through the tube very quickly and will lose its chance for fertilization (20–23).

The presence also of high concentrations of cytokines, especially interleukin-1, could be an important factor in infertility since these cytokines are known to be toxic to the embryo (24).

The direct involvement of the tube with endometriosis is also known. Endometriosis lesions can be found on the wall of the fallopian tube involving the serosa and may be the muscle wall (Figure 11.9). In severe cases, the muscle wall could be seriously affected, which will lead to severe fibrotic reaction and may be obstruction of the lumen of the fallopian tube. Usually, this fallopian tube is patent and the fimbria are not involved except when they are surrounded with peritubal adhesions. This is completely different from the involvement of the fallopian tube in pelvic inflammatory disease. The endosalpinx in cases with tubal endometriosis is usually intact.

MICROSURGERY FOR TUBAL DISEASE

During the past thirty years, the field of reproductive surgery witnessed great advances that have been utilized for correction of pelvic pathology, in general, and tubal obstruction, in particular. Laparoscopy, laser, and microsurgery were added to

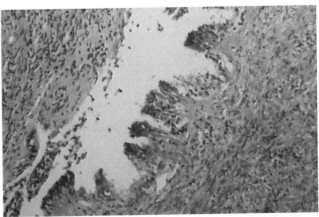

Figure 11.7. Microscopic section of fallopian tube stump removed during tubal anastomosis following unipolar coagulation for sterilization. Note the absence of tubal mucosa in part of the lumen and fimbriotic changes in tubal wall.

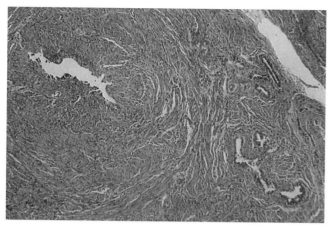

Figure 11.9. Microscopic section of the fallopian tube with ectopic endometrium representing endometriosis.

our specialty, and the use of these technologies improved the outcome for the treatment of infertility in women with pelvic pathology (25, 26).

The principles of microsurgery include proper and gentle handling of the tissues, proper hemostasis using bipolar forceps, intermittent irrigation of the tissues using lactated ringers solution with heparin and hydrocortisone, and the use of non-reactive suture material (15). The implementation of these principles will keep the tissues under normal physiological conditions during surgery and will prevent scar tissue formation. Furthermore, at the end of the surgery, the use of barrier methods to cover the site of surgery adds to the technology for prevention of adhesions. In our division, we use Interecede, which is a reduced oxidized cellulose membrane that adheres to the tissues and then becomes gelatinous and is reabsorbed within one week. During this time, healing would have occurred, and therefore, this barrier technology prevents adhesions between the surgical site and intestines or omentum.

Salpingostomy is a technique used to open the distal end of the fallopian tube. This is mostly in cases of hydrosalpinx (27). Usually, the fimbriated end of the tube is agglutinated. This salpingostomy could be done laparoscopically or by laparotomy. Laparoscopically, we use CO_2 laser to open the tube by a cruciate incision. Following that, the CO_2 laser power is reduced and the laser beam is defocused and the serosal edge near the new osteum is vaporized, thus averting the mucosa over the serosa. Some surgeons may use the harmonic scapel or the bovie to open the tube. The thermal effect is far less with the use of laser and harmonic scapel than using the bovie.

Tubal anastomosis is the procedure used to correct the obstruction resulting from tubal sterilization. In this technology, the obstructed stumps of the tubes are excised and the tubal lumens are tested for patency. The proximal end is tested by using retrograde hydrotubation through a catheter inserted into the uterus preoperatively and connected to a syringe containing indigo carmine. The patency of the distal end of the tube is tested using an angiocatheter connected to an indigo carmine syringe. The angiocatheter is fed through the new opening of the tube and it is then tested. Following establishment of the patency of both ends of the tube, the process of anastomosis begins. Usually, the mesosalpinx is approximated first and, in our division, using 7.0 Prolene interrupted

sutures. Following that the anastomosis of the ends of the tube is done in two layers: the first layer is muscle to muscle using 8.0 nylon sutures in an interrupted fashion at 6, 3, and 9, and 12 o'clock positions and second layer using 8.0 nylon interrupted sutures, seromuscular, to complete the anastomosis. At the end, we do hydrotubation to confirm that the tube, as a whole, is patent. The same procedure is usually done on the other tube if there is enough length.

Usually, in all these cases of tuboplasty, magnification is essential. We use a microscope that has proper soft light and has various control systems for focusing, zooming, and moving it to the proper field. This is usually accomplished by handles attached to the head of the scope and available to the surgeon. In addition, the procedure is televised to monitors in the operating room so both the nursing staff and anesthetist can follow the technique until its end.

Surgical management of endometriosis of the fallopian tube follows the same principles of dealing with endometriosis of the pelvic cavity, and this could be accomplished by the use of CO_2 laser or harmonic scalpel or microcautery. The endometriotic lesions are destroyed or vaporized. Adhesions are lysed. Endometriomas are excised. Raw areas are covered with Intercede as a measure to prevent adhesions (28).

There has been a debate among fertility specialists whether microsurgery for the fallopian tube in the presence of tubal disease is appropriate and can lead to a good success rate. Some colleagues believe that all these cases should go to in vitro fertilization and that will be more cost effective. Unfortunately, in this day and age, the choice of the procedure has been guided by the insurance coverage in the United States. Sometimes, insurance covers surgical reconstruction of the fallopian tube, but in other situations it only covers in vitro fertilization. The reproductive surgeon and the infertility specialist must apply their knowledge and experience in defining those cases that will benefit mostly from reconstructive surgery as compares to cases that will mostly benefit from the application of in vitro fertilization. We also have to be able to counsel our patients properly for the cost, the success rate, complications, and the long-term outcome (29, 30).

The results of surgery for proximal tubal disease showed a pregnancy rate of 34 percent with macrosurgery as compared to 68 percent following microsurgery. It is also noted that among women who wanted to have another pregnancy, about half of them achieved success (31–33).

Proximal tubal disease also could be treated using tubal catheterization, which is a technology in which soft Teflon catheters could be introduced into the cornual and isthmic portion of the fallopian tube through the uterus. This is usually accomplished either by hysteroscopy or by interventional radiology technology. The pregnancy rate after this technology is about 12.8 percent, up to 36 percent (34, 35).

The pregnancy rate after salpingostomy for hydrosalpinx varies between 14.5 and 33 percent. The success rate after fimbrioplasty is better because of the intact fimbria, and the pregnancy rate is up to 51.4 percent (36–38).

It is also to be noted that the ectopic pregnancy rate after tubal surgery for proximal and distal obstruction is high in the range of 10 percent for the proximal tubal obstruction and up to 16.5 percent for the distal tubal obstruction. Certainly, in vitro fertilization in these situations might lead to a better pregnancy rate and reduction in the ectopic pregnancy rate, especially in the cases in which these tubes are removed surgically prior to assisted reproduction. Cochrane studies and meta-analysis studies certainly confirm the fact that pregnancy rate with in vitro fertilization is higher when the *hydrosalpinges* are removed. Furthermore, a unilateral hydrosalpinx that is surgically removed improves the chances of having a spontaneous pregnancy (39, 40). A retrospective study showed a pregnancy rate of 88 percent in an average of 5.6 months following the surgery of unilateral hydrosalpinx (41).

Microsurgical tubal anastomosis following tubal sterilization is very highly successful, with a pregnancy rate of 55–85 percent (42, 43). The pregnancy rate is found to be higher in patients younger than thirty-five years. Most of these cases are done through laparotomy with proper approximation of the segments of the fallopian tube in two layers. Laparoscopic tubal anastomosis has been tried with 70 percent pregnancy rate; however, the number of these cases are small and, therefore, there is no comparison with the laparotomy approach (44).

Lyses of adhesions is usually done with laparoscopy for peritubal and periovarian adhesions. Usually, in these cases, the rest of the fallopian tube with the fimbria are intact. The pregnancy rate has been reported to be up to 50–60 percent (45, 46).

IN VITRO FERTILIZATION FOR TUBAL DISEASE

In vitro fertilization was introduced in the late 1970s as a treatment of tubal factor infertility. The main indication is tubal disease leading to obstruction, with or without prior tuboplasty. With the improved technology for in vitro fertilization, the success rate has improved and many reproductive endocrinologists and fertility specialists use this technology, not only for tubal disease but also for other factors leading to infertility (47). Several studies have shown the success rate of in vitro fertilization to be equivalent or sometimes better for tubal disease compared to surgical correction. Results of in vitro fertilization for tubal disease from Cornell Medical Center revealed a cumulative pregnancy rate for cycles one to four at 32, 59, 70, and 77 percent, respectively. The results also showed that there is a decline in the pregnancy rate with advancing age. The authors of this study stated that the options between microsurgery and the in vitro fertilization should not be regarded as competitive but rather complimentary in order to achieve a successful outcome (29).

Other investigators have the same conclusions regarding the selection of the patients that will benefit most from microsurgery through laparotomy or laparoscopy, and these cases are tubal sterilization reversal and also adhesions without fimbrial damage. In such indications, the live birth rates were reported to be 60–80 percent for the microsurgical tubal anastomosis and 45–65 percent for lyses of adhesions. These authors also stated that such approach certainly will have a high pregnancy rate, but there is also a marked decrease in the risk for ovarian hyperstimulation syndrome and also multiple-birth pregnancies. These are certainly very important aspects that have to be taken into consideration in counseling and treating these patients.

There is also agreement in the literature about the management of hydrosalpinx. These patients will benefit more from in vitro fertilization with a high success rate after removal of these diseased fallopian tubes. The data show that the odds ratio of pregnancy is 1.75 and ongoing pregnancy and live birth is 2.13.

These authors concluded that laparoscopic salpingectomy should be considered before in vitro fertilization for all patients with hydrosalpinx. Furthermore, other studies concluded that salpingectomy for hydrosalpinx was followed by better implantation rate and clinical pregnancy rate in comparison to untreated tubal disease for in vitro fertilization (39).

There have been suggestions that microsurgery for tubal disease is something of the past, and all these patients should go ahead and register for in vitro fertilization. Reviewing all the data in the literature and also my personal experience leads me to the important conclusion that many others in this field have also supported that microsurgery for tubal disease and pelvic pathology is an essential part of our specialty. Certainly, selection of cases based on proper diagnostic methods is important in order to decide which patients will benefit most from microsurgery and which patients will benefit most from in vitro fertilization technology. Both aspects are essential for our specialty, and they are complimenting each other to improve the pregnancy rate for our infertile population (48–51).

KEY POINTS

- Information regarding the anatomy and pathophysiology of the fallopian tube may be obtained by various tests that are essential in the workup of a patient who desires fertility workup. These tests include hysterosalpingogram and laparoscopy. Hysterosalpingogram will lead to the diagnosis of certain pathological conditions such as salpingitis isthmica nodosa and hydrosalpinx. Laparoscopy is an excellent method of diagnosis of other pelvic conditions including peritubal and periovarian adhesions and endometriosis.
- The etiology of tubal obstruction includes tubal sterilization, chronic salpingitis leading to hydrosalpinx, salpingitis isthmica nodosa, and involvement of the fallopian tube with endometriosis as part of the pelvic involvement or rarely specific to the fallopian tube.
- Microsurgery introduced in the 1970s has added a great dimension to the management of tubal disease by reproduction surgeons. The success rate increased. It gave an excellent chance for patients who have chronic tubal disease, and the improvement by the use of microsurgery has been of great dimension. In the 1980s, the use of laser surgery for pelvic disease has also had a positive impact on the outcome of tubal surgery.
- The introduction of in vitro fertilization in the late 1970s certainly added a new dimension to the treatment of the infertile couple, especially those that have tubal disease that failed to respond to surgical interventions or could not be corrected surgically. An example in place is the treatment of a large hydrosalpinx. Microsurgical neosalpingostomy leads to a pregnancy rate less than 30 percent. However, removal of this hydrosalpinx surgically followed by in vitro fertilization leads to a better success rate.
- There has been a debate whether microsurgery is obsolete or an item of the past and all these patients will be treated with in vitro fertilization. It is my opinion and others in the field that both microsurgery and in vitro fertilization should be two methodologies that are available to patients with tubal disease. Assessment of tubal disease is essential, and selection of the cases for either line of treatment is an important duty for the reproductive surgeon and endocrinologist.

REFERENCES

1. Arey LB. Developmental Anatomy, 7th Edition. Philadelphia: WB Saunders, 1965: 295.

2. Warwick R, Williams TL. Gray's Anatomy 35th D. Edition. Philadelphia: WB Saunders, 1973:1354.

3. Pauerstein CJ. The Fallopian Tube—A Reappraisal. Philadelphia: Lea and Febiger, 1974.

4. Hafez ESE, Black DL. The mammalian utero-tubal junction. In Hafez ESE, Blandau RJ (Eds.), The Mammalian Oviduct: Comparative Biology and Methodology. Chicago: The University of Chicago Press, 1969:85.

5. Gordts S, Campo R, Rombauts L, Brosens I. Endoscopic visualization of the process of fimbrial ovum retrieval in the human. Hum Reprod 1998;13:1425–8.

6. Leese HJ, Tay JI, Reischl J, Downing SJ. Formation of fallopian tubal fluid: role of a neglected epithelium. Reproduction 2001; 121:339–346.

7. Surrey ES. Falloposcopy. Obstet Gynecol Cl North America 1999;26:53–62.

8. Donnez J, Casanas-Roux F, Caprasse J, et al. Cyclic changes in ciliation, cell height, and mitotic activity in human tubal epithelium during reproductive life. Fertil Steril 1985;43:554–9.

9. Jansen RPS. Endocrine response in the fallopian tube. Endocr Rev 1984;5:525–51.

10. Patton DL, Moore DE, Spadoni LR, et al. A comparison of the fallopian tube's response to overt and silent salpingitis. Obstet Gynecol 1989;73:622–30.

11. Vasquez G, Winston RML, Boeckx W, et al. The epithelium of human hydrosalpinges: a light optical in the scanning microscopic study. Br J Obstet Gynecol 1983;90:764–70.

12. Blazar AS, Hogan JW, Seifer DB, Frishman GN, Wheeler CA, Haning RV. The impact of hydrosalpinx on successful pregnancy in tubal factor infertility treated by in-vitro fertilization. Fertil Steril 1997;67:517–20.

13. Vandromme J, Chasse E, LeJeune B, VanRysselberg M, Delvigne A, LeRoy F. Hydrosalpinges in in-vitro fertilization unfavorable prognostic feature. Hum Reprod 1995;10:576–9.

14. Copperman AB, Wells V, Luna M, Kalir T, Sandler B, Mukherjee T. Presence of hydrosalpinx correlated to endometrial inflammatory response in-vivo. Fertil Steril 2006;85(4):972–6.

15. Rizk B, Abdalla H. Tubal factor and fertility. In Rizk B, Abdalla H (Eds.), Infertility and Assisted Reproductive Technology. Chapter I.3. Oxford, UK: Health Press, 2008, 60–1.

16. Jenkins CS, Williams SR, Schmidt GE. Salpingitis isthmica nodosa: a review of the literature, discussion of clinical significance and consideration of patient management. Fertil Steril 1993;60:599–607.

17. McComb PF, Rowe TC. Salpingitis isthmica nodosa: evidence—it is a progressive disease. Fertil Steril 1989;51:542–4.

18. Hillis SD, Marchbanks PA, Taylor LR, Peterson HB. Post sterilization regret: findings from the United States Collaborative Review of Sterilization. Obstet Gynecol 1999;93:889–95.

19. Rizk B, Abdalla H. Epidemiology and pathogenesis. In Rizk B, Abdalla H (Eds.), Endometriosis. Chapter 1. Abingdon, Oxford: Health Press Limited, 2003; 9–12.

20. Badawy SZA, Marshall L, Cuenca V. Peritoneal fluid prostaglandins in various stages of the menstrual cycle: role in infertile patients with endometriosis. Int J Fertil 1985;30(2):48–52.

21. Badawy SZA, Cuenca V, Marshall L et al. Cellular components in peritoneal fluid in patients with and without endometriosis. Fertil Steril 1984;42:704.

22. Badawy SZA, Marshall L, Gabal AA et al. The concentration of 13, 14-dihydro-15- keto prostaglandin F2alpha and prostaglandin E2 in peritoneal fluid of infertile patients with and without endometriosis. Fertil Steril 1982;38:166.

23. Rizk B, Abdalla H (2003). Endometriosis and fertility. In Endometriosis. Abingdon, Oxford: Health Press Limited, 2003; chapter 2, 32–40.

24. Fakih H, Baggett B, Holtz G et al. Interleukin-1: a possible role in the infertility associated with endometriosis. Fertil Steril 1987;47:213–17.

25. Gomel V. Tubal reanastomosis by microsurgery. Fertil Steril 1977;28:59–65.

26. Winston RM. Microsurgical tubocornual anastomosis for reversal of sterilization. Lancet 1977;1:284–5.

27. Dubuisson JB, Chapron C, Morice P, Aubriot FX, Foulot H, deJoliniere JB. Laparoscopic salpingostomy: fertility results according to the tubal mucosal appearance. Hum Reprod 1994;9:334–9.

28. Rizk B, Abdalla H. Surgical treatment of endometriosis. In Rizk B, Abdalla H (Eds.), Endometriosis. Abingdon, Oxford, United Kingdom: Health Press Limited, 2003; chapter 2, 71–80.

29. Benadiva CA, Kligman I, Davis O, Rosenwaks Z. In-vitro fertilization versus tubal surgery: is pelvic reconstructive surgery obsolete? Fertil Steril 1995;64(6):1051–61.

30. Novy MJ. Tubal surgery of IVF-making the best choice in the 1990s. Int J Fertil Menopausal Stud 1995;40(6):292–7.

31. Honore GM, Holden AEC, Schenken RS. Pathophysiology and management of proximal tubal blockage. Fertil Steril 1999; 71:785–95.

32. Dubuisson JB, Chapron C, Ansquer Y, Vacher-Lavenui MC. Proximal tubal occlusion: is there an alternative to microsurgery? Hum Reprod 1997;12:692–8.

33. Gillett WR, Clarke RH, Herbison GP. First and subsequent pregnancies after tubal microsurgery: evaluation of the fertility index. Fertil Steril 1997;68:1033–42.

34. Woolcott R, Petchpud A, O'Donnell P, Stanger J. Differential impact on pregnancy rate of selective salpingography, tubal catheterization and wire guide recanulization in the treatment of proximal fallopian tube obstruction. Hum Reprod 1995;10:1423–6.

35. Lang EK, Dunaway HH. Recanalization of the obstructed fallopian tube by selective salpingography and transvaginal bougie dilatation outcome and cost analysis. Fertil Steril 1996;66:210–15.

36. Aboulghar MA, Mansour RT, Serour GI. Controversies in the modern management of hydrosalpinx. Hum Reprod Update 1998;98:637–42.

37. Winston RML, Margara RA. Microsurgical salpingectomy is not an obsolete procedure. Br J Obstet Gynecol 1991;98:637–42.

38. Andeburt AJM, Pouly JL, Theobold PV. Laparoscopic fimbrioplasty: an evaluation of 35 cases. Hum Reprod 1998;13:1496–9.

39. Johnson NP, Mak W, Sowter MC. Surgical treatment for tubal disease in women due to undergo in-vitro fertilization. Cochrane Data Base Syst Rev 2001;(3):CD002125.

40. Mardesic T, Muller P, Huttelova R, Zvarova J, Hulvert J, Voboril J, Becvarova V, Mikova M, Landova K, Jirkovsky M. Effect of salpingectomy on the results of IVF in women with tubal sterility—prospective study. Ceska Gynekol 2001;66(4):259–64.

41. Sagoskin AW, Lessey BA, Mottla GL, et al. Salpingectomy or proximal tubal occlusion of unilateral hydrosalpinx increases the potential for spontaneous pregnancy. Hum Reprod 2003;18:2634–7.

42. Hanafi MM. Factors affecting pregnancy rate after microsurgical reversal of tubal ligation. Fertil Steril 2003;80:434–40.

43. Kim SH, Shin CJ, Kim JG, Moon SY, Lee JY, Chang YS. Microsurgical reversal of tubal sterilization: a report on 118 cases. Fertil Steril 1997;68(5):865–70.

44. Bissonnette F, Lapense L, Bowzayen R. Outpatient laparoscopic tubal anastomosis and subsequent fertility. Fertil Steril 1997; 72(3):542–52.

45. Hull MGE, Fleming CF. Tubal surgery versus assisted reproduction: assessing their role in infertility therapy. *Curr Opin Obstet Gynecol* 1995;7:160–7.

46. Milingos S, Kallipoliis G, Loukradis D, et al. Adhesions: laparoscopic surgery versus laparotomy. *Am NY Acad Sci* 2000; 900:272–85.

47. Rizk B, Abdalla H. In vitro fertilization. In Rizk B, Abdalla H (Eds.), Infertility and Assisted Reproductive Technology. Chapter III.1. Oxford, UK: Health Press, 2008; 160–2.

48. Palagiano A. Female infertility: the tubal factor. *Minerva Ginecol* 2005;57(5):537–43.

49. El-Mowafi DM, Ngoh NN. Management of tubal obstructions. *Surg Technol Int* 2005;14:199–212.

50. Strandell A, Lindhard A, Eckerlund I. Cost-effectiveness analysis of salpingectomy prior to IVF, based on a randomized controlled trial. *Hum Reprod* 2005;20(12):3284–92.

51. Gomel V, McComb PF. Microsurgery for tubal infertility. *J Reprod Med* 2006;51(3):177–84.

12

THE FUTURE OF OPERATIVE LAPAROSCOPY FOR INFERTILITY

Camran Nezhat, Bulent Berker

CURRENT TRENDS

There is little consensus regarding the composition of the ideal evaluation of the couple experiencing infertility. Validation of the most cost-effective, productive, and minimally invasive means of completing the infertility evaluation is an evolving art requiring a critical eye, willingness to learn new techniques, and a desire to best serve the interests of our patients. A diagnosis of unexplained infertility is usually made only after it has been demonstrated that the female partner ovulates regularly, has patent Fallopian tubes, shows no evidence of peritubal adhesions, fibroids or endometriosis, and has a partner with normal sperm production and function. Only when all standard clinical investigations yield normal results should the diagnosis of unexplained infertility be raised (1). This means that for an optimal evaluation of an infertile woman, optimal assessment of the morphology of the pelvic cavity, uterus, and the tubes demands the utilization of laparoscopy. The principal options for the evaluation of the morphology of the uterus and tubes are hysterosalpingography (HSG) and laparoscopy with hydrotubation. The two techniques are complementary, but there is considerable pressure to simplify the investigation and the cost/benefit calculation tends to favor hysterosalpingography (2). Whereas, one should keep in mind that, in infertile couples, laparoscopy reveals abnormal findings in twenty one to sixty eight percent of cases with a normal HSG (3).

Laparoscopy allows for the comprehensive evaluation of the pelvis and uterus including confirmation of tubal patency and evaluation of tubo-ovarian relationships. Although there is a tendency to leave out the laparoscopy during the infertility workup, pelvic adhesions, endometriosis, and tubal disease can be assessed and, in most circumstances, simultaneously treated in a relatively noninvasive outpatient procedure during laparoscopic approach (4). The additional value of laparoscopy over a normal HSG depends not only on the prevalence of disclosed pathology but also on the contribution of the diagnostic laparoscopy with regard to the decision of which treatment should be applied. Although time is of the essence in many clinical cases, the installation of laparoscopic treatment into the management of infertility early on could alleviate the need to continually expose patients to fertility medicines by altering the treatment strategy. This approach may also improve the results of assisted reproductive treatment (5).

Has the obituary of laparoscopy for infertility surgery been written? Although we agree that the sun has set on laparotomy for infertility surgery, a role for laparoscopy in the treatment of infertility unquestionably remains. Clearly, artificial reproductive technology (ART) represents an effective treatment option for the treatment of infertility. However, concerns exist regarding ART outcomes. In view of these concerns, other treatment strategies that obviate ART may be more desirable for appropriately selected couples. In particular, laparoscopy represents an effective alternative to ART for women with tubal disease/hydrosalpinx, leiomyoma, endometriosis, and/or unexplained infertility.

IVF AND ICSI CONCERNS

Increasingly, with the advances made in the ART, there is a move away from a "diagnostic workup" toward a "prognosis-orientated approach" to the investigation and treatment of infertility. Unfortunately, however, ART are sometimes used to treat incompletely evaluated patients; women are recommended to proceed to ART following an accelerated and often incomplete workup. Because of the remarkable progress in the availability and success of IVF-embryo transfer, it has been assumed that more liberal use of this and other ART is warranted as part of routine infertility treatment. Consequently, irrespective of the fact that certain conditions dictate the use of advanced therapy early in the workup, IVF increasingly is being used as the prime intervention in newly established infertility approaches. By current estimates, 1 percent of infants born in the United States are conceived through ART. Yet, there are concerns associated with ART. Several investigators have reported increased complications associated with ART conceptions, to include an odds ratio of 2.2 for congenital anomaly and an odds ratio of 1.6 for intrauterine growth restriction. Additionally, a recent meta-analysis revealed an increased risk of preterm delivery (OR 1.95) and perinatal mortality (OR 2.19) in singleton gestations conceived via ART (6). These obstetric and neonatal risks are even greater for multiple gestations, an occurrence reaching epidemic proportion in ART conceptions. Of more than 31,000 pregnancies reported in the 2003 SART database, 29 percent were twin gestations and 5.9 percent were gestations with triplets or higher.

In designing practices and policies to improve the success of IVF, at a minimum, providers and patients need to be educated about the risks and adverse outcomes. Multiple gestations and ovarian hyperstimulation syndrome (OHSS) are known complications of ART. The National Center for Health

Statistics recently reported a dramatic increase in multiple births during the past decade (7). From 1995 to 1996 alone, the number of live triplet and higher-order births increased 19 percent and was increased 344 percent since 1980. The report indicates that this increase is due, in part, to an increase in the use of treatments to enhance fertility, such as the use of ovulation stimulation medications and IVF. More than 1.3 million fertility drug prescriptions are filled annually at a cost of $230 million. Data published by the Centers for Disease Control and Prevention indicate that greater than 30 percent of ART births are multiples compared with 2 percent in the general population (8). In addition, 58 percent of multiples are delivered by women who use fertility drugs, with another 22 percent born to women undergoing IVF (7). This increase in the birth of multiples poses significant medical, social, and financial risks.

It is a common belief that multiple pregnancies are a failure rather than a success of the IVF enterprise. The reasons higher-order multiple births are not considered to be a success are many. Medical risks to the mother and the children are significant, and the birth of multiples also may pose psychological, economical, and social harms. Many medical complications result from the fact that multiples are often born prematurely. As a result, many multiples require treatment and extended care in neonatal intensive care units. Multiples may also suffer long-term medical and developmental problems. Multiple births also pose long- and short-term medical risks to women. The maternal risks of a multiple pregnancy include premature labor, premature delivery, pregnancy-induced hypertension, toxemia, gestational diabetes, and vaginal-uterine hemorrhage (9). Gestating multiples may require a woman to spend extended periods of time on bed rest, hospitalization, administration of medication to prevent preterm labor, and even a minor surgical procedure known as cerclage in which the cervix is sewn closed to prevent preterm dilation.

OHSS is another serious complication of ovulation induction. It can vary from being a mild illness to a severe, life-threatening disease requiring hospitalization. Thromboembolic events are a devastating complication of severe OHSS that can occur despite appropriate therapy and can ultimately lead to death. Although the prevalence of the severe form of OHSS is small, it is important to remember that OHSS is usually an iatrogenic complication of a nonvital treatment.

The risk of birth defects in infants born following ART treatment is a controversial question. Most publications examining the prevalence of birth defects in ICSI and IVF infants compared to spontaneously conceived infants have serious methodological limitations; despite this, most researchers have concluded that there is no increased risk. Hansen et al. carried out a systematic review to identify all papers published by March 2003 with data relating to the prevalence of birth defects in infants conceived following IVF and/or ICSI compared with spontaneously conceived infants (10). According to this review, pooled results from all suitable published studies suggest that children born following ART are at increased risk of birth defects compared with spontaneous conceptions. This information should be made available to couples seeking ART treatment.

Controlled ovarian hyperstimulation exposes the ovaries to supraphysiological levels of gonadotropins to result in multiple follicular development for assisted conception. Long-term effect of hormonal fertility treatments on cancer is unknown. In particular, concerns have been raised by some investigators regarding the risk of ovarian malignancy during or after ovarian stimulation. The studies that have adjusted for the effects of confounding factors such as duration of oral contraceptive use and number of pregnancies have noted an increased risk of ovarian cancer among infertile women who remain childless despite long periods of unprotected intercourse (11–13). Whether such women are at risk due to the primary basis for their infertility or factors such as ovulation-inducing drugs has been the subject of several studies. To date, the findings on ovarian cancer risk associated with fertility drug treatment are reassuring, but not definitive. A stronger association has been observed between fertility drug use and borderline tumors of the ovary (14).

Conclusively, the novelty of IVF has attracted a large number of studies on the health of the newborn but less is known about the long-term health effects of IVF on children or about the health effects on the women. Given these concerns, alternatives for the optimization of fertility, where appropriate, deserve consideration. Surgery has demonstrated benefit in the management of a variety of conditions associated with infertility. Laparoscopy has effectively replaced laparotomy in the management of these conditions. This minimally invasive technique is associated with improved cosmesis, less postoperative pain, shorter hospital stay, decreased cost, lower incidence of infectious complications, and lower incidence of de novo adhesion formation.

BENEFITS OF LAPAROSCOPY DURING INFERTILITY WORKUP

Recent advances in endoscopic surgical techniques and the increased sophistication of surgical instruments have offered new operative methods and techniques for the gynecologic surgeon (15). Recent years have witnessed a marked increase in the number of gynecologic endoscopic procedures performed, mainly as a result of technological improvements in instrumentation. The addition of a small video camera to the laparoscope (videolaparoscopy) greatly enhanced the popularity of operative endoscopy because of the possibility of operating in a comfortable, upright position and using the magnification capabilities of the camera (16, 17). Currently, laparoscopy is perceived as a minimally invasive surgical technique that both provides a panoramic view of the pelvic organs and allows surgery at the time of diagnosis. Laparoscopy has become an integral part of gynecologic surgery for the diagnosis and treatment of abdominal and pelvic disorders of the female reproductive organs, including infertility. Endoscopic reproductive surgery intended to improve fertility may include surgery on the uterus, ovaries, pelvic peritoneum, and the Fallopian tubes.

Traditionally, laparoscopy has been the final diagnostic procedure used in infertility investigations. However, as the success rates with IVF improve, clinicians increasingly believe that turning to the ART is appropriate, even without laparoscopy. Also, with the option of IVF, it is often hard to persuade a woman with a normal HSG to undergo an invasive procedure, for example, laparoscopy. It has been stressed that these women often prefer to have IVF, with a good chance of pregnancy (6, 18). However, it is our impression that laparoscopy should be considered before ART cycles, if the procedure diagnoses and treats a pelvic pathology at the same time and if laparoscopic intervention increases the chance of pregnancy following these cycles.

In respect of infertility, the most common pelvic pathologies are adhesions, endometriosis, and hydrosalpinx. However, women with polycystic ovary syndrome and ovarian transposition deserve additional attention. It is the reality that the impatience of treated couples and considerations of health-care cost are of utmost importance and influence the type of diagnostic tools or treatments selected by couples. Omitting laparoscopy from the infertility workup when HSG is normal can increase the cost of fertility treatment without increasing success rates.

Even when tubal patency has been demonstrated by HSG, laparoscopy has been suggested as a mandatory step to rule out the existence of peritubal adhesions as well as endometriosis as causes of infertility. Tanahatoe et al. reported that diagnostic laparoscopy before intrautarine insemination (IUI) revealed some pelvic abnormalities that could result in changing the treatment plan in 25 percent of women with normal hysterosalpingography (19). Twenty-one percent of these pelvic pathologies were stage I or II endometriosis and periadnexal adhesions, which were treated by laparoscopy, followed by IUI. Similarly, Capelo et al. recently evaluated the laparoscopic findings in a group of patients who failed to achieve pregnancy after ovulation induction with clomiphene citrate (20). They found that 35 percent of these patients had stage III or IV endometriosis, pelvic adhesions, or tubal disease, whereas 29 percent had stage I or II endometriosis.

Based on our experience and findings, we recommend the diagnostic approach of laparoscopy in the evaluation of female infertility. Diagnostic laparoscopy combined with operative endoscopic procedures allow prompt and complete identification of all contributory factors, helping the physician to institute appropriate therapy, and will help ensure higher conception rates over shorter intervals. In the recent era of evidence-based medicine, it is recommended that a multicentric prospective randomized study is needed to prove the efficacy of laparoscopic evaluation in predicting the fertility outcome in patients experiencing infertility.

BENEFITS OF LAPAROSCOPY: CURRENT SURGICAL APPLICATIONS

Infertility Outcomes after Laparoscopic Surgical Management of Adhesions

Adhesions may cause infertility by distorting pelvic anatomy and by preventing normal blood supply to the pelvic structures. Periovarian adhesions may constrict the ovarian blood supply and prevent adequate delivery of gonadotrophins and growth factors to the developing follicle (21). In fact, the number of oocytes recovered has been shown to be negatively correlated with the severity of periovarian adhesions. Patients with severe periovarian adhesions have low pregnancy rates and respond poorly to gonadotrophin stimulation during IVF treatment. Although no previous studies have shown the beneficial effects of adhesiolysis prior to IVF, laparoscopic adhesiolysis may have a role in assuring initial access to the ovaries during oocyte recovery and in improving subsequent attempts (22).

The decision to treat adhesions to increase fertility rates may be based on certain prognostic factors associated with future fecundity. Regardless of whether it was performed via microsurgical techniques or via laparoscopy, data show that the removal of filmy adhesions is associated with improved fecundity. In one study, 176 patients with pelvic adhesions suffering from inability to conceive underwent operative laparoscopy and CO_2 laser adhesiolysis (23). According to the severity of adhesions, the patients were categorized by diagnostic laparoscopy as mild, group I; moderate, group II; and severe, group III. After laparoscopic adhesiolysis, all patients were followed for one year. Pregnancy occurred in fifty one (70.8 percent), twenty eight (48.3 percent), and eight (21.6 percent) patients in groups I, II, and III, respectively. Laparoscopic adhesiolysis still remains a useful and effective procedure for infertile couples with pelvic adhesions. This suggests that adhesiolysis might be associated with higher spontaneous pregnancy rates. However, whether laparoscopic adhesiolysis also enhances pregnancy rates after IUI has never been studied. Assuming that the pathophysiological mechanism of peritubal adhesions is based on impaired ovum pickup due to decreased tubal motility, it is likely that laparoscopic adhesiolysis might increase spontaneous pregnancy rates as well as pregnancy rates after IUI (24).

In addition to the severity of the preexisting disease, postoperative adhesion formation is the most important determinant of the success of infertility surgery and is largely responsible for the majority of failures associated with these procedures. An inverse relationship exists between the grade of adhesions and pregnancy rates, regardless of the condition of the adnexa. Increased rate of adhesion formation has been reported in the majority of patients who underwent reproductive surgery by laparotomy (25, 26). When performed by laparotomy, reproductive pelvic surgery procedures are frequently complicated not only by adhesion reformation but also by de novo adhesion formation. However, endoscopic surgery fulfills the important microsurgical principles of gentle handling of tissue, constant irrigation, meticulous hemostasis, and precise tissue dissection without the need for laparotomy, which itself is a significant invasion of the peritoneal cavity. In one of their study, Nezhat et al. demonstrated that endoscopic reproductive surgery was very effective in reducing peritoneal adhesions, was associated with a low frequency of postoperative adhesion recurrence, and almost completely avoided the formation of de novo adhesions (27).

Infertility Outcomes after Laparoscopic Surgical Management of Hydrosalpinx

As it is well known that hydrosalpinx is a chronic pathological condition of the Fallopian tube and is a major cause of infertility. In most patients, the fimbriated end of the tube adjacent to the ovary is occluded and the distal half of the tube is distended with fluid (28). This embryotoxic fluid then seeps proximally into the endometrial cavity where it has deleterious effects on embryo survival and implantation. Clinically, the presence of a hydrosalpinx has negative consequences in terms of implantation, pregnancy, and delivery rates. The observed reduction in pregnancy rates is not ameliorated by ART. The presence of hydrosalpinx can be diagnosed by hysterosalpingogram or by laparoscopy with or without chromopertubation. A meta-analysis of all the studies comparing hysterosalpingography to the gold standard of laparoscopy with chromopertubation showed the hysterosalpingogram to have a sensitivity of 65 percent in the diagnosis of tubal obstruction and a specificity of 83 percent (29, 30). Laparoscopy provides both the certain diagnosis and the treatment of hydrosalpinx at the same session.

Distal tubal occlusion with a hydrosalpinx has been reported to be associated with a lower implantation rate per embryo as well as with a lower clinical pregnancy rate. One meta-analysis demonstrated the deleterious effects of hydrosalpinx on achieving pregnancy in women undergoing IVF. It was shown that the clinical pregnancy rate was about 50 percent lower and the miscarriage rate was more than twofold higher in patients with hydrosalpinx (1,144 IVF cycles) than in the patients without hydrosalpinx (5,569 IVF cycles) (31). In addition, a randomized multicentre trial in Scandinavia on salpingectomy prior to the first cycle of IVF/embryo transfer indicated that clinical pregnancy rates per included patient were 36.6 percent in the salpingectomy group and 23.9 percent in the nonintervention group ($P = 0.067$) and the ensuing delivery rates were 28.6 and 16.3 percent ($P = 0.045$) (32). Finally, patients with a hydrosalpinx have shown significantly lower implantation rates and significantly higher miscarriage and ectopic pregnancy rates than normal controls in donor oocyte cycles (33). There may be a direct effect on embryos as well as an alteration in uterine implantation. The proposed mechanism by which embryo toxicity occurs begins with a leakage of the fluid from the hydrosalpinx into the uterine cavity. This fluid may not only be harmful to embryos but may also have an effect on uterine receptivity and implantation mechanisms. In addition to improving overall pregnancy rates by removal of the diseased tubes, it has been suggested that treatment decreases the rate of miscarriage compared with those with untreated hydrosalpinges (34).

Shelton et al. were the first to conduct a prospective study that demonstrated a positive impact on pregnancy rates in patients with repeated IVF failures by removing the hydrosalpinges (35). Fifteen patients with unilateral or bilateral hydrosalpinges with a history of repeated IVF failures underwent laparoscopic excision of the affected tubes. Because the patients undergoing surgical excision served as their own control, the ongoing pregnancy rate per transfer was 0 percent presalpingectomy. After salpingectomy, the ongoing pregnancy per transfer rate was 25 percent. Improved pregnancy rates were noted for both the fresh and the frozen embryo transfers after surgery. Pregnancy rates can be improved by removal of the hydrosalpinx prior to IVF. A Cochrane review confirmed that the odds of pregnancy were increased with laparoscopic salpingectomy for hydrosalpinges prior to IVF (OR = 1.75, 95 percent CI 1.07 to 2.86), as were the odds of ongoing pregnancy/live birth (OR = 2.13, 95 percent CI 1.24–3.65) (36). All these data demonstrate that laparoscopic salpingectomy for hydrosalpinges is the preferred procedure for improving pregnancy rates. The accumulated clinical evidence led the ASRM Clinical Practice Committee to conclude, "Salpingectomy performed for hydrosalpinx prior to IVF improves subsequent pregnancy, implantation and live birth rates" (37). Consensus exists in the role for laparoscopy in the management of hydrosalpinx-associated subfertility.

Infertility Outcomes after Laparoscopic Surgical Management of Myomas

Uterine leiomyomas are the most common tumor of the female reproductive tract and affect 30–40 percent of reproductive-age women. Although they are seldom the sole cause of infertility, myomas have been linked to fetal wastage and premature delivery. Several elements indicate that myomas are responsible for infertility. For example, pregnancy rate is lower in patients with myomas, and in cases of medically assisted procreation, the implantation rate is lower in patients presenting with interstitial myomas. There are other indirect evidences supporting a negative impact, including lengthy infertility before surgery (unexplained by other factors), and rapid conception after myomectomy. Approximately 50 percent of women who have not previously conceived become pregnant after myomectomy (38).

Additionally, few studies have evaluated the effect of myoma uteri on the pregnancy rate after ART. Eldar-Geva et al. (39) compared 106 ART cycles in patients with uterine fibroids with 318 ART cycles in age-matched patients without fibroids and concluded that implantation and pregnancy rates were significantly lower in patients with intramural or submucosal fibroids, even those with no deformation of the uterine cavity. Stovall et al. (40) showed that even after patients with submucosal fibroids are excluded, the presence of fibroids reduces the efficacy of ART. Therefore, if women with unexplained infertility have a better chance of conception after myomectomy and if the main factors in treatment success are patient age and duration of infertility, this conservative operation should not be postponed for too long.

Since medically treated fibroids tend to grow back or recur, most fibroids that cause symptoms are managed surgically. Depending on their number and their location, myomas with mostly intracavity development should be dealt with by hysteroscopy. Interstitial and subserous myomas can be operated either by laparotomy or by laparoscopy. Technological advancements in endoscopic instrumentation, equipment, and the surgeon's expertise have lead to an ever-increasing number of informed women choosing the advantages of the new and innovative techniques utilizing hysteroscopy and laparoscopy. Laparoscopy is most often employed in women that are diagnosed early when their fibroids are small and more suited to laparoscopic removal. However, new surgical devices called morcellators allow the safe and efficient removal of fibroid tumors much larger than could have been accomplished in the past.

As fertility preservation is one of the primary goals of myomectomy, the marked reduction of adhesion formation by laparoscopic myomectomy (LM) gives it a distinct advantage over laparotomy. The incidence of adhesions following laparotomic myomectomy and laparoscopic myomectomy is nearly 100 percent and 36–67 percent, respectively (41–45). These adhesions can adversely affect fertility, cause pain, and increase the risk of ectopic pregnancy. The factors responsible for prolonged surgical times in LM are the need to morcellate large or multiple fibroids for removal through the trocar and suture repair of the myometrium. In 1994, Nezhat et al. first described laparoscopically assisted myomectomy (LAM) where myoma enucleation was done laparoscopically or through a 5-cm Pfannenstiel minilaparotomy, following which the uterus could be exteriorized for palpation and multilayered open suturing (46). This technique combines the advantages of increased exposure, visibility, and magnification provided by the laparoscope (especially for evaluation of the posterior cul-de-sac and under the ovaries) with the ease of adequate uterine repair and removal of specimen that is associated with minilaparotomy. LAM is a safe alternative to LM and is less difficult and less time consuming. This technique can be used for large (greater than 8 cm), multiple, or deep intramural myomas. Using a combination of laparoscopy and a 2- to 4-cm abdominal incision, uterine defect can be closed in two or three layers to reduce the risk of uterine dehiscence, fistula, and adhesion formation. Women who desire future fertility and require myomectomy for an intramural tumor may benefit from LAM to ensure proper closure of the myometrial incision.

Infertility Outcomes after Laparoscopic Surgical Management of Endometriosis

Although the elucidation of the relationship between infertility and endometriosis is beyond the scope of this chapter, it is well known that endometriosis is frequently associated with infertility. Indeed, 30–70 percent of infertile women have been reported to have endometriosis (47). In 1986, we reported our results for the treatment of endometriosis-associated infertility patients with videolaseroscopy (48). The carbon dioxide laser has been used laparoscopically for the removal of endometriotic implants, excision of endometrioma capsules, and lysis of adnexal adhesions in 102 patients. Of 102 patients presenting with infertility attributed to endometriosis, 60.7 percent conceived within 24 months after laser laparoscopy. The rates of conception after surgery were as follows: 75 percent for patients with mild endometriosis, 62 percent for patients with moderate endometriosis, 42.1 percent for patients with severe endometriosis, and 50 percent for patients with extensive endometriosis. Controversy remains regarding the benefit of surgical treatment of endometriosis in respect of improvement in fecundity at the time of laparoscopy (49, 50). However, because of the progressive nature of the disease in many patients, combined with the largest prospective, randomized trial demonstrating improved fecundity with therapy at the time of surgery, it appears prudent to ablate endometriotic lesions at the time of endoscopic surgery in patients with minimal and mild endometriosis (51–53). Since there are no prospective, randomized studies yet, we are unable to draw any conclusions as to whether endoscopic treatment of advanced endometriosis will improve reproductive outcome; however, there is no reason to be pessimistic. Hence, if the multiple aspects of the reproductive cycle are found to be impaired in women with endometriosis or endometriomas as some investigators claim, it can be normalized by surgery. Supporting this, a 50 percent pregnancy rate was obtained after laparoscopic management in a series of 814 women with endometriomas (54). It could be that the removal or destruction of endometriomas provides further than simply restoring the normal anatomy and ovarian structure.

However, it has been suggested that ovarian surgery in cases of ovarian endometriomas could be deleterious for the residual normal ovarian tissue either by removing ovarian stroma with oocytes together with the capsule or by thermal damage provoked by coagulation. In a case-controlled study, Aboulghar et al. reported that the outcome of IVF in stage IV endometriosis with previous surgery was significantly lower compared with an age-matched group of tubal factor infertility (55). Some investigators reported a marked reduction in the number of both dominant follicles and retrieved oocytes in the operated ovary (56–58). In contrast, others failed to observe this difference (47, 59). The results from randomized trials comparing laser vaporization and stripping enucleation for the treatment of endometrioma are warranted to draw definitive conclusions on this topic. The decreased ovarian response may not be related to the surgical procedure. In this regard, based on histological analysis, it has been reported recently that the ovarian tissue surrounding the cyst wall in endometriomas is morphologically altered and possibly not functional, thus suggesting that a functional disruption may already be present before surgery (60). Therefore, the decreased ovarian response, which may be observed in patients previously treated for a large ovarian endometrioma, may also be a consequence of the disease. This needs to be taken into account when proposing the nonsurgical management of these patients.

With the advances obtained in IVF, a large number of patients, especially when age is a factor, opt to proceed with IVF, without undergoing adequate surgical evaluation and treatment of endometriosis. Although IVF is one of the options that can be offered to an infertile couple with endometriosis, its success rate is lower compared with that of women undergoing IVF for other indications. Numerous studies have compared IVF outcome in terms of fertilization rate, embryo development, and implantation and pregnancy rates in women with endometriosis with other diagnostic entities. The question of whether the presence of endometriosis affects the outcome of women undergoing IVF has not been resolved, with some authors noting negative associations and others noting no association. Recently, in a meta-analysis, Barnhart et al. investigated the IVF outcome for patients with endometriosis (61). It was demonstrated that patients with endometriosis have more than 50 percent reduction in pregnancy rate after IVF compared with women with tubal factor infertility. Multivariate analysis also demonstrated a decrease in fertilization and implantation rates and a significant decrease in the number of oocytes retrieved for endometriosis patients. These data, therefore, suggest that the presence of endometriosis affects multiple aspects of the reproductive cycle, including oocyte quality, embryogenesis, and/or the receptivity of the endometrium. Thus, it is unlikely that the effect of endometriosis is due solely to alterations of normal pelvic anatomy, and an effect on the developing follicle, oocyte, and embryo is suggested. Further evidence of poor oocyte quality, and thus reduced implanting ability of embryos, is strengthened by studies showing no adverse effect on implantation rates in women with endometriosis using donated oocytes, and recipients of oocytes from donors with endometriosis may result in lower implantation rates (52, 53, 62).

However, it is still unclear whether treatment of endometriosis will improve IVF outcomes or not since there are no prospective, randomized, double-blind controlled studies. Published studies are almost exclusively retrospective and observational, which may be affected by bias and confounding. Recently, Donnez et al. have demonstrated that endometrioma surgery did not interfere with the fertilization rate. Also, in the same study, a second analysis was performed on patients with unilateral endometriomas, whereby a paired comparison was made between the ovary that had encountered the vaporization procedure and the contralateral normal ovary of the same patient. No difference in ovarian stimulation was observed (47). However, several studies have concluded that laparoscopic removal of endometriomas before IVF does not improve fertility outcomes (63–65). For example, in their retrospective study, Garcia-Velasco et al. have found that laparoscopic cystectomy for endometriomas before commencing an IVF cycle did not improve fertility outcomes (64). Studies addressing the impact of endometriosis on IVF outcome often fail to take into account the intrinsic diagnostic limitations of ultrasound (66). The resolution obtained with current ultrasound techniques is inadequate to detect smaller endometriomas, and most smaller endometriomas are "true" endometriomas and require complete excision (67, 68), not partial treatment by coagulation (64), if we are expecting the best results. Ultrasound can be used by the clinician to help establish a presumptive diagnosis of ovarian involvement with endometriosis, but laparoscopy is necessary to confirm the diagnosis (69).

Currently, in advanced endometriosis cases, there are no randomized, controlled trials comparing the outcome of endoscopic infertility surgery and IVF to definitively lead us to a conclusion. On the bases of the accumulated data, we believe that laparoscopic diagnosis and treatment of endometriosis will be useful in increasing the probability of conception either spontaneously or with IVF treatment. This should be also valid for patients with multiple IVF failures. Since it is a well-known fact that endometriosis is more prevalent in the setting of infertility, with proper patient selection, a meticulously performed laparoscopic surgery is an excellent option that provides these patients the potential to achieve repeated future pregnancies. Furthermore, patients with previously treated endometriosis prior to IVF may still benefit from endoscopic reevaluation and complete therapy. In a retrospective analysis, we reported our experience with patients who have failed IVF treatment and underwent laparoscopic evaluation and management (70). In our study, twenty two of twenty nine patients (76 percent) achieved pregnancy after laparoscopic treatment for endometriosis. This suggests that, even in the setting of multiple IVF failures, laparoscopic management of endometriosis remains a viable option. It is likely that in many of these women, IVF can still be successful despite the presence of untreated endometriosis. However, bypassing the pelvic factor may not always be sufficient to achieve optimal success. It is our stance that complete and thorough microsurgical eradication of endometriosis allows many patients to conceive without further IVF therapy and may help optimize success for those who require subsequent IVF cycles. Still, many will agree that the use of laparoscopy to diagnose and potentially treat endometriosis in patients who suffer from infertility has been superseded by IVF and sometimes oocyte donation, especially in older patients. The findings of our study add another dimension to management of endometriosis in the setting of infertility and emphasize the importance of keeping laparoscopy in the infertility management equation.

Last but not the least, since it is a well-known fact that endometriosis is more prevalent in the setting of infertility, with proper patient selection, a meticulously performed laparoscopic surgery is an excellent option that provides these patients the potential to achieve repeated future pregnancies. The inability to thoroughly treat the endometriosis might have also been a contributing factor to the contradictory results of the studies. Patients with endometriomas have increased rate of accompanying peritoneal endometriosis also and should be thoroughly treated in those who desire to get pregnant. Another important point is the declining number of endoscopic surgeries being performed in response to the increasing numbers of patients opting for IVF. This phenomenon results in fewer physicians who develop adequate proficiency in performing these technically advanced procedures.

CONCLUSIONS

It is generally thought to be a good clinical practice to establish a diagnosis prior to therapy. Infertility treated with ART alone does not address underlying pelvic pathology. Laparoscopy can diagnose significant pathology and avoid unnecessary treatments. Laparoscopy can treat this pathology and improve spontaneous and IVF pregnancy rates. As always in medicine, the primary saying should be "primum non nocere" ("do no harm"), and we should, therefore, try to avoid two major complications of IVF, namely OHSS and multiple pregnancies.

In the past, no workup of an infertility problem was complete without a diagnostic laparoscopy. More recently, it has been proposed that laparoscopy has its place in certain infertile couples, but not in all. It is not easy to construct algorithms determining the exact place of laparoscopy, but suffice it to say that in couples where the conception is thought possible through ovulation induction or intrauterine insemination, laparoscopy is necessary in all cases where the medical history is suggestive of endometriosis or tubal disease or when the result of tubal patency screening is abnormal.

Careful selection of patients based on clinical history as well as physical examination and noninvasive laboratory techniques will identify those patients most likely to benefit from endoscopic examination for their infertility evaluation. With proper patient selection, laparoscopic infertility surgery is an excellent option that provides patients the potential to achieve repeated future pregnancies.

Technological advances have resulted in a great expansion in the endoscopic techniques available to the reproductive surgeon for the evaluation of the woman with infertility. Advances in endoscopy have revolutionized our approaches to gynecologic surgery. Among reproductive operations, most of them could and should be done by laparoscopy. The variety of conditions indicative of surgery demonstrates the importance of maintaining surgical skills in the reproductive medicine practice, so that patients can be offered the most appropriate treatment. Traditional laparoscopic techniques have not been replaced but rather are complemented by the addition of tubal endoscopy, hysteroscopy, and possibly transvaginal hydrolaparoscopy. Validation of the most cost-effective, productive, and minimally invasive means of completing the infertility evaluation is an evolving art requiring a critical eye, willingness to learn new techniques, and a desire to best serve the interests of our patients. It appears that endoscopic surgery for infertility patients, when performed by an experienced endoscopist, is efficacious and can produce better results than other approaches. Endoscopic surgery is surgery for today and for the future and will continue to create profound changes in the field of reproductive surgery.

KEY POINTS

- ■ Has the obituary of laparoscopy for infertility surgery been written? Although we agree that the sun has set on laparotomy for infertility surgery, a role for laparoscopy in the treatment of infertility unquestionably remains.
- ■ Increasingly, with the advances made in the ART, there is a move away from a "diagnostic workup" toward a "prognosis-orientated approach" to the investigation and treatment of infertility.
- ■ There are concerns associated with ART including increased obstetric and neonatal risks.
- ■ Currently, epidemiological data do not show a link between invasive ovarian cancer risk and gonadotropin use. However, an association does exist between borderline ovarian tumor risk and gonadotropin use.

- Laparoscopy represents an effective alternative to ART for women with tubal disease/hydrosalpinx, leiomyoma, endometriosis, and/or unexplained infertility.
- Salpingectomy performed for hydrosalpinx prior to IVF improves subsequent pregnancy, implantation, and live birth rates. Consensus exists in the role for laparoscopy in the management of hydrosalpinx-associated subfertility.
- The available evidence suggests an important role for pre-ART laparoscopic myomectomy in the management of fibroid-associated infertility.
- It is a well-known fact that endometriosis is more prevalent in the setting of infertility; with proper patient selection, a meticulously performed laparoscopic surgery is an excellent option that provides these patients the potential to achieve repeated future pregnancies.
- Infertility treated with ART alone does not address underlying pelvic pathology. Laparoscopy can diagnose significant pathology and avoid unnecessary treatments. Laparoscopy can treat this pathology and improve spontaneous and IVF pregnancy rates.
- It appears that endoscopic surgery for infertility patients, when performed by an experienced endoscopist, is efficacious and can produce better results than other approaches.
- Endoscopic surgery is surgery for today and for the future and will continue to create profound changes in the field of reproductive surgery.

REFERENCES

1. Fatum M, Laufer N, Simon A. Investigation of the infertile couple: should diagnostic laparoscopy be performed after normal hysterosalpingography in treating infertility suspected to be of unknown origin? *Hum Reprod* 2002;17(1):1–3.
2. Crosignani PG, Rubin BL. Optimal use of infertility diagnostic tests and treatments. The ESHRE Capri Workshop Group. *Hum Reprod* 2000;15(3):723–32.
3. Corson SL, Cheng A, Gutmann JN. Laparoscopy in the "normal" infertile patient: a question revisited. *J Am Assoc Gynecol Laparosc* 2000;7(3):317–24.
4. Surrey ES. Endoscopy in the evaluation of the woman experiencing infertility. *Clin Obstet Gynecol* 2000;43(4):889–96.
5. Nezhat C, Littman ED, Lathi RB, Berker B, Westphal LM, Giudice LC, Milki AA. The dilemma of endometriosis: is consensus possible with an enigma? *Fertil Steril* 2005;84(6):1587–8.
6. Jackson RA, Gibson KA, Wu YW, Croughan MS. Perinatal outcomes in singletons following in vitro fertilization: a meta-analysis. *Obstet Gynecol* 2004;103(3):551–63.
7. Elster N. Less is more: the risks of multiple births. The Institute for Science, Law, and Technology Working Group on Reproductive Technology. *Fertil Steril* 2000;74(4):617–23.
8. Centers for Disease Control. 1997 assisted reproductive technology success rates, national summary and fertility clinic reports, Centers for Disease Control, Atlanta (1999).
9. Ayres A, Johnson TR. Management of multiple pregnancy: prenatal care-part I. *Obstet Gynecol Surv.* 2005;60(8):527–37.
10. Hansen M, Bower C, Milne E, de Klerk N, Kurinczuk JJ. Assisted reproductive technologies and the risk of birth defects—a systematic review. *Hum Reprod* 2005;20(2):328–38.
11. Ness RB, Cramer DW, Goodman MT. Infertility, fertility drugs, and ovarian cancer a pooled analysis of case-control studies. *Am J Epidemiol* 2002;155:217–24.
12. Parazzini F, Pelucchi C, Negri E, Franceschi S, Talamini R, Montella M. Use of fertility drugs and risk of ovarian cancer. *Hum Reprod* 2001;16:1372–5.
13. Kashyap S, Moher D, Fung MF, Rosenwaks Z. Assisted reproductive technology and the incidence of ovarian cancer a meta-analysis. *Obstet Gynecol* 2004;103:785–94.
14. Mahdavi A, Pejovic T, Nezhat F. Induction of ovulation and ovarian cancer: a critical review of the literature. *Fertil Steril* 2006;85(4):819–26.
15. Nezhat C, Winer WK, Cooper JD, Nezhat F, Nezhat C. Endoscopic infertility surgery. *J Reprod Med* 1989;34(2):127–34.
16. Nezhat C, Hood J, Winer W, Nezhat F, Crowgey SR, Garrison CP. Videolaseroscopy and laser laparoscopy in gynaecology. *Br J Hosp Med* 1987;38(3):219–24.
17. Nezhat C, Nezhat F, Nezhat CH, Admon D. Videolaseroscopy and videolaparoscopy. *Baillieres Clin Obstet Gynaecol* 1994;8(4):851–64.
18. Hovav Y, Hornstein E, Almagor M, Yaffe C. Diagnostic laparoscopy in primary and secondary infertility. *J Assist Reprod Genet* 1998;15(9):535–7.
19. Tanahatoe S, Hompes PG, Lambalk CB. Accuracy of diagnostic laparoscopy in the infertility work-up before intrauterine insemination. *Fertil Steril* 2003;79:361–6.
20. Capelo FO, Kumar A, Steinkampf MP, Azziz R. Laparoscopic evaluation following failure to achieve pregnancy after ovulation induction with clomiphene citrate. *Fertil Steril* 2003;80:1450–3.
21. Nagata Y, Honjou K, Sonoda M, et al. Peri-ovarian adhesions interfere with the diffusion of gonadotrophin into the follicular fluid. *Hum Reprod* 1998;13:2072–6.
22. Daniell JF, Pittaway DE, Maxson WS. The role of laparoscopic adhesiolysis in an in vitro fertilization program. *Fertil Steril* 1983;40:49–52.
23. El Sahwi S. Laparoscopic pelvic adhesiolysis using CO_2 laser. *J Am Assoc Gynecol Laparosc* 1994;1(4):10–1.
24. Tanahatoe SJ, Hompes PG, Lambalk CB. Investigation of the infertile couple: should diagnostic laparoscopy be performed in the infertility work up programme in patients undergoing intrauterine insemination? *Hum Reprod* 2003;18(1):8–11.
25. Risberg B. Adhesions: preventive strategies. *Eur J Surg* Suppl 1997;577:32–9.
26. Brill AI, Nezhat F, Nezhat CH, Nezhat C. The incidence of adhesions after prior laparotomy: a laparoscopic appraisal. *Obstet Gynecol* 1995;85(2):269–72.
27. Nezhat CR, Nezhat FR, Metzger DA, Luciano AA. Adhesion reformation after reproductive surgery by videolaseroscopy. *Fertil Steril* 1990;53(6):1008–11.
28. Mansour R, Aboulghar M, Serour GI. Controversies in the surgical management of hydrosalpinx. *Curr Opin Obstet Gynecol* 2000;12(4):297–301.
29. Mol BWJ, Swart P, Bossuyt PMM, van Beurden M, van der Veen F. Reproducibility of the interpretation of hysterosalpingography in the diagnosis of tubal pathology. *Hum Reprod* 1996;11:1204–8.
30. Swart P, Mol BWJ, van der Veen F, van Beurden M, Radekop WK, Bossuyt PMM. The accuracy of hysterosalpingography in the diagnosis of tubal pathology, a meta-analysis. *Fertil Steril* 1995;64:486–91.
31. Zeyneloglu HB, Arici A, Olive DL. Adverse effects of hydrosalpinx on pregnancy rates after in vitro fertilization-embryo transfer. *Fertil Steril* 1998;70:492.
32. Strandell A, Lindhard A, Waldenström U, et al. Hydrosalpinx and IVF outcome: a prospective, randomized multicentre trial in Scandinavia on salpingectomy prior to IVF. *Hum Reprod* 1999;14:2762–9.

33. Cohen MA, Lindheim SR, Sauer MV. Hydrosalpinges adversely affect implantation in donor oocyte cycles. *Hum Reprod* 1999;14: 1087–9.

34. Spielvogel K, Shwayder J, Coddington CC. Surgical management of adhesions, endometriosis, and tubal pathology in the woman with infertility. *Clin Obstet Gynecol* 2000;43(4):916–28.

35. Shelton KE, Butler L, Toner JP, Oehninger S, Muasher SJ. Salpingectomy improves the pregnancy rate in in-vitro fertilization with hydrosalpinx. *Hum Reprod* 1996;11:523–5.

36. Johnson NP, Mak W, Sowter MC. Laparoscopic salpingectomy for women with hydrosalpinges enhances the success of IVF: a Cochrane review. *Hum Reprod* 2002;17:543.

37. American Society for Reproductive Medicine Clinical Practice Committee. Salpingectomy for hydrosalpinx prior to in vitro fertilization. *Fertil Steril* 2006;86(Suppl. 5):S200–1.

38. Verkauf BS. Myomectomy for fertility enhancement and preservation. *Fertil Steril* 1992;58:1–15.

39. Eldar-Geva T, Meagher S, Healy DL, MacLachlan V, Breheny S, Wood C. Effect of intramural, subserosal, and submucosal uterine fibroids on the outcome of assisted reproductive technology treatment. *Fertil Steril* 1998;70:687–91.

40. Stovall DW, Parrish SB, Van Voorish BJ, Hahn SJ, Sparks AET, Syrop CH. Uterine leiomyomata reduce the efficacy of assisted reproduction cycles: results of a matched follow-up study. *Hum Reprod* 1998;13:192–7.

41. Tulandi T, Murray C, Guralnick M. Adhesion formation and reproductive outcome after myomectomy and second-look laparoscopy. *Obstet Gynecol* 1993;82:213–15.

42. Nezhat C, Nezhat F, Silfen SL. Laparoscopic myomectomy. *Int J Fertil* 1991;36:275–80.

43. Hasson HM, Rotman C, Rana N. Laparoscopic myomectomy. *Obstet Gynecol* 1992;80:884–8.

44. Mais V, Agossa S, Guerriero S, Mascia M, Solla E, Melis GB. Laparoscopic versus abdominal myomectomy: a prospective, randomized trial to evaluate benefits in early outcome. *Am J Obstet Gynecol* 1996;174:654–8.

45. Dubuisson JB, Fauconnier A, Chapron C, Krieker G, Norgaard C. Second look after laparoscopic myomectomy. *Hum Reprod* 1998;13:2102–6.

46. Nezhat C, Nezhat F, Bess O, et al. Laparoscopically assisted myomectomy: a report of a new technique in 57 cases. *Int J Fertil* 1994;39:34–44.

47. Donnez J, Wyns C, Nisolle M. Does ovarian surgery for endometriomas impair the ovarian response to gonadotropin? *Fertil Steril* 2001;76(4):662–5.

48. Nezhat C, Crowgey SR, Garrison CP. Surgical treatment of endometriosis via laser laparoscopy. *Fertil Steril* 1986;45(6): 778–83.

49. Hughes EG, Fedorkow DM, Collins JA. *Fertil Steril* 1993;59: 963–70.

50. Parazzini F. Ablation of lesions or no treatment in minimal-mild endometriosis in infertile women: a randomized trial. Gruppo Italiano per lo Studio dell'Endometriosi. *Hum Reprod* 1999;14: 1332–4.

51. Marcoux S, Maheux R, Berube S. Laparoscopic surgery in infertile women with minimal or mild endometriosis. Canadian Collaborative Group on Endometriosis. *N Engl J Med* 1997;337: 217–22.

52. Buyalos RP, Agarwal SK. Endometriosis-associated infertility. *Curr Opin Obstet Gynecol* 2000;12(5):377–81.

53. Winkel CA. Evaluation and management of women with endometriosis. *Obstet Gynecol* 2003;102:397–408.

54. Donnez J, Nisolle M, Gillet N, Smets M, Bassil S, Casanas-Roux F. Large ovarian endometriomas. *Hum Reprod* 1996;11:641–6.

55. Aboulghar MA, Mansour RT, Serour GI, Al-Inany HG, Aboulghar MM. The outcome of in vitro fertilization in advanced endometriosis with previous surgery: a case-controlled study. *Am J Obstet Gynecol* 2003;188:371–5.

56. Nargund G, Cheng WC, Parsons J. The impact of ovarian cystectomy on ovarian response to stimulation during in-vitro fertilization cycles. *Hum Reprod* 1996;11:81–3.

57. Ho HY, Lee RK, Hwu YM, Lin MH, Su JT, Tsai YC. Poor response of ovaries with endometrioma previously treated with cystectomy to controlled ovarian hyperstimulation. *J Assist Reprod Genet* 2002;19:507–11.

58. Somigliana E, Ragni G, Benedetti F, Borroni R, Vegetti W, Crosignani PG. Does laparoscopic excision of endometriotic ovarian cysts significantly affect ovarian reserve? Insights from IVF cycles. *Hum Reprod* 2003;18(11):2450–3.

59. Loh FH, Tan AT, Kumar J, Ng SC. Ovarian response after laparoscopic ovarian cystectomy for endometriotic cysts in 132 monitored cycles. *Fertil Steril* 1999;72:316–21.

60. Muzii L, Bianchi A, Croce C, Manci N, Panici PB. Laparoscopic excision of ovarian cysts: is the stripping technique a tissue-sparing procedure? *Fertil Steril* 2002;77:609–14.

61. Barnhart K, Dunsmoor-Su R, Coutifaris C. Effect of endometriosis on in vitro fertilization. *Fertil Steril* 2002;77(6):1148–55.

62. Elsheikh A, Milingos S, Loutradis D, Kallipolitis G, Michalas S. Endometriosis and reproductive disorders. *Ann N Y Acad Sci* 2003;997:247–54.

63. Surrey ES, Schoolcraft WB. Does surgical management of endometriosis within 6 months of an in vitro fertilization–embryo transfer cycle improve outcome? *J Assist Reprod Genet* 2003; 20:365–70.

64. Garcia-Velasco JA, Majutte NG, Corona J, Zuniga V, Giles J, Arici A, et al. Removal of endometriomas before in vitro fertilization does not improve fertility outcomes a matched, case-control study. *Fertil Steril* 2004;81:1194–7.

65. Strandell A. Surgery in contemporary infertility. *Curr Womens Health Rep* 2003;3:367–74.

66. Brosens I. Endometriosis and the outcome of in vitro fertilization. *Fertil Steril* 2004;81:1198–200.

67. Nezhat C, Siegler A, Nezhat F, Nezhat C, Seidman D, Luciano A. Laparoscopic treatment of endometriosis. In C. Nezhat (Editor), Operative Gynecologic Laparoscopy Principles and Techniques (2nd ed.), McGraw-Hill, New York, 2000; 169–209.

68. Nezhat F, Nezhat C, Allan CJ, Metzger DA, Sears DL. A clinical and histologic classification of endometriomas implications for a mechanism of pathogenesis. *J Reprod Med* 1992;37:771–6.

69. The Practice Committee of the American Society for Reproductive Medicine. Endometriosis and infertility. *Fertil Steril* 2004;81:1441–6.

70. Littman E, Giudice L, Lathi R, Berker B, Milki A, Nezhat C. Role of laparoscopic treatment of endometriosis in patients with failed in vitro fertilization cycles. *Fertil Steril* 2005;84(6): 1574–8.

13

OPERATIVE HYSTEROSCOPY FOR UTERINE SEPTUM

Mohamed F. M. Mitwally, Mostafa Abuzeid

INTRODUCTION

This chapter presents a comprehensive review of the reproductive problems that could be associated with uterine septum. We believe that this topic has significant amount of controversy regarding its diagnosis and treatment due to the paucity of comprehensive evidence-based data on female congenital anomalies, in particular uterine septum. This resulted in the lack of a consensus on how the presence of a uterine septum might affect female reproduction. We will discuss the available data aiming at providing a balanced appraisal that can help the reproductive medicine specialists to better counsel patients about their reproductive potentials when a uterine septum is discovered.

Development

During the embryo development, the uterus forms from fusion of the paramesonephric ducts (Müllerian ducts), which join in the midline around the "tenth" week of gestation to form the unified body of the uterus. In the absence of Müllerian-inhibiting substance, the Müllerian ducts develop into the uterus and fallopian tubes (and possibly the upper part of the vagina) (1–4). It is interesting to note that the Müllerian ducts can develop into two distinct types of tissue: the smooth muscle tissue of the uterus and the fibrous tissue of the cervix (3). We believe this explains the various structural subtypes of uterine septum when it comes to different proportion of fibrous and muscle structure, that is, some uterine septa may contain more fibrous (cervical differentiation) component, while others contain more muscular (uterine differentiation) component. Such structural disparity might have implications on the mechanism of reproductive failure associated with uterine septum, as we will explain later.

A uterine septum results when there is incomplete resorption of the adjacent walls of the two Müllerian ducts. The resulting fibromuscular structure can range from a slight midline septum in the fundus of the uterus to complete midline division of the endometrial cavity. Even segmental septa can exist, resulting in partial communications of a partitioned uterus (4). Apoptosis has recently been proposed as the mechanism by which the fused portions of the two Müllerian tubes normally regress. Bcl-2, a protein involved with regulating apoptosis, was found to be absent from the septa of four uteri using a monoclonal antibody for Bcl-2 and immunohistochemical analysis. The absence of Bcl-2 may result in failure of resorption of the septum (5).

Reports of cases of complete vaginal septum associated with different degrees of uterine septum ranging from complete uterine septum with cervical duplication (6) to incomplete septum (subseptate uterus) (7, 8) challenged the classic theory of unidirectional (caudal to cranial) Müllerian development. We recently operated on a patient who had a complete longitudinal vaginal septum, but completely normal uterine cavity with no septum or bicornuate uterus (unpublished data). Therefore, an alternative "bi-directional" theory was proposed, which suggested that fusion and resorption begin at the isthmus of the uterus and proceed simultaneously in both the cranial and caudal directions (9).

Epidemiology

Although uterine anomalies have been reported in 0.1–2 percent of all women, in 4 percent with infertility and in up to 15 percent of those with recurrent miscarriage, their true incidence is not known (9a, 9b). Pedro Acien suggested that the variability in the reported incidence of uterine anomalies is due to the fact that it depends on five variables: 1) the population studied; 2) the study design and physician interest and awareness to find or reject an uterine anomaly; 3) the diagnostic method used; 4) the classes included as congenital uterine anomalies in the different studies, for example, hypoplastic uterus, T-shaped anomalies, and arcuate uterus frequently not included; and 5) the criteria and diagnostic tools used to classify the different types of uterine malformation (9b).

In 1998, a meta-analysis study that included a Medline search and standard reference tracing has located forty-seven studies from fourteen countries regarding the prevalence and distribution of uterine anomalies. In a pooled sample of more than 50,000 women from all included studies, the author calculated a prevalence of uterine anomalies in the general population of about 1 in 200 women (0.5 percent). The distribution of those anomalies was 39 percent bicornuate, 34 percent septate, 11 percent didelphic, 7 percent arcuate, 5 percent unicornuate, and 4 percent the remaining types including hypoplastic/aplastic/solid and other forms (10).

Comparable prevalence rate has been reported in a prospective study (11). In a cohort of girls and women who were evaluated for reasons unrelated to the presence of uterine anomalies, Byrne et al. (11) used standard ultrasound examinations to establish the prevalence of Müllerian duct abnormalities. The authors did prospective ultrasound examinations for nonobstetric indications in 2,065 consecutive girls and women (aged eight to ninety-three years). They found Müllerian anomalies in eight girls and women, that is, about 1 in 250 women (0.4 percent) with 95 percent confidence interval 1.67–7.62. The anomalies included bicornuate uterus, septate uterus, and double uterus.

Other investigators reported higher prevalence (12–16). Grimbizis et al. reported that in a review of five relatively recent studies (9b, 12–18) (between 1988 and 1997) and about 3,000 cases, the mean overall incidence of uterine malformation in the general population and/or the population of fertile women was 4.3 percent (18). In a report on more than 3,000 women that included family planning and contraception clients or patients undergoing infertility evaluation, Raga et al. (11) have found the frequency of uterine malformations in fertile patients (family planning and contraception clients) to be 3.8 percent, while the prevalence in infertile patients (with history of recurrent miscarriage or preterm delivery) was almost twice as high (6.3 percent), a difference that was statistically significant. The authors included various modalities for the diagnosis of Müllerian anomalies including HSG and/or surgery (laparoscopy/laparotomy). Both uterine septum (33.6 percent) and arcuate uterus (32.8 percent) were the most common malformations observed.

In a selected group of women undergoing hysteroscopy for abnormal uterine bleeding, Maneschi et al. (13) assessed the prevalence of uterine anomalies and compared the reproductive outcome in women with Müllerian anomalies to those in women with a normal uterine cavity. The authors found Müllerian anomalies in about 10 percent of women. Their findings were similar to those reported in studies dealing with the frequency of diagnosis of uterine anomalies in women undergoing tubal sterilization investigated by HSG, when septate and bicornuate and arcuate uteri were found in 1.9 and 3.6 percent and 11.5 percent, respectively, of women with no history of reproductive problems (14, 15).

Higher prevalence was also reported by other investigators who found that the overall prevalence of Müllerian defects was 5 percent among women with normal reproductive histories, 3 percent among infertile women, 5–10 percent among women with first-trimester recurrent miscarriages (excluding women with hypoplastic and arcuate uterus), and greater than 25 percent among women with late first-trimester/early second-trimester miscarriages and preterm labor (9b). Despite the discrepancy in the reported figures on the prevalence of Müllerian anomalies, almost all studies agreed upon the very high proportion of uterine septum anomaly among the other Müllerian anomalies. Uterine septum (complete or partial) has been the most common (34–48 percent) type of structural uterine anomaly (12, 17, 18). The significance of the uterine septum comes from the fact that it is the form of Müllerian anomaly that is believed to be associated with the poorest reproductive outcome including low fetal survival rates of 6–28 percent and high rates of spontaneous miscarriages (19).

Types

The classification of uterine anomalies divides the uterine septum into complete (septate) or partial (subseptate) groups, according to whether the septum approaches the internal os or not, respectively (20). The complete septum that divides both the uterine cavity and the endocervical canal may be associated with a longitudinal vaginal septum (1). However, the

Table 13.1: Buttram and Gibbons Classification of Müllerian Anomalies (20)

Uterine morphology	Fundal contour	External contour
Normal	Straight or convex	Uniformly convex or with indentation <10 mm
Arcuate	Concave fundal indentation with central point of indentation at obtuse angle	Uniformly convex or with indentation <10 mm
Subseptate	Presence of septum that does not extend to cervix, with central point of septum at an acute angle	Uniformly convex or with indentation <10 mm
Bicornuate	Two well-formed uterine cornua, with a convex fundal contour in each	Fundal indentation >10 mm dividing the two cornua

presence or absence of a longitudinal vaginal septum is not considered in the classification (20). Different classification systems were proposed for Müllerian anomalies with the early classification systems criticized for their confusion, incompleteness, or irrelevant details. In 1979, Buttram and Gibbons (20) introduced a classification system of Müllerian anomalies shown in Table 13.1. The American Fertility Society (currently known as the American Society for Reproductive Medicine or the ASRM) revised the Buttram and Gibbons's classification system of Müllerian anomalies (21) with the aim to make it an easy-to-use reporting system that would allow clinicians to classify patients better, so that data could be accumulated more readily concerning the incidence of fetal wastage and obstetric complications for these malformations (Box 13.1 and Figure 13.1).

As shown in Drawing 13.1 and Figures 13.2–13.5, the uterine septum has three parts: *base* (where it attaches to the fundus), *body* of the septum that extends down from the fundus all the way toward the cervix (complete septum) as shown in Figure 13.5 or stops somewhere between the fundus and the cervix (subseptate or short septum) as shown in Figures 13.2 and 13.3, and *apex* of the septum (the cervical end of the septum).

In addition to the regular classification into long (complete) or short (incomplete) subtypes, as shown in Drawings 13.2 and 13.3, in our experience, we observed two different subtypes of the short uterine septum based on the width of the uterine septum and the symmetry between the two uterine cavities on either side of the septum: broad-based (sometimes has a broad apex too) and asymmetrical (unequal sided) septa as shown in Figure 13.5B (usually has a broad base too), in Drawings 13.4 and 13.5, respectively. We noticed those subtypes to be frequently encountered in infertile patients and in patients with poor reproductive outcomes including assisted reproductive technology (ART) failure, pregnancy loss (unpublished data). Another investigator using Three-dimensional (3D) ultrasonography (US) and saline sonogram with 3D US has

Box 13.1: American Fertility Society Classification of Congenital Uterine Anomalies (21)

1. Agenesis: vagina, cervix, uterine fundus, fallopian tube, or any combination thereof

2. Unicornuate uterus

   – Connected

   – Not connected

   – Without a cavity

   – Without a horn

3. Uterus didelphys (double uterus and cervix)

4. Bicornuate uterus (complete, partial, or arcuate)

5. Septate uterus

   – Complete

   – Partial

6. Arcuate

7. DES drug related, e.g., T-shaped uterus resulting from diethylstilbestrol exposure

observed similar subtypes of the short uterine septum, which he named "wide-shallow septum" and "irregular septum." This author also reported a special type, which he called "T-shaped-shallow septum." The latter type was also observed by our group using 3D US (unpublished data).

We believe that the diagnosis of those two subtypes of short septum (broad based and asymmetrical) may be missed or at least confused with the diagnosis of arcuate uterus. This is particularly true when only HSG is relied upon without further evaluation by ultrasonography, especially 3D US and hysteroscopy. This confusion could explain the controversy in the literature regarding the association of reproductive problems (pregnancy loss and preterm labor) and arcuate uterus, as will be discussed later.

Structure

The high rate of spontaneous abortion in patients with uterine septa has been related to a specific histological feature of the septum, in which there is less vascularity and inadequate endometrial development that results in abnormal placentation (22). It has also been claimed that during hysteroscopic excision of the septum when bleeding appears, the natural wall of the uterus (because of its increasing vascularity) has been reached and further excision is not needed (22, 23).

Classically, the uterine septum structure has been described as a "fibroelastic" tissue that has three main features: first, very little amount of muscle tissue (22, 23); second, mainly formed of fibroelastic tissue (24); and third, very scanty vasculature (avascular) (25, 26).

Interestingly, contrary to the classic description of the uterine septum Dabirashrafi et al. (27) reported opposite findings

of significantly less connective tissue in the septum and higher amount of muscle tissue and vasculature when compared to posterior uterine muscle away from the septum. In a group of sixteen patients with uterine septum undergoing Tompkins technique abdominal metroplasty, the authors compared three biopsies obtained from the septum to a fourth biopsy obtained from the posterior uterine wall away from the septum. The three septum biopsies were obtained from the septum as follows: first biopsy obtained from the septum near the serosal layer (base, as shown in Drawing 13.1), second biopsy from the midpoint of the septum (body, as shown in Drawing 13.1), and third biopsy from the tip (apex, as shown in Drawing 13.1) of the septum. The authors examined thirteen characteristics in those specimens by calculating the mean ridit analysis and Bonferroni criteria for multiple comparisons in relation to three outcomes: first amount of connective tissues (four characteristics), second amount of muscles (four characteristics), and third amount of blood vessels (five characteristics) (27). The authors concluded that their findings challenged the classic theory about the cause of fetal wastage associated with uterine septum (avascularity of the septum). They proposed two other mechanisms for the increased pregnancy loss: first the poor decidualization and placentation due to reduced connective tissue and the second, the higher noncoordinated contractility in the uterine septum due to the higher amounts of interlacing muscle tissue (27). Kupesic and Kurjak using color and pulsed Doppler sonographic studies of the septal areas reported vascularity in 71 percent of patients. Therefore, this study suggests that uterine septum can be made of muscular tissue in some patients and primarily of fibroelastic tissue in others (28).

DIAGNOSIS

It is very important to distinguish between the bicornuate uterus and the septate uterus. This is crucially important because the bicornuate uterus is infrequently associated with reproductive problems, whereas the septate uterus is frequently associated with reproductive problems such as pregnancy failure that usually require further intervention (28). It is also important to differentiate between arcuate uterus and short incomplete septum and between complete septum with cervical duplication and longitudinal vaginal septum and uterus didelphys.

Imaging

Although surgery (hysteroscopy, alone or with laparoscopy) constitutes the gold standard for the diagnosis of uterine septum, various imaging tools including hysterosalpingography (HSG), ultrasonography, and magnetic resonance imaging (MRI) have great value in the diagnosis with high level of accuracy.

Hysterosalpingography

HSG provides *valuable* information about tubal patency in addition to *some* information about the uterine cavity. However, its usefulness is limited in identifying uterine anomalies including the uterine septum because it does not provide definitive information about the external contour of the uterus. Other imaging modalities including ultrasonography and MRI have been shown to be useful complementary tools in characterizing and delineating more clearly the exact nature of the Müllerian anomalies (30). This is particularly true for the distinction between the uterine septum and bicornuate uterus that cannot be

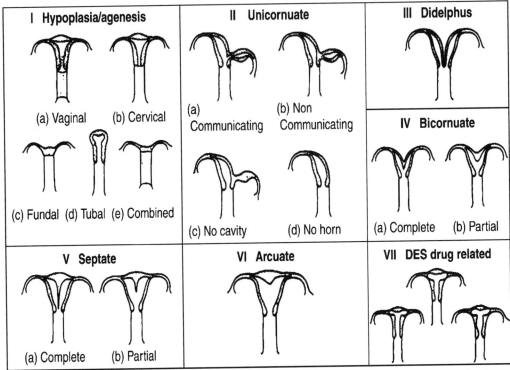

Figure 13.1. American Fertility Society (recently American Society for Reproductive Medicine) classification of congenital uterine anomalies (21).

made definitely by examination of a hysterogram (during HSG) because the image of the cavities may be exactly the same (28).

Ultrasonography

Ultrasonography has the advantages of minimal invasiveness, relatively low cost, and ease of performance. Although transabdominal two-dimensional (2D) US was the first ultrasound technique used for identifying uterine cavity disorders, transvaginal ultrasonography has become the modality of choice replacing the transabdominal approach. This is because of its ability to be closer to the uterus that allows better anatomical delineation, in addition to its higher resolution associated with high frequency of the ultrasound beam that provides images with better contrast and resolution (29).

Despite the advantages of the transvaginal 2D US, it has a fairly low sensitivity as a screening test of uterine anomalies (~70 percent) (31). In addition, sometimes the distinction between different types of anomalies is often impossible. Another problem is that a transverse or oblique transverse view of the uterus is not optimal in diagnosing uterine abnormalities, particularly when the uterine body has a retroverted position. Furthermore, ultrasound is operator dependent, and hard-copy images can be difficult for a third party to interpret (29).

SONOHYSTEROGRAPHY

Optimal imaging of the endometrium and myometrium may require distension of the uterine cavity with saline to separate the walls of the uterus to make it clear to outline the endometrial contour and to detect endoluminal lesions, that is, lesions protruding into the uterine cavity or uterine septum. This procedure is frequently called sonohysterography (SHG) or saline infusion sonohysterography.

Preparing the patient for the SHG is more or less similar to HSG, that is, ensuring that the patient is not pregnant or there is any evidence of active pelvic infection or other less likely contraindications to the procedure such as allergy to the ultrasound contrast medium. In addition, conventional transvaginal ultrasound examination should be done before the SHG to assess the appearance of the uterus before fluid instillation into the uterine cavity and to determine the orientation of the uterus to facilitate insertion of a catheter into the cervical canal for instillation of the saline or the ultrasound contrast medium (29). Performing the procedure during the follicular phase has the advantages of avoiding the risk of disturbing an early pregnancy. It is preferable to use a balloon-bearing catheter to occlude the internal os to allow adequate distension of the uterine cavity (29). However, this has the disadvantages of being more uncomfortable to the patient and its shadow might obscure lesions present in the lower uterine segment or the cervical canal.

SHG is thought to have 100 percent sensitivity and specificity when compared with the gold standard, that is, surgery (32). Another study (33) found SHG having the same diagnostic accuracy as the gold standard for polypoid lesions and endometrial hyperplasia. The overall belief by the experts in the area of ultrasonography of uterine cavity disorders is that SHG or HSG are highly sensitive in the diagnosing of major uterine malformations; however, it is not sufficiently sensitive in the diagnosis of minor uterine abnormalities (29). A recent report suggests the use of a very small volume of viscous gel with impressive results (29a).

THREE-DIMENSIONAL ULTRASONOGRAPHY

Transvaginal 3D US is a noninvasive imaging technique with the ability to generate accurate images of the endometrial

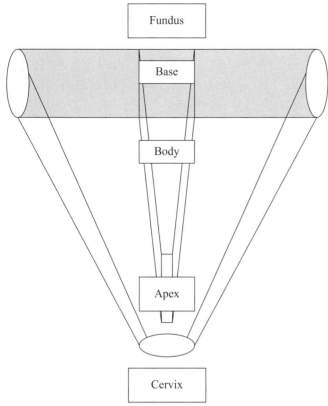

Drawing 13.1. Shows the different parts of the uterine septum in relation to the uterine walls: base of the septum where it meets the fundus, body of the septum that extends down dividing the uterine cavity into two sides, and apex of the septum that is the lower most part of the septum.

cavity and of the external contour of the uterus (34, 35). A major advantage of the 3D US is the ability to obtain the coronal views of the uterus, which is usually not obtainable by the 2D US because of anatomical limitations (the vaginal probe has limited mobility within the confines of the vagina).

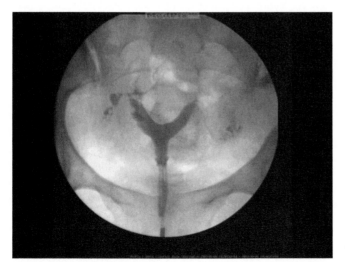

Figure 13.2. Hysterosalpingogram shows incomplete uterine septum. This type of uterine septum is much commoner than the complete one (septum that extends all the way down to the cervix).

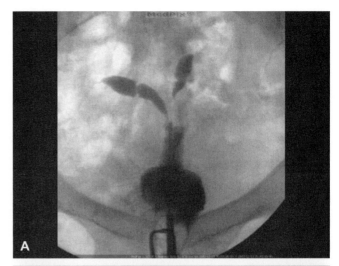

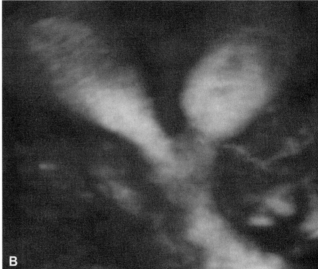

Figure 13.3. The figure shows two hysterosalpingograms of complete uterine septum (A) and bicornuate uterus (B). Notice the wider angle between the two sides of the uterine cavity in the hysterosalpingogram picture of the uterine septum. Such an angle is much smaller in case of the bicornuate uterus.

These coronal views show the relationship between the endometrium and the myometrium at the uterine fundus, delineate the entire cervical canal, and depict the corneal angles. This enables the operator to measure the depth of uterine septum and the distance between the apex of the septum and the internal os. In addition, the use of 3D US enables us to diagnose new types of uterine septum, for example, unequal sides (35a, 35b). Furthermore, 3D US can differentiate between arcuate uterus and a short incomplete septum. Another major advantage is that with 3D US, a volume of ultrasonographic data is rapidly stored and made available for later analysis. This is particularly helpful in case of SHG. The ability to store data would shorten the amount of time during which the uterine cavity must remain distended (36). Obviously, it is a major advantage of 3D US because all of the original ultrasonographic data are contained in the saved volume without loss of information, as might occur when only selected static images are available for interpretation, which is the case with 2D US (37). Even if the

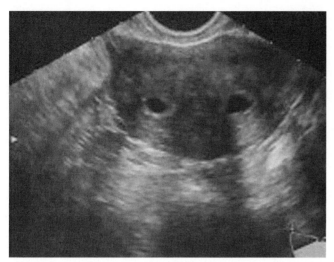

Figure 13.4. Sonohysterogram showing uterine septum. A transverse section through transvaginal ultrasonography shows both sides of the uterine cavity distended with fluid injected through the procedure of sonohysterography. The two sides of the cavity are separated with the septum.

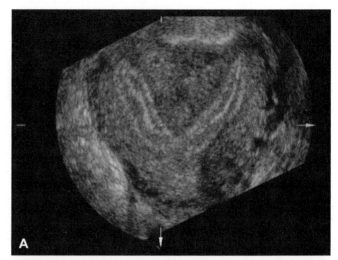

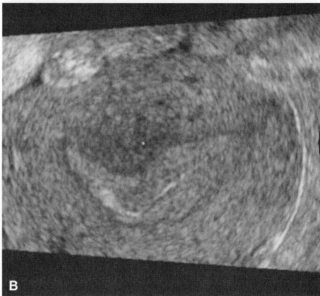

Figure 13.5. Three-dimensional transvaginal ultrasonography showing incomplete uterine septum (A), and the subtype of the incomplete uterine septum that we call as asymmetrical, incomplete uterine septum (B). Notice the advantages of this ultrasound technique in visualizing the dimensions of the septum, relationship to different parts of the uterine cavity, as well as the external contour of the uterus.

ultrasonographic procedure is videotaped, findings remain operator dependent, and any observation not clearly documented on the tape would be lost. The multiplanar capability of 3D US permits an unlimited number of scan planes to be obtained from the original data set, an advantage that would significantly reduce the operator-dependant bias. This data set is available for interactive review at any time after the patient has been discharged or before surgical intervention. Additional findings not initially detected during the real-time examination can be made by "scrolling" through the volume data. Clearly, this can be accomplished without inconveniencing the patient by prolonged or repeated vaginal scanning (37). Clearly, combining SHG with 3D US can add to the accuracy of both procedures (38).

A disadvantage of 3D US is the time required to learn to manipulate the 3D volume data, although this decreases with experience. Also, shadowing caused by the uterine fibroids, irregular endometrial lining, or thickened endometrial lining (as seen during the periovulatory period), as well as the decreased volume of the uterine cavity (in cases of intrauterine adhesions), are obvious limitations of 3D US (29).

Three-dimensional US was reported to have a sensitivity and specificity of 100 percent in diagnosing arcuate uteri compared with 67 and 94 percent, respectively, for transvaginal 2D US. Interestingly, in diagnosing major Müllerian anomalies, while the sensitivity and specificity of transvaginal 3D US were both 100 percent compared with 100 percent sensitivity and 95 percent specificity for transvaginal 2D US, the positive predictive value was 100 percent for the 3D US but only 50 percent for 2D US (34). Because of the higher accuracy of the 3D US in diagnosing Müllerian disorders, higher prevalence (~6 percent) was reported when 3D US was applied for detecting those disorders (35).

DOPPLER ULTRASONOGRAPHY

Evaluating the septum vascularity by Doppler ultrasonography is believed to provide important information about its structure and the risk of reproductive problems. Kupesic and Kurjak (35c) attempted to evaluate the combined use of trans-

vaginal 2D US, transvaginal color and pulsed Doppler ultrasonography, HSG, and transvaginal 3D US in the preoperative diagnosis of uterine septum in a group of 420 infertile patients undergoing operative hysteroscopy. Two hundred and seventy-eight patients had an intrauterine septum (66.2 percent of all patients) that was corrected surgically. In forty-three patients with a uterine septum, there was a history of repeated spontaneous miscarriage, and seventy-one had had one spontaneous miscarriage (fifty-six in the first trimester and fifteen in the second trimester). Each patient underwent transvaginal ultrasound and transvaginal color Doppler examination during the luteal phase of their cycle. Color and pulsed Doppler were superimposed to visualize intraseptal and myometrial vascularity in each patient. It is interesting that although the authors did not find correlation between septal length or the septal

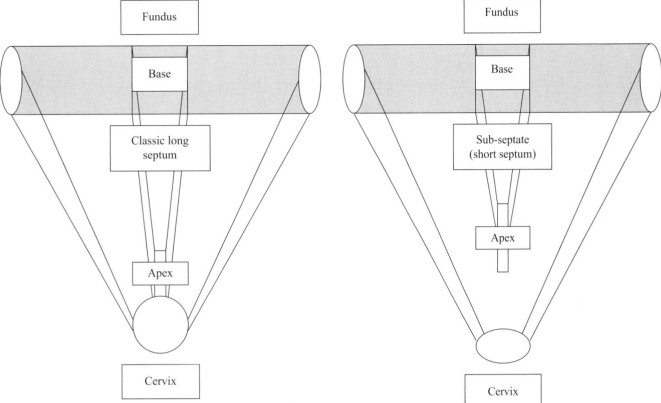

Drawing 13.2. Shows the complete or long septum type (septate uterus). In this type of the uterine septum, the body of the septum extends all the way down from the fundus to the cervix, completely separating the uterine cavity into two sides.

Drawing 13.3. Shows the incomplete short type of the uterine septum (subseptate uterus). In this type, the apex of the septum stops somewhere below the fundus before reaching the cervix.

thickness, and occurrence of obstetric complications, they found the septal vascularity to correlate significantly with those complications. The authors extrapolated from those data that that this might reflect an increased amount of muscle in the septum, producing local uncoordinated myometrial contractility resulting in adverse obstetric outcomes (39).

Magnetic Resonance Imaging

MRI can delineate both internal and external uterine architecture, which provides an interesting alternative diagnostic method for the evaluation of Müllerian tract anomalies. However, several disadvantages make it difficult to apply for routine practice including high cost, being not suitable for office practice, and, most important, the extreme high accuracy of the 3D US that can provide very comparable information to MRI while having the advantages of low cost, suitability for office practice, and even more information including Doppler examination of the vascularity. However, MRI is mandatory for differentiating between uterus didelphys and long, complete uterine septum with cervical duplication and a vertical vaginal septum.

Surgery

Hysteroscopy allows both direct visualization of the uterine cavity and operative intervention when uterine septa are encountered. However, as is the case with HSG, hysteroscopy cannot evaluate the external contour of the uterus. However, an advantage of hysteroscopy is the direct visualization of the endometrium and that it can be performed as an outpatient procedure, but one should be aware of the risk of surgical complications, for example, perforation, infection, and bleeding. Concurrent laparoscopy is essential for evaluation of the external contour of the uterus mainly to differentiate between uterine septum and bicornuate uterus, which cannot be surgically corrected through the hysteroscopic approach if even surgical correction is warranted. In addition, laparoscopy is helpful for assessing the extent of hysteroscopic resection of uterine septa and identifying and repair of uterine perforation promptly should it occur (29). Furthermore, laparoscopy should be mandatory if hysteroscopic metroplasty is performed in a patient with history of infertility to rule out endometriosis, pelvic adhesions, and subtle fimbrial pathology (39a). This is particularly the case in view of recent data suggesting an association between uterine septum and endometriosis (39b).

REPRODUCTIVE PROBLEMS ASSOCIATED WITH UTERINE SEPTUM

Congenital uterine anomalies vary in frequency and are usually estimated to be present in up to 5 percent in the general population, although less than half of those affected have clinical symptoms (2). Various clinical problems have been reported including pregnancy failure and other obstetric complications, for example, preterm labor and placental abruption. Other reproductive problems, especially infertility, have been suggested,

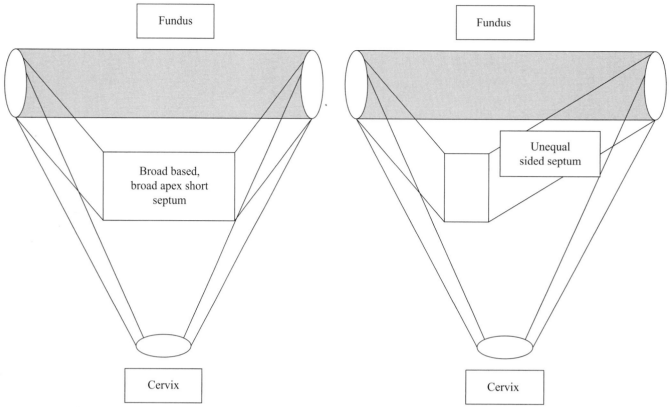

Drawing 13.4. Shows a subtype of the short septum. We call it broad-based short septum. In this type, the base of the septum is very broad, extending between almost the whole distance between the two tubal ostia. The base in this subtype is usually broad.

Drawing 13.5. Shows another subtype of the short septum (asymmetrical). In this type, the two sides of the uterine cavity are unequal. The apex of the septum is deviated more toward one side.

though not universally accepted. Other conditions, for example, endometriosis and urinary tract anomalies and even malignancy have been thought to be associated with congenital uterine malformation.

Pregnancy Loss and Obstetric Complications

Congenital uterine malformations, particularly uterine septum, have been associated with poor reproductive outcome including an increased risk of first- and second-trimester miscarriage, preterm delivery, placental abruption, intrauterine growth restriction, fetal distress, and fetal and maternal death (39–42). It is estimated that 36 percent of uterine malformations have an associated cervical insufficiency. Although congenital uterine malformations are associated with poor reproductive performance, each type may have a different impact on reproduction (23). Pregnancy loss in patients with uterine septa has been reported to be as high as 90 percent, after other causes for miscarriage have been excluded (23, 43, 44). During the first trimester of pregnancy, the risk of spontaneous miscarriage in patients with uterine septum has been reported between 28 and 45 percent, whereas the frequency of spontaneous miscarriage during the second trimester in these patients is approximately 5 percent (44, 45).

Buttram (46) reported a 67 percent miscarriage rate, 33 percent prematurity rate, and 28 percent live birth rate in patients with uterine septum. In a pooled cohort of pregnancies

that were reported in thirteen studies, Kupesic calculated the incidence of pregnancy loss and preterm labor in a total of 1,304 pregnancies achieved in women with untreated uterine septum. She found an incidence of 81.9 and 9.6 percent for pregnancy loss and preterm labor, respectively (29). However, such figures should be carefully interpreted as those studies possibly excluded reports on women with uterine septum associated with normal reproductive outcome.

With the exception of the arcuate uterus, which some believe to have no adverse impact on reproductive outcome (although this is not universally accepted) (47, 48), it is interesting that an inverse relationship has been seen between the extent of the vertical Müllerian duct fusion defect and the risk of pregnancy loss (miscarriage). The less severe the vertical Müllerian duct fusion defect (the shorter the septum), the higher the spontaneous miscarriage rate (49). Therefore, the frequency of pregnancy loss was found to be highest, in descending order, in a partial uterine septum, followed by bicornuate uterus, followed by a complete uterine septum, and finally the didelphic uterus (50). Unfortunately, these conclusions are drawn from studies that suffered from having small numbers, no control population, and different diagnostic criteria for determining the Müllerian anomaly. However, recently with the introduction of 3D US, consistent and strict criteria can be used to define particular Müllerian anomalies (1). Recently, however, Kupesic and Kurjak (29) could not find such a correlation to exist between risk of pregnancy loss and length of the uterine septum or its thickness.

A prospective study looked, over a period of three years, at reproductive outcomes in 106 women with congenital uterine anomalies detected, *incidentally*, by 3D US screening. Compared to a matching control group that included 983 women with normal uterine cavity, confirmed sonographically, at the same period of follow-up, women with uterine cavity anomalies were found to have significantly more adverse obstetric outcomes (51). The authors found women with uterine septum (twenty-eight women) had a significantly higher proportion of first-trimester loss ($Z = 4.68$, $P < 0.01$) compared with women with a normal uterus. Interestingly, women with an "arcuate" uterus (seventy-two women) had a significantly greater proportion of second-trimester loss ($Z = 5.76$, $P < 0.01$) and preterm labor ($Z = 4.1$, $P < 0.01$) (51), opposite to what is believed to be the case in the reported literature (52, 53). It is worth mentioning here that there was no correlation between the depth of fundal indentation in the arcuate uteri and percentage of first-trimester miscarriages ($r = -0.18$, $P = 0.126$), second-trimester miscarriages ($r = 0.1$, $P = 0.398$), or preterm labor ($r = -0.63$, $P = 0.6$), while in women with a subseptate uterus, the first-trimester miscarriage rate appeared to "decrease" with "increasing" length of uterine septum. However, this finding did not reach statistical significance ($r = -0.46$, $P = 0.702$). Furthermore, there was no correlation between septum length and second-trimester miscarriage ($r = 0.211$, $P = 0.273$) or preterm labor ($r = 0.117$, $P = 0.298$) (51). Later, the same team examined the uterine cavity in 509 women with a history of unexplained recurrent miscarriage and 1,976 low-risk women for the presence of congenital uterine anomalies by 3D US. Although the authors found no significant difference in relative frequency of various anomalies or depth of fundal distortion between the two groups, in women with both arcuate and subseptate uteri, the "length" of the remaining uterine cavity was significantly "shorter" ($P < 0.01$) and the "distortion ratio" was significantly higher ($P < 0.01$) in the recurrent miscarriage (54).

Recently, Tomazevic et al. challenged the concept that arcuate uterus or small uterine septum does not compromise reproductive function (54a). This was an observational study that included 826 singleton deliveries to 730 women with history of hysteroscopic resection of uterine septum. They compared the perinatal outcome before and after hysteroscopic resection in two groups of women: women with a small uterine septum (Group A) and those with larger uterine septum (Group B) (54a). The preterm birth rate and the very preterm birth rate in Group A ($n = 420$) were 33.9 and 12.5 percent before and 7.2 and 3.1 percent after hysteroscopic resection, respectively ($P < 0.001$). Similarly, the preterm birth rate and the very preterm birth rate in Group B were 36.5 and 15.0 percent before and 8.0 and 2.9 percent after hysteroscopic resection, respectively ($P < 0.001$). They concluded that similar to a large uterine septum arcuate or small uterine septum is an important hysteroscopically preventable risk variable for preterm birth.

We believe, as supported by the above literature, that the type, extent, and shape of the uterine cavity are important determinants of the reproductive outcomes rather than the simple diagnosis of uterine cavity anomaly. It appears that the shorter and more distorted the uterine cavity (e.g., when the septum distorts that uterine cavity unequally), the more the likelihood of having adverse reproductive outcomes including pregnancy loss (early or mid-trimester), preterm labor, or even placental complications such as placental abruption.

Termination of Pregnancy

The presence of uterine abnormalities may increase both the failure and complications of the procedure including higher risk of uterine perforation and adhesion formation. This advocates the use of transvaginal ultrasonography during pregnancy termination in patients affected with a uterine anomaly (55).

Mechanism of Adverse Obstetric Outcomes in Association with Uterine Septum

Although no studies attempted to elucidate the underlying mechanisms why some women with uterine septa suffer from reproductive loss while others have normal pregnancies, several mechanisms have been suggested including increasing intrauterine pressure with relative cervical incompetence and a poor blood supply to the endometrium through the septum. Another suggested mechanism is the luteal defect associated with uterine septum that could be a result of the local vascular insufficiency and not a hormonal deficiency (56). Fedele in a small study of twelve pregnancies in eight patients suggested that miscarriage is related to septal implantation (56a).

However, according to the most widely accepted theory, the septum is thought to consist of fibroelastic tissue with inadequate vascularization and altered relations between myometrial and endometrial vessels. The poor response to estrogen of the endometrial mucosa covering the septum, including irregular differentiation and estrogenic maturation, is probably because of the scanty vascularization of the septal connective tissue (57, 58). As a result, implantation may be compromised and decidual and placental growth inadequate, resulting in early pregnancy loss and infertility. In addition, impaired fetal growth and placental abruption may occur as a result of an already poorly vascularized placenta and distorted uterine cavity, causing second- and third-trimester complications. Therefore, removing the septum may eliminate an unsuitable site for implantation, improve endometrial function, expand uterine capacity, and dramatically enhance reproductive outcome in selected patients.

Contrary to this classic concept, Dabirashrafi et al. (27) (as discussed earlier) found significantly less connective tissue, a greater proportion of muscle tissue, and more vessels in the septum. They, therefore, suggested that pregnancy wastage is caused by poor decidualization and placentation due to the reduced amounts of connective tissue, as well as by higher or uncoordinated contractility due to the increased muscle content (27). It also has been suggested that estrogen and progesterone receptor deficiency in the endometrium of malformed uteri may further increase abnormal uterine contractions that lead to fetal wastage (57, 58). Pellerito et al. (59) performed MRI of patients with a septate uterus and found a muscular septal component (differentiated from fibrous tissue by its higher signal intensity). This was confirmed by histological examination of biopsy specimens. Another investigator used MRI to assess the composition of the septa in twenty-nine patients and showed that all of them had myometrial tissue with histological confirmation in four of them (59a).

Infertility and ART Failure

The incidence of uterine defect in infertile women has been estimated to be approximately 3 percent, which is similar to the prevalence of approximately 4 percent found in the general population and/or in fertile women (18). The incidence of uterine malformations in infertile women varies between 0.5 and 26 percent (16, 53, 59b–d). In a report by Hinckley and Amin on 1,000 routine office hysteroscopies in infertility patients undergoing IVF treatment, they reported that 0.5 percent of patients were found to have uterine septum (59b). Tulandi et al. also reported a low incidence of uterine anomalies in 2,240 infertile women (1.03 percent), with 78.3 percent having primary infertility (59c). However, other reports indicated that there might be a higher prevalence of uterine anomalies in infertility patient from 16 to 26 percent (16, 59d, e). Raga et al. in 1996 reported a prevalence of 26 percent in a rather small, selected group of patients (59e). Similar results (24 percent) were reported in a small study (59d). Interestingly, Raga et al. in 1997 published a much larger study on 1,024 women, but this time the prevalence was only 2.4 percent (53). However, Acien in 1997 reported an incidence of 16 percent in a large study of 1,200 infertile women. Our group reported recently similar results in a study on 1,011 infertile patients who underwent hysteroscopy and laparoscopy for diagnosis and treatment of infertility (59f). The overall incidence of uterine septum in all infertile patients studied was 17.6 percent, with 15 and 2.5 percent being short incomplete uterine septum and long incomplete uterine septum, respectively (59f). We believe that the variability in the reported incidence of uterine anomalies depends on similar variables as suggested by Acien on the incidence in general/fertile population especially the diagnostic methods used and physician interest and awareness to find or reject uterine anomaly (9b). This topic will remain controversial until a well-designed prospective multicenter study utilizing 3D US and/or hysteroscopy is completed.

Patients with secondary infertility usually have a history of spontaneous miscarriages, while patients with primary infertility have no such history. In those primary infertility patients, when uterine septum is detected, there is more controversy as regards whether to treat the uterine septum or not than with the secondary infertility group that has a poor reproductive history (29). Obviously, future studies would be difficult as resection of uterine septum is so simple and efficacy so dramatic that randomized trials would be ethically questionable (28).

Despite the paucity of data concerning the contribution of the uterine septum to infertility, hysteroscopic resection of uterine septum is recommended before initiation of treatment in women undergoing ART (60). In support for that, Kirsop et al. (61) reported improved results with ART after hysteroscopic treatment of uterine abnormalities among 144 women who had preclinical miscarriage after ART. Dicker et al. (62) found uterine abnormalities (mainly uterine septa) in 14 cases (9.7 percent) and surmised that an incomplete uterine septum may be an important factor predisposing to early pregnancy wastage. In addition, Syrop et al. (63) showed higher prevalence of uterine anomalies (18.2 percent) in patients with repeated ART failure.

Contrary to the above data supporting the recommendation to treat uterine anomalies, in particular short uterine septum in women before undergoing ART treatment, other investigators did not find the presence of uterine anomalies to reduce the chance of pregnancy after ART treatment (64, 65). However, those studies suffered from several methodological problems including small sample size and retrospective analysis (64), as well

as mixing different types of uterine malformations and failure to control significant confounding factors that might affect the outcome of ART treatment.

Endometriosis

Endometriosis is a frequent reproductive disorder that is associated with pelvic pain and infertility. A correlation between retrograde menstruation and likelihood of endometriosis has been shown with a significantly higher prevalence of endometriosis in patients with Müllerian anomalies in comparison with women without such anomalies (controls) (66, 67). However, no difference between nonobstructive anomalies (e.g., uterine septum) and controls was found (68).

Most recently, higher incidence of endometriosis in patients with a uterine septum was reported in a retrospective study that included 120 patients with a uterine septum compared to a control group of 486 consecutive infertile patients with a normal hysteroscopy and laparoscopy. The authors found the incidence of endometriosis significantly higher in patients with uterine septum (25.8 versus 15.2 percent, $P = 0.006$) (69).

In addition, our own data suggest an association between uterine septum and endometriosis (39b).

Interestingly, uterine dysperistalsis was suggested to be the mechanical cause of endometriosis rather than retrograde menstruation (70). One could imagine that uterine anomalies irrespective of their obstructive or nonobstructive character could be associated with a disturbed uterine peristalsis as a risk factor of endometriosis (69). However, further studies are needed.

Urinary Problems

A small percentage of patients (usually less than 10 percent) with a "symmetric" malformation of the uterus have abnormalities of the urinary tract, usually congenital absence of a single kidney. For that reason, urological evaluation is recommended for patients with uterine anomalies uterus, particularly with the more severe uterine anomalies (28).

Polycystic Ovarian Syndrome

The association between polycystic ovary (PCO) appearance on ultrasound and uterine Müllerian anomalies was suggested when PCO was found in 29.9 percent of women with Müllerian anomalies (167 women) compared to a prevalence of 20.1 percent in a control group of 3,165 women with normal uterine cavity (a statistically significant difference) (71). Interestingly, when the Müllerian anomalies were further grouped according to the American Fertility Society classification (21), patients with septate uteri and bicornuate uteri malformations had a statistically higher prevalence of PCO than the controls. While the difference was much more significant with the septate uterus subgroup, it was insignificant in patients with unicornuate and didelphic uteri compared to controls (71).

Malignancy

It is believed that uterine malformations including uterine septum, with its different forms, do not predispose a patient to the development of a malignancy (72, 73).

MANAGEMENT OF UTERINE SEPTUM

Treatment of uterine septum has come full circle that started in 1919, with successful transcervical therapy (74, 75) that was replaced by abdominal approach (e.g., Jones and Tompkins procedures). This approach turned almost obsolete with the consensus now back to the transcervical approach (hysteroscopic metroplasty). Hysteroscopic resection is favored due to its simplicity compared with the abdominal metroplasty that is performed through a laparotomy (76). However, abdominal approach has been advised for extremely wide uterine septum, but transcervical approach can still be accomplished in most cases, although a second attempt might be necessary in certain instances to completely incise the septum (28).

Which Septum Needs Resection?

The answer to which septum needs resection depends on the reproductive history rather than the type of the septum itself, that is, hysteroscopic metroplasty is obviously recommended for patients with a history of recurrent pregnancy loss or bad obstetric history. However, it is important to evaluate patients with pregnancy loss who also have uterine septa, to rule out additional underlying etiologies (77).

Other reasonable indications include women with history of adverse obstetric outcomes including second-trimester losses, abnormal presentation, preterm deliveries, or antepartum hemorrhage when associated with a uterine septum. Again, it is important to reiterate it that it is the history of reproductive problems rather than the extent of the uterine septum that should determine the decision to resect it or not. Age is another consideration because older women may benefit from prompt treatment to optimize outcome. Choe and Baggish (78) suggested that the uterine septum should be corrected as early as possible, especially in patients older than thirty-five years of age, to increase fecundity.

When a uterine septum is an incidental finding in a woman without a history of reproductive problems that are known to be associated with uterine septum, it is still a controversial issue whether prophylactic metroplasty should be done to prevent those complications. Limited data suggest that metroplasty is not indicated for treatment of infertility because primary infertility patients conceived after metroplasty at a similar rate as infertile counterparts without septa (79). In women with the incidental diagnosis of uterine cavity disorders at the time of abdominal or pelvic surgery performed for other reasons, successful pregnancy was achieved in the majority of patients with didelphys, bicornuate, and septate uteri with success rates of 93, 84, and 78 percent (80). Such findings support believes of other investigators that surgical corrections of all uterine defects are not indicated unless patients do poorly on a repetitive basis. In addition some investigators have reported better reproductive outcome among women with a septate uterus not subjected to surgical interventions (47, 82, 83) favoring the opinion that hysteroscopic incision of the uterine septum is not absolutely necessary in these patients, excluding those with recurrent miscarriage (83). However, the achieved pregnancies could simply reflect the draw of luck that the implanting embryo found its way at a place away from the defective endometrium, that is, away from the uterine septum (56a).

However, in our hands (unpublished data), we have extensive experience with a large number of cases (more than 300 cases) in which short uterine septum was diagnosed as an incidental finding during routine infertility workup (~50 percent with primary infertility). After diagnosis, patients with primary infertility were counseled regarding the two options of prophylactic metroplasty versus proceeding with infertility interventions (ovarian hyperstimulation with intrauterine insemination [COH + IUI] and ART when insemination is not successful) without surgical correction of the uterine septum. The majority of these patients opted to undergo hysteroscopic metroplasty. We observed an increased fecundity rate, excellent pregnancy rates after COH + IUI and ART, and good obstetric outcome (unpublished data). Interestingly in patients with secondary infertility, hysteroscopic metroplasty has reversed previous poor outcomes and the majority of those patients achieved full-term deliveries spontaneously or after receiving their infertility intervention following hysteroscopic metroplasty (unpublished data). These findings prompted us to believe and recommend in favor of routine resection of uterine septum (irrespective to its extent) before undergoing infertility interventions (ovarian stimulation with insemination or ART) or even when patients want to continue to try to achieve pregnancy spontaneously (79). Moreover, the simplicity of hysteroscopic treatment and low morbidity have argued for prophylactic hysteroscopic metroplasty particularly in women with unexplained infertility, before ART treatment, or even for removal of the septum at the time of diagnosis to increase fecundity and to prevent miscarriages and obstetric complications (81).

It is also interesting to mention that recently a large series of complete septate uterus with longitudinal vaginal septum has not been found to be associated with increased risk of primary infertility, and pregnancy was reported to progress successfully without surgical treatment. Those results do not support elective hysteroscopic incision of the septum in asymptomatic patients or before first pregnancy. However, that study suffered from several problems including being a descriptive study covering a very long period (almost four decades), which makes the comparison between surgically treated and untreated patients difficult. In addition, the study is associated with many limitations such as absence of a control group and thus no comparative analysis and changes in clinical strategies during the long period. However, that the particular malformation of a complete uterine and vaginal longitudinal septum is so rare and its hysteroscopic surgical correction requires more expertise make the data provided by the study still valuable information (73). Interestingly, we see the findings of this study support what has been previously reported regarding higher risk of reproductive problems with shorter uterine septum than longer ones as discussed earlier.

Other important variables can explain the controversy that some investigators did not find prophylactic resection of uterine septum to be necessary to improve reproductive performance include two major flaws: first those investigators failed to control for important variables that affect reproductive performance in particular age and presence of other infertility factors. Clearly, the presence of uterine septum is not an absolute reason for reproductive failure. It is one factor among several others, all determining reproductive performance, that is, achievement and maintenance of pregnancy until full term. The second, failure to control for the type and extent of the uterine septum. As we mentioned before, there seems to be an inverse relationship between the length and extent of the uterine septum and reproductive failure (not university accepted). Worse outcomes were associated with shorter uterine septum than longer ones. Because it is usually easier to detect and diagnose more extensive (longer) uterine septum than shorter ones, this could have caused a selection bias in earlier studies. Those studies have included more women with longer uterine septum. Those women already have an overall much lower chance of poor reproductive outcome. So exposing them to surgical treatment or not would not be expected to make a significant difference (a huge sample size would be required to show statistical significance). In our experience, the longer the septum, the more vascular it was compared to the shorter septum. This observation was noticed during hysteroscopic metroplasty. This could explain why Dabirashrafi et al. (27) found higher amount of muscle tissue and vasculature in biopsies obtained from patients with uterine septum undergoing Tompkins procedure. Presumably, the majority of these patients had significant septum to warrant abdominal metroplasty.

Preoperative Preparation

Timing of Surgery

It is advisable to perform surgery early during the follicular phase, or patients are preoperatively treated with a gonadotropin-releasing hormone analog, to eliminate the possibility of endometrium, diminishing clarity of view during surgery. We have fairly good experience with endometrial preparation with few weeks of combined oral contraceptives. It is interesting to mention here a novel approach for preparing the endometrial cavity before hysteroscopic metroplasty (and other forms of hysteroscopic surgeries) that benefit from achieving thin endometrium. This novel approach is using one of the new third-generation aromatase inhibitors, for example, anastrozole or letrozole. By shutting off estrogen production, the use of aromatase inhibitors for few days before hysteroscopic surgery is expected to result in a thin endometrium that will facilitate the performance of the surgery (84).

Preoperative Preparation

Preoperative antibiotics are often empirically given, despite the lack of strong evidence to support it (28). In our practice, we do not routinely administer any antibiotics either preoperatively or postoperatively.

Operative Technique

Before proceeding into the detailed description of the surgical management of uterine septum (septum resection), it is important to clarify the misnomer of the word "resection." This is because surgical management of the uterine septum actually involves its "incision" and not "resection." Some prefer the word "lyse" rather than "resect" to describe the surgical management of the uterine septum.

As explained earlier, uterine septum results from the incomplete fusion between the two Müllerian ducts. Anatomically, the two ducts are side to side. So the incomplete fusion results in the persistence of the wall between the two tubes (the uterine septum) that extends anteroposteriorly (sagittal axis). For that reason, the uterine septum extends between the "anterior" and "posterior" walls of the uterus. Hence, the septum should be incised transversely. Every effort should be taken to make the

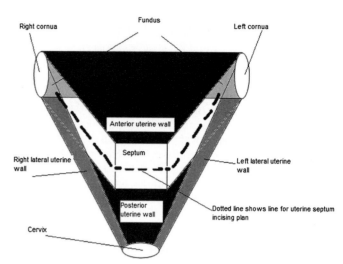

Drawing 13.6. Shows the technique of hysteroscopic incision of the uterine septum. The hallmark of success of this procedure lies in incising the septum in the right plan, that is, the middle of the septum (as shown by the dotted line), avoiding too much digging into the anterior or the posterior wall of the uterus or into the fundus.

transverse incision equidistant between the anterior and posterior uterine wall up to the fundus, without entering the fundal myometrium. The septum should be transected systematically in the midline, avoiding drifting to the posterior or anterior wall.

There are three important tools to help marinating the systematic resection of the septum in the midline (as illustrated in Drawing 13.6): 1) following the symmetry of both uterine tubal openings, 2) observing the rich myometrial vascularization when cutting through the uterine wall, and 3) observing the uniform translucency of the hysteroscopic light laparoscopically.

When the junction between the septum and myometrium is reached, small arteries may be seen pulsating. If these are cut, they bleed upon division, indicating that the septum has been transected completely. With the symmetric visual view of the uterotubal junctions and the laparoscopic uniform translucency of the hysteroscopic light, the hysteroscopist can safely transect the uterine septum without danger of perforation (77).

At the completion of the procedure, the intrauterine pressure produced by the distending fluid may be lowered to less than 50 mmHg. This helps in identifying areas of bleeding. Usually, small bleeders stop on their own, but if the number of active arterial bleeders is significant, these can be individually coagulated with a pinpoint electrode (26, 85–87).

Scissors Versus Resectoscope

As explained earlier, observing fundal bleeding helps in determining the depth of the resection (how close into the uterine fundus). Observing such fundal bleeding suggests transition to the vascular myometrium from the avascular tissue of the septum. For that reason, some surgeons prefer using sharp scissors without applying energy (as in the case with resectoscope) to be able to determine the extent of fundal bleeding the depth of cutting through the base of the uterine septum. However, in the hands of experienced hysteroscopic surgeons, the problem of identifying the depth of the base of the uterine septum and where to stop does not seem to be a problem.

Surgeons favoring sharp scissors than the resectoscope believe that the scissors have the advantage of avoiding greater cervical dilation that is necessary for introduction of the resectoscope into the uterine cavity. Also, when uterine perforation occurs with the resectoscope, it is mandatory to explore potential thermal damage beyond the uterine wall, that is, bowel thermal injury. This is because electrical current can spread a few millimeters beyond the point of contact of the electrode.

Some surgeons tried flexible microscissors. However, they are difficult to direct due to their flexibility and can be tedious with a large septum. However, rigid microscissors mounted on the sheath do not allow resection of a wide septum. The recommended scissors are those semirigid ones. Beside the advantage of watching for fundal bleeding to determine the depth of incision into the base of the uterine septum, semirigid scissors are simple and usually able to resect at a variable distance from the tip of the hysteroscope.

The resectoscope has the advantage of coagulation-resection, which is most beneficial when dealing with a very broad septa. A special straight knife or a loop oriented forward can be used for this purpose, using the blended current for simultaneous cutting and coagulation. Care should be taken not to overcorrect the defect because bleeding may not be a warning sign of invading myometrium when blended current (cutting/coagulating) is used (77). It is important also to realize that the extent of thermal damage is usually few millimeters distal to the damage observed visually. Thermal damage beyond the base of the septum into the myometrium could at least, theoretically, increase the risk of uterine rupture during subsequent pregnancy.

Concomitant laparoscopy was suggested to confirm the diagnosis of the uterine septum and monitor the extent of the depth of incising the base of the uterine septum. Concomitant laparoscopy also allows visualization of the transilluminated uterus by the hysteroscope light. By decreasing the intra-abdominal lighting, the laparoscopist can advice the hysteroscopist when a unified uterine cavity is achieved. Intraoperative ultrasound monitoring is a possibility and needs to be explored clinically. This is specially the case when hysteroscopic metroplasty is performed without concomitant laparoscopy. The availability of the modern 3D US that can very accurately distinguish between different uterine anomalies, especially bicornuate uterus versus uterine septum and can precisely determine the extent of the uterine septum.

The uterine cavity may be distended with several different solutions. Obviously, when energy is used such as electric energy with the hysteroscope, an electrolyte-free solution is necessary. However, with the use of sharp scissors, simple, safer distension media (such as normal saline) can be adequate (1).

Technique of Resecting a Complete Uterine Septum

In patients in whom the uterine is complete, that is, extending from the fundus to the cervix, hysteroscopic resection is still a safe and effective procedure. It may be completed after placing a Foley catheter into one cavity while the other cavity is distended with the distension media through the hysteroscope (76). Incision of the septum should begin "above" the level of the internal cervical os, which can be assisted by creating a window at the level of the internal os with the help of an ancillary probe inserted from the opposite cervical canal and then be continued superiorly until the septum is completely incised until the level of the fundus. It is important to stress here that the lower portion of the septum that lies "below" the level of

the internal cervical os has been suggested to be left without incising it (76). This is because it is believed that the cervical portion of the septum should be preserved to avoid disturbance of the internal os sphincter mechanism (88). However, conserving the cervical part of the complete septum is thought to increase the risk for cesarean section. In addition, it appears that the incidence of cervical incompetence after removal of the complete septum is rare (88a, b). Furthermore, a recent report suggested that resection of the cervical portion of the complete septum makes the procedure safer, easier, and less complicated than on preserving it, without impairment of reproductive outcome (88c).

Postoperative Care

After the procedure, uterine bleeding may be controlled using a Foley catheter to tamponade the cavity. It is important to ensure the patient's ability to void on her own before discharge home. Pain medications are usually administered in the form of mild analgesics. The use of strong analgesics is particularly important when a Foley catheter is left inside the uterine cavity. Some may insert an intrauterine device to prevent intrauterine adhesion formation (synechiae). However, other surgeons may opt to leave the uterine cavity empty. Hormonal therapy is often prescribed after the procedure to promote rapid epithelialization and decrease the risk of intrauterine synechiae. Estrogens are usually given in the form of conjugated estrogens and progesterone such as medroxyprogesterone acetate after estrogen course is completed. At the completion of hormonal treatment, after completing a withdrawal bleeding, SHG with 3D US is performed to assess the results of the hysteroscopic treatment by evaluating the uterine cavity. If the uterine cavity is satisfactory, the patient is allowed to conceive. Once pregnancy is achieved, consideration should be given to cervical cerclage versus careful monitoring of the cervical length with frequent transvaginal ultrasound. Attempts at pregnancy should be postponed for two months after surgery because postoperative hysteroscopy with biopsy has shown the uterine cavity to be normal at eight weeks after surgery (89).

Postoperative Ultrasonography

There have been some pathological studies showing that residual septa on the anterior and posterior walls, after septal incision, retract underneath the endometrium, and then the endometrium overgrows the area (29). Traditionally, most gynecologists are very conservative while performing hysteroscopic metroplasty for fear of uterine perforation or subsequent uterine rupture during pregnancy. Some noted that postoperative HSG always showed a residual septum (89a). Others found that the reproductive performance was not adversely affected by residual septum by up to one centimeter (89b). However, a recent report challenges that concept and suggests that women with a residual uterine septum have an increased chance of successful pregnancy with improved obstetric outcome after normalization of the uterine cavity (90).

OUTCOME OF SURGICAL EXCISION OF UTERINE SEPTUM

Grimbizis et al. (91) reported that all patients with recurrent miscarriage and normal fertility who were trying to become pregnant conceived spontaneously at least once after their treatment. Daly et al. (92) have reported normal postoperative monthly fecundity rates. This confirms that the application of hysteroscopic metroplasty does not impair the fertility potential of women with a history of recurrent miscarriages.

Grimbizis et al. (91) found significant improvement in pregnancy outcomes following hysteroscopic resection of the uterine septum including a drop in the miscarriage rate to 25 percent and increase in term delivery rate to 63.7 percent (although 4.5 percent of the pregnancies were still ongoing at the time of their publication). Other investigators have also described a significant improvement in pregnancy outcome after hysteroscopic metroplasty. Postoperative miscarriage rates between 5 and 20 percent and live birth rates between 73 and 87 percent were reported (22, 23, 26, 78, 87, 93, 94). However, these reports had significant limitations including the retrospective design and absence of control groups (patients served as their own historical control in some). Interestingly, data are more impressive in women with uterine septum undergoing ART. While pregnancy rates achieved after ART treatment done before and after hysteroscopic resection of the septum were comparable, the improvement of pregnancy outcome was very impressive (29). In a review of the literature, an overall term delivery rate of about 50 percent in patients with untreated uterine malformations was achieved, while the term delivery rate after hysteroscopic treatment was about 75 percent. The rate of pregnancy wastage in the post-treatment group was 15 percent compared with 96.3 percent in the pre-treatment group. The authors concluded that hysteroscopic septum resection can be applied as a therapeutic procedure in symptomatic patients and also as a "prophylactic" procedure in asymptomatic patients in order to improve their chances of a successful delivery (91, 95).

Patients with a previous hysteroscopic metroplasty or complicated hysteroscopy should be aware of the potential risks for uterine rupture during pregnancy. In a recent review of the literature to identify predictors of uterine rupture following operative hysteroscopy, the authors found a history of uterine perforation and/or the use of electrosurgery increase this risk but was not considered an independent risk factor. The authors concluded that uncomplicated hysteroscopic surgery did not alter obstetrical outcome and that apart from favorable use of scissors for hysteroscopic metroplasty, no accurate method to prevent or detect impending ruptures in subsequent pregnancies was found (96). In another series, two cases of uterine rupture during the delivery of twin pregnancies after hysteroscopic metroplasty led the investigators to suggest cesarean section to be performed for multiple pregnancy (97). In our experience, we did not have any patients who experienced uterine rupture in a subsequent pregnancy following hysteroscopic resection of the uterine septum (98).

SUMMARY AND FUTURE RESEARCH

There is significant controversy concerning diagnosis and management of uterine septum. The technology of 3D US constitutes a major breakthrough in evaluating the uterine cavity. This is particularly true when the assessment is complemented by both color Doppler examination and distension of the uterine cavity with saline or ultrasound contrast medium (SHG).

There are enough data supporting the routine surgical excision of the uterine septa, irrespective of their types, in women with poor reproductive history, in particular, recurrent preg-

nancy loss. However, in asymptomatic patients, the prophylactic excision of incidentally discovered uterine septum in asymptomatic patient is still controversial. In women undergoing ART treatment, surgical excision of an incidentally discovered uterine septum is more universally accepted. In infertility patients, we believe that incidentally discovered uterine septum and even arcuate uterus should be corrected hysteroscopically prior to any infertility treatment to enhance reproductive outcome.

The hysteroscopic approach for surgical resection of uterine septum is a safe and effective approach (77, 98). While generally it is an operator preference whether to utilize ablative energy, for example, electrical diathermy or laser, or to utilize sharp scissors without energy, the outcome of treatment is comparable as regards complication and reproductive performance after surgery.

For women with incidentally discovered uterine septum, there is a need for randomized prospective trials comparing pregnancy rate and pregnancy outcome in a treated and an untreated group. In such studies, accurate diagnosis of the extent and structure of the uterine septum can provide extremely valuable information about which septum subtypes correlate significantly with the different reproductive outcomes.

KEY NOTES

- The reproductive implications associated with the presence of uterine septa are a matter of significant controversy in the literature.
- There is a consensus on a relationship between uterine septa and various reproductive problems. However, the nature and extent of this relationship is still a big dilemma.
- Significant part of this dilemma is due to variation in the literature as regards the methods of diagnosis, treatment, and follow-up of women with uterine septa.
- The technology of 3D US constitutes a major breakthrough in evaluating the uterine cavity disorders, including uterine septa.
- While there are enough data supporting the routine surgical excision of the uterine septa, irrespective of their types, in women with recurrent pregnancy loss, in asymptomatic patient, the prophylactic excision of incidentally discovered uterine septum is still controversial. However, before assisted reproduction, surgical excision of an incidentally discovered uterine septum is more universally accepted.
- In infertility patients, we believe that incidentally discovered uterine septum and even arcuate uterus should be corrected hysteroscopically prior to any infertility treatment to enhance reproductive outcome.
- While the hysteroscopic approach for surgical resection of uterine septum is a safe and effective approach, the choice of surgical technique (using sharp scissors or electrocautery) is an operator preference.
- For women with incidentally discovered uterine septum, there is a need for randomized prospective trials, comparing reproductive performance in a treated and an untreated group.

REFERENCES

1. Lin PC, Bhatnagar KP, Nettleton GS et al. (2002). Female genital anomalies affecting reproduction. *Fertil Steril.* **78**: 899–915.

2. Ulfelder H, Robboy SJ. (1976). The embryologic development of the human vagina. *Am J Obstet Gynecol.* **126**:769–76.

3. Mossman HW. (1973). The embryology of the cervix. In (Blandau RJ, Moghissi K, (Eds.), *The biology of the cervix.* Chicago: University of Chicago Press, pp. 13–22.

4. Patton PE. (1994). Anatomic uterine defects. *Clin Obst Gynecol* **37**:705–21.

5. Lee DM, Osathanondh R, Yeh J. (1998). Localization of Bcl-2 in the human fetal Müllerian tract. *Fertil Steril* **70**:135–40.

6. McBean JH, Brumsted JR. (1994). Septate uterus with cervical duplication: a rare malformation. *Fertil Steril* **62**:415–17.

7. Ergun A, Pabuccu R, Atay V et al. (1997). Three sisters with septate uteri: another reference to bidirectional theory. *Hum Reprod* **12**:140–2.

8. Balasch J, Moreno E, Martinez-Romans S et al. (1996). Septate uterus with cervical duplication and longitudinal vaginal septum: a report of three new cases. *Eur J Obstet Gynecol Reprod Biol* **65**:241–3.

9. Muller PP, Musset R, Netter A et al. (1967). Etat du haut appareil urinaire chez les porteuses de malformations uterines: etude de 133 observations. *La Presse Med* **75**:1331–6.

9a. March C.M. (1990) Mullerian anomalies. *Fertil News* 24/1 *Endocrine Fertil Forum* **13**:1–5.

9b. Acien P. (1997). Incidence of Müllerian defects in fertile and infertile women. *Hum Reprod* **12**:1372–6.

10. Nahum GG. (1998). Uterine anomalies: how common are they, and what is their distribution among subtypes? *J Reprod Med* **43**:877–87.

11. Byrne J, Nussbaum-Blask A, Taylor WS Rubin A et al. (2000). Prevalence of Müllerian duct anomalies detected at ultrasound. *Am J Med Genet* **94**:9–12.

12. Raga F, Bauset C, Remohi J et al. (1997). Reproductive impact of congenital Müllerian anomalies. *Hum Reprod* **12**:2277–81.

13. Maneschi F, Zupi E, Marconi D et al. (1995). Hysteroscopically detected asymptomatic Müllerian anomalies. *J Reprod Med* **40**: 684–8.

14. Ashton D, Amin HK, Richart RM et al. (1988). The incidence of asymptomatic uterine anomalies in women undergoing transcervical tubal sterilization. *Obstet Gynecol* **72**:28–30.

15. Simon C, Martinez L, Pardo F et al. (1991). Müllerian defects in women with normal reproductive outcome. *Fertil Steril* **56**: 1192–3.

16. Nasri MN, Setchell ME, Chard T. (1990). Transvaginal ultrasound for the diagnosis of uterine malformations. *Br J Obstet Gynecol* **97**:1043–5.

17. Heinonen PK. (1997). Reproductive performance of women with uterine anomalies after abdominal or hysteroscopic metroplasty or no surgical treatment. *J Am Assoc Gynecol Laparosc* **4**:311–17.

18. Grimbizis GF, Camus M, Tarlatzis BC et al. (2001). Clinical implications of uterine malformations and hysteroscopic treatment results. *Hum Reprod Update* **7**:161–74.

19. Homer HA, Cooke TC, Li ID. (2000). The septate uterus a review of management and reproductive outcome. *Fertil Steril* **73**:1–14.

20. Buttram VC, Gibbons WE. (1979). Muellerian anomalies: a proposed classification (An analysis of 144 cases). *Fertil Steril* **32**:40–6.

21. The American Fertility Society. (1988). The American Fertility Society classifications of adnexal adhesions, distal tubal occlusion, tubal occlusion secondary to tubal ligation, tubal pregnancies, Müllerian anomalies and intrauterine adhesions. *Fertil Steril* **49**:944–55.

22. Fayez JA. (1986). Comparison between abdominal and hysteroscopic metroplasty. *Obstet Gynecol* **68**:399–403.

23. Daly DC, Maier D, Soto-Albors C. (1989). Hysteroscopic metroplasty: six years' experience. *Obstet Gynecol* **73**:201–5.

24. March CM. (1983). Hysteroscopy as an aid to diagnosis in female infertility. *Clin Obstet Gynecol* **26**:302–12.

25. Worthen N, Gonzalez F. (1984). Septate uterus: sonographic diagnosis and obstetric complications. *Obstet Gynecol* **64**:345–85.

26. Perino A, Mencaglia L, Hamou J et al. (1987). Hysteroscopy for metroplasty of uterine septa: report of 24 cases. *Fertil Steril* **48**: 321–3.

27. Dabirashrafi H, Bahadori M, Mohammad K et al. Septate uterus: new idea on the histologic features of the septum in this abnormal uterus. *Am J Obstet Gynecol* **172**:1.

28. Kupesic S, Kurjak A. (1998). Septate uterus: detection and prediction of obstetrical complications by different forms of ultrasonography. *J Ultrasound Med* **17**(10):631–6.

29. Kupesic S. (2001). Clinical implications of sonographic detection of uterine anomalies for reproductive outcome. *Ultrasound Obstet Gynecol* **18**:387–400.

29a. Exalto N, Stappers C, van Raamsdonk LA, Emanuel MH. (2007). Gel instillation sonohysterography: first experience with a new technique. *Fertil Steril* **87**:152–5.

30. Carrington BM, Hricak H, Nuruddin RN et al. (1990). Müllerian duct anomalies: magnetic resonance imaging evaluation. *Radiology* **176**:715.

31. Nicolini U, Bellotti M, Bonazzi B et al. (1987). Can ultrasound be used to screen uterine malformations? *Fertil Steril* **47**:89–93.

32. Keltz MD, Olive DL, Kim AH et al. (1997). Sonohysterography for screening in recurrent pregnancy loss. *Fertil Steril* **67**:670–4.

33. Soares SR, Barbosa dos Reis MMB, Camargos AF. (2000). Diagnostic accuracy of sonohysterography, transvaginal sonography, and hysterosalpingography in patients with uterine cavity diseases. *Fertil Steril* **73**:406–11.

34. Jurkovic D, Geipel A, Gruboeck K et al. (1995). Three-dimensional ultrasound for the assessment of uterine anatomy and detection of congenital anomalies: a comparison with hysterosalpingography and two-dimensional sonography. *Ultrasound Obstet Gynecol* **5**:233–7.

35. Jurkovic D, Gruboeck K, Tailor A et al. (1997). Ultrasound screening for congenital uterine anomalies. *Br J Obstet Gynaecol* **104**:1320–1.

35a. Abuzeid OM, Sakhel K, Abuzeid MI. (2005). Diagnosis of various type of uterine septum in infertile patients. *J Minim Invasive Gynecol* **12**(5 Suppl. 1).

35b. Hartman A. (2006). Uterine imaging—malformations, fibroids and adenomyosis, Thirty-Ninth Annual Postgraduate Program, Course 17 Reproductive Imaging—How to Improve the Outcome of Assisted Reproductive Technology, October 22, 2006, New Orleans, Louisana, sponsored by ASRM.

35c. Kupesic S, Kurjak A. (1998). Diagnosis and treatment outcome of the septate uterus. *Croat Med J* **39**:185–90.

36. Weinraub Z, Maymon R, Shulman A et al. (1996). Three-dimensional saline contrast hysterosonography and surface rendering of uterine cavity pathology. *Ultrasound Obstet Gynecol* **8**:277–82.

37. Lev-Toaff AS, Pinheiro LW, Bega G et al. (2001). Three-dimensional multiplanar sonohysterography. *J Ultrasound Med* **20**:295–306.

38. Ayida G, Kennedy S, Barlow D et al. (1996). Contrast sonography for uterine cavity assessment: a comparison of conventional two-dimensional with three-dimensional transvaginal ultrasound: a pilot study. *Fertil Steril* **66**:848–50.

39. Toaff ME, Lev-Toaff AS. (1984). Communicating uteri: review and classification of two previously unreported types. *Fertil Steril* **41**:661–79.

39a. Abuzeid M, Mitwally MF, Ahmed A et al. (2007). The prevalence of fimbrial pathology in patients with early stages of endometriosis. *J Minim Invasive Gynecol* **14**:49–53.

39b. Abuzeid MI, Sakhel K, Khedr M et al. (2003). The association of endometriosis and uterine septum. *Hum Reprod Suppl.* 1: P-610.

40. Kamm ML, Beernik HE. (1962). Uterine anomalies in habitual abortion and premature labor. *Obstet Gynecol* **20**:713–18.

41. Greiss FC, Mauzy CH. (1961). Genital anomalies in women: an evaluation of diagnosis, incidence, and obstetric performance. *Am J Obstet Gynecol* **82**:330–9.

42. Lewis BV, Brant HA. (1966). Obstetric and gynecologic complications associated with Müllerian duct abnormalities. *Obstet Gynecol* **28**:315–22.

43. Acien P. (1993). Reproductive performance of women with uterine malformations. *Hum Reprod* **8**:122–6

44. Goldenberg M, Sivian E, Sharabi Z et al. (1995). Reproductive outcome following hysteroscopic management of intrauterine septum and adhesions. *Hum Reprod* **10**:2663–5.

45. Homer HA, Tin-Chiu L, Cooke ID. (2000). The septate uterus: a report of management and reproductive outcome. *Fertil Steril* **73**:1–14.

45a. Gaucherand P, Awada A, Rudigoz RC et al. (1988). Obstetrical prognosis of septate uterus: a plea for treatment of the septum. *Eur J Obstet Gynecol Scand* **54**:109–12.

46. Buttram CV. (1983). Müllerian anomalies and their management. *Fertil Steril* **40**:159–63.

47. Heinonen PK, Saarkisoski S, Pystynen P. (1982). Reproductive performance of women with uterine anomalies. *Acta Obstet Gynecol Scand* **61**:157–62.

48. Sorensen SS, Trauelsen AG. (1987). Obstetric implication of Müllerian anomalies in oligomenorrheic women. *Am J Obstet Gynecol* **156**:1112–18.

49. Fenton AN, Singh BP. (1952). Pregnancy associated with congenital abnormalities of the female reproductive tract. *Am J Obstet Gynecol* **63**:744–8.

50. Rock JA, Jones HW. (1977). The clinical management of the double uterus. *Fertil Steril* **28**:798–806.

51. Woelfer B, Salim R, Banerjee S. (2001). Reproductive outcomes in women with congenital uterine anomalies detected by three-dimensional ultrasound screening. *Obstet Gynecol* **98**(6): 1099–103.

52. Lin PC. (2004). Reproductive outcomes in women with uterine anomalies. *J Womens Health (Larchmt)* **13**(1):33–9.

53. Raga F, Bauset C, Remohi J et al. (1997). Reproductive impact of congenital Müllerian anomalies. *Hum Reprod* **10**:2277–81.

54. Salim DR, Regan L,Woelfer B et al. (2003). A comparative study of the morphology of congenital uterine anomalies in women with and without a history of recurrent first trimester miscarriage. *Hum Reprod* **18**(1):162–6.

54a. Tomazevic T, Ban-Frangez H, Ribic-Pucelj M et al. (2006). Small uterine septum is an important risk variable for preterm birth. *Eur J Obstet Gynelcol* 2006. [Epub ahead of print.]

55. Jermy K, Oyelese O, Bourne T. (1999). Uterine anomalies and failed surgical termination of pregnancy: the role of routine preoperative transvaginal sonography. *Ultrasound Obstet Gynecol* **14**:431–3.

56. White MM. (1960). Uteroplasty in infertility. *Proc R Soc Med* **53**:1006.

56a. Fedele L, Dorta M, Brioschi D et al. (1989). Pregnancies in septate uteri: outcome in relation to site of uterine implantation as determined by sonography. *AJR* **152**:781–4.

57. Candiani GB, Fedele L, Zamferletti D et al. (1983). Endometrial patterns in malformed uteri. *Acta Eur Fertil* **14**:311–18.

58. Fedele L, Bianchi S, Marchini M et al. (1996). Ultrastructural aspects of endometrium in infertile women with septate uterus. *Fertil Steril* **65**:750–2.

59. Pellerito JS, McCarthy SM, Doyle MB et al. (1992). Diagnosis of uterine anomalies: relative accuracy of MR imaging, endovaginal sonography, and hysterosalpingography. *Radiology* **183**:795–800.

59a. Zreik TG, Troiano RN, Ghoussoub RA. (1998). Myometrial tissue in uterine septum. *J Am Assoc Gynecol Laparosc* **5**:155–60.

59b. Hinckley MD, Milki A. (2004). 1000 office-based hysteroscopies prior to in vitro fertilization: feasibility and findings. *JSLS* **8**:103–7.

59c. Tulandi T, Arronet GH, McInnes RA. (1980). Arcuate and bicornuate uterine anomalies and infertility, *Fertil Steril* **34**:362–4.

59d. Sorensen SS. (1981). Minor Mullerian anomalies and oligomenorrhea in infertile women. *Am J Obstet Gynecol* **140**:636–44.

59e. Raga F, Bonilla-Musoles F, Blanes J, Osborne NG. (1996). Congenital Mullerian anomalies: diagnostic accuracy of three dimensional ultrasound. *Fertil Steril* **65**:523–8.

59f. Abuzeid M, Sakhel K, Ashraf M et al. (2005). The association between uterine septum and infertility. *Fertil Steril* **84**(Suppl. 1): S472.

60. Lavergne N, Aristizabal J, Zarka V et al. (1996). Uterine anomalies and in-vitro fertilization: what are the results? *Eur J Obstet Gynecol Reprod Biol* **68**:29–34.

61. Kirsop R, Porter R, Torode H et al. (1991). The role of hysteroscopy in patients having failed IVF/GIFT transfer cycles. *Aust NZ J Obstet Gynaecol* **31**:263–4.

62. Dicker D, Ashkenazi J, Dekel A et al. (1996). The value of hysteroscopic evaluation in patients with preclinical in-vitro fertilisation abortions. *Hum Reprod* **11**:730–1.

63. Syrop CH, Sahakian V. (1992). Transvaginal sonography detection of endometrial polyps with fluid contrast augmentation. *Obstet Gynecol* **79**:1041–3.

64. Marcus S, Al-Shawaf T, Brinsden P. (1996). The obstetric outcome of in vitro fertilization and embryo transfer in women with congenital uterine malformation. *Am J Obstet Gynecol* **175**:85–9.

65. Testart J, Plachot M, Mandelbaum J et al. (1992). World collaborative report on IVF/ET and GIFT; 1989 results. *Hum Reprod* **7**:362–9.

66. Olive DL, Henderson DY. (1987). Endometriosis and mullerian anomalies. *Obstet Gynecol* **69**:412–15.

67. Ugur M, Turan C, Mungan T et al. (1995). Endometriosis in association with Müllerian anomalies. *Gynecol Obstet Invest* **40**:261–4.

68. Fedele L, Bianchi S, Di Nola G et al. (1992). Endometriosis and nonobstructive Müllerian anomalies. *Obstet Gynecol* **79**:515–17.

69. Nawroth F, Rahimi G, Nawroth C et al. (2006) Is there an association between septate uterus and endometriosis? *Hum Reprod* **2**:542–4. [Epub ahead of print.]

70. Leyendecker G, Kunz G, Herbertz M et al. (2004). Uterine peristaltic activity and the development of endometriosis. *Ann NY Acad Sci* **1034**:338–55.

71. Ugur M, Karakaya S, Zorlu G et al. (1995). Polycystic ovaries in association with Müllerian anomalies. *Eur J Obstet Gynecol Reprod Biol* **62**(1):57–9.

72. Noumoff JS, Heyner S, Farber M. (1986). The malignant potential of congenital anomalies of the paramenonephric ducts. *Sem Reprod Endocrinol* **4**:67–73.

73. Heinonen P. (2006). Reproductive surgery: complete septate uterus with longitudinal vaginal septum. *Fertil Steril* **85**(3):700–5.

74. Hirst BC. The operative treatment of uterus subseptus or semipartus with a case report. *Trans Obstet Soc Phila* **1919**:891–2.

75. Luikart R. (1936). Technic of successful removal of the septum uterine septus and subsequent deliveries at term. *Am J Obstet Gynecol* **31**:797–9.

76. Rock JA, Lippincott JB. (1992). Surgery for anomalies of the Müllerian ducts. In Thompson JD, Rock JA, (Eds.) *Te Linde's operative gynecology*. Seventh Edition. Philadelphia, pp. 603–46.

77. Rizk B (Ed.) (2008). Ultrasonography in reproductive medicine and infertility. Cambridge: United Kingdom, Cambridge University Press, (in press).

78. Choe KJ, Baggish SM. (1992). Hysteroscopic treatment of septate uterus with neodymium-YAG laser. *Fertil Steril* **57**:81–4.

79. Daly DC, Maier D, Soto-Albors C. (1989). Hysteroscopic metroplasty: six years experience. *Obstet Gynecol* **73**:201–5.

80. Lin BL, Iwata Y, Miyamoto N et al. (1987). Three contrast methods: an ultrasound technique for monitoring transcervical operations. *Am J Obstet Gynecol* **56**:469–72.

81. Mencaglia L, Tantini C. (1996). Hysteroscopic treatment of septate and arcuate uterus. *Gynaecol Endosc* **5**:151–4.

82. Thompson JP, Smith RA, Welch JS. (1966). Reproductive ability after metroplasty. *Obstet Gynecol* **28**:363–8.

83. Acién P. (1993). Reproductive performance of women with uterine malformations. *Hum Reprod* **8**:122–6.

84. Mitwally MF, Casper RF, Diamond MP. (2005). The role of aromatase inhibitors in ameliorating deleterious effects of ovarian stimulation on outcome of infertility treatment. *Reprod Bio Endocrinol* **3**:54.

85. Daly DC, Waiters CA, Soto-Albors CE et al. (1983). Hysteroscopic metroplasty: surgical technique and obstetric outcome. *Fertil Steril* **39**:623.

86. Valle RF, Sciarra JJ. Hysteroscopic treatment of the septate uterus. *Obstet Gynecol* **676**:253–986.

87. March CM, Israel R. (1987). Hysteroscopic management of recurrent abortion caused by septate uterus. *Am J Obstet Gynecol* **156**:834.

88. Rock JA, Roberts CP, Hesla JS. (1999). Hysteroscopic metroplasty of the class Va uterus with preservation of the cervical septum. *Fertil Steril* **72**:942.

88a. Vercellini P, De Giorgi O, Cortesi I et al. (1996). Metroplasty for the complete septate uterus: does cervical sparing matter? *J Am Assoc Gynecol Laparosc* **3**:509–14.

88b. Parsanezhad ME, Alborzi S. (2000). Hysteroscopic metroplasty: section of the cervical septum does not impair reproductive outcome. *Int J Gynaecol Obstet* **69**:165–6.

88c. Parsanezhad ME, Alborzi S, Zarei A et al. (2006). Hysteroscopic metroplasty of the complete uterine septum, duplicate cervix, and vaginal septum. *Fertil Steril* **85**:1473–7.

89. Candiani GB, Vercellini P, Fedele L, et al. (1990). Repair of the uterine cavity after hysteroscopic septal incision. *Fertil Steril* **54**:991.

89a. Nisolle M, Donnez J. (1996). Endoscopic treatment of uterine malformations. *Gynaecol Endosc* **5**:155–60.

89b. Fedele L, Bianchi S, Marchini M et al. (1996). Residual uterine septum of less than 1 cm after hysteroscopic metroplasty does not impair reproductive outcome. *Hum Reprod* **11**:727–9.

90. Kormanyos Z, Molnar BG, Pal A. (2006). Removal of a residual portion of a uterine septum in women of advanced reproductive age: obstetric outcome. *Hum Reprod* **4**:1047–51.

91. Grimbizis G, Camus M, Clasen K et al. (1998). Hysteroscopic septum resection in patients with recurrent abortions or infertility. *Hum Reprod* **13**:1188–93.

92. Daly DC, Maier D, Soto-Albers C. (1989). Hysteroscopic metroplasty: six years' experience. *Obstet Gynecol* **73**:201–5.

93. Fedele L, Arcaini L, Parazzini F et al. (1993). Reproductive prognosis after hysteroscopic metroplasty in 102 women: life table analysis. *Fertil Steril* **59**:768–72.

94. Jacobsen IJ, DeCherney A. (1997). Results of conventional and hysteroscopic surgery. *Hum Reprod* **12**:1376–81.

95. Preutthipan S, Linasmita V. (2001). Reproductive outcome following hysteroscopic treatment of the septate uterus: a result of 28 cases at Ramathibodi Hospital. *J Med Assoc Thai* **84**:166–70.

96. Sentilhes L, Sergent F, Roman H et al. (2005). Late complications of operative hysteroscopy: predicting patients at risk of uterine rupture during subsequent pregnancy. *Eur J Obstet Gynecol Reprod Biol* **120**:134–8.

97. Nisolle L, Donnez J. (1996). Endoscopic treatment of uterine malformations. *Gyaecol Endosc* **5**;155–60.

98. Abuzeid M, Mitwally MFM. (2008). Modern evaluation and management of uterine septum. In Rizk B, (Ed.) Ultrasonography in reproductive medicine and infertility. Cambridge: United Kingdom, Cambridge University Press, chapter 28, pp. 282–4.

14

Laser in Subfertility

John Erian, Anastasios Pachydakis

INTRODUCTION

The use of laser for fertility-conserving and fertility-enhancing surgery has gone through extensive debate during the past two decades. Most of the arguments against was the lack of concrete evidence for its superiority in the form of multicenter randomized trials that would justify the cost of this highly efficient precise surgical instrument (1). However, the efficacy and the ease of use have made the laser one of fertility surgeon's favorite. As with all surgical procedures, the most suitable is the one the surgeon is most comfortable with. Which tool a surgeon should use for the operation remains the subject of randomized trials to be conducted. In this chapter, we are going to give a brief description of the physical principles and the applications of the most commonly used lasers in subfertility surgery and provide evidence when it is available.

PHYSICS

Laser stands for light amplification by stimulated emission of radiation. The principle of the production of a laser beam is based on Einstein's theory of stimulated emission; an atom can be stimulated by an energy form – heat, electrical discharge, or photon bombardment – and stays stimulated for a calculated period of time. It then returns to its unstimulated state by emitting a photon, which is practically a light wave packet, one wave of light characteristic of the quality of the atom that was stimulated. Einstein stated that if the same kind of photon that would be normally emitted from a specific atom meets this atom, then the atom can produce another photon immediately, before the end of its calculated stimulated lifetime. The produced photon will be traveling in the same direction with the initial photon.

Imagine a tube that allows only the photons that travel in one direction to escape, while the other ones are reflected back into the tube. The reflected photons are forced to stimulate the production of more photons by changing traveling direction when they meet the walls of the tube in a snooker-like fashion. The result is many more photons – an "amplified" beam to exit the end of the tube traveling parallel to each other as the filter at the end of the tube is selective. If the atoms inside the tube are identical to each other, the photons produced will be identical – they have all the same wavelength – therefore, the beam will be "monochromatic" as opposed, for example, to the sunlight, which consists of photons produced by many particles and therefore can be analyzed during a rainbow phenomenon to many different beams – polychromatic. By using a lens, one can change the course of many photons – waves that travel parallel to each other – to make them all hit the same spot or area. The smaller the area, the more photons will hit the same point, therefore, the more energy will be delivered on a specific spot. If we change the distance between the lens and the beam, then it becomes defocused and the area affected is larger but smaller packets of energy are delivered in the area (Figure 14.1). So a laser that is used from a distance (no-touch method) to vaporize a peritoneal area can be used in close proximity or in contact to cut through the peritoneal surface. As the Nd:YAG laser is more penetrating, it is considered to be safer to use in a contact method only.

Depending on the atoms stimulated to produce a laser beam, the wavelength varies between ultraviolet, visible, or infrared (Nd:YAG and CO_2 lasers). Nonvisible lasers are usually coupled with a helium-neon laser beam that points the direction of the operating beam. Depending also on the wavelength is the percentage of the beam absorption in water or blood, for example, KTP laser is fully absorbed in 1 mm of blood, while CO_2 laser is fully absorbed in 1 mm of water.

PRACTICAL ASPECTS

As we discussed before, different beams have different properties, different absorption patterns, and therefore different potential (Table 14.1).

CO_2 lasers (Figure 14.2) are quickly absorbed in water and, therefore, are suitable for superficial treatments and unsuitable for hysteroscopic surgery as the fluid-filled cavity would quickly fill with bubbles and the energy would not reach the target. For this same reason, it is unsuitable to seal vessels as once it penetrates the vessel wall, it would be absorbed by the blood in the vessel's lumen and leave the opposite wall intact and therefore the vessel open.

The Nd:YAG laser is not absorbed by water, which makes it ideal for hysteroscopic surgery. When Nd:YAG meets the uterine wall, it scatters laterally, creating a crater of 3–5 mm in size, which may affect lateral structures (i.e., tubal ostia) Figure 14.3.

The Ho:YAG (holmium) laser is pulsed, creating a burst of microbubbles in the tissue as it is absorbed by water. This is making it especially useful in the dissection of planes Figure 14.4.

ENDOMETRIOSIS

Stages I–II

The most common application of laser in subfertility surgery is endometriosis. The use of a single puncture laparoscope that

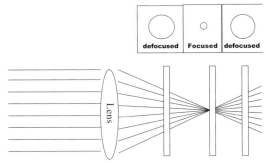

Figure 14.1. Change of focus with changing distance of target.

Table 14.1: Properties of Lasers Commonly Used in Subfertility

	Penetration (mm)	H_2O absorption	Application
CO_2	0.1	Great	C/NC
KTP	1–2	Medium	C/NC
Nd:YAG	4–5	Small	C/NC

admits an optic fiber allows a two port laparoscopy with ablation of the lesions in early-stage disease, while in advanced-stage disease it allows vaporization and coagulation with absolute precision. As there is clear evidence that destruction of early lesions is improving fertility rates and pelvic pain and in the absence of evidence that excision is superior to ablation, this should be considered adequate treatment. The use of a laser at low power permits ablation of nodules in proximity of bladder and the ureters as it is accurately directed, there is minimal lateral damage to the tissues, and the depth of maximum absorption for Nd:YAG (Figure 14.3), for example, between 500 μm and 1 mm (2). As with all coagulating methods, excellent knowledge of anatomy and familiarity with the equipment and the immediate or delayed damage it may cause to tissues is of paramount importance.

The surgeon has to keep in mind that if a lesion is overlying the ureter, for example, the actual depth of tissue at the end of the vaporization of the lesion may be less than 1 mm. Injection of normal saline behind the lesion has been suggested by various authors (3) as a solution to this problem; the water absorbs the remaining energy of the laser protecting the underlying structure, given that the laser used is absorbed by water. However, complications do arise when surgery is extending in the retroperitoneal space and the rectouterine septum. The complication rate can be as high as 6 percent, involving bowel, ureter, and uterine artery perforation (4).

It has been demonstrated that laser is as effective in minimal to moderate disease, while it is more efficient than laparotomy in advanced disease (5) regarding fecundity and pregnancy rates. In the same study, the pregnancy rates between early moderate and severe disease were comparable, reaching 65 percent while later studies suggested that pregnancies after laser treatment occur sooner than after electrosurgery (6). It has to be noted though that this is a trend only and these studies where largely uncontrolled.

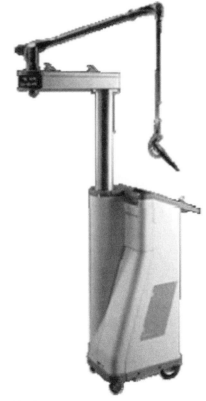

Figure 14.2. CO_2 Laser.

Endometriosis Stages III–IV

The role of extensive surgery to treat deeply infiltrating endometriosis is debatable (5) with the exception of endometriomas (6) where excision seems to be superior to ablation regarding spontaneous pregnancy rate. This does not apply to patients with pelvic pain, where the consensus is that excision is effective in the treatment of the symptoms. The use of assisted reproduction technologies may be the most effective way of improving the pregnancy rates of these patients as the peritoneal factor is bypassed. As the internal surface of chocolate cysts is the external surface of the ovary, and regardless of the debate about the depth of invasion of the endometrionas (7), a surgeon should keep in mind that when ablating the cyst base, ovarian tissue is sacrificed. The accuracy of the laser beam vaporization and the selectivity and limited penetration of the laser, especially the CO_2, may aid the maximal preservation of ovarian tissue. However, experts have favored KTP for ovarian endometriomas in the past (4); in a mixed series of moderate and severe endometriosis, the cumulative pregnancy rates were 80 percent but the miscarriage rate was in the region of 31 percent, reflecting the high pregnancy failure rate related to endometriosis (8). Recent developments in coagulating instruments like the helium thermoablator fall outside the scope of this chapter.

ADHESIONS

Intraperitoneal

There is no evidence of the superiority of laser versus other methods of coagulation or blunt dissection for the treatment

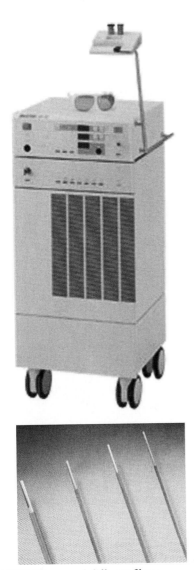

Figure 14.3. NdYAG Laser and different fibres.

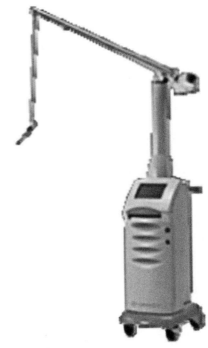

Figure 14.4. Ultrapulse Laser.

of subfertility. Indeed, before embarking into adventurous adhesiolysis, a surgeon should keep in mind that the evidence for the benefits of adhesiolysis to fertility is not robust (9). In our experience, filling the abdomen with normal saline to prevent inadvertent organ damage and use of an operative laparoscope with a second port to introduce grasping forceps are the minimum requirements to perform an adhesiolysis. The CO_2 laser allows accurate dissection planes with minimal lateral damage. The main advantage is the layer-by-layer destruction of the connective tissue, with minimal charring as vaporization occurs before charcoal formation. This phenomenon allows the visualization of the underlying tissue. Another advantage is that there is no concern about electrical current being transferred to adjacent structures. However, when CO_2 laser is used, hemostasis in large vessels is not possible to be achieved; therefore, it is not appropriate for vascular adhesions.

Treatment is through a nonconduct coagulation, which allows fast movement from plane to plane without the probe adhering to the coagulating tissue. Care should be taken for the probe not to dip in the irrigating fluid as its temperature is high and it may be damaged. It has been demonstrated that

there is no difference in pregnancy rates or recurrence between adhesiolysis performed with the CO_2 laser and that done with electrocautery (10,11). The overall intrauterine pregnancy rate after salpingoovariolysis is 51–62 percent, and the rate of ectopic pregnancy is 5–8 percent. No de novo adhesions after treatment of endometriotic adhesions were reported in one series (12). The argon laser has been used with good results, but the instrument-related complication rate including breakage and melting of the tip is reported to be as high as 8 percent (13).

Intrauterine

The treatment of intrauterine adhesions secondary to trauma or infection is imperative to offer a suitable environment for implantation. However, no method is guaranteeing normal placentation and the risk of placenta accreta is present. The Nd:YAG laser has been used successfully to treat intrauterine adhesions with encouraging reproductive outcomes. The obvious benefits are the use of normal saline as distending medium, which is circulated to flush the carbon debris, accurate division with minimal lateral damage, and good access to all sites in the cavity as the optic fiber is extending through the tip of the hysteroscope and therefore can reach difficult angles (13). A two-stage procedure has been suggested when the distortion of the anatomy is preventing identification of normal myometrium (14).

FIBROIDS

Hysteroscopic Myomectomy

The Nd:YAG laser has been widely used for hysteroscopic myomectomies as one- or two-stage procedure. KTP has also been used successfully. In all cases, the uterus must be away from all organs as there is a marked thermal effect with the touch technique. A new solution to the problem is intra-abdominal sonography, (1) but only early reports are available. In case of large fibroids, a two-stage procedure has been suggested where the intracavitary part of the fibroid is dissected with an Nd:YAG laser and subsequently the intramural part is treated with interstitial laser. In a second procedure, the remaining fibroid (if any) can be excised. The absence of a dissecting plane should raise the suspicion of a stromal tumor, which is reported in 1.2 percent of cases of hysteroscopic myomectomy by Donnez and Nicole (15). There is no evidence regarding the safety and the subsequent pregnancy outcomes of the two-stage procedure.

Laparoscopic and MRI/TVUS-Guided Interstitial Myolysis

Interstitial myolysis using a bare optic fiber of KTP, YAG, or diode laser (16) has been reported as resolving symptoms and leaving a uterus capable of child bearing. The MRI technique has the advantage of providing thermal mapping, which allows more accurate distribution of the energy. However, subsequent reports of uterine rupture (17) have led authorities in the field to recommend this procedure only for women who are forty years or older and do not wish to continue further pregnancies (18). All women who had a repeat laparoscopy in the same series of laparoscopic myolysis had extensive adhesions probably secondary to the necrosis.

This is a minimally invasive technique using needles passed through the abdominal wall or the vagina. The optic fiber is subsequently passed through the needles to the core of the fibroid resulting in devascularization and necrosis of the fibroid (18).

- There is clear evidence that surgical treatment of endometriosis improves pelvic pain and fecundity rates.
- There is no proven difference in pregnancy rates or recurrence between adhesiolysis performed with the CO_2 laser versus electrocautery.
- Newer techniques involve use of laser fibers under transvaginal ultrasound or MRI guidance.

MULLERIAN FUSION DEFECTS

The KTP or the Nd:YAG is the laser of choice for uterine septums, and the CO_2 is used for vaginal septums. Division or conservation of the cervical portion of the septum to prevent incompetence is still under debate (19). The vaporization of the septum is continued until the ostia are seen at the same level. The septum is usually avascular; therefore, hemostasis problems should raise suspicion. Simultaneous laparoscopy may help prevent perforation. There is no evidence to support the use of cyclical hormonal treatment or of a intrauterine device postoperatively.

OVARIAN DRILLING

Laparoscopic or transvaginal ovarian drilling using Nd:YAG or CO_2 laser is possible . Results from the transvaginal approach are comparable with the laparoscopic electrosurgery; however, larger series are awaited. The transvaginal route is possible as the fiber is guided through a needle, and the energy is delivered at the tip of the fiber under direct ultrasound control. The tip is embedded in the stroma, and the craters are visible on ultrasound (20).

OTHER APPLICATIONS

Although laser-assisted hatching in IVF cycles seemed a promising new technique, neither laser-assisted hatching nor laser-assisted ICSI showed any advantage when tested in controlled trials (21).

Hair removal in PCOS patients can be achieved through multiple applications of laser. The effect is long lasting but not necessarily permanent, and it appears that the best results are achieved with Nd:YAG laser applied on dark hair in fair skin tone patients (17).

KEY POINTS

- The best instrument is the one the surgeon is familiar with.
- Different types of laser have different qualities and different applications.
- CO_2 laser is better for accurate dissection.
- Nd:YAG and KTP are better for hysteroscopic procedures and sealing vessels.

REFERENCES

1. Kaseki H et al. Laser hysteroscopic myomectomy guided by laparoscopically assisted intra-abdominal sonohysterography (LHMY-GLAIS): a preliminary report. 2001;17(3): 79–86.
2. Bellina JH, Hemmings R, Voros IJ et al. Carbon dioxide laser and electrosurgical wound study with an animal model. A comparison of healing pattern and tissue damage in peritoneal tissue. *Am J Obstet Gynecol* 148:327.
3. Nehzat C, Crowgey SR, Garrison CP. Surgical treatment of endometriosis via laser laparoscopy. *Fertil Steril* 45:778–83.
4. Sutton C. Lasers in infertility. *Rev Hum Reprod* 1993;8(1): 133–46.
5. Green Top Guideline No 24. The Investigation and management of Endometriosis RCOG, October 2006.
6. Hart RJ, Hickey M, Maouris P, Buckett W, Garry R. Excisional surgery versus ablative surgery for ovarian endometriomata (Cochrane Review). *Cochrane Lib* 2006;(3).
7. Garry R. The endometriosis syndromes: a clinical classification in the presence of aetiological confusion and therapeutic anarchy. *Hum Reprod* 2004;19:760–8.
8. Sutton C. Laser laparoscopy in the treatment of endometriosis. A 5-year study. *Br J Obstet Gynaecol* 1990;97(2):181–5.
9. Ahmad G, Watson A, Vandekerckhove P et al. Techniques for pelvic surgery in subfertility. *Cochrane Database Syst Rev.* 2006;(2).
10. Mecke H. Pelviscopic adhesiolysis in chronic pelvic pain—laser versus conventional techniques. *Geburtshilfe Frauenheilkd* 1992; 52(1):47–50.
11. Ahmad G, Watson A, Vandekerckhove P, Lilford R. Techniques for pelvic surgery in subfertility (Cochrane Review). *Cochrane Database Syst Rev* 2006; (2).
12. Nezhat C, Nezhat FR, Metzger DA, Luciano AA. Adhesion reformation after reproductive surgery by videolaseroscopy. *Fertil Steril* 1990;53:1008.
13. Badawy SZ. Argon laser laparoscopy for treatment of pelvic endometriosis associated with infertility and pelvic pain. *J Gynecol Surg* 1991;7(1):27–32.
14. Chapman R. The value of two stage laser treatment for severe Asherman's syndrome. *Br J Obstet Gynaecol* 1996;103(12): 1256–8.

15. Donnez J. Gillerot S, Bourgonjon D, Clerckx F, Nisolle M. Neodymium: YAG laser hysteroscopy in large submucous fibroids. *Fertil Steril* 1990;54:999–1003.

16. Chapman R. New therapeutic technique for treatment of uterine leiomyomas using laser-induced interstitial thermotherapy (LITT) by a minimally invasive method. *Lasers Surg Med* 1998; 22(3):171–8.

17. Sanchez LA, Perez M. Laser hair reduction in the hirsute patient: a critical assessment. *Hum Reprod Update* 2002;8(2):169–81.

18. Donnez J. Laparoscopic myolysis. *Hum Reprod Update* 6(6): 609–13.

19. Rock JA. Hysteroscopic metroplasty of the Class Va uterus with preservation of the cervical septum. *Fertil Steril* 1999;72(5): 942–5

20. Zhu L. Transvaginal, ultrasound-guided, ovarian, interstitial laser treatment in anovulatory women with clomifene-citrate-resistant polycystic ovary syndrome. *BJOG* 2006;113(7): 810–16.

21. Richter K et al. No advantage of laser assisted hatching over conventional intracytoplasmic sperm injection; a randomized controlled trial. *J Exp Clin Assist Reprod Biomed Central.*

15

ULTRASONOGRAPHY OF THE ENDOMETRIUM FOR INFERTILITY

Richard Palmer Dickey

INTRODUCTION

Ultrasound (US) measurement of the endometrium is now an indispensable part of ovulation induction monitoring and assisted reproductive technologies (ART). It also has a role in evaluation of unexplained infertility. Before ultrasound, the condition of the endometrium could only be evaluated by progesterone challenge to induce withdrawal bleeding or by invasive procedures, biopsy, curettage, and hysteroscopy. Endometrial physiology and implantation have recently been reviewed by Strowitzki et al. (1). This chapter will describe the use of US in the evaluation of infertility and monitoring ovulation induction for ART and for relations or artificial insemination.

ENDOMETRIAL EVALUATION

Endometrial Pattern

Evaluation of the endometrium in infertility was initially focused on its appearance or pattern and only later was the importance of endometrial thickness fully appreciated. Smith et al. (2) first reported use of the appearance and thickness of the endometrium to decide when to administer human chorionic gonadotropin to initiate ovulation (hCG). They classified endometrial patterns as Type A, a multilayered "triple-line" endometrium consisting of a prominent outer and central hyperechogenic line and inner hypoechogenic or black regions; Type B, an intermediate isoechogenic pattern, with the same reflectivity as the surrounding myometrium and a nonprominent or absent central echogenic line; and Type C, an entirely homogenous endometrium without a central echogenic line. Subsequently, Gonan et al. (3, 4) reversed the ABC order. The ABC classification is infrequently used in current literature. When endometrial pattern is reported, it is usually described as triple-line or "homogenous," the two most common endometrial patterns (5, 6). A third term "postovulation" may be used to describe the bright hyperechogenic pattern seen normally in the midluteal phase.

Endometrial Thickness

Endometrial thickness is customarily measured from outside to inside in an anterior-posterior view at the widest point; if measured inside to outside, the difference can be as much as 2 mm. The difference in how thickness is measured can explain some of the difference values critical for successful implantation reported in the literature. Endometrial thickness measured by transvaginal US correlates well with histological endometrial maturation according to Hofmann et al. (7). However, others (8, 9) found no relationship between endometrial thickness and histological dating of endometrial tissue obtained by biopsy.

Endometrial waves

Endometrial wavelike activity is often seen on US throughout spontaneous cycles and during ovulation induction with human menopausal gonadotropin (hMG) or follicle-stimulating hormone (FSH) (10–15). The highest rate of activity is seen during the periovulatory period when opposing waves from the fundus to the cervix and from the cervix to the fundus occur in 30–40 percent of spontaneous cycles at a rate of three to four waves per minute (15). Endometrial wavelike activity was found in 100 percent of hMG cycles at the time of ovulation. No waves from the fundus to the cervix occurred during the midluteal phase of hMG cycles. The clinical importance of endometrial waves is undetermined. No relationship between the presence or absence of endometrial waves and the outcome of ovulation induction (OI) or in vitro fertilization (IVF) has been reported.

ENDOMETRIAL CHANGES DURING SPONTANEOUS CYCLES

In spontaneous cycles, endometrial thickness increases from a mean of 4.6 mm during menstruation, nine to thirteen days before the luteinizing hormone (LH) surge, to 12.4 mm the day of the LH surge (16–18) (Figure 15.1). Although the increase in thickness is generally constant, averaging less than 1 mm per day, thickness may increase by as much as 2 mm a day in the late proliferative phase. Endometrial thickness normally decreases by 0.5 mm the day of LH surge, before beginning to increase again by an additional 2 mm during the luteal phase (16). Endometrial thickness has been found to be significantly thicker five days after egg retrieval in IVF cycles (19). The endometrial pattern develops a triple-line appearance from day 6 before the LH surge until seven days after the LH surge, when the triple-line pattern becomes obscured by the increasingly hyperechogenic pattern of the endometrium (18).

Uterine pathology may affect results of endometrial US scans. Sher et al. (20) reported finding uterine pathology

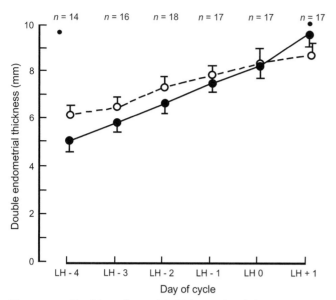

Figure 15.1. Double endometrial thickness (mm) in spontaneous (○) and CC (●) cycles (mean ± SEM). LH-0 = day of onset of LH surge. *$P < 0.05$. From Randall and Templeton (1991). Reproduced with permission of the authors and the publisher, the American Society for Reproductive Medicine (The American Fertility Society).

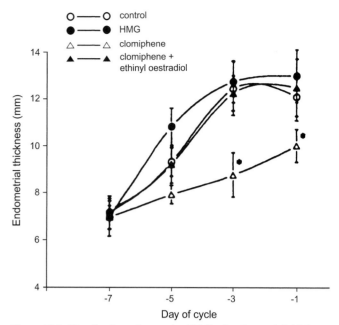

Figure 15.2. Distribution of mean (± SEM) of endometrial thickness at four points in the cycle. ○, controls; ●, human menopausal gonadotropin (HMG); Δ, clomiphene; ▲, clomiphene + ethinyl estradiol. *$P < 0.01$ compared with the control cycle result at the same phase of the cycle. From Yagel et al. (1992). Reproduced with permission of the authors and the publisher, the American Society for Reproductive Medicine (The American Fertility Society).

(leiomyomas, severe uterine synechiae, diethyl stilbestrol DES anomalies, and adenomyosis) in 93.8 percent of patients with homogeneous endometrial patterns, compared to 30 percent of patients with triple-line pattern and endometrial thickness less than 9 mm and 5.8 percent of patients with triple-line pattern and thickness 9 mm or greater.

ENDOMETRIAL CHANGES DURING OI

When clomiphene citrate (CC) is used for ovulation induction, endometrial thickness is often decreased compared to spontaneous cycles during and immediately following the days CC is taken because of its antiestrogen effect (17) (Figure 15.1). During the late proliferative phase, endometrial thickness increases at a faster rate in CC cycles than in spontaneous cycles as it escapes from the antiestrogen and the effect of increased estrogen due to multiple follicle growth becomes manifest. During ovulation induction with hMG and FSH, without CC, endometrial thickness is greater than in spontaneous cycles (21) (Figure 15.2).

During stimulation cycles for IVF, an average increase in length of the endometrial cavity by 3.8 mm and length of the cervical canal by 1.9 mm correlated with increase in endometrial thickness (22).

CRITICAL US VALUES FOR OI

Endometrial Pattern

A triple-line pattern on the day of hCG administration has been reported to be necessary for implantation in controlled ovarian hyperstimulation (COH) cycles, where hMG or FSH is administered, by some authors (23, 24). However, others (6) found

no difference in initial pregnancy rate between a triple-line pattern (10.9 percent) and intermediate pattern (10.2 percent), in CC and COH cycles for OI before intrauterine insemination, but noted a difference in continuing pregnancy rates of 9.4 percent for the triple-line pattern and 7.3 percent for the intermediate pattern.

Endometrial Thickness

Decreased endometrial thickness is linked to failure to conceive and biochemical pregnancy in CC, hMG, and spontaneous cycles (6, 25). In a study of endometrial thickness on the day of hCG administration for timed intrauterine insemination (IUI), optimal pregnancies and birth (continuing pregnancy) rates occurred when endometrial thickness was 9 mm or greater on the day of hCG administration (Table 15.1). No pregnancies occurred when endometrial thickness was less than 6 mm in spontaneous, CC, or hMG cycles (6).

Endometrial thickness was related to the type of OI (Table 15.3). Endometrial thickness was greater than 9 mm in 59.2 percent of HMG cycles, compared to 47.2 percent of clomiphene cycles and 34.8 percent of spontaneous cycles. Endometrial thickness was less than 6 mm in 9.1 percent of CC cycles but was also less than 6 mm in 8.7 percent of spontaneous cycles of donor insemination patients (Table 15.2). By contrast, endometrial thickness on the day of hCG was less than 6 mm in 2.0 percent of patients in hMG cycles. The antiendometrial effect of CC was clearly apparent when CC and hMG (hMG + CC) were used in the same cycle. The finding of decreased endometrial thickness in clomiphene cycles has been confirmed in numerous studies (6, 8, 17, 23, 26–30).

Table 15.1: Endometrial Thickness versus Outcome in OI Intrauterine Insemination Cycles

	Percentage of total pregnancy			Pregnancy/outcome	
Thickness (mm)	Cycle	Rate (%)	Bio. (%)	Clinical Abor. (%)	Term (%)
<6	9.1	0	0	0	0
6–8	43.6	8.1	21.4	15.4	62.5
≥9	47.2	14.0	0	12.2	87.8

Adapted from Dickey et al., 1993a, 1993b. Reproduced with permission of the publisher.

Table 15.2: Endometrial Thickness according to Ovulation Regimen: Percent Cycles

Regimen	No. cycles	<6 mm, % (n)	6–8 mm, % (n)	>9 mm, % (n)
None	23	8.7 (2)	56.5 (12)	34.8 (8)
CC	197	9.1 (18)	43.6 (86)	47.2 (93)
hMG	49	2.0 (1)	38.8 (19)	59.2 (29)
hMG + CC	205	11.2 (23)	55.6 (114)	33.2 (68)

CC, clomiphene. Adapted from Dickey et al., 1993b. Reproduced with permission of the publisher.

Table 15.3: Pregnancy and Continuing Pregnancy per Cycle according to Regimen and Endometrial Thickness

	6–8 mm			>9 mm		
	Cycles (n)	Pregnant, % (n)	Continuing, % (n)	Cycles (n)	Pregnant, % (n)	Continuing, % (n)
None	13	15.4 (2)	7.7 (1)	8	0 (0)	0 (0)
CC	86	8.1 (7)	7.0 (6)	93	14.0 (13)	14.0 (13)
hMG	19	10.5 (2)	0 (0)	29	17.2 (5)	13.8 (4)
hMG + CC	114	9.6 (11)	7.0 (8)	68	14.7 (10)	11.8 (8)

CC, clomiphene. Adapted from Dickey et al., 1993b, Reproduced with permission of the publisher.

CRITICAL US VALUES FOR IVF CYCLES

Endometrial Pattern

Smith et al. (2) who were the first to report the importance of endometrial pattern and thickness to successful outcome in IVF and gamete intra fallopian transfer (GIFT) found that implantation did not occur, or occurred less often, if the endometrium lacked a triple-line pattern on the day of or one day before ovum retrieval in IVF cycles. This finding was later confirmed by others (3–5, 21, 31–36). A triple-line endometrial pattern on the day of hCG administration in IVF cycles is related to serum estradiol level, the number of mature oocytes, and the number of top-quality embryos (5). A triple-line pattern is also important in donor oocyte cycles (37).

Endometrial Thickness

Pregnancy does not occur in IVF cycles presumably because of failure of embryos to implant, if the endometrium it too thin on the day of hCG administration according to the majority of studies (2–5, 22, 38–40); however, others (26, 31–34, 41) have reported no relationship between thickness and pregnancy in IVF cycles. Many of the studies that failed to find a relationship between thickness and outcome compared mean thickness in conception and nonconception cycles, while most studies that found a relationship reported critical or "cutoff" values below which no pregnancies occurred. In most studies, the critical thickness value is reported as 6 mm, but the range is from 4 mm (42) to 7 mm (29). One reason for the different cutoff values is that endometrial thickness can change, either increase or decrease, between the day hCG is administered and the day implantation is presumed to occur, a difference of eight to nine days. Importantly, in all studies of oocyte donation, endometrial thickness on the day of embryo transfer has been found to be critical for implantation (7, 43–45).

As is true for OI and IUI, optimal pregnancy rates and birth rates occur when endometrial thickness on the day of hCG administration is equal to or greater than 9 mm (6, 21, 39, 43) or 10 mm (30, 38, 44), respectively.

It has been suggested that an endometrium that is too thick, 14 mm or greater, on the day of hCG administration may result in reducing the chance of a clinical pregnancy (46). Biochemical pregnancies were found to be more frequent in IVF cycles when endometrial thickness was less than 9 mm or greater than 13 mm (5). No relationship between endometrial thickness on the day of hCG and biochemical pregnancy in IVF was observed in another study (47). An excessively thick endometrium may have its origins in the previous cycle. It is common practice not to start hMG or FSH stimulation for an IVF cycle if endometrial thickness is greater than 6 mm.

Other US Findings

Pregnancy rates are significantly lower when hydrosalpinges are present at the time of transfer (48, 49). Pregnancy rates were doubled, when hydrosalpinges were removed before IVF (49) and when hydrosalpinges were aspirated at the time of oocyte retrieval (50). Implantation does not occur when endometrial fluid is present on US the day of embryo transfer, even when the fluid is aspirated (51). Endometrial polyps less than 2 cm do not decrease pregnancy rates, but there is a trend toward increased pregnancy (52).

PRECLINICAL MISCARRIAGE (BIOCHEMICAL PREGNANCY)

Preclinical miscarriage, also referred to as biochemical pregnancies, in which quantitive hCG levels initially indicate pregnancy but decrease before a gestational sac can be seen on ultrasound, and clinical miscarriage of embryos with karyotype may be the result of inadequate endometrial development. Because there are no products of conception (POC) for chromosome analysis in biochemical pregnancy, the reason for failure cannot be determined. However, because POC karyotypes are normal in 52 percent of spontaneous miscarriages (53), it is reasonable to hypothesize that inadequate endometrial development is responsible for at least some cases of early pregnancy loss. In a study of the relationship of endometrial thickness and pattern to pregnancy outcome following OI cycles for IUI, 21.9 percent of pregnancies were biochemical pregnancies if endometrial thickness was 6–8 mm at the time of hCG administration, compared to none when thickness was 9 mm or greater (25). The incidence of clinical abortion after a gestational sac had been seen on US was 15.6 percent when endometrial thickness was 6–8 mm, compared to 12.2 percent when thickness was 9 mm or greater. On statistical analysis, biochemical pregnancies were significantly related to endometrial thickness and pattern and were unrelated to maternal age or number of previous spontaneous abortions. By contrast, clinical abortions were significantly related to maternal age and previous abortion and were unrelated to endometrial thickness or pattern. In an earlier study of IVF and GIFT outcome, a triple-line endometrial pattern was significantly related to the number of mature oocytes and best-quality embryos in addition to being related to serum estradiol levels (5).

KEY POINTS

■ For optimal pregnancy and birth results, endometrial thickness should be 9 mm or thicker on, at the time of spontaneous LH surge, or when hCG is administered, OI cycles for relations or IUI and when hCG is administered in IVF cycles. When endometrial thickness is less than 9 mm but 6 mm or greater, or if there is fluid in the endometrial cavity, three treatment options are available.

■ Administration of HCG can be delayed to allow thickness to increase and fluid to disappear. Delay in administering HCG is particularly useful in CC cycles because during the late proliferative phase endometrial thickness increases at a faster rate as it escapes from the antiestrogen effect of clomiphene than in spontaneous cycles (17) (Figure 15.1). If delay is not possible because a spontaneous LH surge is starting or because estrogen levels are rising too rapidly, there are still two treatment options.

■ The cycle OI or IVF cycle can be canceled and a different regimen of follicle recruitment used in a latter cycle or, in the case of IVF, hCG and all embryos cryopreserved for transfer at a latter time. If it has been a CC cycle, in sub-

sequent cycles endometrial thickness may be improved by starting CC earlier in the cycle or on menstrual day 3 instead of 5 (6) because the antiestrogen effect of CC lasts no more than three to four days after the last dose, by taking a lower dose of CC, by giving estrogen along with CC (21) (Figure 15.2), or by switching to tamoxifen, an antiestrogenic that is structurally similar to CC but that has less antiestrogen effect on the endometrium and cervical mucus. When tamoxifen is used in place of CC, a dose of 20–25 mg is approximately equal to 50 mg of CC in OI effectiveness. If it has been an hMG or FSH cycle, the dose of gonadotropin can be increased in a subsequent cycle in the expectation, not always realized, that estrogen levels will be higher and result in a better endometrial pattern and thickness.

■ The OI or IVF cycle can be allowed to proceed and estrogen given in the expectation that endometrial thickness will increase by the time implantation occurs or embryos are transferred. In the case of IVF, embryos can be cryopreserved if endometrial thickness does not increase.

■ A potential disadvantage of estrogen administration in nongonadotropin cycles is that high doses may suppress natural FSH secretion or block a spontaneous LH surge. Therefore, estrogen should not be started until after hCG is given or a LH surge has occurred. When oral estrogen is given before an LH surge or hCG, low doses should be taken two to four times a day, instead of a single large dose once a day, to minimize serum levels. An alternative method of administrating estrogen in clomiphene cycles is to start a regimen of four times a day and step down one tablet a day. The rational for this approach is that it takes approximately three days to induce endometrial changes in response to estrogen. The type of estrogen is not important, but highest effectiveness is achieved if the estrogen is administered vaginally. An alternative to oral estrogen is administration by injection, skin patches, or vaginally. In the author's clinic, a 2-mg micronized estradiol tablet, ordinarily taken orally once daily for menopause symptoms, is prescribed for insertion vaginally twice a day.

■ Low-dose aspirin (80–81 mg daily) has been reported to increase the incidence of triple-line pattern (54) and pregnancy rates (54–57) but without a significant increase in endometrial thickness (54, 56). An initial report in 2000 on increased endometrial thickness pregnancy in three of four patients with previous IVF failure, treated with sildenafil, a type 5–specific phosphodiesterase inhibitor that augments the vasodilatory effects of nitrous oxide donor, was not confirmed (58, 59).

REFERENCES

1. Strowitzki T, Germeyer A, Popovici R, von Wolff M (2006) The human endometrium as a fertility-determining factor. *Hum Reprod Update* 12, 617–30.
2. Smith B, Porter R, Ahuja K, Craft I (1984) Ultrasonic assessment of endometrial changes in stimulated cycles in an in vitro fertilization and embryo transfer program. *J IVF-ET* 1, 233–8.
3. Gonen Y, Casper RF, Jacobson W, Blankier J (1989) Endometrial thickness and growth during ovarian stimulation: a possible predictor of implantation in in vitro fertilization. *Fertil Steril* 52, 466–50.

4. Gonen Y, Casper R (1990) Prediction of implantation by the sonographic appearance of the endometrium during controlled ovarian stimulation for in vitro fertilization. *J IVF-ET* 7, 146–52.

5. Dickey RP, Olar TT, Curole DN, Taylor SN, Rye PH (1992) Endometrial pattern and thickness associated with pregnancy outcome after assisted reproduction technologies. *Hum Reprod* 7, 418–21.

6. Dickey RP, Olar TT, Taylor SN, Curole DN, Matulich EM (1993B) Relationship of endometrial thickness and pattern to fecundity in ovulation induction cycles: effect of clomiphene citrate alone and with human menopausal gonadotropin. *Fertil Steril* 59, 756–60.

7. Hofmann GE, Thie J, Scott RT, Navot D 1996 Endometrial thickness is predictive of histologic endometrial maturation in women undergoing hormone replacement for ovum donation. *Fertil Steril* 66, 380–3.

8. Rogers PAW, Polson D, Murphy CR, Hosie M, Susil B, Leoni M (1991) Correlation of endometrial histology, morphometry, and ultrasound appearance after different stimulation protocols for in vitro fertilization. *Fertil Steril* 55, 583–7.

9. Sterzik K, Abt M, Grab D, Schneider V, Strehler E (2000) Predicting the histologic dating of an endometrial biopsy specimen with the use of Doppler ultrasonography and hormone measurements in patients undergoing spontaneous ovulatory cycles. *Fertil Steril* 73, 94–8.

10. Abramowicz J, Archer DF (1990) Uterine endometrial peristalsis—a transvaginal ultrasound study. *Fertil Steril* 54, 451–4.

11. De Vries K, Lyons EA, Ballard G, Levi CS, Lindsay D (1990) Contraction of the inner third of the myometrium. *Am J Obstet Gynecol* 162, 679–82.

12. Lyons EA, Taylor PJ, Zheng XH, Ballard G, Levi CS, Kredentser JV (1991) Characterization of subendometrial myometrial contractions throughout the menstrual cycles in normal fertile women. *Fertil Steril* 55, 771–4.

13. Chalubinski K, Deutinger J, Bernaschek G (1993) Vaginosonography for recording of cycle-related myometrial contractions. *Fertil Steril* 59, 225–8.

14. Ijland MM, Evers JLH, Dunselman GAJ, van Katwijk C, Lo CR, Hoogland HJ (1996) Endometrial wavelike movements during the menstrual cycle. *Fertil Steril* 65, 746–9.

15. Ijland MM, Evers JLH, Dunselman GAJ, Hoogland HJ (1998) Endometrial wavelike activity, endometrial thickness, and ultrasound texture in controlled ovarian hyperstimulation cycles. *Fertil Steril* 70, 279–83.

16. Randall JM, Fisk MM, McTavish A, Templeton AA (1989) Transvaginal ultrasonic assessment of endometrial growth in spontaneous and hyperstimulated menstrual cycles. *Br J Obstet Gynaecol* 96, 954–9.

17. Randall JM, Templeton A (1991) Transvaginal sonographic assessment of follicular and endometrial growth in spontaneous and clomiphene citrate cycles. *Fertil Steril* 56, 208–12.

18. Bakos O, Lundkvist O, Bergh T (1993) Transvaginal sonographic evaluation of endometrial growth and texture in spontaneous ovulatory cycles—a descriptive study. *Hum Reprod* 8, 799–806.

19. Chien LW, Lee WS, Au HK, Tzeng CR (2004) Assessment of changes in utero-ovarian arterial impedance during the peri-implantation period by Doppler sonography in women undergoing assisted reproduction. *Ultrasound Obstet Gynecol* 23, 496–500.

20. Sher G, Herbert C, Maassarani G, Jacobs MH (1991) Assessment of the late proliferative phase endometrium by ultrasonography in patients undergoing in-vitro fertilization and embryo transfer. *Hum Reprod* 6, 232–7.

21. Yagel S, Ben-Chetrit A, Anteby E, et al. (1992) The effect of ethinyl estradiol on endometrial thickness and uterine volume during ovulation induction by clomiphene citrate. *Fertil Steril* 57, 33–6.

22. Strohmer H, Obruca A, Radner KM, Feichtinger W (1994) Relationship of the individual uterine size and the endometrial thickness in stimulated cycles. *Fertil Steril* 61, 972–5.

23. Bohrer MK, Hock DL, Rhoads GG, Kemmann E (1996) Sonographic assessment of endometrial pattern and thickness in patients treated with human menopausal gonadotropins. *Fertil Steril* 66, 244–7.

24. Tsai HD, Chang CC, Hsieh YY, Lee CC, LO HY (2000) Role of endometrial thickness and pattern, of vascular impedance of the spiral and uterine arteries, and of the dominant follicle. *J Reprod Med*, 44, 195–200.

25. Dickey RP, Olar TT, Taylor SN, Curole DN, Harrigill K (1993A) Relationship of biochemical pregnancy to preovulatory endometrial thickness and pattern in patients undergoing ovulation induction. *Hum Reprod* 8, 327–330.

26. Fleischer AC, Herbert CM, Sacks GA, Wentz AC, Entman SS, Jeames AE (1986) Sonography of the endometrium during conception and nonconception cycles of in vitro fertilization and embryo transfer. *Fertil Steril* 46, 442–7.

27. Imoedemhe DA, Shaw RW, Kirkland A, et al. (1987) Ultrasound measurement of endometrial thickness on different ovarian stimulation regimens during in vitro fertilization. *Hum Reprod* 2, 545–7.

28. Eden JA, Place J, Carter GD, et al. (1989) The effect of clomiphene citrate on follicular phase increase in endometrial thickness and uterine volume. *Obstet Gynecol* 73, 187–90.

29. Shoham Z, De Carlo C, Patel A, Conway GS, Jacobs HS (1991) Is it possible to run a successful ovulation induction program based solely on ultrasound monitoring? The importance of endometrial measurements. *Fertil Steril* 56, 836–41.

30. Isaacs JD, Wells CS, Williams DB, Odem RR, Gast MJ, Strickler RC (1996) Endometrial thickness is a valid monitoring parameter in cycles of ovulation induction with menotropins alone. *Fertil Steril* 65, 262–6.

31. Glissant A, de Mouzon J, Frydman R (1985) Ultrasound study of the endometrium during in vitro fertilization cycles. *Fertil Steril* 44, 786–90.

32. Welker BG, Gembruch U, Diedrich K, Al-Hasani S, Krebs D (1989) Transvaginal sonography of the endometrium during ovum pickup in stimulated cycles for in vitro fertilization. *J Ultrasound Med* 8, 549–53.

33. Ueno J, Oehninger S, Bryzski RG, Acosta AA, Philput B, Muasher SJ (1991) Ultrasonographic appearance of the endometrium in natural and stimulated in-vitro fertilization cycles and its correlation with outcome. *Hum Reprod* 6, 901–04.

34. Serafini P, Batzofin J, Nelson J, Olive D (1994) Sonographic uterine predictors of pregnancy in women undergoing ovulation induction for assisted reproductive treatments. *Fertil Steril* 62, 815–22.

35. Sharara FI, Lim J, McClamrock D (1999) Endometrial pattern on the day of oocyte retrieval is more predictive of implantation success than the pattern or thickness on the day of hCG administration. *J Assist Reprod Genet* 16, 523–28.

36. Fanchin R, Righini C, Ayoubi JM, Olivennes F, de Ziegler D, Frydman R (2000) New look at endometrial echogenicity: objective computer-assisted measurements predict endometrial receptivity in in vitro fertilization-embryo transfer. *Fertil Steril* 74, 274–81.

37. Coulam CB, Bustillo M, Soenksen DM, Britten ST (1994) Ultra-sonographic predictors of implantation after assisted reproduction. *Fertil Steril* 62, 1004–10.

38. Check JH, Nowroozi K, Choe J, Dietterich C (1991) Influence of endometrial thickness and echo patterns on pregnancy rates during in vitro fertilization. *Fertil Steril* 56, 1173–5.

39. Noyes N, Liu HC, Sultan K, Schattman G, Rosenwaks Z (1995) Endometrial thickness appears to be a significant factor in embryo implantation in in-vitro fertilization. *Hum Reprod* 10, 919–22.

40. Oliveira JBA, Baruffi RLR, Mauri AL, Petersen CG, Borges MC, Franco JG (1997) Endometrial ultrasonography as a predictor of pregnancy in an in-vitro fertilization programme after ovarian stimulation and gonadotropin-releasing hormone and gonadotropin. *Hum Reprod* 12, 2515–18.

41. Rabinowitz R, Laufer N, Lewin A, Navot D, Bar I, Margalioth EJ (1986) The value of ultrasonographic endometrial measurement in the prediction of pregnancy following in vitro fertilization. *Fertil Steril* 45, 824–8.

42. Sundstrom P (1998) Establishment of a successful pregnancy following in-vitro fertilization with an endometrial thickness of no more than 4 mm. *Hum Reprod* 13, 1550–2.

43. Antinori S, Versaci C, Gholami GH, Panci C, Caffa B (1993) Oocyte donation in menopausal women. *Hum Reprod* 8, 1487–90.

44. Check JH, Nowroozi K, Choe J, Lurie D, Dietterich C (1993) The effect of endometrial thickness and echo pattern on in vitro fertilization outcome in donor oocyte-embryo transfer cycle. *Fertil Steril* 59, 72–5.

45. Abdalla HI, Brooks AA, Johnson MR, Kirkland A, Thomas A, Studd JWW (1994) Endometrial thickness: a predictor of implantation in ovum recipients. *Hum Reprod* 9, 363–5.

46. Weissman A, Gotlieb L, Casper RF (1999) The detrimental effect of increased endometrial thickness on implantation and pregnancy rates and outcome in an in vitro fertilization program. *Fertil Steril* 71, 147–9.

47. Krampl E, Feichtinger W (1993) Endometrial thickness and echo patterns. *Hum Reprod* 8, 1339.

48. Camus E, Poncelet C, Goffinet FG, Wainer B, Merlet F, Nisand I, Philippe HJ (1999) Pregnancy rates after in-vitro fertilization in cases of tubal infertility with and without hydrosalpinx: a meta-analysis of published comparative studies. *Hum Reprod* 14, 1243–9.

49. Nackley AC, Muasher SJ (1998) The significance of hydrosalpinx in in vitro fertilization. *Fertil Steril* 69, 373–84.

50. Van Voorhis BJ, Sparks ET, Syrop CH, Stovall DW (1998) Ultrasound-guided aspiration of hydrosalpinges is associated with improved pregnancy and implantation rates after in-vitro fertilization cycles. *Hum Reprod* 13, 736–9.

51. Mansour RT, Aboulghar MA, Serour GI, Riad R (1991) Fluid accumulation of the uterine cavity before transfer: a possible hindrance for implantation. *J IVF-ET* 8, 157–9.

52. Lass A, Williams G, Abusheikha N, Brinsden P (1999) The effect of endometrial polyps on outcomes of in vitro fertilization cycles. *J Assist Reprod Genet* 16, 410–15.

53. Boué J, Boué A, Lazar P (1973) Retrospective and prospective epidemiological studies of 1500 karyotyped spontaneous human abortions. *Teratology* 12, 11–26.

54. Hsieh YY, Tsal HD, Chang CC, Lo HY, Chen CL (2000) Low-dose aspirin for infertile women with thin endometrium receiving intrauterine insemination: a prospective randomized study. *J Assist Reprod Genet* 17, 174–7.

55. Wada I, Hs CC, Williams G, Macnamee MC, Brinsden PR (1994) The benefits of low-dose aspirin therapy in women with impaired uterine perfusion during assisted conception. *Hum Reprod* 9, 1954–7.

56. Weckstein LN, Jacobson A, Galen D, Hampton K, Hammel J (1997) Low-dose aspirin or oocyte donation recipients with a thin endometrium: prospective, randomized study. *Fertil Steril* 68, 927–30.

57. Rubinstein M, Marazzi A, de Fried EP (1999) Low-dose aspirin treatment improves ovarian responsiveness, uterine and ovarian blood flow velocity, implantation, and pregnancy rates in patients undergoing in vitro fertilization: a prospective, randomized double-blind placebo-controlled assay. *Fertil Steril* 71, 825–9.

58. Sher G, Fisch JD (2000) Vaginal sildenafil (Viagra): a preliminary report of a novel method to improve uterine artery blood flow and endometrial development in patients undergoing IVF. *Hum Reprod* 13, 806–9.

59. Dickey RR (2008) Ultrasonography of the endometrium. In Rizk B (Ed.) Ultrasonography in reproductive medicine and infertility. Cambridge: United Kingdom, Cambridge University Press, chapter 14, 112–4.

16

Ultrasonography of the Cervix

Mona Aboulghar, Botros R. M. B. Rizk

INTRODUCTION

Ultrasound is an essential diagnostic tool in gynecologic and obstetric practice and is of special importance for management of infertile patients. With the advancement of ultrasound technology and ultrasound machines and with introduction of 3D technology as well, detailed examination of the uterine cervix, anatomy, and accurate measurements have become possible (1). This has broadened the uses of sonographic examination in infertile patients as well as in pregnancy, mainly due to the importance of uterine cervix examination for prediction of preterm labor (2).

MORPHOLOGY OF THE UTERINE CERVIX

The cervix is the cylindrical portion of the uterus, which enters the vagina and lies at right angles to it. It measures 2–4 cm in length. The point of junction to the uterus is called the isthmus. Branches of the uterine arteries are situated lateral to the cervix and can be seen by color Doppler at transvaginal ultrasound (3).

By transvaginal ultrasound, the cervix is seen in the sagittal plane as a cylindrical, moderately echogenic structure with a central canal (Figure 16.1). The internal os is better identified during pregnancy. The cervical mucus is more prominent during pregnancy, facilitating the recognition of the cervical canal (Figure 16.2). The cervical gland area is an area surrounding the cervical canal, which is either hypo- or hyperechoic; its absence has been related to preterm labor (4–6).

ROUTE OF ULTRASOUND EVALUATION OF THE CERVIX

The transvaginal route is the preferred route to examine the cervix whether in nonpregnant or pregnant states. Rizk et al (1990) demonstrated that the transvaginal route is superior to the transabdominal route as confirmed by other investigators (7a–d).

It avoids limitations of the transabdominal route, which include difficulties due to maternal habitus and need for a full bladder (8). In addition, the cervical length may be falsely increased by the transabdominal route (9).

Transperineal Route

Comparing transvaginal and transperineal route for assessment of cervix (in pregnancy) found good agreement and very similar measurements of cervical length for both routes (10–13), except for one study (14).

The need for evaluating possibility of the transperineal (translabial) route arose since some authors argued against transvaginal ultrasound in some conditions, as in patients with threatened preterm labor, patients with ROM for fear of chorioamnionitis, and risk of bleeding in patients with placenta previa; however, it has been shown that these are not true clinical risks (15, 16). In our practice, we have not found this to be a contraindication to transvaginal ultrasonography; in patients with ROM, a sterile sheath is used.

TECHNIQUE OF TRANSVAGINAL ULTRASOUND

The patient should be examined in the supine position with hips abducted and an empty bladder. A high-frequency probe, 3.5- to 8-MHz transvaginal transducer covered with a condom is inserted midway between introitus and cervix.

In the pregnancy state, the entire length of the cervical canal should be measured from the internal os (demarcated by the junction with amniotic membrane) and the external os.

Benign gynecologic conditions seen by US in nonpregnant state: include Nabothian cysts, cervical polyps, fibroids and Mullerian anomalies (17).

Nabothian Cysts

They represent a reparative upward growth of squamous epithelium, causing obstruction of the ducts of the end cervical glands. Retention of mucus within these glands results in nabothian cysts. They are very common and could be single or multiple and by ultrasound appear as anechoic cysts within cervical tissue (3) (Figures 16.3 and 16.4.)

Cervical Polyps

Cervical Polyps are common findings, in most cases, difficult to distinguish from cervical mucus. A large polyp could be seen as an echogenic mass in the cervical canal, and this could be made easier by saline infusion (sonohysterography).

Evaluation of the cervical anatomy is of importance during investigation of infertility as surgical procedures might be needed (polypectomy) before embarking on treatment as IUI and IVF (Figure 16.5) difficulties might be encountered during catheter introduction (18). It is our routine practice to have an

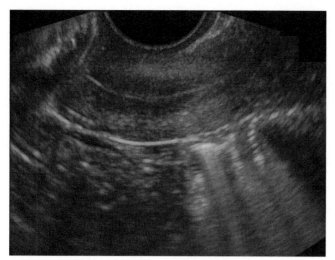

Figure 16.1. Normal cervix—nonpregnant state.

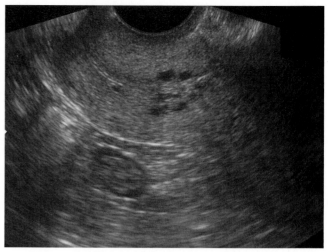

Figure 16.3. Nabothian cysts (small).

ultrasound image of the cervical canal and uterus, measuring cervical length and uterine body length, to assist during embryo transfer.

Cervical Fibroids

Most commonly, fibroids are arising from the uterine body extending into the cervical canal, that is, pedicled fibroid, or rarely arising primarily from the cervix. In both instances, sonohysterography enhances visualization of the fibroid and its exact origin (19, 20) (Figure 16.6).

Mullerian Anomalies

Prevalence of Mullerian anomalies is reported in various studies to be in the range of 1–26 percent of infertile females (21). Two-dimensional ultrasound is a good screening test with high sensitivity for detection of Mullerian uterine anomalies (22, 23). However, 2D US has limited ability to distinguish different types of uterine abnormalities and is operator dependant (23–25). So 3D US is now used extensively, carrying a greater advantage due

its ability to demonstrate the coronal view of the uterus and cervix. It can, therefore, differentiate different Mullerian anomalies with good reported sensitivity and specificity (26, 27). This is of course of importance in infertile patients with asymmetrical division, vaginal septae, and uterine horns, especially if IVF is to be performed with ET to be done in the correct body (Figures 16.7–16.10).

Assessment of cervical length in this specific group of patients is of importance due to higher incidence of preterm labor; it was found that a short cervical length on transvaginal ultrasonography in women with uterine anomalies had a Thirteen fold risk for preterm birth. Among all Mullerian anomalies, unicornuate uterus had the highest rate of cervical shortening and preterm delivery (28).

ULTRASOUND EXAMINATION OF CERVIX IN PREGNANCY

It is well documented in the literature that pregnancy following ART has a higher risk of adverse outcomes. A meta-analysis comparing IVF with spontaneous conceptions showed that IVF singleton pregnancies had significantly higher odds of perinatal

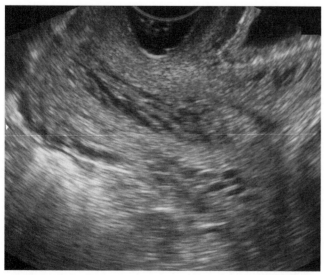

Figure 16.2. Cervix in pregnancy.

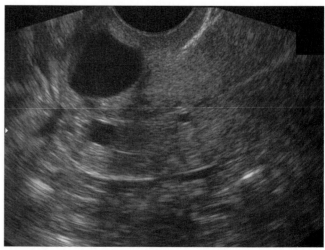

Figure 16.4. Nabothian cyst (large).

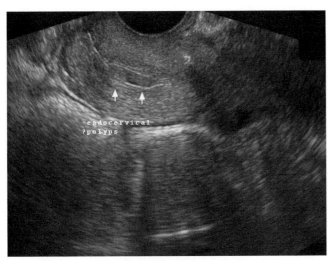

Figure 16.5. Endocervical polyps.

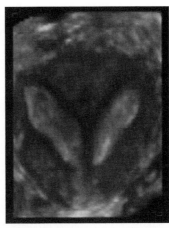

Figure 16.7. Mullerian anomaly, 3D image of uterus didelphys.

mortality [odds ratio (OR) 2.2; 95 percent confidence interval (CI) 1.6–3.0], preterm delivery (OR 2.0; 95 percent CI 1.7–2.2), low birth weight (OR 1.8; 95 percent CI 1.4–2.2), very low birth weight (OR 2.7; 95 percent CI 2.3–3.1), and small for gestational age (OR 1.6; 95 percent CI 1.3–2.0) (29–31).

Similarly, IVF/ICSI twins had a Ten fold increased age- and parity-adjusted risk of delivery before thirty-seven completed weeks (OR 9.9; 95 percent CI 8.7–11.3) and a 7.4-fold increased risk of delivery before thirty-two completed weeks (OR 7.4; 95 percent CI 5.6–9.8) compared with singletons. Correspondingly, ORs of birth weight greater than 2,500 g and birth weight greater than 1,500 g in twins were 11.8 (95 percent CI 10.3–13.6) and 5.4 (95 percent CI 4.1–7.0), respectively (30, 31).

Even spontaneous pregnancies of untreated but infertile women are reported to have a higher risk for obstetrical complications and perinatal mortality than spontaneous pregnancies in fertile women (31).

Prediction of preterm labor is thus important in this specific group of patients. Although no literature has been published studying the cervix of pregnancies following ART, we have unpublished data confirming that cervical length is a good predictor of preterm labor, both in ICSI singleton and twin

pregnancies as cervical length was significantly shorter in singleton and twin ICSI pregnant patients who delivered preterm compared to those who delivered at term (Aboulghar MM unpublished data 2006).

CERVICAL ASSESSMENT AT MIDTRIMESTER

Sonographic assessment of cervical length is better than digital examination in screening for preterm delivery, in low-risk patients as well as high-risk patients (32–36). Shortened cervical length in comparison with high Bishop score was found to have twelvefold higher positive likelihood ratio for preterm delivery in a low-risk population (37.4; 95 percent CI 8.2–170.7 vs. 3.2; 95 percent CI 1.1–9.2) (32).

Cervical length measurement by ultrasound proved to be the most important predictor of preterm labor. The relative risk of preterm delivery increased as the length of the cervix decreased (37).

CERVICAL FUNNELING

Funneling is described as dilatation of internal os so that cervical canal changes in shape, with bulge of the bag of membranes through the dilated cervix into cervical canal. The funnel

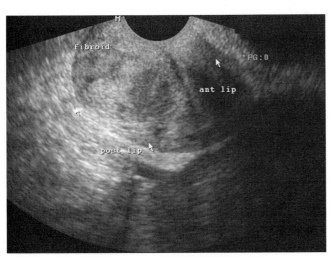

Figure 16.6. Cervical fibroid.

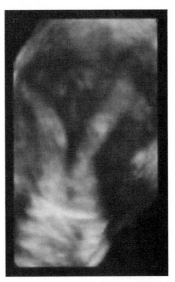

Figure 16.8. 3D image of uterus didelphys.

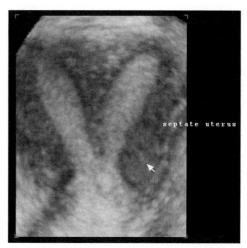

Figure 16.9. 3D image of septate uterus.

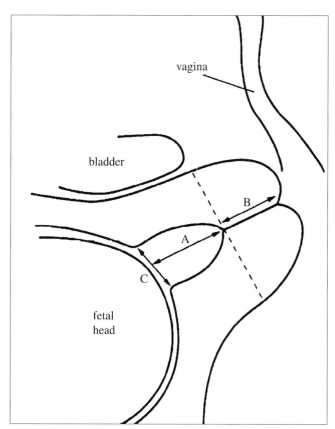

Diagram 16.1. Cervical funneling. By permission Berghella et al. (42).

has a width, length, and usually residual cervical length is measured as well (Diagram 16.1). Care must be taken as funneling can be falsely noted when bladder is overdistended, during contractions or with undue vaginal pressure with probe on the cervix. It is always advised to keep vaginal probe midway between introitus and cervix and also to wait for three to five minutes before assessing cervical length and morphology as it might change (38, 39). Most of studies found funneling to be of significance in predicting preterm labor in addition to a short cervical length (40–42).

However, To et al. found cervical length to be of more significance (43).

The finding of a dynamic cervix occurs more frequently in patients at risk for preterm labor; in these cases, the residual cervical length is of importance to be measured (38, 44, 45).

The measurement of cervical length was also shown to be of benefit in patients presenting with threatened preterm labor. Sonographic measurement of cervical length helps to avoid overdiagnosis of preterm labor in women with preterm contractions, and to distinguish between true and false labor, a cut-off of 15 mm was reported in two studies to be the best for prediction of delivery, within seven days from admission and ultrasound evaluation of the cervix. Logistic regression analysis demonstrated that the only significant contributor in the prediction

of delivery within seven days was cervical length greater than 15 mm (OR = 101; 95 percent CI 12–800, $P < 0.0001$) (46, 47).

TIMING OF ULTRASOUND EXAMINATION OF THE CERVIX DURING PREGNANCY: WHEN TO PERFORM THE CERVICAL ULTRASOUND ASSESSMENT?

Early (between eleven and fourteen weeks) ultrasound assessment of the cervix was not found to be a reliable screening method in prediction of spontaneous preterm delivery (48). Comparing early eleven- to fourteen-weeks assessment with midtrimester assessment at twenty-two to twenty-four weeks showed that cervical length early at eleven to fourteen weeks was not significantly different when compared between the groups that delivered at term and preterm. However, at the twenty-two-week to twenty-four-week evaluation, cervical length was significantly shorter in the group that had a preterm delivery than that in those who had a term delivery ($P = 0.0001$). This confirms that there is a spontaneous shortening in the pregnant cervix from the first to the second trimester of pregnancy, and thus, this is the best timing for screening of the cervix (49).

ULTRASOUND-GUIDED EMBRYO TRANSFER (ET)

Transabdominal Ultrasound-Guided ET, Importance of Uterocervical Angle

Ultrasound-guided ET has been introduced and studied by several authors, and many of them found an increase in pregnancy

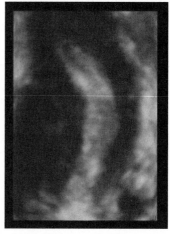

Figure 16.10. 3D image of unicornuate uterus.

rates (50, 51), while others found it to be equivalent to clinical touch transfers (52). However, two recent meta-analysis, one by our group (53), found a higher live birth, ongoing pregnancy, clinical pregnancy and implantation rates, and easier transfers with ultrasound-guided technique (54).

The advantage of transabdominal ultrasound-guided transfer with a full bladder is mainly attributed to straightening of uterocervical angle. Facilitating entry of catheter into uterine cavity, however, carries disadvantage of patient discomfort. Obesity and retroversion of the uterus might cause inadequate visualization of the endometrial cavity. A study done to compare empty bladder with full bladder at time of transabdominal ultrasound-guided ET had comparable results for all three groups of full bladder and empty bladder, both guided transabdominally or clinical touch ET (55).

Another study examined the effect of molding the ET catheter to the uterocervical angle (measured by transabdominal ultrasound). Molding the ET catheter according to the uterocervical angle significantly increased clinical pregnancy (OR 1.57; 95 percent CI 1.08–2.27) and implantation rates (OR 1.47; 95 percent CI 1.10–1.96) compared with the "clinical touch" method. It also significantly reduced difficult transfers (OR 0.25; 95 percent CI 0.16–0.40) and blood during transfers (OR 0.71; 95 percent CI 0.50–0.99). Patients with large angles (>60 degrees) had significantly lower pregnancy rates compared with those with no angle (OR 0.36; 95 percent CI 0.16–0.52) (56). This confirms the need for assessment of the cervix as regards angle, length, and body length with ultrasound before ET (18).

Placenta Previa

The incidence of placenta previa is 1:200 and increases with parity. Maternal mortality has decreased to less than 1 percent and perinatal mortality to 5 percent with modern treatment. It is essential therefore to diagnose placenta previa during pregnancy and to determine its type and need for C-section according to relation of the placenta to the internal os. The incidence of placenta previa is reported to be higher in pregnancies following ART. A sixfold increased risk of placenta previa was found, when compared to naturally conceived pregnancies (57).

Ultrasound is the main tool used for diagnosing placenta previa and for follow-up as well. Diagnosing placenta previa in second trimester of pregnancy showed that with ultrasound follow-up, approximately 85 percent of cases ended up with a normally situated placenta (58).

Comparing route of ultrasound for confirmation of placenta previa and determination of its exact relation to internal cervical os, transvaginal ultrasound appears to be a superior method than transabdominal ultrasound (59–64) in addition to being a safe route without increased risk of vaginal bleeding (16, 62, 63) (Figure 16.11).

The importance of transvaginal ultrasound in diagnosing placenta previa lies also in the ability by transvaginal ultrasound to determine exact distance of placental edge from internal os, which will consequently determine mode of delivery. Studies support that a distance of 2 cm or greater from internal cervical os to placental edge warrants safe vaginal delivery (65–67). As for placentas lying at a distance of 1–2 cm, management differs; however, probability of C-section is very high and reached 40 percent in one of the studies (66), while in another study all patients underwent C-section (65, 67).

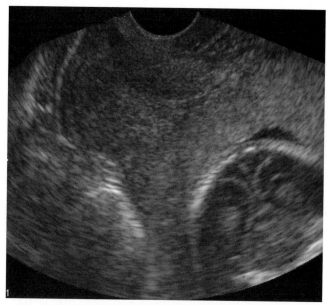

Figure 16.11. Placenta previa.

Vasa Previa

It is defined as fetal vessels coursing within the membranes between the presenting part and cervix (Figure 16.12).

Incidence

1:1,200 to 1:5,000 pregnancies (68–70).

Anatomical Variants

The vessels over the cervix can lead from the placenta to a velamentous cord insertion or connect the main bulk of the placenta to a succenturiate lobe.

Vasa previa carry a high fetal morbidity and mortality since fetal vessels within the membranes are unprotected by Wharton's jelly, they are prone to compression during labor and may tear when the membranes rupture, resulting in fetal exsanguination.

The classic presentation is rupture of membranes followed by painless, dark vaginal bleeding associated with profound fetal distress or fetal demise. Vasa previa can cause abnormal intrapartum fetal heart rate patterns including sinusoidal

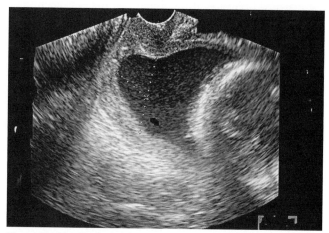

Figure 16.12. Fetal vessels crossing over cervix [by permission Catanzarite et al. (74)].

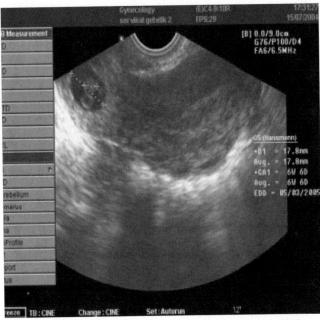
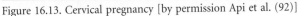

Figure 16.13. Cervical pregnancy [by permission Api et al. (92)]

tracings (71) and severe variable decelerations (72). Clinically, the diagnosis is occasionally made based on the palpation of fetal vessels within the (intact) membranes at the time of vaginal examination and can also be made by amnioscopy (73).

However, more recently, it is diagnosed by ultrasound, both abdominal and transvaginal and in some occasions a combination of both (74, 75). In addition, color and power Doppler studies are essential in confirming vasa previa (74).

An attempt to visualize the cord insertion in the placenta and a sweep across the lower uterine segment to look for velamentous vessels has been recommended. And if a low-lying succenturiate lobe is seen, to examine the region over the cervix using color Doppler. Serial sonograms should be done and in case of confirmed vasa previa, maternal rest, and close monitoring are advised, and delivery by C-section after confirmation of fetal lung maturity is advised.

Evaluating the outcomes and predictors of neonatal survival in pregnancies complicated by vasa previa, comparing outcomes in prenatal diagnosed cases of vasa previa with those not diagnosed prenatal, it was found that the only significant predictors of neonatal survival were prenatal diagnosis of vasa previa ($P < .001$) and gestational age at delivery ($P = .01$). The overall perinatal mortality reported was high (36 percent), and this was reduced in cases diagnosed prenatal and when C-section was done early in cases of rupture of membranes, labor, or significant bleeding (76).

Some reports indicate that there could be increased incidence of vasa previa in pregnancies following IVF due to a suggested higher incidence of velamentous and marginal insertions of the umbilical cord (77). Also, disturbed orientation of the blastocyst at implantation, a contributing factor to vasa previa, is probably related to the IVF-ET procedure (78).

CERVICAL PREGNANCY

Cervical pregnancy is a rare ectopic pregnancy, defined as implantation of gestation sac in the endocervix (78–80). Rizk and Brindsen (1990) suggested that ART may be associated with an increased risk of ectopic pregnancy (81–82).

Ultrasound is the main diagnostic tool (Figure 16.13). It is reported to have improved pretreatment diagnosis up to 81.8 percent. Obligatory sonographic criteria of cervical pregnancy include endocervical localization of the gestational sac and trophoblastic invasion (83).

Doppler is a very important tool as well; to confirm viability, up to 60 percent of cervical ectopic pregnancies are viable (83).

Due to its difficult diagnosis, it should be differentiated from the cervical stage of spontaneous abortion and nabothian cyst and cervical choriocarcinoma.

The risks of cervical pregnancy are mainly severe hemorrhage, necessitating hysterectomy in many situations, and it usually occurs in nulliparous or low-parity women, adding to the dilemma of management.

Management of cervical pregnancy is mainly conservative (Figure 16.13). Giving methotrexate systemically and in some cases curettage, curettage and Foley catheter tamponade, cervical cerclage, ligation of the descending branches of uterine arteries, or ligation of hypogastric arteries. Intraamniotic injection of methotrexate (or potassium chloride) has also been described with success and with excellent postrecovery (84–92).

KEY POINTS

■ Advancement in ultrasound technology, especially 3D, has allowed good imaging of the uterine cervix, both in nonpregnant and pregnant states. The cervix is visual well by transvaginal ultrasound especially during pregnancy when cervical mucus makes cervical canal prominent and demarcates the internal os well, when measurement of cervical length needs to be done.

■ Ultrasound examination of the cervix is best done by transvaginal ultrasound, rather than the transabdominal route. The transperineal route is also an option in cases of bleeding or PROM.

- Benign gynecologic findings seen by ultrasound include nabothian cysts, cervical polyps, cervical fibroids, and Mullerian anomalies. In the latter case, 3D imaging provides higher sensitivity and specificity. In addition, Mullerian anomalies should be diagnosed before IVF trials, so as not to face problems during embryo transfer. An image of the cervical canal and uterine body and measurements of length of each are very helpful in clinical touch technique of embryo transfer.

- Cervical length at midtrimester is the best predictor for preterm labor. The relative risk of preterm labor increases with decrease in cervical length. This is of special importance in pregnancies following ART; as this group of patients is known to have higher incidence of adverse perinatal outcomes, preterm labor is one of those risks. Cervical funneling and dynamic cervix both are predictors of preterm labor. In both cases, the residual cervical length is of importance.

- Transabdominal guided ET in IVF increases pregnancy rates; the advantage is straightening of the uterocervical angle. Moulding of the ET catheter to fit the uterocervical angle increases pregnancy rates as well.

- Placenta previa occurs six times more frequently in pregnancies following ART.

- Mortality and morbidity due to placenta previa has decreased with modern management. An essential part of it being ultrasound diagnosis, especially transvaginal ultrasound, which is superior to abdominal ultrasound. It confirms the diagnosis of placenta previa and gives accurate measurements of distance from placental edge to internal cervical os. This will determine the mode of delivery, so that a placenta more than 2 cm from cervical os allows safe vaginal delivery.

- Incidence of vasa previa is reported higher in pregnancies following ART.

- Vasa previa is diagnosed by transvaginal and transabdominal ultrasound and with Doppler flow studies. The main significant predictor of neonatal survival is prenatal diagnosis of vasa previa. Delivery before ROM decreases perinatal mortality. Cervical pregnancy, defined as implantation in the endocervix, has a higher risk in ART pregnancies. The diagnosis is essentially by ultrasound, and the management is conservative, giving methotrexate whether systemically or transvaginally, ultrasound guided. The conservative management aims at reducing the risks of hemorrhage and need for hysterectomy.

REFERENCES

1. Sladkevicius P, Campbell S. Advanced ultrasound examination in the management of subfertility. *Curr Opin Obstet Gynecol* 2000;**12**(3):221–5.

2. Kagan K, To M, Tsoi E, Nicolaides K. Preterm birth: the value of sonographic measurement of cervical length. *BJOG* 2006;**113**(s3):5–56.

3. Di Saia PJ. Disorders of uterine cervix. In Scott JR, DiSaia P, Hammond CB, et al. (Eds.): Danforth's Obstetrics and Gynecology, 7th ed. Philadephia: JB Lippincott, 1994.

4. Sekyia T, Yoshimatsu K, et al. Detection rate of the cervical gland area during pregnancy by transvaginal sonography in the assessment of cervical maturation. *Ultrasound Obstet Gynecol* 1998;**12**:328.

5. Yoshimatsu K, Sekiya T, Ishihara K, Fukami T, Otabe T, Araki T. Detection of the cervical gland area in threatened preterm labor using transvaginal sonography in the assessment of cervical maturation and the outcome of pregnancy. *Gynecol Obstet Invest* 2002;**53**(3):149–56.

6. Pires CR, Moron AF, Mattar R, Diniz AL, Andrade SG, Bussamra LC. Cervical gland area as an ultrasonographic marker for preterm delivery. *Int J Gynaecol Obstet* 2006;**93**(3):214–19.

7a. Rizk B, Steer C, Tan SL, Mason BA. Vaginal versus abdominal ultrasound guided oocyte retrieval in IVF. *British Journal of Radiology* 1990;**63**:638.

7b. Steer C, Rizk B, Tan SL, Mason BA, Campbell S. Vaginal versus abdominal ultrasound for obtaining uterine artery Doppler flow velocity waveforms. *British Journal of Radiology* 1990;**63**:398–9.

7c. Steer C, Rizk B, Tan SL, Mason BA, Campbell S. Vaginal color doppler assesment of uterine artery impedance in a subfertile population. *British Journal of Radiology* 1990;**63**:638.

7d. Qureshi IA, Ullah H, Akram MH, Ashfaq S, Nayyar S. Transvaginal versus transabdominal sonography in the evaluation of pelvic pathology. *J Coll Physicians Surg Pak* 2004;**14**(7):390–3.

8. To MS, Skentou C, Cicero S, Nicolaides KH. Cervical assessment at the routine 23-weeks' scan: problems with transabdominal sonography. *Ultrasound Obstet Gynecol* 2000;**15**(4):292–6.

9. Andersen HF. Transvaginal and transabdominal ultrasonography of the uterine cervix during pregnancy. *J Clin Ultrasound* 1991;**19**(2):77–83.

10. Raungrongmorakot K, Tanmoun N, Ruangvutilert P, Boriboonhirunsarn D, Tontisirin P, Butsansee W. Correlation of uterine cervical length measurement from transabdominal, transperineal and transvaginal ultrasonography. *J Med Assoc Thai* 2004;**87**(3):326–32.

11. Cicero S, Skentou C, Souka A, To MS, Nicolaides KH. Cervical length at 22-24 weeks of gestation: comparison of transvaginal and transperineal-translabial ultrasonography. *Ultrasound Obstet Gynecol* 2001;**17**(4):335–40.

12. Kurtzman JT, Goldsmith LJ, Gall SA, Spinnato JA. Transperineal ultrasonography: a blinded comparison in the assessment of cervical length at midgestation. *Am J Obstet Gynecol* 1998;**179**(4):852–7.

13. Ozdemir I, Demirci F, Yucel O. Transperineal versus transvaginal ultrasonographic evaluation of the cervix at each trimester in normal pregnant women. *Aust N Z J Obstet Gynaecol* 2005;**45**(3):191–4.

14. Carr DB, Smith K, Parsons L, Chansky K, Shields LE. Ultrasonography for cervical length measurement: agreement between transvaginal and translabial techniques. *Obstet Gynecol* 2000;**96**(4):554–8.

15. Carlan Sj, Richmond LB, O'brien WF. Randomized trial of endovaginal ultrasound in preterm premature rupture of membranes. *Obstet Gynecol* 1997;**89**:458–461.

16. Timor-Tritsch IR, Yunis RA. Confirming the safety of transvaginal sonography in patients suspected of placenta previa. *Obstet Gynecol* 1993;**81**:742.

17. Bajo J, Moreno-Calvo FJ, Uguet-de-Resayre C, Huertas MA, Mateos F, Haya J. Contribution of transvaginal sonography to the evaluation of benign cervical conditions. *J Clin Ultrasound* 1999;**27**(2):61–4.

18. Mansour RT, Aboulghar MA. Optimizing the embryo transfer technique. 2002;**17**(5):1149–53.

19. Wongsawaeng W. Transvaginal ultrasonography, sonohysterography and hysteroscopy for intrauterine pathology in patients with abnormal uterine bleeding. *J Med Assoc Thai.* 2005;**88** (Suppl. 3):S77–81.

20. Leone FP, Lanzani C, Ferrazzi E. Use of strict sonohysterographic methods for preoperative assessment of submucous myomas. *Fertil Steril* 2003;**79**(4):998–1002.

21. Grimbizis GF, Camus M, Tarlatzis BC, Bonis JN, Devroey P. Clinical implication of uterine malformations and hysteroscopic treatment results. *Hum Reprod Update* 2001;7(2):161–74.

22. Valdes C, Malini S, Malikanak LR. Ultrasound evaluation of female genital tract anomalies: a review of 64 cases. *Am J Obstet Gynecol* 1984;47:89–93.

23. Nicolini U, Bellotti M, Bonazzi B, Amberletti D, Candini GB. Can ultrasound be used to screen uterine malformations? *Fertil Steril* 1987;47:89–93.

24. Reuter KL, Daly DC, Cohen SM. Septate versus bicornuate uteri: errors in imaging diagnosis. *Radiology* 1989;172:749–52.

25. Randoph JF Jr., Ying YK, Maier DB, Schmidt CL, Riddick DH, Randolph JR Jr. Comparison of real time ultrasonography, hysterosalpingography, and laparoscopy/hysteroscopy in the evaluation of uterine abnormalities and tubal patency. *Fertil Steril* 1986;5:828–32.

26. Raga F, Bonilla-Musoles F, Blanes J, Osborne NG. Congenital Mullerian anomalies: diagnostic accuracy of three-dimensional ultrasound. *Fertil Steril* 1996;65:523–8.

27. Wu MH, Hsu CC, Huang KE. Detection of congenital Mullerian duct anomalies using three-dimensional ultrasound. *J Clin Ultrasound* 1997;25:487–92.

28. Airoldi J, Berghella V, Sehdev H, Ludmir J. Transvaginal ultrasonography of the cervix to predict preterm birth in women with uterine anomalies. *Obstet Gynecol* 2005;106(3):553–6.

29. Jackson RA, Gibson KA, Wu YW, Croughan MS. Perinatal outcomes in singletons following in vitro fertilization: a meta-analysis. *Obstet Gynecol* 2004;103(3):551–63.

30. Pinborg A, Loft A, Nyboe Andersen A. Neonatal outcome in a Danish national cohort of 8602 children born after in vitro fertilization or intracytoplasmic sperm injection: the role of twin pregnancy. *Acta Obstet Gynecol Scand* 2004;83(11):1071–8.

31. Allen VM, Wilson RD, Cheung A. Pregnancy outcomes after assisted reproductive technology. *J Obstet Gynaecol Can* 2006;28(3):220–50.

32. Matijevic R, Grgic O, Vasilj O. Is sonographic assessment of cervical length better than digital examination in screening for preterm delivery in a low-risk population? *Acta Obstet Gynecol Scand* 2006;85(11):1342–7.

33. Guzman ER, Walters C, Ananth CV, O'Reilly-Green C, Benito CW, Palermo A, Vintzileos AM. A comparison of sonographic cervical parameters in predicting spontaneous preterm birth in high-risk singleton gestations. *Ultrasound Obstet Gynecol* 2001;18(3):204–10.

34. Heath VC, Southall TR, Souka AP, Elisseou A, Nicolaides KH. Cervical length at 23 weeks of gestation: prediction of spontaneous preterm delivery. *Ultrasound Obstet Gynecol.* 1998;12(5):312–17.

35. Leung TN, Pang MW, Leung TY, Poon CF, Wong SM, Lau TK. Cervical length at 18-22 weeks of gestation for prediction of spontaneous preterm delivery in Hong Kong Chinese women. *Ultrasound Obstet Gynecol* 2005;26(7):713–17.

36. Cook CM, Ellwood DA. The cervix as a predictor of preterm delivery in 'at-risk' women. *Ultrasound Obstet Gynecol* 2000;15(2):109–13.

37. Iams JD, Goldenberg RL, Meis PJ, Mercer BM, Moawad A, Das A, Thom E, McNellis D, Copper RL, Johnson F, Roberts JM. The length of the cervix and the risk of spontaneous premature delivery. National Institute of Child Health and Human Development Maternal Fetal Medicine Unit Network. *N Engl J Med* 1996;334(9):567–72.

38. Kikuchi A, Kozuma S, Marumo G, et al. Local dynamic changes of the cervix associated with incompetent cervix before and after Shirodkar's operation. *J Clin Ultrasound* 1998;26:371.

39. Parulekar SG, Kiwi R. Dynamic incompetent cervix uteri: sonographic observations. *J Ultrasound Med* 1988;7(9):481–5.

40. Rust OA, Atlas RO, Kimmel S, Roberts WE, Hess LW. Does the presence of a funnel increase the risk of adverse perinatal outcome in a patient with a short cervix? *Am J Obstet Gynecol* 2005;192(4):1060–6.

41. Vayssiere C, Favre R, Audibert F, Chauvet MP, Gaucherand P, Tardif D, Grange G, Novoa A, Descamps P, Perdu M, Andrini E, Janse-Marec J, Maillard F, Nisand I. Cervical length and funneling at 22 and 27 weeks to predict spontaneous birth before 32 weeks in twin pregnancies: a French prospective multicenter study. *Am J Obstet Gynecol* 2002;187(6):1596–604.

42. Berghella V, Kuhlman K, Weiner S, Texeira L, Wapner RJ. Cervical funneling: sonographic criteria predictive of preterm delivery. *Ultrasound Obstet Gynecol* 1997;10(3):161–6.

43. To MS, Skentou C, Liao AW, Cacho A, Nicolaides KH. Cervical length and funneling at 23 weeks of gestation in the prediction of spontaneous early preterm delivery. *Ultrasound Obstet Gynecol* 2001;18(3):200–3. Comment in: *Ultrasound Obstet Gynecol* 2001;18(3):195–9.

44. Bergelin I, Valentin L. Cervical changes in twin pregnancies observed by transvaginal ultrasound during the latter half of pregnancy: a longitudinal, observational study. *Ultrasound Obstet Gynecol* 2003;21(6):556–63.

45. Bergelin I, Valentin L. Normal cervical changes in parous women during the second half of pregnancy—a prospective, longitudinal ultrasound study. *Acta Obstet Gynecol Scand* 2002;81(1):31–8.

46. Tsoi E, Akmal S, Rane S, Otigbah C, Nicolaides KH. Ultrasound assessment of cervical length in threatened preterm labor. *Ultrasound Obstet Gynecol* 2003;21(6):552–5.

47. Fuchs IB, Henrich W, Osthues K, Dudenhausen JW. Sonographic cervical length in singleton pregnancies with intact membranes presenting with threatened preterm labor. *Ultrasound Obstet Gynecol* 2004;24(5):554–7.

48. Conoscenti G, Meir YJ, D'Ottavio G, Rustico MA, Pinzano R, Fischer-Tamaro L, Stampalija T, Natale R, Maso G, Mandruzzato G. Does cervical length at 13-15 weeks' gestation predict preterm delivery in an unselected population? *Ultrasound Obstet Gynecol* 2003;21(2):128–34.

49. Carvalho MH, Bittar RE, Brizot ML, Maganha PP, Borges da Fonseca ES, Zugaib M. Cervical length at 11-14 weeks' and 22-24 weeks' gestation evaluated by transvaginal sonography, and gestational age at delivery. *Ultrasound Obstet Gynecol* 2003;21(2):135–9.

50. Coroleu B, Carreras O, Veiga A, Martell A, Martinez F, Belil I, Hereter L, Barri PN. Embryo transfer under ultrasound guidance improves pregnancy rates after in-vitro fertilization. *Hum Reprod* 2000;15(3):616–20.

51. Matorras R, Urquijo E, Mendoza R, Corcostegui B, Exposito A, Rodriguez-Escudero FJ. Ultrasound-guided embryo transfer improves pregnancy rates and increases the frequency of easy transfers. *Hum Reprod* 2002;17(7):1762–6.

52. Flisser E, Grifo JA, Krey LC, Noyes N. Transabdominal ultrasound-assisted embryo transfer and pregnancy outcome. *Fertil Steril* 2006;85(2):353–7.

53. Abou-Setta AM, Mansour RT, Al-Inany HG, Aboulghar MM, Aboulghar MA, Serour GI. Among women undergoing embryo transfer, is the probability of pregnancy and live birth improved with ultrasound guidance over clinical touch alone? A systemic review and meta-analysis of prospective randomized trials. *Fertil Steril.* 2007;88(2):333–41.

54. Brown JA, Buckingham K, Abou-setta A, Bucket W. Ultrasound versus clinical touch for catheter guidance during embryo transfer in women (Review). *Cochrane Library* 2007; (1).

55. Lorusso F, Depalo R, Bettocchi S, Vacca M, Vimercati A, Selvaggi L. Outcome of in vitro fertilization after transabdominal ultrasound-assisted embryo transfer with a full or empty bladder. *Fertil Steril* 2005;**84**(4):1046–8.

56. Sallam HN, Agameya AF, Rahman AF, Ezzeldin F, Sallam AN. Ultrasound measurement of the uterocervical angle before embryo transfer: a prospective controlled study. *Hum Reprod* 2002;**17**(7):1767–72.

57. Romundstad LB, Romundstad PR, Sunde A, von During V, Skjaerven R, Vatten LJ. Increased risk of placenta previa in pregnancies following IVF/ICSI; a comparison of ART and non-ART pregnancies in the same mother. *Hum Reprod* 2006;**21**(9): 2353–8.

58. Chama CM, Wanonyi IK, Usman JD. From low-lying implantation to placenta praevia: a longitudinal ultrasonic assessment. *J Obstet Gynaecol* 2004;**24**(5):516–18.

59. Smith RS, Lauria MR, Comstock CH, Treadwell MC, Kirk JS, Lee W, Bottoms SF. Transvaginal ultrasonography for all placentas that appear to be low-lying or over the internal cervical os. *Ultrasound Obstet Gynecol* 1997;**9**(1):22–4.

60. Ghorab S. Third-trimester transvaginal ultrasonography in placenta previa: does the shape of the lower placental edge predict clinical outcome? *Ultrasound Obstet Gynecol* 2001;**18**(2):103–8.

61. Heer IM, Muller-Egloff S, Strauss A. Placenta praevia—comparison of four sonographic modalities. *Ultraschall Med* 2006;**27**(4):355–9.

62. Tan NH, Abu M, Woo JL, Tahir HM. The role of transvaginal sonography in the diagnosis of placenta praevia. *Aust N Z J Obstet Gynaecol* 1995;**35**(1):42–5.

63. Sunna E, Ziadeh S. Transvaginal and transabdominal ultrasound for the diagnosis of placenta praevia. *J Obstet Gynecol* 1999;**19**(2):152–4.

64. Chen JM, Zhou QC, Wang RR. Value of transvaginal sonography in diagnosis of placenta previa. *Hunan Yi Ke Da Xue Xue Bao* 2001;**26**(3):289–90.

65. Bhide A, Prefumo F, Moore J, Hollis B, Thilaganathan B. Placental edge to internal os distance in the late third trimester and mode of delivery in placenta praevia. *BJOG* 2003;**110**(9):860–4.

66. Dawson WB, Dumas MD, Romano WM et al. Translabial ultrasonography and placenta praevia: does measurement of the os-placenta distance predict outcome? *J Ultrasound Med* 1996;**15**:441.

67. Opeheimer LW, Farine D, Ritchie JW, et al. What is a low lying placenta. *AM J Obstet Gynecol* 1991;**165**:1036.

68. Fung TY, Lau TK. Poor perinatal outcome associated with vasa previa: is it preventable? A report of three cases and review of literature.

69. Nomiyama M, Toyota Y, Kawano H. Antenatal diagnosis of velamentous umbilical cord insertion and vasa previa with color Doppler imaging. *Ultrasound Obstet Gynecol* 1998;**12**: 426–9.

70. Pent D. Vasa previa. *Am J Obstet Gynecol* 1979;**134**:151–5.

71. Antoine C, Youn BK, Silverman F, Greco MA, Alvarez SP. Sinusoidal fetal heart rate pattern with vasa previa in twin pregnancy. *J Reprod Med* 1982;**27**:295–300.

72. Codero DR, Helgott AW, Landy HJ, Reik R, Medina C, O'sullivan MJA. Nonhemorrhagic manifestation of vasa previa. A clinicopathologic case. *Obstet Gynecol* 1993;**82**:689–701.

73. Young M, Yu N, Barham K. The role of light and sound technologies in the detection of vasa previa. *Reprod Fertil Dev* 1991;**3**:439–51.

74. Catanzarite V, Maida C, Thomas W, Mendoza A, Stanco L, Piacquadio KM. Prenatal sonographic diagnosis of vasa previa: ultrasound findings and obstetric outcome in ten cases. *Ultrasound Obstet Gynecol* 2001;**18**(2):109–15.

75. Baschat AA. Ante- and intrapartum diagnosis of vasa praevia in singleton pregnancies by colour coded Doppler sonography. *Eur J Obstet Gynecol Reprod Biol* 1998;**79**(1):19–25.

76. Oyelese Y, Catanzarite V, Prefumo F, Lashley S, Schachter M, Tovbin Y, Goldstein V, Smulian JC. Vasa previa: the impact of prenatal diagnosis on outcomes. *Obstet Gynecol* 2004;**103**(5 Pt 1): 937–42.

77. Burton G, Saunders DM. Vasa praevia: another cause for concern in in vitro fertilization pregnancies. *Aust N Z J Obstet Gynaecol* 1988;**28**(3):180–1.

78. Englert Y, Imbert MC, Van Rosendael E, Belaisch J, Segal L, Feichtinger W, Wilkin P, Frydman R, Leroy F. Morphological anomalies in the placentae of IVF pregnancies: preliminary report of a multicentric study. *Hum Reprod* 1987;**2**(2):155–7.

79. Pyrgiotis E, Sultan KM, Neal GS, Liu HC, Grifo JA, Rosenwaks Z. Ectopic pregnancies after in vitro fertilization and embryo transfer. *J Assist Reprod Genet* 1994;**11**(2):79–84.

80. Ginsburg ES, Frates MC, Rein MS, Fox JH, Hornstein MD, Friedman AJ. Early diagnosis and treatment of cervical pregnancy in an in vitro fertilization program. *Fertil Steril* 1994; **61**(5):966–9.

81. Rizk B, Brinsden PR. Embryo migration responsible for ectopic pregnancies, 1990;**163**(4):1639.

82. Aboulghar M, Rizk B. Ultrasonography of the Cervix. In: Rizk B (Ed.) Ultrasonography in reproductive medicine and infertility. Cambridge: United Kingdom, Cambridge University Press, 2009, chapter 12.

83. Ushakov FB, Elchalal U, Aceman PJ, Schenker JG, Gembruch U. Cervical pregnancy: past and future. *Obstet Gynecol Surv* 1997;**52**(1):45–59.

84. Kim TJ, Seong SJ, Lee KJ, Lee JH, Shin JS, Lim KT, Chung HW, Lee KH, Park IS, Shim JU, Park CT. Clinical outcomes of patients treated for cervical pregnancy with or without methotrexate. *J Korean Med Sci* 2004;**19**(6):848–52.

85. Doekhie BM, Schats R, Hompes PG. Cervical pregnancy treated with local methotrexate. *Eur J Obstet Gynecol Reprod Biol* 2005; **122**(1):128–30.

86. Sherer DM, Lysikiewicz A, Abulafia O. Viable cervical pregnancy managed with systemic Methotrexate, uterine artery embolization, and local tamponade with inflated Foley catheter balloon. *Am J Perinatol* 2003;**20**(5):263–7.

87. Mitra AG, Harris-Owens M. Conservative medical management of advanced cervical ectopic pregnancies. *Obstet Gynecol Surv* 2000;**55**(6):385–9.

88. Pascual MA, Ruiz J, Tresserra F, Sanuy C, Grases PJ, Tur R, Barri PN. Cervical ectopic twin pregnancy: diagnosis and conservative treatment: case report. *Hum Reprod* 2001;**16**(3): 584–6.

89. Hassiakos D, Bakas P, Creatsas G. Cervical pregnancy treated with transvaginal ultrasound-guided intra-amniotic instillation of methotrexate. *Arch Gynecol Obstet* 2005;**271**(1):69–72

90. Yildizhan B. Diagnosis and treatment of early cervical pregnancy: a case report and literature review. *Clin Exp Obstet Gynecol* 2005;**32**(4):254–6.

91. Kirk E, Condous G, Haider Z, Syed A, Ojha K, Bourne T. The conservative management of cervical ectopic pregnancies. *Ultrasound Obstet Gynecol* 2006;**27**(4):430–7.

92. Api O, Unal O, Api M, Ergin B, Alkan N, Kars B, Turan C. Ultrasonographic appearance of cervical pregnancy following successful treatment with methotrexate. *Ultrasound Obstet Gynecol* 2006;**28**:845–7.

17

TRANSRECTAL ULTRASONOGRAPHY IN MALE INFERTILITY

Levent Gurkan, Andrew C. Harbin, Wayne J. G. Hellstrom

MALE INFERTILITY: PREVALENCE, CLINICAL PRESENTATION, AND DIAGNOSTIC STEPS

Infertility is a clinical problem affecting approximately 15 percent of all couples. Despite the common misperception that females are the major cause of conception difficulties, male factor is present in at least half of the cases (1).

The standard evaluation of male infertility includes complete medical history, focused physical examination, laboratory testing (including semen analysis and determination of the hormone profile), and, in certain situations, selective imaging. Male infertility may be caused by abnormalities in the normal development or fertilization capacity of spermatozoa (e.g., vascular, genetic, hormonal, or immunological) or interference in the transport of spermatozoa from the testis to the prostatic urethra (e.g., agenesis or obstruction).

Azospermia is defined as the complete absence of spermatozoa in the ejaculate, and is found in 5 percent of all infertile couples presenting to infertility clinics (2,3). Azospermia from obstructive causes can be categorized as partial or complete. Complete obstruction, accounting for about 1 percent of cases of azospermia, is localized to the epididymis in 30–67 percent and to the testis in 15 percent of cases. Distal ejaculatory duct obstruction occurs in only 1–3 percent of patients with obstructive azospermia (4). However, partial obstruction of the ejaculatory tract accounts for another 5 percent of male factor infertility (5). Functional obstruction of the distal seminal ducts, which is hypothesized to be related to local neuropathy, has also been reported (6).

Patients suffering from obstructive infertility may provide a specific clinical history including hematospermia, postejaculatory pain, current or previous urethritis or prostatitis, obstructive or irritative urinary symptoms, previous scrotal swelling, infection or pain, prior scrotal surgery, previous inguinal herniorrhaphy, trauma, or chronic sinopulmonary infections (4). Physical examination in such patients reveals at least one normal testis with a volume greater than 15 ml, although in rare situations small testes signifying testicular failure can occur in man with obstructive azospermia and concomitant testicular failure. Other possible physical findings related to obstructive infertility are an enlarged or indurated epididymis, nodules in the epididymes or vas deferens, absence or partial atresia of the vas deferens, signs of urethritis, or prostatic abnormalities. While serum follicle-stimulating hormone (FSH) levels are usually normal in patients with obstructive infertility, normal FSH levels do not exclude azospermia of testicular origin. In fact, serum FSH levels are normal in at least 40 percent of men with primary spermatogenic failure. Inhibin B, a negative feedback signal molecule produced by the Sertoli cells, may have a greater predictive value for the presence of normal spermatogenesis (7).

The importance of the history and physical exam in the majority of these patients should be emphasized, as many physicians focus primarily on semen analysis and imaging. A physical examination should precede any type of radiological or laboratory study. For example, congenital bilateral absence of the vas deferens is easily detected by examination of the scrotal contents and in such circumstances further radiological examination of genital structures is not indicated (though an abdominal ultrasound may be required to rule out concurrent kidney abnormalities). In this subgroup of patients, the optimal therapy is assisted reproduction technologies (ART) involving open or percutaneous retrieval of gametes from the epididymis or testis. Hence, a proper physical examination will circumvent the false hope of natural conception and the significant emotional and financial burden of unnecessary imaging.

Ultrasonographic evaluation of patients suspected of having obstructive infertility includes scrotal and transrectal ultrasound. Scrotal ultrasound is mainly used to evaluate the testis and epididymes, with special attention paid to anatomic structure and echogenicity. Transrectal ultrasound (TRUS) evaluates the distal components of the ejaculatory duct system including the ampullae of the vas deferens, the seminal vesicles, ejaculatory ducts, and the prostate.

CANDIDATES FOR TRUS IMAGING

The classic candidate for TRUS evaluation produces a semen analysis consistent with complete distal ejaculatory obstruction; namely low ejaculate volume (usually <1.5 ml), azospermia, low pH (<7), and absence of fructose. Patients should have at least one palpable vas deferens and will usually have normal sex hormone profiles. Patients with partial distal obstruction may also be candidates for TRUS evaluation. These patients usually present with low-volume ejaculate, severe oligoasthenospermia (low count and low motility), and/or painful ejaculation. In contrast to complete obstruction, however, patients with partial obstruction will have borderline normal fructose levels in the ejaculate and no obvious physical or hormonal abnormalities (4).

ESSENTIALS OF TRUS IMAGING

Transrectal ultrasound follows the same principles as other ultrasonographic evaluations. Sound waves are emitted by a transducer, and the reflected waves are converted into computer-generated images. The quality of the image depends mostly on the frequency of sound generated by the probe. Higher frequency probes generate higher quality images, but they have the disadvantage of having a lower ability to penetrate tissue. The transrectal approach requires limited tissue depth, allowing the operator to use a higher frequency biplane probe (7.0–7.5 mHz). Although the frequency used is lower than that for the superficial examination of the scrotum and penis (10 mHz), the close proximity of the probe to the prostate, ejaculatory ducts, and seminal vesicles provides adequate detailed anatomical information about these structures (1).

Technically, TRUS is minimally invasive and easy to perform. In most cases, it can be performed as an outpatient procedure without the need for anesthesia. Prior to the procedure, rectal examination should be performed to exclude any structural abnormalities, which could contraindicate or complicate TRUS examination. The examination can be performed with the patient in the lithotomy, knee-chest, or lateral decubitus position. Lateral decubitus position is the preferred position as this provides easy access for the operator and less discomfort for the patient. The probe is inserted 8–9 cm after the anal verge with adequate lubrication. The ampullae of the vas deferens, seminal vesicles, ejaculatory ducts, prostate, and surrounding structures are systematically examined in both transverse and sagittal planes. For medical and legal purposes, multiple images of these structures are captured and properly labeled with the patient's name, the structure in the image, and the date. The operator is responsible for proper storage of these materials.

EMBRYOLOGICAL AND ANATOMICAL CONSIDERATIONS RELATED TO TRUS IMAGING

In order to understand the normal and pathological appearance of the ejaculatory structures on TRUS, it is important to appreciate their anatomical relationships and embryological origins.

As the vas deferens approaches the base of the prostate from a posterolateral direction, the distal end joins the seminal vesicle to form the ejaculatory duct. The ejaculatory duct drains into the posterior urethra, lateral to the verumontanum. It constitutes the common urethral entry point for both spermatozoa from the vas deferens and the seminal fluid from the seminal vesicles.

The ureters are derived embryonically from the Wolffian (mesonephric) ducts. During the seventh week of the embryological development, the Wolffian ducts transform into the distal vas deferens and the ejaculatory ducts. This common origin is significant as pathological findings in the vas deferens may predict more significant congenital abnormalities in the ureter and kidney (8). The ejaculatory ducts on sagittal TRUS are as seen as tubular structures less than 2 mm in diameter running in posterolateral to anteromedial direction. The sagittal plane is preferred as the identification of ejaculatory ducts on transverse plane is somewhat difficult.

The prostatic utricle may be seen at the verumontanum between the openings of the ejaculatory ducts. The embryonic origin of the prostatic utricle has been the subject of much debate, with some authorities claiming it to be of endodermal origin (5), while others believe it to be a small remnant of the Mullerian duct (8). Others suggest it is a combination of the Mullerian duct and urogenital sinus epithelium (9). The true identity, as well as the clinical relevance, of the utricle's embryonic origin remains to be determined. While the size of the prostatic utricle varies, it is normally less than 6 mm on TRUS. However, in 10 percent of cases, it is greater than 10 mm.

The seminal vesicles are located behind the posterior wall of the bladder, superior to the prostate. Around the thirteenth week of embryologic development, the seminal vesicles branch from the distal Wolffian ducts, just proximal to their entry into the prostate. Abnormalities in other structures of Wolffian origin, involving the vas deferens or ureters, are frequently associated with seminal vesicle malformations. On TRUS examination, the seminal vesicles appear as hypoechoic areas with fine septations. Anteroposterior diameter up to 15 mm is considered normal.

TRUS AS A DIAGNOSTIC TOOL

Traditionally, vasography after vasopuncture was used to evaluate the patency of the ejaculatory ducts. The procedure involves transscrotal cannulation of the vas deferens and injection of a solution containing a dye (e.g., methylene blue) or a radio-opaque substance, followed by cystoscopy or X-ray imaging, respectively (10). Although vasography is still the gold standard, its use has been supplanted by TRUS. The primary concerns of vasography are its invasive nature, inherent costliness, high risk of iatrogenic stricture and vasal occlusion, and relative risks of anesthetic and radiation exposure (5). Today, the major use of vasography is during definitive surgery for ejaculatory duct obstructions.

Magnetic resonance imaging (MRI) and computerized tomography (CT) have also been proposed for the evaluation of the ejaculatory system.

Because of its low resolution, CT has been shown to have limited value in evaluating the ejaculatory ducts and surrounding structures. MRI with the use of an endorectal coil has proven to be valuable on T2 sequence imaging. Because of its multiplanar nature and high resolution, MRI is superior to TRUS in the diagnosis of small prostatic cysts, evaluation of cyst content, and inspection of the surrounding tissues. However, MRI has restricted use in these circumstances because of its high cost and low availability. Additionally, the low visibility of calcium on MRI makes the diagnosis of calcification problematic. Calcification and stone formation is recognized as one of the major causes of ejaculatory duct obstruction.

Because of its noninvasive nature, reasonable cost, low rate of complications, and high diagnostic efficacy, TRUS is the preferred tool for the diagnosis of ejaculatory duct obstruction. It should be noted that in a recent study, TRUS findings correlated poorly with those obtained by definitive invasive studies (11). Obstruction on TRUS was confirmed in only 52, 48, and 36 percent of vesiculography, seminal vesicle aspiration, and duct chromotubation studies, respectively. If the investigators in this study relied on TRUS findings alone, the authors claim 52 percent of patients would have undergone unnecessary surgical intervention (11).

PATHOLOGICAL FINDINGS ON A DIAGNOSTIC TRUS PROCEDURE

The types of pathologies found on a TRUS evaluation include agenesis or hypoplasia of urogenital structures, cysts, dilatations, calcifications, and stones.

Agenesis of the vas deferens is seen in 1–2.5 percent of infertile men and 4.4–17 percent of azospermic men and is frequently accompanied by seminal vesicle agenesis. Ultrasonographic evaluation of the ipsilateral kidney is indicated in cases of unilateral vas deferens agenesis as ipsilateral renal anomalies may be found in as many as 91 percent of cases (12). This association, as already noted, is because both ureters and vas deferens arise embryologically from the Wolffian ducts. Genetic counseling is advised for infertile males with congenital agenesis of the vas deferens as mutations in genes related to cystic fibrosis are observed in 82 percent of these patients (13).

Seminal vesicle cysts are rare and can be either congenital or acquired. Congenital seminal vesicle cysts are frequently accompanied by ipsilateral renal agenesis or an ectopic ureter. In the latter cases, the ureter is frequently attached to a dysplastic kidney with entry into the seminal vesicle. Seminal vesicle cysts only cause seminal vesicle duct obstruction if they are medially located and reach sufficient size (14).

Prostatic cysts can be classified by location, sperm content, and embryological origin. Non–sperm-containing cysts are found in a midline location and are called either utricular cysts or Mullerian duct cysts. The degree to which these two cysts differ, and the nature of that difference, remains to be determined. Some authors maintain that utricular cysts are of endodermal origin and are located near the verumontanum, while Mullerian duct cysts are of mesodermal origin and are located closer to the prostatic base (5). Other authorities argue that cysts of Mullerian duct origin do not truly exist, and all such cysts derive from the prostatic utricle (9). Whatever the embryonic origin, their appearance on TRUS is nearly identical. Sperm-containing cysts, called Wolffian or ejaculatory duct cysts, are far less common than utricular/Mullerian duct cysts (15). They are usually noted in a more paramedian location rather than strictly midline (16). Sperm may be absent from Wolffian cysts in the setting of concomitant epididymal obstruction or after long-term ejaculatory duct obstruction. This can make differentiation of Wolffian cysts from utricular cysts difficult (17,18). Other cystic formations that can be detected during a TRUS evaluation are congenital and prostatic retention cysts and local abscess formations. These cysts are less likely to cause obstruction because they are frequently located more laterally.

Fibrosis and calcification of the distal ejaculatory ducts occurs secondarily to inflammation or infection. These lesions commonly appear on TRUS as hyperechoic regions. Importantly, TRUS can reveal the anatomical relationship between ejaculatory channels and calcifications. It can also detect proximal dilatation of the ejaculatory tract, which indirectly implies the presence of a distal obstruction. However, it is important to note that obstruction because of excessive fibrosis may occur without any apparent dilatation of the ejaculatory duct. If there is no history of infection or surgical procedure, a subclinical infection is implicated in such situations (16).

DIAGNOSTIC CRITERIA FOR DISTAL EJACULATORY DUCT OBSTRUCTION

Distal ejaculatory duct obstruction (EDO) is strongly suspected in cases of azospermia in which TRUS reveals dilated seminal vesicles with an anteroposterior length greater than 15 mm or ejaculatory ducts with diameters greater than 2.3 mm (19). (Figure 17.2) However, in cases of incomplete ejaculatory obstruction or without sufficient dilatation of the seminal vesicles

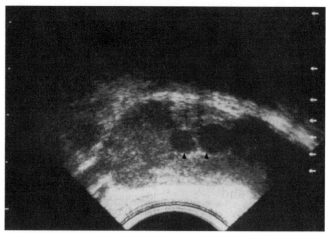

Figure 17.1. Transverse image of the prostate revealing dilated ejaculatory ducts (arrowheads).

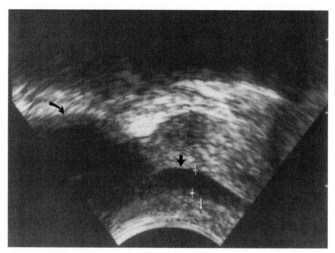

Figure 17.2. Longitudinal image of the junction of the seminal vesicle (curved arrow) and prostate revealing dilated ejaculatory duct (arrow) that measured 3.6 mm.

or ejaculatory ducts (e.g., in cases of excessive fibrosis), it may be difficult to make a definitive diagnosis based on TRUS findings alone. In such atypical presentations, verification of distal obstruction can be confirmed by transrectal aspiration of the seminal vesicles. Diagnosis of distal obstruction is supported by the presence of three or more motile spermatozoa per high-powered field in the aspirate. The sample is obtained two hours after ejaculation since normal seminal vesicles will contain no motile spermatozoa at this time (20) (Figure 17.1).

THERAPEUTIC APPLICATIONS OF TRUS

If TRUS evaluation reveals obstruction of the ejaculatory ducts secondary to fibrosis or calcification or compression by a superficial midline cyst, the preferred therapy is transurethral resection or unroofing of the ejaculatory ducts (TURED) (21). The procedure varies based on the pathological findings, but it may involve resection of the distal portion of the duct, unroofing of any cysts present, or a combination of both (22). In TURED, because there are no guides to identify the ejaculatory ducts, the resection depth and the exact location of the obstructed lesion is not easily determined. Furthermore, complications such as rectal wall, external sphincter, and bladder neck injury can theoretically occur more frequently because of the small prostate volumes in these young infertile men. Concurrent TRUS can be used to monitor resection depth during TURED to prevent complications and also to monitor the efficacy of the procedure. Dye (for direct visualization with cystoscopy) or a combination of dye and echo-enhancing contrast agent (for visualization with TRUS) is injected into the seminal vesicles, using TRUS to identify the ejaculatory ducts (23,24).

TRUS can also be used for therapeutic aspiration and reduction in the size of obstructive cysts. This method is preferred for deep cysts, which are inaccessible by TURED. While this is a simple and noninvasive method of cyst reduction, it is not always curative and the cystic fluid often reaccumulates (15).

TRUS may also be employed in azospermic men with an obstruction distal to the seminal vesicles for sperm retrieval by seminal vesicle aspiration. The sperm retrieved by this method can subsequently be used for ART. Although described as successful in the literature, this approach is not a commonly performed as testicular extraction or epididymal aspiration is more commonly used for sperm retrieval. TRUS-guided aspiration of the seminal vesicles may be suitable for patients undergoing concurrent TRUS-guided aspiration of midline cysts (2, 25, 26).

KEY POINTS

- Infertility is a common problem affecting 15 percent of couples; male factor infertility accounts for about half of these cases.
- Obstructive infertility can present with a wide range of clinical scenarios including azospermia, which is the absence of sperm in the ejaculate.
- Obstructive azospermia is seen in 5 percent of infertile men; ejaculatory duct obstruction accounts for 1–3 percent of cases of obstructive azospermia.
- The standard clinical evaluation of an infertile male includes history, physical examination, semen analysis, hormone profile, and selective imaging. Imaging should not be performed before the earlier steps are completed.
- Transrectal ultrasound is a useful tool for imaging the distal structures of the ejaculatory system (including the ampulla of the vas deferens, the seminal vesicles, the ejaculatory ducts, and the prostate) and for diagnosis of EDO.
- Although it has a low sensitivity, TRUS is currently preferred over MRI, CT, and vasography for diagnosis of ejaculatory duct obstruction because of its minimal risk, reasonable cost, infrequent complications, and diagnostic efficacy.
- Pathological findings on TRUS include prostatic and seminal vesicle cysts, dilatations of the seminal vesicles and ejaculatory ducts, stones, and fibrosis or calcification of the ejaculatory duct region.
- TRUS findings suggestive of EDO include dilated seminal vesicles with an anteroposterior length greater than 15 mm, dilated ejaculatory ducts with a diameter greater than 2.3 mm, and the presence of spermatozoa in the seminal vesicle aspirate two hours after ejaculation.

- TRUS can be applied therapeutically for ART. It can also be used concurrently with TURED, aspiration and reduction of midline cyst, and aspiration of seminal vesicles.

REFERENCES

1. Zahalsky M. and Nagler H. Ultrasound and infertility: diagnostic and therapeutic uses. *Curr Urol Rep* (2001), **2**, 437–42.
2. Cerruto M.A., Novella G., Antoniolli S.Z. and Zattoni F. Use of transperineal fine needle aspiration of seminal vesicles to retrieve sperm in a man with obstructive azoospermia. *Fertil Steril* (2006), **86**, 1764.e7–9.
3. Irvin D.S. Epidemiology and etiology of male infertility. *Hum Reprod* (1998), **13**, Suppl. 1:33–44.
4. Dohle G.R., Colpi G.M., Hargreave T.B., Papp G.K., Jungwirth A. and Weidner W. The EAU Working Group on Male Infertility. EAU guidelines on male infertility. *Eur Urol* (2005), **48**, 703–11.
5. Goluboff E.T., Stifelman M.D. and Fisch H. Ejaculatory duct obstruction in the infertile male. *Urology* (1995), **45**, 925–31.
6. Colpi G.M., Casella F., Zanollo A., Ballerini G., Balerna M., Campana A. and Lange A. Functional voiding disturbances of the ampullo-vesicular seminal tract: a cause of male infertility. *Acta Eur Fertil* (1987), **18**, 165–79.
7. Pierik F.H., Vreeburg J.T., Stijnen T., De Jong F.H. and Weber R.F. Serum inhibin B as a marker of spermatogenesis. *J Clin Endocrinol Metab* (1998), **83**, 3110–4.
8. Veltri R. and Rodriquez R. The molecular biology, endocrinology, and physiology of the prostate and seminal vesicles. In *Wein: Campbell-Walsh Urology: Ninth Edition*, Chapter 85: ed. Wein A.J. et al. (Philadelphia, PA: Saunders Company, 2007).
9. Kato H., Hayama M., Furuya S., Kobayashi S., Islam A.M. and Nishizawa O. Anatomical and histological studies of so-called Mullerian duct cyst. *Int J Urol* (2005), **12**, 465–8.
10. Weintraub M.P., De Mouy E. and Hellstrom W.J.G. Newer modalities in the diagnosis and treatment of ejaculatory duct obstruction. *J Urol* (1993), **150**, 1150–4.
11. Purohit R.S., Wu D.S., Shinohara K. and Turek P.J. A prospective comparison of 3 diagnostic methods to evaluate ejaculatory duct obstruction. *J Urol* (2004), **171**, 232–5.
12. Schlegel P.N., Shin D. and Goldstein M. Urogenital anomalies in men with congenital absence of the vas deferens. *J Urol* (1996), **155**, 1644–8.
13. Chillon M., Casals T., Mercier B., et al. Mutations in the cystic fibrosis gene in patients with congenital absence of the vas deferens. *N Engl J Med* (1995), **332**, 1475–80.
14. Shabsigh R., Lerner S., Fishman I.J. and Kadmon D. The role of transrectal ultrasonography in the diagnosis and management of prostatic and seminal vesicle cysts. *J Urol* (1989), **141**, 1206–9.
15. Elder J.S. and Mostwin J.L. Cyst of the ejaculatory duct/urogenital sinus. *J Urol* (1984), **132**, 768–771.
16. Kuligowska E. and Fenlon H.M. Transrectal US in male infertility: spectrum of findings and role in patient care. *Radiology* (1998), **207**, 173–81.
17. Silber S.J. Ejaculatory duct obstruction. *J Urol* (1980), **124**, 294–7.
18. Patterson L. and Jarow J.P. Transrectal ultrasonography in the evaluation of the infertile man: a report of three cases. *J Urol* (1990), **144**, 1469–71.
19. Nguyen H.T., Etzell J. and Turek P.J. Normal human ejaculatory duct anatomy: a study of cadaveric and surgical specimens. *J Urol* (1996), **155**, 1639–42.
20. Orhan I., Onur R., Cayan S., Koksal I.T. and Kadioglu A. Seminal vesicle sperm aspiration in the diagnosis of ejaculatory duct obstruction. *BJU Int* (1999), **84**, 1050–3.

21. Fisch H., Kang Y.M., Johnson C.W. and Goluboff E.T. Ejaculatory duct obstruction. *Curr Opin Urol* (2002), **12**, 509–15.

22. Schroeder-Printzen I., Ludwig M., Kohn F. and Weidner W. Surgical therapy in infertile men with ejaculatory duct obstruction: technique and outcome of a standardized surgical approach. *Hum Reprod* (2000), **15**, 1364–8.

23. Halpern E.J. and Hirsch I.H. Sonographically guided transurethral laser incision of a Mullerian duct cyst for treatment of ejaculatory duct obstruction. *Am J Roentgenol* (2000), **175**, 777–8.

24. Apaydin E., Killi R.M., Turna B., Semerci B. and Nazli O. Transrectal ultrasonography-guided echo-enhanced seminal vesiculography in combination with transurethral resection of the ejaculatory ducts. *BJU Int* (2004), **93**, 1110–2.

25. Boehlem D. and Schmid H.P. Novel use of fine needle aspiration of seminal vesicles for sperm retrieval in infertile men. *Urology* (2005), **66**, 880.

26. Hellstrom W.J.G. and Gurkan L. Ultrasonography in male infertility. In Rizk B. (Ed.) Ultrasonography in Reproductive Medicine and Infertility. Cambridge University Press, 2008, Chapter 22, pp. 268–72.

18

The Basic Semen Analysis: Interpretation and Clinical Application

T. F. Kruger, S. C. Oehninger

INTRODUCTION

It is estimated that male subfertility is present in up to 40–50 percent of infertile couples, alone or in combination with female factors (1).

The correct approach for male infertility evaluation should include a rational program composed of the careful evaluation of the patient's history, a complete physical examination, laboratory tests of basic/extended semen analysis, and an urological, endocrinological, and genetic workup, as appropriate (2).

Several semen parameters are used to discriminate the fertile male from the subfertile male. The most widely used parameters are sperm concentration, motility, progressive motility, and sperm morphology. All of these parameters are important and must not be used alone to make clinical decisions or seen in isolation. Sperm morphology is, however, the single sperm indicator most widely debated in the literature. A large number of classification systems have been used to describe which cellular features constitute a morphologically normal/abnormal spermatozoon. The most widely accepted classification systems for sperm morphology are the World Health Organization (WHO) criteria of 1987 and 1992 (3, 4) and the Tygerberg strict criteria, now also used by the WHO since 1999 (5–8).

Although there is a positive correlation between normal semen parameters and male fertility potential, the threshold values for fertility/subfertility according to WHO criteria 1987 and 1992 (3, 4) are of little clinical value in discriminating between the fertile and subfertile male (9–13). If these criteria were applied, a great number of fertile males (partners having had pregnancies shortly before, after, or at the time of a spermiogram) were classified as subfertile. The predictive values of sperm morphology using strict criteria in in vitro fertilization (IVF) and intrauterine insemination (IUI) have been reviewed recently and proved to be useful (12, 14). Much less has been published on the use of this criterion regarding in vivo fertility (15, 16).

THE USE OF SEMEN PARAMETERS IN IVF AND IUI PROGRAMS (15, 16)

The percentage of normal sperm morphology (strict criteria) has a positive predictive value in IVF and IUI programs. In a structured literature review (meta-analysis), it was unequivocally shown that normal sperm morphology cutoff values resulted in positive predictive values for IVF success when using the 5 and the 14 percent thresholds, respectively, with the overall fertilization rate and overall pregnancy rates significantly higher in the group with normal morphology greater than or equal to 5 percent as compared with the less than 5 percent group (12, 16).

A meta-analysis of the data on IUI programs showed a significantly higher pregnancy rate per cycle in the group with normal sperm morphology of greater than or equal to 5 percent compared with the group with less than 5 percent normal forms (14). In the group with normal sperm morphology less than 5 percent, other semen parameters proved to be predicting IUI success (14). In the IUI analysis, motility (17) and concentration (18) also played a role in some of the studies evaluated, while others (19) stated that sperm morphology alone was enough to predict the prognosis. Because of the high cost of assisted reproduction (IVF/ICSI), in males with semen parameters where at least one million motile spermatozoa per milliliter can be retrieved after wash and swim-up, IUI can be offered as a treatment option with good results over at least four insemination cycles (18). Conversely, males with a poor fertility potential should be identified and referred to assisted reproduction programs.

FERTILITY/SUBFERTILITY THRESHOLDS FOR SPERM CONCENTRATION, SPERM MOTILITY/ PROGRESSIVE MOTILITY, AND SPERM MORPHOLOGY USING TYGERBERG STRICT CRITERIA (15, 16)

In an effort to establish fertility/subfertility thresholds for the above-mentioned parameters, we identified four articles in the published literature (20–23). These articles compared the different semen parameters of a fertile and a subfertile group. They used either the classification and regression tree analysis or the receiver operating characteristic (ROC) curve analysis to estimate thresholds for the different semen parameters. The ROC curve was also used to assess the diagnostic accuracy of the different parameters and their ability to classify subjects into fertile and subfertile groups.

In these four articles (20–23), the predictive power of the different parameters were calculated as its AUC using the ROC curve. The AUC for sperm morphology ranged from 66 to 78.2 percent, confirming the high predictive power of sperm morphology. In fact, it had the best performance of the different semen parameters in two articles (22, 23). The threshold calculated in these two articles were 10 and 9 percent, respectively,

Table 18.1: Possible Lower Thresholds for the General Population to Distinguish between Subfertile and Fertile Men, Based on the Assumed Incidences of Subfertile Males in Their Populations (Siebert et al. from Clinical Gynaecology: Diagnosis and treatment)

Author	Morphology (%)	Motility (%)	Progressive motility (%)	Concentration (10^6/ml)
Menkveld et al. (16)	3	20		20
Günalp et al. (15)	5	30	14	9
Ombelet et al. (14)	5	28		14.3

while Gunalp et al. (20) calculated a threshold of 12 percent using sensitivity and specificity to analyze their data; the fourth study calculated a 4 percent predictive cutoff point value (21). Although sensitivity and specificity for the values are relatively high, the positive predictive values are not. This will result in classifying fertile males as subfertile, therefore probably leading to a degree of anxiety and an unnecessary and costly infertility treatment. A second and much lower threshold was calculated in three of the four articles (22). Ombelet et al. calculated their second and much lower threshold by using the 10th percentile of the fertile population, while (21) screened the population with the positive predictive value as indicator and Menkveld et al. (21) assumed a 50 percent prevalence of subfertility in their study population. The lower threshold ranged from 3 to 5 percent (Table 18.1). These lower thresholds have a much higher positive predictive value than the higher thresholds with the negative predictive value not much lower (15, 16).

As suggested by WHO in 1999 (7), each tertiary center should develop their own thresholds based on the population they are working in. It seems as if the sperm morphology threshold of 0–4 percent normal forms indicates a higher risk group for subfertility and fits the IVF and IUI data calculated previously (14). A concentration of below fifteen million per ml and percent motility below 30 percent also reflect parameters in the subfertile range. The four articles discussed in the latter half of this chapter showed the same trends and can serve as guidelines to distinguish fertile from subfertile males (20–23).

EXTENDED SEMEN ANALYSIS/SPERM FUNCTIONAL ASSAYS

It was recently stated by Arslan et al. (2) that there is a need for other specific and critical sperm functional capacities that can be more reliably examined in vitro. These functions include motility, competence to achieve capacitation, zona pellucida binding, and acrosome reaction. The assessment of these features is what is typically considered as sperm functional testing.

The extended semen analysis should include the preferential examination of these essential sperm functional attributes. These assays have been categorized into 1) tests that examine defective sperm functions indirectly through the use of biochemical means (i.e., measurement of the generation of reactive oxygen species or evidence of peroxidative damage,

measurement of enzyme activities such as creatine phosphokinase and others) 2) bioassays of gamete interaction (i.e., the heterologous zona-free hamster oocyte test and the homologous sperm-zona pellucida–binding assays) and induced acrosome reaction scoring and 3) computer-aided sperm motion analysis (CASA) for the evaluation of sperm motion characteristics (2).

Oehninger et al. reported an objective, outcome-based examination of the validity of the currently available assays based upon the results obtained from 2,906 subjects evaluated in thirty-four published and prospectively designed, controlled studies. The aim was carried out through a meta-analytical approach that examined the predictive value of four categories of sperm functional assays (CASA, induced acrosome reaction testing, sperm penetration assay or SPA, and sperm-zona pellucida–binding assays) for IVF outcome (24).

Results of this meta-analysis demonstrated a high predictive power of the sperm-zona pellucida binding and the induced acrosome reaction assays for fertilization outcome under in vitro conditions (24). However, the findings indicated a poor clinical value of the SPA as predictor of fertilization and a real need for standardization and further investigation of the potential clinical utility of CASA systems. Although this study provided objective evidence in which clinical management and future research may be directed, the analysis also pointed out to limitations of the current tests and the need for standardization of present methodologies and development of novel technologies.

CLINICAL MANAGEMENT

We suggest that the lower threshold should be used to identify males with the lowest potential for a pregnancy under in vivo conditions. Values above the lower threshold should be regarded as normal. These findings, especially on normal sperm morphology, are in keeping with previous publications by Coetzee et al. (12) (IVF data) and Van Waart et al. (14) (IUI data), which showed a significantly lower chance of successful pregnancies in males with normal morphology below their calculated thresholds.

It is, however, important to realize that patients with lower semen thresholds can, occasionally, still impregnate their partners spontaneously. These thresholds are there to assist the clinician in handling the patient correctly. The principle is to always repeat an abnormal semen analysis and abnormal sperm functional tests. Another valuable practical guide is a simple swim-up with help the clinician in making sound treatment suggestions. As stated before, an IUI must always be considered if sufficient spermatozoa are retrieved after swim-up, taking the indicated thresholds into consideration.

As stated by Arslan et al. recently (2), the treatment plan should be constructed based upon a complete identification of both male and female factors. In the presence of pure male infertility (no identifiable female factors), the appropriate indicated therapeutic management could be 1) medical (endocrine such as in hypogonadism or hyperprolactinemia, antibiotics in case of infection), 2) urological (surgical or nonsurgical treatments, such as conventional, microsurgical, or laparoscopic surgery, including correction of varicocele and epididymo- and vaso-vasostomy and modern approaches for ejaculatory disorders), and/or 3) low- or high-complexity assisted reproductive techniques (ARTs). The severity of male subfertility and some important prognostic risk factors in the female (e.g., age, duration of infertility, presence of endometriosis, and other pathologies) may accelerate the indication for ART (2).

We are in agreement with Arslan et al. who recommend the following course of action if no medical or urological treatment is indicated: "low-complexity" IUI therapy, "standard" IVF and embryo transfer, and IVF augmented with ICSI. If the female partner is older than thirty-five years, typically four to six cycles of IUI using husband's sperm in combination with controlled ovarian hyperstimulation are recommended as a simple (low complexity) ART approach, particularly if more than one million motile sperm can be recovered (18, 25). Preliminary data suggest that in order to increase cost-efficiency and loss of valuable time, IUI should not be performed if the total motile recoverable fraction is low, if the hemizona index is less than 31 percent (24), if the calcium ionophore–induced acrosome reaction is 22 or less (27), if the zona pellucida–induced acrosome reaction is less than 16 percent (26), and/or if the proportion of sperm depicting DNA fragmentation is greater than 12 percent (28). In all these cases, ICSI is the method of choice. Standard or conventional IVF should be limited to cases with acceptable recovery of motile sperm with borderline morphology scores. In addition, it was recently reported that ICSI with testicular spermatozoa provides the first-line ART option for men with high levels of DNA damage in ejaculated sperm (29). In this instance, more studies are needed to clinically validate the methods to assess DNA damage and the impact of DNA abnormalities on clinical outcomes.

KEY POINTS FOR CLINICAL PRACTICE

■ It is estimated that ICSI should be indicated when male infertility is properly diagnosed based upon a state-of-the-art extended evaluation of the male partner and also in cases with previous failed fertilization (2).

■ It is of utmost importance to evaluate the male clinically, and by doing a good semen analysis, valuable information will be obtained to make sound clinical decisions.

■ Swim-up and sperm functional tests must be encouraged to assist clinicians in the day-to-day handling of male factor infertility and be of immense help to make a good decision on a specific male problem.

■ Consequently, to perform ICSI in all cases on a purely pragmatic basis appears to be a significant departure from principles of evidence-based medicine (Arslan 2006).

REFERENCES

1. Irvine DS. Declining sperm quality: a review of facts and hypotheses. *Baillieres Clin Obstet Gynaecol* 1997;11:655.
2. Arslan M, Oehninger S, Kruger TF. Clinical management of male infertility. In: Male Infertility: Diagnosis and Treatment; Oehninger, Krugers editors, Informa Health Care, London: 2006, 305–18.
3. World Health Organization. WHO Laboratory Manual for the Examination of Human Semen and Semen-Cervical Mucus Interaction, edn. 2. Cambridge, Cambridge University Press, 1987.
4. World Health Organization. WHO Laboratory Manual for the Examination of Human Semen and Sperm-Cervical Mucus Interaction, edn. 3. Cambridge, Cambridge University Press, 1992.
5. Kruger TF, Acosta AA, Simmons KF, Swanson RJ et al. Predictive value of abnormal sperm morphology in *in vitro* fertilization. *Fertil Steril* 1988;49:112–17.
6. Kruger TF, Menkveld R, Stander FS, Lombard CJ et al. Sperm morphologic features as a prognostic factor in *in vitro* fertilization. *Fertil Steril* 1986;46:1118–23.
7. Menkveld R, Stander FSH, Kotze TJ et al. The evaluation of morphological characteristics of human spermatozoa according to stricter criteria. *Hum Reprod* 1990;5:586–92.
8. World Health Organization. WHO Laboratory Manual for the Examination of Human Semen and Sperm-Cervical Mucus Interaction, edn 4. Cambridge, Cambridge University Press, 1999.
9. Barratt CL, Naceeni M, Clements S et al. Clinical value of sperm morphology for in-vivo fertility: comparison between World Health Organization criteria of 1987 and 1992. *Hum Reprod* 1995;10:587–93.
10. Blonde JP, Ernst E, Jensen TK et al. Relation between semen quality and fertility: a population-based study of 430 first-pregnancy planners. *Lancet* 1998;352:1172–7.
11. Chia SE, Tay SK, Lim ST. What constitutes a normal seminal analysis? Semen parameters of 243 fertile men. *Hum Reprod* 1998;13:3394–8.
12. Coetzee K, Kruger TF, Lombard CJ. Predictive value of normal sperm morphology: a structured literature review. *Hum Reprod Update* 1998;4:73–82.
13. Ayala C, Steinberger E, Smith DP. The influence of semen analysis parameters on the fertility potential of infertile couples. *J Androl* 1996;17:718–25.
14. Van Waart J, Kruger TF, Lombard CJ et al. Predictive value of normal sperm morphology in intrauterine insemination (IUI): a structured literature review. *Hum Reprod Update* 2001;7:495–500.
15. Siebert TI, van der Merwe FH, Kruger TF et al. How do we define male subfertility and what is the prevalence in the general population. In Male Infertility: Diagnosis and Treatment. Informa Health Care, London, 2006; 269–76.
16. van der Merwe FH, Kruger TF, Oehninger S. The use of semen parameters to identify the subfertile male in the general population. *Gynecol Obstet Invest* 2005;59:86.
17. Montanaro Gauci M, Kruger TF, Coetzee K et al. Stepwise regression analysis to study male and female factors impacting on pregnancy rate in an intrauterine insemination programme. *Andrologia* 2001;33:135–41.
18. Ombelet W, Vandeput H, Van de Putte G et al. Intrauterine insemination after ovarian stimulation with clomiphene citrate: predictive potential of inseminating motile count and sperm morphology. *Hum Reprod* 1997;12:1458–65.
19. Linheim S, Barad D, Zinger M et al. Abnormal sperm morphology is highly predictive of pregnancy outcome during controlled ovarian hyperstimulation and intrauterine insemination. *J Assist Reprod Genet* 1996;13:569–72.
20. Günalp S, Onculoglu C, Gürgan T et al. A study of semen parameters with emphasis on sperm morphology in a fertile population: an attempt to develop clinical thresholds. *Hum Reprod* 2001;16:110–14.
21. Menkveld R, Wong WY, Lombard CJ et al. Semen parameters, including WHO and strict criteria morphology, in a fertile and infertile population: an effort towards standardization of *in vivo* thresholds. *Hum Reprod* 2001;16:1165–71.
22. Ombelet W, Bosmans E, Janssen M et al. Semen parameters in a fertile versus sub-fertile population: a need for change in the interpretation of semen testing. *Hum Reprod* 1997;12:987–93.
23. Guzick DS, Overstreet JW, Factor-Litvak P et al. Sperm morphology, motility, and concentration in fertile and infertile men. *N Engl J Med* 2001;345:1388–93.

24. Oehninger S et al. Sperm function assays and their predictive value for fertilization outcome in IVF therapy: a meta-analysis. *Hum Reprod Update* 2000;6:160.

25. Duran HE et al. Intrauterine insemination: a systematic review on determinants of success, *Hum Reprod Update* 2002b;8:373.

26. Bastiaan HS, Windt ML, Menkveld R, Kruger TF, Oehninger S, Franken DR. Relationship between zona pellucida-induced acrosome reaction, sperm morphology, sperm-zona pellucida binding, and in vitro fertilization. *Fertil Steril.* 2003;79(1):49–55.

27. Katsuki T et al. Prediction of outcomes of assisted reproduction treatment using the calcium ionophore-induced acrosome reaction. *Hum Reprod* 2005;20:469.

28. Duran EH et al. Sperm DNA quality predicts intrauterine insemination outcome: a prospective cohort study. *Hum Reprod* 2002a;17:3122.

29. Greco E et al. Efficient treatment of infertility due to sperm DNA damage by ICSI with testicular spermatozoa. *Hum Reprod* 2005;20:226.

19

EVALUATION OF SPERM DAMAGE: BEYOND THE WHO CRITERIA

Nabil Aziz, Ashok Agarwal

INTRODUCTION

For over twenty-five years, the World Health Organization (WHO) has served to provide a standardized approach to the assessment of the fertility potential of semen sample. These standards are concerned with measurable parameters such as the physical properties of an ejaculate, estimating the count of its cellular content be it sperm or leukocytes, grading sperm morphology and motility, and examining a possible immune interaction between sperm and the content of seminal plasma or the preovulatory mucus produced by the uterine cervix. The adoption of these standards worldwide has been enhanced through local schemes of quality control measures leading to andrology laboratory accreditation and certification. The first andrology laboratory manual published by the WHO in 1981 was the culmination of clinical experience and research in the previous eighty years (1). In its successive editions, the WHO manual portrayed stricter criteria in assessing parameters of interest and as a result values that were thought to be compatible with normal male fertility were modified (2,3). The resounding success of the WHO criteria is met by call for further scrutiny of sperm quality to address numerous concerns born from clinical and research work carried out in more recent years. First, the results of semen analyses can be very subjective and prone to intra- and interobserver variability (4). Second, although the traditional, manual-visual light microscopic methods for evaluating semen quality maintain their central role in assessment of male fertility potential, often a definitive diagnosis of male fertility cannot be made as a result of basic semen analysis (5). Conventional semen analysis per se cannot cover the diverse array of biological properties that the spermatozoon expresses as a highly specialized cell (6,7). Third, there has been growing awareness that the predictive power of the cutoff values of different sperm parameters is not absolute and that there is some degree of overlap between fertile and infertile male populations. As a result, many infertile couples with no detectable abnormalities are labeled with the clinically vague diagnosis of idiopathic infertility. On a different front, further modification of the cutoff points compatible with fertility has been advocated. Fourth, we now have a better understanding of the impact of processes such as the sperm capacitation and the acrosome reaction, sperm oxidative stress and apoptosis on sperm-egg interaction, and the fertilizing ability of sperm, both in vivo and in vitro. The assessment of these aspects of sperm function and physiology are beyond the current remit of the WHO manual. Last but not least, numerous studies in the literature have demonstrated that semen quality is declining and that the incidence of testicular cancers is increasing (8). These observations have been attributed to damage in sperm chromatin. During in vivo reproduction, the natural selection process ensures that only spermatozoon with normal genomic material fertilizes an oocyte. However, some assisted reproduction technologies (ART) bypass this natural selection process, leading to the possibility that an abnormal spermatozoa is selected to fertilize the oocyte.

This chapter reviews the clinical significance of sperm chromatin abnormalities, oxidative stress (OS), apoptosis, and microwave hazards for male gametes highlighting the laboratory methods available to assess these aspects of sperm structure and function.

HUMAN SPERM CHROMATIN

Human Sperm Chromatin Structure and Packaging

Chromatin packaging refers to the highly complex and specific structure into which ejaculated sperm DNA is folded in order to properly deliver the genetic information to the egg. Unlike the relatively loose structure of chromatin (DNA and nuclear proteins) in somatic cells, sperm chromatin is tightly compacted because of the unique associations between the DNA and sperm nuclear proteins (predominantly highly basic proteins known as protamines) (9,10). In the later stages of spermatogenesis, the spermatid nucleus is remodeled and condensed, a process that involves among other things the displacement of histones by transition proteins and then by protamines that have half the size of histones molecule (11). The DNA strands are tightly wrapped around the protamine molecules (about 50 kb of DNA per protamine), forming tight and highly organized loops (toroids) (10). Inter- and intramolecular disulfide cross-links between the cysteine-rich protamines are responsible for the compaction and stabilization of the sperm nucleus. It is thought that this nuclear compaction is important to protect the sperm genome from external stresses such as oxidation or temperature elevation that may be encountered in the sperm trajectory in the male and female genital tracts (12).

It is estimated that 85 percent of sperm chromatin is tightly packaged by protamines, but up to 15 percent of the DNA remains packaged by histones at specific DNA sequences associated with the nuclear periphery and with telomeres (13,14).

The histone-bound DNA sequences that are less tightly compacted and placed at the periphery suggest that these DNA sequences or genes may be involved in fertilization and early embryo development (13). An excess of nuclear histones (>15 percent) results in poorer chromatin compaction and a subsequent increased susceptibility to external stresses (e.g., oxidation or temperature elevation in the female reproductive tract) (12).

In comparison with other species (15), human sperm chromatin packaging is exceptionally variable, both within and between men. This variability has been mostly attributed to its basic protein component. Infertile men, as compared with fertile controls, have an increased sperm histone:protamine ratio (11,16,17). Moreover, in contrast to mammals whose spermatozoa contain only one type of protamine (P1), human spermatozoa contain a second type of protamine (P2), which is deficient in cysteine residues (18). Consequently, the disulfide cross-linking responsible for more stable packaging is diminished in human sperm as compared to species containing P1 alone (19). Aberrant P1/P2 ratios arise from an abnormal concentration of P1 and/or P2, either of which is associated with male infertility (20–28). Prior to this chromatin rearrangement, recombination is essential for spermatogenesis to occur; as seen in studies using animal knockout models, decreased recombination is associated with diminished spermatogenesis (29).

The main bulk of the sperm DNA is in the nucleus and only a small fraction is of mitochondrial origin within the sperm midpiece. The sperm mitochondrial DNA is a small, circular DNA that is not bound to proteins (30), which exhibits a high rate of mutation (31). Sperm motility is related to the mitochondrial volume within the sperm midpiece, and mutations or deletions in the mitochondrial DNA have been associated with reduced sperm motility (31). Although inheritance of mitochondrial DNA is primarily maternal, paternal transmission of mitochondrial DNA mutations has been reported (32). The examination of mitochondrial DNA may gain some importance in the evaluation of male infertility, particularly in relation to assisted reproductive technologies.

Types and Mechanisms of DNA Damage

Defects in the genomic material in mature sperm may take the form of packaging or nuclear maturity defects, DNA fragmentation (single-strand nicks or double-strand breaks), DNA integrity defects, or sperm chromosomal aneuploidies (33). These sperm chromatin defects have been associated with a diversity of disease conditions, environmental stress factors, and life-style issues. These include cancer, drug use, high fever, and infections, elevated testicular temperature (e.g., use of hot baths, saunas, down-filled blankets, laptop computers, and prolonged periods of driving), varicocele, air pollution, cigarette smoking, alcohol, and advanced age (34–37). These conditions exert their effect through recognized molecular mechanisms of DNA damage. Scientists agree on four distinct mechanisms by which DNA can be compromised or damaged, although there may be others: defective sperm chromatin condensation, apoptosis (38,39), oxidative stress (40,41), and genetic lesions (42–44). It is likely that multiple of these mechanisms are involved in causing DNA damage in any one disease (45).

The two main components of abnormal chromatin packaging are defective histone-protamine replacement (discussed above) and chromatin fragmentation. DNA fragmentation is particularly frequent in the ejaculates of subfertile men (46).

Physiological and environmental stress, as well as gene mutations and chromosomal abnormalities, can all disturb the highly refined biochemical events that occur during spermatogenesis. This disruption can ultimately lead to abnormal chromatin structure that is incompatible with fertility. Stress can also cause sperm chromatin fragmentation by inducing chromatin structural problems through apoptosis or necrosis (47). In addition, chromatin fragmentation can arise during spermiogenesis if the DNA nicking and ligating activities of the endogenous nuclease, DNA topoisomerase II (topo II), are abnormal. High levels of both topo II and DNA nicks are present in elongating spermatids (42,48). The presence of DNA nicks may reflect the need to relieve torsional strain resulting from negative supercoiling associated with the displacement of nucleosomal histones by protamines and modification of tertiary structure in elongating spermatids (42,49,50). Therefore, in elongating spermatids, the presence of nicks is likely a physiological necessity. These nicks are not deleterious when they are ligated by topo II prior to the completion of spermiogenesis and ejaculation (42). However, if topo II ligating activity is abnormal or blocked by exposure to topo II inhibitors (51), nicks may not be repaired properly, and they may remain in otherwise mature, morphologically normal, ejaculated spermatozoa. Oocytes and early embryos have been shown to repair sperm DNA damage (52). Consequently, the biological effect of abnormal sperm chromatin structure depends on the combined effects of sperm chromatin damage and the capacity of the oocyte to repair it.

Genetic lesions are another mechanism that create insults or gaps within the genome and may yield effects ranging from minimal to catastrophic (53). They can be divided into three classes, based on the type of impact they present (54). The first class consists of chromosomal aneuploidies and rearrangements, where batteries of genes on specific chromosomes have changes in expression dosages or changes in their normal genomic environments. The second class encompasses submicroscopic deletions (microdeletions), where deletions or rearrangements of multiple genes mapped in a molecular environment have changes in their expression patterns. The third class embodies single-gene defects where expression of a single gene (or key element) is changed or lost, causing male infertility. These lesions can affect all of the human chromosomes, including any of the 300 genes estimated to be involved in male fertility. They can occur within introns as well as exons, making their impact difficult to predict (53).

The Detection of Nuclear Chromatin Abnormalities

Detection of Chromosome Aneuploidy

During metaphase I or II of meiosis, nondisjunction can occur, resulting in sperm with an abnormal complement of chromosomes. Fluorescent in situ hybridization (FISH) in interphase sperm cells affords convenient evaluation of sperm chromosome ploidy (55) and has revealed that aneuploidy occurs in humans at a much higher rate than in other organisms (56–60). A typical probe is designed to recognize a relatively large section of a particular chromosome (usually 0.2–2 Mb) and then labeled with fluorochrome. After hybridization of the probe with a sample of the sperm, the labeled portion of the chromosome appears as a fluorescent domain within the sperm nucleus and can be identified using fluorescence microscopy. There are multiprobe assays for different chromosome combination to allow the distinction between isolated chromosome disomy and diploidy.

Table 19.1: Various Methods for Assessing Sperm Chromatin Abnormalities.

Assay	Parameter measured	Method of analysis
Acridine orange (68,69)	DNA denaturation (acid)	Fluorescent microscopy
		Flow cytometry
Toluidine blue stain (70)	DNA fragmentation	Optical microscopy
Acidic aniline blue (71)	Nuclear maturity (DNA protein composition)	Optical microscopy
Chromomycin A3 (72)	Nuclear maturity (DNA protein composition)	Fluorescent microscopy
Sperm chromatin dispersion (73)	DNA fragmentation	Fluorescent microscopy
DNA breakage detection–fluorescent in situ hybridization (74)	DNA fragmentation (ssDNA)	Fluorescent microscopy
In situ nick translation (75)	DNA fragmentation (ssDNA)	Fluorescent microscopy
		Flow cytometry
TUNEL (76)	DNA fragmentation	Optical microscopy
		Fluorescent microscopy
		Flow cytometry
Comet (neutral) (77)	DNA fragmentation (dsDNA)	Fluorescent microscopy
Comet (alkaline) (78)	DNA fragmentation (ssDNA/dsDNA)	Fluorescent microscopy
Sperm chromatin structure assay (79)	DNA denaturation (acid/heat)	Flow cytometry
OHdG measurement (39)	8-OHdG	High-performance liquid chromatography

8-OHdG, 8-hydroxy-2-deoxyguanosine; dsDNA, double-stranded DNA; ssDNA, single-stranded DNA.

Due to the limitation of the eye for detecting color differences, assays are limited to three or four probes at a time.

Men with severe oligozoospermia, asthenozoospermia, and/or teratozoospermia have been shown to have increased sperm aneuploidy rates, and this is the likely cause of their abnormal WHO sperm parameters (61–64). There is evidence that there is no selection against aneuploid sperm during fertilization or embryo development to the first cell division (65). However, it is still unknown to what extent increased aneuploidies in sperm contribute to adverse outcomes in assisted reproduction and natural conception (66). The risk includes the chance of spontaneous abortion or delivery of a child with a congenital abnormality. Thus, probes for chromosomes X, Y, 13, 18, and 21 allow us to detect sperm that may lead to various important aneuploidy syndromes: triple X, Klinefelter, Turner, XYY, Patau, Edwards, or Down's syndrome. A screening program in which men with severe teratozoospermia and severe oligozoospermia undergoing assisted reproduction, in combination with an investigation of the chromosomal status of embryos, will help clarify the likelihood of paternal transmission of aneuploidies and its effect on embryogenesis (67).

Although the test has high specificity, it is labor intensive requiring close attention to strict scoring criteria to ensure precision and minimize intertechnician variability. So far, the lack of automation has limited the number of studies that employed this technique in reproductive medicine.

Detection of Sperm Nuclear DNA Damage

Several assays have been developed to evaluate sperm chromatin integrity, and their capability to assess male fertility potential has been under active scrutiny (Table 19.1). In general,

all assays can be divided into three groups: 1) sperm chromatin structural probes, 2) tests for direct assessment of sperm DNA fragmentation, and 3) sperm nuclear matrix assays. Other methods less frequently used include high-performance liquid chromatography.

Chromatin Structural Probes Using Nuclear Dyes

Chromatin structural probes using nuclear dyes are both sensitive and simple to use and therefore attractive for clinical utilization. Their cytochemical bases, however, are rather complex because several factors may influence the staining of the chromatin: 1) secondary structure of DNA, 2) regularity and density of chromatin packaging, and 3) binding of DNA to chromatin proteins.

Detection of DNA Secondary Structure and Conformation Defects

Even a single DNA strand break causes conformational transition of the DNA loop domain from a supercoiled state to a relaxed state. Supercoiled DNA avidly takes up intercalating dyes [like acridine orange (AO)] because this reduces the free energy of torsion stress (orthochromasy: monomeric AO binds to DNA and fluoresces green). In contrast, the affinity for intercalation is low in relaxed DNA and is lost in fragmented or denatured DNA. In this case, an external mechanism of dye binding to DNA phosphate residues and dye polymerization is favored (metachromasy, aggregated AO binds to DNA, and fluoresces red) (80,81). Since the 1960s, it has been known that fragmented DNA is easily denatured (82,83). Tejada et al. (68) introduced the microscopic AO assay, a simplified fluorescent microscopic method using acid fixative that does not require flow cytometry equipment. The AO assay may be used in conjunction with flow cytometry. It has been demonstrated that staining with AO assay shows a significant difference between fertile and infertile males. The "cutoff" value for normal chromatin percentage that is compatible with natural fertility varies between 80 and 50 percent (green fluorescence) (84,85). It has been shown that sperm with excess single-stranded DNA (ssDNA) that is detected by a low-incidence green fluorescence (<50 percent) negatively affects the fertilization process in a standard IVF program. However, no correlation was found with pregnancy rate and live births achieved by ICSI, except in patients having 0 percent of spermatozoa with ssDNA, in whom the pregnancy rate was significantly high (86).

Toluidine blue is another basic nuclear dye used for metachromatic and orthochromatic staining of chromatin (70). It becomes heavily incorporated in the damaged dense chromatin. This stain is a sensitive structural probe for DNA structure as well as packaging. Sperm head with good chromatin integrity stain light blue. Abnormal nuclei (purple sperm heads) have been shown to be correlated with counts of red-orange sperm heads as, revealed by the AO method (87).

Chromatin Packaging Density

Chromatin proteins in sperm nuclei with impaired DNA packaging appear to be more accessible to binding with the acidic dye, as found by the aniline blue (AB) test (88). An increase in the ability to stain sperm by acid AB (blue color) indicates a looser chromatin packaging and increased accessibility of the basic groups of the nucleoprotein due to the presence of excess residual histones (89). This large, bulky dye is unable to bind to the densely packaged chromatin of normal sperm (with its full complement of protamines). Results of acid AB sperm assessment correlate well with the AO test (90) and have shown a clear association between abnormal sperm chromatin and male infertility (91). However, the correlation between the percentage of AB-stained spermatozoa and other sperm parameters remains controversial (92). Most important is the finding that chromatin condensation as visualized by aniline blue staining is a good predictor for IVF outcome, although it cannot determine the fertilization potential, cleavage, and pregnancy rate following ICSI (93).

Chromatin Proteins

Similar to the AO test, the Chromatin Structure Assay (SCSA^{TM}) (94) measures the susceptibility of sperm nuclear DNA to acid-induced conformational transition in situ by quantifying the metachromatic shift of AO fluorescence from green (native DNA) to red (denatured or relaxed DNA or RNA). It is an indirect indicator of DNA damage because it measures the amount of ssDNA after treatments that normally do not denature sperm DNA (heat or acid PH). SCSA uses flow cytometry to measure the relative amount of red versus green fluorescence on a per sperm basis, in large number of sperm (typically 5,000 to 10,000 per sample) in only a few minutes. Each sperm is classified as normal or abnormal based on the amount of ssDNA it contains, and the percentage of abnormal cells is calculated for each semen sample. A threshold was established that identifies samples compatible with pregnancy (<30 percent sperm cell damage). This cutoff point has been shown to have a predictive value for both in vivo and

in vitro fertilization (95–97). A recent review indicated that in a meta-analyses, SCSA infertility test was significantly predictive for reduced pregnancy success using in vivo, IUI, and routine IVF and to a lesser extent ICSI fertilization (98). It is claimed that because the SCSA is more constant over prolonged periods of time than routine WHO semen parameters, it may be used effectively in epidemiological studies of male infertility (99).

The prohibitive cost of running flow cytometry assay to many laboratories and the stringent quality control required meant that this test is available through central laboratories to which semen samples should be sent for testing. The SCSA is less specific relative to the DNA damage tests described below in that it may detect alterations in protamine content and disulfide cross-linkage within the protamine, as well as sperm DNA damage. Indeed, SCSA data include 1) the percentage of sperm with undetectable, medium, and high levels of DNA fragmentation, 2) the percentage of sperm with a high level of DNA stainability (immature chromatin with less protamines); and 3) relative amounts of seminal debris, bacteria, and broken cells since native semen is used for the analysis (100). This lower specificity can be an advantage when predicting infertility since sperm that are defective in one or more ways will be detected (100).

Chromomycin-A$_3$ (CMA$_3$) is another slide-staining technique, which has been used as a measure of sperm chromatin condensation anomalies. CMA$_3$ is a fluorochrome specific for GC-rich sequences and is believed to compete with protamines for association with DNA. The extent of staining is, therefore, related to the degree of protamination of mature spermatozoa (72,101). On balance, the most widely used techniques for sperm chromatin structure assessment are the SCSA, AO, and TB tests. The later two are simple to perform but are labor intensive and subject to inter- and intraobserver variability compared to the former.

Tests for Direct Assessment of Sperm DNA Fragmentation

The most widely used of these tests are in situ nick translation assays, terminal deoxynucleotidyl transferase-mediated dUTP nick end-labeling assay (TUNEL), and single-cell gel electrophoresis assay (COMET). Their basic principles are summarized in Table 19.1. Nick translation (75) is a relatively simple assay for fluorescence microscopy that quantifies the incorporation of biotinylated dUTP at SSDNA breaks in a reaction catalyzed by the template-dependent enzyme, DNA polymerase I. The TUNEL assay quantifies the same incorporation at breaks in double-stranded DNA using a reaction catalyzed by terminal deoxynucleotidyl transferase. TUNEL can be assessed using bright-field, fluorescence microscopy, or flow cytometry (Figure 19.1). Several reports have demonstrated that an increased fraction of human spermatozoa showing DNA strand breaks has a negative impact on the success rate of assisted fertilization techniques (102,103). These assays are specific in that they detect DNA strand breaks, but the origin of the breaks is not always clear. In somatic cells, TUNEL has been reported to be more selective in detecting DNA degradation typical of apoptosis, whereas nick translation is thought to be indicative of necrosis (104).

The COMET assay quantifies ssDNA and/or double-stranded DNA breaks (dependant on the pH conditions, see

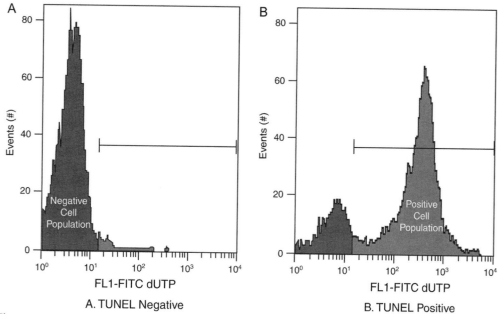

Figure 19.1. TUNEL assay fluorescent activated cell sorting (FACS) histograms with markers (|————|) for detection of fluorescence set at 650 nm. (A) A semen sample with low percentage of sperm DNA fragmentation; (B) a semen sample with high percentage of sperm DNA fragmentation.

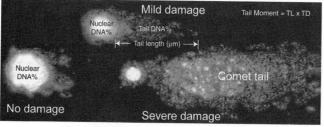

Figure 19.2. COMET assay uses the electro gel electrophoresis principle to assess the DNA damage. After DNA extraction and gel electrophoresis, damaged DNA looks like a "comet." The level of DNA fragmentation is measured using special software after transferring a live video image of the microscopic field into the computer. One of the indices used is "tail moment," which is a relation between the size and density (DNA percent) of the comet head and tail [= TL (tail length) × TD (tail density)]. The tail moment lies in one of three levels: mild, moderate, and severe, and their percentage in the sample are given.

Table 19.1), using single-cell electrophoresis of spermatozoa stained with a fluorescent DNA-binding dye (Figure 19.2). It is, therefore, suggested as a very sensitive assay for DNA damage evaluation. The COMET assay has been shown to correlate significantly with TUNEL and SCSA assays (105). It is simple to perform, has a low intraassay coefficient of variation, and a low performance cost (106). Because it is based on fluorescent microscopy, the assay requires an experienced observer to analyze the slides and interpret the results. Similar to SCSA test, the COMET assay has been successfully used in the evaluation of DNA damage after cryopreservation (107). It may also predict embryo development after IVF and ICSI, especially in couples with unexplained infertility (108,109).

Although the assay seems simple in principle, applying it to spermatozoa is not straightforward mainly because it is first necessary to open up the highly compact sperm nucleus so that the DNA is releasable during electrophoresis (100). This requires harsh chemical treatment with detergents, enzymes (RNase and/or proteinase K), and/or disulfide-reducing agent that may induce DNA breaks. Furthermore, the stainability of sperm DNA is dynamic, increasing as the sperm DNA opens up and its associated proteins (protamine) are degraded and removed. Therefore, direct comparisons between the amounts of DNA remaining in the sperm (comet) head with that moving into the comet tails are difficult to make. Additionally, many protocol variations have been reported, with differences not only in pH but also in composition of the cell lysis solution, the timing and conditions of the electrophoresis, and the introduction of new chromatin dyes. Once comets are generated, they have been measured in different ways and with different software programs. Finally, the outcome(s) has been reported differently: some labs calculate the percentage of sperm-forming comets, and others report average measures of the extent of DNA migration for a given sperm population (8,46,110). Thus, the method is still evolving, and standardization is lacking causing difficulty in comparing results across laboratories.

Sperm Nuclear Matrix Assays

Two similar assays have been described that can be allocated to this group. The sperm nuclear matrix stability assay and the sperm chromatin dispersion test are based on the ability of intact DNA deprived of chromatin proteins to loop around the sperm nucleus carcass (73,111,112). Published data show that germline mutations in the nuclear matrix protein may lead to deficient DNA repair and chromatin organization (113), so matrix pathologies can impair fertility and should be considered in future.

OXIDATIVE STRESS

Reactive oxygen species (ROS) in low, controlled levels in the extracellular space play an important physiological role, modulating gene and protein activities vital for sperm proliferation, differentiation, and function. OS is defined as a cellular condition associated with an imbalance between the production of free radicals, mainly ROS, and their scavenging capacity by antioxidants. When the production of ROS exceeds the available antioxidant defense, significant oxidative damage occurs to many cellular organelles by damaging lipids, proteins, DNA, and carbohydrates, thus ultimately leading to cell death.

It is reported that up to 40 percent of infertile men have high seminal ROS levels (114,115). Moreover, high ROS production has been found to be inversely correlated with the outcome of IVF (116). Infertile males that produce high levels of ROS have a fivefold less chance of initiating a pregnancy than infertile males that produce low levels of ROS (117). High levels of seminal ROS have also been correlated with poor sperm morphology and high sperm deformity index (41).

ROS represent a broad category of molecules that includes a collection of radical and nonradical oxygen derivatives (Table 19.2) (118). In addition, there are other classes of free radicals that are nitrogen derived called reactive nitrogen species and lipid derived called reactive lipid species (Table 19.2) (119,120).

Table 19.2: Types of Reactive Oxygen Species That Exist as Radicals and Free Radicals in Living Organisms

Radicals		Nonradicals	
Hydroxyl	OH′	Peroxynitrite	ONOO⁻
Superoxide	O₂′	Hypochloric acid	HOCl
Nitric oxide	NO′	Hydrogen peroxide	H₂O₂
Thyl	RS′	Singlet oxygen	⁻¹O₂
Peroxyl	RO₂′	Ozone	O₃
Lipid peroxyl	LOO′	Lipid peroxide	LOOH

Origin of ROS in Male Reproductive System

Sperm-Produced ROS

Following spermiation, spermatozoa extrude cytoplasm. Since cytoplasm is the major source of antioxidants, lack of cytoplasm causes a deficiency in antioxidant defense (Figure 19.3).

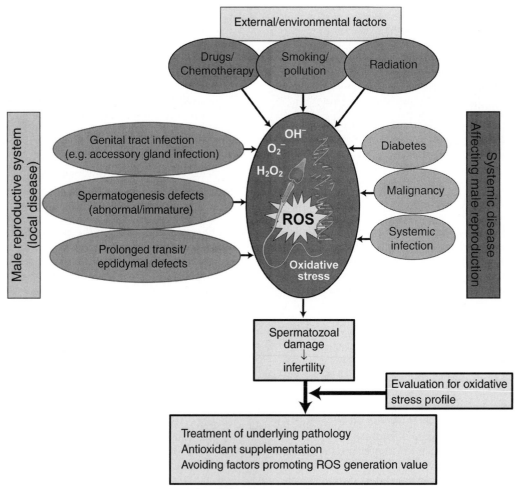

Figure 19.3. Etiology and management of oxidative stress. Many factors, including primary pathological condition of male reproductive system, systemic disorders, and environmental factors, increase oxidative stress status, which causes spermatozoa dysfunction leading to infertility.

Ironically, when this process is hindered, residual cytoplasm forms a cytoplasmic droplet in the sperm midregion, exhibiting high rates of ROS generation (121–123), which may be related to the enhanced presence of glucose-6-phosphate dehydrogenase. This enzyme fuels the generation of NADPH that, in turn, stimulates the production of ROS (122,124). Independent reports have also demonstrated that biochemical markers of the cytoplasmic space, such as creatine kinase, are positively correlated with the induction of peroxidative damage (121,125). Spermatozoa with cytoplasmic droplet, usually referred to as immature spermatozoa, appear more frequently in human semen compared with other animals. This has been attributed to inefficient human spermiogenesis that involves fewer steps, leading to less rigorous quality control (126). The increased presence of residual cytoplasm in infertile males suggests the control of spermiogenesis is even less efficient than that observed under normal conditions. This results in the release of significantly higher numbers of immature spermatozoa with cytoplasmic retention into the seminiferous tubules.

In addition to this major source of ROS production, there are three other possible sources of excess ROS generation from within the human sperm itself (53). The first is through leakage of electrons from the mitochondrial transport chain (127). This was proposed because of tests performed on rat spermatozoa, indicating increased translocation of mitochondrial free radicals into the sperm genome. However, this was not demonstrated in human spermatozoa (36). The second proposed source is through NADPH-oxidase in sperm. This theoretical oxidase would serve to transfer electrons from NAD(P)H to ground-state oxygen to create the superoxide anion. It is known that NAD(P)H in leukocytes helps to contribute to ROS production in rat spermatozoa, but it has yet to be demonstrated in humans (127,128). The third proposed intracellular source of ROS production is through the generation of nitric oxide (NO) in the postacrosmal and equatorial regions of the sperm (129–131).

External Sources

1) Leukocytes, particularly neutrophils and macrophages, have been associated with excessive ROS production, and they ultimately cause sperm dysfunction (132–136). ROS produced by leukocytes forms the first line of defense in any infectious process. DNA and structural damage can be found in spermatozoa from leukocytospermic patients (41,137,138). Leukocytes act either directly by synthesizing ROS or indirectly by inducing other neighboring white cells via soluble factors as cytokines (139). The scavenging effect of antioxidants is greatly diminished under such infectious conditions (140).
2) Female genital tract tissues or fluids may be the source of ROS including NO (141).
3) Environmental and lifestyle factors: this source of OS lies outside of the host's body and includes xenobiotic agents such as organophosphorous pesticides that disrupt the endocrine system (Figure 19.3). These agents possess estrogenic properties, capable of inducing ROS production by male germ cells (128,142). Cigarette smoking is also known to increase ROS levels through increased leukocyte generation and increased seminal leukocytes (143). Infertile smokers are known to harbor increased levels of seminal oxidative stress compared to infertile nonsmokers (144).

Finally, scrotal heat stress was demonstrated in stallions and mouse model to damage sperm chromatin structure, possibly by oxidative stressors (145,146). Raised testicular heat may explain raised seminal ROS in infertile patients with varicocele (147). Increase in scrotal temperature in laptop computer users has been reported (148).

ROS and Sperm Physiological Functions

It is now recognized that low, controlled levels of extracellular ROS produced by spermatozoa are involved in sperm capacitation and acrosome reaction (149,150). The mechanism by which ROS regulates these processes is unclear but may involve tyrosine phosphorylation of sperm proteins (124). Low concentrations of NO', a free radical with a relatively long half-life (7 s), promotes capacitation (151) and zona pellucida binding (152) by regulating cyclic adenosine monophosphate concentration and adenyl cyclase activity.

Pathological Effects of ROS on Sperm Function

Due to the unique structural composition, high ROS levels in seminal plasma have been associated with inhibition of sperm function and viability due to the peroxidation of membrane polyunsaturated fatty acids (153). This leads to loss of sperm membrane fluidity required for sperm adhesion and oocyte fusion. High levels of ROS including NO' have detrimental effect on sperm kinetics through effecting a reduction in adenosine triphosphate (154).

DNA bases pyridines and purines and deoxyribose sugar are most susceptible to OS. Oxidation of the sugar by the hydroxyl radical is the main cause for DNA strand breaks. Oxidative damage can cause base degradation, DNA fragmentation, and cross-linking to protein (155). In addition, incorporation of oxidized deoxyribonucleoside triphosphate causes gene mutation or altered gene expression (156). The rate of DNA fragmentation is increased in the ejaculate of infertile men (157–161) as indicated by the high level of 8-OHdG, which is a product of DNA oxidation (Table 19.1). Sperm DNA is normally protected from oxidative insult by two factors: the antioxidants present in seminal plasma and the characteristic tight packaging of the DNA. ROS-induced oxidative damage also plays an important role in initiating programmed cell death, apoptosis.

Assessment of OS

To accurately quantify OS, levels of ROS and antioxidants should be measured in fresh samples. Direct methods such as pulse radiolysis and electron-spin resonance spectroscopy have been useful for other systems of the body. However, the relatively low volume of the seminal plasma, short life span of ROS, and need to evaluate in fresh samples have led to nonusage of direct methods for the male reproductive system (162).

One of the most widespread methods of measuring ROS is the chemiluminescence assay, which uses sensitive probes such as luminol and lucigenin for quantification of redox activities of the spermatozoa (163). Although the sensitivity of these probes is high, they are susceptible to interference. Leukocyte contamination is a major confounder. Also, the time of analysis after collection (less than one hour) and the high sperm count requirement ($>1 \times 10^6$/ml) are some of the drawbacks to this technique. Moreover, the source of ROS in semen is not identified (162).

Another method of measuring intracellular ROS inside the cell is by flow cytometery. Different probes such as 2′, 7′-dichlorofluorescin-diacetate hydroethidine are used (164). Sperm cells are exposed to the probes that react with ROS to emit a red fluorescence (164). The assay is highly sensitive and requires a relatively low number of cells but is more expensive and requires expertise to handle sophisticated equipment (165). The colorimetric technique is also widely used for indirectly quantifying ROS. It is based on the principle of spectrophotometry and measures lipid peroxide end-products such as malondialdehyde, lipid hydroperoxides, and isoprostanes among others.

Antioxidant Measuremet

The presence of low antioxidant in the seminal plasma is another important reason for increased OS, leading to male infertility. Hence, it is important to measure the total antioxidant capacity (TAC) of the semen. Different methods such as oxygen radical absorption capacity (166), ferric reducing ability of plasma (167), and phycoerythrin fluorescence–based assay are available for measuring TAC. However, the most widely used method for measuring TAC in semen is enhanced chemiluminescence. This method requires expensive instrumentation and is cumbersome and time consuming. Another emerging method for measurement of TAC is the colorimetric assay. First described by Miller et al. in 1993, this method gained its popularity as simple, rapid, and inexpensive alternative to enhanced chemiluminescence method (168).

To accommodate for the variations in ROS and TAC values, the concept of combined ROS-TAC score was proposed (169). ROS-TAC score was computed using principal component analysis. ROS-TAC scores were calculated from proven fertile men with low levels of ROS. The composite ROS-TAC scores from these men were representative of the fertile group and any score less than thirty was considered infertile.

APOPTOSIS

Apoptosis is a mode of programmed cellular death based on a genetic mechanism that induces a series of cellular, morphological, and biochemical alterations, leading the cell to suicide without eliciting an inflammatory response, pain, or scaring distinguishing apoptosis from necrosis (170). Apoptosis is required for normal spermatogenesis in mammals and is believed to ensure cellular homeostasis and maintain the delicate balance between germ cells and Sertoli cells. Its second role is for the depletion of abnormal spermatozoa (43,171).

Features and Mechanisms of Apoptosis

Morphologically, apoptosis is characterized by chromatin aggregation, cytoplasmic condensation, and indentation of nuclear and cytoplasmic membranes in apoptotic cells. Finally, the nucleus undergoes fragmentation and the whole cell blebs and fragments into apoptotic bodies (172).

In general, somatic cell apoptosis can be induced through extrinsic mechanisms acting at the plasma membrane, mitochondrial, or nuclear level (Figure 19.4) (173). The plasma membrane–dependent mechanism is typified by the interaction of the Fas receptor (CD95) and a Fas ligand that can proceed

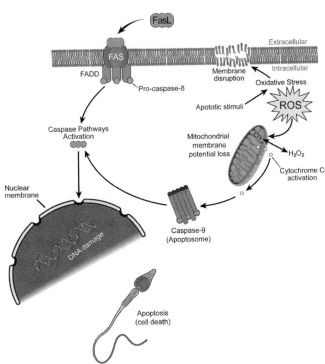

Figure 19.4. ROS-induced apoptosis. ROS (apoptotic stimulus) trigger mitochondria to release cytochrome *c*, initiating a caspase cascade. Interaction between Fas and Fas ligand is also necessary in apoptotic mechanism. DNA fragmentation occurs as a result of activation of effector caspases (caspases 3, 6, and 9), eventually causing apoptosis.

through two pathways (174). The type I pathway is mitochondria independent, involving an adaptor protein to recruit caspase-8 to the cytoplasmic domain of the Fas receptor to form a death-induced signaling complex and activation of caspase-8. The type II pathway is mitochondria dependent and involves the release of cytochrome c from the mitochondria, inducing the activation of caspase-9 -3, -6, and/or -7 (Figure 19.4) (175). At the cytoplasmic level, several stimuli, including the activation of the mitochondrial membrane Bax (a member of the pro-apoptotic Bcl-2 family of proteins) lead to the release of cytochrome *c* (173). In the cytosol, cytochrome *c* stimulates a cascade of events leading to activation of caspase-3. The outer mitochondrial membrane is permeabilized releasing apoptosis-inducing factor (AIF) and/or cytochrome *c*. AIF directly translocates to the nucleus where it provokes large-scale DNA fragmentation and initial chromatin condensation. At the nuclear level, the genome contains genes that are transcribed as a response to apoptotic stimuli. For example, p53 functions normally as a regulator of the cell cycle and a tumor suppressor in vivo. Following DNA damage, p53 induces apoptosis by upregulation of the expression of the pro-apoptotic Bax gene and simultaneous downregulation of Bcl-2 expression, a sensitive regulator-inhibitor of apoptosis (176). During apoptosis, phosphatidylserine, normally present on the cytoplasmic face of the plasma membrane, is allowed to migrate to the outer leaflet, thus marking the cells for destruction by phagocytes (177,178).

Apoptosis may be initiated by ROS-induced oxidative damage of mitochondria membrane resulting in the release of cytochrome c that activates the caspases family. Too much OS can terminate apoptosis by inactivating the caspase enzyme cascade (181,182). Antioxidants can either suppress or facilitate

Table 19.3: Reported Studies That Correlated the Presence of Apoptotic Markers in Semen and the WHO Semen Parameters Including the Sperm Deformity Index (SDI)

WHO sperm parameter	Relationship with sperm apoptotic markers
Sperm viability and motility	Negative correlation (39,164,191,198–200)
Sperm normal morphology	Negative correlation (201,202)
	No correlation (203)
SDI	Positive correlation (204)

apoptosis (182). Infertile men have been shown to have high levels of cytochrome c in the seminal plasma indirectly reflecting significant mitochondrial damage caused by high levels of ROS. Levels of ROS in infertile men are correlated positively with apoptosis, which in turn is negatively correlated with conventional semen parameters (118,162).

Apoptosis and Male Infertility

Mature sperm cells have been reported to express distinct markers of terminal apoptosis-related cell damage (38,183–186), although they lack transcriptional activity and have a very small amount of cytoplasm (187,188). Externalization of PS activated caspase-3, loss of the integrity of the mitochondrial membrane potential (MMP), and DNA fragmentation and membrane-bound death receptor Fas are markers of terminal apoptosis expressed by varying proportions of ejaculated sperm (189).

There is an established consensus on the implication of apoptosis in male infertility (184,190–192)and poor WHO semen parameters (Table 19.3); however, the exact mechanisms of its involvement remains to be elucidated (143). Relatively high rates of apoptosis have been reported in testicular biopsies from infertile men with different degrees of testicular insufficiency (194). The proportions of apoptotic sperm is reported to be higher in ejaculated semen samples from infertile men compared to healthy men (191). Moreover, sperm caspases become more activated in patients with infertility than in healthy donors during cryopreservation (189,195). Although apoptosis is considered a mechanism to ensure selection of sperm cells with undamaged DNA, sperm with DNA damage that are not eliminated by apoptosis may fertilize an ovum (108,186). Poor chromatin packaging and/or damaged DNA have been implicated in the failure of sperm decondensation after intracytoplasmic sperm injection, resulting in fertilization failure (196,197).

To date, it is not clear whether the apoptotic markers detected in spermatozoa are residues of an abortive apoptotic process started before ejaculation (38,192,205–207) or whether they result from apoptosis initiated in the postejaculation period (189). During faulty sperm development, the elimination of aberrant germ cells by apoptosis may be deranged leading to the release of surviving immature cells with activated caspase-3 in the cytoplasmic droplet (204,208). It is suggested that the presence of antiapoptotic Bcl-$_{XL}$ protein provides protection against activated caspase-3 (208). It is also proposed that apoptosis may be reflective of mechanisms related to endocrinopathies, varicoceles, and inflammation/infection and involves OS as initiator of apoptosis (118,190). Also, because spermatozoa are terminally differentiated cells, like neutrophils, they may exhibit a defined ex vivo lifetime that could be inherent to mature spermatozoa or could be related to anoikis, which is programmed cell death when cells are not anchored to an extracellular matrix (189,209).

Magnetic-activated cell sorting (MACS) using annexin V–conjugated superparamagnetic microbeads can effectively separate nonapoptotic spermatozoa from those with deteriorated plasma membranes based on the externalization of PS. MACS separation of sperm yields two fractions: annexin V negative (intact membranes and nonapoptotic) and annexin V positive (externalized PS and apoptotic) (210,211). A sperm preparation protocol that combines MACS with double-density centrifugation has been described to provide spermatozoa of higher quality in terms of motility, viability, and apoptosis indices compared with other conventional sperm preparation methods (203). It has been suggested that the protocol can also be used to improve cryosurvival rates following freezing and thawing and to enhance ART outcome (212,213).

Assessment of Apoptosis in Ejaculated Sperm

Sperm expression of apoptotic markers both in semen and sperm preparation has been examined applying a diversity of techniques including:

- PS externalization using a monoclonal mouse anti-human PS antibody (39,41,203,204,214).
- Caspase-3 activation using fluorescein-labeled inhibitor of caspase, which is cell permeable and noncytotoxic and which binds covalently to active caspase-3 (41,203,204,215–219).
- MMP integrity using a lipophilic cationic dye (5,50,6,60-tetrachloro-1,10,3,30-tetraethylbenzimi-dazolyl carbocyanine chloride) to detect intact MMP in spermatozoa (41, 203,204,216).
- Chromatin fragmentation (201,202,207,220).
- Membrane-bound death receptor Fas and p53 (205,207).

MICROWAVE SPERM DAMAGE

Microwaves can affect reproductive function via an electromagnetic wave (EMW)–specific effect, thermal molecular effect, or combination of the two (221). Increase in tissue or body temperature on exposure to EMW is known to cause reversible disruption of spermatogenesis (222,223). Various investigators have addressed the concern that use of devices emitting microwaves might have adverse impacts on sperm function.

Animal Studies

It was demonstrated that application of radiofrequency waves of 869–894 MHz (five days a week for four weeks) in a population of twenty rats resulted in a decrease in seminiferous tubular diameter and epithelial thickness (224). Similarly, a time-dependent rise in the germ cell apoptosis of the rat testis after exposure to high power microwave (HPM) radiation of 10 MW/cm^2 was reported (225). The same study found that only five minutes of

HPM exposure was sufficient to cause testicular germ-cell damage. Saunders et al. studied the thermal effects of microwave radiation on mice spermatogenic epithelium. In their study involving 2.45 GHz microwaves exposure, thirty minutes daily for six days to male mice testis, they found 39°C as a threshold effect for the depletion of the spermatocytes (226). In another experiment, Lebovitz et al. found a modest decline in daily sperm production after exposure of Sprague-Dawley rats to 1.3 GHz of pulse-modulated microwave radiation for ninety minutes (227). In this study, the mean intratesticular temperature of 40°C as a result of exposure to microwave radiation lead to primary spermatocytes damage.

Human Studies

It was reported that in 371 men undergoing infertility evaluations, the duration of possession, and the daily transmission time of cell phones correlated negatively with the proportion of rapidly progressive motile sperms (228). This suggested that prolonged exposure to microwaves emitting devices might have negative effects on the sperm motility. In another prospective study involving thirteen men with normal semen analysis, it was found that using GSM phones for six hours a day for five days decreased the rapid progressive motility of spermatozoa (229). Similarly, a decrease in sperm motility in semen samples of twenty-seven men exposed to 900 MHz cell phone for five minutes was reported (230). A recent study from Cleveland Clinic involving 361 men attending an infertility clinic reported that the use of cell phones adversely affect the quality of semen by decreasing the sperm counts, motility, viability, and morphology in a use-dependent manner (231).

In spite of the these startling revelations, most of these studies had some limitations, such as the inability to analyze covariates such as life style issues, occupational history, and radiofrequency radiation (RFR) exposure from other sources like radio towers, PDA's Bluetooth devices, and computers. However, despite the limitations of previous studies, they have revealed important findings that have started an intense debate on this topic, thus necessitating the need for further studies to determine whether spermatogenesis, sperm function, sperm quality, and sperm fertilizing potential are affected by the exposure to devices emitting radiofrequency microwaves.

Association between DNA Damage, Apoptosis, OS, and Microwave Sperm Damage

Although microwaves have been suggested to cause sperm damage, the mode of action is still unclear. DNA damage and OS are among the most commonly studied mechanisms. Spermatozoa are extremely vulnerable to DNA damage as they lose their cytoplasm containing antioxidant enzymes and their capacity for DNA repair (232). Lai and Singh first reported DNA strand breaks from low-intensity microwave radiofrequency radiations in rat brain cells. In their study, two hours exposure to 2,450 MHz continuous and pulsed RFR produced a dose-dependent increase in ssDNA and double-strand DNA breaks (233). More recently, Aitken et al. found significant damage to mitochondrial and nuclear genome in epididymal spermatozoa of rats with radio frequency EMW exposure of 900 MHz twelve hours per day for seven days (234). Although there is no evidence of the adverse affects of RFR on human sperm DNA, investigators have found evidence of EMW-induced DNA

damage in other human tissues. In vitro exposure of human cultured diploid fibroblasts to 1,800 MHz RFR for sixteen hours induced ssDNA and double-stranded DNA breaks (235).

However, whether RFR is capable of inducing oxidative stress, which would lead to sperm cell damage, is still debatable. Musaev et al. found that high-intensity microwave exposure stimulated basal lipid peroxidation levels in rat hypothalamus (236). However, Hook et al. did not find any alteration in the level of intracellular oxidants and antioxidant defenses in mouse macrophage cells on exposure to RFR fields (237). Conflicting studies have also been published regarding the effect of EMW exposure on the secretion of an antioxidant melatonin (18–20,238–240).

Studies analyzing the effects of radiofrequency radiation on apoptosis failed to find any significant effect. An exposure of 1,800 MHz signal for twelve hours failed to induce apoptosis in human Mono Mac 6 cells (241). Similarly, no evidence of apoptosis has been detected after exposing human leukemia cells in vitro to RFR waves twenty-five times higher than the reference levels set by the International Commission on Non-Ionizing Radiation Protection) (242). The effects of RFR on human sperm cell apoptosis have not been evaluated yet.

Rizk and Abdalla (2008) highlighted that given the vulnerability of spermatozoa to genotoxic and oxidative damage, and the clinical significance of this damage in terms of fertility, pregnancy, and childhood health, studies are urgently needed on the impact of RF microwaves on OS and DNA damage in the male germ line (243).

CONCLUSIONS

OS, sperm DNA damage, and apoptosis are clearly implicated in the pathogenesis of male infertility. These interlinked molecular events are associated with various clinical and laboratory manifestations that may be present in infertile males. It has been suggested that EMW and RFR may induce OS and DNA damage in the male germ line. In view of this evolving understanding of sperm molecular structure and function, additional assessment of sperm damage beyond the WHO criteria may serve to provide a definitive diagnosis of the underlying causes of idiopathic male fertility. This may also identify the group of men and their offspring that through techniques such as intracytoplasmic sperm injection may perpetually propagate their genetic complement linked to male infertility. Strategies required to handle this risk should encompass the standardization of the laboratory techniques required to test for sperm damage. It is conceivable that the WHO next task is to provide the required standards to achieve this goal. In doing so, the WHO would provide standardized two-level approach for male-fertility assessment. Level one should be adequately served by the criteria and standards included in its current manual, with the objective of offering initial screening for men presenting within an infertile relationship. Level two testing has the objective of offering definitive diagnosis for men with abnormal findings in level one assessment and for those who are offered intracytoplasmic sperm injection.

KEY POINTS

- OS, sperm DNA damage, and apoptosis are clearly implicated in the pathogenesis of male infertility.

- Although standardized assays for diagnosing these conditions need to be improved, assessment is advised in selected cases where the exact diagnosis is suspected.
- Identifying the exact nature of the defect will help in selecting proper management, which in turn will improve natural and assisted reproduction success rates and help to ensure healthy offspring.
- We have to continually be aware of the possible deleterious impact of new technological advances such as those using EMW and RFR on human fertility.

REFERENCES

1. Morice P, Josset P, Chapron C, Dubuisson JB. History of infertility. *Hum Reprod Update* 1995;1:497–504.
2. Kruger TF, Acosta AA, Simmons KF, Swanson RJ, Matta JF, Oehninger S. Predictive value of abnormal sperm morphology in in vitro fertilization. *Fertil Steril* 1988;49:112–17.
3. Aziz N, Buchan I, Taylor C, Kingsland CR, Lewis-Jones I. The sperm deformity index: a reliable predictor of the outcome of oocyte fertilization in vitro. *Fertil Steril* 1996;66:1000–8.
4. Keel B, Webster B. The standard semen analysis. In: Webster B (ed.), CRC Handbook of the Laboratory Diagnosis and Treatment of Infertility. Boca Raton, FL: CRC Press, 1990:27–69.
5. Nallella KP, Sharma RK, Aziz N, Agarwal A. Significance of sperm characteristics in the evaluation of male infertility. *Fertil Steril* 2006;85(3):629–34.
6. Zini A, Kamal K, Phang D, et al. Biologic variability of sperm DNA denaturation in infertile men. *Urology* 2001;58:258–61.
7. Evenson D, Larson K, Jost L. Sperm chromatin structure assay: its clinical use for detecting sperm DNA fragmentation in male infertility and comparisons with other techniques. *J Androl* 2002;23:25–43.
8. Aitken RJ, Koopman P, Lewis SE. Seeds of concern. *Nature* 2004;432:48–52.
9. Ward WS, Coffey DS. DNA packaging and organization in mammalian spermatozoa: comparison with somatic cells. *Biol Reprod* 1991;44:569–74.
10. Brewer LR, Corzett M, Balhorn R. Protamine induced condensation and decondensation of the same DNA molecule. *Science* 1999;286:120–3.
11. Steger K, Pauls K, Klonisch T, et al. Expression of protamine-1 and -2 mRNA during human spermiogenesis. *Mol Hum Reprod* 2000;6:219–25.
12. Kosower NS, Katayose H, Yanagimachi R. Thiol-disulfide status and acridine orange fluorescence of mammalian sperm nuclei. *J Androl* 1992;13:342–8.
13. Gatewood JM, Cook GR, Balhorn R et al. Sequence-specific packaging of DNA in human sperm chromatin. *Science* 1987;236:962–4.
14. Gineitis AA, Zalenskaya IA, Yau PM et al. Human sperm telomere-binding complex involves histone H2B and secures telomere membrane attachment. *J Cell Biol* 2000;151:1591–8.
15. Lewis JD, Song Y, de Jong ME, Bagha SM, Ausio J. A walk through vertebrate and invertebrate protamines. *Chromosoma* 1999;111:473–82.
16. Bench GS, Friz AM, Corzett MH, Morse DH, Balhorn R. DNA and total protamine masses in individual sperm from fertile mammalian subjects. *Cytometry* 1996;23:263–71.
17. Oliva R. Protamines and male infertility. *Hum Reprod Update* 2006;12:417–35.
18. Corzett M, Mazrimas J, Balhorn R. Protamine 1: protamine 2 stoichiometry in the sperm of eutherian mammals. *Mol Reprod Dev* 2002;61:519–27.
19. Jager S. Sperm nuclear stability and male infertility. *Arch Androl* 1990;25:253–9.
20. Balhorn R, Reed S, Tanphaichitr N. Aberrant protamine 1/protamine 2 ratio in sperm of infertile human males. *Experientia* 1988;44:52–5.
21. de Yebra L, Ballesca JL, Vanrell JA, Bassas L, Oliva R. Complete selective absence of protamine P2 in humans. *J Biol Chem* 1993;268:10553–7.
22. Bench G, Corzett MH, De Yebra L, Oliva R, Balhorn R. Protein and DNA contents in sperm from an infertile human male possessing protamine defects that vary over time. *Mol Reprod Dev* 1998;50:345–53.
23. de Yebra L, Ballesca JL, Vanrell JA, Corzett M, Balhorn R, Oliva R. Detection of P2 precursors in the sperm cells of infertile patients who have reduced protamine P2 levels. *Fertil Steril* 1998;69:755–9.
24. Carrell DT, Liu L. Altered protamine 2 expression is uncommon in donors of known fertility, but common among men with poor fertilizing capacity, and may reflect other abnormalities of spermiogenesis. *J Androl* 2001;22:604–10.
25. Carrell DT, Emery BR, Hammoud S. Altered protamine expression and diminished spermatogenesis: what is the link? *Hum Reprod Update* 2007; advance online access:1–15.
26. Mengual L, Ballesca JL, Ascaso C, Oliva R. Marked differences in protamine content and P1/P2 ratios in sperm cells from percoll fractions between patients and controls. *J Androl* 2003;24:438–47.
27. Nasr-Esfahani MH, Salehi M, Razavi S et al. Effect of protamine-2 deficiency on ICSI outcome. *Reprod Biomed Online* 2004;9:652–8.
28. Aoki VW, Liu L, Carrell DT. Identification and evaluation of a novel sperm protamine abnormality in a population of infertile males. *Hum Reprod* 2005;20:1298–306.
29. Carrell DT, De Jonge C, Lamb DJ. The genetics of male infertility: a field of study whose time is now. *Arch Androl* 2006;52:269–74.
30. Anderson S, Bankier AT, Barrell BG, et al. Sequence and organization of the human mitochondrial genome. *Nature* 1981;290:457–65.
31. Kao SH, Chao HT, Wei YH. Multiple deletions of mitochondrial DNA are associated with the decline of motility and fertility of human spermatozoa. *Mol Hum Reprod* 1998;4:657–66.
32. Schwartz M, Vissing J. Paternal inheritance of mitochondrial DNA. *N Engl J Med* 2002;347:576–80.
33. Perreault SD, Aitken RJ, Baker HW et al. Integrating new tests of sperm genetic integrity into semen analysis: breakout group discussion. *Adv Exp Med Biol* 2003;518:253–68.
34. Jung A, Schill WB, Schuppe HC. Genital heat stress in men of barren couples: a prospective evaluation by means of a questionnaire. *Andrologia* 2002;34:349–55.
35. Zini A, Libman J. Sperm DNA damage: clinical significance in the era of assisted reproduction. *Can Med Assoc J* 2006;175:495–500.
36. Erenpreiss J, Spano M, Erenpreisa J, Bungum M, Giwercman A. Sperm chromatin structure and male fertility: biological and clinical aspects. *Asian J Androl* 2006;8:11–29.
37. Agarwal A, Allamaneni SS. Sperm DNA damage assessment: a test whose time has come. *Fertil Steril* 2005;84:850–3.
38. Sakkas D, Mariethoz E, Manicardi G, Bizzaro D, Bianchi PG, Bianchi U. Origin of DNA damage in ejaculated human spermatozoa. *Rev Reprod* 1999;4:31–7.
39. Shen H, Ong C. Detection of oxidative DNA damage in human sperm and its association with sperm function and male infertility. *Free Radic Biol Med* 2000;28:529–36.

40. Agarwal A, Saleh RA, Bedaiwy MA. Role of reactive oxygen species in the pathophysiology of human reproduction. *Fertil Steril* 2003;79:829–43.

41. Said TM, Aziz N, Sharma RK, Lewis-Jones I, Thomas AJ Jr., Agarwal A. Novel association between sperm deformity index and oxidative stress-induced DNA damage in infertile male patients. *Asian J Androl* 2005;7,121–6.

42. McPherson SM, Longo FJ. Nicking of rat spermatid and spermatozoa DNA: possible involvement of DNA topoisomerase II. *Dev Biol* 1993;158:122–30.

43. Sharma RK, Said T, Agarwal A. Sperm DNA damage and its clinical relevance in assessing reproductive outcome. *Asian J Androl* 2004;6:139–48.

44. Lewis SEM, Aitken RJ. DNA damage to spermatozoa has impacts on fertilization and pregnancy. *Cell Tissue Res* 2005;322:33–41.

45. Agarwal A, Said TM. Role of sperm chromatin abnormalities and DNA damage in male infertility. *Hum Reprod Update* 2003;9:331–45.

46. Irvine DS, Twigg JP, Gordon EL, Fulton N, Milne PA, Aitken RJ. DNA integrity in human spermatozoa: relationships with semen quality. *J Androl* 2000;21:33–44.

47. Darzynkiewicz Z, Juan G, Li X, Gorczyca W, Murakami T, Traganos F. Cytometry in cell necrobiology: analysis of apoptosis and accidental cell death (necrosis). *Cytometry* 1997;27:1–20.

48. Roca J, Mezquita C. DNA topoisomerase II activity in nonreplicating, transcriptionally inactive, chicken late spermatids. *Embo J* 1989;8:1855–60.

49. Balhorn R. A model for the structure of chromatin in mammalian sperm. *J Cell Biol* 1982;93:298–305.

50. Risley MS, Einheber S, Bumcrot DA. Changes in DNA topology during spermatogenesis. *Chromosoma* 1986;94:217–27.

51. Morse-Gaudio M, Risley MS. Topoisomerase II expression and VM-26 induction of DNA breaks during spermatogenesis in Xenopus laevis. *J Cell Sci* 1994;107:2887–98.

52. Genesca A, Caballin MR, Miro R, Benet J, Germa JR, Egozcue J. Repair of human sperm chromosome aberrations in the hamster egg. *Hum Genet* 1992;89:181–6.

53. Marchesi DE, Feng HL. Sperm DNA integrity from sperm to egg. *J Androl*. Published ahead of print.

54. Vogt PH. Molecular genetic of human male infertility: from genes to new therapeutic perspectives. *Curr Pharm Design* 2004; 10:471–500.

55. Martin RH, Ko E, Chan K, Rademaker AW. Detection of aneuploidy in human interphase spermatozoa by fluorescence in situ hybridization (FISH). *Cytogenet Cell Genet* 1993;64:23–6.

56. Griffin DK. The incidence, origin, and etiology of aneuploidy. *Int Rev Cytol* 1996;167:263–96.

57. Spriggs EL, Rademaker AW, Martin RH. Aneuploidy in human sperm: the use of multicolor FISH to test various theories of nondisjunction. *Am J Hum Genet* 1996;58:356–62.

58. Hassold TJ. Nondisjunction in the human male. *Curr Top Dev Biol* 1998;37:383–406.

59. Martin RH, Rademaker AW. Nondisjunction in human sperm: comparison of frequencies in acrocentric chromosomes. *Cytogenet Cell Genet* 1999;86:43–5.

60. Lamb NE, Hassold TJ. Nondisjunction: a view from ringside. *N Engl J Med* 2004;351:1931–4.

61. Lewis-Jones I, Aziz N, Seshadri S, Douglas A, Howard P. Sperm chromosomal abnormalities are linked to sperm morphologic deformities. *Fertil Steril* 2003;79:212–15.

62. Martin RH, Rademaker AW, Greene C, Ko E, Hoang T, Barclay L, Chernos J. A comparison of the frequency of sperm chromosome abnormalities in men with mild, moderate, and severe oligozoospermia. *Biol Reprod* 2003;69:535–9.

63. Calogero AE, De Palma A, Grazioso C et al. Aneuploidy rate in spermatozoa of selected men with abnormal semen parameters. *Hum Reprod* 2001;16:1172–9.

64. Burrello N, Vicari E, Shin P et al. Lower sperm aneuploidy frequency is associated with high pregnancy rates in ICSI programmes. *Hum Reprod* 2003;18:1371–6.

65. Carrell DT, Wilcox AL, Lowy L et al. Elevated sperm chromosome aneuploidy and apoptosis in patients with unexplained recurrent pregnancy loss. *Obstet Gynecol* 2003;101:1229–35.

66. Benjamin R, Emery BR, Carrell DT. The effect of epigenetic sperm abnormalities on early embryogenesis. *Asian J Androl* 2006;8:131–42.

67. Escudero T, Abdelhadi I, Sandalinas M, Munne S. Predictive value of sperm fluorescence in situ hybridization analysis on the outcome of preimplantation genetic diagnosis for translocations. *Fertil Steril* 2003;79 (Suppl. 3):1528–34.

68. Tejada RI, Mitchell JC, Norman A, Marik JJ, Friedman S. A test for the practical evaluation of male fertility by acridine orange (AO) fluorescence. *Fertil Steril* 1984;42:87–91.

69. Darzynkiewicz Z. Acid-induced denaturation of DNA in situ as a probe of chromatin structure. *Methods Cell Biol* 1994;41: 527–41.

70. Erenpreisa J, Freivalds T, Slaidina M et al. Toluidine blue test for sperm DNA integrity and elaboration of image cytometry algorithm. *Cytometry* 2003;52:19–27.

71. Baker H, Liu D. Assessment of nuclear maturity. In: Acosta A, Kruger T, eds. Human Spermatozoa in Assisted Reproduction. London: CRC Press, 1996:93–203.

72. Manicardi G, Bianchi P, Pantano S et al. Presence of endogenous nicks in DNA of ejaculated human spermatozoa and its relationship to chromomycin A3 accessibility. *Biol Reprod* 1995; 52:864–7.

73. Fernandez J, Muriel L, Rivero M et al. The sperm chromatin dispersion test: a simple method for the determination of sperm DNA fragmentation. *J Androl* 2003;24:59–66.

74. Fernandez J, Vazquez-Gundin F, Delgado A et al. DNA breakage detection–FISH (DBD–FISH) in human spermatozoa: technical variants evidence different structural features. *Mutat Res* 2000;253:77–82.

75. Gorczyza W, Gong J, Darzynkiewics Z. Detection of DNA strand breaks in individual apoptotic cells by the in situ terminal deoxynucleotidyl transferase and nick translation assays. *Cancer Res* 1993;53:1945–51.

76. Barroso G, Morshedi M, Oehninger S. Analysis of DNA fragmentation, plasma membrane translocation of phosphatidylserine and oxidative stress in human spermatozoa. *Hum Reprod* 2000;15:1338–44.

77. Singh N, McCoy M, Tice R et al. A simple technique for quantification of low levels of DNA damage in individual cells. *Exp Cell Res* 1988;175:184–91.

78. Singh N, Danner D, Tice R, McCoy MT, Collins GD, Schneider EL. Abundant alkali-sensitive sites in DNA of human and mouse sperm. *Exp Cell Res* 1989;184:461–70.

79. Evenson D, Jost L, Baer R, Turner TW, Schrader SM. Individuality of DNA denaturation patterns in human sperm as measured by the sperm chromatin structure assay. *Reprod Toxicol* 1991;5:115–25.

80. Erenpreisa EA, Zirne RA, Zaleskaia ND, S'iakste TG. Effect of single-stranded breaks on the ultrastructural organization and cytochemistry of the chromatin in tumor cells. *Biull Eksp Biol Med* 1988;106:591–3.

81. Erenpreisa EA, Sondore OIu, Zirne RA. Conformational changes in the chromatin of tumor cells and the phenomenon of nuclear achromasia. *Eksp Onkol* 1988;10:54–7.

82. Rigler R, Killander D, Bolund L, Ringertz NR. Cytochemical characterization of deoxyribonucleoprotein in individual cell nuclei. Techniques for obtaining heat denaturation curves with the aid of acridine orange microfluorimetry and ultraviolet microspectrophotometry. *Exp Cell Res* 1969;55:215–24.

83. Darzynkiewicz Z, Traganos F, Sharpless T, Melamed MR. Thermal denaturation of DNA in situ as studied by acridine orange staining and automated cytofluorometry. *Exp Cell Res* 1975;90: 411–28.

84. Evenson D, Jost L, Marshall D et al. Utility of the sperm chromatin structure assay as a diagnostic tool in the human fertility clinic. *Hum Reprod* 1999;14:1039–49.

85. Zini A, Fischer M, Sharir S, Shayegan B, Phang D, Jarvi K. Prevalence of abnormal sperm DNA denaturation in fertile and infertile men. *Urology* 2002;60:1069–72.

86. Variant-Klun I, Tomazevic T, Meden-Vrtovec H. Sperm single-stranded DNA, detected by acridine orange staining, reduces fertilization and quality of ICSI-derived embryos. *J Assist Reprod Genet* 2002;19:319–28.

87. Erenpreiss J, Bars J, Lipatnikova V, Erenpreisa J, Zalkalns J. Comparative study of cytochemical tests for sperm chromatin integrity. *J Androl* 2001;22:45–53.

88. Auger J, Mesbah M, Huber C, Dadoune JP. Aniline blue staining as a marker of sperm chromatin defects associated with different semen characteristics discriminates between proven fertile and suspected infertile men. *Int J Androl* 1990;13:452–62.

89. Terquem T, Dadoune JP. Aniline blue staining of human spermatozoa chromatin. Evaluation of nuclear maturation. In: Adre J, ed. The Sperm Cell. The Hague: Martinus Nijhoff Publishers; 1983.

90. Liu DY, Baker HW. Sperm nuclear chromatin normality: relationship with sperm morphology, sperm-zona pellucida binding, and fertilization rates in vitro. *Fertil Steril* 1992;58: 1178–84.

91. Foresta C, Zorzi M, Rossato M, Varotto A. Sperm nuclear instability and staining with aniline blue: abnormal persistence of histones in spermatozoa in infertile men. *Int J Androl* 1992; 15:330–7.

92. Hammadeh M, Zeginiadov T, Rosenbaum P et al. Predictive value of sperm chromatin condensation (aniline blue staining) in the assessment of male fertility. *Arch Androl* 2001;46:99–104.

93. Hammadeh M, Stieber M, Haidl G, Schmidt W. Association between sperm cell chromatin condensation, morphology based on strict criteria, and fertilization, cleavage and pregnancy rates in an IVF program. *Andrologia* 1998;30:29–35.

94. Evenson DP, Darzynkiewicz Z, Melamed MR. Relation of mammalian sperm chromatin heterogeneity to fertility. *Science* 1980;210:1131–3.

95. Evenson DP, Jost LK, Marshall D, Zinaman MJ, Clegg E, Purvis K et al. Utility of the sperm chromatin structure assay as a diagnostic and prognostic tool in the human fertility clinic. *Hum Reprod* 1999;14:1039–49.

96. Spano M, Bonde JP, Hjollund HI, Kolstad HA, Cordelli E, Leter G. Sperm chromatin damage impairs human fertility. The Danish First Pregnancy Planner Study Team. *Fertil Steril* 2000;73: 43–50.

97. Larson-Cook KL, Brannian JD, Hansen KA, Kasperson KM, Aamold ET, Evenson DP. Relationship between the outcomes of assisted reproductive techniques and sperm DNA fragmentation as measured by the sperm chromatin structure assay. *Fertil Steril* 2003;80:895–902.

98. Evenson D, Wixon R. Meta-analysis of sperm DNA fragmentation using the sperm chromatin structure assay. *Reprod Biomed Online* 2006;12:466–72.

99. Spano M, Kolstad A, Larsen S et al. The applicability of the flow cytometric sperm chromatin structure assay in epidemiological studies. *Hum Reprod* 1998;13:2495–505.

100. Perreault SD, Aitken HW, Baker DP et al. Integrating new tests of sperm genetic integrity into semen analysis: breakout group discussion. In: Robaire B, Hales BF, eds. Male-Mediated Developmental Toxicity. Kluwer Academic/Plenum Publisher; 2003:256–66.

101. Bianchi PG, Manicardi GC, Bizzaro D, Bianchi U, Sakkas D. Effect of deoxyribonucleic acid protamination on fluorochrome staining and in situ nick-translation of murine and human mature spermatozoa. *Biol Reprod* 1993;49:1083–8.

102. Sakkas D, Urner F, Bizzaro D, Manicardi G, Bianchi PG, Shoukir Y et al. Sperm nuclear DNA damage and altered chromatin structure: effect on fertilization and embryo development. *Hum Reprod* 1998;13 (Suppl. 4):11–19.

103. Lopes S, Sun JG, Jurisicova A, Meriano J, Casper RF. Sperm deoxyribonucleic acid fragmentation is increased in poor-quality semen samples and correlates with failed fertilization in intracytoplasmic sperm injection. *Fertil Steril* 1998;69: 528–32.

104. Gorczyca W, Traganos F, Jesionowska H, Darzynkiewicz Z. Presence of DNA strand breaks and increased sensitivity of DNA in situ to denaturation in abnormal human sperm cells: analogy to apoptosis of somatic cells. *Exp Cell Res* 1993;207: 202–5.

105. Aravindan GR, Bjordahl J, Jost LK, Evenson DP. Susceptibility of human sperm to in situ DNA denaturation is strongly correlated with DNA strand breaks identified by single cell electrophoresis. *Exp Cell Res* 1997;236:231–7.

106. Chan PJ, Corselli JU, Patton WC, Jacobson JD, Chan SR, King A. Simple comet assay for archived sperm correlates DNA fragmentation. Reduced hyperactivation and penetration of zona-free hamster ocytes. *Fertil Steril* 2001;75:186–92.

107. Duty S, Singh N, Ryan L et al. Reliability of the comet assay in cryopreserved human sperm. *Hum Reprod* 2002;17: 1274–80.

108. Morris I, Ilott S, Dixon L, Brison DR. The spectrum of DNA damage in human sperm assessed by single cell gel electrophoresis (comet assay) and its relationship to fertilization. *Hum Reprod* 2002;17:990–8.

109. Tomsu M, Sharma V, Miller D. Embryo quality and IVF treatment outcomes may correlate with different sperm comet assay parameters. *Hum Reprod* 2002;17:1856–62.

110. Hughes CM, Lewis SE, McKelvey-Martin VJ, Thompson W. A comparison of baseline and induced DNA damage in human spermatozoa from fertile and infertile men, using a modified comet assay. *Mol Hum Reprod* 1996;2:613–19.

111. Ankem MK, Mayer E, Ward WS, Cummings KB, Barone JG. Novel assay for determining DNA organization in human spermatozoa: implications for male factor infertility. *Urology* 2002; 59:575–8.

112. Ward WS, Kimura Y, Yanagimachi R. An intact sperm nuclear matrix may be necessary for the mouse paternal genome to participate in embryonic development. *Biol Reprod* 1999;60:702–6.

113. Sjakste N, Sjakste T. Nuclear matrix proteins and hereditary diseases. *Genetika* 2005;41:293–8.

114. Iwasaki A, Gagnon C. Formation of reactive oxygen species of spermatozoa of infertile patients. *Fertil Steril* 1992;57:409.

115. Sharma RK, Agarwal A. Role of reactive oxygen species in male infertility. *J Urol* 1996;48:835–50.

116. Aitken RJ, Fisher H. Reactive oxygen species generation and human spermatozoa: the balance of benefit and risk. *Bioassays* 1994;16:259–67.

117. Aitken RJ, Irvine DS, Wu FC. Prospective analysis of sperm-oocyte fusion and reactive oxygen species generation as criteria for the diagnosis of infertility. *Am J Obstet Gynecol* 1991;64:542–51.

118. Agarwal A, Ftabakaran SA. Mechanism, measurement, and prevention of oxidative stress in male reproductive physiology. *Indian J Exp Biol* 2003;43:963–74.

119. Darley-Usmar V, Wiseman H, Halliwell B. Nitric oxide and oxygen radicals: a question of balance. *FEBS Lett* 1995;369:131–5.

120. Gutierrez J, Ballinger SW, Darley-Usmar VM, Landar A. Free radicals, mitochondria, and oxidized lipids: the emerging role in signal transduction in vascular cells. *Circ Res* 2006;27;99:924–32.

121. Gomez E, Buckingham DW, Brindle J, Lanzafame F, Irvine DS, Aitken RJ. Development of an image analysis system to monitor the retention of residual cytoplasma by human spermatozoa: correlation with biochemical markers of the cytoplasmic space, oxidative stress, and sperm function. *J Androl* 1996;17:276–87.

122. Gil-Guzman E, Ollero M, Lopez MC, Sharma RK, Alvarez JG, Thomas AJ Jr., Agarwal A. Differential production of reactive oxygen species by subsets of human spermatozoa at different stages of maturation. *Hum Reprod* 2001;16:1922–30.

123. Aziz N, Saleh RA, Sharma RK, Lewis-Jones I, Esfandiari N, Thomas AJ Jr., Agarwal A. Novel association between sperm reactive oxygen species production, sperm morphological defects, and the sperm deformity index. *Fertil Steril* 2004; 81:349–54.

124. Aitken J. Molecular mechanisms regulating human sperm function. *Mol Hum Reprod* 1997;3:169–73.

125. Huszar G, Vigue L. Correlation between the rate of lipid peroxidation and cellular maturity as measured by creatine kinase activity in human spermatozoa. *J Androl* 1994;15:71–7.

126. Clermont Y. The cycle of the seminiferous epithelium in man. *Am J Anat* 1963;112:35–51.

127. Vernet P, Fulton N, Wallace C, Aitken RJ. Analysis of reactive oxygen species generating systems in rat epididymal spermatozoa. *Biol Reprod* 2001;65:1102–13.

128. Baker MA, Aitken RJ. Reactive oxygen species in spermatozoa: methods for monitoring and significance for the origins of genetic disease and infertility. *Reprod Biol Endocrinol* 2005;3:67–75.

129. Balercia G, Moretti S, Vignini A, Magagnini M, Mantero F, Boscaro M et al. Role of nitric oxide concentrations on human sperm motility. *J Androl* 2004;25:245–9.

130. Lewis SEM, Donnelly ET, Sterling ESL, Kennedy MS, Thompson W, Chakrawarthy U. Nitric oxide synthase and nitrite production in human spermatozoa: evidence that endogenous nitric oxide is beneficial to sperm motility. *Mol Hum Reprod* 1996;2:873–8.

131. Herrero MB, Chatterjee S, Lefievre L, de Lamirande E, Gagnon C. Nitric oxide interacts with the cAMP pathway to modulate capacitation of human spermatozoa. *Free Rad Biol Med* 2000;29:522–36.

132. Aitken RJ, Baker HW. Seminal leukocytes: passengers, terrorists or good samaritans? *Hum Reprod* 1995;10:1736–9.

133. Shalika S, Duaan K, Smith RD. The effect of positive semen bacterial and uroplasmal cultures on in vitro fertilization success. *Hum Reprod* 1996;11:2789–92.

134. Aitkin RJ, Fisher HM, Fulton N. Reactive oxygen species generation by human spermatozoa is induced by exogenous NADPH and inhibited by the flavoprotein inhibitors diphenylene iodonium and quinacrine. *Mot Reprad Dev* 1997;47:468–82.

135. Hendin BN, Kolettis PN, Sharma RK, Thomas AJ Jr., Agarwal A. Varicocele is associated with elevated spermatozoal reactive oxygen species production and diminished seminal plasma antioxidant capacity. *J Urol* 1999;161:1831–4.

136. Saleh RA, Agarwal A, Kandirali E, Sharma RK, Thomas AJ Jr., Nada EA et al. Leukocytospermia is associated with increased reactive oxygen species production by human spermatozoa. *Fertil Steril* 2002;78:1215–24.

137. Alvarez JG, Sharma RK, Ollero M, Saleh RA, Lopez MC, Thomas AJ Jr. et al. Increased DNA damage in sperm from leukocytospermic semen samples as determined by the sperm chromatin structure assay. *Fertil Steril* 2002;78:319–29.

138. Aziz N, Agarwal A, Lewis-Jones I, Sharma RK, Thomas AJ Jr. Novel associations between specific sperm morphological defects and leukocytospermia. *Fertil Steril* 2004;82:621–7.

139. Garrido N, Meseguer M, Simon C, Pellicer A, Remohi J. Pro-oxidative and anti-oxidative imbalance in human semen and its relation with male fertility. *Asian J Androl* 2004;6:59–65.

140. Hendin BN, Kolettis PN, Sharma RK, Thomas AJ Jr., Agarwal A. Varicocele is associated with elevated spermatozoal reactive oxygen species production and diminished seminal plasma antioxidant capacity. *J Urol* 1999;161:1831–4.

141. de Lamirande E, Leclerc P, Gagnon C. Capacitation as a regulatory event that primes spermatozoa for the acrosome reaction and fertilization. *Mol Hum Reprod* 1997;3:175–94.

142. Sanchez-Pena LC, Reyes BE, Lopez-Carrillo L, Recio R, Moran-Martinez J, Cebrian ME, Quintanilla-Vega B. Organophosphorous pesticide exposure alters sperm chromatin structure in Mexican agricultural workers. *Toxicol Appl Pharm* 2004;196:108–13.

143. Agarwal A, Said TM. Oxidative stress, DNA damage and apoptosis in male infertility: a clinical approach. *Brit J Urol Int* 2005;95:503–7.

144. Saleh RA, Agarwal A, Sharma RK, Nelson DR, Thomas AJ Jr. Effect of cigarette smoking on levels of seminal oxidative stress in infertile men: a prospective study. *Fertil Steril* 2002;78:491–9.

145. Love CC, Kenney RM. Scrotal heat stress induces altered sperm chromatin structure associated with a decrease in protamines disulfide bonding in the stallion. *Biol Reprod* 1999;60:615–20.

146. Ishii T, Matsuki S, Iuchi Y, Okada F, Toyosaki S, Tomita Y et al. Accelerated impairment of spermatogenic cells in SOD1-knockout mice under heat stress. *Free Radic Res* 2005;39:697–705.

147. Agarwal A, Prabakaran S, Allamaneni SS. Relationship between oxidative stress, varicocele and infertility: a meta-analysis. *Reprod Biomed Online* 2006;12:630–3.

148. Sheynkin Y, Jung M, Yoo P, Schulsinger D, Komaroff E. Increase in scrotal temperature in laptop computer users. *Hum Reprod* 2005;20:452–5.

149. Aitken RJ, Buckingham DW, Harkiss D, Paterson M, Fisher H, Irvine DS. The extragenomic action of progesterone on human spermatozoa is influenced by redox regulated changes in tyrosine phosphorylation during capacitation. *Mol Cell Endocrinol* 1996;117:83–93.

150. De Lamirande E, Tsai C, Harakat A, Gagnon C. Involvement of reactive oxygen species in human sperm acrosome reaction induced by A23187, lysophosphatidylcholine, and biological fluid ultrafiltrates. *J Androl* 1998;19:585–94.

151. Zini A, De Lamirande E, Gagnon C. Low levels of nitric oxide promote human sperm capacitation in vitro. *J Androl* 1995;16:424–31.

152. Sengoku K, Tamate K, Yoshida T, Takaoka Y, Miyamoto T, Ishikawa M. Effects of low concentrations of nitric oxide on the zona pellucida binding ability of human spermatozoa. *Fertil Steril* 1998;69:522–7.

153. Saleh RA, Agarwal A. Oxidative stress and male infertility: from research bench to clinical practice. *J Androl* 2002;23:737–52.

154. Balercia G, Moretti S, Vignini A et al. Role of nitric oxide concentrations on human sperm motility. *J Androl* 2004;25:245–9.

155. Agarwal A, Saleh RA. Role of oxidants in male infertility: rationale, significance, and treatment. *Urol Clin North Am* 2002; 29:817–27.

156. Tominaga H, Kodama S, Matsuda N et al. Involvement of reactive oxygen species (ROS) in the induction of genetic instability by radiation. *J Radiat Res* 2004;45:181–8.

157. Moustafa MH, Sharma RK, Thornton J et al. Relationship between ROS production, apoptosis and DNA denaturation in spermatozoa from patients examined for infertility. *Hum Reprod* 2004;19:129–38.

158. Agarwal A, Allamaneni SS. The effect of sperm DNA damage on assisted reproduction outcomes. *Minerva Ginecol* 2004;56: 235–45.

159. Agarwal A, Said TM. Role of sperm chromatin abnormalities and DNA damage in male infertility. *Hum Reprod Update* 2003;9(45):331.

160. Saleh RA, Agaswat A, Nada EA et al. Negative effects of increased sperm DNA damage in relation to seminal oxidative stress in men with idiopathic and male factor infertility. *Fertil Steril* 2003;79 (Suppl. 3):1597–605.

161. Twigg J, Fuhpa N, Gomez E, Irvine DS, Aitken RJ. Analysis of the impact of intracellular reactive oxygen species generation on the structural and functional integrity of human spermatozoa: lipid peroxidation, DNA fragmentation and effectiveness of antioxidants. *Hum Reprod* 1998;13(6):1429–36.

162. Agarwal A, Prabakaran SA, Sikka S. Clinical relevance of oxidative stress in patients with male factor infertility: evidence-based analysis. *AUA Update* 2007;26:1–12.

163. Aitken RJ, Baker MA, O'Bryan M. Shedding light on chemiluminescence: the application of chemiluminescence in diagnostic andrology. *J Androl* 2004;25:455–65.

164. Marchetti C, Obert G, Deffosez A, Formstecher P, Marchetti P. Study of mitochondrial membrane potential, reactive oxygen species, DNA fragmentation and cell viability by flow cytometry in human sperm. *Hum Reprod* 2002;17:1257–65.

165. Robinson JP, Carter WO, Narayanan PK. Oxidative product formation analysis by flow cytometry. *Methods Cell Biol* 1994; 41:437–47.

166. Cao G, Prior RL. Comparison of different analytical methods for assessing total antioxidant capacity of human serum. *Clin Chem* 1998;44:1309–15.

167. Benzie IF, Strain JJ. The ferric reducing ability of plasma (FRAP) as a measure of "antioxidant power": the FRAP assay. *Anal Biochem* 1996;239:70–6.

168. Miller NJ, Rice-Evans C, Davies MJ et al. A novel method for measuring antioxidant capacity and its application to monitoring the antioxidant status in premature neonates. *Clin Sci (Lond)* 1993;84:407–12.

169. Sharma RK, Pasqualotto FF, Nelson DR et al. The reactive oxygen species-total antioxidant capacity score is a new measure of oxidative stress to predict male infertility. *Hum Reprod* 1999;14:2801–7.

170. Wyllie AH, Kerr JF, Currie AR. Cell death: the significance of apoptosis. *Int Rev Cytol* 1980;68:251–306.

171. Spano M, Seli E, Bizzaro D, Manicardi GC, Sakkas D. The significance of sperm nuclear DNA strand breaks on reproductive outcome. *Curr Opin Obstet Gynecol* 2005;17:255–60.

172. Anzar M, He L, Buhr MM, Kroetsch TG, Pauls KP. Sperm apoptosis in fresh and cryopreserved bull semen detected by flow cytometry and its relationship with fertility. *Biol Reprod* 2002;66:354–60.

173. Gottlieb RA. Mitochondria and apoptosis. *Biol Signals Recept* 2001;10:147–61.

174. Scaffidi C, Fulda S, Srinivasan A, Friesen et al. Two CD95 (APO-1/Fas) signaling pathways. *EMBO J* 1998;7:1675–87.

175. Thornberry NA, Lazebnik Y. Caspases: enemies within. *Science* 1998;281:1312–16.

176. Selivanova G, Wiman KG. p53: a cell cycle regulator activated by DNA damage. *Adv Cancer Res* 1995;66:143–80.

177. Fadok VA, de Catelineau A, Daleke DL, Henson PM, Bratton DL. Loss of phospholipid asymmetry and surface exposure of phospha-tidylserine is required for phagocytosis of apoptotic cells by macrophages and fibroblasts. *J Biol Chem* 2001;276, 1071–7.

178. Hoffmann PR, de Cathelineau AM, Ogden CA et al. Phosphatidylserine (PS) induces PS receptor-mediated macropinocytosis and promotes clearance of apoptotic cells. *J Cell Biol* (2001); 115:649–59.

179. Hampton MB, Fadeel B, Orrenius S. Redox regulation of the caspase during apoptosis. *Am N Y Acad Sci* 1999;854:328–35.

180. Agarwal A, Sharma Bedaiwy MA. Role of reactive oxygen species in the pathophysiology of human reproduction. *Fertil Steril* 2003;79:829–43.

181. Wang X, Sharma RK, Sikka SC, Falcone T, Agarwal A. Oxidative sum iş associated with increased apoptosis leading to spermatime DNA damage in patients with male factor infertility. *Fertil Steril* 2003;80:531–5.

182. Halliwell B. Antioxidant defence mechanisms: from the beginning to the end (of the beginning). *Free Radic Res* 1999;31:261–72.

183. Muratori M, Maggi M, Spinelli S, Filimberti E, Forti G, Baldi E. Spontaneous DNA fragmentation in swim-up selected human spermatozoa during long term incubation. *J Androl* 2003;24: 253–62.

184. Oosterhuis GJ, Mulder AB, Kalsbeek-Batenburg E, Lambalk CB, Schoemaker J, Vermes I. Measuring apoptosis in human spermatozoa: a biological assay for semen quality? *Fertil Steril* 2000;74:245–50.

185. Shen HM, Dai J, Chia SE, Lim A, Ong CN. Detection of apoptotic alterations in sperm in subfertile patients and their correlations with sperm quality. *Hum Reprod* 2002;17:1266–73.

186. Sun JG, Jurisicova A, Casper RF. Detection of deoxyribonucleic acid fragmentation in human sperm: correlation with fertilization in vitro. *Biol Reprod* 1997;56:602–7.

187. Weil M, Jacobson MD, Raff MC. Are caspases involved in the death of cells with a transcriptionally inactive nucleus? Sperm and chicken erythrocytes. *J Cell Sci* 1998;111:2707–15.

188. Grunewald S, Paasch U, Glander HJ, Anderegg U. Mature human spermatozoa do not transcribe novel RNA. *Andrologia* 2005;37:69–71.

189. Paasch U, Sharma RK, Gupta AK, Grunewald S, Mascha EJ, Thomas AJ Jr. et al. Cryopreservation and thawing is associated with varying extent of activation of apoptotic machinery in subsets of ejaculated human spermatozoa. *Biol Reprod* 2004;71: 1828–37.

190. Oehninger S, Morshedi M, Weng SL, Taylor S, Duran H, Beebe S. Presence and significance of somatic cell apoptosis markers in human ejaculated spermatozoa. *Reprod Biomed Online* 2003; 7:469–76.

191. Taylor SL, Weng SL, Fox P, Duran EH, Morshedi MS, Oehninger S, Beebe SJ. Somatic cell apoptosis markers and pathways in human ejaculated sperm: potential utility as indicators of sperm quality. *Mol Hum Reprod* 2004;10:825–34.

192. Sakkas D, Seli E, Bizzaro D, Tarozzi N, Manicardi GC. Abnormal spermatozoa in the ejaculate: abortive apoptosis and faulty nuclear remodelling during spermatogenesis. *Reprod Biomed Online* 2003;7:428–32.

193. Lin WW, Lamb DJ, Wheeler TM, Lipshultz LI, Kim ED. In situ end-labeling of human testicular tissue demonstrates increased apoptosis in conditions of abnormal spermatogenesis. *Fertil Steril* 1997;68:1065–9.

194. Jurisicova A, Lopes S, Meriano J, Oppedisano L, Casper RF, Varmuza S. DNA damage in round spermatids of mice with a targeted disruption of the Pp1cgamma gene and in testicular biopsies of patients with non-obstructive azoospermia. *Mol Hum Reprod* 1999;5:323–30.

195. Grunewald S, Paasch U, Wuendrich K, Glander HJ. Sperm caspases become more activated in infertility patients than in healthy donors during cryopreservation. *Arch Androl* 2005;51:449–60.

196. Sakkas D, Urner F, Bianchi PG, Bizzaro D, Wagner I, Jaquenoud N et al. Sperm chromatin anomalies can influence decondensation after intracytoplasmic sperm injection. *Hum Reprod* 1996;11:837–43.

197. Shoukir Y, Chardonnens D, Campana A, Sakkas D. Blastocyst development from supernumerary embryos after intracytoplasmic sperm injection: a paternal influence? *Hum Reprod* 1998;13:1632–7.

198. Weil M, Jacobson MD, Raff MC. Are caspases involved in the death of cells with a transcriptionally inactive nucleus? Sperm and chicken erythrocytes. *J Cell Sci* 1998;111:2707–15.

199. Pena FJ, Johannisson A, Wallgren M, Rodriguez-Martinez H. Assessment of fresh and frozen-thawed boar semen using an Annexin-V assay: a new method of evaluating sperm membrane integrity. *Theriogenology* 2003;60:677–89.

200. Liu CH, Tsao HM, Cheng TC, Wu HM, Huang CC, Chen CI et al. DNA fragmentation, mitochondrial dysfunction and chromosomal aneuploidy in the spermatozoa of oligoasthenoteratozoospermic males. *J Assist Reprod Genet* 2004;21:119–26.

201. Chen Z, Hauser R, Trbovich AM, Shifren JL, Dorer DJ, Godfrey-Bailey et al. The relationship between human semen characteristics and sperm apoptosis: a pilot study. *J Androl* 2006;27:112–20.

202. Siddighi S, Patton WC, Jacobson JD, King A, Chan PJ. Correlation of sperm parameters with apoptosis assessed by dual fluorescence DNA integrity assay. *Arch Androl* 2004;50:311–14.

203. Said TM, Paasch U, Grunewald S, Baumann T, Li L, Glander HJ, Agarwal A. Advantage of combining magnetic cell separation with sperm preparation techniques. *Reprod Biomed Online* 2005b;10:740–6.

204. Aziz N, Said T, Paasch U, Agarwal A. The relationship between human sperm apoptosis, morphology and the sperm deformity index. *Hum Reprod* 2007;15; [Epub ahead of print].

205. Sakkas D, Mariethoz E, St John JC. Abnormal sperm parameters in humans are indicative of an abortive apoptotic mechanism linked to the Fas-mediated pathway. *Exp Cell Res* 1999;15:350–5.

206. Sakkas D, Mariethoz E, Manicardi G, Bizzarro D, Bianchi PG, Bianchi U. Origin of DNA damage in ejaculated human spermatozoa. *Rev Reprod* 1999;4:31–7.

207. Sakkas D, Moffat O, Manicardi GC, Mariethoz E, Tarozzi N, Bizzaro D. Nature of DNA damage in ejaculated human spermatozoa and the possible involvement of apoptosis. *Biol Reprod* 2002;66:1061–7.

208. Cayli S, Sakkas D, Vigue L, Demir R, Huszar G. Cellular maturity and apoptosis in human sperm: creatine kinase, caspase-3 and Bcl-XL levels in mature and diminished maturity sperm. *Mol Hum Reprod* 2004;10:365–72.

209. Frisch SM, Screaton RA. Anoikis mechanisms. *Curr Opin Cell Biol* 2001;13:555–62.

210. Grunewald S, Paasch U, Glander HJ. Enrichment of non-apoptotic human spermatozoa after cryopreservation by immunomagnetic cell sorting. *Cell Tissue Bank* 2001;2:127–33.

211. Glander HJ, Schiller J, Suss R, Paasch U, Grunewald S, Arnhold J. Deterioration of spermatozoal plasma membrane is associated with an increase of sperm lyso-phosphatidylcholines. *Andrologia* 2002;34:360–6.

212. Said TM, Grunewald S, Paasch U et al. Effects of magnetic-activated cell sorting on sperm motility and cryosurvival rates. *Fertil Steril* 2005;83:1442–6.

213. Said T, Agarwal A, Grunewald S et al. Selection of nonapoptotic spermatozoa as a new tool for enhancing assisted reproduction outcomes: an in vitro model. *Biol Reprod* 2006;74:530–7.

214. Ricci G, Perticarari S, Fragonas E et al. Apoptosis in human sperm: its correlation with semen quality and the presence of leukocytes. *Hum Reprod* 2002;17:2665–72.

215. Ekert PG, Silke J, Vaux DL. Caspase inhibitors. *Cell Death Differ* 1999;6:1081–6.

216. Barroso G, Taylor S, Morshedi M et al. Mitochondrial membrane potential integrity and plasma membrane translocation of phosphatidylserine as early apoptotic markers: a comparison of two different sperm subpopulations. *Fertil Steril* 2006;85:149–54.

217. Paasch U, Grunewald S, Fitzl G, Glander HJ. Deterioration of plasma membrane is associated with activation of caspases in human spermatozoa. *J Androl* 2003;24:246–52.

218. Weng SL, Taylor SL, Morshedi M et al. Caspase activity and apoptotic markers in ejaculated human sperm. *Mol Hum Reprod* 2002;8:984–91.

219. Almeida C, Cardoso F, Sousa M et al. Quantitative study of caspase-3 activity in semen and after swim-up preparation in relation to sperm quality. *Hum Reprod* 2005;20:1307–13.

220. Benchaib M, Braun V, Lornage J et al. Sperm DNA fragmentation decreases the pregnancy rate in an assisted reproductive technique. *Hum Reprod* 2003;18:1023–8.

221. Blackwell RP. Standards for microwave radiation. *Nature* 1979;282:360.

222. Kandeel FR, Swerdloff RS. Role of temperature in regulation of spermatogenesis and the use of heating as a method for contraception. *Fertil Steril* 1988;49:1–23.

223. Saunders R, Sienkiewicz Z, Kowalczuk C. Biological effects of electromagnetic fields and radiation. *J Radiol Prot* 1991;11:27–42.

224. Ozguner M, Koyu A, Cesur G, Ural M, Ozguner F, Gokcimen A et al. Biological and morphological effects on the reproductive organ of rats after exposure to electromagnetic field. *Saudi Med J* 2005;26:405–10.

225. Yu C, Yao Y, Yang Y, Li D. [Changes of rat testicular germ cell apoptosis after high power microwave radiation]. *Zhonghua Nan Ke Xue* 2004;10:407–10.

226. Saunders RD, Kowalczuk CI. Effects of 2.45 GHz microwave radiation and heat on mouse spermatogenic epithelium. *Int J Radiat Biol Relat Stud Phys Chem Med* 1981;40:623–32.

227. Lebovitz RM, Johnson L, Samson WK. Effects of pulse-modulated microwave radiation and conventional heating on sperm production. *J Appl Physiol* 1987;62:245–52.

228. Fejes I, Zavaczki Z, Szollosi J, Koloszar S, Daru J, Kovacs L et al. Is there a relationship between cell phone use and semen quality? *Arch Androl* 2005;51:385–93.

229. Davoudi M, Brossner C, Kuber W. The influence of electromagnetic waves on sperm motility. *Urol Urogynacol* 2002;19: 18–22.

230. Erogul O, Oztas E, Yildirim I, Kir T, Aydur E, Komesli G et al. Effects of electromagnetic radiation from a cellular phone on human sperm motility: an in vitro study. *Arch Med Res* 2006;37:840–3.

231. Agarwal A, Deepinder F, Sharma RK, Ranga G, Li J. Effect of cell phone usage on semen analysis in men attending infertility clinic: an observational study. *Fertil Steril* 2007. In press.

232. Aitken RJ. The Amoroso Lecture. The human spermatozoon—a cell in crisis? *J Reprod Fertil* 1999;115:1–7.

233. Lai H, Singh NP. Single- and double-strand DNA breaks in rat brain cells after acute exposure to radiofrequency electromagnetic radiation. *Int J Radiat Biol* 1996;69:513–21.

234. Aitken RJ, Bennetts LE, Sawyer D, Wiklendt AM, King BV. Impact of radiofrequency electromagnetic radiation on DNA integrity in the male germline. *Int J Androl* 2005;28:171–9.

235. Diem E, Schwarz C, Adlkofer F, Jahn O, Rudiger H. Non-thermal DNA breakage by mobile-phone radiation (1800 MHz) in human fibroblasts and in transformed GFSH-R17 rat granulosa cells in vitro. *Mutat Res* 2005;583:178–83.

236. Musaev AV, Ismailova LF, Gadzhiev AM. [Influence of (460 MHz) electromagnetic fields on the induced lipid peroxidation in the structures of visual analyzer and hypothalamus in experimental animals]. *Vopr Kurortol Fizioter Lech Fiz Kult* 2005; 17–20.

237. Hook GJ, Spitz DR, Sim JE et al. Evaluation of parameters of oxidative stress after in vitro exposure to FMCW- and CDMA-modulated radiofrequency radiation fields. *Radiat Res* 2004;162:497–504.

238. Burch JB, Reif JS, Noonan CW et al. Melatonin metabolite excretion among cellular telephone users. *Int J Radiat Biol* 2002;78:1029–36.

239. de Seze R, Ayoub J, Peray P, Miro L, Touitou Y. Evaluation in humans of the effects of radiocellular telephones on the circadian patterns of melatonin secretion, a chronobiological rhythm marker. *J Pineal Res* 1999;27:237–42.

240. Gavella M, Lipovac V. Antioxidative effect of melatonin on human spermatozoa. *Arch Androl* 2000;44:23–7.

241. Lantow M, Viergutz T, Weiss DG, Simko M. Comparative study of cell cycle kinetics and induction of apoptosis or necrosis after exposure of human mono mac 6 cells to radiofrequency radiation. *Radiat Res* 2006;166:539–43.

242. Port M, Abend M, Romer B, Van Beuningen D. Influence of high-frequency electromagnetic fields on different modes of cell death and gene expression. *Int J Radiat Biol* 2003;79:701–8.

243. Rizk B. (Ed.). Ultrasonography in reproductive medicine and infertility. Cambridge: United Kingdom, Cambridge University Press 2008: (in press).

20

Male Factor Infertility: State of the Art

Frank Comhaire, Ahmed Mahmoud

INTRODUCTION

Andrologists are medical doctors who practice the clinical management of typically male problems, including congenital malformations of the male genital tract, abnormal pubertal development, male infertility, sexual dysfunction, and male aging. In Europe, an andrologist may be a specialist in endocrinology or urology who has acquired and proven his expertise through a well-defined education program sanctioned by an examination before an international jury of the European Academy of Andrology (1).

McLeod has highlighted the importance of the "male factor" in couple infertility in his milestone publications where reference values for "normal" semen quality were established (2). For several decades, male infertility has been considered incurable because the majority of patients were suspected of suffering from an idiopathic condition. Both high-quality clinical research and fundamental biological investigations have revealed that certain diseases may cause male infertility and effective treatments have been developed (3).

The relative importance of the male factor as a cause of couple infertility has become proportionally larger, particularly since biologists and gynecologists using techniques of assisted reproduction detect many more cases with abnormal semen quality. However, the epidemiology of causal factors has changed over time, with particular diseases becoming less frequent (e.g., obstructive azoospermia acquired by infection of the reproductive tract), whereas other diseases are detected more commonly (e.g., varicocele).

DIAGNOSTIC FLOW CHART AND ITS IMPLICATIONS FOR TREATMENT

Rational treatment of the infertile male requires a correct and complete etiological diagnosis. Standardized history taking and physical examination are complemented by scrotal thermography and ultrasound examination of the pelvic organs and the scrotal content, thorough semen analysis, and selected blood tests. Criteria for each diagnosis are clearly defined (3) and are introduced into the flow chart (Table 20.1). There is evidence that lifestyle and environmental factors, such as hormone disrupters, and professional exposure to toxins exert a major influence and may determine whether or not a particular pathological condition will "come to expression" and cause infertility (4). Also, infertility covers a broad scale with different degrees of reduction of the monthly probability of conception.

Treatment should aim at correcting all detectable causes since it has become clear that many patients present a combination of factors that act in synergism (5). Logically, to correct only one contributing factor may not restore fertility in such cases. In addition, treatment may remain unsuccessful because it is incorrectly applied. For instance, treatment of infection of the accessory sex glands may use an ineffective antibiotic that does not penetrate into the affected glands (e.g., tetracyclins) (3) or an inadequate dose and/or insufficient duration of application. Similarly, varicocele treatment that does not completely interrupt the commonly bilateral reflux in the internal spermatic veins will not restore testicular function. The use of antioxidants or other food supplements may not improve sperm function if the choice of substances and dose given are not judicious (6). The selection of cases for IUI and method of sperm preparation will largely define the success rate of this mode of treatment.

In general, meta-analysis cannot take into account these particular aspects that are, in fact, constituting good medical practice. Hence, the conclusions of meta-analyses should be interpreted with great caution. Consensus-based medicine is the preferred approach because decision making includes the understanding of pathophysiology as well as the results of observational and controlled clinical trials.

VARICOCELE

Varicocele results from increased hydrostatic pressure in the intrascrotal pampiniform plexus and in the testicular venules (7). This, together with the reflux of vasoconstrictive catecholamines (8), reduces or blocks the arterial capillary blood supply to the seminiferous tubules and the cells of Leydig. The increased pressure itself is caused by failure of the valves of the internal spermatic veins that, normally, prevent reflux. The reflux may cause visible (grade III) or palpable (grade II) distension of the pampiniform plexus. In grade I varicocele, the distension can be palpated during Valsalva maneuver, whereas reflux can only be detected by means of thermography and/or duplex Doppler examination in patients with subclinical varicoceles (9, 10). The pathogenic mechanisms are equally active in all grades of varicocele and commonly exert their effects bilaterally (11).

Varicocele develops during puberty, and it is the most common cause of male infertility with prevalence varying between

Table 20.1: Flow Chart for the Etiological Diagnosis of the Infertile Male (3)

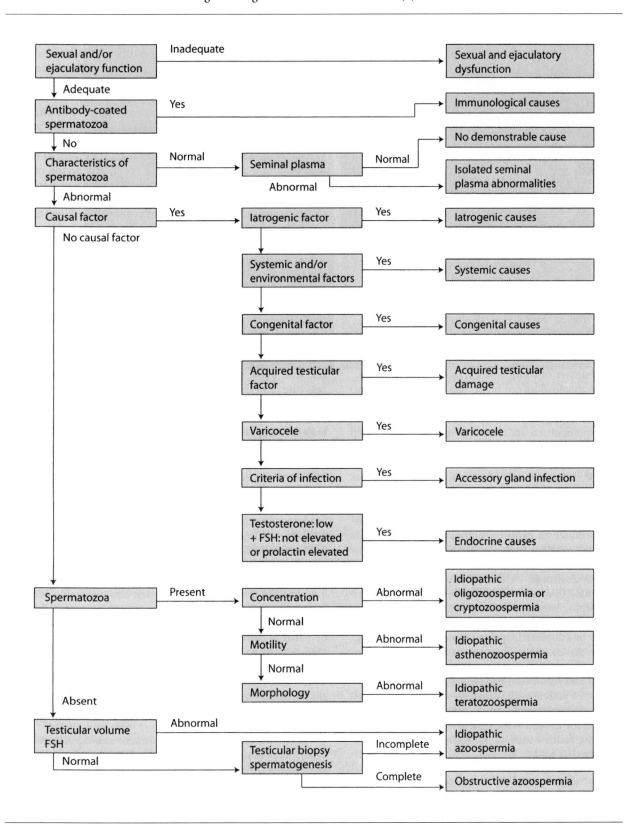

Table 21.1: Pharmaceutical Agents Associated with EjD

Antihypertensive agents

Thiazide diuretics

Prazosin

Phenoxybenamine

Phentolamine

Tamsulosin

Psychiatric agents

MAOIs

Fluoxetine

Paroxetine

Sertaline

Imipramine

Amitriptyline

Clomipramine

Haloperidol

Thioridazine

Reserpine

Nonsteroidal anti-inflammatory agents

Naproxen

Baclofen

Other

Alcohol

Morphine

Methadone

Chlordiazepoxide

via the sympathetic tracts to the bladder neck. Lack of a closed bladder neck may lead to AE or retrograde ejaculation. Spinal cord lesions, whether congenital, acquired, or traumatic, commonly lead to ejaculatory dysfunction. Lesions above T10–T11 are likely to cause anejaculation, whereas lower lesions may merely inhibit the expulsion phase of ejaculation, leaving emission intact. Partial spinal cord injuries may only cause IE. Multiple sclerosis commonly causes a number of sexual dysfunctions, including inability to achieve orgasm or ejaculate, in up to 61 percent of patients (22).

INFECTIOUS

Scarring of the reproductive tract caused by infection can lead to obstruction and subsequent low ejaculate volume. Urethritis from sexually transmitted diseases may cause partial obstruction of the urethra; *Chlamydia* and *Gonorrhea* remain the most prevalent pathogens, particularly when antibiotic therapy is delayed (23). Tuberculosis has an affinity for the genitourinary tract. Atrophy of the seminal vesicles or scarring and obstruction of the epididymal ducts are common occurrences in genitourinary tuberculosis (24), either of which can lead to low ejaculate volume or infertility.

MEDICATIONS

A wide array of medications can induce EjD through a number of different mechanisms (25) (Table 21.1). Antihypertensive medications including alpha-methyl dopa, thiazide diuretics, and clonidine have been implicated. Numerous psychiatric medications from psychotropics to antidepressants, including haloperidol, tricyclic antidepressants, SSRIs, and monoamine oxidase inhibitors, have ejaculatory side effects. When possible, discontinuation of the offending pharmaceutical agent is the best treatment option. Alcohol abuse may also cause AE or IE. Alpha-adrenergic blockers such as tamsulosin were previously believed to lead to retrograde ejaculation; however, it has recently been determined that they cause anejaculation by a central mechanism (26).

Retrograde Ejaculation (RE)

DEFINITION

RE is the misdirected propulsion of semen from the posterior urethra into the bladder instead of antegrade through the anterior urethra and out the urethral meatus (25). RE can either be complete, with a total absence of ejaculate, or partial, with preservation of a minimal amount of antegrade ejaculate. Patients will often present to a urologist with infertility or azospermia.

DIAGNOSIS

For the patient with orgasm but no ejaculation, RE appears very similar to AE, and the diagnosis is left to the urologist; the two conditions, in fact, share many common causes. Like most diseases in medicine, a thorough history and physical examination is the foundation for diagnosis. Patients will report a history of aspermia, and any chronic medical conditions, medications, or previous surgeries must be elucidated. The physical examination includes a digital rectal examination and a complete neurological examination. Postejaculate urinalysis revealing greater than five to ten spermatozoa per high-powered field after centrifugation confirms the diagnosis.

ETIOLOGY

For antegrade ejaculation to occur, the prostate, bladder neck, external sphincter, seminal vesicles, vas deferens, and perineal musculature must all be anatomically and functionally intact (25) and follow a coordinated series of events to propel semen through the urethral meatus.

INCIDENCE

Among all patients presenting for infertility, RE is found as the underlying cause in less than 2 percent of the cases but is more frequent in patients with azospermia, accounting for 18 percent of the latter (27, 28).

CAUSES

Common causes of RE can be categorized as anatomic, neurogenic, pharmacological, or idiopathic in origin (Table 21.2). Many of the underlying processes have the ability to cause either AE or RE.

ANATOMIC

Surgical procedures involving the bladder neck that lead to a compromise of its ability to close and remain closed throughout the expulsion phase of ejaculation are the most common anatomic and iatrogenic causes of RE. TURP procedures

Table 21.2: Retrograde Ejaculation Etiologies

Anatomic

  Congenital

    Bladder neck incompetence

    Abnormal location of ejaculatory duct orifice

    Utricular cyst

    Posterior urethral valve/prolapse

  Acquired

    Prostatectomy

    Trauma

    Bladder neck surgery

    Urethral stricture

    Ureterocele

    Bladder neck fibrosis

Pharmacological

  Alpha-adrenergic blockers

  Antihypertensives

  Antidepressants

  Antipsychotics

Neurogenic

  Neuropathic

    Diabetes mellitus

    Multiple sclerosis

  Acquired

    RPLND

    Sympathectomy

    Aortoiliac surgery

    Abdominal Perineal Resection

Toxic

  Alcohol

  Cocaine

  Morphine

Idiopathic

for treatment of benign prostatic hyperplasia cause RE in up to 75 percent of patients; transurethral incision of the prostate has lower rates (29) but still must be considered as a potential etiology. Urethral trauma, bladder neck surgery, ureterocele excision, urethral stricture repair, and open prostatectomy are other surgical causes of anatomic RE. Congenital anatomic anomalies include posterior urethral valves, ectopic ejaculatory duct openings, epispadias, or utricle cysts and may also cause RE.

NEUROGENIC

Similar to AE, both neuropathies and surgical disruption of sympathetic ganglia and hypogastric plexus and nerves can reduce neural tone to the bladder neck, leading to incompetence and RE. Attempts to preserve nerves during RPLND have led to decreased rates of RE following surgical treatments of testicular tumors (30).

IDIOPATHIC

When no offending medication, anatomic abnormality, or neurological cause can be found as the cause of RE, it is considered idiopathic, possibly psychogenic, in nature and accounts for a large percentage of all cases. Fortunately, idiopathic RE responds well to treatment, with medical therapy alone leading to success rates of 78 percent.

TREATMENT

Treatment of RE can be aimed either at simply restoring antegrade ejaculation or allowing for fertility and reproduction. Restoring antegrade ejaculation focuses on increasing sympathetic tone of the bladder neck or decreasing parasympathetic activity. If successful, the return of antegrade ejaculation may be sufficient to allow for natural conception or may provide enough good quality sperm to use with ARTs. Imipramine, given as a daily dose of 25–50 mg for seven days prior to planned intercourse, has been successfully used to treat RE, with a return of antegrade ejaculation in 65–100 percent of patients and a 40 percent rate of spontaneous pregnancy (31). Anticholinergics, alpha-adrenergic agonists, or similar combinations may be used to modulate bladder neck activity but are not as effective as imipramine, which should be considered the first-line therapeutic agent for RE.

SPERM RECOVERY

If medical management fails to return antegrade ejaculation, then attempts can be made to harvest sperm from urine for later use with ART. Since the acidity and high osmolarity or urine is detrimental to spermatozoa motility and viability, two different techniques are commonly employed to adjust the urine within the bladder. The first involves drainage of the bladder by urethral catheter and instillation of isotonic buffer solution that will prevent damage to the sperm. The patient masturbates, and then voids to recover sperm. A less invasive method involves alkalinization of the urine by drinking sodium bicarbonate solutions until the urine has a pH of 7.6–8.1 and an osmolarity of 300–500 mOsm/l. Once again, the patient masturbates and the urine is collected for sperm harvesting.

SUMMARY/KEY POINTS FOR CLINICAL PRACTICE

Ejaculatory dysfunction is the most common male sexual dysfunction, afflicting a high percentage of men and causing both the patient and their partner significant levels of distress. Despite this fact, ejaculatory difficulties are frequently underdiagnosed, undertreated, and underresearched. Premature ejaculation is the most common form of ejaculatory dysfunction, affecting up to one in three men at some point in their lives. Although standardization for PE of a common definition is lacking, most clinical definitions rely on subjective criteria and cutoff points for intravaginal latency time up to two minutes. Although not approved by the FDA for this indication, PE responds well to the SSRI class of medications, administered either on a daily or on an as-needed basis. Paroxetine has been demonstrated to have the least number of adverse events and to be the most effective of this class of medications. PE does not interfere with fertility as long as intravaginal ejaculation occurs. In cases of severe PE, collection devices are useful for achieving fertility when used in conjunction with ART. Retrograde ejaculation, anejaculation, and inhibited ejaculation share many common causes and similar treatments. At the root of RE is the failure of the bladder neck to close during the expulsion phase of ejaculation, which allows semen to travel retrograde into the urinary bladder. Urological and general surgical procedures may often lead to IE, AE, or RE and must be discussed frankly with patients prior to surgery while obtaining informed consent. Medications to treat both AE and RE aim to increase sympathetic tone of the bladder neck and can successfully return normal antegrade flow and allow for spontaneous pregnancy. The success of ED medications and its public awareness has opened the door for more patients to inquire about other sexual dysfunctions, including EjD, and actively seek out medical care. The study of EjD remains in its preliminary stages, with many pathophysiological pathways and pathogenic concepts waiting to be identified and related treatments to be introduced.

REFERENCES

1. Lauman EO, Paik A, Rosen RC. Sexual dysfunction in the United States. *JAMA* 1999;281:537–44.
2. Brooks JD. Chapter 2. Anatomy of the lower urinary tract and male genitalia. In: Wein: Campell-Walsh Urology, 9th ed. Edited by Wein AJ. Saunders (Philadelphia, PA), 2007.
3. Sigman M, Jarow JP. Chapter 19. Male infertility. In: Wein: Campell-Walsh Urology, 9th ed. Edited by Wein AJ. Saunders (Philadelphia, PA), 2007.
4. Veltri R, Rodriguez R. Chapter 85. The molecular biology, endocrinology, and physiology of the prostate and seminal vesicles. In: Wein: Campell-Walsh Urology, 9th ed. Edited by Wein AJ. Saunders (Philadelphia, PA), 2007.
5. American Psychiatric Association. Diagnostic and Statistical Manual of Mental Disorders, 4th ed. Washington, D.C.: American Psychiatric Pub, Inc. 2000.
6. Montague DK, Jarow J, Broderick GA, Dmochowski RR, Heaton JPW, Lue TF, et al. AUA guideline on the pharmacologic management of premature ejaculation. *J Urol* 2004;172:290.
7. Waldinger MD, Schweitzer DH. Changing paradigms from a historical DSM-III and DSM-IV view toward an evidence-based definition of premature ejaculation. Part II—proposals for DSM-V and ICD-11. *J Sex Med* 2006;3:693–705.
8. Waldinger M, Hengeveld M, Zwinderman A, Olivier B. An empirical operationalization of DSM-IV diagnostic criteria for premature ejaculation. *Int J Psychiat Clin Pract* 1998;2:287–93.
9. Spanier G. Measuring dyadic adjustment: new scales for assessing the quality of marriage and similar dyads. *J Marriage Fam* 1976;38:15.
10. Grenier G, Byers S. Operationalizing early or rapid ejaculation. *J Sex Res* 2001;38:369.
11. Schuster TG, Ohl DA. Diagnosis and treatment of ejaculatory dysfunction. *Urol Clin North Am* 2002;29(4):939–48.
12. Reading A, Wiest W. An analysis of self-reported sexual behavior in a sample of normal males. *Arch Sex Behav* 1984;13(1):69–83.
13. Carson CC, Glasser DB, Laumann EO, West SL, Rosen RC. Prevalence and correlates of premature ejaculation among men aged 40 years and older: a United States nationwide population-based study. *J Urol Suppl* 2003;169:321, abstract 1249.
14. Aschka C, Himmel W, Ittner E, Kochen MM. Sexual problems of male patients in family practice. *J Fam Pract* 2001;50:773.
15. Althof SE. Prevalence, characteristics and implications of premature ejaculation/rapid ejaculation. *J Urol* 2006;175(3):842–8.
16. Shamloul R, El Nashaar A. Chronic prostatitis in premature ejaculation: a cohort study in 153 men. *J Sex Med* 2006;3(1):150–4.
17. Waldinger M, Hengeveld MW, Zwinderman AH, Olivier B. Effect of SSRI antidepressants on ejaculation: a double-blind, randomized, placebo-controlled study with fluoxetine, fluvoxamine, paroxetine, and sertraline. *J Clin Psychopharmacol* 1998;18(4):274–81.
18. McMahon CG, Touma K. Treatment of premature ejaculation with paroxetine hydrochloride as needed: 2 single-blind placebo controlled crossover studies. *J Urol* 1999;161:1826.
19. Salonia A, Maga T, Colombo R, et al. A prospective study comparing paroxetine alone versus paroxetine plus sildenafil in patients with premature ejaculation. *J Urol* 2002;168(6):2486–9.
20. Geboes K, Steeno O, De Moor P. Primary anejaculation: diagnosis and therapy. *Fertil Steril* 1975;26:1018.
21. Dunsmuir WD, Emberton M. Surgery, drugs, and the male orgasm: informed consent can't be assumed unless effects on orgasm have been discussed. *BMJ* 1997;314(7077):319–20.
22. Mattson D, Petrie M, Srivastava DK, McDermott M. Multiple sclerosis: sexual dysfunction and its response to medications. *Arch Neurol* 1995;52(9):862–8.
23. Hargreave T. Male fertility disorders. *Endocrinol Metab Clin North Am* 1998;27(4):765–82, vii–viii.
24. Paick J, Kim SH, Kim SW. Ejaculatory duct obstruction in infertile men. *Br J Urol Int* 2000;85:720–4.
25. Kendirci M, Hellstrom WJG. Retrograde ejaculation: etiology, diagnosis, and management. *Curr Sex Health Rep* 2006;3:133–8.
26. Hellstrom WJG, Sikka SC. Effects of acute treatment with tamsulosin versus alfuzosin on ejaculatory function in normal volunteers. *J Urol* 2006;176:10.
27. Yavetz H, Yogev L, Hauser R, et al. Retrograde ejaculation. *Hum Reprod* 1994;9:381–6.
28. Van der Linden PJQ, Nan PM, te Velde ER, et al. Retrograde ejaculation: successful treatment with artificial insemination. *Obstet Gynecol* 1992;79:126.
29. AUA Practice Guidelines Committee. AUA Guideline on Management of Benign Prostatic Hyperplasia (2003). Chapter 1. Diagnosis and treatment recommendations. *J Urol* 2003;170(2 Pt 1):530–47.
30. Solsona E. Preservation of antegrade ejaculation in retroperitoneal lymphadenectomy due to residual masses after primary chemotherapy for testicular carcinoma. *Eur Urol* 1994;25(3):199–203.
31. Ochsenkühn R, Kamischke A, Nieschlag E. Imipramine for successful treatment of retrograde ejaculation caused by retroperitoneal surgery. *Int J Androl* 1999;22(3):173–7.

■ 22 ■

OVULATION INDUCTION

Evert J. P. Van Santbrink, Bart C. J. M. Fauser

INTRODUCTION

Primary treatment of patients presenting with infertility and chronic anovulation aims at restoring normal physiology, that is, selection of a single dominant follicle followed by mono-ovulation (ESHRE Capri Workshop Group, 2003). This process is generally referred to as "ovulation induction." Alternative protocols for ovarian stimulation used in fertility treatment are (controlled) ovarian hyperstimulation used for intrauterine insemination or in vitro fertilization (IVF). These treatment protocols are aimed at the development of multiple instead of one dominant follicle and thereby result in a nonphysiological condition.

Anovulation is a relatively common problem in the infertility population (approximately, 21 percent of fertility couples; Hull et al., 1985), and it may be considered an absolute factor to prevent pregnancy. Treatment results may be expected to be very good when normoovulatory cycles are restored, in the absence of concomitant fertility problems.

Classification of anovulation is generally based on the combination of a menstrual cycle disturbance (oligo- or amenorrhea) and laboratory findings (Insler et al., 1968; Rowe et al., 1993). The majority of anovulatory patients (about 80 percent, Rowe et al., 1993) will have normal serum concentrations of estradiol (E_2) and follicle-stimulating hormone (FSH) and a small proportion (approximately 10 percent) decreased concentrations of both hormones (WHO2 and WHO1, respectively according to the WHO-classification). The remaining group (approximately 10 percent) may be classified as WHO3 and they present with elevated FSH combined along with decreased E_2 concentrations resulting in anovulation caused by (imminent) ovarian failure or premature ovarian aging. Whereas ovulation induction can be regarded as a useful treatment option in the WHO1 (hypogonadotropic hypo-estrogenic anovulatory patients) and WHO2 (normogonadotropic normo-estrogenic anovulatory patients) population, treatment options in the WHO3 group (hypergonadotropic hypo-estrogenic anovulatory patients) are limited to IVF (combined with oocyte donation) or adoption programs. Within the WHO2 population a subgroup can be identified, well known as the polycystic ovary syndrome (PCOS). For many years there was much confusion about the definition of this syndrome (van Santbrink et al., 1997a) until in 2003 a consensus meeting was held in Rotterdam, The Netherlands (PCOS consensus, 2004). For the definition of PCOS two of the following criteria are required: 1) oligo- or anovulation,

2) clinical and/or biochemical signs of hyperandrogenism, and 3) polycystic ovaries on ultrasound. Other etiologies of these criteria should be excluded.

Body weight is considered to have a significant impact on ovarian function (Kiddy et al., 1992; Clark et al., 1998) and nearly 50 percent of WHO2 patients are obese [body mass index (BMI = length/weight^2) > 25 m/kg^2]. Since this negative effect of overweight is reversible, weight reduction should be advised before any treatment is started.

After patient selection, ovulation induction may be started using various interventions. Traditionally, first-line treatment of WHO2 patients consists of antiestrogenic therapy, in case of treatment failure followed by FSH. Recently introduced alternative interventions such as insulin-sensitizing drugs (Nestler et al., 1998), aromatase inhibitors (Mitwally and Casper, 2003), laparoscopic ovarian electrocautery (LEO) (Greenblatt and Casper, 1987), or combinations of the above mentioned may be introduced in this sequence, when proven effective (Figure 22.1; van Santbrink et al., 2000b).

Multiple follicle development associated with multiple pregnancy and ovarian hyperstimulation syndrome (OHSS) remain the major complication, although the use of low-dose FSH protocols and extensive ovarian monitoring during the stimulation and (Fauser and van Heusden, 1997) may considerably reduce these risks (Rizk and Aboulghar, 1991; Rizk and Smitz, 1992; Aboulghar and Mansour, 2006; Rizk, 2006).

Efforts to improve treatment outcome of ovulation induction are increasingly focused on patient characteristics instead of treatment characteristics. Hopefully, this will enable us to develop a more "patient-tailored" approach in which an ideal selective use of the various interventions in an optimal sequence can be offered for each individual patient. This may result in more patient convenience, better treatment results, and less complications.

PHYSIOLOGICAL FOLLICULAR DEVELOPMENT

A continuous flow of primordial follicles from a resting to a growing stage can be observed throughout life. During the first (intra-uterine) period of life, follicle depletion starts at a very high rate, and approximately 2 million primordial follicles remain at birth (Fauser and van Heusden, 1997). After birth, this process decelerates and when reproductive life starts at menarche, approximately 0.5 million primordial follicles are present. Initiation of follicle growth occurs continuously and independent of the menstrual cycle. Development from primordial to

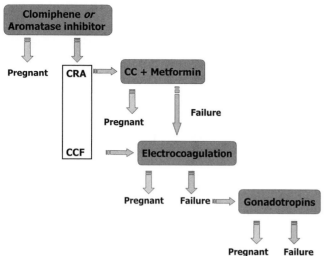

Figure 22.1. A possible future treatment algorithm for ovulation induction: first-line treatment with clomiphene (CC) or aromatase inhibitor, followed by metformin or LEO, and finally after treatment failure patients will receive gonadotropins. Initial patient characteristics will predict the optimal individual treatment sequence. CRA = clomiphene resistant anovulation; CCF = clomiphene treatment failure.

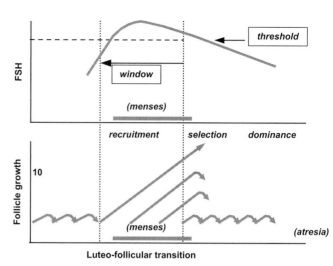

Figure 22.2. The FSH threshold/window concept. In the physiological situation (left panel), early follicular phase increase in serum FSH concentration above the FSH threshold induces follicular growth; when followed by FSH decrease (narrow FSH window), this prevents selection of multiple follicles (left panel). In ovarian hyperstimulation, intentional multiple follicle development results from absence of FSH decrease (upper line, right panel).

a pre-ovulatory follicle takes at least 85 days and only the last part of follicle development is gonadotropin dependent. In a lifetime, approximately 400 follicles will reach full maturation and ovulate. The remaining follicles become atretic before reaching maturity. Most of the involved regulatory processes remain unknown.

When a follicle reaches the stage of gonadotropin responsiveness during the women's early follicular FSH rise, this follicle is stimulated to continue growing (recruited). It must be considered that at every time point, there are many follicles in slightly different developmental stages that are ready to be recruited. They will go into atresia when there is not sufficient gonadotropin exposure. By exposure to gonadotropins, inside the growing follicle, cholesterol will be converted to androstenedione in the theca-cells and this will be aromatized to E_2 in the granulosa cells. This is referred to as the "two-cell two-gonadotropin" theory (McGee and Hsueh, 2000).

As all follicles are in a (slightly) different developmental stage and the fact that a larger follicle needs less FSH to continue growing, it is postulated that in the early follicular phase serum FSH concentrations increase until the FSH "threshold" for ongoing follicle growth is surpassed (Brown, 1978; van Santbrink et al., 1995). This results in follicle recruitment and initiation of production of large amounts of E_2 by the growing follicles (Figure 22.2). Due to negative feedback of the rising inhibin B and E_2 serum concentrations at the hypothalamic-pituitary level, FSH serum concentrations will decrease in response. Since each follicle has its own FSH threshold and this changes when the follicle becomes bigger, only the largest follicle that needs the smallest amount of FSH is able to continue growing and becomes the dominant follicle. The time that the FSH threshold is surpassed is called the FSH-window (Fauser and van Heusden, 1997). When the window is narrow, only one follicle becomes dominant. When the window is wider, more follicles may become dominant (multi follicular growth).

INTERVENTIONS FOR OVULATION INDUCTION

Hypogonadotropic Anovulation

Anovulation in hypogonadotropic hypo-estrogenic (WHO1) patients may result from a hypothalamic or pituitary problem. To distinguish between these two, a gonadotropin-releasing hormone (GnRH) stimulation test can help. The pulsatile administration of GnRH will cause an increase in serum gonadotropins, when the pituitary gland is functional. Fertility treatment may consist of a pulsatile GnRH pump or direct stimulation of the ovaries with exogenous gonadotropins (FSH and LH). Whereas continuous GnRH administration results in pituitary "down regulation" that is used in IVF procedures to prevent a premature LH rise (Filicori, 1994), pulsatile GnRH administration may restore ovulation including a physiological feedback loop in patients with inadequate hypothalamic function. In case of FSH stimulation it must be considered that a corpus luteum insufficiency will occur in absence of a functional LH-pulse generator (hypothalamic dysfunction) in this patient group. This luteal insufficiency can be prevented by administration of "luteal support" by providing human chorionic gonadotropin (hCG) or progesterone during the period from ovulation until sufficient hCG production is provided by the trophoblast cells (Beckers et al., 2006).

Normogonadotropic Anovulation

Although the classical treatment sequence for normogonadotropic anovulation (WHO2) is clomiphene citrate followed by FSH, a number of new interventions are proven to be useful for these patients. Still, it is unclear if and at what point they would be of additional value in the classical sequence.

Weight Reduction

Body weight is considered to have a significant impact on ovarian function (Kiddy et al., 1992; Clark et al., 1998) and nearly 50 percent of WHO2 patients are obese (BMI = length/weight^2 >25 m/kg^2). Insulin resistance and concomitant increase in serum insulin concentrations are considered to play a keyrole in the pathophysiology of adverse health effects coinciding obesity. These effects may not only include increased chances on cycle disturbance (anovulation), early pregnancy loss, and various disorders during pregnancy (hypertension, pregnancy diabetes, and less favorable neonatal outcome) but also increased long-term health risks as diabetes mellitus and cardiovascular disease (Norman et al., 2002). Moreover, during treatment for anovulation, overweight and obese patients are prone for less favorable outcome. During treatment with antiestrogens, obesity is correlated with anovulation and decreased live birth rates (Imani et al., 2002), while during FSH ovulation induction more ampoules of FSH needed, increased cycle cancellation rates, and persistent anovulation are reported (White et al., 1996; Mulders et al., 2003).

Lifestyle modification resulting in weight reduction is reported to result in restoration of the endocrine milieu: improving insulin sensitivity and hyperandrogenism (Kiddy et al., 1992). This also may have beneficial effects not only on return of menstrual cyclicity and spontaneous pregnancy rates but also on outcome parameters of fertility treatment (Clark et al., 1998). Since this negative effect of overweight may be reversible, weight reduction should be strongly advised before any treatment is started (Hoeger, 2006).

A very low BMI (<19 m/kg^2) may also cause cycle disturbances and anovulation. Women exposed to excessive exercise or suffering from anorexia or bulimia are prone to develop a hypogonadotropic, hypo-estrogenic amenorrhea (WHO1). When in these patients the metabolic state is normalized reflected by a normal BMI (>20 m/kg^2), a regular menstrual cycle will be restored in the majority of patients (Stafford, 2005).

Dopamine Agonists

Introduction: The most common cause of hyperprolactinemia is a prolactin secreting (micro)adenoma of the pituitary. The preferred imaging method of these adenomas is by magnetic resonance imaging (MRI). They are arbitrarily classified as microadenoma (<1 cm) and macroadenoma (>1 cm) and clinical signs may be galactorrhea, amenorrhea, headache, and bitemporal hemianopia. Patients presenting with oligo- or amenorrhea due to hyperprolactinemia may be effectively treated with dopamine agonists (see Chapter 29).

Working mechanism: Dopamine agonists inhibit prolactine secretion.

Treatment schedule: Bromocriptine is started in a dosage of half a tablet (2.5 mg) daily and the dosage may be increased when prolactin concentrations are not decreasing to a maximum of two to three times daily, 2.5 mg.

Treatment results: Return of a regular ovulatory menstrual cycle occurs in about 80 percent of treated patients, and assuming there are no other factors decreasing fertility, pregnancy chances are returning to normal.

Complications: Side effects of dopamine agonists may be syncope, nausea, and vomiting. Bromocriptine is the most widely used dopamine agonist and no adverse effects are reported

for this drug when used during pregnancy, while less is known for more recently developed preparations as cabergoline (the manufacturer advises discontinuation at least one month before pregnancy) and quinagolide.

Antiestrogens

Clomiphene Citrate (CC)

Introduction: Antiestrogens have been used since the early 1960s for ovulation induction. They are effective, safe, easy to use, and cheap and therefore first-line treatment in normogonadotropic anovulation (see Chapter 23).

Working mechanism: The non-selective E$_2$ receptor antagonist CC interferes with endogenous estrogen feedback at the hypothalamic-pituitary level causing increased gonadotropin release by the pituitary gland.

Treatment schedule: After a spontaneous or progestagen induced withdrawal bleeding, CC is generally started on day 3 and continued for five days with a daily dose of 50 mg. The daily dose may be increased in two steps to a maximum of 150 mg in case of persistent anovulation. Several studies reported effect of the chosen starting day: when clomiphene treatment was started on day 5 rather than day 1, this resulted in a decreased ovulation and pregnancy rate (Debahsi et al., 2006).

Treatment results: Restoration of ovulation will occur in about 80 percent of treated patients and a cumulative live birth rate of about 40 percent may be expected (Imani et al., 1998). Most pregnancies will occur in the first six ovulatory cycles and after twelve cycles pregnancy is unlikely (Koustra et al., 1997).

Complications: Hot flushes and nausea are reported but uncommon side effects. Multiple follicular development has been often described. A multiple pregnancy rate between 2 and 13 percent is reported. Severe ovarian hyperstimulation syndrome has not been reported following CC treatment (Homburg, 2005). A possible increased risk of ovarian cancer after use of CC longer that twelve months together with decreased pregnancy chances after this period may result in a recommendation to not to use this drug more than 12 months (Rossing et al., 1994).

Tamoxiphene (TMX)

Introduction: Comparable to CC but less popular in ovulation induction, possible advantage over CC may be less antiestrogenic effect on endometrium and cervical mucus (Roumen et al., 1984).

Working mechanism: A nonselective estrogen receptor modulator, developed for the treatment of breast cancer but used for ovulation induction for many years.

Treatment schedule: After a spontaneous or progestagen-induced withdrawal bleeding, TMX is generally started on day 3 and continued for five days with a daily dose of 20 mg. The daily dose may be increased in two steps to a maximum of 60 mg in case of persistent anovulation.

Treatment results: In a prospective randomized trial, the efficacy of CC and TMX were compared in 86 normogonadotropic anovulatory patients and no significant differences in ovulation and pregnancy rates were reported (Boostanfar et al., 2001).

Complications: No specific complications are reported but it may be comparable with CC.

Insulin Sensitizers (metformin)

Introduction: It is generally accepted that insulin resistance plays an important role in the pathogenesis of normogonadotropic anovulation (PCOS consensus, 2004). Hyperinsulinemia causes hyperandrogenism by increasing ovarian androgen production and decreasing sex steroid – binding globulin serum concentrations, resulting in an increased bio availability of androgens. Moreover, hyperinsulinemia facilitates an estrogen hyperresponse on FSH stimulation resulting in an early FSH drop. This causes follicle growth arrest in the early follicular phase and the classic polycystic image of the ovaries on ultrasound. As obese patients may benefit insulin sensitizers most (Lord et al., 2003), it may be important to realize that weight reduction by lifestyle modification is a primary solution for this problem and insulin sensitizers alone will not cause weight reduction (Lord et al., 2003).

Working mechanism: Insulin sensitizers are reported to restore the endocrine milieu: lowering insulin resistance and hyperandrogenism normalizes ovarian FSH responsiveness and thereby promotes restoration of ovulatory cycles (Coffler et al., 2003).

Treatment schedule: metformin is started in a daily dose of $2–3 \times 500$ mg to a maximum daily dose of 2000 mg.

Treatment results: First-line treatment with metformin is not superior to CC (Lord et al., 2003), neither is combined use of metformin and CC (Moll et al., 2006). In contrast, second-line treatment of patients presenting with clomiphene resistant anovulation (CRA) and a BMI > 25 kg/m^2 by additional metformin to CC results in a 50 percent ovulation rate (Lord et al., 2003). Addition of metformin to gonadotropin ovulation induction may result in a more physiological ovarian response (less hyperstimulation) and reduced amounts of FSH needed, especially in obese and hyperandrogenic subjects (Yarali et al., 2002; van Santbrink et al., 2005a). Unfortunately, data available on this topic are inconclusive due to limited patient numbers included.

Complications: Severe gastrointestinal complaints are reported: nausea, vomiting, and diarrhea. These side effects will diminish when metformin is used for a longer period. Metformin may reduce risk of gestational diabetes and it may be safe using it during pregnancy (Glueck et al., 2004), but convincing evidence is lacking. Always discuss with patients that metformin is not licensed for ovulation induction.

Aromatase Inhibitors

Introduction: Although the action of aromatase inhibitors (inhibition of negative feedback by blocking estrogen synthesis) may be comparable to anti-estrogens, the advantage could be the lack of antiestrogenic effects on target organs as the endometrium and cervical mucus (see Chapter 24). Unfortunately, only small and uncontrolled studies have been conducted in mostly normal ovulating women (Fisher et al., 2002), and recently, potential fetal toxicity was reported for Letrozole, resulting in an official warning by the producer (Novartis Pharmaceuticals) to avoid using it for this indication.

Working mechanism: Inhibition of aromatase activity in the granulosa cells prevents conversion of androgens into estrogens and thereby inhibits negative feedback on the hypothalamic-pituitary level.

Treatment schedule: After a spontaneous or progestagen-induced withdrawal bleeding, Letrozole is generally started on day 3 and continued for five days with a daily dose of 2.5 mg.

Treatment results: In a prospective randomized trial the efficacy of CC 100 mg and Letrozole 2.5 mg, administered from days 3 to 7, were compared in seventy four PCOS patients that had no former fertility treatment. Although decreased E$_2$

concentration were reported in the Letrozole group on the day of hCG administration, comparable ovulation and pregnancy rates were reported (Bayar et al., 2006).

Complications: Recently, potential fetal toxicity was reported for Letrozole resulting in a official warning by the producer, although the short half-life and use during the early follicular phase may limit the possibilities of substantial influence on fetal organogenesis (Tiboni, 2004).

Laparoscopic Electrocautery of the Ovaries

Introduction: From the classic wedge resection described by Stein and Leventhal (1935), the surgical approach to ovulation induction evolved to laparoscopic electrocautery and laser treatment. The major advantage is that there is no increased risk for multiple pregnancies (see Chapter 31).

Working mechanism: Electrocautery of the ovarian surface has been demonstrated to decrease hyperandrogenism and may restore ovulation in normogonadotropic anovulatory patients by an unknown mechanism.

Treatment schedule: Laparoscopic electrocoagulation of the ovarian surface.

Treatment results: LEO was compared to CC/FSH ovulation induction in normogonadotropic CRA patients (Bayram et al., 2004). The LEO group received CC/FSH co-treatment after six months. Follow-up after one year reported equal ovulation and pregnancy rates, but reduced multiple pregnancy rates in the LEO group. LEO alone resulted in less than 50 percent ovulatory cycles and time to pregnancy was doubled in the LEO group. LEO was also compared to metformin treatment in a placebo-controlled randomized trial in overweight normogonadotropic patient remaining anovulatory during CC treatment. metformin was more effective in treatment results as well as health economics (Palomba et al., 2004).

Complications: Laparoscopic surgical complications have to be discussed, but are rare.

Gonadotropins

Introduction: Gonadotropins are available from the early 1960s. At first, gonadotropins were extracted from urine of postmenopausal women (human menopausal gonadotropin) in a 1:1 ratio of LH and FSH. To improve batch-to-batch variability, nonactive proteins were removed resulting in highly purified urinary preparations. The urinary extraction process needed large amounts of postmenopausal urine and the increasing demands for gonadotropins compromised the possibilities to guarantee a consistent supply of the medication worldwide. When in the 1990s recombinant DNA technology made it possible to produce human FSH in Chinese hamster ovary cell lines, this production problem was solved. Moreover, these recombinant preparations offer improved purity and consistency. Batch-to-batch variation may be limited by using protein weight instead of bioactivity to determine the amount of active protein per unit. This resulted in a more general use of recombinant instead of urinary gonadotropins for ovulation induction in the past 15 years. Patients remaining anovulatory or failing to conceive after first-line treatment with antiestrogens, antiestrogens combined with metformin, aromatase inhibitors, or LEO are generally treated with exogenous gonadotropins. Individual differences in the required daily amount of FSH to induce ongoing follicle growth (the FSH response dose) have been suggested to be the main factor in hyperresponsiveness and severe complications during gonadotropin ovulation induction

(Fauser and van Heusden, 1997). This resulted in mainly two different approaches: the "step-up" and "step-down" protocols.

Working mechanism: Direct stimulation of follicle growth in the ovary.

Treatment schedule: The step-up protocol is aimed at increasing the initial low daily FSH dose (37.5–50 IU) by small increments (37.5–50 IU), until finally the FSH threshold is surpassed, resulting in ongoing follicle growth and ovulation. The step-down protocol is aimed at a starting dose of FSH that equals the response dose and thereby directly will cause ongoing follicle growth (van Santbrink and Fauser, 1997b). Thereafter, the daily FSH dose can be decreased (37.5–50 IU) every three days resulting in the development of a single dominant follicle. Although the step-down protocol mimics the physiological serum FSH profile more closely and dominant follicle growth is established more quickly, it appears that for a considerable percentage of patients treated according to a step-up protocol the FSH starting dose appears to be the response dose (van Santbrink and Fauser, 1997; Christin Maitre and Hugues, 2003). When those easy-responding patients (with a low FSH threshold) will be treated according to a step-down protocol, the starting dose would be too high resulting in multifollicular growth. To determine the individual FSH response dose, a dose-finding step-up cycle can be used and consecutive treatment cycles can be performed according to the step-down protocol, unless the starting dose equals the response dose. In that case, a fixed dose regimen can be used (van Santbrink et al., 2005b).

Frequent monitoring of ovarian response by ultrasonography is the most important tool to prevent multifollicular development because the duration of the FSH threshold being surpassed determines whether there will be mono- or multi follicular growth (Fauser and van Heusden, 1997). hCG is used to trigger ovulation when at least one follicle with a diameter of 16 mm is present. Stimulation is canceled when more than three follicles larger than 12 mm in diameter are present.

Treatment results: Cumulative ovulation rate of 82 percent, ongoing pregnancy rate of 58 percent, single live birth rate of 43 percent, and multiple birth rate of 5 percent (Mulders et al., 2003).

Complications: Although the overall multiple pregnancy rates after gonadotropin ovulation induction seems to be acceptable, the contribution of ovulation induction to higher order multiple pregnancies is substantial (Fauser et al., 2005). Chances for OHSS and multiple pregnancy after gonadotropin ovulation induction are related to frequent monitoring and strict cancellation criteria (Aboulghar and Mansour, 2003; Rizk, 2006).

Opioid Antagonists (Naltrexon)

Introduction: The hypothalamic pulse generator that controls GnRH secretion is inhibited by endogenous opioids (Dobson et al., 2003). Opioid receptor antagonists have been shown to increase GnRH pulsatility and thereby pulsatile LH secretion in the pituitary (Yen et al., 1985). In the 1990s, opioid receptor antagonists were explored to elucidate if they could be used to treat anovulation in hypo- and normogonadotropic anovulation (WHO1 and WHO2).

Working mechanism: Opioid receptor antagonists that inhibit hypothalamic GnRH secretion.

Treatment schedule: Daily dose of 50–100 mg in two gifts are reported.

Table 22.1: Pregnancy Rates of 240 Normogonadotrophic Anovulatory Infertility Patients (WHO2) Treated with CC and FSH Including Combined Sequential Cumulative Treatment Results. (Reproduced with permission from van Santbrink, 2005b.)

	Cumulative pregnancy rate (%)	Cumulative singleton live birth rate
CC	47	37
FSH	58[a]	43
CC + FSH	78	71

[a]Cumulative ongoing pregnancy rate.

Treatment results: Conflicting data on treatment success are reported in hypothalamic anovulation patients (WHO1); this was explained by the fact that gonadal steroids may enhance opioid modulation (Couzinet et al., 1995). Others combined opioid receptor antagonists with CC in patients with clomiphene-resistant anovulation in normogonado tropic anovulation (WHO2) this small study resulted in an 86 percent ovulation rate (Roozenburg et al., 1997). Unfortunately, no randomized controlled studies are published yet to prove the additional value of opioid antagonists in ovulation induction.

Complications: Data on safe use of opioid receptor antagonists during pregnancy are not available.

Ovulation Induction in Practice

Results of Ovulation Induction

In a large prospective, follow-up study, 259 patients, after first referral to a fertility clinic, with normogonadotropic anovulatory infertility were treated according to the classic algorithm starting with CC (Imani et al., 1998). This resulted in an 80 percent ovulation rate and a cumulative live birth rate of 41 percent. The patients remaining anovulatory (CRA) or failing to conceive were treated with exogenous FSH. This resulted in an 89 percent ovulation rate and a 58 percent cumulative conception rate after six ovulation induction cycles (see Table 22.1). The total classic treatment sequence of CC followed by exogenous FSH in case of treatment failure resulted after a 24-month follow-up in a 71 percent cumulative singleton live birth rate (Eykemans et al., 2003). Alternative interventions for ovulation induction have been introduced during recent years. Their effectiveness compared to the classic sequence has been evaluated for subgroups of patients and will be discussed subsequently. As discussed before, first-line treatment with the insulin sensitizer metformin alone or combined with CC is not superior to CC. But in obese patients (BMI > 25 kg/m2) who remain anovulatory despite the highest dose of CC, co-treatment with insulin sensitizers with a 56 percent ovulation rate compared to 35 percent in the placebo group (Costello and Eden, 2003). LEO has also been evaluated as possible second-line ovulation induction therapy after CRA (Bayram et al., 2004). Laparoscopic electrocautery of the ovaries was compared to CC/FSH ovulation induction. Ovulation and pregnancy rates were comparable in both groups but multiple pregnancy rates were lower in the LEO group. In a placebo-controlled randomized trial, LEO and metformin were compared directly as second-line ovulation induction treatment intervention (Palomba et al., 2004). Metformin was more effective as well in treatment results as in costs.

Complications of Ovulation Induction

The major complication of ovulation induction is development of multiple follicles resulting in increased chances of multiple pregnancy and OHSS (Aboulghar and Mansour, 2003). Because a distinct variability exists in intra- and interindividual ovarian response to treatment compounds and regimens, intensive ultrasound monitoring is mandatory to prevent unrestricted follicle growth.

Multiple pregnancy rate after CC treatment is reported between 2 and 13 percent and mainly twin pregnancies are reported (Imani et al., 1998; Homburg, 2003). For gonadotropin induction of ovulation, multiple pregnancy rates between 5 and 20 percent are reported (Fauser and van Heusden, 1997). Although the contribution of ovulation induction to the reported frequency of all multiple pregnancies is relatively small, the contribution to higher order multiple pregnancies is at least substantial (Figure 22.3; Fauser et al., 2005). This may be due to suboptimal monitoring utilities in smaller fertility clinics (see Chapter 28).

In OHSS, the following symptoms and signs may be determined: gross enlargement of the ovaries (>6 cm diameter), ascites and sometimes pleural effusion caused by increased vascular permeability, thromboembolism, liver function abnormalities, renal failure, adult respiratory stress syndrome, and shock. Symptoms may be abdominal discomfort, nausea, vomiting, diarrhea, and dyspnoea. Treatment may include maintenance of intravascular volume, thrombosis prophylaxis, function of ascites, and suppletion of plasma albumin. Mild and severe OHSS is hardly seen after CC ovulation induction, and in gonadotropin treatment, frequencies reported are between 2 and 5 percent (Fauser and van Heusden, 1997).

PERSPECTIVES OF OVULATION INDUCTION

Individualized Treatment Protocol in Ovulation Induction

The conventional treatment of normogonadotropic anovulatory infertility is anti-estrogens followed by exogenous gonadotropins, in case of treatment failure. This algorithm may be effective, as discussed earlier, but is associated with complications related to limited control of follicle growth. Due to individual differences in treatment response, multiple follicle development instead of maturation of a single oocyte occurs, which may result in multiple pregnancy and OHSS. Efforts to improve treatment outcome and decrease complication of ovulation induction were mainly directed at purification of compounds and alternative dose regimens. Evidence accumulates that factors determining ovarian response are initial patient characteristics instead of treatment regimens. This implies that prognostic models using these initial patient characteristics may be able to predict for an individual patient the chances on success and complication for every compound available. Before clinical application of these prognostic models is allowed, they should be developed and validated for every intervention and population in which it is used. Prognostic models have been developed for spontaneous pregnancy chances (Snick et al., 1997; Hunault et al., 2005), CC (Imani et al., 2002b; Figure 22.4), gonadotropins (Imani et al., 2002a;

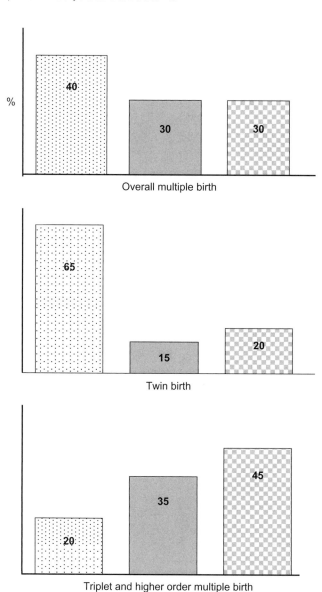

Figure 22.3. Contribution (percent) of ovarian stimulation and IVF to overall multiple birth (upper panel), twin pregnancies (middle panel), and triplet and higher order pregnancies (lower panel).

Mulders et al., 2003), and LEO (Amer et al., 2004). Prognostic models are able to identify patients who will not respond effectively to a certain treatment modality. Moreover, an optimal individual treatment sequence (Figure 22.1) may be discussed before treatment is started with every patient, reducing complications and improving treatment outcome and health economics (Eijkemans et al., 2005).

Recommendations

Although ovulation induction aims at restoration of monofollicular development and ovulation, major complications result from limited control of follicle growth. Multiple pregnancies and OHSS are the price to pay. Intensive monitoring by experienced professionals may decrease the risk on these complications. Inter- and intraindividual variation of ovarian response

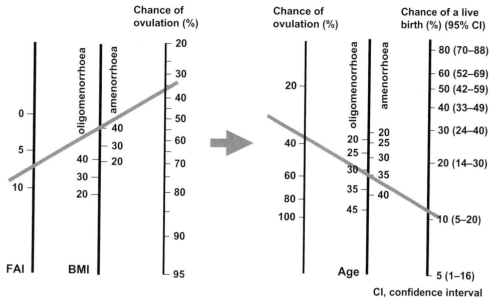

Figure 22.4. A nomogram predicting live birth after CC treatment in normogonadotropic anovulatory infertility, based on initial patient characteristics cycle history (oligo or amenorrhea), BMI (= weight [kg] divided by squared height [m]), free-androgen index (FAI = testosterone [T] × 100/sex-binding globulin and age. (Reproduced with permission from Imani et al. 2002b.)

to stimulation is hard to predict in this heterogeneous group of patients. New compounds or strategies such as insulin sensitizers, aromatase inhibitors, and LEO should be compared to traditional compounds in patient subgroups with various characteristics. Multivariate prognostic models using initial patient characteristics will be able to help identify these subgroups that have favorable treatment outcome with a certain intervention. This strategy may enable professionals to propose a treatment plan for every individual patient based on initial patient characteristics. Chances for success and complications may be discussed in advance. This will reduce complications and benefit patient and doctors convenience.

KEY POINTS FOR CLINICAL PRACTICE

- Ovulation induction aims at restoration of monofollicular development and mono-ovulation.
- Intensive monitoring is mandatory to prevent complications.
- Conventional ovulation induction (CC followed by FSH) is a highly effective treatment sequence (cumulative singleton live birth rate 71 percent after twenty four months follow-up).
- Treatment response is determined by individual patient characteristics.
- Patient-tailored treatment sequences may be able to further optimize the results of ovulation induction.

REFERENCES

Aboulghar M.A. and Mansour R.T. (2006). Ovarian hyperstimulation syndrome: classifications and critical analysis of preventive measures. *Human Reproduction Update*, 9, 275–289.

Amer S.A., Li T.C. and Ledger W.L. (2004). Ovulation induction using laparoscopic ovarian drilling in women with PCOS: predictors of success. *Human Reproduction*, 19, 1719–1724.

Bayar U., Basaran M., Kiran S., Coskun A. and Gezer S. (2006). Use of an aromatase inhibitor in patients with polycystic ovary syndrome: a prospective randomized trial. *Fertility and Sterility*, 86, 1447–1451.

Bayram N., van Wely M., Kaayk E.M., Bossuyt P.M. and van der Veen F. (2004). Using an electrocautery strategy or recombinant follicle stimulating hormone to induce ovulation in polycystic ovary syndrome: randomised controlled trial. *British Medical Journal*, 328, 192–195.

Beckers N.G., Platteau P., Eijkemans M.J., Macklon N.S., de Jong F.H., Devroey P. and Fauser B.C. (2006). The early luteal phase administration of estrogen and progesterone does not induce premature luteolysis in normo-ovulatory women. *European Journal of Endocrinology*, 155, 355–363.

Boostanfar R., Jain J.K., Nishell D.R. and Paulson R.J. (2001). A prospective randomized trial comparing clomiphene citrate with tamoxifen citrate for ovulation induction. *Fertility and Sterility*, 75, 1024–1026.

Brown J.B. (1978) Pituitary control of ovarian function – concepts derived from gonadotropin therapy. *The Australian and New Zealand Journal Obstetrics and Gynecology*, 18, 47–54.

Christin-Maitre S. and Hugues J.N. (2003). A comparative randomized multicentric study comparing the step-up versus step-down protocol in polycystic ovary syndrome. *Human Reproduction*, 18, 1626–1631.

Clark A.M., Thornley B., Tomlinson L., Galletley C. and Norman R.J. (1998). Weight loss in obese infertile women results in improvement of reproductive outcome for all forms of fertility treatment. *Human Reproduction*, 13, 1502–1505.

Coffler M.S., Patel K., Dahan M.H., Yoo R.Y., Malcom P.J. and Chang R.J. (2003). Enhanced granulosa cell responsiveness to FSH during insulin infusion in women with PCOS treated with pioglitazone. *Journal of Clinical Endocrinology and Metabolism*, 88, 5624–5631.

Costello M.F. and Eden J.A. (2003). A systematic review of the reproductive system effects of metformin in patients with PCOS. *Fertility and Sterility*, 79, 1–13.

Couzinet B., Young J., Brailly S., Chanson P. and Schaison G. (1995). Even after priming with ovarian steroids or pulsatile gonadotropin-releasing hormone administration, naltrexon is unable to induce ovulation in women with functional hypothalamic amenorrhea. *Journal of Clinical Endocrinology and Metabolism*, 80, 2102–2107.

Dehbashi S., Vafaei H., Parsanezhad M.D. and Alborzi S. (2006). Time of initiation of clomiphene citrate and pregnancy rate in polycystic ovarian syndrome. *International Journal of Gynaecology and Obstetrics*, 93, 44–48.

Dobson H., Ghuman S., Prabhakar S. and Smith R. (2003). A conceptual model of the influence of stress on female reproduction. *Reproduction*, 125, 151–163.

Eijkemans M.J., Imani B., Mulders A.G., Habbema J.D. and Fauser B.C. (2005). High singleton live birth rate following classical ovulation induction in normogonadotropic anovulatory infertility. *Human Reproduction*, 18, 2357–2362.

Eijkemans M.J., Polinder S., Mulders A.G., Laven J.S., Habbema J.D. and Fauser B.C. (2005). Individualized cost-effective conventional ovulation induction treatment in normogonadotrophic anovulatory infertility (WHO₂). *Human Reproduction*, 20, 2830–2837.

ESHRE Capri Workshop Group. (2003). Mono-ovulatory cycles: a key goal in profertility programmes. *Human Reproduction Update*, 9, 263–274.

Fauser B.C. and van Heusden A.M. (1997). Manipulation of human ovarian function: physiological concepts and clinical consequences. *Endocrine Reviews*, 18, 71–106.

Fauser B.C., Devroey P. and Macklon N.S. (2005). Multiple birth resulting from ovarian stimulation for subfertility treatment. *Lancet*, 365, 1807–1816.

Filicori M. (1994). Gonadotrophin releasing hormone agonists. A guide to use and selection. *Drugs*, 48, 41–58.

Fisher S.A., Reid R.L., van Vught D.A. and Casper R.F. (2002). A randomized double blind comparison of the effects of CC and the aromatase inhitor letrozole on the ovulatory function in normal women. *Fertility and Sterility*, 78, 280–285.

Glueck C.J., Goldenberg N., Pranikoff J., Loftspring M., Sieve L. and Wang P. (2004). Height, weight and motor-social development during the first 18 months of life in 126 infants born to 109 mothers with polycystic ovary syndrome who conceived on and continued metformin through pregnancy. *Human Reproduction*, 19, 1323–1330.

Greenblatt E. and Casper R.F. (1987). Endocrine changes after laparoscopic ovarian cautery in polycystic ovary syndrome. *American Journal of Obstetrics and Gynecology*, 156, 279–285.

Hoeger K.M. (2006). Role of lifestyle modification in the management of polycystic ovary syndrome. *Best Practice and Research in Clinical Endocrinology and Metabolism*, 20, 293–310.

Homburg R. (2005). Clomiphene citrate-end of an era? A mini review. *Human Reproduction*, 20, 2043–2051.

Hull M.G., Glazener C.M., Kelly N.J., Conway D.I., Foster P.A., Hinton R.A., Coulson C., Lambert P.A., Watt E.M. and Desai K.M. (1985). Population study of causes, treatment, and outcome of infertility. *British Medical Journal*, 291, 1693–1697.

Hunault C.C., Laven J.S., van Rooij I.A., Eijkemans M.J., te Velde E.R. and Habbema J.D. (2005). Prospective validation of two models predicting pregnancy leading to live birth among untreated subfertile couples. *Human Reproduction*, 20, 1636–1641.

Imani B., Eijkemans M.J., te Velde E.R., Habbema J.D. and Fauser B.C. (1998). Predictors of patients remaining anovulatory during clomiphene citrate induction of ovulation in normogonadotropic oligoamenorrheic infertility. *Journal of Clinical Endocrinology and Metabolism*, 83, 2361–2365.

Imani B., Eijkemans M.J., Faessen G., Bouchard P., Giudice L.C. and Fauser B.C. (2002a). Prediction of the individual FSH-threshold for gonadotrophin induction of ovulation in anovulatory infertility: an approach to minimize multiple gestation, ovarian hyperstimulation, and treatment expense. *Fertility and Sterility*, 77, 83–90.

Imani B., Eijkemans M.J., te Velde E.R., Habbema J.D. and Fauser B.C. (2002b). A nomogram to predict the probability of live birth after clomiphene citrate induction of ovulation in normogonadotropic oligoamenorrheic infertility. *Fertility and Sterility*, 77, 91–97.

Insler V., Melmed H., Mashiah S., Monselise M., Lunenfeld B. and Rabau E. (1968). Functional classification of patients selected for gonadotropic therapy. *Obstetrics and Gynecology*, 32, 620–626.

Kiddy D.S., Hamilton-Fairley D., Bush A., Short F., Anyaoku V., Reed M.J. and Franks S. (1992). Improvement in endocrine and ovarian function during dietary treatment of obese women with polycystic ovary syndrome. *Journal of Clinical Endocrinology and Metabolism*, 36, 105–111.

Koustra E., White D.M. and Franks S. (1997). Modern use of CC in induction of ovulation. *Human Reproduction Update*, 3, 359–365.

Lord J.M., Flight I.H.K. and Norman R.J. (2003). Metformin in polycystic ovary syndrome: systematic review and meta-analysis. *British Medical Journal*, 327, 951–953.

McGee E.A. and Hsueh A.J. (2000). Initial and cyclic recruitment of ovarian follicles. *Endocrine Reviews*, 21, 200–214.

Mitwally M.F. and Casper R.F. (2003). Aromatase inhibitors for the treatment of infertility. *Expert Opinion on Investigational Drugs*, 12, 353–371.

Moll E., Bossuyt P.M., Korevaar J.C., Lambalk C.B. and van der Veen F. (2006). Effect of clomifene citrate plus metformin and clomifene citrate plus placebo on induction of ovulation in women with newly diagnosed polycystic ovary syndrome: randomised double blind clinical trial. *British Medical Journal*, 332, 1485.

Mulders A.G., Eijkemans M.J., Imani B. and Fauser B.C. (2003). Prediction of chances for success or complications in gonadotrophin ovulation induction in normogonadotrophic anovulatory infertility. *Reproductive Biomedicine Online*, 7, 48–56.

Nestler J.E., Jakubowicz D.J., Evans W.S. and Pasquali R. (1998). Effects of metformin on spontaneous and clomiphene-induced ovulation in the polycystic ovary syndrome. *New England Journal of Medicine*, 338, 1876–1880.

Norman R.J., Davies M.J., Lord J. and Moran L.J. (2002). The role of lifestyle modification in polycystic ovary syndrome. *Trends in Endocrinology and Metabolism*, 13, 251–257.

Palomba S., Orio F., Nardo L.G., Falbo A., Russo T., Corea D., Doldo P., Lombardi G., Tolino A., Colao A. and Zullo F. (2004). Metformin administration versus laparoscopic ovarian diathermy in clomiphene citrate-resistant women with PCOS: a prospective parallel randomized double-blind placebo-controlled trial. *Journal of Clinical Endocrinology and Metabolism*, 89, 4801–4809.

PCOS consensus (2004a). The Rotterdam ESHRE/ASRM-Sponsored PCOS consensus workshop group. Revised 2003 consensus on diagnostic criteria and long-term health risks related to polycystic ovary syndrome (PCOS). Human Reproduction, 19, 41–47.

PCOS consensus (2004b). The Rotterdam ESHRE/ASRM-Sponsored PCOS consensus workshop group. Revised 2003 consensus on diagnostic criteria and long-term health risks related to polycystic ovary syndrome (PCOS). *Fertility and Sterility*, 81, 19–25.

Roozenburg B.J., van Dessel H.J., Evers J.L. and Bots R.S. (1997). Successful induction of ovulation in normogonadotrophic clomiphene resistant anovulatory women by combined naltrexon and clomiphene citrate treatment. *Human Reproduction*, 12, 1720–1722.

Rossing M.A., Daling J.R., Weiss N.S., Moore D.E. and Self S.G. (1994). Ovarian tumors in a cohort of infertile women. *New England Journal of Medicine*, 33, 771–776.

Roumen F.J., Doesburg W.H. and Rolland R. (1984). Treatment of infertile women with a deficient postcoital test with two antiestrogens: clomiphene and tamoxifen. *Fertility and Sterility*, 41, 237–243.

Rowe P.J., Comhaire F.H., Hargreave T.B. and Mellows H. (1993). WHO manual for the standardized investigation and diagnosis of the infertile couple. Cambridge University Press.

Rizk B. Aboulghar (1991). Modern management of Ovarian Hyperstimulation Syndrome. *Human Reproduction*, 6(8), 1092–1097.

Rizk B. and Smitz J. (1992). Ovarian Hyperstimulation Syndrome after superovulation for IVF and related procedures. *Human Reproduction*, 7, 320–327.

Rizk B. (2006). Epidemiology of ovarian hyperstimulation syndrome. In Rizk B. (Ed.) Ovarian Hyperstimulation Syndrome. Cambridge: United Kingdom, Cambridge University Press, chapter 2, 10–42.

Snick H.K., Snick T.S., Evers J.L. and Collins J.A. (1997). The spontaneous pregnancy prognosis in untreated subfertile couples: the Walcheren primary care study. *Human Reproduction*, 12, 1582–1588.

Stafford D.E. (2005). Altered hypothalamic-pituitary-ovarian axis function in young female athletes: implications and recommendations for management. *Treatments in Endocrinology*, 4, 147–154.

Stein I.F. and Leventhal M.L. (1935). Amenorrhea associated with bilateral polycystic ovaries. *American Journal of Gynecology*, 29, 181–191.

Tiboni G.M. (2004). Aromatase inhibitors and teratogenesis. *Fertility and Sterility*, 81, 1158–1159.

van Santbrink E.J., Hop W.C., van Dessel H.J., de Jong F.H. and Fauser B.C. (1995). Decremental FSH and dominant follicle development during the normal menstrual cycle. *Fertility and Sterility*, 64, 37–43.

van Santbrink E.J., Hop W.C. and Fauser B.C. (1997). Classification of normogonadotrophic anovulatory infertility: polycystic ovaries diagnosed by ultrasound versus endocrine characteristics of polycystic ovary syndrome. *Fertility and Sterility*, 67, 453–458.

van Santbrink E.J. and Fauser B.C. (1997). Urinary follicle-stimulating hormone for normogonadotropic clomiphene-resistant anovulatory infertility: prospective, randomized comparison between low-dose step-up and step-down dose regimens. *Journal of Clinical Endocrinology and Metabolism*, 82, 3597–3602.

van Santbrink E.J., Hohmann F.P., Eijkemans M.J., Laven S.J. and Fauser B.C. (2005a). Does metformin modify ovarian responsiveness during exogenous FSH ovulation induction in normogonadotrophic anovulation? A placebo controlled double blind assessment. *European Journal of Endocrinology*, 152, 611–617.

van Santbrink E.J., Eijkemans M.J., Laven S.J. and Fauser B.C. (2005b). Patient-tailored conventional ovulation induction algorithms in anovulatory infertility. *Trends in Endocrinology and Metabolism*, 16, 381–389.

Van Wely M., Bayram N., van der Veen F. and Bossuyt P.M. (2005). Predictors for treatment failure after laparoscopic electrocautery of the ovaries in women with clomiphene citrate resistant PCOS. *Human Reproduction*, 20, 900–905.

White D.M., Polson D.W., Kiddy D., Sagle P., Watson H., Gilling-Smith C., Hamilton-Fairly D. and Franks S. (1996). Induction of ovulation with low-dose gonadotropins in polycystic ovary syndrome: an analysis of 109 pregnancies in 225 women. *Journal of Clinical Endocrinology and Metabolism*, 81, 3821–3824.

Yarali H., Yildiz B.O., Demirol A., Zeyneloglu H.B., Yigit N., Bukulmez O. and Koray Z. (2002). Co-administration of metformin during rFSH treatment in patients with clomiphene citrate-resistant polycystic ovarian syndrome: a prospective randomized trial. *Human Reproduction*, 17, 289–294.

Yen S.S., Quigley M.E., Reid R.L., Ropert J.F. and Cetel N.S. (1985). Neuroendocrinology of opioid peptides and their role in the control of gonadotropin and prolactin secretion. *American Journal of Obstetrics and Gynecology*, 152, 485–493.

Clomiphene Citrate for Ovulation Induction

Richard Palmer Dickey

INTRODUCTION

Clomiphene revolutionized the management of infertility in 1967 when it was approved for treatment of anovulation due to polycystic ovaries (PCO). The clinical introduction of clomiphene followed six years of research (Greenblatt et al., 1961; Tyler et al., 1962; Vorys et al., 1964; Dickey et al., 1965; Kistner, 1966) cumulating in a report of results in 3,220 patients and 1,032 conceptions (Table 23.1) (Macgregor et al., 1967; Macgregor et al., 1968). Today, clomiphene remains the first-line treatment for WHO Group II anovulation in which ovarian activity can be demonstrated by withdrawal bleeding from progesterone. In addition to treatment of anovulation, clomiphene is now also used alone and in combination with human menopausal gonadotropin (HMG) and follicle-stimulating hormone (FSH) to increase the number of preovulatory follicles in patients with unexplained infertility (Melis et al., 1987; Deaton et al., 1990; Glazener et al., 1990), in patients requiring husband or donor intrauterine insemination (IUI) (Shalev et al., 1989; Dickey et al., 1992), and to increase progesterone in patients with luteal insufficiency (Hammond and Taubert, 1982; Fukuma et al., 1983; Dickey, 1984; Guzick and Zeleznik, 1990). The advantages of clomiphene over gonadotrophin for ovulation induction include low incidence of multiple pregnancies, low cost, ease of treatment, absence of need for daily cycle monitoring, and low incidence of ovarian hyperstimulation syndrome (OHSS) (Rizk, 2006, 2008; Rizk and Dickey 2008).

PHARMACOKINETICS AND PHARMACODYNAMICS

The pharmacokinetics and pharmacodynamics of clomiphene explain its characteristic actions. Clomiphene, chemical name 1-[p(β-diethylaminoethoxy)phenyl]-1,2-diphenylchloroethylene (Holtkamp et al., 1960), is related to other trianyl ethylene compounds chlorotrianisene, triparanol (a cholesterol inhibitor), and tamoxifen, a class of drugs called *selective estrogen receptor modulators* (Figure 23.1) and is distantly related to the nonsteroidal estrogen diethylstilbestrol. Clomiphene has strong antiestrogenic activity and weak estrogenic activity and is therefore a competitive antagonist of estrogen. The two unsubstituted phenyl groups are responsible for both its weak estrogenic activity, compared to estradiol, and prolonged retention at estrogen receptor sites where it blocks the attachment of more active estrogens. Because of its diethylamino ethoxy side chain on the third phenyl group, clomiphene has

been called a catechol estrogen. However, the catecholamino side chain is inert and only the diphenyl portions are active. Clomiphene is sold under different names throughout the world: Clomid, Clomphid, Clomivid, Clostilbegyt, Dyneric, Ikaclomine, and Serophene.

Clomiphene acts as a competitive antagonist of 17β-estradiol at the level of the cytoplasmic nuclear receptor complex in the hypothalamus, pituitary, and elsewhere (Clark and Markaverich, 1988). Blockade of estrogen receptors in the hypothalamic arcuate nucleus leads to an increase in gonadotropin-releasing hormone (GnRH) and to an increase in LH, and presumably FSH, pulse frequency but not in pulse amplitude (Kerin et al., 1985). Additionally, clomiphene increased pituitary sensitivity to GnRH in a fashion similar to estradiol (Hsueh et al., 1978). As a result of these actions, serum concentrations of FSH and LH secretions are increased three- to fourfold during clomiphene administration (Dickey et al., 1965). The increased FSH stimulates folliculogenesis, whereas LH stimulates steroidogenesis. In clomiphene cycles unlike gonadotropin cycles, monofollicular development is facilitated and multiple follicular development is attenuated because FSH is downregulated by negative feedback of estradiol during the follicular phase.

Because it acts as an antiestrogen, induction of ovulation with clomiphene requires an intact hypothalamic-pituitary-ovarian axis and estrogen. Due to its site of action, the total daily dose of clomiphene must be taken at one time to optimize entry into the hypothalamic and central nervous system receptor sites.

Clomiphene occurs in two isomers, enclomiphene (formerly called transclomiphene) and zuclomiphene (formerly called cisclomiphene) (Ernst et al., 1976; Holtkamp, 1987). Clomiphene available in the United States, Canada, and England contain a mixture of approximately 38 percent zuclomiphene and 62 percent enclomiphene. Zuclomiphene is mildly estrogenic, as well as antiestrogenic, while enclomiphene is entirely antiestrogenic. There is controversy about which isomer is more important for ovulation. Glasier et al. (1989) concluded that enclomiphene was the active isomer in inducing ovulation and that zuclomiphene was inactive. Young et al. (1991) determined zuclomiphene to be five times as potent as enclomiphene in inducing ovulation. Charles et al. (1969) found enclomiphene to be superior to and zuclomiphene to be equal to the racemic mixture in inducing ovulation, while Murthy et al. (1971) and Connaughton et al. (1974) found enclomiphene to have less activity than the racemic mixture.

Table 23.1: Response to Clomiphene in 3,220 Patients with Ovulatory Dysfunction[a,b]

Treatment cycle no.	No. of patients ovulating	No. of conceptions	% Clinical pregnancies
1	1,750	373	21.3
2	1,321	279	21.1
3	876	176	20.1
4	488	101	20.7
5	234	46	19.7
6	158	23	14.6
7	98	16	16.3
8	74	10	13.5
9	37	5	13.5
10	21	3	14.3
Total	5,057	1,032	20.4

[a]Adapted from Macgregor et al. (1967). Reproduced with permission of the authors.
[b]Average rate of pregnancy for cycles 1–6 was 20.7% and for cycles 7–10 was 14.8%.

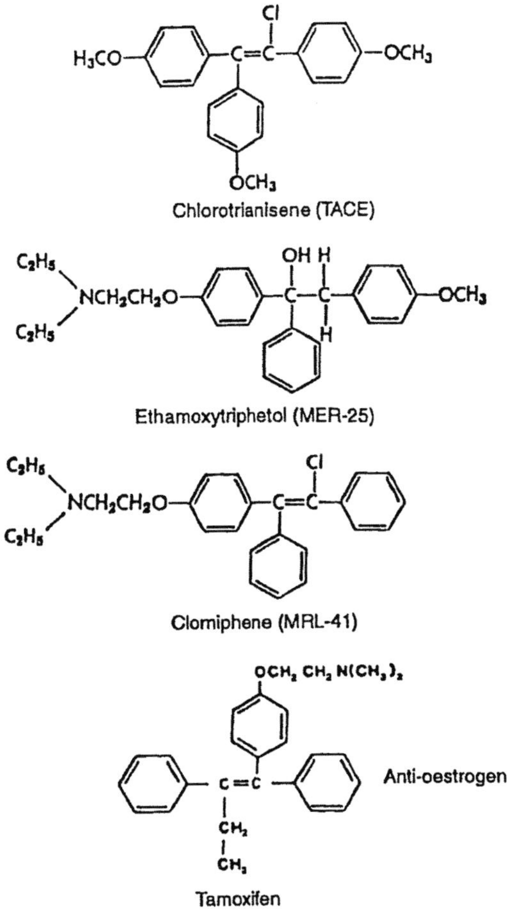

Serum concentration of zuclomiphene peak six hours after oral administration of 50 mg (Figure 23.2; Mikkelson et al., 1986). A steady state, approximately 25 percent, of peak concentration is reached at forty-eight hours and remains constant for the next fourteen days. Serum half-lives of zuclomiphene vary from 14.2 to 33.4 days and of enclomiphene from 2.5 to 11.8 days, (Harman and Blackman, 1981). Variability is, in part, related to body weight (Shepard et al., 1979). For this reason, the dose of clomiphene necessary to induce ovulation or increase luteal phase progesterone is proportional to body weight (Shepard et al., 1979; Dickey et al., 1997). Five days after oral administration, 51 percent of clomiphene has been excreted principally through the intestines. Serum concentrations of zuclomiphene remain at least 10 percent of peak levels twenty-eight days after ingestion of a single 50-mg tablet, and some clomiphene continues to be excreted for at least six weeks. The effect of repeated administration of a single 50-mg tablet at twenty-eight-day intervals is cumulative, with basal levels of zuclomiphene increasing by 50 percent per month (Mikkelson et al., 1986; Figure 23.3). Owing to the accumulation of zuclomiphene, clomiphene may be more or less effective in inducing ovulation during the second and later cycles of treatment, even though the dose administered remains the same. Also, because of the continuing presence of zuclomiphene, ovulation as a result of clomiphene may occur in the first one or two cycle following discontinuation of treatment.

After ovulation induction with clomiphene, serum progesterone and estradiol serum levels are increased during the luteal phase of the cycle in a direct dose-response relationship (Hammond and Talbert, 1982; Fukuma et al., 1983). Following conception, serum progesterone levels are 200–300 percent greater than those measured in spontaneous pregnancies until the eleventh postovulation week, after which they decrease but

Figure 23.1. Chemical structures of antioestrogens of the triphenylethylene type. Reproduced with permission of the author and publisher.

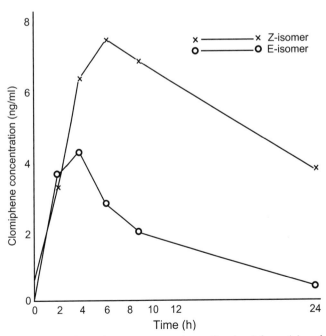

Figure 23.2. Mean plasma concentrations of zyclomiphene (x) and enclomiphene (○) after oral administration of one 50-mg tablet of clomiphene (n = 23). From Mikkelson et al. (1986). Reproduced with permission of the authors and the publisher, American Society for Reproductive Medicine (The American Fertility Society).

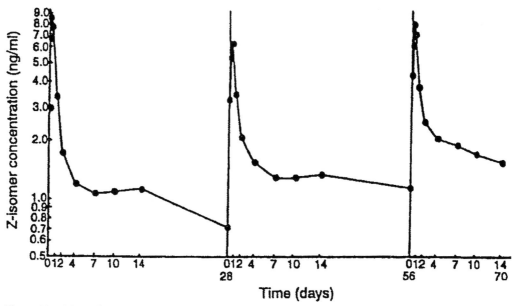

Figure 23.3. Mean plasma concentration of zuclomiphene after administration of one 50-mg tablet of clomiphene at twenty-eight-day intervals. From Mikkelson et al. (1986). Reproduced with permission of the authors and the publisher, the American Society for Reproductive Medicine (The American Fertility Society).

continue to be 75 percent greater than spontaneous pregnancies through at least the sixteenth gestational week (Dickey, 1984; Dickey and Hower, 1995; Figure 23.4). Serum estrogen levels, approximately 66 percent greater in spontaneous pregnancies, continue through at least the sixteenth gestational week. Uterine artery volume of blood flood is increased approximately 25 percent in clomiphene pregnancies during the first eight gestational weeks due to the combined effect of increased estrogen and progesterone (Dickey and Hower, 1995).

Antiestrogenic Effects

Antiestrogenic effects of clomiphene caused by competitive antagonism of estrogen receptors outside the hypothalamic-pituitary axis important to management of infertility patients are decreased endometrial thickness and decreased quantity and/or quality of cervical mucus. Other antiestrogen effects include hot flashes and scintillating scotoma (moving, flashing lights). Hot flashes and scintillating scotoma are limited to the days clomiphene tablets are taken and are managed by reducing the dose of clomiphene. Clomiphene should be discontinued when scintillating scotoma occurs but may be restarted at a lower dose in a subsequent cycle.

Endometrial Thickness

Endometrial thickness is decreased in clomiphene cycles (Fleisher et al., 1984; Imoedemhe et al., 1987; Eden et al., 1989; Randall and Templeton, 1991; Rogers et al., 1991; Dickey et al., 1993a, 1993b). Decreased endometrial thickness is linked to failure to conceive and biochemical pregnancy in clomiphene, gonadotropin, and spontaneous cycles (Table 23.2 Dickey et al., 1993a, 1993b). In a study of endometrial thickness on the day of HCG administration for timed intrauterine insemination (IUI), no pregnancies occur when endometrial thickness was less than 6 mm compared to a 9.4 percent pregnancy rate when thickness was 6–8.9 mm and a 14.1 percent

pregnancy rate when thickness was 9 mm or greater. No biochemical pregnancies occurred, and the clinical abortion rate was 12 percent when thickness was 9 mm or greater. When thickness was 6–8.9 mm, the biochemical pregnancy rate was 22 percent and clinical abortion rate was 16 percent (Dickey 2008).

Cervical Mucus

Clomiphene decreases cervical mucus quality and quantity as seen by decreased ferning and spinnbarkeit formation (Macgregor et al., 1967; Pildes, 1965; Van Campenhout et al., 1968; Marchini et al., 1989; Acharya et al., 1993). Poor cervical mucus quality or quantity and fewer than five motile sperm was found in 39 of 100 patients referred for gonadotropin ovulation induction and/or IUI because of failure to become pregnant after three to eighteen clomiphene cycles (Dickey 2006; Table 23.3).

CLINICAL MANAGEMENT

A minimal requirement for safe clinical use of clomiphene is the availability of ultrasound.

Indications

Clomiphene is indicated for treatment of infertility in WHO type II oligomenorrhic and anovulatory women who have evidence of significant estrogen production. Evidence of estrogen production may be withdrawal bleeding after a progesterone challenge, serum estrogen levels greater than menopausal (20 pg/mL), or endometrial thickness 6 mm or greater than. Clomiphene is ineffective in women whose ovaries do not produce estrogen because of lack of FSH due to hypothalamic-pituitary disorders WHO type I) or ovarian failure. Macgregor et al. (1967) reported the results of ovulation induction with clomiphene in 4,098 patients according to type of anovulatory disorder. Ovulation occurred in 80 percent with oligomenorrhea and menses every one to six months, 76 percent with PCOS, 75

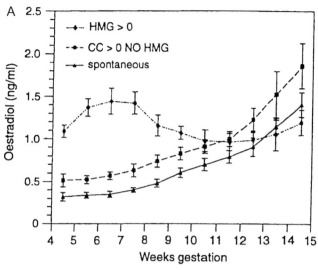

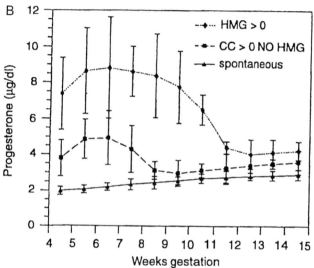

Figure 23.4. (A) Serum 17 β-oestsradiol and (B) serum progesterone concentrations during the first fifteen weeks of pregnancy, following spontaneous ovulation (group I, ▲), clomiphene citrate (CC) without HMG (group II, ■) or CC followed by HMG (group III, ♦). Values shown are mean ± SE. From Dickey and Hower (1995).

Table 23.2: Pre-Ovulation US Endometrial Thickness versus Outcome

Thickness (mm)	% of Clomiphene cycle	Pregnancy rate (%)	Bio. (%)	Pregnancy/ outcome clinical abortions (%)	Term (%)
<6	9.1	0	0	0	0
6–8	43.6	8.1	21.4	15.4	62.5
≥9	47.2	14.0	0	12.2	87.8

Adapted from Dickey et al. (1993a, 1993b). Reproduced with permission of the publisher.

Table 23.3: Additional Diagnosis of 100 Points Referred for Clomiphene Failure*

Cervical factor	39%
Endometriosis	31%
Male factor	25%
Tubal factor	24%
Type II DM	12%
Hypothyroid	5%

*Fertility Institute of New Orleans 2001. Adapted from Dickey (2003).

percent with postcontraceptive amenorrhea, 60 percent with psychogenic amenorrhea, 53 percent with oligo-ovulation and menses less frequently than every six months, 42 percent in lactation-amenorrhea syndrome, and 0 percent with pituitary disorders amenorrhea.

Clomiphene is used, alone and in combination with HMG and FSH, to increase the number of preovulatory follicles in patients with unexplained infertility and in patients requiring husband or donor IUI (Shalev et al., 1989; Deaton et al., 1990; Glazener et al., 1990; Dickey et al., 1992) and to increase progesterone concentration in patients with luteal insufficiency (Hammond and Talbert, 1982; Downs and Gibson, 1983; Fukuma et al., 1983; Dickey, 1984; Huang K-E, 1986). However, when used alone without gonadotropins in normo-ovulatory patients without luteal insufficiency, clomiphene may decrease the probability of pregnancy in patients requiring artifical insemination due to its antiendometrial effect.

Clomiphene may be necessary for ovulation in patients with hyperprolactinemia amenorrhea treated with bromocriptine-type drugs, in patients with insulin resistance and type II diabetes treated with metformin, and in patients with mild adrenal hyperplasia treated with low-dose corticosteroids.

Starting Dose of Clomiphene

Clomiphene is manufactured in 50-mg tablets, grooved to facilitate splitting into 25-mg halves. Clomiphene is administered orally for five days beginning the third to seventh cycle day. The total daily clomiphene dose is taken at one time. The starting dose of clomiphene can be 50 mg with a plan to increase the dose in 50-mg increments in the same or subsequent cycle if ovulation does not occur, or the initial dose can be based on body weight and, when used for luteal insufficiency, on progesterone level.

Starting Day

Clomiphene is ineffective if started too soon, before estradiol levels are 45–60 pg/mL. Follicle sizes are 6 mm or greater when estradiol is in this range. Estradiol levels and follicle sizes often reach these parameters on the third cycle day but may require seven days or longer. When estradiol levels and follicle sizes are known, these can be used to determine the best day to start; otherwise clomiphene should be started on the third cycle day for women with regular menstrual cycles to decrease the effect on endometrial thickness and cervical mucus.

Table 23.4: Relationship of Clomiphene Dose to Weight at Conception[a]

Clomiphene dose (mg)	Total no. (%) patients	No. (%) of patients in each weight group at conception				
		<45 kg/<100 lb	45–59 kg/100–131 lb	60–74 kg/132–164 lb	75–89 kg/165–197 lb	90 kg/198 lb
25	54(3.2)	4(9.1)	27(3.4)	23(3.9)	0(0.0)	0(0.0)
50	784(46.6)	25(56.8)	430(54.4)	248(42.6)	56(36.3)	25(24.5)
100	596(35.5)	12(27.3)	245(31.0)	220(37.2)	70(45.4)	49(48.0)
>100	247(14.7)	3(6.8)	88(11.1)	100(16.9)	28(18.2)	28(27.4)
150	197(11.7)	3(6.8)	73(9.2)	83(14.0)	21(13.6)	17(16.7)
200	44(2.7)	0(0.0)	14(1.8)	17(2.9)	5(3.2)	8(7.3)
250	6(0.4)	0(0.0)	1(0.1)	0(0.0)	2(1.3)	3(2.9)
Total	1,681	44	790	591	154	102

Adapted from Dickey et al. (1997) reproduced with permission of the publishers.

Weight

Clomiphene is not sequestered in fat cells as occurs for natural steroids, but because blood volume constitutes 15 percent of total body weight, serum levels of clomiphene are related to body weight. An analysis of the clomiphene dose taken during the cycle of conception illustrates the relationship between weight and effective dose (Table 23.4; Dickey et al., 1997). Sixty-six percent of women who weighed less than 100 lb (45 kg) became pregnant on 50 mg per day, compared to 24 percent of women who weighed 198 lb (90 kg) or more. Doses of 100 mg or more were taken for the cycle of conception by 42 percent of women weighing 100–131 lb (45–59 kg), 54 percent of women weighing 132–164 lb (60–74 kg), and 64 percent of women weighing 165–197 lb (75–89 kg). There was a positive relationship between clomiphene dose and the number of follicles, but no relationship to multiple pregnancies or abortion. Because of clomiphene's antiestrogen effects on endometrium thickness (Dickey et al., 1993a), and mucus, the starting dose should not be greater than 50 mg for women who weigh less than 132 lb (60 kg). A starting dose of 100 mg is recommended for use in women who weigh 165 lbs (75 kg) or more, providing that endometrial thickness and cervical mucus are monitored.

Midluteal Progesterone Levels

When clomiphene is used for treatment of luteal insufficiency, the dose of clomiphene may be selected based on the midluteal progesterone level (see below, Monitoring Progesterone level). A starting dose of 100 mg is recommended if the deficiency of progesterone is greater than 1,000 ng/dL (10 pg/mL) providing weight is at least 132 lbs (60 kg).

Tests Required or Recommended before Initiating Treatment

Ultrasound

Ultrasound of the ovaries should always be performed before initiating clomiphene treatment for the first time to rule out preexisting ovarian neoplasm, endometriomas, and persistent corpus luteum cysts to evaluate the number and size of antral follicles. Ovarian neoplasms even when benign, and endometriomas, may inhibit follicle development by pressure. Endometrio-mas may expand and rupture during stimulation. Active hemorrhagic and nonhemorrhagic corpus luteum and simple cysts inhibit follicle development on the ipsolateral side by reason of estrogen and progesterone production. Antral follicle counts greater than eight to ten per ovary are diagnostic of PCO and increase the possibility of triplet or higher order pregnancy.

Ultrasound of the ovaries should be performed during the midluteal phase of the first cycle or before initiating the second clomiphene cycle to rule out hemorrhagic and nonhemorrhagic corpus luteum and simple cysts.

Ultrasound of the uterine fundus, endometrium, and fallopian tubes is necessary to rule out correctable uterine abnormalities (fibroids and septate uterus), endometrial pathology (polyps and hyperplasia), hydrosalpinx, and pregnancy. Submucosal uterine fibroids, septate uterus, endometrial polyps, and hydrosalpinx visible on ultrasound should be evaluated and treated by customary methods before initiating ovulation induction.

Clomiphene should not be started while endometrial thickness is greater than 6 mm because follicle response will be poor and implantation will be impaired. In most cases, a too thick endometrium will decrease to less than 6 mm, and high progesterone levels due to still active corpus luteum will decrease to less than 60 ng/dL (0.6 pg/mL) by waiting two to three days.

Management of Ovarian Cysts

Ovarian cysts larger than 4 cm should be explored surgically and removed, not drained. Smaller cysts without cancer characteristics of wall thickness 3 mm or greater or inclusions may either be followed until they resolve or suppressed with oral contraceptives. Progesterone alone is ineffective, and GnRH agonists may cause functional cysts to grow larger. The best oral contraceptives (OCs) for the purpose of cyst suppression are those containing 50 mcg of estrogen (Dickey, 2006) but are no longer available in many countries and may cause a delay in return to ovarian activity. OCs containing 30 mcg estrogen may be used, and the dose doubled to two per day in a second cycle if they fail to suppress or new cysts appear. Rest cycle or suppression is unnecessary if cysts are clear and less than 1 cm or if serum progesterone concentration is less than 60 ng/dL (0.6 pg/mL).

Baseline Estradiol and Progesterone Levels

Serum estradiol and progesterone levels are recommended if results can be rapidly available. Serum estrogen levels will show if it is too early to start clomiphene. Progesterone levels will resolve whether ovarian cysts are active or inactive and unable to interfere with follicle development. Clomiphene will be ineffective if estradiol levels are less than 45–60 pg/mL. This may occur following OC suppression and sometimes occurs in PCOS patients. Estradiol levels increase at a rate of 50 percent per day, doubling every two days during the follicular phase of the cycle. Before deciding that a patient is unresponsive to clomiphene treatment, estradiol levels should be measured on the customary start day to determine if clomiphene has been started too soon.

Other Endocrine Tests

Thyroid-stimulating hormone (TSH) levels 4.5 mIU/mL or higher are diagnostic of subclinical hypothyroidism. However, TSH levels 2.5 mIU/mL or higher may cause menstrual dysfunction. Treatment is levothyroxine. When pregnant TSH should be repeated, levels less than 2.0 mIU/mL are desirable during pregnancy.

Fasting insulin levels greater than 20 μU/mL and a fasting glucose to fasting insulin ratio less than 4.5 (Legro et al., 1998) indicate possible insulin resistance (IR), a common endocrine abnormality in women with PCO (see III 1 Legro, and III 2 Tulandi). Due to wide variability among different ethnic groups [in some groups a ratio less than 7.2 indicates IR (Kauffman et al., 2002)], the two-hour glucose/insulin response to a 75 g glucose load is considered more reliable. A two-hour insulin level of 100–150 μU/mL indicates probable IR, 150–300 μU/mL is diagnostic for IR, and greater than 300 μU/mL indicates severe IR. A two-hour glucose of 140–199 mg/dL indicates impaired glucose tolerance; 200 mg/dL indicates noninsulin-dependent diabetes (type II diabetes). The first line of treatment for women with borderline and mild IR should be weight loss. Metformin 1,000–2,000 mg day is indicated for anovulatory women who continue to have elevated insulin levels and who do not ovulate with clomiphene alone.

Dehydroepiandrosterone sulfate (DHEAS) levels greater than 180 μg/dL may indicate nonclassical adrenal hyperplasia in women with symptoms of mild androgen excess and anovulation. Treatment is low-dose corticosteroid treatment (0.5 mg dexamethasone or 5 mg prednisone at bedtime). The addition of clomiphene is often necessary for ovulation. Corticosteroids should be discontinued after ovulation due to the risk of birth defects.

Prolactin levels greater than 25 mIU/mL may benefit from bromocriptine and similar drugs. Women with anovulation due to hyperprolactinemia often require addition of clomiphene in order to ovulate.

Monitoring

Although monitoring is not required to use clomiphene, it shortens the time to and improves the chances of pregnancy. Monitoring is performed before ovulation, five to seven days after the last tablet, with ultrasound, postcoital test, and serum or urine LH, to evaluate follicular development, endometrial thickness, and sperm-mucus interaction and to time intercourse or IUI. Monitoring is performed five to seven days postovulation with progesterone to confirm ovulation and ascertain that the dose is adequate.

Follicle Development

The number and size of preovulatory follicles predict the chance of pregnancy and multiple pregnancy and of the number of days until ovulation. Follicles destined to ovulate ordinarily increase in diameter at a rate of 1 mm per day until they reach 10 mm, then at a rate of 2 mm per day until ovulation (Steinkampf, 2008). In clomiphene cycles, the lead follicles is usually 20–24 mm the day of ovulation and 18–20 mm the day of spontaneous LH surge. Pregnancy rates in clomiphene cycles are most closely related to the number of follicles 15 mm or larger and multiple pregnancy rates to the number of follicles 12 mm or larger on the day of spontaneous LH surge or HCG injection (Dickey et al., 1992, 2001; Table 23.5). The highest pregnancy rates occur when there are four follicles 15 mm or larger and are not increased when there were five or more follicles. When HCG is used to trigger ovulation, highest pregnancy rates are achieved when the lead follicle is 16 mm. All follicles 12 mm or larger (vs. ≥10 mm in gonadotropin cycles) may ovulate and contribute to a multiple pregnancy (Dickey et al., 1991, 1992, 2001).

Failure of Follicle Development

If no developing follicles 10 mm or larger are present five to seven days after the last clomiphene tablet and serum estradiol levels or endometrial thickness (a measure of estrogen activity) are unchanged, clomiphene can be repeated immediately at a 50 mg higher dose. If 10- to 14-mm follicles are present, it should be repeated in two to four days to confirm continued growth.

Endometrial Thickness

Endometrial thickness should be at least 6 mm and preferably 9 mm or greater on preovulatory ultrasound (Table 23.3; Dickey et al., 1993a, 1993b; Dicky, 2008). Endometrial thickness increases at a faster rate in clomiphene cycles than in spontaneous cycles during the late proliferative phase as it escapes from the antiestrogen effect of clomiphene (Randall and Templeton, 1991; Figure 23.5). If the endometrial is too thin on preovulation ultrasound, administration of HCG should be delayed. Estradiol taken concurrently with clomiphene (Yagel et al., 1992; Figure 23.6) or following clomiphene will increase thickness. Taubert and Dericks-Tan (1976) have shown that high does of estradiol do not interfere with the ovulation-inducing effects of clomiphene; nevertheless, high doses of estrogen should be given in divided orally four times a day or vaginally two times a day. In subsequent cycles, endometrial thickness may be improved by taking a lower dose of clomiphene or switching to tamoxifen.

Postcoital Test

Unless IUI is already planned, a postcoital test is necessary to confirm the presence of adequate numbers of motile sperm. Five progressively motile sperm are considered sufficient for conception; however, higher numbers are desirable and result in greater pregnancy rates, and pregnancies can occur when fewer or no sperm are seen. A poor postcoital result due to mucus quality or quantity will improve as estrogen levels increase and antiestrogen effect of clomiphene decreases; therefore, the test can be usefully repeated closer to ovulation. A poor test despite good mucus quality indicates a possible male factor and IUI should be considered.

Serum or Urine LH

An increase in serum LH to twice baseline level predicts ovulation within twenty-four hours. Urine LH predicts

Table 23.5: Relationship of Follicle Number to Pregnancy and Multiple Implantations, All Patients Age Less Than Forty-three without Tubal Factor

	Clomiphene citrate (CC)					HMG					CC + HMG				
No. foll	Cycles no.	Pregnancy[a] no. (%)	Imp[b] fol %	Multi-implants[c] 2	≥ 3	Cycles no.	Preg no. (%)	Imp fol %	Multi-implants 2	≥ 3	Cycles no.	Preg no. (%)	Imp fol %	Multi-implants 2	≥ 3
Follicles ≥12 mm															
1	281	20(7.1)	7.1	0(0.0)	0(0.0)	61	6(9.8)	9.8	0(0.0)	0(0.0)	67	3(4.5)	4.5	0(0.0)	0(0.0)
2	424	49(11.6)	6.2	2(4.1)	1(2.0)	97	7(7.2)	4.1	1(14.2)	0(0.0)	100	14(14.0)	10.5	5(35.7)	1(7.1)
3	301	41(13.6)	5.5	9(22.0)	0(0.0)	116	18(15.5)	6.6	3(16.7)	1(5.6)	118	16(13.6)	5.9	3(18.8)	1(6.2)
4	182	22(12.1)	3.2	2(9.1)	0(0.0)	111	26(23.4)	7.4	5(19.2)	1(3.8)	97	16(16.5)	6.4	6(37.5)	1(6.2)
5	74	8(10.8)	2.4	1(12.5)	0(0.0)	112	24(21.4)	4.5	1(4.2)	0(0.0)	53	12(22.6)	5.7	0(0.0)	1(8.3)
6	31	7(22.6)	4.8	0(0.0)	1(14.3)	63	14(22.2)	5.0	1(7.1)	2(14.3)	43	12(27.9)	5.0	1(8.3)	0(0.0)
7–8	24	4(16.7)	2.2	0(0.0)	0(0.0)	95	20(21.0)	4.3	3(15.0)	2(10.0)	51	10(19.6)	4.2	1(10.0)	2(20.0)
9–10	10	3(30.0)	5.3	0(0.0)	1(33.3)	58	15(25.9)	4.2	1(6.7)	3(20.0)	30	8(26.7)	3.9	1(12.5)	1(12.5)
>10	4	2(50.0)	4.2	0(0.0)	0(0.0)	90	24(26.7)	2.3	3(12.5)	2(8.3)	35	8(22.8)	2.2	3(37.5)	0(0.0)
Total	1,333	155(11.6)	4.8	14(9.0)	3(1.9)	803	154(19.2)	4.3	18(11.7)	11(7.1)	594	99(16.7)	5.0	20(20.2)	7(7.2)
Follicles ≥15 mm															
0[d]	86	8(9.4)	0.0	3(37.5)	0(0.0)	21	3(14.2)	0.0	1(33.3)	0(0.0)	29	4(13.8)	0.0	1(25.0)	0(0.0)
1	531	44(8.3)	9.2	1(2.3)	2(4.5)	167	26(15.6)	19.2	2(7.7)	2(7.7)	153	18(11.8)	14.4	4(22.2)	0(0.0)
2	411	55(13.4)	7.2	4(7.3)	0(0.0)	172	25(14.5)	8.4	4(16.6)	0(0.0)	149	23(15.4)	10.7	4(17.4)	2(8.7)
3	194	27(13.9)	5.3	4(14.8)	0(0.0)	144	30(20.8)	8.8	4(13.3)	2(6.7)	109	18(16.5)	7.6	3(16.6)	2(11.1)
4	73	14(19.2)	5.5	2(14.3)	0(0.0)	119	26(21.8)	6.9	3(11.5)	1(3.8)	55	13(23.6)	8.3	4(30.8)	1(7.7)
5–6	28	5(17.8)	3.4	0(0.0)	0(0.0)	93	24(25.8)	7.2	2(8.3)	4(16.6)	61	17(27.9)	8.2	3(17.6)	2(11.8)
7–8	7	1(14.3)	6.1	0(0.0)	1(1.0)	45	7(16.3)	3.0	1(14.2)	1(14.2)	24	3(12.5)	2.3	1(33.3)	0(0.0)
> 8	3	1(33.3)	3.0	0(0.0)	0(0.0)	42	13(31.7)	3.4	1(7.7)	1(7.7)	14	3(21.4)	1.7	0(0.0)	0(0.0)
Total	1,333	155(11.6)	7.0	14(9.0)	3(1.9)	803	154(19.2)	7.2	18(11.7)	11(7.1)	594	99(16.7)	8.1	20(20.2)	7(7.2)
Follicles ≥18 mm															
0[e]	329	29(8.8)	0.0	4(13.8)	1(3.4)	164	29(17.7)	0.0	5(17.2)	1(3.4)	149	23(15.4)	0.0	9(39.1)	1(4.3)
1	583	58(9.9)	10.6	2(3.4)	1(1.7)	224	35(15.6)	19.6	3(8.6)	3(8.6)	161	22(13.7)	16.1	2(9.1)	1(4.5)
2	319	46(15.1)	7.8	4(8.7)	0(0.0)	176	34(19.3)	13.1	7(20.6)	2(5.9)	139	26(18.7)	12.2	4(15.4)	2(7.7)
3	97	11(11.7)	5.2	4(36.3)	0(0.0)	114	24(21.0)	8.5	1(4.2)	1(4.2)	72	16(22.7)	10.6	5(31.2)	1(6.2)
4	31	11(35.4)	10.5	0(0.0)	1(9.1)	58	12(20.7)	7.8	1(8.3)	2(16.7)	41	6(15.0)	5.5	0(0.0)	1(16.7)
> 4	14	1(7.1)	1.1	0(0.0)	0(0.0)	67	20(31.2)	5.7	1(5.0)	2(10.0)	32	6(18.8)	4.4	0(0.0)	1(16.7)
Total	1,333	155(11.6)	10.2	14(9.0)	3(1.9)	803	154(19.2)	12.4	18(11.7)	11(7.1)	594	99(16.7)	13.3	20(20.2)	7(7.2)

[a]Pregnancy: number, percent per cycle.
[b]Implantations, percent per follicle ≥18 mm.
[c]Multiple implantations: number, percent of pregnancies.
[d]No follicles ≥15 mm were present.
[e]No follicles ≥18 mm were present.
Significance, χ^2 with 4 d.f.; CC $P < .003$, HMG $P < .05$, CC + HMG $P = .62$.
Adapted from Dickey et al. (2001). Reproduced with permission of the publishers.

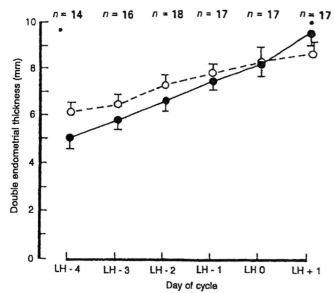

Figure 23.5. Double endometrial thickness (mm) in spontaneous (O) and clomiphene citrate (●) cycles (mean ± SEM). LH-0 = day of onset of LH surge. *P < 0.05. From Randall and Templeton (1991). Reproduced with permission of the authors and the publisher, the American Society for Reproductive Medicine (The American Fertility Society).

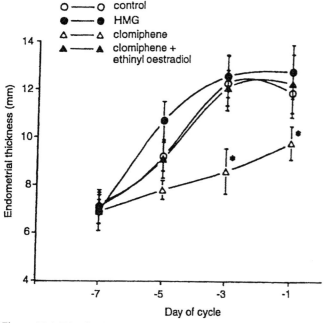

Figure 23.6. Distribution of mean (±SEM) of endometrial thickness at four points in the cycle. O, controls; ●, HMG; △, clomiphene; ▲, clomiphene + ethinyl oestradiol. *P < 0.01 compared with the control cycle result at the same phase of the cycle. From Yagel et al. (1992). Reproduced with permission of the authors and the publisher, the American Society for Reproductive Medicine (The American Fertility Society).

ovulation within twelve hours. Pregnancy rates can be improved by timing intercourse or IUI to the spontaneous LH surge. Administration of 5,000–10,000 IU HCG after one or more follicles are at least 16 mm can be used to time intercourse or IUI. HCG does not increase pregnancy or multiple pregnancy rates. Couples who choose to not use LH or HCG timing should be instructed to have intercourse every other day from cycle days 12 through 18.

Progesterone

Progesterone is used to confirm ovulation to determine if the dose of clomiphene is sufficient. It should be measured in the midluteal phase five to seven days after ovulation, to coincide with the day of embryo implantation. Progesterone levels in the midluteal phase of clomiphene cycles that result in term pregnancies average 3,700 ng/dL (37 pg/mL), compared to 2,200 ng/dL (22 pg/mL) in spontaneous cycles (Dickey, 1984; Dickey and Hower, 1995). Dickey (1984) observed that there were no term pregnancies when midluteal progesterone levels were less than 1,500 ng/dL (15 pg/mL). When progesterone levels are less than 1,800 ng/dL (18 pg/mL), progesterone supplementation should be considered in the current cycle and the dose of clomiphene should be increased as 50-mg increments until progesterone levels are 2,000 ng/dL (20 pg/mL) or higher in subsequent cycles.

Midluteal Ultrasound

A repeat ultrasound in the midluteal phase to confirm ovulation is useful but not mandatory if ultrasound is performed at the beginning of the second cycle. Partial ovulation is common when there are multiple follicles of various sizes at the time of LH surge or HCG administration. It is usually the smaller 8- to 10-mm follicles that fail to ovulate but may continue to grow that result in cysts.

Serum FSH: The Clomiphene Challenge Test

In the clomiphene challenge test, FSH levels are measured before and after administration of 100 mg, five times a days. FSH levels 11 mIU/mL or higher either before or after the clomiphene challenge signify decreased ovarian reserve (Scott and Hofmann, 1995). Women with decreased ovarian reserve were observed to have a reduced possibility of spontaneous pregnancy during the next twenty-four months with pregnancy rates from 13 percent for age less than thirty years to 0 percent for age greater than or equal to forty years compared to 66 percent for age less than thirty years and 10 percent for age greater than or equal to forty years for women with "normal" ovarian reserve.

Methods to Increase Pregnancy Rates in Clomiphene Cycles

Pregnancy rates may be increased in clomiphene cycles by increasing the number of follicles that develop, by improving endometrial conditions and cervical mucus, and by IUI when numbers of sperm on a postcoital test are low or absent. Maximum pregnancy rates in clomiphene cycles occur when there are four preovulatory follicles 15 mm or greater (Dickey et al., 2001; Table 23.4).

Methods to Increase Follicle Numbers

Increasing the Dose of Clomiphene

When 50 mg clomiphene is taken, the average number of follicles 12 mm or larger, 15 mm or larger, and 18 mm or larger is 2.4, 1.7, and 1.2, respectively (Dickey et al., 1997). Increasing the dose of clomiphene in subsequent cycles has a minimal effect. When 100 mg is taken, the average number of follicles 12 mm or larger, 15 mm or larger, and 18 mm or larger is 2.6, 1.9, and 1.3, respectively. The number of follicles did not increase with 150 mg, 200 mg, or 250 mg clomiphene. Marrs et al. (1984) reported that administration of 150 mg of clomiphene for five days significantly increased the number of preovulatory follicles available for IVF and that the final number of follicles was not affected by the cycle day on which clomiphene was started. Quigley et al. (1984), however, found no difference between administration of 50 mg of clomiphene and 150 mg of clomiphene in recruitment of follicles 15-mm diameter for IVF. Shalev et al. (1989) reported an increase in the average number of follicles larger than 15-mm diameter from 1.0 for 50 mg of clomiphene to 2.4 for 200 mg. The benefit of increasing the dose of clomiphene must be balanced against the possibility of increasing the antiestrogen effect on the endometrium and cervical mucus.

Extending the Number of Days Clomiphene Is Taken

Extending the number of days that 50 mg of clomiphene is taken to eight or even ten days has been shown to result in ovulation in patients who did not respond to 200 mg or even 250 mg for five days in small series (Adams et al., 1972; Lobo et al., 1982a). The benefit of prolonging the dose of clomiphene must be balanced against the possibility of extending the antiestrogen effect on the endometrium and cervical mucus.

Addition of Dexamethasone

Adding dexamethasone to clomiphene can result in a significant improvement in pregnancy rate with and without increased DHEAS levels (Beck et al., 2005). The traditional method has been to use low-dose dexamethasone (0.5 mg at bed time) for one month or until six days after ovulation (Lobo et al., 1982a; Daly et al., 1984; Hoffman and Lobo, 1985; Trott et al., 1996; Isaacs et al., 1997). Recently, use of high-dose dexamethasone (2.0 mg) from days 5 to 14 has been reported to provide equally good results with no serious side effects (Parasanezhad et al., 2002; Elnashar et al., 2006). An added beneficial effect of dexamethasone is that when added to clomiphene, it appears to negate the antiestrogen effect on the endometrium (Trott et al., 1996; Parasanezhad et al., 2002). In view of the potential risk of high-dose dexamethasone and the absence of studies showing that it is more effective than low-dose therapy, it seems prudent to use the lower dose.

Addition of Metformin

The combination of metformin with clomiphene increases the rate of ovulation in women who do not ovulate with clomiphene alone. While metformin improves ovulation principally in women with insulin resistance and hyperandrogenism associated with PCOS resistant to clomiphene alone (Nestler et al., 1998; Vandermolen et al., 2000; Kocak et al., 2002), its low incidence of side effects indicate that it may be used empirically in other women. Metformin may also improve cervical mucus in clomiphene cycles (Kocak et al., 2002). The usual dose of 1,000–2,000 mg per day can be administered in a single or divided dose with meals.

Addition of Gonadotropin following Clomiphene

Addition of gonadotropin 75 mIU for three to four days following the last clomiphene tablet increases the number of follicles 12 mm or larger and 18 mm or larger that develop to 3.9 and 1.7, respectively, and doubles the pregnancy rates per cycle but also increases the risk of twin and triplet or higher order pregnancy to the same level as in gonadotrophin-only cycles (Table 23.5; Dickey et al., 1991, 1993c).

Intrauterine Insemination

Use of clomiphene to improve pregnancy rates in IUI cycles has had mixed success. Several groups reported increased pregnancies (Corson et al., 1983; Kemmann et al., 1987; DiMarzo et al., 1992). Others found no improvement in IUI pregnancy rates when clomiphene was added (Melis et al., 1987; Martinez et al., 1990). Use of IUI to improve pregnancy rates in patients receiving clomiphene for ovulatory disorders has not been studied as often. Pregnancy rates increase in proportion to the total sperm count in initial semen specimen used for IUI from 4.2 percent when there were ten to forty million to 8.9 percent when there were ninety million or more (Dickey et al., 1993b). The upper value is more than double the WHO criterion for normal male fertility of forty million. This suggests IUI should be considered for women whose partner's sperm only meet minimal standards for normal as well as women who have mucus abnormalities.

Unexplained Infertility

Use of clomiphene to increase preovulation estrogen levels and postovulation progesterone levels, alone or combined with IUI, has been shown to be an effective first-line treatment for "unexplained infertility" (Melis et al., 1987; Deaton et al., 1990; Glazener et al, 1990; Dickey 2006). Many cases of unexplained infertility (regular "ovulatory" cycles, normal sperm count, and open fallopian tubes) can be explained by luteal insufficiency and mucus or endometrial factors. Luteal insufficiency is often the result of inadequate FSH stimulation in the follicular phase. The diagnosis of luteal insufficiency can be missed if it is assumed that a progesterone level of 500 pg/dL (5 ng/mL) is normal. In fact progesterone levels average need to be 1,500 ng/dL (15 pg/mL) or higher for term pregnancy and average 2,200 ng/dL (22 pg/mL) in spontaneous cycles ending in term pregnancy (Dickey et al., 1984). Diagnosis of mucus factor and endometrial factor require preovulatory postcoital testing and ultrasound, which have not been performed in many studies of the so-called unexplained infertility.

Treatment Results

In the first report of a large-scale study, the pregnancy rate averaged 21.8 percent through the first five cycles and 14.7 percent during cycles six through ten for patients who ovulated (Table 23.1; Macgregor et al., 1967). These results have never been equaled in part because of the way in which ovulation was defined. In a later report in which all cycles were reported, the pregnancy rate averaged 8.9 percent (Macgregor et al., 1968). All the patients reported by Macgregor were receiving clomiphene for treatment of anovulation, and although age was not reported, it can be assumed that most were aged less than thirty-five.

Hammond et al. (1983) reported average pregnancy rates of 13.3 percent through the first five cycles and 16.0 percent during cycles six through ten in mostly anovulatory patients but

Table 23.6: Clomiphene Citrate IUI: Cumulative and per Cycle Pregnancy Rates

Cycle	No. of patients starting cycle	No. of pregnancies	Not pregnant	Monthly pregnancy rate (%)	Cumulative pregnancy rate (%)
1	1,624	169	1,455	10.4	10.4
2	887	81	806	9.1	19.5
3	461	41	420	8.9	28.4
4	207	18	189	8.6	37.0
5	93	2	91	2.2	39.2
6	52	2	50	3.8	43.0
>7	57	0	57	0.0	43.0
Total	3,381	313	3,068		

Adapted from Dickey et al. (2002). Reproduced with permission of the publishers.

noted pregnancy rates were reduced 50 percent in patients with endometriosis. In a study of clomiphene use in IUI cycles, pregnancy rates averaged 6.1 percent through six cycles with none in thirty-five and seventh and later cycles (DiMarzo et al., 1992).

In a review of 3,381 clomiphene IUI cycles with HCG timing, pregnancy rates per cycle decreased slowly through the first four cycles and then were markedly lower in cycles five and six, with no pregnancies in fifty-seven latter cycles (Table 23.6; Dickey et al., 2002).

How Many Cycles of Clomiphene Should be Performed?

The number of clomiphene cycles that should be performed before recommending other addition of gonadotropins, switching to gonadotropins entirely, or switching to IVF depends on follicle response, whether or not there are other infertility factors such as endometriosis, tubal factor, or severe husband factor, whether donor or husband IUI were performed, and patients age (Dickey et al., 2002).

The most accurate information about the effect of different factors on pregnancy rates come from HCG-timed IUI cycles because the number of mature follicles and the presence of sufficient sperm in the uterus and fallopian tube at the time of ovulation are known with certainty. When clomiphene IUI cycles in which results were controlled for confounding factors of age, sperm quality, number of follicles, and diagnosis, pregnancy rates per cycle through the first four cycles ranged from a highs of 20.4 percent for luteal insufficiency, 16.5 percent for donor IUI, 14.6 percent for age less than thirty, and 13.3 percent for PCO, to lows of less than 4 percent for age greater than or equal to forty-three and low-quality sperm (Table 23.7; Dickey et al., 2002).

Cumulative pregnancy rates after six cycles of clomiphene IUI reach 75 percent in women receiving donor sperm and 65 percent in women treated with clomiphene for ovulatory dys-

function if they were younger than forty-two years, used sperm of satisfactory quality, and did not have endometriosis or tubal factor (Figure 23.7A–D; Dickey et al., 2002).

Diagnosis

Pregnancy rates remained constant through six cycles of clomiphene IUI, reaching 75 percent after six cycles in patients with ovulatory disorders (Figure 23.7A; Dickey et al., 2002). For patients with endometriosis, tubal factor, and other diagnoses except male factor, few or no pregnancies occurred after the fourth cycle. Unless a surgically correctable condition is present, clomiphene should not be continued beyond four cycles with the exception that, if not done previously, laparoscopy should be performed after the fourth cycle, and clomiphene can be continued for at least two additional cycles, if there are no findings. If endometriosis or minor tubal disease is discovered and can be treated, four additional cycles of clomiphene are justified.

Age

Age is a factor in how long clomiphene should be used at the extremes of reproductive life (Figure 23.7B; Dickey et al., 2002). Nearly all women younger than thirty who are going to become pregnant will do so in the first four cycles because of their high rate of fecundity per ovulation. Women forty-three years and older with a much lower rate of fecundity rarely become pregnant after the third cycle. All other age groups from age thirty through forty-two can become pregnant through at least the sixth cycle, with a decreased pregnancy rate after the fourth cycle.

Male Factor

The source and quality of sperm is a significant factor in how rapidly patient's pregnancy occurs and the eventual pregnancy rate per patient; but when sperm is of extremely low quality, it does not depend on how long clomiphene should be used (Figure 23.7C; Dickey et al., 2002). When donor sperm was used for IUI, pregnancy rates were constant through six cycles and reached a cumulative rate of 75 percent, confirming previous reports of high pregnancy rates when donor IUI is performed. When husband IUI was performed with initial sperm numbers of least five million motile sperm and 30 percent progressive motility, minimal values necessary for IUI (Dickey et al., 1999) pregnancy rates were constant through at least six cycles although the 55 percent pregnancy rate per patient after six cycles was lower than for donor sperm. When husband IUI was performed using less than five million motile sperm or when motility was less than 30 percent, no pregnancies occurred after the third cycle and pregnancy rate per patient was only 10 percent at that time.

Follicle Number

The number of preovulatory follicles affect how rapidly patients became pregnant but may not affect their chance of becoming pregnant if treatment is continued long enough (Figure 23.7D; Dickey et al., 2002). Patients with three or more follicles 15 mm or larger achieved a cumulative pregnancy rate of 65 percent in five cycles. Patients who developed two follicles per cycle reached almost the same pregnancy rate (60 percent) after six cycles, and the rate may have gone higher if treatment had been continued. Patients who developed only one follicle per cycle had an average pregnancy rate of 9 percent per cycle

Table 23.7: Patient Factors: Mean Pregnancy Rates Cycles 1–4

	Cycles	Pregnancies (%)	Odds ratio (95% CI)	P-values
Diagnosis[a]				
Ovulatory dysfunction	1,075	157(14.6)	1.01(0.86–1.44)	NS
Polycystic ovaries	884	118(13.3)	—	—
Luteal insuffiency	191	39(20.4)	1.67(1.12–2.49)	.017
Endometriosis	1,102	89(8.1)	0.57(0.43–0.76)	.0002
Wo tubal invol.	797	63(7.9)	0.56(0.40–0.77)	.0004
W tubal invol.	305	26(8.5)	0.60(0.39–0.94)	.034
Tubal factor no endo	279	16(5.7)	0.39(0.27–0.59)	.0008
Other	354	37(10.4)	0.76(0.51–1.12)	NS
Age[b] (years)				
<30	431	63(14.6)	—	—
30–34	604	84(13.9)	0.94(0.66–1.34)	NS
35–37	221	26(11.8)	0.78(0.48–1.27)	NS
38–42	173	21(12.1)	0.81(0.48–1.37)	NS
≥43	53	2(3.8)	0.29(0.07–1.23)	NS
Semen[c]				
WHO	410	53(12.9)	—	—
IUI threshold	527	60(11.4)	0.86(0.58–1.28)	NS
Sub-IUI threshold	186	6(3.2)	0.22(0.10–0.53)	.0004
Donor	492	81(16.5)	1.32(0.91–1.93)	NS
Number follicles >15 mm[d]				
1	377	37(9.8)	—	—
2	286	41(14.3)	1.54(0.96–2.47)	NS
≥3	215	38(17.7)	1.97(1.21–3.12)	.008

[a]Patient's age greater than or equal to forty-three and cycles with total initial motile sperm count less than five million or motility <30 percent excluded.

[b]Patients with endometriosis, tubal impairment, and cycles with total initial motile sperm count less than five million or motility <30 percent excluded.

[c]Patient's age greater than or equal to forty-three and patients with endometriosis and tubal factor excluded.

[d]Patients age greater than or equal to forty-three, patients with endometriosis and tubal factor, and cycles with total initial motile sperm count less than five million or motility <30 percent excluded.

Endo: endometriosis; Invol: involvement; IUI threshold: initial sperm quality less than WHO criteria but greater than or equal to five million total motile sperm and greater than or equal to 30 percent initial motility; NS: not significant; Sub-IUI threshold: initial motile sperm count less than five million or motility <30 percent; w: with; WHO: initial sperm quality greater than or equal to World Health Organization criteria of twenty million concentration, forty million total count, 50 percent progressive motility, 30 percent normal forms; wo: without.

Adapted from Dickey et al. (2002). Reproduced with permission of the publishers.

through four cycles; none of the twelve who tried became pregnant after the fourth cycle.

These results and those of large series by Macgregor et al. (1967) and Hammond et al. (1983) for clomiphene intercourse and DiMarzo et al. (1992) for clomiphene IUI differ markedly from those of a small series, which did not report per cycle pregnancy rates or use life-table analysis (Gysler et al., 1982),

that has been cited by gonadotropin manufacturers as showing that patients should be switched to gonadotropins after the third failed clomiphene cycle. As the above studies demonstrate, clomiphene can be continued for a minimum of four cycles (three cycles for severe sperm factor or age greater than or equal to forty-three) before recommending gonadotropins or IVF. Clomiphene can usefully be continued

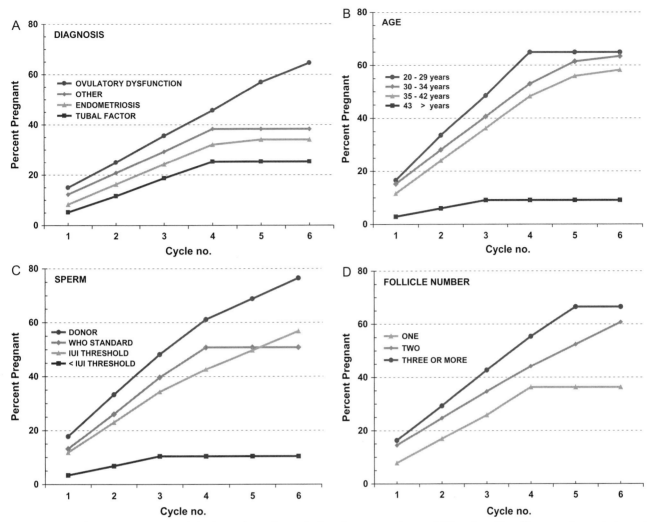

Figure 23.7. Cumulative pregnancy rate. (A) Diagnosis: ovulatory dysfunction = anovulatory, PCO, or luteal insuffiency; endometriosis = with or without tubal involvement; tubal factor = unilateral tubal obstruction or tubal adhesions without endometriosis; other = cervical factor, male factor, or unexplained infertility and normal cycles without endometriosis or tubal factor. Patient's age greater than or equal to forty-three and cycles with total initial motile sperm count less than five million or motility <30 percent excluded. (B) Age, patients with endometriosis, tubal impairment, and cycles with total initial motile sperm count less than five million or motility <30 percent excluded. (C) Sperm, WHO: initial sperm quality greater than or equal to World Health Organization (1992) criteria of twenty million concentration, forty million total count, 50 percent progressive motility, 30 percent normal forms. IUI threshold; initial sperm quality less than WHO criteria but greater than or equal to five million total motile sperm and ≥ 30 percent initial motility. Sub-IUI threshold: initial motile sperm count less than five million or motility <30 percent. Patient's age greater than or equal to forty-three, and patients with endometriosis and tubal factor excluded. (D) Follicle number, patient's age greater than or equal to forty-three, and patients with endometriosis and tubal factor, and cycles with total initial motile sperm count less than five million or motility <30 percent excluded. Adapted from Dickey et al. (2002). Reproduced with permission of the publishers.

for at least six cycles in patients aged thirty to forty-two, without endometriosis, tubal factor, or severe male factor. Treatment longer than four cycles may also be indicated when timed intercourse or IUI is not used due to the possibility that sperm was not present at the time of ovulation in all cycles.

Multiple Pregnancy

In the premarket study conducted during the 1960s (Macgregor et al., 1968), 123 of the 1,201 live births (10.2 percent) were twins

and 13 (1.1 percent) were triplets or higher order, including quadruplets and quintuplets. Multiple pregnancy rates are related to the number of follicles 12 mm or larger in clomiphene cycles. In a review of 1,333 clomiphene IUI cycles and 803 gonadotropin IUI cycles, there were an average 2.7 follicles 12 mm or larger in clomiphene cycles and 5.4 follicles 12 mm or larger in gonadotropin cycles (Table 23.5; Dickey et al., 2001). For clomiphene, two or more follicles 12 mm or larger were present in 79 percent of cycles, three or more follicles in 47 percent of cycles, and six or more follicles in 5 percent of cycles. For gonadotropin, two or more follicles 12 mm or larger were present in 92 percent

Table 23.8: Clomiphene Citrate

	Age <35					Age ≥35				
		Multiple implantation					Multiple implantation			
		2 Sacs		> 3 Sacs			2 Sacs		> 3 Sacs	
	Pregnancies per cycle (%)	Per pregnancy (%)	Per cycle (%)	Per pregnancy (%)	Per cycle (%)	Pregnancies per cycle (%)	Per pregnancy (%)	Per cycle (%)	Per pregnancy (%)	Per cycle (%)
Estradiol										
<500 pg/ml	14.3	4.5	0.65	0.0	0.0	10.2	0.0	0.0	0.0	0.0
≥500 pg/ml	16.5	11.1	1.84	0.0	0.0	6.0	0.0	0.0	0.0	0.0
Follicles ≥12 mm										
<6	11.2	11.8	1.3	1.0	0.1	8.9	6.2	0.5	0.0	0.0
≥6	24.5[b]	0.0		15.3[a]	3.8[a]	12.5	0.0	0.0	0.0	0.0
Follicles ≥15 mm										
<4	10.9	8.0	0.9	2.3	0.2	12.0	5.0	0.6	0.0	0.0
≥4	22.2[c]	11.1	2.5	5.6	1.2	10.0	0.0	0.0	0.0	0.0
Follicles ≥18 mm										
<2	9.2	10.3	0.9	3.4	0.3	11.2	0.0		0.0	0.0
≥2	17.4[d]	10.9	1.9	1.8	0.3	10.6	14.3	1.5	0.0	0.0

Fishers exact test: [a]P < .05
[b]P < .02
[c]P < .01
[d]P < .001
Adapted from Dickey et al. (2001). Reproduced with permission of the publishers.

of cycles, three or more follicles in 80 percent of cycles, and six or more follicles in 38 percent of cycles. The number of follicles 15 or larger or 18 mm or larger did not predict twin or triplet pregnancies. There was no difference between clomiphene and gonadotropins in the implantation rate per follicle.

The triplet pregnancy rate for patients aged more than thirty-five was 15 percent, when there were six or more follicles 12 mm or larger compared to 1.0 percent when there were fewer than six follicles of this size (Table 23.8; Dickey et al., 2001). No triplet pregnancies occurred in patients aged thirty-five or older. The twin pregnancy rate was 4 percent when there were two follicles 12 mm or larger, compared to 14 percent when there were three or more than follicles 12 mm or larger. The twin pregnancy rate was twice as high when serum estradiol level was 500 pg/mL as when it was less. Multiple pregnancies were unrelated to clomiphene dose; all triplets occurred in patients taking 50 mg clomiphene. Due to spontaneous loss of one or more gestations, 25 percent of initial twin pregnancies end in single births and 50 percent of initial triplet pregnancies end in either singleton or twin births (Dickey et al., 2002). Consideration should be given to canceling clomiphene cycles due to increased risk of high-order multiple pregnancy when six or more follicles 12 mm or larger are present or when two or more follicles 12 mm or larger are present and patients wish to avoid twins for medical or personal reasons.

Clomiphene and Cancer

A 1992 meta-analysis that suggested past use of clomiphene was associated with an increase in ovarian cancer (Whittemore et al., 1992). A subsequent cohort study concluded that increase in ovarian cancer after use of ovulation induction drugs is limited to women who use drugs for more than twelve cycles without becoming pregnancy (Rossing et al., 1994).

Clomiphene, Miscarriage, and Birth Defects

Reports that clomiphene causes an increase in spontaneous abortion come from mostly small inadequately controlled studies without a comparable group of infertile women not taking clomiphene (Goldfarm et al., 1968; Roland, 1970; Garcia et al., 1977). One study found the frequency of chromosomal anomalies in clinical abortions was increased in clomiphene-initiated pregnancies (Boue and Boue, 1973). A large prospective five-year multihospital study compared outcomes in 1,034 pregnancies conceived following clomiphene, 186 pregnancies conceived following HMG and 29,900 spontaneous conceptions. Abortion rates were not significantly different for clomiphene (14.8 percent) than for spontaneous ovulation (13.9 percent) but were higher following HMG (19.4 percent; Kurachi et al., 1983).

Table 23.9: Percentage of Male Births by Drug and Technique in Singleton Pregnancies and the Effect of Clomiphene on Birth and Sex Ratio[a]

Source[a]	Treatment	Total births	Known outcome	Total births	No. (%) female births	No. (%) male births	Sex ratio male/female
Holtkamp (1984) cited in Corson et al. (1984)	Clomiphene, No IUI	2,155	2,026	1,568	777(49.5)	791(50.5)	1.018
Sampson et al. (1983)	No clomiphene, donor IUI	195	187	162	64(39.5)	98(60.5)	1.531
	Clomiphene, donor IUI	123	119	89	48(53.9)	41(46.1)	0.854
Dickey et al. (1995)	No clomiphene, no IUI	2,715	2,346	1,885	963(51.1)	922(48.9)	0.957
	Clomiphene, no IUI	1,186	1,133	904	453(50.1)	451(49.9)	0.996
	Husband/donor IUI, no clomiphene	76	75	59	26(44.1)	33(55.9)	1.269
	Clomiphene, husband/donor IUI	191	187	149	80(53.7)	69(46.3)	0.862

Adapted and revised from Dickey et al. (1995). Reproduced with permission from publisher.

A twenty-year infertility clinic prospective study reported spontaneous biochemical and clinical abortion rates combined of 23.7 percent for 1,738 pregnancies initiated with clomiphene, 20.4 percent for 3,471 spontaneous pregnancies, and 36.4 percent for 107 HMG- or FSH-initiated pregnancies (Dickey et al., 1996). The incidence of biochemical pregnancies in clomiphene compared to spontaneous pregnancies was higher for patients older than 30 years (8.0 percent compared to 4.9 percent), while the incidence of clinical abortion was higher for patients older than 30 years (15.9 versus 11.2 percent). For all ages combined, the incidence of biochemical pregnancy was 3.9 percent in spontaneous pregnancy, 5.8 percent in clomiphene-initiated pregnancy, and 11.2 percent in HMG or FSH pregnancy.

In a total of 2,369 births reported to the manufacturer, the incidence of birth defects was 2.4 percent compared to a 2.7 percent incidence in the population at large (Asch and Greenblatt, 1976). Of the fifty-eight infants with birth defects, eight were born to mothers who inadvertently took clomiphene during the first six weeks of pregnancy.

Ectopic Pregnancy

Reports that the rate of ectopic pregnancies is increased following use of clomiphene in cycles of coitus (Powell-Phillips, 1979; Chaukin, 1982; Marchbanks et al., 1986) or when clomiphene is used in combination with HMG for IVF (Cohen et al., 1986; Snyder and del Castillo, 1988) were not controlled for endometriosis or tubal disease. In an analysis of 2,086 spontaneous and 1,391 clomiphene pregnancies following intercourse or IUI, at a single clinic, the incidence of ectopic pregnancy was increased only in women who had preexisting tubal disease or endometriosis (Dickey et al., 1989). Ectopic pregnancy occurred in 3.0 percent of spontaneous pregnancies and 3.4 percent of clomiphene pregnancies if endometriosis was present, compared to 1.4 percent of spontaneous pregnancies and 0.8 percent of clomiphene pregnancies if there was no endometriosis or tubal disease.

LACK OF CLOMIPHENE EFFECT ON SEX RATIO

The papers most often cited as evidence of decreased male births are James (1980) and James (1985). These papers include many cases in which HMG, not clomiphene, was used. The majority of patients in James' 1980 report had received HMG and 43 percent of those births were male, which negates his argument for a clomiphene-specific effect. His 1985 meta-analysis which reported 496 singleton births of which 48.4 percent were male included both clomiphene and HMG pregnancies and did not investigate the effect of IUI. James' conclusions are contravened by other larger studies from single sources (Corson et al., 1983; Holtcamp cited in Corson et al., 1984; Dickey et al., 1995a, 1995b; Table 23.9). In the largest series of clomiphene births (Holtkamp, 1984, cited in Corson et al., 1984), 50.5 percent of 1,568 singleton births were male. In a series of 904 consecutive singleton births following clomiphene without IUI, 49.9 percent were males compared to 48.9 percent males following spontaneous ovulation (Dickey, 1995a). The male birth rate was 55.9 percent following IUI without clomiphene or HMG and 46.3 percent when clomiphene was used before IUI. Sampson et al. (1983) in a smaller series reported 60.5 percent male births following spontaneous ovulation and donor insemination, compared to 46.1 percent male births when clomiphene was used before donor insemination.

The most that can be concluded are the following: the male birth rate following intercourse is not affected by clomiphene; male births may be increased by IUI, but this may only occur with donor sperm; clomiphene may cause decreased male births when used before IUI, but this may be due to poor quality of husband sperm; and the differences are too small to be clinically significant. The timing of IUI may also be a factor in whether male or female births are greater.

CONCLUSIONS

Clomiphene is the first-line treatment for WHO Group II anovulation in which ovarian activity can be demonstrated by withdrawal bleeding from progesterone. In addition to treatment of anovulation, clomiphene is also used alone and in combination with HMG and FSH to increase the number of preovulatory follicles in patients with unexplained infertility, in patients requiring husband or donor IUI, and to increase progesterone in patients with luteal insufficiency. The advantages of clomiphene over gonadotrophin for ovulation induction include low incidence of multiple pregnancies, low cost, ease of treatment, absence of need for daily cycle monitoring, and low incidence of OHSS. Both pregnancy rates and multiple pregnancy rates are related to number of preovulatory follicles and age. Pregnancy rates are related to the number of follicles 15 mm or larger, diagnosis, and sperm quality, but are relatively unaffected by age until the age of forty-three. Pregnancy rates per cycle remain constant through four cycles of clomiphene, and treatment should be continued for at least that long, for all patients except those older than forty-three or when sperm quality is extremely poor. Cumulative pregnancies reach 65 percent after four to six cycles in patients older than thirty years for ovulatory dysfunction, and 75 percent for donor IUI, provided there is no endometriosis or tubal disease. Triplet and higher order pregnancies are related to number of follicles greater than or equal to 12 mm and age. They can be reduced by use of preovulatory ultrasound and cancellation of the 5 percent of cycles in which six or more follicles develop.

KEY POINTS FOR CLINICAL PRACTICE

■ Clomiphene is indicated for induction of ovulation in WHO type II oligomenorrhic and anovulatory women who have evidence of significant estrogen production and to increase progesterone concentration in patients with luteal insufficiency.

■ A minimal requirement for safe clinical use of clomiphene is the availability of ultrasound. Pelvic ultrasound should be performed before initiating the first cycle of clomiphene to rule out ovarian cysts and ovulation during the first cycle to determine the number of preovulatory follicles and endometrial thickness.

■ Clomiphene is started on cycle day 3 in women with regular menstrual cycles in order to minimize the antiestrogen effect on the endometrium and cervical mucus. Oligomenorrhic and amenorrheic women who menstruate every 60–180 days may be given progesterone 100 mg in oil to initiate menses and clomiphene may be started on cycle days 5–7.

■ For the best results, serum estradiol and progesterone should be measured the day clomiphene is started. Clomiphene is ineffective if estradiol is less than 45–60 pg/mL. Follicular development is retarded if progesterone levels are greater than 80–90 ng/dL. If either of these levels are found, waiting one or two days to start clomiphene will result in a much better response. Estradiol levels double every two days and progesterone levels fall by 50 percent per day at the start of the cycle.

■ The starting dose of clomiphene is usually 50 mg per day for five days, but because the response to clomiphene is weight dependent, the starting dose can be increased to 100 mg in women who weigh 165 lb (75 kg) or more and can be reduced to 25 mg in women who weigh less than 110 lb (45 kg).

■ The dose of clomiphene is increased until ovulation occurs and the midluteal phase progesterone level is at least 1,800 ng/dL (18 pg/mL).

■ A postcoital test should be performed during the first cycle of clomiphene to determine if intrauterine insemination is required.

■ Pregnancy rates are related to the number of preovulatory follicles 15 mm or larger and remain constant through the four to six cycles of clomiphene in women who do not have tubal factor infertility or endometriosis.

■ Twin and higher order pregnancies are related to the number of preovulatory follicles 12 mm or larger and age. Consideration should be given to canceling clomiphene cycles due to increased risk of high-order multiple pregnancy when six or more follicles 12 mm or larger are present or when two or more follicles 12 mm or larger are present and patients wish to avoid twins for medical or personal reasons.

REFERENCES

Acharya U, Irvine DS, Hamilton MP, Templeton AA (1993) The effect of three anti-oestrogen drugs on cervical mucus quality and in-vitro sperm-cervical mucus interaction in ovulatory women. *Hum Reprod* 8:437–41.

Adams R, Mishell DR, Israel R (1972) Treatment of refractory anovulation with increased and prolonged duration of cyclic clomiphene citrate. *Obstet Gynecol* 39:562–6.

Adashi EY (1996) Ovulation induction: clomiphene citrate. In Adashi EY, Rock JA, Rosenwaks, eds. *Reproductive Endocrinology, Surgery, and Technecology*. Chapter 59. Lippincott-Raven Publishers, Philadelipha, pp. 1181–206.

Adashi EY, Rock JA, Sapp KC, et al. (1979) Gestational outcome of clomiphene-related conceptions. *Fertil Steril* 31:620–6.

Asch RH, Greenblatt RB (1976) Update on the safety and efficacy of clomiphene citrate as a therapeutic agent. *J Reprod Med* 17: 175–80.

Bergqvist C, Nillius SJ, Wide L (1983) Human gonadotropin therapy. II. Serum estradiol and progesterone patterns during nonconceptual cycles. *Fertil Steril* 39:766–71.

Boue Boue (1973) Increased frequency of chromosomal anomalies in abortions after induced ovulation. *Lancet* 1:679–80.

Charles D, Klein T, Lunn SF, Loraine JA (1969) Clinical and endocrinological studies with isomeric components of clomiphene citrate. *J Obstet Gynaecol Br Commonw* 76:1100–10.

Chaukin W (1982) The rise in ectopic pregnancy exploration of possible reasons. *Int J Gynecol Obstet* 20:341–50.

Clark JH, Markaverich BM (1988) Actions of ovarian steroid hormones. In Knobil E, Neill J et al., eds. *The Physiology of Reproduction*. Raven Press, New York, pp. 675–723.

Connaughton JF, Garcia C-R, Wallach EE (1974) Induction with cisclomiphene and a placebo. *Obstet Gynaceol* 43:697–701.

Corson SL, Batzer DR, Otis C, Corson J (1983) Clomiphene citrate: nuances of clinical application. *Clin Reprod Fertil* 2:1–17.

Corson SL, Batzer FR, Alexander NG, et al. (1984) Sex selection by sperm separation and insemination. *Fertil Steril* 42:756–60.

Daly DC, Walters CA, Soto-Albors CE, et al. (1984) A randomized study of dexamethasone in ovulation induction with clomiphene citrate. *Fertil Steril* 41:844–8.

Deaton JL, Gibson M, Blackmer KM, et al. (1990) A randomized controlled trial of clomiphene citrate and intrauterine insemination in couples with unexplained infertility or surgically corrected endometriosis. *Fertil Steril* 54:1083–8.

Dickey RP (1984) Evaluation and management of threatened and habitual first trimester abortion. In Osofsky H., ed. *Advances in Clinical Obstetrics and Gynecology*, Vol. 2, Chapter 2. Yearbook Medical Publishers, Chicago, pp. 329–88.

Dickey RP (2003) Superovulation/IUI rather than IVF should be the primary management for patients with unexplained infertility. Presented at 2003 ASRM Annual Meeting, San Antonio, TX, Oct. 2003.

Dickey RP (2006) *Managing Oral Contraceptive Pill Patients*, 13th edn. EMIS Dallas, Texas.

Dickey RP (2008) Ultrasonography of the endometriosis. In Rizk B. (ed.), Ultrasonography in Reproductive Medicine and Infertility. Cambridge: United Kingdom, Cambridge University Press, (in press).

Dickey RP, Hower JF (1995) Effect of ovulation induction on uterine blood flow and oestradiol and progesterone concentrations in early pregnancy. *Hum Reprod* 10:2875–9.

Dickey RP, Matis R, Olar TT, et al. (1989) The occurrence of ectopic pregnancy with and without clomiphene citrate use in assisted and non-assisted reproductive technology. *J In Vitro Fertil Embryo Transfer* 6:294–7.

Dickey RP, Olar TT, Curole DN, et al. (1990) The probability of multiple births when multiple gestational sacs or viable embryos are diagnosed at first trimester ultrasound. *Hum Reprod* 5:880–2.

Dickey RP, Olar TT, Taylor SN, et al. (1991) Relationship of follicle number, serum estradiol, and other factors to birth rate and multiparity in human menopausal gonadotropin-induced intrauterine insemination cycles. *Fertil Steril* 56:89–92.

Dickey RP, Olar TT, Taylor SN, et al. (1992) Relationship of follicle number and other factors to fecundability and multiple pregnancy in clomiphene citrate-induced intrauterine insemination cycles. *Fertil Steril* 57:613–19.

Dickey RP, Olar TT, Taylor SN, et al. (1993a) Relationship of biochemical pregnancy to preovulatory endometrial thickness and pattern in ovulation induction patients. *Hum Reprod* 8:327–30.

Dickey RP, Olar TT, Taylor SN, et al. (1993b) Relationship of endometrial thickness and pattern to fecundity in ovulation induction cycles: effect of clomiphene citrate alone and with human menopausal gonadotropin. *Fertil Steril* 59:756–60.

Dickey RP, Olar TT, Taylor SN, et al. (1993c) Sequential clomiphene citrate and human menopausal gonadotropin for ovulation induction: comparison to clomiphene citrate alone and human menopausal gonadotropin alone. *Hum Reprod* 8:56–9.

Dickey RP, Taylor NN, Lu PY, Sartor MM, Rye PH, Pyrzak R (2002) Effect of diagnosis, age, sperm quality, and number of preovulatory follicles on the outcome of multiple cycles of clomiphene citrate-intrauterine insemination. *Fertil Steril* 78:1088–95.

Dickey RP, Taylor SN, Curole DN, et al. (1995) Male birth rates are influenced by the insemination of unselected spermatozoa and not by clomiphene citrate. *Hum Reprod* 10:761–4.

Dickey RP, Taylor SN, Curole DN, et al. (1996) Incidence of spontaneous abortion in clomiphene pregnancies. *Hum Reprod* 11:2623–8.

Dickey RP, Taylor SN, Curole DN, et al. (1997) Relationship of dose and weight to successful outcome in clomiphene pregnancy. *Hum Reprod* 12:449–53.

Dickey RP, Taylor SN, Lu PY, et al. (2002). Spontaneous reduction of multiple pregnancy: incidence and effect on outcome. *Am J Obstet Gynecol* 186:77–83.

Dickey RP, Taylor SN, Lu PY, Sartor BM, Pyrzak R (2004) Clomiphene citrate intrauterine insemination (IUI) before gonadotropin IUI affects the pregnancy rate and the rate of high-order multiple pregnancies. *Fertil Steril* 81:545–50.

Dickey RP, Taylor SN, Rye PH, Lu PY, Pyrzak R (1999) Comparison of sperm quality resulting in successful intrauterine insemination to World Health Organization threshold values for normal sperm. *Fertil Steril* 71:684–9.

Dickey RP, Vorys N, Stevens VC, Hamwi G, Ullery JC (1965) Observations on the mechanism of action of clomiphene (MRL 41). *Fertil Steril* 16:485–94.

DiMarzo SJ, Kennedy JF, Young PE, et al. (1992) Effect of controlled ovarian hyperstimulation on pregnancy rates after intrauterine insemination. *Am J Obstet Gynecol* 166:1607–13.

Downs KA, Gibson M (1983) Clomiphene citrate therapy for luteal phase defect. *Fertil Steril* 39:34.

Eden JA, Place J, Carter GD, et al. (1989) The effect of clomiphene citrate on follicular phase increase in endometrial thickness and uterine volume. *Obstet Gynecol* 73:187–90.

Elnashar A, Abdelageed E, Fayed M, et al. (2006) Clomiphene citrate and dexamethasone in treatment of clomiphene citrate-resistant polycystic ovary syndrome: a prospective placebo-controlled study. *Hum Reprod* 7:1805–8.

Ernst S, Hite G, Cantrell JS, et al. (1976) Stereochemistry of geometric isomers of clomiphene: a correction of the literature and a reexamination of structure-activity relationships. *J Pharmacol Sci* 65:148–50.

Fleisher AC, Pittaway DE, Beard LA, et al. (1984) Sonographic depiction of endometrial changes occurring with ovulation induction. *J Ultrasound Med* 3:341–6.

Fukuma K, Fukushima T, Matsuo I, et al. (1983) A graduated regimen of clomiphene citrate: its correlation to glycogen content of the endometrium and serum levels of estradiol and progesterone in infertile patients at the midluteal phase. *Fertil Steril* 39: 780–4.

Garcia J, Jones GS, Wentz AC (1977) The use of clomiphene citrate. *Fertil Steril* 28:707–17.

Glasier AF, Irvine DS, Wickings EJ, et al. (1989) A comparison of the effects on follicular development between clomiphene citrate, it's two separate isomers and spontaneous cycles. *Hum Reprod* 4:252–6.

Glazener CM, Coulson C, Lambert PA, et al. (1990) Clomiphene treatment for women with unexplained infertility: placebo-controlled study of hormonal responses and conception rates. *Gynecol Endocrinol* 4:75–83.

Gleicher N, Oleske DM, Tur-Kaspa I, Vidali A, Karande V (2000) Reducing the risk of high-order multiple pregnancy after ovarian stimulation with gonadotropins. *N Engl J Med* 343:2–7.

Greenblatt RB, Barfield WE, Jugck EC, et al. (1961) Induction of ovulation with MRL/41, Preliminary Report. *J Am Med Assoc* 178:101–4.

Groll M (1984) Analysis of 700 clomiphene citrate pregnancies. *Infertility* 7:1–12.

Guzick DS, Zeleznik A (1990) Efficacy of clomiphene citrate in the treatment of luteal phase deficiency: quantity versus quality of preovulatory follicles. *Fertil Steril* 54:206–10.

Gysler M, March CM, Misell DR Jr., et al. (1982) A decade's experience with an individualized clomiphene treatment regimen including its effect on the postcoital test. *Fertil Steril.* 37:161–7.

Hammond MG, Halme JK, Taubert LM (1983) Factors affecting the pregnancy rate in clomiphene citrate induction of ovulation. *Obstet Gynecol* 62:196–202.

Hammond MG, Taubert LM (1982) Clomiphene citrate therapy of infertile women with low luteal phase progesterone levels. *Obstet Gynecol* 59:275–9.

Harman PJ, Blackman GL (1981) High-performance liquid chromatographic determination of clomiphene using post-column online photolysis and fluorescence detection. *J Chromatogr* 225;131–8.

Hoffman D, Lobo RA (1985) Serum dehydroepiandrosterone sulfate and the use of clomiphene citrate in anovulatory women. *Fertil Steril* 43:196–9.

Holtkamp DE (1984) Cited in Corson SL, Batzer FR, Alexander NJ, et al. (1984). Sex selection by sperm separation and insemination. *Fertil Steril* 42:756–60.

Holtkamp DE (1987) Research and development of clomiphene citrate. In Asch RH et al. eds. *Recent Advances in Human Reproduction*. Fondazione Per Gli Studi Sulla Riproduzione Umana, Stampato d'alla, Maggio, Italy, pp. 17–27.

Holtkamp DE, Greslin JG, Root CA, et al. (1960) Gonadotropin inhibiting and anti-fecundability effects of chloramiphene. *Proc Soc Exp Biol Med* 105:197–201.

Hsueh AJW, Erickson GF, Yen SSC (1978) Sensitization of pituitary cells to luteinizing hormone releasing hormone by clomiphene citrate in vitro. *Nature* 273:57–9.

Huang K-E (1986) The primary treatment of luteal phase inadequacy: progesterone versus clomiphene citrate. *Am J Obstet Gynecol* 155:824–8.

Imoedemhe DA, Shaw RW, Kirkland A, et al. (1987) Ultrasound measurement of endometrial thickness on different ovarian stimulation regimens during in vitro fertilization. *Hum Reprod* 2:545–7.

Isaacs JD Jr., Lincoln SR, Cowan BD (1997) Extended clomiphene citrate (CC) and prednisone for the treatment of chronic anovulation resistant to CC alone. *Fertil Steril* 67:641–3.

James WH (1980) Gonadotropin and the human secondary sex ration. *Br Med J* 281:711–12.

James WH (1985) The sex ratio of infants born after hormonal induction of ovulation. *Br J Obstet Gynecol* 92:299–301.

Jansen RPS (1982) Spontaneous abortion incidence in the treatment of infertility. *Am J Obstet Gynecol* 143:451–73.

Kauffman RP, Baker VM, DiMarino P, et al. (2002) Polycystic ovarian syndrome and insulin resistance in white and Mexican American women: a comparison of two distinct populations. *Am J Obstet Gynecol* 187:1362–9.

Kemman E, Bohrer M, Shelden R, et al. (1987) Active ovulation management increases the monthly probability of pregnancy occurrence in ovulatory women who receive intrauterine insemination. *Fertil Steril* 48:916–20.

Kerin JF, Liu JH, Phillipou G, Yen SSC (1985) Evidence for a hypothalamic site of action of clomiphene citrate in women. *J Clin Endocrinol Metab* 61:265–8.

Kistner RW (1966) Use of clomiphene citrate, human chorionic gonadotropins and human menopausal gonadotropins for induction of ovulation in the human female. *Fertil Steril* 17;569–83.

Kocak M, Caliskan E, Simsir C, et al. (2002) Metformin therapy improves ovulatory rates, cervical scores and pregnancy rates in clomiphene citrate resistant women with polycystic ovary syndrome. *Fertil Steril* 77:101–6.

Kurachi K, Aono T, Minagawa J, et al. (1983) Congenital malformations of newborn infants after clomiphene-induced ovulation. *Fertil Steril* 40:187–9.

Legro RS, Finegood D, Dunaif A (1998) A fasting glucose to insulin ratio is a useful measure of insulin sensitivity in women with polycystic ovary syndrome. *J Clin Endocrinol Metab* 83;2694–8.

Lobo RA, Granger LR, Davajan V, Mishell DR (1982a) An extended regimen of clomiphene citrate in women unresponsive to standard therapy. *Fertil Steril* 37:762–6.

Lobo RA, Paul W, March CM, et al. (1982b) Clomiphene and dexamethasone in women unresponsive to clomiphene alone. *Obstet Gynecol* 60:497–501.

Macgregor AH, Johnson JE, Bunde CA (1967) Induction of ovulation with clomiphene citrate. Presented at the 14th Annual Meeting of the Canadian Society for the Study of Fertility, Montreal, June 19–21.

Macgregor AH, Johnson JE, Bunde CA (1968) Further clinical experience with clomiphene citrate. *Fertil Steril* 19:616–22.

Maclin VM, Radwanska E, Binor Z, et al. (1990) Progesterone: estradiol ratios at implantation in ongoing pregnancies, abortions, and nonconception cycles resulting from ovulation induction. *Fertil Steril* 54:238–44.

Marchbanks PA, Coulam CB, Annegers JF (1986) An association between clomiphene citrate and ectopic pregnancy: a preliminary report. *Fertil Steril* 44:268–70.

Marchini M, Dorta M, Bombelli F, et al. (1989) Effects of clomiphene citrate on cervical mucus: analysis of some influencing factors. *Int J Fertil* 34:154–9.

Marrs RP, Vargas JM, Shangold GM, et al. (1984) The effect of time of initiation of clomiphene citrate on multiple follicle development for human in vitro fertilization and embryo replacement procedures. *Fertil Steril* 41:682–5.

Martinez AR, Bernardus RE, Voorhorst FJ, et al. (1990) Intrauterine insemination does and clomiphene citrate does not improve fecundity in couple with infertility due to male or idiopathic factors: a prospective, randomized, controlled study. *Fertil Steril* 53: 847–53.

Melis GB, Paoletti AM, Strigini F, et al. (1987) Pharmacologic induction of multiple follicular development improves the success rate of artificial insemination with husband's semen in couples with male-related or unexplained infertility. *Fertil Steril* 47:441–5.

Mikkelson TJ, Kroboth PD, Cameron WJ, et al. (1986) Single-dose pharmacokinetics of clomiphene citrate in normal volunteers. *Fertil Steril* 46:392–6.

Murthy YS, Parekh MC, Arronet GH (1971) Experience with clomiphene and cisclomiphene. *Int J Fertil* 16:66–74.

Nestler JE, Jakubowics DJ, Evans WS, et al. (1998) Effects of metformin on spontaneous and clomiphene-induced ovulation in the polycystic ovary syndrome. *N Engl J Med* 338:1876–80.

Palopoli FP, Feil VJ, Allen RE et al. (1967) Substituted aminoalkoxytriarylhodoethylenes. *J Med Chem* 10:84–7.

Parsanezhad ME, Albozi S, Motazedian S, et al. (2002) Use of dexamethasone and clomiphene citrate in the treatment of clomiphene citrate-resistant patients with polycystic ovary syndrome and normal dehydroepiandrosterone sulfate levels; a prospective, double-blind, placebo-controlled trial. *Fertil Steril* 78:1001–4.

Pildes RB (1965) Induction of ovulation with clomiphene. *Am J Obstet Gynecol* 91:466–73.

Powell-Phillips WD (1979) Clomiphene citrate induced concurrent ovarian and intrauterine pregnancy. *Obstet Gynecol* 53:37–9.

Quigley MM, Berkowitz AS, Gilbert SA, et al. (1984) Clomiphene citrate in an in vitro fertilization program; hormonal comparisons between 50- and 150-mg dosages. *Fertil Steril* 41:809–15.

Randall JM, Templeton AT (1991) Transvaginal sonographic assessment of follicular and endometrial growth in spontaneous and clomiphene citrate cycles. *Fertil Steril* 56:208–12.

Rizk B (2006) Epidemiology of ovarian hyperstimulation syndrome. In Rizk B. (ed.), Ovarian Hyperstimulation Syndrome. Cambridge: United Kingdom, Cambridge University Press, chapter 2, 10–42.

Rizk B (Ed.) (2008) Ultrasonography in Reproductive Medicine and Infertility. Cambridge: United Kingdom, Cambridge University Press, (in press).

Rizk B, Dickey RP (2008) Ovarian Hyperstimulation Syndrome. In Dickey RP, Brinsden PR Pyrzak R (Eds.) Intrauterine Insemination. Cambridge: United Kingdom, Cambridge University Press, (in press).

Rogers PA, Polson D, Murphy CR, et al. (1991) Correlation of endometrial histology, morphometry, and ultrasound appearance after different stimulation protocols for in vitro fertilization. *Fertil Steril* 55:583–7.

Rossing MA, Daling JR, Weiss NS, et al. (1994) Ovarian tumors in a cohort of infertile women. *N Engl J Med* 331:771–6.

Schneider L, Bessis R, Simmonet T (1979) The frequency of ovular resorption during the first trimester of twin pregnancy. *Acta Genet Med Gemollol* 28:271–2.

Scott RT, Hofmann GE (1995) Prognostic assessment of ovarian reserve. *Fertil Steril* 63:1–11.

Shalev J, Goldenberg M, Kukia E, et al. (1989) Comparison of five clomiphene citrate dosage regimens: follicular recruitment and distribution in the human ovary. *Fertil Steril* 52:560–3.

Shepard MK, Balmaceda JP, Leija CG (1979) Relationship of weight to successful induction of ovulation with clomiphene citrate. *Fertil Steril* 32:641–5.

Steinkampf (2008) Ultrasonography for Computing Controlled Ovarian Hyperstimulation. In Rizk B. (ed.), Ultrasonography in Reproductive Medicine and Infertility. Cambridge: United Kingdom, Cambridge University Press, (in press).

Sterzik K, Dallenbach C, Scneider V, et al. (1988) In vitro fertilization: the degree of endometrial insufficiency varies with the type of ovarian stimulation. *Fertil Steril* 50:457–62.

Taubert HD, Dericks-Tan JSE (1976) High doses of estrogens do not interfere with the ovulation-inducing effect of clomiphene citrate. *Fertil Steril* 27:375–82.

Trott EA, Plouffe LJr., Hansen K, et al. (1996) Ovulation induction in clomiphene resistant anovulatory women with normal dehydroepiandrosterone sulfate levels; beneficial effects of the addition of dexamethasone during the follicular phase. *Fertil Steril* 66:484–7.

Tyler ET, Winer J, Gotlib M, et al. (1962) Effects of MRL-41 in human male and female fertility studies (Abstr). *Clin Res* 10:119.

Van Campenhout J, Simard R, Leduc B (1968) Antiestrogen effect of clomiphene in the human being. *Fertil Steril* 19:700–6.

Vandermolen DT, Ratts VS, Evans WS, et al. (2000) Metformin increases the ovulatory rate and pregnancy rate from clomiphene citrate in patients with polycystic ovary syndrome who are resistant to clomiphene citrate alone. *Fertil Steril* 75: 310–15.

Vorys N, Gantt CL, Hamwi IGJ, et al. (1964) Clinical utility of chemical induction of ovulation. *Am J Obstet Gynecol* 88:425–32.

Whittemore AS, Harris R, Intyre J, et al. (1992) Characteristics relating to ovarian cancer risk: collaborative analysis of 12 US case-control studies. *Am J Epidemiol* 136:1184–203.

World Health Organization (1992) World Health Organization Laboratory Manual for the Examination of Human Sperm-Cervical Mucus Interaction. Cambridge University Press, Cambridge, pp. 43–44.

Yagel S, Ben-Chetrit A, Anteby E, et al. (1992) The effect of ethinyl estradiol on endometrial thickness and uterine volume during ovulation induction by clomiphene citrate. *Fertil Steril* 57:33–6.

Yanagimachi R, Sato A (1986) Effects of a single oral administration of ethinyl estradiol on early pregnancy in the mouse. *Fertil Steril* 19:787–801.

Young RL, Goldzieher JW, Elkind-Hirsch K, et al. (1991) A short-term comparison of the effects of clomiphene citrate and conjugated equine estrogen in menopausal/castrate women. *Int J Fertil* 36:167–71.

▪ 24 ▪

AROMATASE INHIBITORS FOR ASSISTED REPRODUCTION

Mohamed F. M. Mitwally, Robert F. Casper

This chapter discusses the potential role of the new group of medications called "aromatase inhibitors" in assisted reproduction. In the past few years, aromatase inhibitors have emerged as promising agents for infertility treatment, particularly ovarian stimulation. We reported the first series in the literature of the successful application of an aromatase inhibitor for induction of ovulation in women with polycystic ovarian syndrome (PCOS) (1) and ovarian stimulation in women with ovulatory infertility, for example, unexplained infertility (2). Following this report, we showed the success of aromatase inhibition for controlled ovarian hyperstimulation (COH) (3–5), whether as a single- or multiple-dose administration (6), and suggested the potential application in various infertility treatments including assisted reproduction (7–13), with data on safety of the pregnancy outcome (14).

Since these first reports, more than a hundred clinical trials have been presented in international meetings, confirming our original findings, by investigators from all over the globe. Many peer-reviewed manuscripts (15–33) have already confirmed the success of aromatase inhibitors in various infertility applications. Currently, several multicenter clinical trials are running testing the clinical efficacy of aromatase inhibitors for infertility treatment including ovarian stimulation. In this chapter, we will discuss the potential role of aromatase inhibitors for assisted reproduction, presenting the theoretical benefits and the available evidence.

AROMATASE INHIBITORS

Blocking estrogen production by inhibiting the enzyme catalyzing its synthesis from androgens (aromatase enzyme) is a treatment modality that has been in clinical application for more than half a century since the development of the first generations of aromatase inhibitors including aminoglutethimide. However, the successful applications of aromatase inhibitors in managing estrogen-dependant disorders, particularly malignancies such as breast cancer, have not achieved significant success and popularity until recently. This was due to several problems encountered with the clinical use of the early generations of the aromatase inhibitors. Those problems could be overcome to a great extent by the development of the third generation of aromatase inhibitors. Table 24.1 summarizes the different generations of the aromatase inhibitors, while Boxes 24.1 and 24.2 summarize the significant problems associated with the early generations of the aromatase inhibitors and the advantages of the third-generation aromatase inhibitors, respectively.

The Aromatase Enzyme

Aromatase or "estrogen synthase" is the enzyme that catalyzes the rate-limiting step in estrogen synthesis, that is, the conversion of androgens (androstenedione and testosterone) into estrogens (estrone and estradiol, respectively). Many tissues express aromatase activity, in particular the ovaries, brain, adipose tissue, muscle, liver, breast tissue, and malignant tumors, for example, breast tumors. During the reproductive age (premenopausal women), the main source of circulating estrogens is the ovaries, while most of the circulating estrogen comes from the adipose tissue in women after menopause (34).

Aromatase Inhibitors

Being a terminal step in the cascade of steroidogenesis, aromatase is a good target for selective inhibition. A large number of aromatase inhibitors have been developed over the past five decades with the third-generation aromatase inhibitors licensed for suppressing estrogen synthesis in postmenopausal women with breast cancer in the past decade. The third-generation aromatase inhibitors were developed after the clinical failure of the earlier generations of aromatase inhibitors, as explained above in Boxes 24.1 and 24.2 (34, 35).

HYPOTHETICAL ROLE OF AROMATASE INHIBITORS FOR ASSISTED REPRODUCTION

We postulated that aromatase inhibitors can play a major role in the practice of assisted reproduction, both as ovarian stimulation agents as well as adjuvant agents that can enhance the outcome of assisted reproduction. Aromatase inhibitors can improve sensitivity to FSH and reduce complications such as severe ovarian hyperstimulation while lowering the overall cost of assisted reproduction. This section of the chapter is a hypothetical discussion of the underlying scientific justification supporting the application of aromatase inhibitors for assisted reproduction.

Mechanisms of Aromatase Inhibition for Ovarian Stimulation

Several years have now passed since the first report of the success of aromatase inhibition for ovarian stimulation. However, the underlying mechanisms behind the success of aromatase

Table 24.1: Different Generations of Aromatase Inhibitors

Generation	Nonsteroidal aromatase inhibitors	Steroidal aromatase inhibitors (sometimes called suicidal inhibitors of the aromatase enzyme)
	Work by temporary (reversible) inactivation of the aromatase enzyme	Work by permanent (irreversible) inactivation of the aromatase enzyme
First generation	Aminoglutethimide (Cytadren®)	NA
Second generation	Rogletimide	Formestane
	Fadrozole	
Third generation	Letrozole (Femara®, 2.5 mg/tablet)	Exemestane (Aromasin®, 25 mg/tablet)
	Anastrozole (Arimidex®, 1 mg/tablet)	
	Vorozole	

Box 24.1: Problems Associated with Early Generations Aromatase Inhibitors

PHARMACODYNAMIC ADVANTAGES:

1   Low potency in inhibiting the aromatase enzyme, particularly in premenopausal women (very low potency)

2   Lack of specificity in inhibiting the aromatase enzyme with significant inhibition of other steroidogenesis enzymes, leading to medical adrenalectomy

PHARMACOKINETIC ADVANTAGES:

1   Not all members are available orally (some require parenteral administration)

2   Variable bioavailability after oral administration

3   Variable half-life that changes with the period of administration due to induction of its metabolism

CLINICAL ADVANTAGES:

1   Poorly tolerated on daily administration, with more than a third of patients discontinuing treatment due to adverse effects

2   Significant side effects related to both the aromatase inhibitors, for example, drowsiness, morbilliform skin rash, nausea and anorexia, and dizziness and side effects secondary to the steroids used for replacement therapy, for example, glucocorticoids

3   Interaction with alcohol with significant potentiation of its action

4   Significant interactions with other medications, for example, coumarin and warfarin

5   Need for replacement therapy due to medical adrenalectomy, for example, glucocorticoid and mineralocorticoid replacement

6   Long-term possible carcinogenesis (at least in animals)

inhibition for ovarian stimulation have not been completely elucidated. We believe that several mechanisms, both central (at the level of the brain) and peripheral (at the level of the ovaries and the uterus), function together, with one or more mechanisms more important than the others in certain infertile subgroups.

Central Mechanisms

Centrally, blocking estrogen synthesis in the brain as well as lowering circulating estrogens by reducing whole-body estrogen synthesis would release the hypothalamus and/or pituitary from the estrogen-negative feedback on the production and release of gonadotropins (without depletion of estrogen receptors as occurs with antiestrogens, e.g., clomiphene citrate). The resultant increase in gonadotropin secretion will stimulate the growth of the ovarian follicles. Withdrawal of estrogen centrally also increases activins, which are produced by a wide variety of tissues including the pituitary gland (36) and will stimulate synthesis of FSH by a direct action on the gonadotropes (37).

Peripheral Mechanisms

Peripherally, aromatase inhibition may increase ovarian follicular sensitivity to FSH stimulation. This could result from temporary accumulation of intraovarian androgens since conversion of those androgen substrates to estrogens is blocked by inhibition of the aromatase enzyme. This assumption is based on data supporting a stimulatory role for androgens in early follicular growth in primates (38) mediated directly through testosterone augmentation of follicular FSH receptor expression (39, 40) and indirectly through androgen stimulation of

Box 24.2: Advantages of Third-Generation Aromatase Inhibitors

PHARMACODYNAMIC ADVANTAGES:

1 Extreme potency in inhibiting the aromatase enzyme (up to thousand times potency of the first-generation aminoglutethimide)

2 Very specific in inhibiting the aromatase enzyme without significant inhibition of the other steroidogenesis enzymes. This is true even at high doses

3 Absence of estrogen receptor depletion

PHARMACOKINETIC ADVANTAGES:

1 Orally administered (other routes of administration are also possible, e.g., vaginal and rectal)

2 Almost 100 percent bioavailability after oral administration

3 Rapid clearance from the body due to short half-life (approximately eight hours for the Aromasin® to approximately forty-five hours for the Femara® and Arimidex®)

4 Absence of tissue accumulation of the medications or any of their metabolites

5 No significant active metabolites

CLINICAL ADVANTAGES:

1 Well tolerated on daily administration for up to several years (in postmenopausal women with breast cancer) with few adverse effects

2 Few mild side effects

3 Very safe without significant contraindications

4 Absence of significant interactions with other medications

5 Very wide safety margin (toxic dose is several thousand times higher than recommended efficacious therapeutic dose)

6 Relatively inexpensive

---

insulin-like growth factor I (IGF-I), which may synergize with FSH to promote folliculogenesis (41, 42).

Reducing the Detrimental Effects of High Estrogen Levels Associated with COH

In women undergoing COH for assisted reproduction, supraphysiological levels of estrogen are inevitably attained due to the growth of multiple mature ovarian follicles. Whether such very high estrogen levels have detrimental effects on the outcome of assisted reproduction is still a matter of debate (10). Several explanations for the controversy include the different methodologies applied for assessing estrogen production during COH and the probability that different infertility subgroups are more vulnerable than others to the supraphysiological levels of estrogen (4, 44). A complete discussion of this issue is not within the scope of this chapter but the reader is referred to our recent review of the issue (10). Box 24.3 summarizes a list of potential mechanisms that have been postulated for detrimental effects of supraphysiological levels of estrogen on the outcome of infertility treatment including assisted reproduction (10).

When an aromatase inhibitor is applied during COH, estrogen production per growing ovarian follicle has been found to be significantly lower than when aromatase inhibitors are not used (about 40–60 percent less) (3–5). This makes sense as estrogen synthesis is significantly reduced by inhibiting the aromatase enzyme. We believe that the milder elevation in the levels of estrogen associated with aromatase inhibitor use dur-

ing COH might improve the treatment outcome by reducing possible detrimental effects of supraphysiological estrogen levels that would be attained without aromatase inhibitors. This might be especially important in subgroups of patients who are probably more vulnerable to the high estrogen levels, for example, PCOS and women with endometriosis-associated infertility and in women with breast cancer (Oktay references) (22, 50, 51).

Reducing the Risk of Severe Ovarian Hyperstimulation Syndrome

Although there is a lack of consensus on the role of high estrogen levels in the pathophysiology and development of severe ovarian hyperstimulation syndrome (45), lowering the supraphysiological levels of estrogen by aromatase inhibitors seems to be a potential method of preventing or at least ameliorating the severity of severe ovarian hyperstimulation syndrome. Further investigation of this speculation is required.

In Vitro Maturation

The use of aromatase inhibitors for in vitro maturation is an exciting application that can involve a brief aromatase inhibitor–induced rise in endogenous gonadotropin secretion leading to multiple ovarian follicles, followed by retrieval of immature oocytes. Currently, there are no available data for such an application.

Box 24.3: Possible Detrimental Effects of the Supraphysiological Estrogen Levels Attained during Ovarian Stimulation and Assisted Reproduction

---

STRONG EVIDENCE:
Effect on the endometrium and implantation

1 Defective steroid hormones receptor development in particular estrogen, progesterone, and androgen receptors

2 Dyssynchronization of the stromal/epithelial endometrial development

3 Dyssynchronization between implantation window (advanced endometrial development while delayed in vitro development of the transferred embryos)

4 Abnormal temporal expression of the endometrial pinopodes (temporarily distant from the embryo transfer time)

5 Impaired endometrial blood flow (both subendometrial and possibly uterine blood flow)

6 Abnormal expression of the endometrial integrins and other adhesion molecules

REASONABLY STRONG EVIDENCE:
Effect on the developing gametes and embryos

1 Effect on chromosomal and cytogenetic integrity of the developing oocyte

2 Defective mitochondrial function in the oocyte

3 Effect on the sperm causing possible premature acrosome reaction and deactivation

4 Effect on the developing embryo and blastocyst hatching

LESS STRONG EVIDENCE:

1 Effect on the ovaries and pituitary (defective corpus luteum function and luteal phase) due to defective LH secretion, LH surge, and LH tonic pulse release

2 Other probable targets:

    a Abnormal leptin production
    b Excessive activation of the coagulation system
    c Defective development of placenta

Benefits in Particular Patient Groups

As mentioned earlier, both lowering supraphysiological levels of estrogen during COH and improving response to COH by enhancing endogenous gonadotropin production and increasing the ovarian follicular sensitivity to gonadotropin stimulation could be of benefit in particular groups of patients, for example, poor responders, endometriosis-associated infertility, PCOS, and survivors of estrogen-dependant malignancies, for example, breast cancer.

Poor Responders

As discussed in the sections of the mechanism of ovarian stimulation by aromatase inhibitors, administering aromatase inhibitors is expected to increase endogenous gonadotropin production and increase the sensitivity of the ovarian follicles to FSH stimulation according to the central and peripheral hypotheses, respectively. This would obviously be expected to enhance the response to COH in poor responders with accumulating evidence supporting this idea (3, 20). However, one should be cautious here as a good proportion of women with poor response to gonadotropins have depletion of the ovarian follicular reserve and early ovarian failure. Such a group of poor responders would not be expected to respond to any modality of COH, and their best chance for pregnancy lies in donor oocyte-assisted reproduction.

Endometriosis

The expression of the aromatase enzyme in endometriotic tissues and the significant role played by locally produced estrogen in endometriosis progression (4, 46, 47) suggests a benefit of aromatase inhibitors in endometriosis-related infertility. The inhibition of local estrogen production in endometrial implants and the lower peripheral estrogen levels associated with the use of aromatase inhibition for ovarian stimulation are expected to possibly protect against progression of endometriosis and may improve the outcome of assisted reproduction in this group of women. However, this idea still awaits confirmation by clinical trials.

Polycystic Ovarian Syndrome

Women with PCOS are at high risk of complications during COH and assisted reproduction, particularly severe ovarian hyperstimulation syndrome. As discussed earlier, those women could benefit from lowering estrogen levels by aromatase inhibition and possibly reduce the risk of severe OHSS.

Interestingly, aromatase inhibition can play a role at the level of the endometrium in those patients. Estrogen has been shown to decrease the level of its own receptor by stimulating ubiquitination of estrogen receptors. This results in rapid degradation of the receptors. In the absence of estrogen, ubiquitination is decreased allowing upregulation of the estrogen receptors and increasing sensitivity to subsequent estrogen administration (48). This could increase endometrial response to estrogen, resulting in more rapid proliferation of endometrial epithelium and stroma and improved blood flow to the uterus and endometrium (49). As a result, normal endometrial development should occur despite the observed lower estrogen concentrations in aromatase inhibitor–treated cycle.

Survivors of Estrogen-Dependant Malignancies

Estrogen-sensitive cancers such as breast cancer can affect women in the reproductive age-group. Those women usually suffer from ovarian failure following chemotherapy particularly with alkylating agents. With the recent success of different fertility preservation options such as oocyte cryopreservation, some women may opt to freeze oocytes or embryos for later use by themselves or a gestational carrier. Oktay et al. reported the success of aromatase inhibition for COH in women undergoing assisted reproduction before receiving cancer treatment. Following COH, patients were followed for almost two years, during which the cancer recurrence rate was similar for patients who received aromatase inhibitor COH and those who had no ovarian stimulation (control patients) (50, 51).

AVAILABLE EVIDENCE FOR POTENTIAL ROLE OF AROMATASE INHIBITORS FOR ASSISTED REPRODUCTION

Evidence is accumulating to confirm the success of aromatase inhibitors as adjuvant agents to enhance the outcome of assisted reproduction. However, larger clinical trials are still needed to confirm and quantify the nature and extent of the benefits from adding aromatase inhibitors to COH stimulation protocols.

Reducing the Dose of Gonadotropins Required for COH and Improving Response in Poor Responders

A significant reduction in the gonadotropin dose required was found (45–55 percent reduction) when the aromatase inhibitor, letrozole, was added to gonadotropin COH treatment (3–5). Because gonadotropin injections constitute a significant part of the cost of infertility treatment, especially during assisted reproduction, we believe that aromatase inhibitors will markedly reduce the cost of infertility treatment by decreasing the gonadotropin dose required for optimum ovarian stimulation. This could make assisted reproductive technology available to a larger group of infertile couples. Moreover, such reduction in the gonadotropin dose observed by combining letrozole with gonadotropins encouraged us to explore the value of aromatase inhibition in improving ovarian response to gonadotropins in poor responders.

In a randomized, controlled study that included poor responders undergoing COH for assisted reproduction, Goswami et al. (20) compared letrozole plus gonadotropin protocol with a standard GnRH agonist and gonadotropin protocol. The study was a small pilot study that included thirty-eight patients. The authors found that adding the aromatase inhibitor, letrozole, to a small dose of gonadotropin (150 IU; two injections of 75 IU on cycle days 3 and 8) resulted in a similar number of oocytes retrieved, embryos transferred, and pregnancy rate as observed in the women on the standard protocol. Interestingly, the group that received the standard protocol had a mean

($\pm$SEM) total gonadotropins dose of 2865 $\pm$ 228 IU, that is, almost twenty times the total amount of gonadotropins received by the letrozole group.

In a more recent and larger study, Garcia-Velasco et al. (21) used the aromatase inhibitor, letrozole, as an adjuvant to gonadotropins in 147 poor responder patients undergoing COH for assisted reproduction. The patients had at least one previous assisted reproduction cycle that was canceled due to poor response to COH. The study was prospective but not randomized. The women were divided into a control group of seventy-six patients treated with high-dose gonadotropins in a GnRH-antagonist regimen. The experimental group included seventy-one patients who received the aromatase inhibitor, letrozole, at a dose of 2.5 mg plus gonadotropins for the first five days of stimulation followed by the same gonadotropin/antagonist regimen. The authors found women who received letrozole had higher numbers of oocytes retrieved with a higher implantation rate despite receiving the same doses of gonadotropins as the control group. Interestingly, both testosterone and androstenedione concentrations were significantly increased in the follicular fluid in the experimental group compared to the control group. These findings are consistent with our peripheral hypothesis that aromatase inhibition, by blocking androgen to estrogen conversion, increases intraovarian androgens and follicular FSH receptor expression and sensitivity to FSH administration.

Most recently, Verpoest et al. (33) in a pilot study randomized patients to receive letrozole (group A; $n = 10$), versus no letrozole (group B; $n = 10$) in an ovarian stimulation protocol with recombinant FSH 150 IU/day starting on day 2 of the cycle and gonadotropin-releasing hormone antagonist 0.25 mg/day starting on day 6 of the cycle. The authors found significantly higher LH concentrations in group A versus group B during letrozole administration. Group A (the letrozole group) was also associated with lower estradiol concentrations but higher serum FSH, testosterone, and androstenedione concentrations compared to group B, throughout the follicular phase. However, the differences were not statistically significant. Median endometrial thickness was significantly higher in group A (letrozole) on the day of human chorionic gonadotropin administration. Pregnancies were higher in the letrozole group. However, the small sample size did not allow the difference to reach statistical significance. The authors concluded that their pilot study supported the idea that aromatase inhibitors can contribute to normal implantation and follicular response, without having negative antiestrogenic effects (33).

Safety Concerns about Aromatase Inhibitors for Ovarian Stimulation

With the short period of clinical experience with aromatase inhibitors for infertility treatment, caution needs to be applied and proper patient consent is necessary for full approval of the ovarian stimulation indication to be attained.

Side Effects of Aromatase Inhibitors

Most of the data about side effects associated with clinical use of aromatase inhibitors come from clinical trials involving postmenopausal women with breast cancer. In this group of patients, third-generation aromatase inhibitors were generally well tolerated. The main side effects are hot flushes and gastrointestinal events (nausea and vomiting) and leg cramps. In those trials, very few patients withdrew from first- or second-line comparative phase III trials because of drug-related adverse events with aromatase inhibitors (50–52). Obviously, these adverse effects were observed in older women with advanced breast cancer who received aromatase inhibitors daily over a long period of time for several months up to few years. Obviously, fewer adverse effects are expected in women who would receive aromatase inhibitors while undergoing assisted reproduction. Those women are usually healthier and younger and would receive the aromatase inhibitors for a short course of few days. In our clinical experience with the use of aromatase inhibitors for ovarian stimulation and in patients undergoing assisted reproduction, we have observed few side effects such as hot flushes and PMS-type symptoms. Interestingly, most of the patients who had a history of treatment with clomiphene citrate found treatment with an aromatase inhibitor to be better tolerated with fewer side effects compared to the clomiphene citrate (53). However, so far, there are no clinical trials that compared the adverse effects associated with the use of aromatase inhibitors for ovarian stimulation with other ovarian stimulation agents.

Low Estrogen Levels Associated with Aromatase Inhibitor Treatment

As expected, aromatase inhibition results in estrogen levels that are significantly lower when compared to serum estrogen levels at midcycle seen with treatment with other ovarian stimulation agents such as gonadotropins or clomiphene citrate. Midcycle estradiol levels per mature follicle were around half that found without aromatase inhibitors treatment (3–5). The question whether low or very low intrafollicular estrogen is compatible with follicular development, ovulation, and corpus luteum formation has been reviewed before and markedly reduced to even absent intrafollicular concentrations of estrogen are known to be compatible with follicular "expansion," retrieval of fertilizable oocytes, and apparently normal embryo development (54). However, the rapid clearance of the aromatase inhibitors due to their relatively short half-life (around two days), the reversible nature of enzyme inhibition, and elevated levels of FSH, which induces new expression of aromatase enzyme, are factors that result in increasing estrogen production that has been demonstrated to be relatively normal at the time of ovulation; (21).

Outcome of Pregnancy Achieved after Treatment by Aromatase Inhibitors

Animal embryonic safety studies have found the aromatase inhibitor, anastrozole, to have no teratogenic or clastogenic effect, whereas there have been some concerns regarding teratogenic effects of letrozole if administered unintentionally during pregnancy (55). The short half-life of aromatase inhibitors, together with their administration in the early follicular phase, several days before ovulation, should result in their clearance before implantation takes place.

We reported the clinical outcome of early pregnancies achieved after the use of the aromatase inhibitor, letrozole, for ovulation induction or COH for IUI (14). In this non-randomized cohort study, the outcome of pregnancies achieved after letrozole were compared along with the outcome of pregnancies achieved with other ovarian stimulation treatments with a control group of pregnancies spontaneously conceived without ovarian stimulation. In three tertiary referral centers over a two-year period, there were 394 pregnancy cycles in 345 infertile couples (133 pregnancies with 2.5 mg or 5 mg letrozole alone or with gonadotropins, 113 pregnancies with CC alone or with gonadotropins, 110 pregnancies with gonadotropins alone, and 38 pregnancies achieved without ovarian stimulation). Pregnancies conceived after IUI treatment were associated with comparable miscarriage and ectopic pregnancy rates compared to all other groups including the spontaneous conceptions. In addition, letrozole use was associated with a significantly lower rate of multiple gestation compared to CC consistent with the hypothesis of intact central estrogen negative-feedback mechanism on gonadotropin secretion.

A more recent multicenter study (56) that included 911 babies, 514 born after letrozole treatment, and 397 after CC treatment did not find any increase in the rates of major and minor malformations in babies conceived after letrozole treatment. Both groups (letrozole and clomiphene citrate) included infertility patients who received ovulation induction followed by IUI or timed intercourse. The study found seven newborns in the CC group (1.8 percent) and only one in the letrozole group (0.2 percent) to have congenital cardiac anomalies ($P = 0.02$). The incidence of cardiac anomalies in the letrozole group was slightly lower than the rate of congenital cardiac anomalies reported among all births (0.4–1.2 percent), and the CC rates were slightly higher. Ventricular septal defect was the predominant cardiac anomaly (five of eight newborns with cardiac anomalies), similar to the findings in spontaneously conceived pregnancies (57). These findings suggest that congenital cardiac anomalies are less frequent in the letrozole group than in the CC group and the general population.

REFERENCES

1. Mitwally MFM, Casper RF. Aromatase inhibition: a novel method of ovulation induction in women with polycystic ovarian syndrome. *Reprod Technol* 2000; 10: 244–7.
2. Mitwally MFM, Casper RF. Use of an AI for induction of ovulation in patients with an inadequate response to clomiphene citrate. *Fertil Steril* 2001; 75: 305–9.
3. Mitwally MFM, Casper RF. Aromatase inhibition improves ovarian response to follicle-stimulating hormone in poor responders. *Fertil Steril* 2002; 774: 776–80.
4. Mitwally MF, Casper RF. Aromatase inhibition reduces gonadotrophin dose required for controlled ovarian stimulation in women with unexplained infertility. *Hum Reprod* 2003; 188: 1588–97.
5. Mitwally MF, Casper RF. Aromatase inhibition reduces the dose of gonadotropin required for controlled ovarian hyperstimulation. *J Soc Gynecol Investig* 2004; 11: 406–15.
6. Mitwally MFM, Casper RF. Single dose administration of the aromatase inhibitor, letrozole: a simple and convenient effective method of ovulation induction. *Fertil Steril* 2005; 83: 229–31.
7. Mitwally MF, Casper RF. Potential of aromatase inhibitors for ovulation and superovulation induction in infertile women. *Drugs* 2006; 66(18) 66(17): 2149–60.
8. Mitwally MFM, Casper RF. Letrozole for ovulation induction. *Exp Rev Obstet Gynecol* 2006; 1(1): 15–27.
9. Casper RF, Mitwally MF. Review: aromatase inhibitors for ovulation induction. *J Clin Endocrinol Metab* 2006; 91: 760–71.
10. Mitwally MF, Casper RF, Diamond MP. The role of aromatase inhibitors in ameliorating deleterious effects of ovarian

stimulation on outcome of infertility treatment. *Reprod Biol Endocrinol* 2005; 3: 54.

11. Mitwally MF, Casper RF. Aromatase inhibitors in ovulation induction. *Semin Reprod Med* 2004; 22(1): 61–78.

12. Mitwally MF, Casper RF. Aromatase inhibitors for the treatment of infertility. *Expert Opin Investig Drugs* 2003; 12(3): 353–71.

13. Mitwally MF, Casper RF. Aromatase inhibition for ovarian stimulation: future avenues for infertility management. *Curr Opin Obstet Gynecol* 2002; 14(3): 255–63.

14. Mitwally MFM, Casper RF. Pregnancy outcome after the use of an AI for induction of ovulation. *Am J Obstet Gynecol* 2005; 192: 381–6.

15. Healey S, Tan SL, Tulandi T, Biljan MM. Effects of letrozole on superovulation with gonadotropins in women undergoing intrauterine insemination. *Fertil Steril* 2003; 806: 1325–9.

16. Cortinez A, De Carvalho I, Vantman D, et al. Hormonal profile and endometrial morphology in letrozole-controlled ovarian hyperstimulation in ovulatory infertile patients. *Fertil Steril* 2005; 83(1): 110–5.

17. Fatemi HM, Kolibianakis E, Tournaye H, et al. Clomiphene citrate versus letrozole for ovarian stimulation: a pilot study. *Reprod Biomed Online* 2003; 75: 543–6.

18. Al-Omari WR, Sulaiman WR, Al-Hadithi N. Comparison of two AIs in women with clomiphene-resistant polycystic ovary syndrome. *Int J Gynaecol Obstet* 2004; 853: 289–91.

19. Al-Fozan H, Al-Khadouri M, Tan SL, Tulandi T. A randomized trial of letrozole versus clomiphene citrate in women undergoing superovulation. *Fertil Steril* 2004; 82: 1561–3.

20. Goswami SK, Das T, Chattopadhyay R, et al. A randomized single-blind controlled trial of letrozole as a low-cost IVF protocol in women with poor ovarian response: a preliminary report. *Hum Reprod* 2004; 19: 2031–5.

21. Garcia-Velasco JA, Moreno L, Pacheco A, et al. The aromatase inhibitor, letrozole increases the concentration of intraovarian androgens and improves in vitro fertilization outcome in low responder patients: a pilot study. *Fertil Steril* 2005; 84: 82–7.

22. Oktay K, Buyuk E, Libertella N, Akar M, Rosenwaks Z. Fertility preservation in breast cancer patients: a prospective controlled comparison of ovarian stimulation with tamoxifen and letrozole for embryo cryopreservation. *J Clin Oncol* 2005; 23: 4347–53.

23. Bayar U, Tanrierdi HA, Barut A, et al. Letrozole vs. clomiphene citrate in patients with ovulatory infertility. *Fertil Steril* 2006; 85: 1045–8.

24. Elnashar A, Fouad H, Eldosoky M, et al. Letrozole induction of ovulation in women with clomiphene citrate-resistant polycystic ovary syndrome may not depend on the period of infertility, the body mass index, or the luteinizing hormone/follicle stimulating hormone ratio. *Fertil Steril* 2006; 85: 161–4.

25. Atay V, Cam C, Muhcu M, et al. Comparison of letrozole and clomiphene citrate in women with polycystic ovaries undergoing ovarian stimulation. *J Int Med Res* 2006; 34: 73–6.

26. Sohrabvand F, Ansari S, Bagheri M. Efficacy of combined metformin-letrozole in comparison with metformin-clomiphene citrate in clomiphene-resistant infertile women with polycystic ovarian disease. *Hum Reprod* 2006; 21: 1432–5.

27. Sipe CS, Davis WA, Maifeld M, Van Voorhis BJ. A prospective randomized trial comparing anastrozole and clomiphene citrate in an ovulation induction protocol using gonadotropins. *Fertil Steril* 2006; Sep 26; [Epub ahead of print].

28. Bayar U, Basaran M, Kiran S, Coskun A, Gezer S. Use of an aromatase inhibitor in patients with polycystic ovary syndrome: a prospective randomized trial. *Fertil Steril* 2006; 86(5): 1447–51.

29. Barroso G, Menocal G, Felix H, Rojas-Ruiz JC, Arslan M, Oehninger S. Comparison of the efficacy of the aromatase inhibitor letrozole and clomiphene citrate as adjuvants to recombinant follicle-stimulating hormone in controlled ovarian hyperstimulation: a prospective, randomized, blinded clinical trial. *Fertil Steril* 2006; 86(5): 1428–31.

30. Grabia A, Papier S, Pesce R, Mlayes L, Kopelman S, Sueldo C. Preliminary experience with a low-cost stimulation protocol that includes letrozole and human menopausal gonadotropins in normal responders for assisted reproductive technologies. *Fertil Steril* 2006; 86(4): 1026–8.

31. Jee BC, Ku SY, Suh CS, Kim KC, Lee WD, Kim SH. Use of letrozole versus clomiphene citrate combined with gonadotropins in intrauterine insemination cycles: a pilot study. *Fertil Steril* 2006; 85(6): 1774–7.

32. Bedaiwy MA, Forman R, Mousa NA, Al Inany HG, Casper RF. Cost-effectiveness of aromatase inhibitor co-treatment for controlled ovarian stimulation. *Hum Reprod* 2006; 21(11): 2838–44.

33. Verpoest WM, Kolibianakis E, Papanikolaou E, Smitz J, Van Steirteghem A, Devroey P. Aromatase inhibitors in ovarian stimulation for IVF/ICSI: a pilot study. *Reprod Biomed Online* 2006; 13(2): 166–72.

34. Cole PA, Robinson CH. Mechanism and inhibition of cytochrome P-450 aromatase. *J Med Chem* 1999; 33: 2933–44.

35. Buzdar A, Howell A. Advances in aromatase inhibition: clinical efficacy and tolerability in the treatment of breast cancer. *Clin Cancer Res* 2001; 7: 2620–35.

36. Roberts V, Meunier H, Vaughan J, et al. Production and regulation of inhibin subunits in pituitary gonadotropes. *Endocrinology* 1989; 124: 552–4.

37. Mason AJ, Berkemeier LM, Schmelzer CH, et al. Activin B: precursor sequences, genomic structure and in vitro activities. *Mol Endocrinol* 1989; 3: 1352–8.

38. Weil SJ, Vendola K, Zhou J, et al. Androgen receptor gene expression in the primate ovary: cellular localization, regulation, and functional correlations. *J Clin Endocrinol Metab* 1989; 837: 2479–85.

39. Weil S, Vendola K, Zhou J, et al. Androgen and follicle-stimulating hormone interactions in primate ovarian follicle development. *J Clin Endocrinol Metab* 1999; 848: 2951–6.

40. Vendola KA, Zhou J, Adesanya OO, et al. Androgens stimulate early stages of follicular growth in the primate ovary. *J Clin Invest* 1998; 10112: 2622–9.

41. Vendola K, Zhou J, Wang J, et al. Androgens promote oocyte insulin-like growth factor I expression and initiation of follicle development in the primate ovary. *Biol Reprod* 1999; 612: 353–7.

42. Giudice LC. Insulin-like growth factors and ovarian follicular development. *Endocr Rev* 1992; 13: 641–69.

43. Mitwally MF, Bhakoo HS, Crickard K, Sullivan MW, Batt RE, Yeh J. Estradiol production during controlled ovarian hyperstimulation correlates with treatment outcome in women undergoing in vitro fertilization-embryo transfer. *Fertil Steril* 2006; 86(3): 588–96.

44. Mitwally MF, Bhakoo HS, Crickard K, Sullivan MW, Batt RE, Yehl J. Area under the curve for estradiol levels do not consistently reflect estradiol levels on the day of hCG administration in patients undergoing controlled ovarian hyperstimulation for IVF-ET. *J Assist Reprod Genet* 2005; 22(2): 57–63.

45. Rizk B, Aboulghar M. Modern management of ovarian hyperstimulation syndrome. *Hum Reprod* 1991; 6(8): 1082–7.

46. Bulun SE, Zeitoun KM, Takayama K, Sasano H. Estrogen biosynthesis in endometriosis: molecular basis and clinical relevance. *J Mol Endocrinol* 2000; 1: 35–42.

47. Vignali M, Infantino M, Matrone R, et al. Endometriosis: novel etiopathogenetic concepts and clinical perspectives. *Fertil Steril* 2002; 784: 665–678.

48. Nirmala PB, Thampan RV. Ubiquitination of the rat uterine estrogen receptor: dependence on estradiol. *Biochem Biophys Res Commun* 1995; 2131: 24.

49. Rosenfeld CR, Roy T, Cox BE. Mechanisms modulating estrogen-induced uterine vasodilation. *Vascul Pharmacol* 2002; 382: 115.

50. Oktay K. Further evidence on the safety and success of ovarian stimulation with letrozole and tamoxifen in breast cancer patients undergoing in vitro fertilization to cryopreserve their embryos for fertility preservation. *J Clin Oncol* 2005; 23(16): 3858–9.

51. Oktay K, Buyuk E, Libertella N, et al. Fertility preservation in breast cancer patients: a prospective controlled comparison of ovarian stimulation with tamoxifen and letrozole for embryo cryopreservation. *J Clin Oncol* 2005; 23(19): 4347–53.

52. Hamilton A, Piccart M. The third-generation nonsteroidal AIs: a review of their clinical benefits in the second-line hormonal treatment of advanced breast cancer. *Ann Oncol* 1999; 10: 377–84.

53. Goss PE. Risks versus benefits in the clinical application of aromatase inhibitors. *Endocr Relat Cancer* 1999; 6: 325–32.

54. Palter SF, Tavares AB, Hourvitz A, et al. Are estrogens of importance to primate/human ovarian folliculogenesis? *Endocr Rev* 2001; 223: 389–424.

55. Tiboni GM. Aromatase inhibitors and teratogenesis. *Fertil Steril* 2004; 81: 1158–9.

56. Tulandi T, Al-Fadhli R, Kabli N, et al. Congenital malformations among 911 newborns conceived after infertility treatment with letrozole or clomiphene citrate. *Fertil Steril* 2006; 85(6): 1761–5.

57. Hoffman JIE. Incidence of congenital heart disease: I. Postnatal incidence. *Pediatr Cardiol* 1995; 16: 103.

25

PHARMACODYNAMICS AND PHARMACOKINETICS OF GONADOTROPHINS

A. Michele Schuler, Jonathan G. Scammell

INTRODUCTION

Exogenous hormone supplementation has been used to treat infertility for nearly 100 years (1). Compounds extracted from urine and serum have been used in pharmacotherapeutic preparations as the mainstay of exogenous hormone supplementation until recently. These preparations enabled clinicians to manipulate the hypothalamic-pituitary-ovarian axis to induce follicular recruitment and subsequent ovulation in otherwise anovulatory infertile patients. A resurgence of interest in the treatment of infertility occurred with the birth of the first infant following successful in vitro fertilization (IVF), baby Louise Brown. It is interesting that this pregnancy did not result from exogenous hormone supplementation but rather from a non-induced ovulation (2). Nevertheless, with this successful pregnancy came renewed interest in treatment of infertility. This interest has resulted in the development of new technologies for the production of better, safer, and more affordable treatment options for the infertile female patient.

Ovulation of a single healthy oocyte in a natural cycle is a carefully orchestrated event modulated by secretion of several glycoproteins that act on the ovary and other reproductive tissues to stimulate changes in functional morphology and to stimulate steroidogenesis (Table 25.1). Follicle-stimulating hormone (FSH) is secreted from the anterior pituitary gland in response to the secretion of gonadotropin-releasing hormone from the hypothalamus. Circulating FSH stimulates follicular growth in the ovary by acting on specific FSH receptors in the cell membranes of granulosa cells. Initially, during endogenous secretion of FSH, an antral follicle emerges and exhibits autocrine feedback to increase sensitivity to FSH, luteinizing hormone (LH), and chorionic gonadotropin (CG) through an increase in the receptors to these hormones. As the antral follicle grows and continues to secrete estradiol, the remaining follicles in the ovary undergo atresia. This single follicle becomes a *mature* follicle, which will ovulate in response to a surge in LH. LH is also secreted from the anterior pituitary gland. Prior to ovulation, it acts on specific LH receptors in ovarian thecal cells to stimulate oocyte maturation. After ovulation, it stimulates corpus luteum formation and supports corpus luteum function. Ovulation of the mature oocyte occurs as a result of an LH surge (Figure 25.1) (3).

After fertilization, the developing blastocyst secretes CG, which supports implantation by the developing embryo (4). CG is later secreted in large quantities by the placenta. The major function of CG is to prevent regression of the corpus luteum, thus ensuring adequate progesterone secretion during the first trimester of pregnancy. After the first trimester, the secretion of CG diminishes and the corpus luteum begins to regress. This regression corresponds to an increase of placental progesterone in the maternal circulation.

FSH, LH, and CG are used pharmacologically in fertility induction protocols. For a long time, these hormones were purified from various sources, including pituitary extracts, animal serum, or human urine. The use of these purified materials has several drawbacks including uncertainty of biological activity, local injection reactions, and sensitization (5). Controlled ovarian stimulation protocols have been greatly improved by the advent of recombinant technology. This technology allows for the production of large quantities of highly purified protein from cell culture. There are now recombinant products commercially available for FSH, LH, and CG (Table 25.2). The use of these recombinant products is now considered to be the standard of care for the infertile patient. In this chapter, we will highlight what is known about these recombinant products, including their pharmacokinetics and pharmacodynamics. We will also briefly summarize current research regarding FSH, LH, and CG in animal models as these models have important implications in the study and treatment of human infertility.

STRUCTURE AND PHARMACOKINETICS OF FSH

FSH is administered during the first part of the controlled ovarian stimulation protocol in an effort to stimulate follicular recruitment in infertile women. FSH is a glycoprotein made up of two subunits, α and β, that are noncovalently linked. The α-subunit is identical to the α-subunits of LH and CG. The β-subunits differ for these glycoproteins and confer their specific biological activities. The β-subunit of human FSH is 111 amino acids in length and is glycosylated at two sites (6).

Recombinant human FSH (r-hFSH) is expressed in Chinese hamster ovary (CHO) cells in large-volume (15 L) bioreactors (6). These cells are transfected with both α- and β-subunit vectors and have "continuous and reproducible" production of FSH (6). FSH produced from these cells is purified through a series of comprehensive steps designed to remove contaminants such as proteins introduced from the culture medium and degraded FSH. The purification process yields relatively large amounts of high-potency, high-quality r-hFSH (6).

Table 25.1: Glycoproteins Secreted during a "Natural" Cycle and Their Actions

Glycoprotein	Secreted by	Action(s)
FSH	AP	Stimulates follicular growth
		Stimulates secretion of estradiol from the dominant follicle
LH	AP	Prior to ovulation, stimulates oocyte maturation
		Surge stimulates ovulation
		After ovulation, supports corpus luteum formation and function
CG	Blastocyst	Supports early embryo implantation
	Placenta	Prevents regression of the corpus luteum

AP, anterior pituitary gland.

Table 25.2: Examples of Recombinant Products Approved by the United States Food and Drug Administration for Ovulation Induction Protocols

Product	Trade name	Company	FDA approval
r-hFSH	Follistim®	Organon	September 1997
	Gonal-F®	Serono	September 1997
r-hLH	Luveris®	Serono	May 2005
r-hCG	Ovidrel®	Serono	September 2000

r-hCG, recombinant human chorionic gonadotropin; r-hLH, recombinant human-luteinizing hormone.

PHARMACODYNAMICS OF FSH

FSH has its action through binding to the FSH receptor (FSHR), a G-protein–coupled receptor (7). The FSHR is leucine rich and is characterized by seven transmembrane helices (Figure 25.2). Binding occurs through a hand-clasp binding model (8). As the name suggests, a hand-clasp binding model resembles the appearance of two hands clasped together: the FSH molecule fits into a notch in the curved receptor, and the receptor itself wraps around the middle of the FSH molecule. FSH in complex with the FSHR has recently been crystallized (Figure 25.3). Upon binding of FSH to the FSHR in the ovary, the receptor is activated and signal transduction occurs through

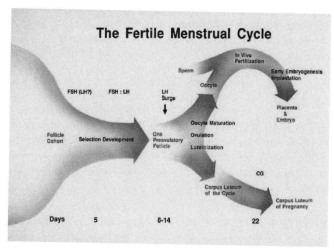

Figure 25.1. Diagram of the events occurring in the ovary and reproductive tract during the initial three weeks of the fertile menstrual cycle leading to natural reproduction in primates. From: Stouffer and Zelinski-Wooten: *Reproductive Biology and Endocrinology* 2: 32, 2004. http://www.rbej.com/content/2/1/32.

Biological activity is determined through an in vivo assay that measures and quantifies an increase in ovarian mass in rats.

The half-life of r-hFSH has been calculated to be approximately seventeen hours, and the volume of distribution to be 11 L as measured by immunoradiometric assay (6). FSH has a relatively long serum half-life. Clearance is 0.5 L per hour and occurs primarily through glomerular filtration and hepatic metabolism. r-hFSH can be administered either intramuscularly or subcutaneously. Half-life and clearance are similar for both routes of administration. Body mass index has an inverse relationship with absorption: the higher the index, the lower the absorption (6). Therefore, a higher dose of r-hFSH may be needed in obese patients.

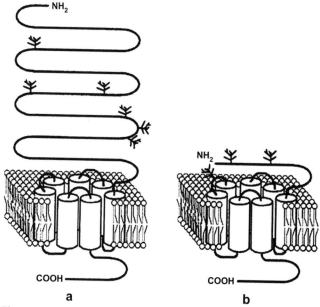

Figure 25.2. A schematic of a plasma membrane G-protein–coupled receptor. G-protein–coupled receptors have an extracellular N-terminus, an intracellular C-terminus, and seven α-helical transmembrane domains. (A) The long N-terminus is typical of a glycoprotein G-protein receptor (such as the FSHR or LHR) (B) The shorter N-terminus is typical of other G-protein–coupled receptors. From: Wheatley and Hawtin: *Human Reproduction Update* 5: 356–364, 1999. Oxford University Press.

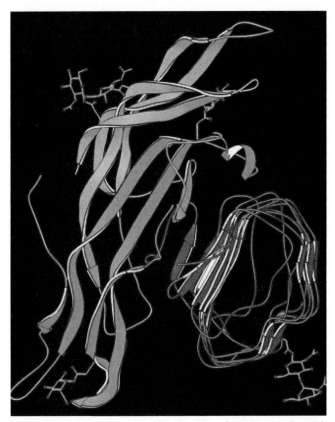

Figure 25.3. Ribbon diagram of the structure of FSH in complex with the FSHR. FSH α-chains are in green. FSH β-chains are in blue. FSHR is in red. N-linked glycosylation sites (of both the FSH molecule and the FSHR) are in yellow. From: Fan and Hendrickson: *Nature* 433: 269–277, 2005. Macmillan Publishers Ltd.

a G-protein cascade of events. This culminates in the activation of adenylate cyclase and the production of cAMP that, in turn, stimulates the secretion of estradiol from the follicle. Circulating estradiol then provides negative feedback to the pituitary and results in a decrease in FSH secretion. In studies where murine L*tk*⁻ cells (L cells) were transfected with recombinant rat FSHR, cAMP accumulates in response to FSH. This cell culture system has been used as a highly sensitive method to determine the bioactivity of FSH in human patient samples (9). The regulation of FSH receptor expression is very complex and is beyond the scope of this chapter; it is discussed in detail by Gromoll and Simoni (10).

r-hFSH AND CONTROLLED OVARIAN STIMULATION IN PRIMATES

r-hFSH has been shown to be effective in follicular recruitment in humans and various species of non-human primates including macaques. Administration of r-hFSH to women can induce oocyte development in multiple follicles (3). Therefore, r-hFSH is frequently the treatment of choice for infertile women (6). r-hFSH is also the treatment of choice for controlled ovarian stimulation in macaques. It is highly effective in ovarian stimulation and produces multiple oocytes from a single animal in a single cycle. In addition, it does not appear to induce the production of antibodies against r-hFSH as was observed for

pregnant mare serum gonadotropin (PMSG), another preparation used for controlled ovarian stimulation in non-human primates (3, 11). PMSG has both FSH and LH activity and is effective in inducing follicular recruitment for a limited number of cycles in macaques. However, macaques secrete antibodies against PMSG with exposure to this preparation (11). We have attempted to use both r-hFSH and PMSG in ovarian stimulation protocols in squirrel monkeys. Unlike macaques and humans, squirrel monkeys respond more robustly to PMSG than to r-hFSH (12). The structure of the squirrel monkey FSHR has yet to be determined. It is possible that the squirrel monkey FSHR differs structurally from the human FSHR and does not bind r-hFSH with high affinity.

STRUCTURE AND PHARMACOKINETICS OF LH

LH is a recent addition to controlled ovarian stimulation protocols. It is used to augment follicular recruitment and can induce oocyte maturation. Although it can also be used to stimulate an endogenous LH surge, human CG (hCG) remains the preparation of choice for ovulation induction. Like FSH and CG, LH is a glycoprotein made up of two subunits, α and β. The β-subunit of LH is 121 amino acids in length and is glycosylated at one site (13, 14). Glycosylation of the β-subunit of LH is N-linked. LH binds to the LH/CG receptor, a receptor that is acted on by both LH and CG in humans (15, 16).

Recombinant human LH (r-hLH) is also made in CHO cells, which secrete LH into the culture medium (13, 14). It is then purified through chromatography. When r-hLH is administered to human subjects, the half-life is reported to be ten hours. Volume of distribution is approximately 14 L, and clearance has been calculated to be 1.7 L per hour, occurring primarily through hepatic metabolism. Renal filtration plays a very small role in clearance. r-hLH can be administered either intramuscularly or subcutaneously. Half-life is shorter when administered intramuscularly but is still adequate for pharmacological action (13, 14).

PHARMACODYNAMICS OF LH

LH and CG bind with high affinity to the LH receptor (LHR), a glycoprotein G-protein–coupled receptor with seven transmembrane domains (Figure 25.2). Binding to the LHR not only results in a cascade of events in adenylate cyclase–mediated signaling but also in phosphoinositide-mediated signaling (15). Both CG and LH bind with high affinity to the LHR and can activate the LHR (16). Activation of the LHR in the ovary supports follicular maturation, induces ovulation, and/or stimulates corpus luteum formation/function, depending on the stage of the cycle and hormonal interactions at that time (17). Ultimately, LH binding to the LHR supports the secretion of progesterone from the corpus luteum. Cell-surface expression of the LHR is regulated by a number of factors and is detailed by Menon et al. (18). A discussion of the regulation of LHR is beyond the scope of this chapter.

r-hLH AND CONTROLLED OVARIAN STIMULATION

r-hLH can be used in controlled ovarian stimulation protocols to promote follicular maturation when used in conjunction with r-hFSH. Typically, ovarian response to r-hFSH can be augmented by the administration of r-hLH and the number of recruited follicles will be maximized (3). In addition, it is thought that the quality of retrieved oocytes (to be used for IVF) is better when FSH is supplemented with LH (19). LH can also be used for induction of ovulation in FSH primed patients (17).

STRUCTURE AND PHARMACOKINETICS OF CG

hCG is administered during controlled ovarian stimulation protocols to induce oocyte maturation. It can be administered prior to oocyte retrieval to mimic an endogenous LH surge if the oocytes will be used for IVF or prior to intrauterine insemination if fertilization is attempted in the patient's uterus. It is also administered after fertilization to support the function of the corpus luteum. The β-subunit of hCG is 145 amino acids. Homology between the β-subunits of human CG and human LH is approximately 80 percent (20), with CG possessing a C-terminal extension of twenty-four amino acids. The β-subunit of CG is glycosylated at six sites, four are O-linked and two are N-linked (20). O-linked glycosylation in the C-terminus protects CG from degradation. The oligosaccharide chains form a physical barrier, protecting the protein core. If these chains are removed, the protein core becomes susceptible to protease degradation (21).

Like r-hFSH, r-hCG is also made in a CHO cell culture system (22). This system yields highly purified product without many of the contaminants observed in urinary origin hCG. The pharmacodynamics of recombinant hCG (r-hCG) are similar to the pharmacodynamics of urinary hCG, but r-hCG is more potent than urinary hCG. The half-life is biphasic; the longer phase is reported to be approximately twenty-four to thirty-three hours (22). The steady-state volume of distribution is reported to be approximately 5–7 L, depending on the dose and route of administration (22). Both the liver and kidneys play a role in clearance. Clearance is reported to be 0.3 L per hour (22). The liver metabolizes approximately 80 percent of cleared hCG (20). Unmetabolized hCG is excreted in the urine.

PHARMACODYNAMICS OF CG

CG binds to the CG/LH receptor (LHR). Like the FSHR, the LHR is also a G-protein–coupled receptor (Figure 25.2). A more complete description of the LHR appears in the section *Pharmacodynamics of LH*.

R-hCG AND CONTROLLED OVARIAN STIMULATION

R-hCG can be used in controlled ovarian stimulation protocols to induce maturation of the oocyte and can improve pregnancy outcome (23). In addition, r-hCG has significant advantages over urinary CG including a higher serum hCG concentration, higher serum progesterone concentration, and a reduction in local reactions. Exogenously administered CG in controlled ovarian stimulation has also been shown to increase endometrial receptivity to the early embryo (20).

LESSONS FROM NEW WORLD MONKEYS

A fascinating variation on this theme is seen in New World primates (infraorder Platyrrhini). New World primates are thought to have separated from Old World anthropoids about thirty-five million years ago (24). Living New World primates, which include primate species such as marmosets, squirrel monkeys, and owl monkeys, likely appeared fifteen to twenty million years ago and are distributed from Central to South America. In 1997, Zhang et al. cloned and sequenced the LHR from common marmoset testis (25). They found that, unlike human LHR mRNA that is transcribed from eleven exons, the LHR in marmoset testis lacks exon 10 at the mRNA level. More recent studies indicate that 1) the absence of LHR exon 10 mRNA is also seen in testicular RNA from other New World primates including squirrel monkeys (26), 2) exon 10 sequences are present in genomic DNA from New World primates (26), and 3) the skipping of exon 10 results from alterations in nucleotides in the New World primate genes leading to failure of the splicing machinery (27). This form of the receptor has been termed the type II LHR. Expression of the type II LHR lacking exon 10 has also been observed in humans (28).

The activity of the type II LHR was subsequently compared to that of wild-type LHR in vitro and found to be impaired in several aspects of receptor function. First, the type II receptor was transported less efficiently to the plasma membrane than wild-type LHR (29). Once expressed at the cell surface, however, the type II LHR binds both natural ligands LH and CG normally (30). The second defect in the type II receptor involves signal transduction. Whereas LH and CG are equipotent in generating the intracellular signal cyclic AMP in COS-7 cells transfected with wild-type receptor, activation of type II LHRs by LH was significantly impaired compared to CG. These results suggest that type II LHRs are refractory to stimulation by LH, but respond normally to CG. This is supported by a study of a patient with Leydig cell hypoplasia secondary to homozygous deletion of exon 10. This patient failed to respond to highly elevated serum LH levels, but treatment with CG achieved an increase in testosterone biosynthesis, an increase in testicular volume, and complete spermatogenesis (28).

The question arises immediately: how does LH complete its functions in New World primates if these primates naturally express an LH receptor type that is refractory to LH? The answer is simply that New World primates do not express LH, but rather CG is the relevant pituitary gonadotropin. Attempts to amplify by reverse-transcriptase polymerase chain reaction the β-subunit of LH from marmoset pituitaries were unsuccessful. Rather, it was discovered that the β-subunit of CG is highly expressed in marmoset pituitaries (26, 31). We have found that squirrel monkey and owl monkey pituitary glands similarly express CG, but not LH, β-subunit (32). Thus, CG is the only gonadotropin with luteinizing function in the pituitaries of New World primates. Furthermore, New World primate CG possesses an amino acid sequence that may result in in vivo behavior different from human CG. As mentioned above, the carboxyl-terminal extension of the β-subunit of human CG possesses four O-linked glycosylation sites that are thought to confer a long circulating half-life, approximately thirty hours (33, 34). Using the NetOGlyc 3.1 Server online program, none of these four sites are predicted to be O-linked glycosylated in New World primate CGβ (Figure 25.4), although Amato et al. reported that the carbohydrate composition of marmoset CGβ suggested the presence of one O-linked site (35). One of the O-linked sites in New World

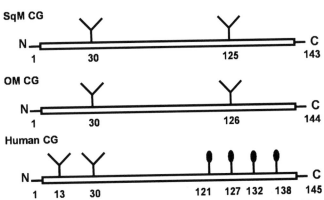

Figure 25.4. Schematic showing predicted glycosylation sites in New World squirrel monkey and owl monkey CG (SqM CG and OM CG, respectively). Human CG possesses N-linked oligosaccharide chains at positions 13 and 30 and O-linked oligosaccharide chains at positions 121, 127, 132, and 138. No sites for O-linked glycosylation are predicted to exist in squirrel monkey or owl monkey CG. Rather, New World primate CGs have gained a unique recognition sequence for N-linked glycosylation in the C-terminus.

primate CGβ is a recognition site for N-linked glycosylation (31, 32, 36, 37). The different glycosylation pattern of New World primate CGβ could result in a shorter half-life, which would be appropriate for a pituitary gonadotropin released in a pulsatile manner. Further studies are required to determine the relative half-lives of human and New World primate CG and indeed to determine within New World primates whether patterns of glycosylation (and hence half-life) of placental CG are different from pituitary CG.

LESSONS FROM KNOCKOUT MICE

Knockout mice have been made for FSHβ, FSHR, LHβ, and LHR (38–42). These animal models have been invaluable for the understanding of the activities/actions of LH, FSH, LHR, and FSHR. FSHβ knockout female mice are infertile with small ovaries. These mice have no circulating FSH but have higher than expected circulating LH. Interestingly, these female mice can be "rescued" with the administration of PMSG (39). This suggests that the ovaries remain "competent" in these knockout mice and can be stimulated to respond when an FSH analog is administered. Like the FSHβ knockout female mice, FSHR knockout mice also are infertile. But, unlike FSHβ knockout female mice, these mice cannot be rescued (40). Circulating FSH and LH are elevated in these mice because of a lack of feedback to the anterior pituitary. The ovaries in these animals lack ovulatory competence and cannot respond to exogenous FSH. This suggests that FSHR expression is necessary for normal ovarian function. LHβ knockout female mice are also infertile but can be rescued in the short-term through administration of human CG (41). Ovarian histology revealed normal primary and secondary follicles. However, antral follicles contained degenerating oocytes. This suggests that in the absence of circulating LH, the follicles develop relatively normally but then do not ovulate as the endogenous LH surge is absent. When exogenous CG is administered, the ovaries have the capability to respond with ovulation. Finally, LHR knockouts are also infer-

tile and have structural multiple defects in the reproductive tract (42). These mice are unable to respond to exogenous hormone administration; fertility cannot be restored. This is in part due to the severity of structural defects in the reproductive tract but is also due to the complete absence of antral follicles in the ovary. These mouse models are important resources in the study of human anovulatory infertility and can be used to study novel treatment regimens.

KEY POINTS FOR CLINICAL PRACTICE

■ The pharmacokinetics and pharmacodynamics of pharmacotherapeutic preparations must be considered when selecting agents for use in controlled ovarian stimulation. There are several recombinant products available for use in controlled ovarian stimulation protocols that offer high purity and high-potency alternatives to urine- or serum-derived gonadotropins. These products are effective in follicular recruitment and oocyte maturation and can simulate an endogenous LH surge to induce ovulation. They also lack many of the side effects of urine- or serum-derived compounds such as uncertainty of biological activity, local injection reactions, and sensitization (5). Clinicians should consider the use of these products when developing a treatment plan for the infertile female patient.

ACKNOWLEDGMENTS

Work performed in the authors' laboratories and reported here was supported by grants K01 RR021971 (A.M. Schuler), R24 RR 13200 (J.G. Scammell), and R24 RR 20052 and P40 RR 01254 (C.R. Abee) from the National Center for Research Resources (NCRR), NIH. The content of this chapter is solely the responsibility of the authors and does not necessarily represent the official views of the NCRR or NIH.

REFERENCES

1. Ludwig M, Diedrich K. Follow-up of children born after assisted reproductive technologies. *Reprod Biomed Online* 2002; 5: 317–22.
2. Steptoe PC, Edwards RG. Birth after the reimplantation of a human embryo. *Lancet* 1978; 2: 366.
3. Stouffer RL, Zelinski-Wooten MB. Overriding follicle selection in controlled ovarian stimulation protocols: quality vs quantity. *Reprod Biol Endocrinol* 2004; 2: 32.
4. Srisuparp S, Strakova Z, Fazleabas AT. The role of chorionic gonadotropin (CG) in blastocyst implantation. *Arch Med Res* 2001; 32: 627–34.
5. Ludwig M, Doody KJ, Doody KM. Use of recombinant human chorionic gonadotropin in ovulation induction. *Fertil Steril* 2003; 79: 1051–9.
6. [No authors listed]. Recombinant follicle stimulating hormone: development of the first biotechnology product for the treatment of infertility. Recombinant Human FSH Product Development Group. *Hum Reprod Update* 1998; 4: 862–81.
7. Wheatley M, Hawtin SR. Glycosylation of G-protein-coupled receptors for hormones central to normal reproductive functioning: its occurrence and role. *Hum Reprod Update* 1999; 5: 356–64.

8. Fan QR, Hendrickson WA. Structure of human follicle-stimulating hormone in complex with its receptor. *Nature* 2005; 433: 269–77.

9. Gudermann T, Brockmann H, Simoni M, Gromoll J, Nieschlag E. In vitro bioassay for human serum follicle-stimulation hormone FSH based on L cells transfected with recombinant rat FSH receptor: validation of a model system. *Endocrinology* 1994; 135: 2204–13.

10. Gromoll J, Simoni M. Genetic complexity of FSH receptor function. *Trends Endocrinol Metab* 2005; 16: 368–73.

11. Bavister BD, Dees C, Schultz RD. Refractoriness of rhesus monkeys to repeated ovarian stimulation by exogenous gonadotropins is caused by nonprecipitating antibodies. *Am J Reprod Immunol Microbiol* 1986; 11: 11–16.

12. Schuler AM, Westberry JM, Scammell JG, Abee CR, Kuehl TJ, Gordon JW. Ovarian stimulation of squirrel monkeys (*Saimiri boliviensis boliviensis*) using pregnant mare serum gonadotropin. *Comp Med* 2005; 56: 12–6.

13. le Cotonnec JY, Porchet HC, Beltrami V, Munafo A. Clinical pharmacology of recombinant human luteinizing hormone: Part I. Pharmacokinetics after intravenous administration to healthy female volunteers and comparison with urinary human luteinizing hormone. *Fertil Steril* 1998; 69: 189–94.

14. le Cotonnec JY, Porchet HC, Beltrami V, Munafo A. Clinical pharmacology of recombinant human luteinizing hormone: Part II. Bioavailability of recombinant human luteinizing hormone assessed with an immunoassay and an in vitro bioassay. *Fertil Steril* 1998; 69: 195–200.

15. Dufau ML. The luteinizing hormone receptor. *Annu Rev Physiol* 1998; 60: 461–96.

16. Segaloff DL, Ascoli M. The lutropin/chorionic gonadotropin receptor...4 years later. *Endocr Rev* 1993; 14: 324–47.

17. Filicori M, Cognigni GE, Pocognoli P, Ciampaglia W, Bernardi S. Current concepts and novel applications of LH activity in ovarian stimulation. *Trends Endocrinol Metab* 2003; 14: 267–73.

18. Menon KM, Munshi UM, Clouser CL, Nair AK. Regulation of luteinizing hormone/human chorionic gonadotropin receptor expression: a perspective. *Biol Reprod* 2004; 70: 861–6.

19. Huirne JA, Lambalk CB, van Loenen AC, Schats R, Hompes PG, Fauser BC, Macklon NS. Contemporary pharmacological manipulation in assisted reproduction. *Drugs* 2004; 64: 297–322.

20. Stenman UH, Tiitinen A, Alfthan H, Valmu L. The classification, functions and clinical use of different isoforms of hCG. *Hum Reprod Update* 2006; 12: 769–84.

21. Fares F. The role of O-linked and N-linked oligosaccharides on the structure-function of glycoprotein hormones: development of agonists and antagonists. *Biochim Biophys Acta* 2006; 1760: 560–7.

22. Trinchard-Lugan I, Khan A, Porchet HC, Munafo A. Pharmacokinetics and pharmacodynamics of recombinant human chorionic gonadotrophin in healthy male and female volunteers. *Reprod Biomed Online* 2002; 4: 106–15.

23. Griesinger G, Diedrich K, Devroey P, Kolibianakis EM. GnRH agonist for triggering final oocyte maturation in the GnRH antagonist ovarian hyperstimulation protocol: a systematic review and meta-analysis. *Hum Reprod Update* 2006; 12: 159–68.

24. Schrago CG. On the time scale of New World primate diversification. *Am J Phys Anthropol* 2007; 132: 344–54.

25. Zhang FP, Rannikko AS, Manna PR, Fraser HM, Huhtaniemi IT. Cloning and functional expression of the luteinizing hormone receptor complementary deoxyribonucleic acid from the marmoset

26. monkey testis: absence of sequences encoding exon 10 in other species. *Endocrinology* 1997; 138: 2481–90.

26. Gromoll J, Wistuba J, Terwort N, Godmann M, Muller T, Simoni M. A new subclass of the luteinizing hormone/chorionic gonadotropin receptor lacking exon 10 messenger RNA in the New World monkey (*Platyrrhini*) lineage. *Biol Reprod* 2003; 69: 75–80.

27. Gromoll J, Lahrmann L, Godmann M, Muller T, Michel C, Stamm S, Simoni M. Genomic checkpoints for exon 10 usage in the luteinizing hormone receptor type 1 and type 2. *Mol Endocrinol* 2007; 21: 1984–96.

28. Gromoll J, Eiholzer U, Neischlag E, Simoni M. Male hypogonadism caused by homozygous deletion of exon 10 of the luteinizing hormone (LH) receptor: differential action of human chorionic gonadotropin and LH. *J Clin Endocrinol Metab* 2000; 85: 2281–6.

29. Zhang FP, Kero J, Huhtaniemi I. The unique exon 10 of the human luteinizing hormone receptor is necessary for expression of the receptor protein at the plasma membrane in the human luteinizing hormone receptor, but deleterious when inserted into the human follicle-stimulating hormone receptor. *Mol Cell Endocrinol* 1998; 142: 165–74.

30. Muller T, Gromoll J, Simoni M. Absence of exon 10 of the human luteinizing hormone (LH) receptor impairs LH, but not human chorionic gonadotropin action. *J Clin Endocrinol Metab* 2003; 88: 2242–9.

31. Muller T, Simoni M, Pekel E, Luetjens CM, Chandolia R, Amato F, Norman RJ, Gromoll J. Chorionic gonadotrophin beta subunit mRNA but not luteinising hormone beta subunit mRNA is expressed in the pituitary of the common marmoset (*Callitrix jacchus*). *J Mol Endocrinol* 2004; 32: 115–28.

32. Scammell JG, Funkhouser JD, Moyer FS, Gibson SV, Willis DL. Molecular cloning of pituitary glycoprotein α-subunit and follicle stimulating hormone and chorionic gonadotropin β-subunits from New World squirrel monkey and owl monkey. *Gen Comp Endocrinol* 2008; 155(3): 534–41.

33. Matzuk MM, Hsueh AJ, Lapolt P, Tsafriri A, Keen JL, Boime I. The biological role of the carboxyl-terminal extension of human chorionic gonadotropin [corrected] beta-subunit. *Endocrinology* 1990; 126; 376–83.

34. Saal W, Glowania HJ, Hengst W, Happ J. Pharmacodynamics and pharmacokinetics after subcutaneous and intramuscular injection of human chorionic gonadotropin. *Fertil Steril* 1991; 56: 225–9.

35. Amato F, Simula AP, Gameau LJ, Norman RJ. Expression, characterization and immunoassay of recombinant marmoset chorionic gonadotrophin dimer and beta-subunit. *J Endocrinol* 1998; 159: 141–51.

36. Simula AP, Amato F, Faast R, Lopata A, Berka J, Norman RJ. Luteinizing hormone/chorionic gonadotropin bioactivity in the common marmoset (*Callithrix jacchus*) is due to a chorionic gonadotropin molecule with a structure intermediate between human chorionic gonadotropin and human luteinizing hormone. *Biol Reprod* 1995; 53: 380–9.

37. Maston GA, Ruvolo M. Chorionic gonadotropin has a recent origin within primates and an evolutionary history of selection. *Mol Biol Evol* 2002; 19: 320–35.

38. Kumar TR. What have we learned about gonadotropin function from gonadotropin subunit and receptor knockout mice? *Reproduction* 2005; 130: 293–302.

39. Kumar TR, Wang Y, Lu N, Matzuk MM. Follicle stimulating hormone is required for ovarian follicle maturation but not male fertility. *Nat Genet* 1997; 15: 201–4.

40. Abel MH, Wootton AN, Wilkins V, Huhtaniemi I, Knight PG, Charlton HM. The effect of a null mutation in the follicle-stimulating hormone receptor gene on mouse reproduction. *Endocrinology* 2000; 141: 1795–803.

41. Ma X, Dong Y, Matzuk MM, Kumar TR. Targeted disruption of luteinizing hormone beta-subunit leads to hypogonadism, defects in gonadal steroidogenesis, and fertility. *Proc Natl Acad Sci USA* 2004; 101: 17294–9.

42. Zhang FP, Poutanen M, Wilbertz J, Huhtaniemi I. Normal prenatal but arrested postnatal sexual development in luteinizing hormone receptor knockout (LuRKO) mice. *Mol Endocrinol* 2001; 15: 172–83.

26

THE FUTURE OF GONADOTROPHINS: IS THERE ROOM FOR IMPROVEMENT?

Marc Princivalle

INTRODUCTION

As described in textbooks and numerous scientific publications, human reproduction is a relatively inefficient process and this paradox is critical for the survival of the species (1, 2). The chance of achieving a spontaneous pregnancy after timed intercourse is about 30 percent. Moreover, up to 30 percent of early human embryos fail to develop into viable fetuses, and this is largely, but not exclusively, due to chromosomal abnormalities, implantation failure, and/or recurrent miscarriage (1–3). Scientists, clinicians, and pharmaceutical companies have tried for more than fifty years to develop methods, molecules, and protocols to improve fertility first in animal models but ultimately for couples with conception difficulties. Despite their efforts they have not yet found the ideal regimen, compounds, and/or protocols to achieve the maximum pregnancy rate expected by these infertile couples (4).

Infertility affects about 15 percent of couples of reproductive age, with infertility defined as one year of unprotected coitus without conception. Previously considered as a female problem, it is now widely accepted that the male factors represent between 40–50 percent of infertility. Female factors are recognized in 25–30 percent of infertile couples, whereas 10–15 percent will ultimately be classified as unexplained infertility (4). In Western countries, infertility is a growing problem; one of the causes is that increasingly couples decide to delay childbearing to an age where they have to deal with the problem of unintended infertility. This problem of life choice is now also emerging in countries like India and China.

Stimulation protocols for recruitment of multiple healthy fertilizable oocytes for the purpose of in vitro fertilization (IVF) have been constantly evolving over the past fifty years. Since the retrieval of a single oocyte during the preovulatory phase of the natural cycle was abandoned in the early 1980s in favor of using gonadotrophins for the stimulation of multiple oocytes, the protocols used have been in a state of dynamic flux, depending on the availability of stimulatory agents. Human menopausal gonadotrophin (hMG), extracted from the urine of postmenopausal women, was the only gonadotrophin available on the market in the early 1980s when Elizabeth Carr, the first IVF baby in the United States, was born on December 28, 1981. Since that time several gonadotrophins preparations have been introduced on the market alongside GnRH agonist and antagonists with the aim of suppressing the LH surge. Table 26.1 is a summary of the available gonadotrophins.

IVF as practiced today is complex, time consuming, and expensive, generating much stress, side effects, and chances for complications (5). Success rates are still low despite improvement over the years, with pregnancy occurring in approximately 25 percent of cycles in recent years. Moreover, awareness is growing throughout the world that the rate of multiple pregnancies – especially triplet and higher order pregnancies – following IVF can no longer be accepted (5). Although gonadotrophin therapy is now taken for granted as an essential component in the routine management of infertility, a great deal of discovery, research, and investment from university and pharmaceutical companies was necessary in order to develop preparations that are safe, of very high quality, and effective for routine clinical use (6). The aim of this chapter is not to review what has been done in the past [a very good review has been written and published recently by our colleague Bruno Lunenfeld (6)] but to focus on the potential future developments in the field of gonadotrophins and to describe where the pharmaceutical companies are focusing their efforts to provide better, cheaper, and safer molecules.

Recent studies have started to clarify what is needed by clinicians to increase pregnancy rates. Bart Fauser et al. (1) have tested whether ovarian stimulation for IVF affects oocyte quality and thus chromosome segregation behavior during meiosis and early embryo development. In a prospective, randomized controlled trial, they compared two ovarian stimulation regimens: mild stimulation with GnRH antagonist cotreatment versus conventional long protocol of high-dose exogenous gonadotrophin cotreatment with a GnRH agonist cotreatment (1). The results were very interesting as the study was terminated prematurely after an unplanned interim analysis found a lower embryo aneuploidy rate following mild stimulation. Compared with conventional stimulation, significantly fewer oocytes and embryos were obtained following mild stimulation; consequently, both regimens generated on an average a similar number of chromosomally normal embryos. Differences in rates of mosaic embryos suggest an effect of ovarian stimulation on mitotic segregation errors. In summary, future ovarian stimulation strategies should ideally avoid maximizing oocyte yield but aim at generating a sufficient number of chromosomally normal embryos by reducing interference with ovarian physiology and possibly more importantly with endometrium receptivity (1). To achieve this, the industry has to provide new therapeutic tools for the clinician with the aim of developing the "perfect" gonadotrophin, providing safety, compliancy, and efficacy.

Table 26.1: Currently Commercially Available Gonadotrophins

	Brand	Molecule	Company
Urinary			
hMG	Repronex	FSH and LH and 95 percent urine proteins	Ferring Pharmaceuticals
hMG	Humegon	FSH and LH and 95 percent urine proteins	Organon
hMG	Pergonal	FSH and LH and 95 percent urine proteins	Serono
Highly purified hMG	Menopur	FSH and LH and <5 percent urine proteins	Ferring Pharmaceuticals
Purified FSH	Metrodin	Urofollitropin and 95 percent urine proteins	Serono
Highly purified FSH	Bravelle	Urofollitropin and <5 percent urine proteins	Ferring Pharmaceuticals
Highly purified FSH	Metrodin HP	Urofollitropin and <5 percent urine proteins	Serono
Human chorionic gonadotrophin (hCG)	Novarel	Choriogonadotropin and <5 percent urine proteins	Ferring Pharmaceuticals
hCG	Profasi	Choriogonadotropin and <5 percent urine proteins	Serono
hCG	Pregnyl	Choriogonadotropin and <5 percent urine proteins	Organon
Recombinant			
FSH	Gonal-F	Follitropin alpha	Serono
FSH	Puregon	Follitropin beta	Organon
LH	Luveris	Lutropin alpha	Serono
hCG	Ovidrel	Choriogonadotropin alpha	Serono

AVAILABLE GONADOTROPHINS

Since the early 1980s, when gonadotrophins were first routinely used in ovarian stimulation regimens, there have been important advances in pharmaceutical product development, leading to the availability today of highly purified and consistent human gonadotrophin preparations. The source of these gonadotrophins could be either from human urinary source or from recombinant technology, but despite the differences between these products, they have resulted in improved cycle management and treatment outcomes. This "evolution" has introduced scientifically robust and "state-of-the-art" processes and equipment to ensure that the product is consistent, pure, and safe. Production and preparation of human proteins whether highly purified or recombinant has resulted in improvements in product purity, consistency, and delivery. These progresses are enabling the industry to design the future generation of gonadotrophins, namely long-acting forms, new formulations, but more importantly orally active small-molecule follicle-stimulating hormone (FSH) agonist [with or without luteinizing hormone (LH) activity]. Table 26.1 summarizes currently available gonadotrophins.

Interestingly, recent papers indicate that researchers are also considering and taking into account the importance of the endometrium as part of a successful protocol, considering the endometrium as a critical member of the complex process (7). As suggested recently by Devroey et al., there is an urgent need to carefully study endometrial changes in the context of IVF, to understand the mechanism involved, and to intensify research in this field (7). The implantation window is defined as the period when the uterus is receptive (eight to ten days after ovulation). Remarkably, confusion still exists regarding the functional normality of the luteal phase after ovarian stimulation. In principle, a functional luteal phase implies a normal hormonal milieu and a normal endometrium (7). Little data are available on this, either after ovulation induction in anovulatory women or after multifollicular ovarian stimulation for IVF in ovulatory women. Luteal phase inadequacy has been described in association with many drug regimens employed to stimulate the ovaries (7).

Despite the fact that recombinant gonadotrophins do represent interesting progress, recombinant gonadotrophins are as efficient but simply more sophisticated and expensive. The choice remains with the physicians according to variable criteria such as the socioeconomic environment of his personal experience. For this reason, research efforts are increasingly toward a milder stimulation and more sophisticated supplementation of the luteal phase during IVF treatment or in the development of new alternatives to injectable gonadotropins.

ALTERNATIVES TO GONADOTROPHINS

FSH-CTP

Exogenous gonadotrophin therapy remains a foundation of treatment for couples having difficulty conceiving. Prolonged therapy is necessary to achieve a therapeutic effect, typically for eight to ten consecutive days to stimulate folliculogenesis in women or in the case of hypogonadotrophic males, as replacement therapy to induce spermatogenesis. Recombinant human FSH (hFSH) or urinary hFSH are administered as an intramuscular (i.m.) or subcutaneous (s.c.) daily injection. Decreasing the frequency of administration would facilitate therapy and render gonadotrophin administration more tolerable.

Two long-acting gonadotrophins developed by fusing the carboxyterminal peptides (CTP) of human chorionic gonadotrophin (hCG) to native recombinant hFSH either as a noncovalently bound heterodimer containing the common α- and β-FSH subunits (8) or as a contiguous peptide (9) have previously been reported (10). hCG is known to have a longer circulating half-life. This has been attributed to the four O-linked glycosylation sites present on the CTP sequence on the β-subunit of hCG. hCG shares a common receptor with hLH and both hormones elicit similar biological activity on binding to the receptor. Relative to hLH, however, the serum half-life of hCG is more than twofold greater (thirty to fifty-six hours as compared with about eleven hours for hLH). Except for the CTP on the β-subunit of hCG (amino acids 113–145), the two hormones share more than 85 percent sequence homology. The CTP thus appears to alter the metabolism of hCG without interfering with receptor binding and signal transduction (9, 10). Alternatively, long-acting FSH may be created by additional glycosylation of the FSH molecule (9, 10). Preclinical research has indicated that FSH-CTP has an in vitro pharmacological activity comparable to recombinant FSH and an anticipated half-life that is two- to threefold longer compared with recombinant FSH (11, 12).

In 2001, the first report of a clinical trial for FSH-CTP was published (11). In this, phase I, nonblind, multicenter study, thirteen hypogonadotrophic hypogonadal male subjects were enrolled to test the safety of FSH-CTP in terms of antibody formation, and to determine the pharmacokinetic profile of this new recombinant protein (11). The use of FSH-CTP is safe and does not lead to detectable formation of antibodies; the pharmacokinetic and pharmacodynamic profile of this new FSH recombinant protein may lead to the development of a new treatment for female infertility (11) (ORG36286). Recent clinical trails in women in an IVF setting (13) and in women with WHO group II anovulatory infertility (14) showed that a single dose of long-acting FSH-CTP was able to induce one or more follicles to grow up to ovulatory sizes, but additional research will be needed to select the optimal FSH-CTP dose and treatment time interval (13). In summary, Organon is developing injectable corifollitropin-α (FSH-CTP), which compared with recombinant FSH, has a two- to threefold longer half-life. Repeated FSH-CTP administration in hypogonadotropic hypogonadal male volunteers appeared to be safe and well tolerated and did not give rise to antibody formation (11). In addition, ongoing pregnancies were obtained in the FSH-CTP groups. However, the optimal dose and regimen has yet to be established through additional studies (4). In July 2006, the company started the 1,700-patients, phase III, LIFE trial program in Europe, United States, Canada, Asia, Latin America, and Australia to evaluate a single injection of corifollitropin-α in women undergoing controlled ovarian stimulation. In September 2006, the phase II results showing that corifollitropin-α effectively sustained multifollicular development were reported. The dose-finding study investigated the response to 60, 100, and 180 mg doses of the drug or Puregon (recombinant hFSH) in 314 patients undergoing controlled ovarian stimulation for IVF. A single s.c. injection of corifollitropin-α followed by a fixed daily dose of Puregon from day 8 induced multiple follicular growth at all doses tested. The primary end point was the number of oocytes retrieved for fertilization. In the 60 mcg group, a mean of 5.2 oocytes was retrieved. A total of 10.3 and 12.5 oocytes were retrieved from the 120 and 180 mcg treatment groups, respectively. The effects were sustained for up to a week. In addition, serum levels of estradiol and inhibin-B also increased. By this strategy, Organon demonstrated the possibility to reduce the number of gonadotrophins injections, increasing patient's compliancy.

Long-Acting FSH Formulation

Serono is currently developing a novel, long-acting formulation of recombinant hFSH. The new formulation is based on Alkermes' ProLeased injectable sustained-release drug delivery technology, which involves the encapsulation of a drug into small polymeric microspheres. These degrade slowly release the encapsulated drug at a controlled rate following s.c. or i.m. injection. The new formulation is designed to offer patients the alternative of a single injection rather than multiple daily injections.

Small-Molecule Gonadotrophin Mimetics

Introduction

FSH purified from urine or prepared through recombinant technology is central to current therapy for infertile couples, and different companies are developing new formulations and new devices to inject the different products. However, the inconvenience and low patient compliance associated with therapeutic proteins that must be administered via s.c. or i.m. injection support research to find alternative molecules capable of fulfilling the role of gonadotrophins. The pharmaceutical industry is following two different routes to achieve a full and complete folliculogenesis, namely, acting on a element downstream of the receptors or by discovering small-molecule agonists that could be taken orally. The ultimate goal of the pharmaceutical industry is to decrease the cost of the treatment, increase the safety profile of these compounds, and more importantly, to increase dramatically the compliancy with the treatment by the patients, with more flexibility for the clinicians. Thus, low–molecular-weight gonadotrophin receptor agonists could form the basis for a new therapeutic approach to infertility.

An alternative approach to solve the pharmacological issue about recombinant and urinary products is the route of small molecule or hormone mimetic. The discovery of a small-molecule agonist for peptide/protein receptors has historically been a great challenge. In the case of FSH and LH, the challenge is even more difficult by the size of FSH of kDa. However, an increasing number of small-molecule agonists for hormone receptors have been identified recently through different chemistry approaches and high-throughput screening. Moreover, this approach may provide a substantial number of advantages, mainly regarding the possibility to formulate a compound responding to the increased need for more controlled delivery. Alternatively, an orally available compound may be a very interesting approach to the problem of compliancy. Effectively, the potential advantages of the small-molecule mimetics of gonadotrophins may be the lack of immunogenicity, fewer drug side effects, and nonparenteral routes of administration. Small molecules might also be less expensive to produce. Disadvantages include shorter half-life compared to hFSH and hCG and differences in potency but medicinal chemistry may help to develop the ideal gonadotrophins.

The discovery of small-molecule agonists and antagonists for receptors that are normally triggered and activated by large endogenous peptides or glycoproteins has always been a huge challenge for medicinal chemists (15). However, new technologies that encompass molecular biology and high-throughput screening technologies (HTS) have massively accelerated the discovery of small-molecule agonists and antagonists for different G-protein–coupled receptors. Over the past few years, various companies have filed different patent applications claiming a variety of small-molecule LH receptor (LHR) and FSH receptor (FSHR) agonists and antagonists. These companies also published papers and pharmacological data providing additional information for these different and interesting compounds. The aim of this chapter is not to review extensively all the work done in the field but to choose relevant examples. For a complete review of the patent, refer to the excellent review written by Guo (16).

LHR Agonist

In a number of different patents and patent applications (17, 18), Organon describes a range of interesting bicyclic heteroaromatic compounds, including new thienopyrimidines as active LHR agonists. Figure 26.1 described two typical examples of this family of LHR agonist. In vitro data performed using the mouse functional testicular Leydig cells assay showed interesting EC50 values of 270 nM for compound 1 and 870 nM

for compound 2. In vivo using the standard ovulation induction model in immature twenty-day-old female mice primed with FSH, compound 1 orally dosed at 50 mg/kg induced ovulation in 40 percent of the animals and in 50 percent of the animals for compound 2, as compared with urinary hCG at 20 IU/kg s.c., which induced 100 percent ovulation. Further medicinal chemistry effort resulted in a lead compound (compound 3, Org41841) as a typical example (19). In the functional assay using mouse testicular Leydig cells, compound 3 gave an EC50 value of 430 nM. More interestingly, in the standard mouse ovulation induction model, compound 3 induced ovulation in 40 percent of the animals orally dosed at 50 mg/kg (19). However, this compound (compound 3) has been described as a starting point for further optimization, which could eventually lead to a selective, orally active drug for ovulation induction in assisted reproduction (19). Moreover, Org41841 has been reported as a partial agonist for thyroid-stimulating hormone receptor, demonstrating its capacity in binding to and activating another glycoprotein hormone receptor via interaction with its transmembrane domain (20). This further medicinal chemistry work from Organon has allowed them to develop another compound from the same series: Org43553, an orally available, low-molecular-weight LHR agonist (Figure 26.1, compound 4). Org43553 was shown

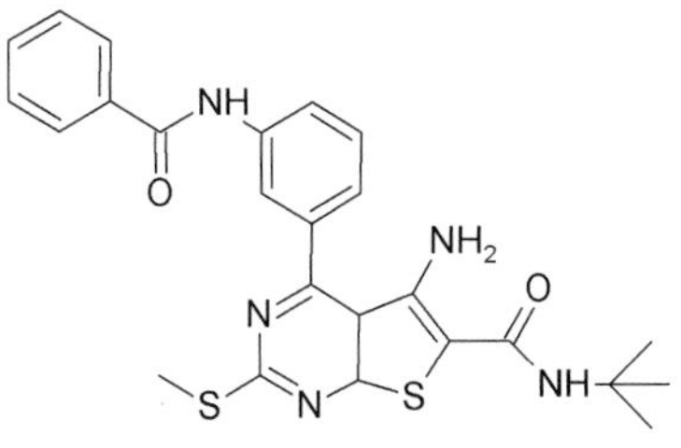

1. mouse Leydig Assay LHR
EC50=270nM

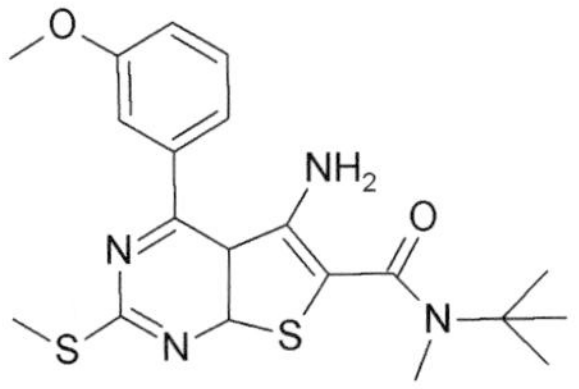

2. mouse Leydig Assay LHR
EC50=870nM

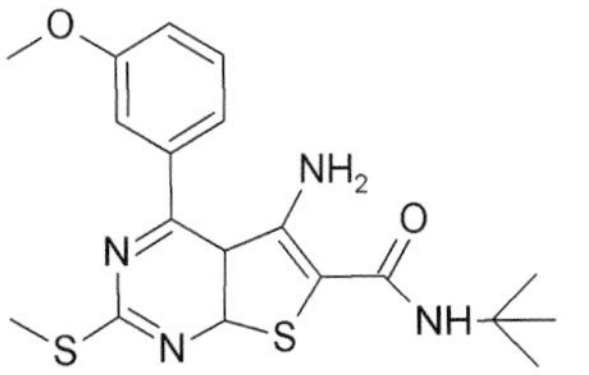

3. Org 41841
Mouse Leydig Assay LHR EC50=430nM
hLHR EC50=20nM
in vivo = 40% ovulation

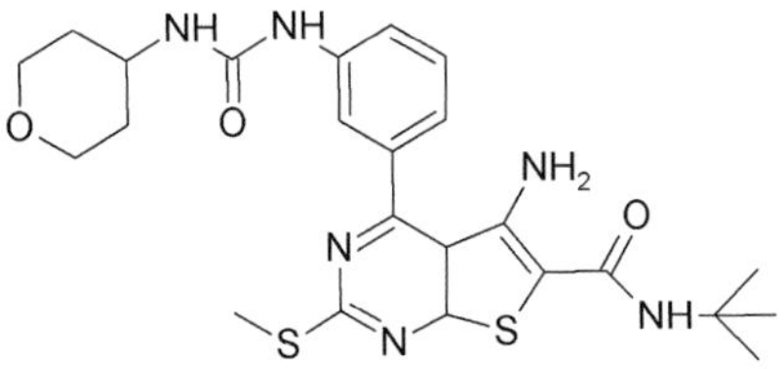

4. Org 43553

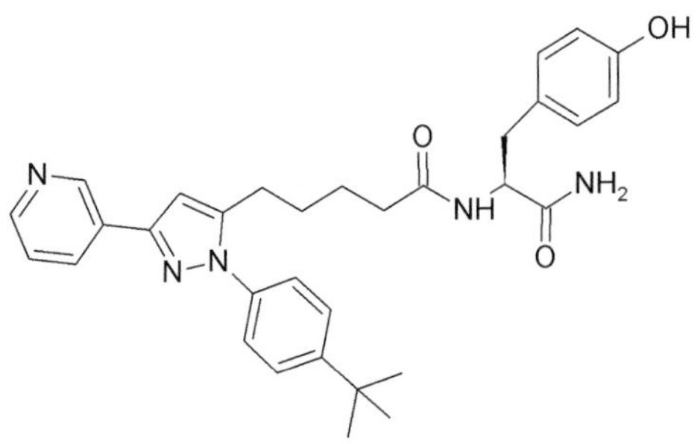

5. hFSHR EC50=130nM (73%)
hLHR EC50=20nM (53%)
rat fonctional assay: EC50=390nM (73%)

Figure 26.1. Examples of small-molecule LH agonists. Compounds 1–4: Organon, compound 5: Serono.

to have a good oral bioavailability of 79 percent in rats and 44 percent in dogs at 50 mg/kg, with respective plasma half-life of 4.5 and 3.5 hours (4). Organon recently reported the first human exposure study using Org43533 in female volunteers (42) of reproductive age. In this study, oral administration of Org43553 up to single doses of 2,700 mg was well tolerated and safe. The mean peak concentration of Org43553 was at 0.5–1 hours, and the mean elimination half-life ($t_{1/2}$) varied between 30 and 47 hours. Based on follicle rupture observed by ultrasound and rises of serum progesterone (>15 nmol/L), treatment with a single oral dose of Org43553 resulted most frequently in ovulation in the 300-mg and 900-mg dose groups. To date, this is the first report on an oral active LHR agonist that appears to be safe and effective in humans (17, 18, 21).

In other patent applications (22), Serono discloses a series of substituted pyrazole derivatives as dual agonists of LHR and FSHR useful for the treatment of infertility. Using the same typical high-throughput screening and medicinal chemistry approach, Serono described different compounds being potent LHR agonists (as exemplified by compound 5, Figure 26.1). This compound has a reported EC50 value of 20 nM (efficacy 53 percent) in a human gene reporter assay for the LHR and an EC50 value of 130 nM (efficacy 73 percent) in a human assay for the FSHR. In vivo, this compound induced testosterone release in male rats after

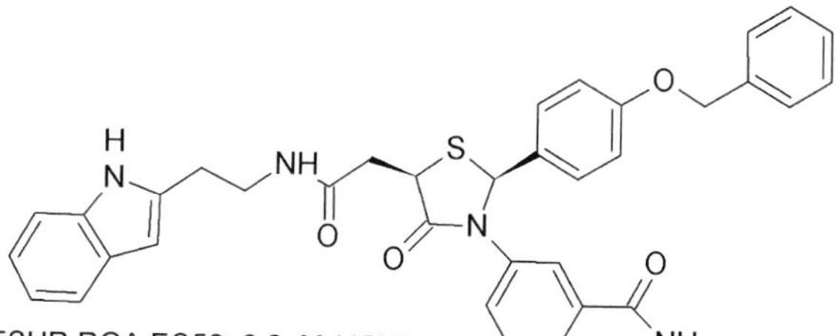

1. hFSHR RGA EC50=6.8nM (45%)
50% diasteromers

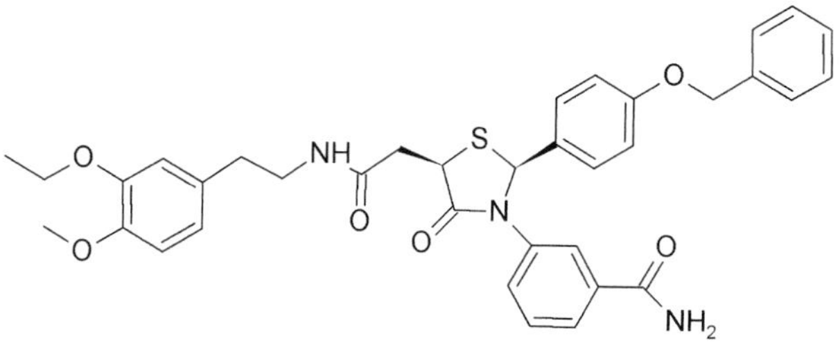

2. hFSHR RGA EC50=14+/-3nM (100%)
hFSHR cAMP EC50= 167+/-117nM (76%)
Granulosa cells assay= 70+/-6nM (77%)
50% diasteromers

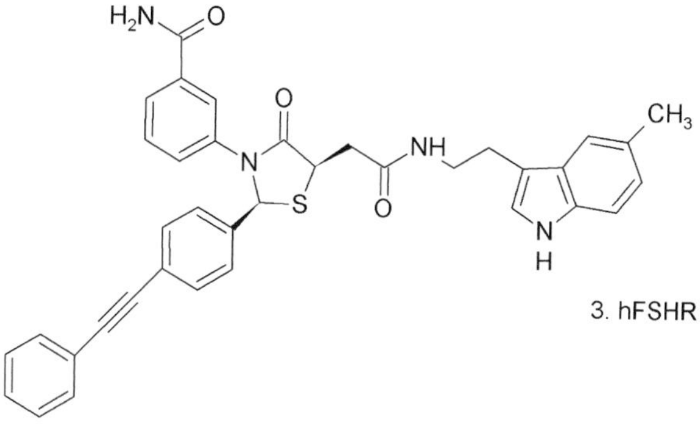

3. hFSHR RGA EC50=3nM (91%)

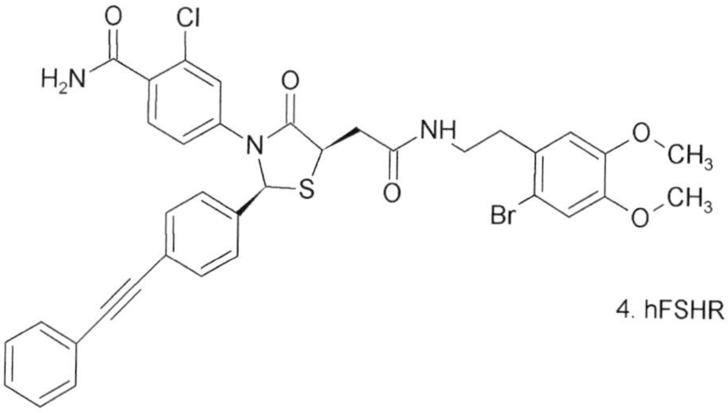

4. hFSHR RGA EC50=1nM (87%)

Figure 26.2. Examples of small-molecule FSH agonists. Compounds 1,2: Affymax Research Institute. Compounds 3,4: Affymax and Weyth.

intraperitoneal dosing. Compound 5 is another example of small molecules activating and mimicking LH activity (16, 22).

FSHR Agonist

Affymax Research Institute released patents on the role of thiazolidinone derivatives as FSHR agonists (23). Compounds 1 and 2 in Figure 26.2 are examples of this series of compounds. Recently, the details of the synthesis of these compounds have been published (24). Affymax have used an interesting combinatorial chemistry and HTS approach. They screened a focused thiazolidinone combinatorial library using HTS hFSHR gene reporter assay in CHO cells (CHO-FSHR-Luc assay). However, only the *cis*-isomers of these compounds are active and need to be purified from the mix as the *trans*-isomers are always produced as the major products. However, the discovery of compounds of

rather weak activity is a common phenomenon in library screening, and optimizing that activity can often be difficult and time-consuming (25). Further work on this series of compounds done by Wyeth in collaboration with Affymax gave more compounds showing FSHR agonist activity in a gene reporter assay with good efficacy (between 91 and 87 percent). Examples are compounds 3 and 4 in Figure 26.2 (26). These compounds appear to function through a novel allosteric mechanism (26).

Pharmacopoeia has also performed interesting work in collaboration with Organon, providing a range of biaryl derivatives as modulators of the FSHR, published (15, 27), patented (28), and discussed (29). Based on two micromolar hits identified from their libraries of about two million compounds in a CHO-FSHR-Luc assay, further work gave seventy-two distinct active compounds. From these early compounds, solid-phase

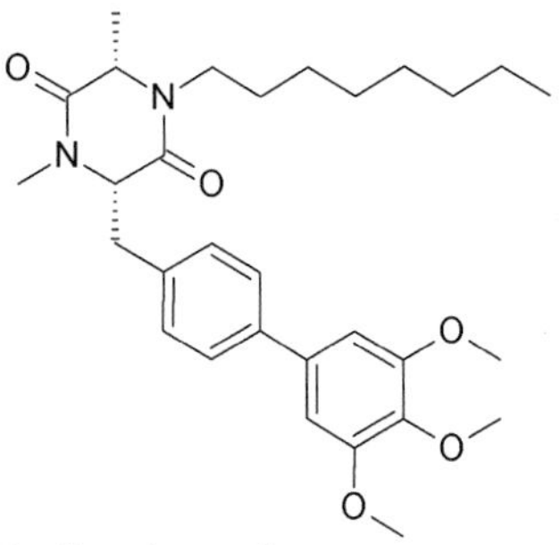

1. Rat Granulosa cells assay
EC50=32nM (47%)

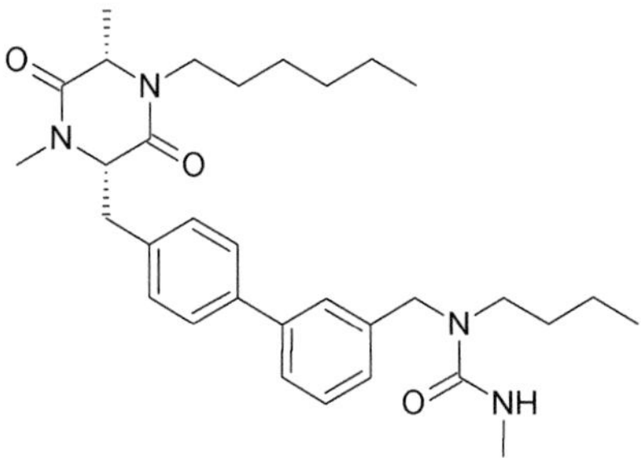

2. Rat Granulosa cells assay
EC50=9.5nM (85%)

3. hFSHR RGA EC50=39nM
Rat Granulosa cells assay EC50=1.4μM

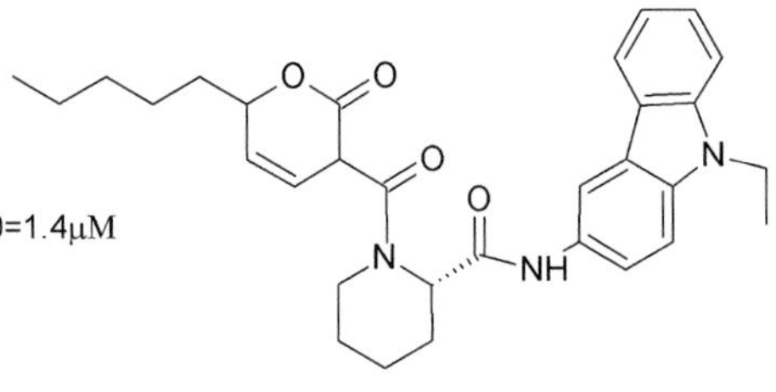

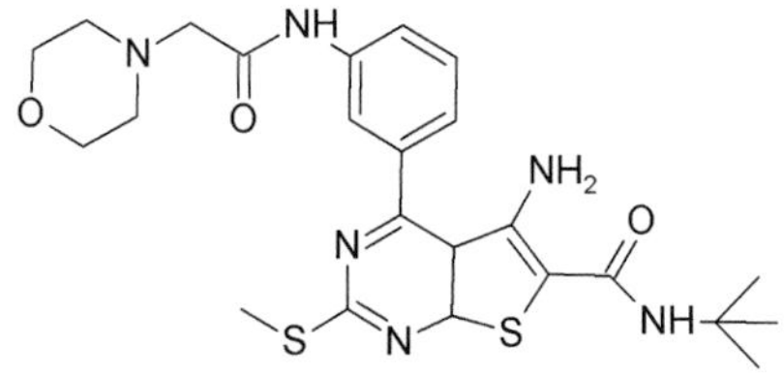

4. hFSHR RGA EC50=8nM (?%)
hLHR RGA EC50=1040nM

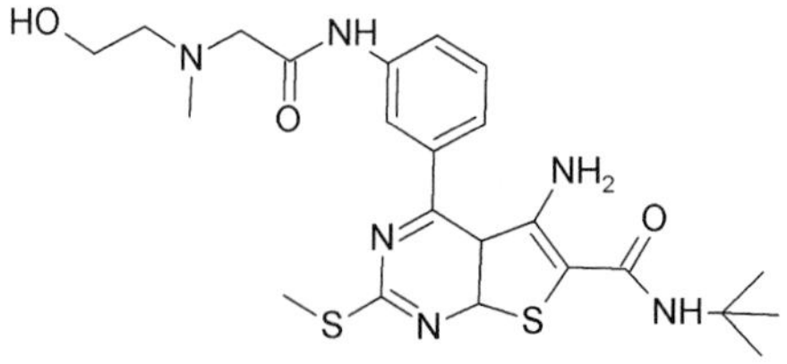

5. hFSHR RGA EC50=2.7nM (?%)
hLHR RGA EC50=57nM

Figure 26.3. Examples of small-molecule FSH agonists. Compounds 1,2: Pharmacopeia and Organon. Compound 3: Serono. Compound 4,5: Organon.

parallel synthesis of more than 300 compounds resulted in the discovery of potent small-molecule FSHR agonists exemplified by compounds 1 and 2 in Figure 26.3. In a functional assay, these compounds exhibited EC50 values of 32 nM (efficacy 47 percent) and 9.5 nM (efficacy 85 percent).

Serono has also patented interesting compounds (30, 31). In the first patent, they described a range of α- and β-amino-carboxamide derivatives with compound 3 as a representative example (Figure 26.3). Compound 3 gave an EC50 value of 39 mM in a CHO-hFSHR-Luc assay gene reporter assay. However, this compound showed poor activity and potency in a rat functional assay measuring estradiol production in rat granulosa cells (EC50 value of 1.4 μM). In another patent (31), Serono details a range of 1-sulfonylpiperazine-2-carboxamide derivatives with FSHR agonist activity with EC50 values reported, for example, at 40 nM in a gene reporter assay.

Interestingly, the first in vivo data are coming for another series of compounds patented by Organon (32, 33) where they described a series of glycine-substituted thienopyrimidines as dual agonists of FSHR and LHR. Compound 4 and compound 5 in Figure 26.3 are representative of this very interesting class of dual agonists. In vitro data gave an EC50 value of 8 nM in a human FSHR reporter gene assay (RGA) and of 1,040 nM in an hLHR RGA showing higher selectivity for the FSH receptor by compound 5 and an EC50 value of 2.7 nM in a human FSHR RGA with 57 nM in a human LHR RGA. More interestingly, using a mouse ovulation model (immature female mice primed with urinary FSH), compounds 4 and 5 at 50 mg/kg orally dosed caused a mean production of twenty and eight oocytes per animal, respectively.

KEY POINTS

- hMG, extracted from the urine of postmenopausal women, was the only gonadotrophin available on the market in the 1980s.
- IVF as practiced today is complex, time consuming, and expensive, generating much stress, side effects, and chances for complications.
- Success rates are still low despite improvement over the years, with pregnancy occurring in approximately 25 percent of cycles in recent years
- Future ovarian stimulation strategies should ideally avoid maximizing oocyte yield but aim at generating a sufficient number of chromosomally normal embryos by reducing interference with ovarian physiology and possibly more importantly with endometrium receptivity.
- Two new long-acting gonadotrophins developed by fusing the CTP of hCG to native recombinant hFSH have been reported.
- Small-molecule gonadotrophin mimetics are currently reported to be in development. The drugability of these small-molecule LHR and FSHR modulators, coupled with their promising in vivo efficacy, makes it highly promising that suitable candidate compounds may soon be discovered and pushed into human clinical investigation.

REFERENCES

1. Baart EB, Martini E, Eijkemans MJ, Van Opstal D, Beckers NGM, Verhoeff A et al. Milder ovarian stimulation for in-vitro fertil-ization reduces aneuploidy in the human preimplantation embryo: a randomized controlled trial. *Hum Reprod* 2007:22,484.
2. Norwitz ER, Schust DJ, Fisher SJ. Implantation and the survival of early pregnancy. *N Engl J Med* 2001;345(19):1400–8.
3. Healy DL, Trounson AO, Andersen AN. Female infertility: causes and treatment. *Lancet* 1994;343(8912):1539–44.
4. Papanikolaou EG, Kolibianakis E, Devroey P. Emerging drugs in assisted reproduction. *Expert Opin Emerg Drugs* 2005;10(2):425–40.
5. Fauser BCJM, Bouchard P, Bennink HJTC, Collins JA, Devroey P, Evers JLH et al. Alternative approaches in IVF. *Hum Reprod Update* 2002;8(1):1–9.
6. Lunenfeld B. Historical perspectives in gonadotrophin therapy. *Hum Reprod Update* 2004;10(6):453–67.
7. Devroey P, Bourgain C, Macklon NS, Fauser BCJM. Reproductive biology and IVF: ovarian stimulation and endometrial receptivity. *Trends Endocrinol Metab* 2004;15(2):84–90.
8. Fares FA, Suganuma N, Nishimori K, LaPolt PS, Hsueh AJ, Boime I. Design of a long-acting follitropin agonist by fusing the C-terminal sequence of the chorionic gonadotropin beta subunit to the follitropin beta subunit. *Proc Natl Acad Sci USA* 1992; 89(10):4304–8.
9. Klein J, Lobel L, Pollak S, Ferin M, Xiao E, Sauer M et al. Pharmacokinetics and pharmacodynamics of single-chain recombinant human follicle-stimulating hormone containing the human chorionic gonadotropin carboxyterminal peptide in the rhesus monkey. *Fertil Steril* 2002;77(6):1248–55.
10. Klein J, Lobel L, Pollak S, Lustbader B, Ogden RT, Sauer MV et al. Development and characterization of a long-acting recombinant hFSH agonist. *Hum Reprod* 2003;18(1):50–6.
11. Bouloux PM, Handelsman DJ, Jockenhovel F, Nieschlag E, Rabinovici J, Frasa WL et al. First human exposure to FSH-CTP in hypogonadotrophic hypogonadal males. *Hum Reprod* 2001;16(8):1592–7.
12. Duijkers IJ, Klipping C, Boerrigter PJ, Machielsen CS, de Bie JJ, Voortman G. Single dose pharmacokinetics and effects on follicular growth and serum hormones of a long-acting recombinant FSH preparation (FSH-CTP) in healthy pituitary-suppressed females. *Hum Reprod* 2002;17(8):1987–93.
13. Devroey P, Fauser BC, Platteau P, Beckers NG, Dhont M, Mannaerts BM. Induction of multiple follicular development by a single dose of long-acting recombinant follicle-stimulating hormone (FSH-CTP, Corifollitropin Alfa) for controlled ovarian stimulation before in vitro fertilization. *J Clin Endocrinol Metab* 2004;89(5):2062–70.
14. Balen AH, Mulders AG, Fauser BC, Schoot BC, Renier MA, Devroey P et al. Pharmacodynamics of a single low dose of long-acting recombinant follicle-stimulating hormone (FSH-Carboxy Terminal Peptide, Corifollitropin Alfa) in women with World Health Organization Group II anovulatory infertility. *J Clin Endocrinol Metab* 2004; 89(12):6297–304.
15. Guo T, Adang AEP, Dolle RE, Dong G, Fitzpatrick D, Geng P et al. Small molecule biaryl FSH receptor agonists. Part 1: Lead discovery via encoded combinatorial synthesis. *Bioorganic Med Chem Lett* 2004;14(7):1713–16.
16. Guo T. Small molecule agonists and antagonists for the LH and FSH receptors. *Expert Opin Therapeutic Patents* 2005;15:1555–64.
17. Gerritsma GG, van Straten NC, Corine R, Adang AE. Bicyclic heteroaromatic compounds useful as LH agonists. *patent WO0061586.* 2000. 2000.
18. Timmers CM, Karstens WJ. Bicyclic heteroaromatic compounds. *patent WO0224703.* 2000. Mar 2000.
19. van Straten NC, Schoonus-Gerritsma GG, van Someren RG, Draaijer J, Adang AE, Timmers CM et al. The first orally active low molecular weight agonists for the LH receptor: thienopyr

(im)idines with therapeutic potential for ovulation induction. *Chembiochem* 2002;3(10):1023–6.

20. Jaschke H, Neumann S, Moore S, Thomas CJ, Colson AO, Costanzi S et al. A low molecular weight agonist signals by binding to the transmembrane domain of thyroid-stimulating hormone receptor (TSHR) and luteinizing hormone/chorionic gonadotropin receptor (LHCGR). *J Biol Chem* 2006;281(15): 9841–4.

21. Mannaerts B. Novel FSH and LH agonists. 4th World Congress on Ovulation Induction. 2004.

22. Shroff H, Reddy AP, El Tayar N, Brugger N, Jorand-Lebrun C. Pharmaceutically active compounds and methods of use. *patent WO0187287*. 2007. 2007.

23. Scheuerman RA, Yanofsky SD, Holmes CP, MacLean D, Ruhland B, Barrett RW et al. Agonist of follicle stimulating hormone activity. *patent WO0209706*. 2007. Feb 2007.

24. MacLean D, Holden F, Davis AM, Scheuerman RA, Yanofsky S, Holmes CP et al. Agonists of the follicle stimulating hormone receptor from an encoded thiazolidinone library. *J Comb Chem* 2004;6(2):196–206.

25. Wrobel J, Jetter J, Kao W, Rogers J, Di L, Chi J et al. 5-Alkylated thiazolidinones as follicle-stimulating hormone (FSH) receptor agonists. *Bioorganic Med Chem* 2006;14(16):5729–41.

26. Yanofsky SD, Shen ES, Holden F, Whitehorn E, Aguilar B, Tate E et al. Allosteric activation of the follicle-stimulating hormone (FSH) receptor by selective, nonpeptide agonists. *J Biol Chem* 2006;281(19):13226–33.

27. Guo T, Adang AEP, Dong G, Fitzpatrick D, Geng P, Ho KK et al. Small molecule biaryl FSH receptor agonists. Part 2: Lead optimization via parallel synthesis. *Bioorg Med Chem Lett* 2004; 14(7):1717–20.

28. Guo T, Ho KK, McDonald E, Dolle RE, Saionz KW. Bisaryl derivatives having FSH receptor modulatory activity. *patent WO02070493*. 2002. Sep 2002.

29. van Straten NC, van Berkel TH, Demont DR, Karstens WJ, Merkx R, Oosterom J et al. Identification of substituted 6-amino-4-phenyltetrahydroquinoline derivatives: potent antagonists for the follicle-stimulating hormone receptor. *J Med Chem* 2005; 48(6):1697–700.

30. El Tayar N, Reddy AB, Buckler DR, Magar S. FSH mimetic for the treatment of infertility. *patent WO0008015*. 2002. Jul 2002.

31. Magar S, Goutopoulos A, Liao YT, Schwarz MK, Russell TJ. Piperazines derivatives and methods of use. *patent WO04031182*. 2004. Apr 2004.

32. Hanssen RG, Timmers CM. Thieno[2,3-D]pyrimidines with combined LH and FSH agonistic activity. patent WO03020726. 2003. Mar 2003.

33. Hanssen RG, Timmers CM, Kelder J. Glycine-substituted thieno [2,3-d]Pyrimidines with combined LH and *FSH agonistic activity*. 2003. Mar 2003.

27

OVARIAN HYPERSTIMULATION SYNDROME

Cristiano E. Busso, Juan A. Garcia-Velasco, Raúl Gomez, Claudio Alvarez, Carlos Simón, Antonio Pellicer

INTRODUCTION

Ovarian hyperstimulation syndrome (OHSS) is an iatrogenic complication of ovulation induction, which may cause serious impact on the patient's health, with 0.1–2 percent of the patients developing severe forms of the syndrome (1). This low incidence is increasing worldwide through the expansion of assisted reproductive techniques (ART) (2). Generally speaking, OHSS is a consequence of exogenous gonadotropin/clomiphene citrate administration for ovulation induction – restoring ovulation in anovulatory patients through pharmacological induction of two or three follicles – and more frequently for aggressive controlled ovarian hyperstimulation (COH) used in ART, trying to increase the cohort of follicles achieving maturation in normal ovulatory women. This potentially life-threatening disorder causes massive extracellular exudate accumulation combined with profound intravascular volume depletion and hemoconcentration, accompanied by ovarian enlargement with exaggerated esteroidogenesis and multiple system failure as end point (3).

There are many hormonal variables that are closely related to the pathophysiology of OHSS syndrome, perhaps the most important of which is whether being exogenous or endogenous (e.g., pregnancy derived) (4,5). Elimination of hCG will prevent the full-blown picture of OHSS. In fact, when hCG was replaced for progesterone as luteal support in ovulation induction (OI) or COH, the incidence of OHSS was reduced, maintaining excellent pregnancy rates (6). If hCG is used for luteal phase support, the risk of OHSS is enhanced.

Rizk (2006) highlighted that some forms of OHSS may present in a different clinical setting than exogenous gonadotropin administration (2). This may occur if an endogenous ovarian stimulus is present, and four different situations have been described:

- Pregnant women with polycystic ovary syndrome, who are known to be more sensitive to gonadotropins and may respond to endogenously released gonadotropin, probably potentiated by certain cytokines or growth factors (7).
- Pregnancies that exhibit abnormally high serum levels of hCG, such as molar pregnancies or triploids, either diandric or digynic (8).
- Women with primary hypothyroidism, in whom the similarity of the binding receptors of thyroid-stimulating hormone (TSH) and FSH, and a hypothetical "hormone-imprinting effect" if the FSH receptor has been perinatally exposed to TSH, may contribute to the spontaneous hyperstimulation in these patients (9).
- Different mutations in the FSH receptor have been described in women presenting spontaneous OHSS (10–14). These women seem to have hypersensitivity to chorionic and some mutations are a cause of familial spontaneous OHSS (11,12).
- Gonadotroph adenoma may induce cosecretion of FSH and LH and consequently a huge rise in E2 levels with ovarian enlargement. Interestingly, no ascites was found in these cases (15).

All of these different clinical settings illustrate how it is the gonadotropin stimulus the essential mechanism by which OHSS is produced.

There are two clear patterns of the onset of OHSS: *early* OHSS (E-OHSS), that generally presents three to seven days after hCG administration and *late* OHSS (L-OHSS), twelve to seventeen days after hCG (2,16). This suggests that there are two mechanisms for the induction of OHSS. E-OHSS is an acute effect of ovulatory hCG, and it can occur in patients who do not become pregnant. However, L-OHSS is induced by endogenous hCG from the trophoblast of the implanting pregnancy. The L-OHSS is known to resolve rapidly if the pregnancy is aborted, which supports this hypothesis.

It is assumed that certain ovarian biosynthetic components produced in excess during induction of ovulation initiate the cascade of events that result in the syndrome. Investigations focused on vasoactive substances because it is clear that profound alterations in the vascular compartment are the major initial changes that lead to the full appearance and maintenance of OHSS. Thus, hCG may induce the release of a mediator that has potent and direct systemic effects on the vascular system and that may be responsible for the pathophysiology and clinical consequences (17).

PATHOPHYSIOLOGY: THE ROLE OF VASCULAR ENDOTHELIAL GROWTH FACTOR (VEGF)

Over the years, many substances involved in the regulation of vascular permeability (VP) have been implicated in causing OHSS (18). Some of them still being under investigation, the list of potential mediators includes estradiol (19), histamines

(20), prostaglandins (1), the ovarian renin-angiotensin system (21), interleukin (IL)-6, IL-2, and IL-8 (22), angiogenin (23), endothelin-1 (24), insulin (25), or the ovarian kinin-kallikrein system (26) among others (27).

Rizk et al. pointed to the importance of VEGF as one of the main angiogenic factors responsible for increased vascular permeability (iVP) leading to extravasation of protein-rich fluid and, subsequently, the full appearance of OHSS. Both its vasoactive properties and its increased ovarian expression during the development of OHSS suggest that VEGF plays a major role in the development of this syndrome (28).

The VEGF was originally described as a tumor-secreted protein, which caused substantial vascular leakage (29). It is a homodimer of Mr about 46,000, which is produced by many cell types (30) including a variety of tumors, folliculostellate cells, macrophages, possibly podocytes, capsular epithelial cells in the renal glomeruli, and granulosa cells (31) among others. VEGF/VPF is a potent enhancer of endothelial permeability, being 50,000 times more potent than histamine (32). VEGF increases capillary and venular leakage, as a result of opening intercellular junctions between neighboring endothelial cells, as well as other morphological modifications that can rapidly occur ten minutes after topical application, like the induction of fenestrae in venular and capillary endothelia that normally are not fenestrated (33).

The human VEGF gene has been mapped to chromosome 6p12 (34) and is made up of eight exons (35). Exons 1–5 and 8 are always present in VEGF mRNA, while the expression of exons 6 and 7 is regulated by alternative splicing. This process allows the formation of various VEGF isoforms differing in length, all VEGF products having a common region. In humans, five different VEGF mRNAs have been detected encoding the isoforms $VEGF_{121}$, $VEGF_{145}$, $VEGF_{165}$, $VEGF_{189}$, and $VEGF_{206}$ (36). Isoforms $VEGF_{121}$ and $VEGF_{165}$ appear to be mainly involved in the process of angiogenesis (37) and are in fact the only ones the ovary is able to secrete (38,39).

The VEGF gene shows the same exonic structure in rodents and humans (40). Murine VEGF-expressed isoforms $VEGF_{120}$, $VEGF_{144}$, $VEGF_{164}$, $VEGF_{188}$, and $VEGF_{205}$ have only one amino acid less in length when compared to human VEGF isoforms, and there is a 95 percent protein homology between these two (41). Similar to that of humans (42–47), hybridization studies in the rat ovary have demonstrated significant VEGF mRNA expression seen mostly after the LH surge (48).

The receptors for VEGF are present on the endothelial cells' surface and belong to the tyrosine kinase receptor family (49). They are also present in the inner theca of human follicles (31,46). Two specific endothelial cell membrane receptors for VEGF have been identified, VEGFR-1 (Flt-1) and VEGFR-2 (Flk1/KDR) (49,50). The receptor Flk1/KDR appears to be mainly involved in regulating VP, angiogenesis, and vasculogenesis (51,52). VEGFR-1 is also produced as soluble receptors (sVEGFR-1) by alternative splicing of the precursor mRNA (53), acting as a modulator of VEGF bioactivity (54). In fact, the soluble molecules compete with the full-length VEGFR-1 for binding VEGF and inhibit vascular permeability (55,56). Targeting the Flk1/KDR receptor has been a goal for researchers working in gynecologic oncology. Different specific VEGFR-2 blockers have been used in animal models, which reduce tumor growth and ascites (57,58). Although the mechanism of ascites formation may be different in neoplasms and OHSS (59), nobody had tried so far to reverse ascites formation

in OHSS targeting the VEGF system, so this has been our main goal during the recent years.

There are several findings that support the role of VEGF in the development of OHSS in humans: serum VEGF levels increase after hCG administration in superovulated women at risk of developing OHSS (17). In fact, a rise in serum VEGF levels has been used as a marker for subsequent development of OHSS (60). Moreover, VEGF plasma levels correlate with the clinical picture of OHSS (61), and the changes of VEGF levels in ascites have been correlated with the clinical course of OHSS (62).

In women who develop OHSS, VEGF is overexpressed and produced by granulosa-lutein cells (42–46) and released into the follicular fluid (42,47,63) in response to hCG (41), inducing increased capillary permeability (42,47,63). HCG induces the expression of VEGF in cultured granulosa-lutein cells of women developing OHSS (64). Similarly, we have shown that hCG stimulates the release of VEGF in human endothelial cells that, in turn, acts in an autocrine manner increasing VP (63). Thus, both the granulosa and the endothelial cells may be involved in the production and release of VEGF in women who develop OHSS, although the concept that granulosa-lutein cells behave as actual endothelial cells has also been proposed (65).

In an attempt to establish the role of VEGF in OHSS, we developed an in vivo rodent model that allows inducing OHSS consistently, including the two main characteristics, ovarian enlargement and increased VP, leading to ascites. In immature rats, the hypothalamic pituitary axis is inactive and, therefore, follicle development is nearly inactive as these animals lack endogenous LH production, but it can be induced by the exogenous administration of gonadotropins. Follicle development was induced with pregnant mare's serum (PMSG) (this is the equivalent to the human menopausal gonadotropin) 10 IU during four consecutive days. On the fifth day, these animals were injected with hCG 30 IU in order to trigger ovulation. In agreement with previous studies from Ujioka (66), OHSS manifestations developed included ascites, enlarged ovaries, and iVP in these animals. Quantification of VP in such animal model can be evaluated objectively with the measurement of the extravasation of a previously injected dye. Time-course experiments were performed to analyze VP by injecting Evans blue (EB) dye into the femoral vein and quantifying the amount of dye recovered after irrigating the abdominal cavity with a fixed volume of saline thirty minutes later (39). The results of these experiments validated the animal model employed because increased VP values during the time course were observed in superovulated animals with PMSG if hCG was administered to trigger ovulation. No OHSS was observed in animals that received PMSG without hCG. Maximal iVP was observed forty-eight hours after hCG administration.

In addition, to the VP experiments, the expression of whole VEGF mRNA in the mesentery and the ovaries employing reverse transcriptase polymerase chain reaction (RT-PCR) was also measured to determine the tissue source(s) of VEGF. The reason to select ovary or mesentery to measure VEGF expression was related to the possible, ovarian or systemic, origin of the syndrome based on the presence of hCG receptors in both the ovary and the endothelial cells. So the ovary and the mesentery as a highly vascularized tissue were selected as representative tissues of an ovarian or systemic origin of the syndrome, respectively. The results of this experiments showed that in narrow correlation to VP, ovarian mRNA VEGF expression increased during the time-course, reaching peak values after forty-eight

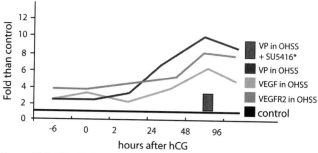

Figure 27.1. VP, VEGF, and VEGFR-2 mRNA expression over time in hyperstimulated rats. The profound effect of a specific VEGFR-2 blocker (SU5416) on VP is also showed in a brown barr. (Adapted from reference 39.)

hours, whereas no significant change in expression was observed in the mesentery (Figure 27.1). To further prove the ovarian origin of VEGF, we showed that VP was not altered when ovariectomized rats were treated with PMSG + hCG (39).

Furthermore, we also analyzed which of the VEGF isoforms were expressed by the ovaries of hyperstimulated animals, with specific primers for conventional RT-PCR. The ovary expressed $VEGF_{120}$ and $VEGF_{164}$ isoforms. Inasmuch, we showed that there was also an increase of VEGF receptor 2 (VEGFR-2) expression in the ovaries, coincidental in time with maximal VP (59), demonstrating the involvement of the VEGF-VEGFR-2 system in OHSS (Figure 27.1). Immunohistochemistry showed VEGF in granulosa and in the zona pellucida of preovulatory and atretric follicles and in granulosa-lutein and endothelial cells of whole corpus luteum (39,67).

In summary, these experiments showed that the VEGF system (ligand and receptor 2) is upregulated in the ovaries of hyperstimulated animals, coincidental in time with maximal VP, clearly suggesting a crucial role for locally (ovary)-produced VEGF in OHSS.

After the relevance of VEGF in establishing VP was demonstrated, a series of blocking experiments were designed through the administration of SU5416, a VEGFR-2 inhibitor, as a new strategy to prevent and treat OHSS in an attempt to prevent increased VP. Since this was a totally new concept, which had been primarily designed to be employed as an anti-angiogenic approach in cancer patients, we attempted several protocols of SU5416 administration in order to block iVP in our OHSS animal models. We found that SU5416 should be administered after hCG, with a single injection being as effective as multiple injections (39). The reasons for this behavior can be found in the fact that the syndrome develops only during corpus luteum formation after the ovulation process (Figure 27.1).

In any case, the ability to reverse hCG action on VP by targeting the VEGFR-2 employing SU5416 was not only reassuring of the key role of VEGF in OHSS but also provided new insights into the development of strategies to prevent and treat the syndrome based on its pathophysiological mechanism, rather than using empirical approaches as we do today. In fact, tumor growth, neoangiogenesis, and ascites formation have been prevented in animals with different ovarian neoplasms targeting the VEGF system (68,69) and specifically the Flk-1 receptor with SU5416 (70).

Our first approach to test the relevance of VEGF in humans was a prospective observational study of women undergoing

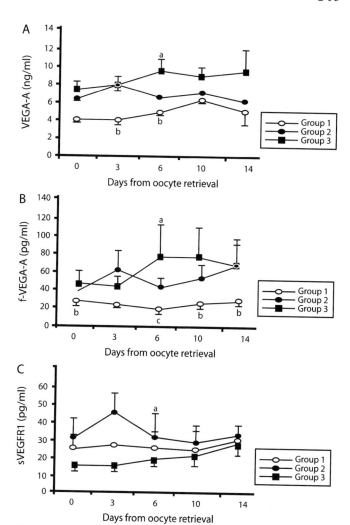

Figure 27.2. VP, VEGF, and VEGFR-2 mRNA expression over time in hyperstimulated rats. The profound effect of a specific VEGFR-2 blocker (SU5416) on VP is also showed in a brown barr. (Adapted from reference 39.)

IVF. The aim was to analyze VEGF dynamics in E-OHSS and L-OHSS (71). In order to study E-OHSS, subjects were divided into three groups: nonpregnant women not at risk for OHSS (group 1) and patients at risk who did not (group 2) and did (group 3) develop severe OHSS. Blood was drawn on day of ovum retrieval (day 0) and on days 3, 6, 10, and 14. L-OHSS patients were divided into women with single pregnancies who did not (group 4) and did (group 5) develop OHSS and compared to a control group of pregnant women after oocyte donation. Blood was drawn weekly (between weeks 4 and 12). Total VEGF (VEGF-A), free VEGF (f-VEGF), and sVEGFR-1 were measured. In E-OHSS group, women who developed OHSS had significantly higher levels of VEGF-A and f-VEGF and significantly lower levels of sVEGFR-1 on day 6 (Figure 27.2). In L-OHSS group, women who developed OHSS secreted higher amounts of VEGF-A at six, nine, and twelve weeks of pregnancy and higher amounts of f-VEGF during weeks 5 and 9. sVEGFR-1 was lower in women who developed OHSS (Figure 27.3). This study shows that the factors that most determinate the future development of E- and L-OHSS is the ability to secrete sVEGFR-1 and to reduce the availability of f-VEGF. It also confirms in humans what we have previously

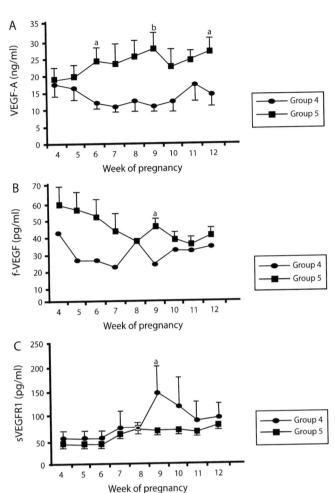

Figure 27.3. Comparison of (A) VEGF-A, (B) f-VEGF, and (C) sVEGFR-1 levels in groups 4 and 5 during the first trimester of pregnancy. [a]$P < 0.05$; [b]$P < 0.01$. Printed with permission from reference 71.

Table 27.1: Characteristics of Patients at Risk of Developing OHSS

1. Before gonadotrophin administration

   Young

   Lean habitus

   PCO (necklace sign)

   PCOD (hyperinsulinemia)

   Allergy (immunoactivation)

2. During or after gonadotrophin administration

   Multiple follicles (>35 in COH, >6 in OI)

   High serum estradiol (>4,000 pg/mL in COH, >1,700 in OI)

   Conception cycles (pregnancy)

   hCG luteal supplementation

   Serum/follicular fluid VEGF levels

seen in mice (39): the entire phenomenon is restricted to the ovaries since women who become pregnant following oocyte donation did not develop OHSS, despite high f-VEGF levels.

We also have recently described the VEGF mechanism of action in humans employing human endothelial cells from umbilical veins. We observed that high levels of VEGF and hCG enhance vascular endothelial cadherin (VEC) release, which leads to endothelial barrier architecture loss. VEC is a transmembrane protein responsible for adhesion, extravasation, recruitment, and activation of endothelial cells. When cells were treated with anti-human VEGF antibodies, VEC concentrations were lower, and when cells were treated with estradiol, no differences in VEC levels were seen. These findings support the theory that estradiol is not directly related to OHSS pathophysiology and gives us insights for new approaches to prevent and treat OHSS targeting VEGF, which, in turn, may decrease VEC production maintaining vascular structure (72).

RISK FACTORS FOR OHSS

Identifying the population at risk is the most important step to reduce the incidence of OHSS (Table 27.1). There are epidemiological, hormonal, ultrasonographic, and biochemical criteria that help to identify patients at risk (18,28). Most studies

agree that young women with lean habitus have a higher tendency to develop OHSS (73). High serum E2 levels is another well-known risk factor, synthesized in the granulosa cells of the multiple immature and intermediate follicles that these patients produce. It is widely accepted that OHSS occurs more frequently in patients with polycystic ovary disease (PCOD), defined as the typical appearance of the ovaries on ultrasound examination and/or the presence of hyperandrogenism, obesity, and elevated serum LH levels (74). Apart from PCOD, patients showing the "necklace sign" in an ovarian ultrasound are at increased risk of developing OHSS. The "necklace" is the ultrasonographic image of multiple, small, early antral follicles under 10 mm in diameter, which are arranged around the periphery of the ovary, with rich stroma in the inner structure of the ovary. Although this finding may be observed in normo-ovulatory women with no clinical signs of PCOD, as the pathophysiology may be different, we have to be cautious when stimulating the ovaries of these patients as the entire cohort of follicles from the necklace may be forced to mature and this multifollicular response may end up in OHSS.

A new risk factor was described in women with PCOD (25). In these patients, the insulinemic pattern may influence the ovarian response to gonadotropin administration, so hyperinsulinemic women – diagnosed by an oral glucose tolerance test – are at greater risk for OHSS than normoinsulinemic patients with PCOD. An epidemiological study described that women who develop OHSS have an increased prevalence of allergy (56 vs. 21 percent), indicating that general immunologic mechanisms may play a role (73). In fact, mast cells are more abundant in the dominant follicle, so they could have a role in ovulation and, thus, hyperreact in this system in the ovary of allergic individuals.

CLINICAL MANIFESTATIONS OF OHSS

The original classification (19) has gone through minor revisions. Rizk and Aboulghar classified OHSS into four stages (75): mild, moderate, severe, and life-threatening forms (Table 27.2). Mild OHSS is characterized by high-serum E2

Table 27.2: Clinical Features (Adapted from Reference 1), Laboratorial Findings and Management of Different Stages of OHSS

	Clinical features	Laboratorial findings	Management
Mild	Abdominal distention/discomfort	No important laboratorial alterations	Analgesia
	Mild nausea/vomiting		Antiemetic
	Diarrhea		Avoid heavy physical activity and sexual intercourse
	Enlarged ovaries		Report to clinic in case of worsening symptoms
Moderate	Mild features	Elevated hematocrit (>41 percent)	Outpatient
	+	Elevated WBC (>15,000)	Overhydration protocol
	Ultrasonographic evidence of ascitis	Hypoproteinemia	Fluid restriction protocol
			Prophylactic anticoagulation if necessary
			i.v. albumin (if necessary)
			Furosemide (if necessary)
Severe/serious illness	Mild + moderate features +	Hemoconcentration (Htc >55 percent)	Hospitalization (intensive care, if necessary)
	Clinical evidence of ascitis	WBC >25,000	Close monitoring
	Hydrothorax	Creatinine clearance <50 mL/min	Close fluid/electrolyte management
	Severe dyspnea	Creatinine >1.6	Prophylactic anticoagulation
	Oliguria/anuria	Hyponatremia (Na$^+$ < 135 mEq/L)	Therapeutic anticoagulation if necessary
	Intractable nausea/vomiting	Hypokalemia (K$^+$ > 5 mEq/L)	
	Tense ascitis	Elevated liver enzymes	
	Low blood/central venous pressure		
	Rapid weight gain (>1 kg in twenty four hours)		
	Syncope		
	Severe abdominal pain		
	Venous thrombosis		
Critical	Anuria/acute renal failure	Worsening of severe findings	Intensive care unit
	Thromboembolism		Multidisciplinary approach
	Arrhythmia		Dopamine
	Pericardial effusion		
	Massive hydrothorax		
	Arterial thrombosis		
	ARDS		
	Sepsis		

and progesterone and mildly enlarged ovaries (<5 cm). In moderate OHSS, besides the hormonal hyperstimulation described, the patient suffers abdominal distension and discomfort, nausea and/or vomiting, and/or diarrhea, with ovaries ranging from 5 to 12 cm in diameter. Severe OHSS features extensive ovarian enlargement (more than 12 cm in diameter), ascites, and less frequently hydrothorax or pericardial effusion.

Renal dysfunction (decreased urine output <600 mL/twenty-four hours, creatinine 1.0–1.5 mg/dL, creatinine clearance ≥50 mL/min) and hemoconcentration (hematrocrit >45 percent) are often found, together with leukocytosis (>15,000). In critical or life-threatening forms, the patient will develop tense ascites with hydrothorax and/or pericardial effusion, severe hemoconcentration (hematrocrit >55 percent), profound leukocytosis

(⩾25,000), and extreme renal damage (oligoanuria, creatinine ⩾1.6 mg/dL, creatinine clearance <50 mL/min, and renal failure). Adult respiratory distress syndrome (ARDS) may appear as well as thromboembolic phenomena. Mild and moderate forms may be managed with home care, while severe and critical forms should be hospitalized and intensive care instituted (Table 27.2).

Abramov et al. (76) reported the clinical features of 209 patients with severe OHSS in a nationwide, ten-year multicenter study. Most commonly, patients complained of dyspnea (92 percent), abdominal discomfort because of the ascites (99 percent), gastrointestinal disturbances (54 percent), and decreased urine output (30 percent). Peripheral edema (13 percent), peritoneal irritation (6 percent), pneumonia – either by uncoordinated lung ventilation or atelectasis – (4 percent), ARDS – consequence of massive hydration – (2 percent), pulmonary embolism – profound hypoxemia without pronounced hydrothorax should alert us – (2 percent), and acute renal failure (1 percent) were infrequent though clinically relevant events, especially to prevent its complications.

It is of interest to note that ovarian enlargement in COH will not be as evident as in OI, mainly due to the thorough follicular aspiration with iatrogenic intrafollicular hemorrhage that appears as a consequence. Ovarian size, therefore, should be interpreted cautiously in patients undergoing COH, and the stage of the OHSS should rely more on the clinical and laboratory parameters (1).

Thromboembolism is the most dangerous manifestation of OHSS (77). The majority are venous in origin (75 percent) (deep venous, internal jugular vein, subclavian vein, and inferior vena cava), being the remaining arterial thromboses (25 percent) (middle cerebral artery, anterior cerebral artery, internal carotid artery, vertebral artery, humeral artery, femoral artery, mesenteric artery, aorta, and subclavian artery).

Liver dysfunction is not an infrequent event in severe OHSS, and abnormal liver function tests are detected in around one-third of patients (78). Several hypotheses have been postulated to justify the cholestatic damage. Progestative treatment and enhanced vascular permeability that could lead to hepatic edema do not seem to explain the liver abnormalities. Among all the cytokine network, IL-6, which mediates leukocytosis and increased vascular permeability, has been implicated in the pathogenesis of liver dysfunction. A more likely hypothesis is the increased estrogen level secondary to administration of gonadotropins (79); as this is the most prominent hormone in OHSS, there is a strong correlation between serum E2 concentrations and the incidence of this syndrome, and it has been described that ultrastructural rearrangements in the liver are designed to enhance the metabolic degradation of the increased estrogen levels, similar to those observed after administration of oral contraceptives.

Abnormal forms of presentation, as described above, have been reported. OHSS may be triggered not only by exogenous gonadotropin administration but also by endogenous stimulation. Endogenous ovarian stimulus may be originated in different clinical settings: patients with PCOD, who are more sensitive to endogenously released gonadotropins, pregnant patients with abnormally high serum levels of hCG such as in molar pregnancies, women with primary hypothyroidism, patients with gonadotroph adenoma that may induce cosecretion of FSH and LH, and patients presenting a mutation in the FSH receptor. Even, the flare-up induced by GnRH-a may provoke OHSS in women with PCOD, without any exogenous gonadotropin. Thus, a thorough differential diagnosis should be performed when enlarged ovaries are observed in the ultrasound, mainly to rule out malignant ovarian disease.

Occasionally, isolated forms of OHSS are observed. Symptoms may appear without the full expression of the syndrome. Hydrothorax as the only clinical manifestation of OHSS has been reported in rare occasions. Probably, it is the result of positive intra-abdominal pressure, negative intrathoracic pressure, diaphragmatic defects that promote the transfer of intra-abdominal fluid into the pleural space, and the transfer of vasoactive substances from the abdomen into the pleural space (80,81).

Other clinical consequences of OHSS are as follows:

- Reduced implantation in humans: it is a proven fact that COH for IVF deteriorates uterine receptivity compared with natural cycles, as supraphysiological levels of steroid hormones induce morphological and biochemical endometrial alterations relevant to uterine receptivity. We have consistently found a lower implantation rate in women who have a high response to gonadotropins (82), as indeed OHSS is a consequence of such a high response. More interestingly, uterine receptivity can be improved when E2 levels are decreased during the preimplantation period using a lower-dose, step-down stimulation protocol (83).
- Reduced quality of oocytes: it has been suggested that OHSS may have a detrimental effect on oocyte quality. A lower maturity and quality, resulting in a lower fertilization rate was reported (84). This may be related with obese, nonhyperandrogenic women with PCO ovaries, as a subgroup of these particular patients with derangement of insulin secretion have a lower fertilization rate of their oocytes and produce embryos that are unable to implant (85).

PREVENTION OF OHSS

Different strategies for preventing OHSS have been proposed, to identify women at risk being the first and most interesting one as previously mentioned. As this is not always possible, there are several options to avoid the development of the full-blown syndrome:

- hCG withholding: There is enough evidence in the literature to support that hCG is the main triggering cause of OHSS, probably through other less known mediators; so withholding hCG administration is a safe alternative to avoid OHSS, postponing the treatment cycle until the ovaries have been rendered quiescent (18). Cycle cancellation has financial and emotional implications, frustrates both patient and physician, and results in cancellation of a high percentage of cycles that would not have progressed to clinical OHSS; but in case we suspect that severe OHSS may be triggered, it is a valid and safe alternative.
- Ovarian electrocautery: Although it is not a first-line option for women at risk, laparoscopic ovarian diathermy after pituitary desensitization has been proposed to prevent OHSS (86). The mechanisms of action are not clear, but it seems to manipulate the intraovarian endocrine environment through rupture of androgen-rich cysts, destruction of androgen-producing stroma, or disruption of the

thickened ovarian capsule (87). Laparoscopic ovarian electrocautery should be reserved for women who have previously had at least one canceled cycle for risk of OHSS.

■ Coasting or drifting: When E2 levels increase rapidly in women undergoing COH with the concomitant administration of gonadotropins and GnRH-a, if gonadotropins – and not GnRH-a – are withheld, as there is no endogenous gonadotropins secretion to sustain follicular growth, a rapid decline in E2 levels will occur (88). Healthy developing follicles tolerate a brief period of gonadotropin deprivation, but granulosa cells of smaller follicles are less tolerant of withholding gonadotropin stimulus. Furthermore, another evidence that could explain the coasting physiology is that VEGF expression and secretion is significantly decreased in coasted patients (89). This is the rationale for coasting in order to reduce the risk/severity of OHSS in a high-risk population (90). In a prospective study, when E2 levels in women undergoing OI exceeded a threshold of 1,800 pg/mL, coasting was initiated until E2 level decreased by at least 25 percent or until at least three follicles were 18 mm or larger, and afterward hCG was administered, reaching an excellent pregnancy rate per cycle of 23 percent (91). Coasting was evaluated also in women undergoing COH for IVF with mature follicles, when E2 levels rose over 3,000 pg/mL, and with immature follicles, when numerous intermediate-sized follicles were observed and E2 levels were over 4,000 pg/mL, and restimulation of follicular growth was reinstituted after E2 levels normalized. Pregnancy rate was similar in these two groups (37 percent per cycle) (91). Interestingly, all patients progressed on to oocyte retrieval. The good results described in this report validate this option as a truly valid alternative to reduce, but not eliminate, the risk of severe OHSS. Coasting or drifting is part of the step-down approach of ovulation induction: the principle of lowering the dose of gonadotropins emulating the physiological pattern in order to select a reasonable number of mature follicles without risk of OHSS (92). The little tolerance of granulosa cells from small follicles to gonadotropin deprivation facilitates that coasting can safely rescue overstimulated OI and IVF cycles without compromising the pregnancy rate.

■ The different stimulation protocols may offer an increased risk or a relative protection. Originally, it was thought that pure FSH preparations would be safer in terms of OHSS, but a high rate of OHSS with pure FSH has been reported (1). Recombinant hormones, due to their higher bioactivity, are not free from complications either (93). Thus, it is much more significant to diagnose patients at risk than the LH/FSH ratio in the medication used in the stimulation protocol.

■ Follicular aspiration before or after hCG: Follicular aspiration at the time of oocyte retrieval might protect against OHSS by causing intrafollicular hemorrhage and granulosa cell aspiration, inducing a decline in the ovarian production of substances responsible for the onset of the syndrome (1,81). Two reports have evaluated the role of early-timed follicular aspiration of one ovary prior to administration of hCG in preventing severe OHSS (94,95). They hypothesized that this approach should prevent or reduce the production of intraovarian factors induced by hCG, as well as alter the corpora lutea arising from such follicles. Although the first observational, retrospective study showed promising results, no beneficial effect was reported later in a prospective, randomized study as no reduction in the occurrence of severe OHSS in women at risk was observed (94). Apart from preventing OHSS, immature oocyte recovery could be developed as a safe approach in women at risk as these oocytes retain their maturational and developmental competence for in vitro maturation and fertilization.

■ Intravenous albumin: Human albumin infusion immediately after oocyte retrieval was proposed a few years ago as a safe, effective, and economical treatment for prevention of severe OHSS in high-risk patients. Minimizing the effects the OHSS is not prevention; that should be considered as a treatment; here, we are considering human albumin infusion as an intervention to reverse or retard the disease process before it appears. Several contradictory reports have been published since then, and no consensus has been reached so far. Excellent reviews on this subject are available, and they do not suggest a role of prophylactic i.v. albumin in severe OHSS according to the published evidence (96). As the incidence of the syndrome is low, most of the published reports are observational studies with a small sample size and not enough power to validate the null hypothesis; so conclusions should be carefully interpreted. Other plasma expanders such as hydroxyethyle starch solution (HES) have been assayed in prevention of severe OHSS (88). König et al. reported a prospective, randomized trial in which 6 percent HES significantly reduced the incidence of moderate-severe OHSS in patients undergoing IVF treatment (97).

Our experience described in a prospective study of 976 patients at risk for OHSS (twenty or more oocytes retrieved) does not show any benefit in using albumin for preventing OHSS (98): the subjects were divided into two groups. The first group received 40 g of intravenous albumin, and the second group received no treatment. Moderate-severe and severe-only OHSS rates were similar. The incidence of hemoconcentration and liver and renal dysfunction seven days after oocyte retrieval was similar in the two groups. In women who developed moderate/severe ($n = 66$) or only severe ($n = 46$) OHSS (Table 27.3), there was no difference based on prior albumin administration between blood parameters or body weight on the day of oocyte retrieval, seven days later, and even when comparing variations between both measurements (Table 27.3). Moreover, the number of patients with paracentesis, hospital admissions, complications, and days of OHSS until resolution did not differ (98).

■ Cryopreservation of embryos: As OHSS syndrome is more common in conception cycles due to the endogenous hCG from the trophoblast of the implanting pregnancy, elective cryopreservation of all embryos has been postulated. Obviously, the main problem with cryopreserving all embryos is that pregnancy rate may be lower than with a transfer of fresh embryos. Several groups (99) reported in observational retrospective reports acceptable pregnancy rates in women who elected to cryopreserve all their embryos in order to prevent the onset of OHSS. The benefits from this approach have been compared to i.v. albumin infusion, and it seems to render higher pregnancy rates, with no differences in preventing OHSS in high-risk patients (100). A possible explanation is that i.v. albumin infusion does not lower the extremely high serum E2 levels, which we know diminish the endometrial receptivity (71), while thawed embryos are transferred in a natural or HRT cycle.

Table 27.3: (A) Number of Subjects and Incidence of OHSS in Albumin and Control Group. (B) Comparison of Abnormal Hematological Parameters of Albumin and Control Group Seven Days after Oocyte Retrieval

	Albumin	Control
A		
n	495	**493**
Moderate + severe OHSS (%)	7.1	**6.7**
Severe OHSS (%)	5.0	**4.7**
B		
n	488	**488**
Hemoglobin ≥15% (n)	29	**19**
Hematocrit ≥45% (n)	16	**13**
Leucocytes ≥20,000/mm^3 (n)	1	**3**
Creatinine >1.2 mg/dL (n)	1	**1**
AST >40 IU/mL (n)	10	**13**
ALT >40 IU/mL (n)	27	**29**

No significant differences were shown in the studied populations ($P \geq 0.05$). ALT, alanine aminotransferase; AST, aspartate aminotransferase (adapted from reference 98).

- Alternatives for women under COH without GnRH-a:
  □ FSH to trigger ovulation: A potential benefit may be obtained from administering a bolus of FSH to replace the midcycle LH/hCG surge and promote periovulatory events in order to avoid hCG administration in women at risk. The reinitiation of oocyte meiosis, fertilization, and granulosa cell luteinization is not due to residual LH contamination in the purified FSH preparations as recombinant FSH is able to induce such changes (101).
  □ GnRH agonists to trigger ovulation: GnRH-a induces surges of endogenous LH and FSH, with similar luteal phase length and progesterone levels than hCG cycles (102,103). It may be an acceptable substitute in cycles of OI to trigger ovulation in women at risk instead of hCG, although it is not applicable to COH protocols with GnRHa suppression (104,105). The relatively short half-life (three to five hours) eliminates the risk of OHSS in nonconception cycles. Ovulation rates close to 75 percent and pregnancy rates around 17 percent have been reported, with a low rate of multiple pregnancy. None of the women developed OHSS in this short series.
  □ Octreotide: Somatostatin analogues reduce insulin, insulin-like growth factor 1, and LH levels, so it was hypothesized that they may lower the risk of OHSS when administered to women at risk. When given to women with PCOD who are resistant to clomiphene citrate, it reduced E2 levels and follicle numbers compared to placebo, so it may be of valuable interest in reducing the incidence of OHSS in these particular patients (106).

- □ GnRH antagonists: As GnRH receptors are expressed in granulosa-lutein cells, this new drug may be a new alternative to not only suppress pituitary function but also exert direct actions at the ovarian level, being able to abort imminent OHSS-lowering serum E2 concentrations and decreasing ovarian size (88,107).
  □ Ketokonazole: Intermittent low doses of ketokonazole during induction of ovulation effectively reduce ovarian estrogen synthesis, which may lower the cancellation rate in women prone to hyperstimulated cycles (108). It has not been proven yet whether the addition of ketokonazole during COH reduces the risk of OHSS.

TREATMENT OF OHSS

Until the pathogenesis of this syndrome is totally understood, the treatment will continue to be largely empiric. However, some pathogenetic enigmas have been partially clarified, and they have provided the basis of the evidence-based treatment (Table 27.2).

- Bed rest: There is a rational basis for strict bed rest in OHSS. If the patient is in an upright position, the renin-angiotensin-aldosterone and sympathetic nervous systems are activated, with a reduction of glomerular filtration rate and sodium excretion and a decreased response to loop diuretics (109).
- Transvaginal ultrasound-guided aspiration of ascitic fluid: When tense ascites develops secondary to the rapid accumulation of ascitic fluid, paracentesis should be performed to provide symptomatic relief (18). The increased intra-abdominal pressure may compromise venous return and, consequently, cardiac output as well as renal edema and possibly thrombosis. So, if tense ascites is detected with oliguria, increasing levels of creatinine, or hemoconcentration unresponsive to medical therapy, ultrasound-guided aspiration of ascitic fluid must be performed using the transvaginal approach suggested by Aboulghar et al. (110). The dramatic improvement in clinical symptoms (rise in urine output and creatinine clearance, decrease in hematocrit, alleviation of dyspnea, and abdominal discomfort) supports this treatment modality as it is safe and exceptionally beneficial (18,75). To prevent the need for multiple paracentesis, which some patients may require, it has been proposed to leave a closed-system Dawson-Mueller catheter with a "simp-loc" locking design to allow continuous drainage of the ascitic fluid (92,111). However, if the patient is hemodynamically unstable, or if hemoperitoneum is suspected, paracentesis should not be performed. A close surveillance of the hemodynamic condition of the patient is mandatory, as rapid mobilization of ascites by paracentesis may be followed by a reduction in effective intravascular volume. Peritoneous shunting for continuous autotransfusion of ascites has proved beneficial in patients with severe OHSS, expanding circulating plasma volume and leading to prompt recovery (112).
- Low-salt albumin: Plasma expanders should be used when a correct fluid balance cannot be restored by crystalloids alone in order to increase the effective arterial blood volume as hypovolemia is a landmark in OHSS. Among all the

volume expanders currently available, low-salt albumin is the preferred one (1): it is the protein that is lost into the third space in this syndrome, it is nontoxic and safe from viral contamination, and it has a longer half life than other volume expanders. Fifty to 100 g of albumin every six to twelve hours is a commonly used and effective dosage.

- Furosemide: Blocking the renal sodium-retaining mechanisms with a potent natriuretic agent such as furosemide will immediately increase urine volume and sodium excretion. Although contraindicated if hypotension or hemoconcentration is present, diuretics will restore the prerenal impairment in renal function, which could progress to acute tubular necrosis and renal failure if untreated. Furosemide is a rapid-acting diuretic with a short half-life, which allows a close control of dosage according to diuresis (10 mg i.v. every four hours). A practical approach is to administer 100 g of albumin followed by 10 mg furosemide i.v. every four hours. The diuretic should be discontinued when normal urine output is obtained (>1,000 mL/day for forty-eight hours) (109).
- Low sodium intake: With the purpose to mobilize the intra-abdominal fluid by creating a negative balance of sodium, a dietary sodium restriction (60 mEq/day) may be a useful measure to improve ascites in patients with severe OHSS (109). However, a low-sodium diet did not influence renal and ovarian renin and prorenin production during ovarian stimulation, so the usefulness of this approach remains controversial.
- Dopamine: The use of low doses of dopamine may be useful in severe OHSS patients. Ferraretti et al. treated seven oliguric patients with low doses of dopamine by peripheral infusion, restricted fluid intake, and protein/salt-rich diet, with regression of illness within twenty-four to forty-eight hours after starting dopamine infusion. No maternal or fetal adverse effects were described (113).
- Careful monitoring of:
  □ Fluid balance and electrolyte concentration: A strict control of intake and output is mandatory. Crystalloids may correct the hypovolemia, but if necessary, volume expanders should be used. Serum sodium, potassium, and chloride are useful indicators of hemodilution or electrolyte imbalance. Potassium supplementation may be needed.
  □ Liver dysfunction: As generalized peripheral arterial vasodilation improves, the tendency toward liver cirrhosis is diminished (3). Simultaneously, high serum E2 level may cause liver dysfunction while trying to enhance the metabolic degradation of these increased estrogen levels. So, biochemical liver parameters should be closely monitored and reestablished.
  □ Blood hemostatic markers: It is useless to test general blood coagulation parameters including clotting time, bleeding time, platelet count, prothrombin time, and fibrinogen as they all will be within the normal limits. A more specific investigation for this severe complication should be performed, and we should look for two sensitive markers of the prothrombotic state: 1) D-dimers, which are considered to be a reliable molecular marker of the fibrinolytic system activation, as this substance is generated as a result of lysis of thrombus, and 2) plasmin-α^2 antiplasmin complexes, a good indicator of activation of

the coagulation of fibrinolytic system (114). Other authors recommend additional molecules to be considered, as thrombin-antithrombin complexes that are also good clinical markers for this procoagulant condition in severe OHSS (3). If any of these markers is altered, heparinization of the patient should be started (5,000 IU/12 h). In the daily clinical practice, hemoconcentration can be used as a parameter to indicate heparinization.

Dopamine Agonists in the Prevention and Treatment of OHSS

In previous experiences, we showed that inhibition of VEGF action was accompanied by reduced VP. However, the use of such strategies employing antiangiogenic drugs has been abandoned in women due to side effects of these compounds (115–117). Aiming to find a specific nontoxic treatment for OHSS, we came back to the beginning of our hypothesis, but this time we turned to the using of array technology in order to look at not only one or few but all the possible genes involved in the development of OHSS. With this idea in mind, we looked at the expression of gene products regulated under OHSS conditions. This approach resulted in the development of new approaches to block the onset of the syndrome by employing dopamine agonists.

We compared ovarian gene expression in animals subjected to different regimens of stimulation, including control animals and stimulated rats developing OHSS (67). Forty-eight hours after hCG, VP was measured and mRNA from ovaries extracted to perform gene expression profiles in macroarray filters containing 14,000 genes. Gene expression showed eighty upregulated and seven downregulated genes in OHSS as compared to mild stimulation and controls. Upregulated genes were grouped in five families: cholesterol synthesis, VEGF signal transduction, prostaglandins synthesis, oxidative stress process, and cell cycle regulation. The downregulation of tyrosine hydroxylase (TH, enzyme responsible for dopamine synthesis) was considered a characteristic of OHSS as well.

Taking together the results described above, we realized that targeting the upregulated genes could compromise basic cellular or physiological processes, like E2 and P4 production and ovulation, or well block unspecific secondary signal transduction pathways shared by many molecules. So we focused on the downregulated genes, in the idea that they could act on the opposite as the upregulated genes, that is, as natural inhibitors of the angiogenic processes that then needed to be enhanced or upregulated.

TH, the key enzyme responsible for dopamine synthesis was downregulated, suggesting that maybe dopamine could act as an antiangiogenic factor in the ovary, so a deficit in its production after PMSG + hCG administration in our OHSS animal (as we observed) model could be involved in the increased VP, which characterizes the syndrome. In fact, several reports had showed that dopamine administration could decrease VP in in vitro (118) and in vivo (119) cancer models by decreasing VEGFR-2 phosphorylation, which is the first step in VEGF downstream signaling leading to iVP after VEGF binding to this receptor (120). Although the mechanism by which dopamine is able to decrease VEGFR-2 phosporylation still remains unknown, we wondered if administering dopamine to our OHSS rats would become as effective, inhibiting iVP as it had been decreasing angiogenesis in the cancer models.

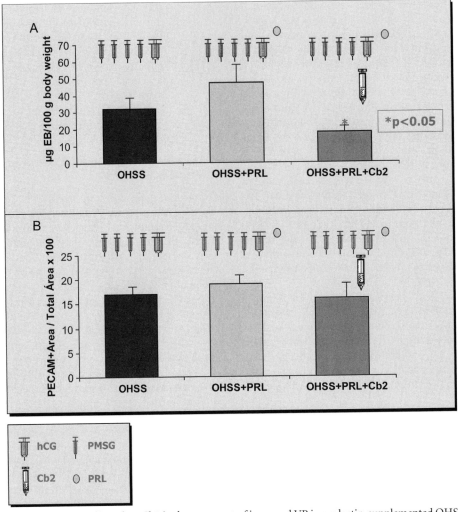

Figure 27.4. The effects of low-dose Cb2 in the treatment of increased VP in prolactin-supplemented OHSS rats. The state of increased vascular permeability (A) (as micrograms of extravasated EB dye per 100 g animal weight) was significantly reversed after Cb2 administration in prolactin-supplemented OHSS rats. These changes in VP in the experimental group were not mediated by luteolytic effects since luteal vascular density (B) (as the percentage of PECAM, a specific endothelial cell marker) was not affected. (Adapted from reference 121.)

Dopamine receptor 2 (Dp-r2) agonists, used in the treatment of human hyperprolactinemia including pregnancy, inhibit VEGFR-2-dependent VP and angiogenesis when administered at high doses in animal cancer models. To test whether VEGFR-2-dependent VP and angiogenesis could be segregated in a dose-dependent fashion with the Dp-r2 agonist cabergoline (Cb2), a well-established OHSS rat model supplemented with prolactin was used. A 100 µg/kg low-dose Dp-r2 agonist Cb2 reversed VEGFR-2-dependent VP without affecting luteal angiogenesis through partial inhibition of ovarian VEGFR-2 phosphorylation levels (Figure 27.4). No luteolytic effects (serum progesterone levels and luteal apoptosis unaffected) were observed. Cb2 administration also did not affect VEGF/VEGFR-2 ovarian mRNA levels (121).

Previous reports in the literature have shown that this approach could be successful. Ferraretti et al. (113) were the first to publish a substantial improvement in urinary output and overall symptoms in seven critically ill patients after intravenous Dp infusion. Two uncontrolled reports of Dp agonists'

use to prevent/treat OHSS followed. Tsunoda et al. administered docarpamine, an oral Dp prodrug, in twenty-seven patients hospitalized and refractory to therapy with albumin. Urinary output was increased and symptoms associated with ascites gradually improved, suggesting a positive effect of Dp agonists on OHSS (122). Similarly, Manno et al. administered Cb2 at a dose of 1 mg every forty-eight hours to twenty patients at risk of hyperstimulation, starting the evening after pickup, and to ten severe hyperstimulated pregnant women after twenty-four- to forty-eight-hour Dp infusion. They reported the absence of OHSS in women at risk and a prompt improvement in hospitalized patients (123).

Moreover, Papaleo et al. described a group of women with PCOD and hyperprolactinemia receiving Cb2 during ovarian stimulation. They observed that these patients had reduced sensitivity of the ovaries, resulting in lower number of follicles developed, lower serum E2 levels, and, most importantly, reduced incidence of OHSS (124). In addition, pituitary adenomas are sometimes associated with plurihormonal production including FSH, inducing spontaneous OHSS (125–127). The symptoms of OHSS have been successfully treated with the dopamine agonist bromocriptine (128) and very recently with Cb2 in two patients (129).

Results in the animal model and the safe clinical profile of Dp-r2 agonists encouraged us to administer Cb2 to oocyte donors at high risk for developing the syndrome. We designed a prospective, randomized, and double-blind study: fifty-four oocyte donors in whom twenty to thirty follicles larger than 12 mm developed and more than twenty oocytes were retrieved. Immediately after hCG administration, patients were allocated in two groups based on a computer randomization: the study group ($n = 29$) received 0.5 mg oral Cb2 daily for eight days; the control group ($n = 25$) received one tablet of placebo during eight days. Women were monitored every forty-eight hours from the day of hCG (day 0) up to day 8. Hemoconcentration and the presence and volume of ascitic fluid were significantly reduced in the study group. The occurrence of OHSS decreased from 65 (controls) to 25 percent (treatment). Dopamine agonists are widely employed in pregnant patients without any adverse effect; the concept should be proven in larger studies and the mechanism of action described (130).

KEY POINTS FOR CLINICAL PRACTICE

■ Ovarian hyperstimulation syndrome is an abnormal response of the ovaries to gonadotropins. It is a broad spectrum of signs and symptoms, usually self-limiting, but sometimes it can become a life-threatening condition. It is caused by changes in the capillary permeability that lead to fluid shift to third-space compartments, causing intravascular volume depletion, ascitis, and hemoconcentration, which may be complicated by thrombosis and/or by renal, hepatic, respiratory, and hematological dysfunction. The OHSS primary prevention is to reduce its incidence, being the most important step to identify patients at risk that will undergo IVF treatment, using a softer stimulation protocol and giving these patients special attention and close monitoring than usual with frequent ultrasound and serum estradiol levels. Secondary prevention consists in identification and early screening of the disease, reducing prevalence, duration, severity, and the appearance of complications. Therefore, it is essential to monitor OHSS patients very closely.

■ Until recently, OHSS treatment was reduced to the management of its complications. New data as the VEGF system studies are providing new insights for prevention and treatment of OHSS. For the first time a physiopathological approach to OHSS is proposed and the use of Cb2 and other dopamine agonists might be a useful tool in the secondary prevention of OHSS.

REFERENCES

1. Navot D., Bergh P.A., Laufer N. Ovarian hyperstimulation syndrome in novel reproductive technologies: prevention and treatment. *Fertility and Sterility* (1992), **58**, 249–61.
2. Rizk B. Epidemiology of ovarian hyperstimulation syndrome: iatrogenic and spontaneous. In Rizk B., (Ed.), *Ovarian Hyperstimulation Syndrome*. Cambridge, New York: Cambridge University Press (2006), Chapter 2, pp. 10–42.
3. Balasch J., Fabregues F., Arroyo V. Peripheral arterial vasodilation hypothesis: a new insight into the pathogenesis of ovarian hyperstimulation syndrome. *Human Reproduction*, (1998) **13**, 2718–30.
4. Rizk B. Pathophysiology of hyperstimulation syndrome. In Rizk B., (Ed.), *Ovarian Hyperstimulation Syndrome*. Cambridge, New York: Cambridge University Press (2006), Chapter 3, pp. 43–78.
5. Rizk B. Ovarian hyperstimulation syndrome. In (Studd J., Ed.), *Progress in Obstetrics and Gynecology*, Volume 11. Edinburgh: Churchill Livingstone (1993a), Chapter 18, pp. 311–49.
6. McClure N., Leya J., Radwanska E., Rawlins R., Haning R.V. Luteal phase support and severe ovarian hyperstimulation syndrome. *Human Reproduction*, (1992) **7**, 758–64.
7. Zalel Y., Orvieto R., Ben-Rafael Z., Homburg R., Fisher O., Insler V. Recurrent spontaneous ovarian hyperstimulation syndrome associated with polycystic ovary syndrome. *Gynecologic Endocrinology*, (1995) **9**, 313–5.
8. Cappa F., Pasqua C., Tobia M., Ventura T. Ascites and hydrothorax due to endogenous hyperstimulation of H.C.G. in a case of hydatidiform mole destruens with secondary irreversible kidney insufficiency due to disseminated intravascular coagulation. *Rivista Italiana di Ginecologia*, (1976) **56**, 363–8.
9. Guvenal F., Guvenal T., Timuroglu Y., Timuroglu T., Cetin M. Spontaneous ovarian hyperstimulation-like reaction caused by primary hypothyroidism. *Acta Obstetricia et Gynecologica Scandinavica*, (2006) **85**, 124–5.
10. Smits G., Olatunbosun O., Delbaere A., Pierson R., Vassart G., Costagliola S. Ovarian hyperstimulation syndrome due to a mutation in the follicle-stimulating hormone receptor. *New England Journal of Medicine*, (2003) **21**, 760–6.
11. Vasseur C., Rodien P., Beau I., Desroches A., Gerard C., de Poncheville L., Chaplot S., Savagner F., Croue A., Mathieu E., Lahlou N., Descamps P., Misrahi M. A chorionic gonadotropin-sensitive mutation in the follicle-stimulating hormone receptor as a cause of familial gestational spontaneous ovarian hyperstimulation syndrome. *New England Journal of Medicine*, (2003) **21**, 753–9.
12. Montanelli L., Delbaere A., Di Carlo C., Nappi C., Smits G., Vassart G., Costagliola S. A mutation in the follicle-stimulating hormone receptor as a cause of familial spontaneous ovarian hyperstimulation syndrome. *The Journal of Clinical Endocrinology and Metabolism*, (2004a) **89**, 1255–8.
13. Montanelli L., Van Durme J.J., Smits G., Bonomi M., Rodien P., Devor E.J., Moffat-Wilson K., Pardo L., Vassart G., Costagliola S. Modulation of ligand selectivity associated with activation of the transmembrane region of the human follitropin receptor. *Molecular Endocrinology*, (2004b) **18**, 2061–73.
14. Delbaere A., Smits G., De Leener A., Costagliola S., Vassart G. Understanding ovarian hyperstimulation syndrome. *Endocrine*, (2005) **26**, 285–90.
15. Kihara M., Sugita T., Nagai Y., Saeki N., Tatsuno I., Seki K. Ovarian hyperstimulation caused by gonadotroph cell adenoma: a case report and review of the literature. *Gynecological Endocrinology*, (2006) **22**, 110–3.
16. Lyons C.A., Wheeler C.A., Frishman G.N., Hackett R.J., Seifer D.B., Haning R.V. Jr. Early and late presentation of the ovarian hyperstimulation syndrome: two distinct entities with different risk factors. *Human Reproduction*, (1994) **9**, 792–9.
17. Pellicer A., Albert C., Mercader A., Bonilla-Musoles F., Remohí J., Simón C. The pathogenesis of ovarian hyperstimulation syndrome: in vivo studies investigating the role of interleukin-1α, interleukin-6, and vascular endothelial growth factor. *Fertility and Sterility*, (1999) **71**, 482–9.
18. Rizk B., Aboulghar M. Modern management of ovarian hyperstimulation syndrome. *Human Reproduction* (1991) **6**, 1082–7.

19. Schenker J.G., Weinstein D. Ovarian hyperstimulation syndrome: a current survey. *Fertility and Sterility*, (1978) **30**, 255–68.

20. Knox G.E. Antihistimine blockade of the ovarian hyperstimulation syndrome. *American Journal of Obstetrics and Gynecology*, (1974) **118**, 992–4.

21. Navot D., Margalioth E.J., Laufer N., Birkenfeld A., Relou A., Rosler A., Schenker J.G. Direct correlation between plasma renin activity and severity of the ovarian hyperstimulation syndrome. *Fertility and Sterility*, (1987) **48**, 57–61.

22. Loret de Mola J.R., Baumgardner G.P., Goldfarb J.E., Friedlander M.A. Ovarian hyperstimulation syndrome: preovulatory serum concentrations of interleukin-6, interleukin-1 receptor antagonist and tumor necrosis factor-α cannot predict its occurrence. *Human Reproduction*, (1996) **7**, 1377–80.

23. Aboulghar M.A., Mansour R.T., Serour G.I., Elhelw B.A., Shaarawy M. Elevated levels of angiogenin in serum and ascitic fluid from patients with severe ovarian hyperstimulation syndrome. *Human Reproduction*, (1998) **13**, 2068–71.

24. Magini A., Granchi S., Orlando C., Vannelli G.B., Pellegrini S., Milani S., Grappone C., De Franco R., Susini T., Forti G., Maggi M. Expression of endothelin-1 gene and protein in human granulosa cells. *The Journal of Clinical Endocrinology and Metabolism*, (1996) **81**, 1428–33.

25. Fulghesu A.M., Villa P., Pavone V., Guido M., Apa R., Caruso A., Lanzone A., Rossodivita A., Mancuso S. The impact of insulin secretion on the ovarian response to exogenous gonadotropins in polycystic ovary syndrome. *The Journal of Clinical Endocrinology and Metabolism*, (1997) **82**, 644–8.

26. Senger D.R., Galli S.J., Dvorak E., Perruzzi C.A., Harvey V.S., Dvorak H.F. Tumor cells secrete a vascular permeability factor that promotes accumulation of ascites fluid. *Science*, (1983) **219**, 983–5.

27. Rizk B. Ovarian hyperstimulation syndrome. In Brindsen P.R., Rainsbury R.A., (Eds.), *A Textbook of In Vitro Fertilization and Assisted Reproduction*. Carnforth, UK: Parthenon Publishing (1992), Chapter 23, pp. 369–84.

28. Rizk B., Aboulghar N.A., Smitz J. et al. The role of vascular endothelial growth factor and interleukins in the athogenesis of severe ovarian hyperstimulation syndrome. *Human Reproduction Update*, (1997) **3**, 255–66.

29. Ujioka T., Matsura K., Tanaka N., Okamura H. Involvement of ovarian kinin-kallicrein system in the pathophysiology of ovarian hyperstimulation syndrome: studies in a rat model. *Human Reproduction*, (1998) **13**, 3009–15.

30. Senger D.R., Van De Water L., Brown L.F., Nagy J.A., Yeo K.T., Yeo T.K., Berse B., Jackman R.W., Dvorak A.M., Dvorak H.F. Vascular permeability factor (VPF, VEGF) in tumor biology. *Cancer Metastasis Reviews*, (1993) **12**, 303–24.

31. Yan Z., Weich H.A., Bernart W., Breckwoldt M., Neulen J. Vascular endothelial growth factor (VEGF) messenger ribonucleic acid (mRNA) expression in luteinized human granulosa cells in vitro. *The Journal of Clinical Endocrinology and Metabolism*, (1993) **77**, 1723–5.

32. Senger D.R., Connolly D.T., Van De Water L., Feder J., Dvorak H.F. Purification and NH_2-terminal amino acid sequence of guinea pig tumor secreted vascular permeability factor. *Cancer Research* (1990) **50**, 1774–8.

33. Roberts W.G., Palade G.E. Increased microvascular permeability and endothelial fenestration induced by vascular endothelial growth factor. *Journal of Cell Science*, (1995) **108**, 2369–79.

34. Wei M.H., Popescu N.C., Lerman M.I., Merrill M.J., Zimonjic D.B. Localization of the human vascular endothelial growth factor gene, VEGF, at chromosome 6p12. *Human Genetics*, (1996) **97**, 794–7.

35. Rizk B. Genetics of ovarian hyperstimulation syndrome. In Rizk B., (Ed.), *Ovarian Hyperstimulation Syndrome*. Cambridge, New York: Cambridge University Press (2006), Chapter 4, pp. 79–91.

36. Neufeld G., Cohen T., Gengrinovitch S., Poltorak Z. Vascular endothelial growth factor (VEGF) and its receptors. *The FASEB Journal*, (1999) **13**, 9–22.

37. Watkins R.H., D'Angio C.T., Ryan R.M., Patel A., Maniscalco W.M. Differential expression of VEGF mRNA splice variants in newborn and adult hyperoxic lung injury. *The American Journal of Physiology*, (1999) **276**, 858–67.

38. Olson T.A., Mohanraj D., Carson L.F., Ramakrishnan S. VP factor gene expression in normal and neoplastic human ovaries. *Cancer Research*, (1994) **54**, 276–80.

39. Gómez R., Simón C., Remohi J., Pellicer A. Vascular endothelial growth factor receptor-2 activation induces vascular permeability in hyperstimulated rats, and this effect is prevented by receptor blockade. *Endocrinology*, (2002) **143**, 4339–48.

40. Shima D.T., Kuroki M., Deutsch U., Ng Y.S., Adamis A.P., D'Amore P.A. The mouse gene for vascular endothelial growth factor. Genomic structure, definition of the transcriptional unit, and characterization of transcriptional and post-transcriptional regulatory sequences. *The Journal of Biological Chemistry*, (1996) **271**, 3877–83.

41. Burchardt M., Burchardt T., Chen M.W., Shabsigh A., de la Taille A., Buttyan R., Shabsigh R. Expression of messenger ribonucleic acid splice variants for the vascular endothelial growth factor in the penis of adult rats and humans. *Biology of Reproduction*, (1999) **60**, 398–404.

42. Neulen J., Yan Z., Raczek S., Weindel K., Keck C., Weich H.A., Marme D., Breckwoldt M. Human chorionic gonadotropin-dependent expression of vascular endothelial growth factor/VP factor in human granulosa cells: importance in ovarian hyperstimulation syndrome. *The Journal of Clinical Endocrinology and Metabolism*, (1995) **80**, 1967–71.

43. Gordon J.D., Mesiano S., Zaloudek C.J., Jaffe R.B. Vascular endothelial growth factor localization in human ovary and fallopian tubes: possible role in reproductive function and ovarian cyst formation. *The Journal of Clinical Endocrinology and Metabolism*, (1996) **81**, 353–9.

44. Otani N., Minami S., Yamoto M., Shikone T., Otani H., Nishiyama R., Otani T., Nakano R. The vascular endothelial growth factor/fms-like tyrosine kinase system in human ovary during the menstrual cycle and early pregnancy. *The Journal of Clinical Endocrinology and Metabolism*, (1999) **84**, 3845–51.

45. Yamamoto S., Konishi I., Tsuruta E., Nanbu K., Mandai M., Kuroda H., Matsushita K., Hamid A.A., Yura Y., Mori T. Expression of vascular endothelial growth factor (VEGF) during folliculogenesis and corpus luteum formation in the human ovary. *Gynecologic Endocrinology*, (1997) **11**, 371–81.

46. Goldsman M.P., Pedram A., Domínguez C.E., Ciuffardi I., Levin E., Asch R.H. Increased capillary permeability induced by human follicular fluid: a hypothesis for an ovarian origin of the hyperstimulation syndrome. *Fertility and Sterility*, (1995) **63**, 268–72.

47. McClure N., Healy D.L., Rogers P.A., Sullivan J., Beaton L., Haning R.V. Jr., Connolly D.T., Robertson D.M. Vascular endothelial cell growth factor as permeability agent in ovarian hyperstimulation syndrome. *Lancet*, (1994) **344**, 235–6.

48. Phillips H.S., Hains J., Leung D.W., Ferrara N. Vascular endothelial growth factor is expressed in rat corpus luteum. *Endocrinology*, (1990) **127**, 965–7.

49. De Vries C., Escobedo J.A., Ueno H., Houck K., Ferrara N., Williams L.T. The fms-like tyrosine kinase, a receptor for vascular endothelial growth factor. *Science*, (1992) **255**, 989–91.

50. Waltenberger J., Claesson-Welsh L., Siegbahn A., Shibuya M., Heldin C.H. Different signal transduction properties of KDR and Flt1, two receptors for vascular endothelial growth factor. *The Journal of Biological Chemistry*, (1994) **269**, 26988–95.

51. Shalaby F., Rossant J., Yamaguchi T.P., Gertsenstein M., Wu X.F., Breitman M.L., Schuh A.C. Failure of blood island formation and vasculogenesis in Flk-1-deficient mice. *Nature*, (1995) **376**, 62–6.

52. Verheul H.M., Hoekman K., Jorna A.S., Smit E.F., Pinedo H.M. Targeting vascular endothelial growth factor blockade: ascites and pleural effusion formation. *Oncologist*, (2000) **5**, (Suppl. 1), 45–50.

53. Kendall R.L., Wang G., Thomas K.A. Identification of a natural soluble form of the vascular endothelial growth factor receptor, flt-1, and its heterodimerization with KDR. *Biochemical and Biophysical Research Communications*, (1996) **226**, 324–8.

54. Hornig C., Behn T., Bartsch W., Yayon A., Weich H.A. Detection and quantification of complexed and free soluble human vascular endothelial growth factor receptor-1 (sVEGFR-1) by ELISA. *Journal of Immunological Methods*, (1999) **226**, 169–77.

55. Kendall R.L., Thoma K.A. Inhibition of vascular endothelial growth factor activity by an endogenously encoded soluble receptor. *Proceedings of the National Academy of Sciences of the United States of America*, (1993) **90**, 10705–9.

56. Roeckle W., Hecht D., Sztajer H., Waltenberger J., Yayon A., Weich H.A. Differential binding characteristics and cellular inhibition by soluble VEGF receptor 1 and 2. *Experimental Cell Research*, (1998) **241**, 161–70.

57. Xu L., Yoneda J., Herrera C., Wood J., Killion J.J., Fidler I.J. Inhibition of malignant ascites and growth of human ovarian carcinoma by oral administration of a potent inhibitor of the vascular endothelial growth factor receptor tyrosine kinases. *International Journal of Oncology*, (2000) **16**, 445–54.

58. Yukita A., Asano M., Okamoto T., Mizutani S., Suzuki H. Suppression of ascites formation and re-accumulation associated with human ovarian cancer by an anti-VPF monoclonal antibody in vivo. *Anticancer Research*, (2000) **20**, 155–60.

59. Kobayashi H., Okada Y., Asahina, Gotoh J., Terao T. The kallikrein-kinin system, but not vascular endothelial growth factor, plays a role in the increased VP associated with ovarian hyperstimulation syndrome. *Journal of Molecular Endocrinology*, (1998) **20**, 363–74.

60. Agrawal R., Tan S.L., Wild S., Sladkevicius P., Engmann L., Payne N., Bekir J., Campbell S., Conway G., Jacobs H. Serum vascular endothelial growth factor concentrations in in-vitro fertilization cycles predict the risk of ovarian hyperstimulation syndrome. *Fertility and Sterility*, (1999) **71**, 287–93.

61. Abramov Y., Barac V., Nisman B., Schenker J.G. Vascular endothelial growth factor plasma levels correlate to the clinical picture in severe ovarian hyperstimulation syndrome. *Fertility and Sterility*, (1997) **67**, 261–5.

62. Chen C.D., Wu M.Y., Chen H.F., Chen S.U., Ho H.N., Yang Y.S. Prognostic importance of serial cytokine changes in ascites and pleural effusion in women with severe ovarian hyperstimulation syndrome. *Fertility and Sterility*, (1999) **72**, 286–92.

63. Albert C., Garrido N., Rao C.V., Remohi J., Simon C., Pellicer A. The role of the endothelium in the pathogenesis of ovarian hyperstimulation syndrome. *Molecular Human Reproduction*, (2002) **8**, 409–18.

64. Wang T.H., Horng S.G., Chang C.L., Wu H.M., Tsai Y.J., Wang H.S., Soong Y.K. Human chorionic gonadotropin-induced ovarian hyperstimulation syndrome is associated with up-regulation of vascular endothelial growth factor. *Journal of Clinical Endocrinology and Metabolism*, (2002) **87**, 3300–08.

65. Antczak M., Van Blerkom J. The vascular character of ovarian follicular granulosa cells: phenotypic and functional evidence for an endothelial-like cell population. *Human Reproduction*, (2000) **15**, 2306–18.

66. Ujioka T., Matsuura E., Kawano T., Okamura H. Role of progesterone in capillary permeability in hyperstimulated rats. *Human Reproduction*, (1997) **12**, 1629–34.

67. Gómez R., Simón C., Remohi J., Pellicer A. Administration of moderate and high doses of gonadotropins to female rats increases ovarian vascular endothelial growth factor (VEGF) and VEGF receptor-2 expression that is associated to vascular hyperpermeability. *Biology of Reproduction*, (2003) **68**, 2164–71.

68. Brekken R.A., Overholser J.P., Stastny V.A., Waltenberger J., Minna J.D., Thorpe P.E. Selective inhibition of vascular endothelial growth factor (VEGF) receptor 2 (KDR/Flk-1) activity by a monoclonal anti-VEGF antibody blocks tumor growth in mice. *Cancer Research*, (2000) **60**, 5117–24.

69. Wedge S.R., Ogilvie D.J., Dukes M., Kendrew J., Curwen J.O., Hennequin L.F., Thomas A.P., Stokes E.S., Curry B., Richmond G.H., Wadsworth P.F. ZD4190: an orally active inhibitor of vascular endothelial growth factor signaling with broad-spectrum antitumor efficacy. *Cancer Research*, (2000) **60**, 970–5.

70. Vajkoczy P., Menger M.D., Vollmar B., Schilling L., Schmiedek P., Hirth K.P., Ullrich A., Fong T.A. Inhibition of tumor growth, angiogenesis, and microcirculation by the novel Flk-1 inhibitor SU5416 as assessed by intravital multi-fluorescence videomicroscopy. *Neoplasia*, (1999) **1**, 31–41.

71. Pau E., Alonso-Muriel I., Gómez R., Novella E., Ruiz A., Garcia-Velasco J.A., Simon C., Pellicer A. Plasma levels of soluble vascular endothelial growth factor receptor-1 may determine the onset of early and late ovarian hyperstimulation syndrome. *Human Reproduction*, (2006) **21**, 1453–60. Epub (2006) Feb 17.

72. Villasante A., Pacheco A., Ruiz A., Pellicer A., Garcia-Velasco J.A. Vascular endothelial cadherin regulates vascular permeability: implications for ovarian hyperstimulation syndrome. *The Journal of Clinical Endocrinology and Metabolism*, (2006) **10**. [Epub ahead of print]

73. Enskog A., Henriksson M., Unander M., Nilsson L., Bränström M. Prospective study of the clinical and laboratory parameters of patients in whom ovarian hyperstimulation syndrome developed during controlled ovarian hyperstimulation for in vitro fertilization. *Fertility and Sterility*, (1999) **71**, 808–14.

74. Rizk B., Smitz J. Ovarian hyperstimulation syndrome after superovulation for IVF and related procedures. *Human Reproduction* (1992) **7**, 320–7.

75. Rizk B., Aboulghar M.A. (1999). Classification, pathophysiology and management of ovarian hyperstimulation syndrome. In Brinsden P., (Ed.), *A Textbook of In-vitro Fertilization and Assisted Reproduction*, Second Edition. Canforth, UK: The Pathenon Publishing Group, Chapter 9, pp. 131–55.

76. Abramov T., Elchalal U., Schenker J.G. Pulmonary manifestations of severe ovarian hyperstimulation syndrome: a multicenter study. *Fertility and Sterility*, (1999) **71**, 645–51.

77. Rizk B. Complications of ovarian hyperstimulation syndrome. In Rizk B., (Ed.), *Ovarian Hyperstimulation Syndrome*. Cambridge, New York: Cambridge University Press (2006), Chapter 5, pp. 92–118.

78. Fábregues F., Balasch J., Ginés P., Manau D., Jiménez W., Arroyo V., Creus M., Vanrell J.A. Ascites and liver test abnormalities during severe ovarian hyperstimulation syndrome. *American Journal of Gastroenterology*, (1999) **94**, 994–9.

79. Balasch J., Carmona F., Llach J., Arroyo V., Jové I., Vanrell J.A. Acute prerrenal failure and liver dysfunction in a patient with severe ovarian hyperstimulation syndrome. *Human Reproduction*, (1990) **5**, 348–51.

80. Gore L., Nawar M.G., Rizk B. et al. Resistant unilateral hydrothorax as the sole manifestation of ovarian hyperstimulation syndrome. *Middle East Fertility Society Journal*, (2002) **7**, 149–53.

81. Kingsland C, Collins JV, Rizk B, Mason B. Ovarian hyperstimulation presenting as acute hydrothorax after in-vitro fertilization. *American Journal of Obstetric and Gynecology*, (1989) **16**, 381–2.

82. Pellicer A., Valbuena D., Cano F., Remohí J., Simón C. Lower implantation rates in high responders: evidence for an altered endocrine milieu during the preimplantation period. *Fertility and Sterility*, (1996) **65**, 1190–5.

83. Simón C., Garcia-Velasco J.A., Valbuena D., Peinado J.A., Moreno C., Remohí J., Pellicer A. Increasing uterine receptivity by decreasing estradiol levels during the preimplantation period in high responders with the use of a follicle-stimulating hormone step-down regimen. *Fertility and Sterility*, (1998) **70**, 234–9.

84. Aboulghar M.A., Mansour R.T., Serour G.I., Ramzy A.M., Amin Y.M. Oocyte quality in patients with severe ovarian hyperstimulation syndrome (OHSS). *Fertility and Sterility*, (1997) **68**, 1017–21.

85. Cano F., García-Velasco J.A., Millet A., Remohí J., Simón C., Pellicer A. Oocyte quality in polycystic ovaries revisited: identification of a particular subgroup of women. *Journal of Assisted Reproduction and Genetics*, (1997) **14**, 254–61.

86. Rimington M.R., Walker S.M., Shaw R.W. The use of laparoscopic ovarian electrocautery in preventing cancellation of in vitro fertilization treatment cycles due to risk of ovarian hyperstimulation syndrome in women with polycystic ovaries. *Human Reproduction*, (1997) **12**, 1443–7.

87. Rizk B., Nawar M.G. Laparoscopic ovarian drilling for surgical induction of ovulation in polycystic ovarian syndrome. In Allahbadia G. (Ed.), *Manual of Ovulation Induction*. Mumbai, India: Rotunda Medical Technologies (2001), Chapter 18, pp. 140–4.

88. Rizk B. Prevention of ovarian hyperstimulation syndrome. In Rizk B., (Ed.), *Ovarian Hyperstimulation Syndrome*. Cambridge, New York: Cambridge University Press (2006), Chapter 7, pp. 130–99.

89. Garcia-Velasco J.A., Zuniga A., Pacheco A., Gómez R., Simon C., Remohi J., Pellicer A. Coasting acts through downregulation of VEGF gene expression and protein secretion. *Human Reproduction*, (2004) **19**, 1530–8.

90. Garcia-Velasco J.A., Isaza V., Quea G., Pellicer A. Coasting for the prevention of ovarian hyperstimulation syndrome: much to do about nothing? *Fertility and Sterility*, (2006) **85**, 547–54.

91. Fluker M.R., Hooper W.M., Yuzpe A.A. Withholding gonadotropins ("coasting") to minimize the risk of ovarian hyperstimulation during superovulation and in vitro fertilization-embryo transfer cycles. *Fertility and Sterility*, (1999) **71**, 294–301.

92. Rizk B. Coasting for the prevention of threatening OHSS: An American Perspective. In Gerris J., Oliveness F., Delvigne A., (Eds.) *Ovarian Hyperstimulation Syndrome*. Tayler and Francis (2006), Chapter 23, pp. 247–67.

93. Rizk B., Thorneycroft I.H. Does recombinant follicle stimulating hormone abolish the risk of severe ovarian hyperstimulation syndrome? *Fertility and Sterility*, (1996) **65**, S151–2.

94. Egbase P.E., Maksheed M., Sharhan M.A., Grudzinskas J.G. Timed unilateral ovarian follicular aspiration prior to administration of human chorionic gonadotrophin for the prevention of severe ovarian hyperstimulation syndrome in in-vitro fertilization: a prospective, randomized study. *Human Reproduction*, (1997) **12**, 2603–6.

95. Tomazevic T., Meden-Vrtovec H. Early timed follicular aspiration prevents severe ovarian hyperstimulation syndrome. *Journal of Assisted Reproduction and Genetics*, (1996)**13**, 282–6.

96. Orvieto R., Ben-Rafael Z. Role of intravenous albumin in the prevention of severe ovarian hyperstimulation syndrome. *Human Reproduction*, (1998) **98**, 3306–9.

97. König E., Bussen S., Sütterlin M., Steck T. Prophylactic intravenous hydroxyethyl starch solution prevents moderate-severe ovarian hyperstimulation in in-vitro fertilization patients: a prospective, randomized, double-blind and placebo-controlled study. *Human Reproduction*, (1998) **13**, 2421–4.

98. Bellver J., Munoz E.A., Ballesteros A., Soares S.R., Bosch E., Simon C., Pellicer A., Remohi J. Intravenous albumin does not prevent moderate-severe ovarian hyperstimulation syndrome in high-risk IVF patients: a randomized controlled study. *Human Reproduction*, (2003) **18**, 2283–8.

99. Awonuga A.O., Dean N., Zaidi J., Pittrof R.U., Bekir J.S., Tan S.L. Outcome of frozen embryo replacement cycles following elective cryopreservation of all embryos in women at risk of developing ovarian hyperstimulation syndrome. *Journal of Assisted Reproduction and Genetics*, (1996) **13**, 293–7.

100. Shaker A.G., Zosmer A., Dean N., Bekir J.S., Jacobs H.S., Tan S.L. Comparison of intravenous albumin and transfer of fresh embryos with cryopreservation of all embryos for subsequent transfer in prevention of ovarian hyperstimulation syndrome. *Fertility and Sterility*, (1996) **65**, 992–6.

101. Zelinski-Wooten M.B., Hutchison J.S., Hess D.L., Wolf D.P., Stouffer R.L. A bolus of recombinant human follicle stimulating hormone at midcycle induces periovulatory events following multiple follicular development in macaques. *Human Reproduction*, (1998) **13**, 554–60.

102. Rizk B. Ovarian hyperstimulation syndrome: prediction, prevention, and management. In Rizk B., Devroey P., Meldrum D.R., (Eds.), *Advances and Controversies in Ovulation Induction*. 34th ASRM Annual Postgraduate Program, Middle East Fertility Society Precongress Course. ASRM, 57th Annual Meeting, Orlando, FL, Birmingham, Alabama: the American Society for Reproductive Medicine (2001), pp. 23–46.

103. Rizk B. Can OHSS in ART be eliminated? In Rizk B., Meldrum D., Schoolcraft W., (Eds.), *A Clinical Step-by-Step Course for Assisted Reproductive Technologies*. 35th ASRM Annual Postgraduate Program, Middle East Fertility Society Precongress Course. ASRM 58th Annual Meeting, Seattle, WA, Birmingham, Alabama: The American Society for Reproductive Medicine (2002), pp. 65–102.

104. Shalev E., Geslevich Y., Ben-Ami M. Induction of pre-ovulatory luteinizing hormone surge by gonadotropin-releasing hormone agonist for women at risk of developing the ovarian hyperstimulation syndrome. *Human Reproduction*, (1994) **9**, 417–19.

105. Rizk B. Nawar M.G. Ovarian hyperstimulation syndrome. In Serhal P., Overton C. (Eds.), *Good Clinical Practice in Assisted Reproduction*. Cambridge, UK: Cambridge University Press (2004), Chapter 8, pp. 146–66.

106. Morris R.S., Karande V.C., Didkiewicz A., Morris J.L., Gleicher N. Octreotide is not useful for clomiphene citrate resistance in patients with polycystic ovary syndrome but may reduce the likelihood of ovarian hyperstimulation syndrome. *Fertility and Sterility*, (1999) **71**, 452–6.

107. de Jong D., Macklon N.S., Mannaerts B.M., Coelingh Bennink H.J., Fauser B.C. High dose gonadotrophin-releasing hormone antagonist (ganirelix) may prevent ovarian hyperstimulation syndrome caused by ovarian stimulation for in-vitro fertilization. *Human Reproduction*, (1998) **13**, 573–5.

108. Gal M., Eldar-Geva T., Margalioth E.J., Barr I., Orly J., Diamant Y.Z. Attenuation of ovarian response by low-dose ketoconazole during superovulation in patients with polycystic ovary syndrome. *Fertility and Sterility*, (1999) **72**, 26–31.

109. Balasch J., Fábregues F., Arroyo V., Jiménez W., Creus M., Vanrell J.A. Treatment of severe ovarian hyperstimulation syndrome by a conservative medical approach. *Acta Obstetricia et Gynecologica Scandinavica*, (1996) **75**, 662–7.

110. Aboulghar M.A., Mansour R.T., Serour G.I., Amin, Y.M. Ultrasonically guided vaginal aspiration of ascites in the treatment of severe ovarian hyperstimulation syndrome. *Fertility and Sterility*, (1990) **53**, 933–5.

111. Al-Ramahi M., Leader A., Claman P., Spence J. A novel approach to the treatment of ascites associated with ovarian hyperstimulation syndrome. *Human Reproduction*, (1997) **12**, 2614–16.

112. Koike T., Araki S., Minakami H., Ogawa S., Sayama M., Shibahara H., Sato I. Clinical efficacy of peritoneovenous shunting for the treatment of severe ovarian hyperstimulation syndrome. *Human Reproduction*, (2000) **15**, 113–7.

113. Ferraretti A.P., Gianaroli L., Diotallevi L., Festi C., Trounson A. Dopamine treatment for severe ovarian hyperstimulation syndrome. *Human Reproduction*, (1992) **7**, 180–3.

114. Kodama H., Fukuda J., Karube H., Matsui T., Shimizu T., Tanaka T. Characteristics of blood hemostatic markers in a patient with ovarian hyperstimulation syndrome who actually developed thromboembolism. *Fertility and Sterility*, (1995) **64**, 1207–9.

115. Marx G.M., Steer C.B., Harper P., Pavlakis N., Rixe O., Khayat D. Unexpected serious toxicity with chemotherapy and antiangiogenic combinations: time to take stock! *Journal of Clinical Oncology*, (2002) **20**, 1446–8.

116. Glade-Bender J., Kandel J.J., Yamashiro D.J. VEGF blocking therapy in the treatment of cancer. *Expert Opinion on Biological Therapy*, (2003) **3**, 263–76.

117. Kuenen B.C., Tabernero J., Baselga J. Efficacy and toxicity of the angiogenesis inhibitor SU5416 as a single agent in patients with advanced renal cell carcinoma, melanoma, and soft tissue sarcoma. *Clinical Cancer Research*, (2003) **9**, 1648–55.

118. Basu S., Nagy J.A., Pal S., Vasile E., Eckelhoefer I.A., Bliss V.S., Manseau E.J., Dasgupta P.S., Dvorak H.F., Mukhopadhyay D. The neurotransmitter dopamine inhibits angiogenesis induced by vascular permeability factor/vascular endothelial growth factor. *Nature Medicine*, (2001) **7**, 569–74.

119. Sarkar C., Chakroborty D., Mitra R.B. Dopamine in vivo inhibits VEGF-induced phosphorylation of VEGFR-2, MAPK, and focal adhesion kinase in endothelial cells. *American Journal of Physiology, Heart and Circulatory Physiology*, (2004) **287**, H1554–60.

120. Quinn T.P., Peters K.G., De Vries C., Ferrara N., Williams L.T. Fetal liver kinase 1 is a receptor for vascular endothelial growth factor and is selectively expressed in vascular endothelium. *Proceedings of the National Academy of Sciences of the United States of America*, (1993) **90**, 7533–7.

121. Gomez R., Gonzalez-Izquierdo M., Zimmermann R.C., Novella-Maestre E., Alonso-Muriel I., Sanchez-Criado J., Remohi J., Simon C., Pellicer A. Low-dose dopamine agonist administration blocks vascular endothelial growth factor (VEGF)-mediated vascular hyperpermeability without altering VEGF receptor 2-dependent luteal angiogenesis in a rat ovarian hyperstimulation model. *Endocrinology*, (2006) **147**, 5400–11.

122. Tsunoda T., Shibahara H., Hirano Y., Suzuki T., Fujiwara H., Takamizawa S., Ogawa S., Motoyama M., Suzuki M. Treatment for ovarian hyperstimulation syndrome using an oral dopamine prodrug, docarpamine. *Gynecolgical Endocrinology*, (2003) **17**, 281–6.

123. Manno M., Tomei F., Marchesan E., Adamo V. Cabergoline: a safe, easy, cheap, and effective drug for prevention/treatment of ovarian hyperstimulation syndrome? *European Journal of Obstetrics, Gynecology, and Reproductive Biology*, (2005) **122**, 127–8.

124. Papaleo E., Doldi N., De Santis L., Marelli G., Marsiglio E., Rofena S., Ferrari A. Cabergoline influences ovarian stimulation in hyperprolactinaemic patients with polycystic ovary syndrome. *Human Reproduction*, (2001) **16**, 2263–6.

125. Shimon I., Rubenek T., Bar-Hava I., Nass D., Hadani M., Amsterdam A., Harel H. Ovarian hyperstimulation without elevated serum estradiol associated with pure follicle-stimulating hormone-secreting pituitary adenoma. *Journal of Clinical Endocrinology and Metabolism*, (2001) **86**, 3635–40.

126. Christin-Maitre S., Rongiéres-Bertrand C., Kottler M.L., Lahlou N., Frydman R., Touraine P., Bouchard P. A spontaneous and severe hyperstimulation of the ovaries revealing a gonadotroph adenoma. *Journal of Clinical Endocrinology and Metabolism*, (1988) **83**, 3450–3.

127. Gómez R., González M., Simón C., Remohi J., Pellicer A. Tyroxine hydroxylase (TH) downregulation in hyperstimulated ovaries reveals the dopamine agonist bromocriptine (Br2) as an effective and specific method to block increased vascular permeability (VP) in OHSS. *Fertility and Sterility*, (2003) **80**, (Suppl. 3), 43–4.

128. Murata Y., Ando H., Nagasaka T., Takahashi I., Saito K., Fukugaki H., Matsuzawa K., Mizutani S. Successful pregnancy after bromocriptine therapy in an anovulatory woman complicated with ovarian hyperstimulation caused by follicle-stimulating hormone-producing plurihormonal pituitary microadenoma. *Journal of Clinical Endocrinology and Metabolism*, (2003) **88**, 1988–93.

129. Knoepfelmacher M., Danilovic D.L., Rosa Nasser R.H., Mendonca B.B. Effectiveness of treating ovarian hyperstimulation syndrome with cabergoline in two patients with gonadotropin-producing pituitary adenomas. *Fertility and Sterility*, (2006) **86**, 719.

130. Alvarez C., Bosch E., Melo M.A.B., Fernández-Sánchez M., Muñoz J., Remohí J., Simón C., Pellicer A. The dopamine agonist cabergoline prevents moderate-severe early ovarian hyperstimulation syndrome (OHSS) in high-risk ART patients. *Human Reproduction*, (2006) **21** (Suppl. 1), i96.

28

REDUCING THE RISK OF HIGH-ORDER MULTIPLE PREGNANCY DUE TO OVULATION INDUCTION

Richard Palmer Dickey

INTRODUCTION

Ovulation induction (OI) that is not part of an *in vitro fertilization* (IVF) cycle is the cause of 40–70 percent of high-order multiple pregnancies (HOMP), pregnancies with three or more conceptus, and 11–21 percent of twins, in countries where modern infertility treatment is practiced (Levene et al., 1992; Corchia et al., 1996; Reynolds et al., 2003; Figure 28.1). The high incidence of HOMP due to OI is primarily due to use of gonadotropins, follicular stimulation hormone (FSH), and human menopausal gonadotropin (HMG), but also occurs with use of clomiphene citrate (CC). In IVF cycles, twin and HOMP pregnancies can be prevented 99 percent of the time by transferring no more than one or two embryos. In OI cycles, twin and HOMP pregnancies can be prevented by canceling cycles when more than one or two preovulatory follicles are present or estrogen levels are too high and by aspirating supernumerary follicles. Recommendations to prevent multiple birth have included withholding human chorionic gonadotropin (hCG) administration when more than six follicles are 12 mm or larger (Valbuena et al., 1996; Dickey et al., 2001); when more than three follicles are 14 mm or larger (Pittrof et al., 1996; Takokoro et al., 1997), or 16 mm or larger (Yovich and Matson, 1988); when more than two (Zikopoulos et al., 1993) or three (Tomlinson et al., 1996; Hughes et al., 1998) follicles are 18 mm or larger; and when E_2 exceeded 400 pg/mL (Kemmann et al., 1987), 600 pg/mL (Schenker et al., 1981), 1,000 pg/mL (Valbuena et al., 1996; Hughes et al., 1998), or 2,000 pg/mL (Vollenhoven et al., 1996; Remohi et al., 1989).

In order to prevent multiple pregnancies, all cycles would have to be canceled whenever two or more preovulatory follicles 10 mm or larger are present in gonadotropin OI cycles (Tur et al., 2001, Dickey et al., 2005) or 12 mm or larger were present in CC cycles (Dickey et al., 2001). Previous authors have reported that canceling cycles failed to prevent all HOMP when six or more follicles were 14 mm or larger (Ragni et al., 1999) or 16 mm (Gleicher et al., 2000). However, in the study conducted by Ragni (1999), the HOMP rate was 1.9 percent, and in that by Gleicher (2000), no HOMP occurred in 3,347 gonadotropin cycles unless ten or more total follicles, 7 mm or larger, were present or estradiol levels were 405 pg/mL or higher. Similarly, aspiration would have to include all supernumerary follicles 10 mm or larger. A least one author has recommended that gonadotropin OI should be abandoned in favor of IVF because of the large percent of cycles that would need to be canceled (Gleicher et al., 2000).

None of the authors who have recommended that gonadotropin OI should be abandoned considered the effect of patient age or previous treatment, more importantly they employed higher doses of gonadotropin than necessary in order to achieve maximum pregnancy rates, a procedure known as controlled ovarian hyperstimulation (COH). This technique was introduced in the United States by Sher et al. in 1984 but was not widely used before a publication in the journal *Fertility and Sterility* in 1987 that advocated COH with intrauterine insemination (IUI) as an alternative to IVF (Dodson et al., 1987). Initially, HMG was used to treat amenorrhea due to FSH deficiency secondary to pituitary or hypothalamic disorders (WHO type I), or anovulation refractory to treatment with CC, and the lowest dose consistent with follicular development was used. This changed to use of HMG in patients with unexplained infertility and to employing high doses of HMG in order to induce multiple follicular development so as to maximize the opportunity for pregnancy during a single cycle. In order to reduce multiple pregnancies due to ovulation induction, it is not enough to cancel cycles when there are excessive numbers of preovulatory follicles, and it is also necessary use the least stimulation that results in follicular development.

TECHNIQUES TO REDUCE HIGH-ORDER MULTIPLE PREGNANCIES

There are three steps necessary to reduce multiple pregnancies due to OI, without decreasing a patients overall chance to become pregnant. They are use of the least amount of stimulation that results in ovulation, continuation of low-dose stimulation for more than three cycles, and selective cancellation of cycles only for patients at significant risk of becoming pregnant with multiple gestations. The first technique requires using CC, low-dose gonadotropin, or pulsatile GnRH to stimulate monofollicular development and may include addition of LH or HCG in the late proliferative phase to inhibit development of preovulatory follicles, coasting, and aspiration of supernumerary follicles. The second requires continuation of stimulation cycles based on a patient's cause of infertility and individual response to stimulation as measured by preovulatory ultrasound. The third requires taking into consideration the patients age, number of previous failed cycles of treatment, inherent fecundity, and ability to carry safely to term if she should conceive twins when deciding whether or not to cancel a cycle.

A

SOURCE OF TWIN BIRTHS 2000

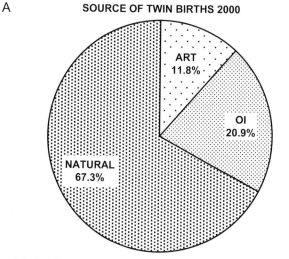

Adapted from Reynolds et.al. 2000, Pediatrics, 111, 1159-1162.

B   **SOURCE OF TRIPLET AND HIGHER ORDER BIRTHS 2000**

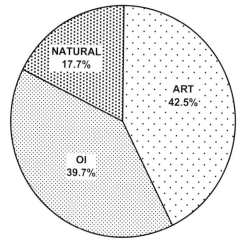

Adapted from Reynolds et.al. 2000, Pediatrics, 111, 1159-1162.

Figure 28.1. (A) Source of twin births, 2000; (B) Source of triplet and higher order births, 2000. ART, assisted reproductive technologies. Adapted from Dickey and Sartor (2005). Reprinted with publisher's permission.

Clomiphene Citrate

CC increases FSH secretion from the pituitary by temporarily blocking the negative feedback of estrogen that is necessary to regulate production and secretion of FSH. It allows FSH levels to decrease in response to rising estrogen production by the developing follicle or follicles, thereby facilitating monofollicular development. The average number of follicles 12 mm or larger is 2.7 compared to 5.4 in gonadotropin cycles (Dickey et al., 2001). Single follicles 12 mm or larger develop in 21 percent of CC cycles, two follicles develop in 32 percent, and three or more follicles develop in 47 percent of CC cycles (Dickey et al., 2001). When two follicles 12 mm or larger are present, the twin pregnancy rate is 4.1 percent. Rarely, follicles as small as 10 mm can result in pregnancy in CC cycles resulting in triplet pregnancy when two follicles 12 mm or larger are present (Dickey et al., 1992). The number of follicles 15 mm or larger and 18 mm or larger cannot be used to predict triplet pregnancy in CC cycles. The triplet pregnancy rate is 4.5 percent when there is

a single follicle 15 mm or larger and 2.3 percent when there are no follicles or a single follicle 18 mm or larger (Dickey et al., 2001). When six or more preovulatory follicles 12 mm or larger are present, the triplet pregnancy rate for patients younger than 35 is 15.3 percent in CC cycles compared to 13.7 percent in gonadotropin cycles. The implantation rate per follicle and estradiol level per follicle are identical in CC and gonadotropin cycles, only the number of preovulatory follicles is different.

When one or two follicles 12 mm or larger develop in CC cycles, stimulation should be continued for longer than the three cycles recommended in the traditional algorithm and will result in additional pregnancies (see Table 23.5, Chapter 23). The number of follicles 15 mm or larger correlates best with pregnancy rates in CC cycles (Dickey et al., 2001; Dickey et al., 2002b). When there is a single follicle 15 mm or larger, the average pregnancy rate per cycle through the first four cycles of CC with intrauterine insemination (IUI) for patients younger than 42 without endometriosis or tubal factor is 9.8 percent (Dickey et al., 2002b). When there are two follicles 15 mm or larger, the average per cycle through the first four cycles is 14.3 percent. Continuing stimulation to six cycles results in pregnancy rates of 60 percent for patients with two follicles 15 mm or larger and ovulatory dysfunction or requiring donor sperm, providing age is less than 43 and sperm quality is satisfactory. For age less than 30, pregnancies do not occur after the fourth cycle in patients with two follicles due to the higher fecundity of younger patients. For patients with single follicles 15 mm or larger, pregnancies did not occur after the fourth cycle due to switching to other regimens.

Gonadotropin Pregnancy Rates after Clomiphene Cycles Fail to Result in Pregnancy

The standard algorithm before COH-IUI became fashionable, which is still used by infertility specialists trained before 1987, was to use CC for three cycles and then, if pregnancy did not occur, switch to gonadotropin cycles with IUI (Karande et al., 1999). The doses of gonadotropin used were generally low, and few HOMP occurred. The rapid rise in HOMP due to OI did not occur in the United States until after the introduction of COH into many practices beginning in 1987 (Tur et al., 2001; Dickey and Sartor, 2005; Figure 28.2). The rationale for using CC for three cycles before COH is that patients, with the highest antral follicle counts or highest fecundity per ovulated oocyte, who are most likely to become pregnant, will do so during the CC cycles when the number of preovulatory follicles is lower than in COH cycles and therefore will be at less risk for twins and HOMP. By the same reasoning, twins and HOMP may be expected to occur more often during the initial cycles of CC or COH and less often in later cycles.

The ability of the standard algorithm in reducing HOMP due to COH was demonstrated in a retrospective analysis, which found that HOMP was inversely related to the number of prior CC-IUI cycles (Dickey et al., 2004b). The incidence of HOMP, during the first three cycles of COH-IUI, was 8.8 percent when there were no prior CC-IUI cycles (Table 28.1). The incidence of HOMP in COH-IUI was 7.5 percent when there had been one CC-IUI cycle without pregnancy, 5.7 percent when there were two CC-IUI cycles, and 0 percent when there were three or more previous CC-IUI cycles without pregnancy. Twin pregnancy rates, unlike HOMP rates, were unrelated to the number of previous CC-IUI cycles. Pregnancy rates per cycle

UNITED STATES TOTAL TWIN AND TRIPLET BIRTHS

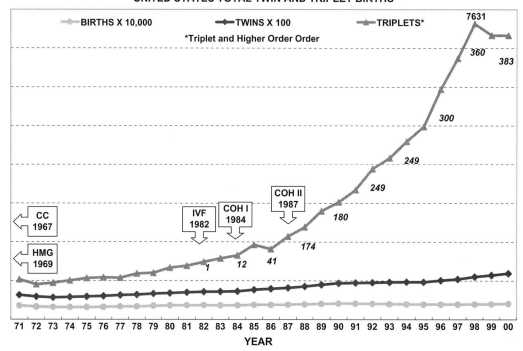

Figure 28.2. Total, twin, and triplet or higher order births, United States 1971–2000. Data show individual births. Italic numbers indicate number of IVF clinics. Adapted from Dickey and Sartor (2005). Reprinted with publisher's permission.

during first three COH-IUI cycles averaged 19–20 percent for patients who had one to four cycles of CC-IUI without pregnancy before being treated with COH-IUI. Patients who failed to become pregnant after four cycles of CC-IUI had a very low chance of becoming pregnant when switched to COH-IUI. Pregnancy rates per COH-IUI cycle decreased to 5 percent when there had been five or more CC-IUI cycles before starting COH-IUI. This illustrates again that when CC is used long enough, nearly all the patients capable of becoming pregnant without IVF, intracytoplasmic sperm injection (ICSI), or other assisted reproductive technology (ART) will do so without the need for COH (Dickey et al., 2002). It is necessary to repeat that the decrease in HOMP occurred when gonadotropin cycles were performed after CC cycles, as distinguished from treatment regimens in which gonadotropin is administered after five days of CC in the same cycle (sequential regimen). When CC and gonadotropin are used in sequential regimens, the number of preovulatory follicles produced and HOMP pregnancy rates are nearly identical to gonadotropin-only cycles (Dickey et al., 1993c, 2001).

An important consideration when using CC is its antiestrogen effects on cervical mucus and the endometrium. In order for a conceptus to implant and develop, the endometrial thickness must be at least 6 mm and for the best possible pregnancy rates should be 9 mm or greater (Dickey et al., 1993a, 1993b). Endometrial thickness can be increased by starting CC earlier in the cycle, by using a lower dose of CC, by adding estrogen (Yagel et al., 1992), or by using the less antiestrogenic selective estrogen receptor modulators (SERM) drug tamoxifen, instead of clomiphene. In order to ensure that sufficient sperm enter the uterus and reach the ampullary fallopian tubes, a postcoital test should be performed in the first CC cycle.

If sperm are not present in numbers four or more progressively motile sperm per 400× field, an IUI should be performed. Pregnancy rates in IUI cycles are markedly reduced when there are fewer than ten million total sperm or less than 30 percent progressive motility before preparation (Dickey et al., 1999). Of the approximately 2,100 CC pregnancies achieved at the author's clinic, 15 percent were the result of IUI. The pregnancy rates quoted above for CC alone and CC cycles before gonadotropin cycles were from cycles in which IUI was performed using husbands or donor sperm.

Minimal Doses of Gonadotropins

"Physicians Information" that was supplied with the Perganol brand of HMG, when it was first sold in the United States, stressed that treatment should be initiated with the lowest dose of gonadotropin that results in ovulation of at least one follicle and continued at that level for a minimum of three cycles before increasing the gonadotropin dose. This excellent recommendation should still be followed. Use of low doses of hMG/FSH has its basis in the threshold hypothesis. The threshold hypothesis proposes that there is a minimum FSH level that needs to be attained in order to initiate an ovarian response and that a very narrow range exists between the threshold for monofollicular growth and a ceiling above which multiple follicular development occurs (Dickey, 2005). The duration and extent to which FSH concentration is above the threshold level determine the number of follicles that reach the final maturation stage (Ben-Rafael et al., 1986).

The threshold level is different for each individual. When gonadotropin is administered IV in a step-up protocol, serum FSH levels greater than 7.8 IU/L are necessary to induce follicular

Table 28.1: Relationship of Number of Previous Cycles of CC-IUI to Pregnancy and Multiple Pregnancy Rates during the First Three Cycles of HMG/FSH-IUI Cycles

Number of CC-IUI cycles	Number of cycles*	Pregnancies per cycle?		Multiple gestation per pregnancy	
		n (%)	OR (95% CI)	2n (%)	≥3n (%)
0	1,459	318 (21.8)	1.00 (—)	61 (19.2)	28 (8.8)
1	408	80 (19.1)	0.88 (0.66–1.15)	15 (18.8)	6 (7.5)
2	268	53 (19.8)	0.83 (0.60–1.16)	10 (18.9)	3 (5.7)
3	130	25 (19.2)	0.83 (0.53–1.31)	5 (20.0)	0 (0.0)
4	57	11 (19.3)	0.84 (0.43–1.64)	2 (18.2)	0 (0.0)
5	23	1 (4.3)	0.16 (0.02–1.19)	0 (0.0)	0 (0.0)
6–12	32	1 (3.1)	0.11 (0.02–0.83)	0.0 (0.0)	0 (0.0)

*Pregnancy rate per cycle: cycles 1–4 (19.6 percent) versus cycles ≥5 (3.6 percent), $p = .006$ Chi square. Reprinted from Dickey et al. (2004) with permission.

growth in hypopituitary-hypothalamic (WHO 1) women and women with normal menstrual cycles suppressed with GnRH analogues, but a variable level ranging from 6.8 to 9.8 IU/L is required in PCO (WHO 2) women (Van Weissenbruch, 1990). Women of similar weights and ages have highly variable ovarian responses to HMG (Benadiva et al. 1988). Because of the narrow therapeutic index for gonadotropin, it is generally recommended that doses be increased by not more than 50 percent at each step up. A common step-up protocol for WHO I women is 35.7 > 50 > 75 > 112.5 > 150 IU. The initial dose of gonadotropin should be continued for five to seven days before determining whether it needs to be increased. Response can be evaluated by estradiol levels or ultrasound. If there is no apparent response, measurement of serum FSH levels is indicated to ensure that threshold levels have been achieved.

After subcutaneous (SC) and intramuscular (IM) administration of FSH, the maximal increases over baseline and elimination half-lives (thirty-seven hours), measured by immunoradiometric assay, are identical (Le Cotonnec et al., 1994). The maximal concentration is reached earlier with the SC route than with the IM route (16 ± 10 hours vs. 25 ± 10 hours), and systemic bioavailability is greater with the SC route compared to the IM route. When SC dosing is continued, a steady state is reached by day 4 at a level three times the single dose peak; thereafter, levels continued to rise about 5 percent per day (Le Cotonnec et al., 1994).

Homburg and Insler (2002) analyzed results from published studies of chronic low-dose gonadotropin treatment in women with PCOS and confirmed the efficacy of low-dose gonadotropin. They concluded that when an initial dose of 75 IU FSH and LH is continued for fourteen days with no increase and then increased in steps of 37.5 IU, 69 percent of cycles were monovulatory, the twin rate was 5 percent, the HOMP rate was 0.7 percent, and the pregnancy rate averaged 20 percent per cycle. Recent studies in which initial low doses of HMG/FSH have been used in 400 or more cycles are shown in Table 28.2. Pregnancy rates in the studies shown range from 10 percent (9.8) to 20 percent per cycle, and HOMP rates are all 2 percent or less. It is important to note that cycles were canceled when there were excessive numbers of preovulatory follicles in all the studies of low-dose gonadotropins in Table 28.2.

Results of Repeated Gonadotropin Cycles When There Are One or Two Preovulatory Follicles

The belief that gonadotropins should not be used for more than three cycles because pregnancy rates decrease markedly after the third cycle (Aboulghar et al., 2001) is true only for patients who develop nine or more preovulatory follicles (Figure 28.3; Dickey et al., 2005). Pregnancies occur after the third cycle of COH-IUI in inverse relation to the number of preovulatory follicles. Patients who developed fewer than nine follicles continue to become pregnant at a reduced rate per cycle after the third cycle. Patients who develop one or two follicles, are younger than thirty-eight years, and do not have tubal factor or severe male factor continue to become pregnant at the same rate through at least five cycles.

Pulsatile GnRH

Pulsatile gonadotropin-releasing hormone (GnRH) administered subcutaneously or intravenously results in pregnancy and multiple pregnancies similar to low-dose gonadotropins (Martin et al., 1990). Both routes of GnRH administration result in greater than 27 percent pregnancy rates per cycle and multiple birth rates of 5–8 percent, primarily of twins. The need for more frequent administration compared to gonadotropin and the lack of clear advantages in the areas of pregnancy and multiple pregnancy have kept GnRH from being more frequently employed in clinical practice.

Low-Dose hCG or rLH During the Late Proliferative Phase

An increasing trend in LH levels for two or more days preceding the LH surge is part of normal unstimulated ovulatory cycles (Hellier, 1994; Dickey, 2005). Addition or substitution of low-dose hCG (50–200 IU/day) in FSH and HMG regimens, after a dominant follicle has been selected, has been shown to impede development of smaller follicles (Arguinzoniz et al., 2000; Loumaye et al., 2000; Filicori et al., 2002a, 2002b). Addition of LH to FSH stimulation protocols for one or two days in the late

Table 28.2: Results of Low-Dose Gonadotropin Stimulation: Studies with 400 or More Cycles

Reference	Type study	Patients	Patients cycles	Initial stimulation	Criteria for hCG	Criteria to cancel	Percent canceled	Clinical pregnancy births					
								Percent/cycle	Twins	≥3 sacs	Percent/cycle	Twins	≥Triplets
Low-dose gonadotropins													
Healy et al. (2003)	Prospective	Failed infertility with ≥1 normal 1 normal tube	234:510	112.5 IU FSH	1 Follicle ≥14 mm	4 Follicle ≥14 mm	2.2	9.8	20	0.2	7.0	10	0.2
Balasch et al. (1996)	Prospective	WHO II CC failures	234:534	75 IU FSH	1 Follicle ≥17	4 Follicle ≥ 14 mm	5.2	17.4	15	0	15.5	N/A	0
Homburg and Howles (1999)	Review:11 studies	WHO II CC failures	717:1391	75 IU FSH	NA	N/A	N/A	20.1	5.0	0.7	N/A	N/A	N/A
White et al. (1996)	Prospective	PCOS	134:505	75 IU FSH	NA	N/A	13.5	11.8	6.7	0	N/A	N/A	N/A
White et al. (1996)	Prospective	PCOS	91:429	52.5 IU FSH	NA	N/A	0	11.4	6.1	0	N/A	N/A	N/A
Wang et al. (2003)	Retrospective	Mixed	824:2,413	37.5 IU FSH	NA	3 Follicle ≥ 16 mm	21.5	20.1	7.4	1.3	N/A	N/A	N/A

Adapted from Dickey (2008).

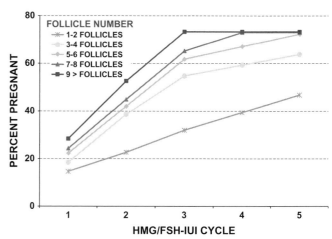

Figure 28.3. Cumulative pregnancy rate in relation to number of preovulatory follicles 10 mm or larger for first five cycles of HMG or FSH–IUI; for patients age <38, without tubal factor, endometriosis, total initial motile sperm count <5 million, or progressive motility <30 percent. Number of follicles as shown on chart. Adapted from Dickey et al. (2005). Reprinted with publisher's permission.

follicular phase, while at the same time reducing or withdrawing FSH, has been proposed as a method of reducing multiple ovulation in patients who require FSH for follicular development but respond with excessive numbers of follicles (Hellier, 1994; Loumaye et al., 1997; Filicori et al., 2002a, 2002b; Shoham, 2002). Because HMG sold for ovarian stimulation contains LH and hCG, use of HMG rather than urinary FSH or recombinant FSH may be result in fewer multiple births (Dickey, 2005). Additional hCG and recombinant LH, which has a longer half-life than urinary LH, are promising methods of reducing HOMP, which require further study.

Coasting

Coasting, delaying hCG administration, and discontinuing stimulation until E_2 levels fall and supernumerary follicles undergo atresia is a common method for rescuing hyperstimulated IVF cycles (Rizk, 2006), but when used in hMG cycles, the multiple pregnancy rates were high. Urman et al. (1992) reported the results of coasting for an average 2.8 days (range 1–8 days), during forty cycles of HMG relations that had become hyperstimulated with average E_2 levels of 9,249 pmol/mL. Clinical pregnancies occurred in ten cases (25 percent), but the multiple pregnancy rate was 50 percent, all twins.

Aspiration of Supernumerary Follicles

Aspiration of supernumerary follicles specifically to reduce multiple pregnancies due to OI was reported first by Ingerslev (1991), and subsequently by others, but only one group has reported results of this technique in more than a few patients. De Geyter et al. (1998) performed aspiration of supernumerary follicles when four or more follicles 14 mm or larger were present before administrating hCG, in 257 of 571 cycles of HMG/FSH-IUI (45 percent), between 1992 and 1996. Pregnancies occurred in 118 cycles (20.7 percent), of which six were ectopic. There were nine sets of twins (7.6 percent) and one set of triplets (1.7 percent) per clinical pregnancy. The results have not been confirmed by other investigators.

Cancellation of Cycles for Excessive Numbers of Preovulatory Follicles or High Estradiol Concentration

A widely used third technique for reducing HOMP during COH-IUI treatment is to withhold hCG administration when excessive numbers of follicles or estradiol (E) concentrations are present (Rizk and Aboulghar, 1991). In a survey of U.S. board–certified reproductive endocrinologists, 82 percent reported that they have withheld hCG in OI cycles in order to decrease the incidence of HOMP (Hock et al., 2002). Two problems with this technique are that there has been no agreement as to what constitutes an excessive number of follicles or an excessive estradiol concentration and, if all cycles with excessive numbers of follicles or estradiol concentrations are canceled, it would eliminate too many patients. Although it is well known from IVF that oocytes from follicles as small as 10 mm on the day of hCG administration are capable of fertilization and may result in a term pregnancy, recognition that follicles 10 mm or larger must be measured in order to predict all cases of HOMP when using COH-IUI was slow to come about. In 1991, Dickey et al. reported that multiple pregnancies in gonadotropin cycles were not predicted by the number of follicles 15 mm or larger or 18 mm but that all multiple pregnancies were predicted by the number of follicles 12 mm or larger (Dickey et al., 2001). They did not investigate the relationship of multiple pregnancies to follicles 10 mm or larger. In 1996, Farhi et al. reported that multiple conceptions differed significantly from singleton conceptions in the total number of follicles larger than 8 mm, on the day of hCG administration. A small earlier study, in which follicles 10 mm or smaller were measured, had not found a relationship between follicle number and multiple births in gonadotropin-IUI cycles, employed abdominal ultrasound, and did not count multiple pregnancies if they resulted in single births (Dodson et al., 1988). Four more recent studies have provided information on a sufficiently large number of cycles to resolve these problems.

Gleicher et al. (2000), already cited, determined that HOMP was related to the total number of preovulatory follicles and estradiol levels. No HOMP occurred in 3,347 gonadotropin cycles unless greater than or equal to ten total follicles, 7 mm or larger, were present but did not provide information about patients' ages or twin pregnancies. When there were ten to fourteen total follicles and estradiol was less than 935 pg/mL by chemiluminescence (CHL) assay, the HOMP rate was 1.8 percent and the pregnancy rate was 11 percent. All together, HOMP occurred in 8.8 percent of 441 pregnancies, 84 percent of the 39 HOMP occurred when there were 15 or greater total follicles and estradiol concentration was 935 pg/mL or higher. If cycles had been canceled when these conditions were present, the HOMP rate would have been 2.7 percent, the pregnancy rate would have been 10 percent in the remaining cycles, and 37 percent of cycles would have been canceled. Because of the natural loss rate in multiple pregnancies, the triplet and higher order birthrate would have been approximately 1.4 percent (Dickey et al., 2002a), providing none of the pregnancies were electively reduced or terminated.

Tur et al. (2001), in an analysis of 1,878 gonadotropin-IUI pregnancies, 107 (5.7 percent) of which were triplet or greater, determined that HOMP was significantly related to the number of follicles 10 mm or larger, estradiol levels, and age. They did not report pregnancy rates per cycle, or twins separately from singleton pregnancies and reported results for only two age groups, lesser than or equal to thirty-two and greater than thirty-two years. When there were more than or equal to six follicles 10 mm or larger and E was higher than 862 pg/mL by radioimmunoassay (RIA), HOMP rates were 18.0 percent for age thirty two or less and 9.4 percent for age greater than thirty two. All together, 80 percent of HOMP in their study occurred when there were more than or equal to four total follicles 10 mm or higher or estradiol level was 935 pg/mL or higher. The authors concluded that hCG should be withheld when either of these conditions was present, without regard to patient age. To do so would have meant canceling 41 percent of gonadotropin-IUI cycles in which pregnancy occurred, and the HOMP rate would still have been 3.9 percent in the uncanceled cycles.

In 2001, Dickey et al. analyzed 1,333 CC-IUI cycles and 155 pregnancies, 3 of which were HOMP, and 1,397 gonadotropin-IUI cycles and 253 pregnancies, 18 of which were HOMP, stratified by number of follicles 12 mm or higher, 15 mm, and 18 mm or higher, estradiol levels; and ages less than thirty five or thirty five or more. They determined that in CC cycles, HOMP was most closely related to follicles 12 mm or higher and pregnancy rate was most closely related to follicles 15 mm or higher, whereas in gonadotropin cycles, both HOMP and pregnancy rate were most closely related to number of follicles 12 mm or higher. Relationships to follicles 10 mm or higher was not examined. When age was less than thirty five years and there were six or more follicles 12 mm or higher, HOMP rates were 13.7 percent in gonadotropin-IUI cycles and 15.3 percent in CC-IUI cycles. When age was thirty five years or more and there were six or more follicles 12 mm or higher, HOMP rates were 1.3 percent in gonadotropin-IUI cycles and 0 percent in CC-IUI cycles. Twin pregnancy rates were unrelated to the number of follicles. They recommended that cycles be canceled when six or more preovulatory follicles 12 mm or higher were present and age was less than thirty five years in both CC and gonadotropin cycles. If this had been done, the HOMP rate for age less than thirty five would have been 4.0 percent in gonadotropin cycles, the pregnancy rate would have been 19.0 percent, and 33.3 percent of cycles would have had to been canceled. For age thirty five or more, the HOMP would be reduced to 0.5 percent, but the pregnancy rate would have been 10.3 percent compared to 24.3 percent when there were six or more follicles. Clearly, a patient's age should be considered when deciding to cancel cycles for excessive numbers of follicles.

In 2005, Dickey et al. reanalyzed their gonadotropin-IUI results using the number of follicles 10 mm or greater and adding additional cycles and additional age groups. They also examined the effect of patient's diagnosis, sperm quality, and number of previous cycles of gonadotropin IUI (Table 28.3). Pregnancy rates were significantly lower for tubal factor alone and endometriosis with tubal involvement, age 38 or more, and poor sperm quality. Pregnancy rates were significantly increased when there were four or more follicles 10 mm or higher, and when E concentration was 1,000 pg/mL or higher. Triplet and higher order pregnancies were significantly increased for ages less than 32, for estradiol 1,000 pg/mL or higher, and when there were seven or more follicles 10 mm or higher. No HOMP occurred for age 38 or more. There was no clinically useful "safe" estradiol concentration below which HOMP did not occur. The lowest E concentration on the day of HCG administration, in a cycle that resulted in HOMP, was 397 pg/mL, measured by CHL (equal to 325 pg/mL by RAI assay). Triplet and higher order pregnancies averaged

Table 28.3. Relationship of Patient Characteristics and Ovarian Response to Clinical Pregnancy and Multiple Pregnancy Rates – Treatment Cycles 1–3

	Cycles, n	Pregnancies, n (%)	OR	95% CI	p-value	Sacs 2, n (%)	⩾3, n (%)	⩾4, n
A. Diagnosis[a]								
Ovulatory dysfunction	1,068	208 (19.5)	—	—	—	41 (19.5)	20 (9.5)	8
Cervical, male, unexp.	553	106 (19.2)	0.98	0.76–1.27	Ns	26 (24.5)	11 (10.4)	2
Endometriosis								
wo tubal invol.	753	121 (16.1)	0.79	0.62–1.01	Ns	26 (21.5)	6 (5.0)	2
w tubal invol.	126	10 (7.9)	0.36	0.18–0.69	.002	1 (10.0)	0 (0.0)	0
Tubal factor wo endo	226	26 (11.5)	0.54	0.35–0.83	.006	4 (15.4)	1 (3.8)	0
B. Age[b] (years)								
<32	1,203	129 (19.0)	—	—	—	46 (20.1)	24 (10.5)	10
32–34	636	120 (19.2)	0.099	0.77–1.26	Ns	28 (23.3)	7 (5.8)	1
35–37	535	86 (16.1)	81	0.62–1.07	Ns	19 (22.1)	6 (7.0)	1
38–40	379	49 (12.9)	0.63	0.45–0.88	.008	5 (10.2)	0 (0.0)	0
41–43	182	11 (6.0)	0.27	0.15–0.51	<.001	1 (9.1)	0 (0.0)	0
C. Sperm[c]								
WHO	1,056	194 (18.4)	—	—	—	43 (22.2)	14 (7.2)	5
IUI threshold	971	164 (16.9)	0.9	0.72–1.14	Ns	37 (22.6)	11 (6.7)	3
Sub-IUI threshold	213	19 (8.9)	0.41	0.25–0.68	<.001	4 (21.0)	0 (0.0)	0
Donor	347	77 (22.2)	1.27	0.94–1.71	Ns	13 (16.9)	12 (15.6)	4
D. Number follicles >10 mm[d]								
1	204	23 (11.3)	—	—	—	0 (0.0)	0 (0.0)	0
2	303	40 (13.2)	1.19	0.69–2.07	Ns	9 (23.2)	0 (0.0)	0
3	334	56 (16.8)	1.58	0.94–2.67	Ns	10 (17.8)	3 (5.4)	0
4	304	60 (19.7)	1.94	1.15–3.25	0.016	14 (23.3)	3 (5.0)	1
5–6	377	82 (21.8)	2.18	1.33–3.60	0.003	16 (19.5)	5 (6.1)	1
7–8	264	58 (22.0)	2.22	1.31–3.74	0.004	10 (16.9)	8 (13.6)	4
⩾9	366	95 (26.0)	2.76	1.67–4.52	<.001	27 (28.4)	18 (18.9)	6
E. Estradiol pg/mL[d]								
<500	538	90 (16.7)	—	—	—	8 (8.9)	4 (4.4)	0
500–999	798	146 (18.3)	1.11	0.84–1.49	Ns	32 (21.9)	8 (5.5)	1
1,000–1,499	401	95 (23.7)	1.54	1.12–2.13	0.01	21 (23.1)	11 (11.6)	4
1,500–1,999	188	43 (22.9)	1.48	0.98–2.22	Ns	9 (20.9)	6 (14.0)	4
⩾2,000	178	45 (25.6)	1.68	1.21–2.53	0.016	14 (31.1)	8 (17.8)	3

[a]Patients' age ⩾38 years and cycles with total initial motile sperm count <5 million or motility <30 percent excluded.
[b]Patients with endometriosis with tubal involvement, tubal factor, and cycles with total initial motile sperm count <5 million or motility <30 percent excluded.
[c]Patients' age ⩾38 years, patients with endometriosis with tubal involvement, and tubal factor excluded.
[d]Patients' age ⩾38 years, patients with endometriosis with tubal involvement, tubal factor, and cycles with total initial motile sperm count <5 million or motility <30 percent excluded.
Endo, endometriosis; invol., involvement; ns, not significant; unex., unexplained; w, with; wo, without.
IUI-threshold, initial sperm quality less than WHO criteria but ⩾5 million total motile sperm and ⩾30 percent initial motility; Sub-IUI threshold, initial motile sperm count <5 million or motility <30 percent; WHO, initial sperm quality ⩾ World Health Organization criteria of 20 million concentration, 40 million total count, 50 percent progressive motility, 30 percent normal forms. Adapted from Dickey et al. (2005) with permission.

5.1 percent when estradiol was lower than 1,000 pg/mL, 12.3 percent when estradiol was 1,000–1,999 pg/mL, and 17.8 percent when estradiol was 2,000 pg/mL or higher. Triplet and higher order pregnancies averaged 5.6 percent when there were three to six follicles compared to 17.0 percent when there were seven or more follicles. Twin pregnancies occurred in all age-groups, but were reduced by half when age was 38 or higher or estradiol was <500 pg/mL.

The combined effect of follicle number, estradiol level, and age are illustrated in Table 28.4. For patients aged thirty eight or more, or thirty two–thirty seven with estradiol levels less than 1,000 pg/mL, there were no triplet and higher order births, and only 3.8 percent HOMP (ages thirty two–thirty seven years). However, triplet pregnancies and births did occur in the larger group of patients aged thirty two–thirty seven years who had three to six follicles. For age less than thirty two years, with seven or more follicles 10 mm or higher, the triplet and higher order birth rate was 18.8 percent, and if the estradiol level was 1,000 pg/mL or higher, more than 67 percent of HOMP were quadruplets or greater. All quadruplet and higher implantations occurred when estradiol concentrations were 1,000 pg/mL or higher. If cycles had been canceled for patients aged less than 32 when there were seven or more preovulatory follicles 10 mm or higher, 34 percent of cycles would have been canceled, but 76 percent of HOMP would be avoided and the HOMP would be 6 percent in the remaining cycles. If cycles had been canceled for patients aged thirty two–thirty seven when there were seven or more preovulatory follicles 10 mm or higher and estradiol was 1,000 pg/mL or higher, 16 percent of cycles would have been canceled, but 80 percent of HOMP would be avoided and the HOMP would be less than 0.4 percent in the remaining cycles. No cycle would have to be canceled for age 38 or more. To avoid all HOMP would have required canceling 78 percent of cycles for age less than 32, and 76 percent of cycles for ages 32–37. Canceling cycles for those patients at highest risk of HOMP because of seven or more preovulatory follicles 10 mm or higher would necessitate canceling 20 percent of all cycles when patient age and estrogen levels are considered, rather than the 37 percent described by Gleicher et al. (2000) or the 41 percent described by Tur et al. (2001).

Effect of the Number of Previous Gonadotropin Cycles on HOMP

The concept introduced in the section Gonadotropin Pregnancy Rates after Clomiphene that patients with the highest follicle counts or highest fecundity per oocyte are more likely to become pregnant during initial treatment cycles and more likely to have multiple pregnancies, and for the same reason HOMP will occur less often during latter cycles, is manifest again in Table 28.5 where HOMP rates in second and latter gonadotropin cycles are presented. No HOMP occurred after the first gonadotropin IUI cycle when there were three to six follicles 10 mm or higher. No HOMP occurred after the second gonadotropin IUI cycle even when there were seven or more follicles. Pregnancy rates also decreased after the first cycle for patients with three to six and seven or more follicles but not for patients with one to two follicles as shown previously in Figure 28.3. The decrease in PR after the first cycle and in HOMP after the second cycle was not the result of patients developing fewer follicles in second and latter cycles but was instead due to a decrease in implantation rate per follicle. The age-adjusted implantation rate per follicle was inversely related to the number of previous cycles (first cycle = 0.051, second cycle = 0.043, third cycle = 0.031, and fourth and later cycles = 0.010). This indicates that it may be safe to increase the gonadotropin dose after the first cycle in patients who respond to initial stimulation by developing one or two follicles and after the second cycle in patients who develop three to six follicles initially.

Twin Pregnancies

Twins occurred at an increased rate in OI cycles compared to spontaneous cycles even when only two preovulatory follicles 10 mm or larger in gonadotropin cycles (Dickey et al., 2005) or 12 mm in CC cycles (Dickey et al., 2001) are present on ultrasound. The 2002 recommendation from the European Society of Human Reproduction and Embryology that the outcome measure of assisted reproductive technology (ART) "singleton live birth rate" (Land and Evers, 2003) could profoundly effect the ability of infertility patients to become pregnant if this recommendation were extended to OI outside of ART. The increased incidence of perinatal mortality, morbidity, and developmental abnormalities in twins compared to singleton births is principally related to a higher incidence of prematurity and low birth weight. These can be ameliorated by rest, good nutrition, and tocolytic medications (Dickey et al., 2004a). Twin pregnancy should be regarded as a necessary but manageable complication of infertility treatment for patients who require OI, who desire more than one child, and who are capable of carrying a twin pregnancy to at least thirty-six weeks. IVF rather than gonadotropins or even CC should be the treatment of choice for women unable to carry a twin pregnancy safely to at least thirty-six weeks due to small stature, uterine anomalies, or poor health.

CONCLUSIONS

High-order multiple pregnancies are positively related to the number of preovulatory follicles 10 mm or larger, estradiol concentration, and use of donor sperm and inversely related to age and number of previous unsuccessful cycles of gonadotropin IUI or clomiphene IUI. High-order multiple pregnancy can be reduced by use of clomiphene IUI before gonadotropin, use of low doses of gonadotropin, and cancellation, when seven or more follicles 10 mm or larger (gonadotropin) or 12 mm (CC) are present. When CC or low-dose gonadotropin stimulation is used, treatment should be continued until the fifth or sixth cycle in patients who develop one or two follicles per cycle. Decisions to cancel cycles should be based on patient's age, estradiol levels, and number of previous CC or gonadotropin cycles in addition to the number of preovulatory follicles. Up to 20 percent of total cycles may need to be canceled, but pregnancy rates in the remaining patients will be 10–20 percent per cycle and high-order multiple pregnancy rates should be less than 2 percent, with high-order multiple births rates less than 1 percent. Ovulation induction should not be attempted, and IVF should be used instead for women who cannot safely carry a twin pregnancy. Lastly, there now is sufficient evidence to support a conclusion that use of COH rather than minimal stimulation in order to increase the probability of pregnancy per cycle is unnecessary and increases the incidence of HOMP without increasing the possibility of pregnancy per patient if low-dose gonadotropins treatment is continued for more than three cycles.

Table 28.4: Pregnancy Rates per Cycle and Multiple Rates per Pregnancy: Relation to Age, Number of Follicles 10 mm or larger, and Estradiol pg/mL (E2), in Gonadotropin IUI Cycles**

Age (years)	1–2 Follicles ≥10 mm					3–6 Follicles >10 mm							≥7 Follicles >10 mm						
	Cycles, n	Pregnancy %	2 Sacs %	Births %	Twins %	Cycles, n	Pregnancy %	2 Sacs %	>3 Sacs % (>4)	Births %	Twins %	Trip % (<4)	Cycles, n	Pregnancy %	2 Sacs %	>3 Sacs % (>4)	Births %	Twins %	Trip % (<4)
≤32	223	14.3	6.2	12.1	7.4	450	22.7	17.6	5.9(2)	18.7	16.7	2.4(1)	344	24.4	20.5	20.5(8)	20.3	15.7	18.8(4)
E2 < 1,000	86	14.5	3.7	12.4	4.3	298	22.1	19.7	6.1(1)	18.1	20.4	1.8(0)	43	18.2	3.8	23.1(0)	13.4	10.5	15.8(0)
E2 ≥ 1,000	37	13.5	20	8.1	33.3	152	23.7	13.9	5.6(1)	19.7	10	3.3(1)	201	28.8	28.1	19.3(8)	25.4	17.6	19.6(4)
32–37	248	11.7	24.1	9.7	16.7	508	18.9	20.8	5.2(0)	14.4	17.6	2.7(0)	272	27.2	27	12.1(2)	22	26.7	6.7(2)
E2 < 1,000	204	10.8	22.7	8.8	11.1	352	18.5	23.1	3.1(0)	13.9	14.3	2.0(0)	106	24.5	23.1	3.8(0)	21.7	17.4	0.0(0)
E2 ≥ 1,000	44	15.9	28.6	13.6	33.3	156	19.9	16.1	9.7(0)	15.4	25	4.2(0)	166	28.9	29.2	16.7(2)	22.3	32.4	10.8(2)
38–43	171	6.4	9.1	4.1	14.3	201	14.9	16.7	0.0(0)	9.4	5.3	0.0(0)	84	16.7	0.0	0.0(0)	10.7	0.0	0.0(0)
E2 <1,000	156	6.7	11.1	3.2	20	184	12.5	17.4	0.0(0)	7.6	7.1	0.0(0)	30	20	0.0	0.0(0)	10	0.0	0.0(0)
E2 ≥ 1,000	15	13.3	0.0	13.3	0.0	61	16	9.1	0.0(0)	8.2	0.0	0.0(0)	54	14.8	0.0	0.0(0)	11.1	0.0	0.0(0)

*Estradiol measured by chemiluminescence (CHL). 1,000 pg/mL by CHL = 820 pg/mL by RIA, and 1,224 pg/ml by monoclonal antibody.**Cycles 1–3: Patients without tubal factor, endometriosis with tubal involvement, or poor sperm quality. Age < thirty two: seven or more follicles vs. three–six follicles; three or more implantations per pregnancy, p = .004; triplet or higher order birth, p = .008. Age thirty eight or more, three or more follicles vs. age less than thirty-eight, three or more follicles; three or more implantations per pregnancy, p = .014. Adapted from Dickey et al. (2005) with permission of the publisher.

Table 28.5: Pregnancy Rates per Cycle and Multiple Rates per Pregnancy: Relation to Cycle Number and Number of Follicles 10 mm or larger in Gonadotropin IUI Cycles*

Cycle	1–2 Follicles ≥10 mm				3–6 Follicles ≥10 mm					≥7 Follicles ≥10 mm				
	Cycles no.	Pregnancy %	2%	≥3%	Cycles no.	Pregnancy %	2%	≥3%	≥4%	Cycles no	Pregnancy %	2%	≥3%	≥4%
One	309	14.6	15.5	0	612	20.8	19.7	7.9	1.6	363	27.5	24.0	15.0	15.0
Two	124	9.7	8.3	0	270	19.2	17.3	0	0	181	24.9	22.2	24.4	11.1
Three	38	10.5	25.0	0	106	17.0	11.1	0	0	72	16.7	33.3	0	0
>Four	28	10.7	0	0	83	6.0	0	0	0	44	2.3	0	0	0

*Patients' age less than thirty eight without tubal factor, or poor sperm quality. Dickey (2007).

KEY POINTS FOR CLINICAL PRACTICE

■ Pregnancy and multiple pregnancies are related to the number of preovulatory follicles, age, and inherent fecundity demonstrated by previous pregnancies.

■ The number of follicles 10 mm or larger are more accurate predictors of multiple pregnancy than the number of 12 mm or larger, 15 mm or higher, or 18 mm or higher.

■ Preovulatory ultrasound should be performed in both clomiphene and gonadotropin cycles in order to determine the risk of multiple pregnancy. All follicles 10 mm or greater must be counted in order.

■ A patient's age should be considered when deciding to cancel cycles for excessive numbers of follicles.

■ High-order multiple pregnancies due to ovulation induction can be reduced by the following steps:

1. Use clomiphene for four to six cycles before switching to gonadotropins.
2. Use lowest dose of gonadotropin that results in ovulation of at least one follicle for three to six cycles before increasing the dose.
3. Cancellation of clomiphene and gonadotropin cycles when there are three or more preovulatory follicles 10 mm or larger.

REFERENCES

Aboulghar M, Mansour R, Serour G, Abdrazek A, Amin Y, Rhodes C. (2001) Controlled ovarian hyperstimulation and intrauterine insemination for treatment of unexplained infertility should be limited to a maximum of three trials. *Fertil Steril* **75**;88–91.

Arguinzoniz M, Duerr-Myers L, Engrand P, Loumaye E. (2000) The efficacy and safety of recombinant human luteinizing hormone for minimizing the number of pre-ovulatory follicles in WHO group I anovulatory women treated with rhFSH. Program of the 15th Annual Meeting of the European Socirty of Human Reproduction and Embryology, Bologna, Italy, Abst. O-176, 2000: pp. 70–1.

Balasch J, Tur R, Alvarez P, Bajo IO, Bosch E, Bruna I, Caballero P, et al. (1996) The safety and effectiveness of stepwise and low-dose administration of follicle stimulating hormone in WHO Group II anovulatory infertile women: evidence from a large multicenter study in Spain. *J Assist Reprod Genet* **13**;551–6.

Benadiva CA, Ben-Rafael Z, Struass JF III, Mastroianni L Jr, Flickinger GL. (1988) Ovarian response of individuals to different doses of human menopausal hormone *Fertil Steril* **49**;997–1001.

Ben-Rafael Z, Struass JF III, Mastroianni L Jr, Flickinger GL. (1986) Differences in ovarian stimulation in human menopausal gonadotropin treated women may be related to follicle stimulating hormone accumulation. *Fertil Steril* **46**;586–92.

Corchia C, Mastroiacovo P, Lanni R, Mannazzu R, Curro V, Fabis C. (1996) What proportion of multiple births are due to ovulation induction? A register-based study in Italy. *Am J Public Health* **86**;851–4.

De Geyter C, De Geyter M, Nieschlag E. (1998) Low multiple pregnancy rates and reduced frequency of cancellation after ovulation induction with gonadotropins, if eventual supernumerary follicles are aspirated to prevent polyovulation. *J Assist Reprod Genet* **15**;111–8.

Dickey RP. (2005) Pharmacokinetics and pharmacodynamics of exogenous gonadotropin administration, *Fourth World Congress on*

Ovulation Induction 2004 From Anovulation to Assisted Reproduction, 1st Edn, Aracne editrice S.r.l., April 2005, pp. 123–157.

Dickey RP. (2008) Strategies to reduce multiple pregnancies due to ovulation induction. *Fertil Steril* (In press).

Dickey RP, Sartor BM. (2005) The impact of ovulation induction and *in vitro fertilization* on the incidence of multiple gestations, in Blickstein I and Keith LG eds. Multiple Gestation; Epidemiology, Gestation & Perinatal outcome, Taylor & Francis Publishers, New York, 2005, chapter 19, pp. 119–139/942.

Dickey RP, Olar TT, Taylor SN, Curole DN, Rye PH, Matulich EM. (1991) Relationship of follicle number, serum estradiol, and other factors to birth rate and multiparity in human menopausal gonadotropin-induced intrauterine insemination cycles. *Fertil Steril* **56**;89–92.

Dickey RP, Olar TT, Taylor SN, Curole DN, Rye PH. (1992) Relationship of follicle number and other factors to fecundability and multiple pregnancies in clomiphene citrate induced intrauterine insemination cycles. *Fertil Steril* **57**;613–9.

Dickey RP, Olar TT, Taylor SN, Curole DN, Harrigill K. (1993a) Relationship of biochemical pregnancy to preovulatory endometrial thickness and pattern in patients undergoing ovulation induction. *Hum Reprod* **8**;327–30.

Dickey RP, Olar TT, Taylor SN, Curole DN, Matulivk EM. (1993b) Relationship of endometrial thickness and pattern to fecundity in ovulation induction cycles: effect of clomiphene citrate alone and with human menopausal gonadotropin. *Fertil Steril* **59**; 756–60.

Dickey RP, Olar TT, Taylor SN, Curole DN, Rye PH. (1993c) Sequential clomiphene citrate and human menopausal gonadotropin for ovulation induction: comparison to clomiphene citrate alone and human menopausal gonadotropin alone. *Hum Reprod* **8**;56–9.

Dickey RP, Taylor SN, Rye PH, Lu PY, Pyrzak R. (1999) Comparison of sperm quality resulting in successful intrauterine insemination to World Health Organization threshold values for normal sperm. *Fertil Steril* **71**;684–9.

Dickey RP, Taylor SN, Lu PY, Sartor BM, Rye PH, Pyrzak R. (2001) Relationship of follicle numbers and estradiol concentrations to multiple implantation of 3608 intrauterine insemination cycles. *Fertil Steril* **75**;69–78.

Dickey RP, Taylor SN, Lu PY, Sartor BM, Storment JM, Rye PH, Pelletier WD, Zender JL, Matulich EM. (2002a) Spontaneous reduction of multiple pregnancy: incidence and effect on outcome. *Am J Obstet Gynecol* **186**;77–83.

Dickey RP, Taylor NN, Lu PY, Sartor MM, Rye PH, Pyrzak R. (2002b) Effect of diagnosis, age, sperm quality, and number of preovulatory follicles on the outcome of multiple cycles of clomiphene citrate-intrauterine insemination. *Fertil Steril* **78**; 1088–95.

Dickey RP, Sartor BM, Pyrzak R. (2004a) What is the most relevant standard of success in assisted reproduction? No single outcome measure is satisfactory when evaluating success in assisted reproduction; both twin births and singleton births should be counted as successes. *Hum Reprod* **19**;783–7.

Dickey RP, Taylor NN, Lu PY, Sartor MM, Pyrzak R. (2004b) Clomiphene citrate intrauterine insemination (IUI) before gonadotropin IUI affects the pregnancy rate and high order multiple pregnancy. *Fertil Steril* **81**;545–50.

Dickey RP, Taylor SN, Lu PY, Sartor BM, Rye PH, Pyrzak R. (2005) Risk factors for high-order multiple pregnancy and multiple birth after controlled ovarian hyperstimulation: results of 4,062 intrauterine insemination cycles. *Fertil Steril* **83**;671–83.

Dodson WC, Hughes CL, Haney AF. (1988) Multiple pregnancies conceived with intrauterine insemination during superovulation: an evaluation of clinical characteristics and monitored parameters of conception cycles. *Am J Obstet Gynecol* **159**;382–5.

Dodson WC, Whitesides DB, Hughes CL, Easley HA, Haney AF. (1987) Superovulation with intrauterine insemination in the treatment of infertility: a possible alternative to gamete intrafallopian transfer and in vitro fertilization. *Fertil Steril* **48**;441–5.

Farhi J, West C, Patel A, Jacobs HS. (1996) Treatment of anovulatory infertility: the problem of multiple pregnancy. *Hum Reprod* **11**;429–34.

Filicori M, Cognigni GE, Samara A, Melappioni S, Perri T, Cantelli B, Parmegiani L, Pelusi G, DeAloysio D. (2002a) The use of LH activity to drive folliculogenesis: exploring uncharted territories in ovulation induction. *Hum Reprod Update* **8**;543–7.

Filicori M, Cognigni GE, Tabarelli C, Pocognoli P, Taraborrelli S, Spettoli D, Ciampaglia W. (2002b) Stimulation and growth of antral ovarian follicles by selective LH activity administration in women. *J Clin Endocrinol Metab* **87**;1156–61.

Fink RS, Bowes LP, Mackintosh CE, Smith WI, Georgiades E, Ginsburg J. (1982) The value of ultrasound for monitoring responses to gonadotropin. *Br J Obstet Gynaecol* **89**;856–61.

Gleicher N, Oleske DM, Tur-Kaspa I, Vidali A, Karande V. (2000) Reducing the risk of high-order multiple pregnancy after ovarian stimulation with gonadotropins. *N Engl J Med* **343**;2–7.

Healy D, Rombauts L, Vollenhoven B, Kovacs, Burmeister. (2003) One triplet pregnancy in 510 controlled ovarian hyperstimulation and intrauterine cycles. *Fertil Steril* **79**;1449–51 [67].

Hellier SG. (1994) Current concepts of the roles of follicle stimulating hormone and luteinizing hormone in follliculogenesis. *Hum Reprod* **9**;188–91.

Hock DL, Seifer DB, Kontopoulos E, Ananth CV. (2002) Practice patterns among board-certified reproductive endocrinologists regarding high-order multiple gestations: a United States National Survey. *Obstet Gynecol* **99**;763–70.

Homburg R, Howles CM. (1999) Low-dose FSH therapy for anovulatory infertility associated with polycystic ovary syndrome: rationale, results reflections and refinements. *Hum Reprod Update* **3**; 493–9.

Homburg R, Insler V. (2002) Ovulation induction in perspective. *Hum Reprod Update* **8**;449–62.

Hughes EG, Collins JA, Gunby J. (1998) A randomized controlled trial of three low-dose gonadotropins protocols for unexplained infertility. *Hum Reprod* **13**;1527–31.

Ingerslev HJ. (1991) Selective follicular reduction following ovulation induction by exogenous gonadotropins in polycystic ovarian disease. A new novel approach to treatment. *Hum Reprod* **6**;682–4.

Karande VC, Korn A, Morris R, Rao R, Balin M, Rinehart J, Dohn K, Gleicher N. (1999) Prospective randomized trial comparing the outcome and cost of in vitro fertilization with that of a traditional treatment algorithm as first-line therapy for couples with infertility. *Fertil Steril* **71**;468–75.

Kemmann E, Bohrer M, Shelden R, Fiasconaro G, Beardsley L. (1987) Active ovulation management increases the monthly probability of pregnancy occurrence in ovulatory women who receive intrauterine insemination. *Fertil Steril* **48**;916–20.

Land JA, Evers JLH. (2003) Risks and complications in assisted reproduction techniques: report of an ESHRE consensus meeting. *Hum Reprod* **18**;455–7.

Le Cotonnec J-Y, Porchet HC, Beltrami V, Khan A, Toon S, Rowland M. (1994) Clinical pharmacology of recombinant human follicle-stimulating hormone. II. Single doses and steady state pharmacokinetics. *Fertil Steril* **61**;679–86.

Levene MI, Wild J, Steer P. (1992) Higher multiple births and the modern management of infertility in Britain. The British

Association of Perinatal Medicine. *Br J Obstet Gynaecol* **99**; 607–13.

Loumaye E, Engrand P, Howles CM, O'Dea L. (1997) Assessment of the role of serum lutenizing hormone and estriol response to follicle-stimulating hormone on in vitro fertilization treatment outcome. *Fertil Steril*, **67**;889–99.

Loumaye E, Duerr-Myers L, Engrand P, Arguinzoniz M. (2000) Minimizing the number of pre-ovulatory follicles in WHO group II anovulatory women over-responding to FSH with recombinant human luteinizing hormone. Program of the 15th Annual Meeting of the European Socirty of Human Reproduction and Embryology, Bologna, Italy, Abst. O-177, 2000: pp. 71.

Martin K, Santoro N, Hall J, Filicore M, Wierman M, Crowley WF. (1990) Clinical review 15: management of ovulatory disorders with pulsatile gonadotropin-releasing hormone. *J Clin Endocrinol Metab* **71**;1081A–G.

Pittrof RU, Shaker A, Dean N, Bekir JS, Campbell S, Tan SL. (1996) Success of intrauterine insemination using cryopreserved donor sperm is related to the age of the woman and the number of preovulatory follicles. *J Assist Reprod Genet* **13**;310–14.

Ragni G, Maggioni P, Guermandi E, Testa A, Baroni E, Colombo M, et al. (1999). Efficacy of double intrauterine insemination in controlled ovarian hyperstimulation cycles. *Fertil Steril* **72**;619–22.

Reynolds MA, Schieve LA, Martin JA, Jeng G, Macaluso M. (2003) Trends in multiple births conceived using assisted reproductive technecology, United States, 1997-2000. *Pediatrics* **111**:1159–62.

Remohi J, Gastaldi C, Patrizio P, Gerli S, Ord T, Asch RH, Balmaceda JP. (1989) Intrauterine insemination and controlled ovarian hyperstimulation in cycles before GIFT. *Hum Reprod* **4**;918–20.

Rizk B. (2006) Prevention of ovarian hyperstimulation syndrome. In Rizk B (Ed.) Ouarvan Hyperstimulation Syndrome. Cambridge: United Kingdom, Cambridge University Press, Chapter 7, 130–99.

Rizk B, Aboulghar M. (1991) Modern Management of ovarian hyperstimulation syndrome. *Hum. Replod* **6**(8);1082–7.

Schenker JG, Yarkoni S, Granat M. (1981) Multiple pregnancies following induction of ovulation. *Fertil Steril* **35**;105–23.

Sher G, Knutzen VK, Stratton CJ, Montakhab MM, Allenson SG. (1984) In vitro sperm capacitation and transcervical intrauterine insemination for the treatment of refractory infertility: phase I. *Fertil Steril* **41**;260–4.

Shoham Z. (2002) The clinical therapeutic window for luteinizing hormone in controlled ovarian stimulation. *Fertil Steril* **77**;1170–7.

Takokoro N, Vollenhoven B, Clark S, Baker G, Kovacs G, Burger H, Healy D. (1997) Cumulative pregnancy rates in couples with anovulatory infertility compared with unexplained infertility in an ovulation induction program. *Hum Reprod* **12**;1939–44.

Tomlinson MJ, Amissah-Arthur JB, Thompson KA, Kasrale JL, Bentick B. (1996) Prognostic indicators for intrauterine insemination (IUI): statistical model for IUI success. *Hum Reprod* **11**;1892–6.

Tur R, Barri PN, Coroleu B, Buxaderas R, Martinez F, Balasch J. (2001) Risk factors for high-order multiple implantation after ovarian stimulation with gonadotropins: evidence from a large series of 1878 consecutive pregnancies in a single center. *Hum Reprod* **16**;2124–9.

Urman B, Pride SM, Ho Yuen B. (1992) Management of overstimulated gonadotropin cycles with a controlled drift period. *Hum Reprod* **7**;213–7.

Valbuena D, Simon C, Romero JL, Remohi J, Pellicer A. (1996) Factors responsible for multiple pregnancies after ovarian stimulation and intrauterine insemination with gonadotropins. *J Asst Reprod Genetics* **13**;663–8.

Van Weissenbruch MM. (1990) Gonadotropins for induction of ovulation, immunological, pharmacological and clinical studies [dissertation], Amsterdam; Free University.

Vollenhoven B, Selub M, Davidson O, Lefkow H, Henault M, Serpa N, Hund TT. (1996) Treating infertility: controlled ovarian hyperstimulation using human menopausal gonadotropin in combination with intrauterine insemination. *J Reprod Med* **41**;658–64.

Wang JX, Kwan M, Davies MJ, Kirby C, Judd S, Norman RJ. (2003) Risk of multiple pregnancy when infertility is treated with ovulation induction by gonadotropins. *Fertil Steril* **80**;664–5.

White DM, Polson DW, Kiddy D, Sagle P, Watson H, Gilling-Smith C, Hamilton-Fairley D, Franks. (1996) Induction of ovulation with low-dose gonadotrophins in polycystic ovary syndrome: an analysis of 109 pregnancies in 225 women. *J Clin Endocrinol Metab* **81**;3821–4.

Yagel S, Ben-Chetrit A, Anteby E, et al. (1992) The effect of ethinyl estradiol on endometrial thickness and uterine volume during ovulation induction by clomiphene citrate. *Fertil Steril* **57**;33–6.

Yovich JL, Matson PL. (1988) The treatment of infertility by the high intrauterine insemination of husband's washed spermatozoa. *Hum Reprod* **3**;939–43.

Zikopoulos K, West CP, Thong PW, Kacser EM, Morrison J, We FCW. (1993) Homologous intrauterine insemination has no advantage over timed natural intercourse when used in combination with ovulation induction for the treatment of unexplained infertility. *Hum Reprod* **8**;563–7.

29

Hyperprolactinemia

Hany F. Moustafa, Ahmet Helvacioglu, Botros R. M. B. Rizk, Mary George Nawar, Christopher B. Rizk, Christine B. Rizk, Caroline Ragheb, David B. Rizk, Craig Sherman

INTRODUCTION

Prolactin is a polypeptide hormone that was discovered more than seventy years ago and is also known as the lactogenic hormone, lactotropin, luteotropic hormone, or luteotropin (1). It was initially thought that it is only produced by the anterior pituitary gland and is mainly involved with lactation, but now there is increasing evidence that there are many other sources of prolactin and that it is involved in diverse essential biological activities (2).

EMBRYOLOGY OF LACTOTROPHS

Prolactin is produced mainly by the pituitary lactotrophs, which normally comprise about 15–25 percent of the anterior pituitary (3). During embryologic development, the anterior pituitary (adenohypophysis) arises from Rathke's pouch (named after German embryologist and anatomist Martin Heinrich Rathke 1793–1860), which is an ectodermal outpouching of the floor of the primitive mouth that grows upwards and later fuses with the postpituitary (neurohypophysis) that develops as a downward extension from the neuroectoderm of the diencephalon (4, 5).

Several home-domain transcription factors are released during the development of the anterior pituitary and are important in the gene activation and cell-lineage differentiation. The most important of which is Pit-1, which is necessary for the activation of prolactin (PRL), growth hormone (GH), growth hormone–releasing hormone (GHRH), and thyroid-stimulating hormone (TSH) genes. Congenital absence of Pit-1 gene causes a syndrome characterized by deficiency of lactotrophs, somatotrophs, and thyrotrophs (6–8).

PROLACTIN BIOSYNTHESIS

Prolactin is a 199–amino acid single polypeptide chain with a very similar structure to that of GH and HPL (human placental lactogen). It is encoded by a single gene located on the short arm of chromosome 6 that has an overall length of approximately 10 kb and consists of five exons separated by four introns. Recently, an additional exon 1a has been described (Figure 29.1).

PRL gene belongs to the PRL/GH/HPL group of genes that are structurally similar to each other and are known as group I helix bundle protein hormones. It is believed that all of them evolved from a common ancestral gene by duplication (9, 10).

Recently, the PRL/GH/HPL family was also linked to another extended family of proteins known as the hematopoietic cytokines, which triggered a controversy on whether PRL should be considered as a cytokine or a hormone. This is based on the fact that the prolactin structure is very similar to the hematopoietic cytokines and its receptor, as will be mentioned later, belongs to the cytokine receptor superfamily, along with the fact that there is evidence that PRL seems to have an immune modulatory effect (11, 12).

The 5′ flanking region contains two independent promoter regions. The proximal 5,000-bp region is known as a pituitary promoter, which directs pituitary-specific expression, while a more upstream promoter region of 3,000 bp is known as the extrapituitary promoter and is responsible for extrapituitary expression (13, 14). Various hormones can bind to and consequently alter the rate of PRL gene expression like estrogen, DA (dopamine), TRH (thyroid releasing hormome), VIP (vasoactive intestinal peptide), and so on. The mature PRL mRNA is only 1 kb long, which undergoes translation to yield the final PRL molecule (15, 16). Further post-translational modifications occur (cleavage, glycosylation, phosphorylation, and polymeration), which is usually detrimental to the PRL molecule as it leads to reduced bioavailability and accelerated proteolytic cleavage (17).

PROLACTIN STRUCTURE

PRL is an all-α-helix protein. The molecule consists of almost 50 percent of α-helices, and the remainder of the protein appears to fold into nonorganized loop structures. The three-dimensional structure of hPRL was recently recognized using the homology-modeling approach, based on the crystallographic coordinates of porcine GH (10, 18, 19) (Figure 29.2).

There is a wide heterogeneity in the final PRL product, but it is mostly in a monomeric form (90 percent), less commonly diametric (8 percent), or seldom polymeric (2 percent). It appears that the most potent biological form of prolactin is the 23-kDa nonglycosylated form, while usually the larger polymers have reduced receptor affinity and lower bioactivity. Macroprolactinemia refers to the condition when most of the elevated prolactin is due to the presence of these large polymers also known as big prolactin (50 kDa) or big-big PRL (>150 kDa) (17). Many patients who have macroprolactinemia were shown to have auto-antibodies to prolactin, which tend to form PRL-antibody aggregates. Even though these polymers have

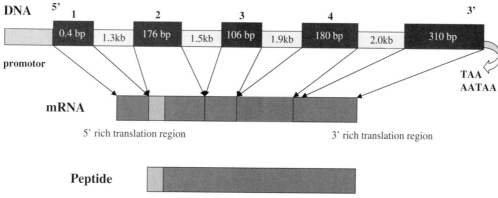

Figure 29.1. Prolactin gene transcription.

reduced in vivo activity, they are still detected by the conventional laboratory assays that explain the normal reproductive functions in many women with macroprolactinemia. Macroprolactinemia is a common condition reported in 10–46 percent of patients with hyperprolactinemia (20–22).

PROLACTIN RECEPTORS

Prolactin receptor is a transmembrane receptor belonging to class 1 of the cytokine receptor superfamily. It is encoded by a gene on chromosome 5p13-14 that contains at least ten exons and has an overall length of 100 kb. It is transcriptionally regulated by three different tissue-specific promoter regions (23).

The receptor has close gross structural semilarity to GH receptors and is composed of an extracellular region (that binds prolactin), a single transmembrane region, and a cytoplasmatic region (24). Numerous prolactin receptor isoforms have been described in different tissues. This includes the long-form activating receptor and at least eight other short variants, which usually vary in the length and composition mostly of their cytoplasmic domain while their extracellular domain is usually identical (25, 26) (Figure 29.3). These various forms of the receptor occur due to alternative splicing of pre-mRNA. In addition to the membrane-anchored prolactin receptors, there is a soluble isoform (known as prolactin receptor–binding protein; PRLRBP) that is generated by proteolytic cleavage of membrane-bound prolactin receptor (27, 28).

Prolactin receptors can bind to other two ligands, which are growth hormone and human placental lactogen, which might explain the less severe phenotypes observed in PRL knockout mice compared to PRLR knockout mice (29).

Prolactin receptors are widely expressed by different cells including the pituitary, breast, liver, pancreas, brain, adrenal cortex, lungs, prostate, epididymus, ovary, and lymphocytes (2).

PROLACTIN SECRETION

PRL release does not depend entirely on the nursing stimulus but is also affected by other stimuli like light, stress, olfaction,

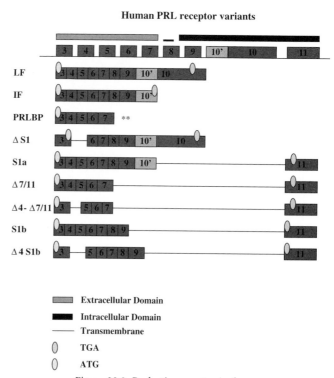

Figure 29.3. Prolactin receptor isoforms.

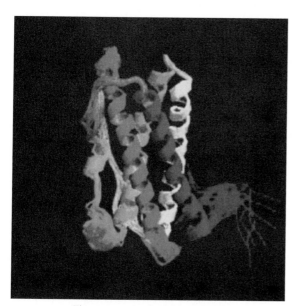

Figure 29.2. Prolactin molecule.

and audition. It is released in a pulsatile pattern with pulse frequency ranging between fourteen pulses per day in the late follicular phase to nine pulses per day in the late luteal phase. Each pulse normally lasts for approximately seventy minutes, with interpulse interval of approximately ninety minutes (30).

There is also a diurnal variation, with the lowest levels occurring the midmorning after the subject awakes and the highest levels during sleep. Levels starts to rise one hour after the onset of sleep and continue to rise until peak values are reached between 5:00 A.M. and 7:00 A.M. (Figure 29.4). Most of the rise occurs in REM sleep and then falls again prior to the next period of REM sleep. This circadian rhythm is generated by the suprachiasmatic nuclei of the hypothalamus. The pulse amplitude of prolactin appears to increase from early to late follicular and luteal phases due to increased levels of estrogens, which promote the release of prolactin (31).

PRL secretion could also be induced by acute stress and exercise just as ACTH and GH. The stress-induced rise usually doubles or triples the PRL basal level for a short period of time and then drops back again within one to two hours. On the contrary, chronic stress and high exercise level do not result in chronic elevation of the PRL basal levels (32, 33).

Due to such variability of secretion along with the inherent limitations of radioimmunoassay, any elevated levels should always be rechecked and specimens should preferably be drawn midmorning and not after stress, venipuncture, breast stimulation, or physical examination, which all increase prolactin levels.

NEUROENDOCRINE REGULATION OF PRL SECRETION

In contrast to other anterior pituitary hormones, which are controlled by hypothalamic-releasing factors, prolactin is normally under the tonic inhibitory effect of DA, which is known as the prolactin inhibitory factor (PIF) (34).

PIF is synthesized in the hypothalamic neurons particularly in the dorsal portion of the arcuate nucleus and the inferior portion of the ventromedial nucleus. It is then transported via neuronal axons, which terminate in the median eminence, a pathway known as the tuberoinfundibular DA pathway

(TIDA). It exerts its effect by binding to D2 receptors on the lactotrophs cell membranes, thus inhibiting the release of prolactin (35).

Prolactin also acts as a negative feedback on its own secretion, either directly through inhibiting the lactotrophs or indirectly through stimulating the neuroendocrine dopaminergic neurons. This might explain why rats with PRLR knockout usually show hyperprolactinemia (36).

One other hormone that possibly has an inhibitory effect on the secretion of PRL is GnRH-associated peptide (GAP), a 56-amino acid peptide chain derived from the carboxyterminal region of the GnRH precursor (37).

In addition to the tonic inhibition by PIF, PRL secretion is positively regulated by other hormones known as the prolactin-releasing factors (PRFs) that include estrogens, TRH, gonadotopin-releasing hormone (GnRH), GHRH, VIP, angiotensin II, and peptide histidine methionine (PHM), which is a VIP precursor with similar structure (38–41).

Estrogens are key regulators of prolactin production as they enhance the growth of prolactin-producing cells and stimulate prolactin production either directly through activating the prolactin gene or indirectly through suppressing DA. It also seems that the stimulatory effect of GnRH on PRL is dependent on the estrogen level as it was shown that the highest response of the lactotrophs is achieved during the periovulatory period. Analysis of PRL and LH secretory pulses showed a high degree of concordance, suggesting a common stimulus that is probably GnRH (42, 43).

Serotonin likely mediates the nocturnal surge of prolactin along with participating in the suckling induced-rise in PRL through the ascending serotonergic pathways from the dorsal Raphe nucleus (40, 44).

VIP has both a paracrine and an autocrine effect on PRL. VIP is synthesized in the paraventricular nucleus of the hypothalamus and is transported via the neuronal axons to the median eminence where it promotes the PRL secretion (paracrine effect), while the autocrine effect is achieved by the VIP that is synthesized by the anterior pituitary itself (41).

Recent studies also revealed the presence of a 31-amino acid peptide, which results in PRL release and hence called PRL-releasing peptide (31). This peptide is released from

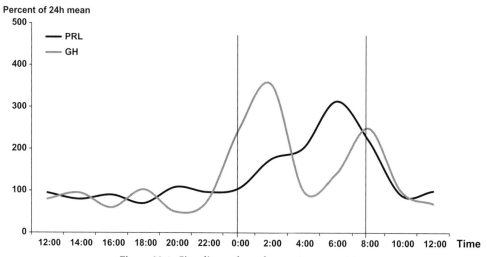

Figure 29.4. Circadian rythm of proactin versus GH.

neurons in the paraventricular and supraoptic nuclei of the hypothalamus and transported via nerve axons to the median eminence (45).

PRIMARY EFFECT OF PROLACTIN

PRL exerts many physiological functions, perhaps the most prominent of which is inducing lobuloalveolar growth of the mammary gland along with stimulation of lactogenesis or milk production after giving birth. Prolactin along with other hormones like cortisol and insulin act to induce the transcription of the genes that encode for milk proteins. This is achieved through increased arginase activity, stimulated ornithine decarboxylase activity, and enhanced rate of transport of polyamines into the mammary gland. All result in increased spermine and spermidine synthesis (polyamines), which are required for milk production. The polyamines stabilize membrane structures, increase transcriptional and translational activities, and regulate enzymes. Prolactin also elicits increased synthesis of casein, spermidine, lactose, and phospholipids, which are all required for lactation (46, 47).

During pregnancy, progesterone interferes with prolactin action at the receptor level. While estrogen and progesterone are required to get full activity of the prolactin receptor, progesterone antagonizes the positive action of prolactin on its receptor by inhibiting upregulation of the prolactin receptor, reducing estrogen binding (lactogenic activity), and competing for binding at the glucocorticoid receptors. Lactation occurs after birth due to the release of progesterone inhibition, which is more rapidly cleared from the maternal serum after delivery in contrast to prolactin. It takes approximately seven days for prolactin to reach nonpregnant levels, while estrogen and progesterone elevations are cleared in three to four days postpartum (48, 49).

In males, prolactin seems to provide the body with sexual gratification after sexual acts and is responsible for the male's refractory period. It is believed that PRL represses the effect of dopamine, which is normally responsible for sexual arousal. Accordingly, the amount of prolactin could be used as an indicator for the amount of sexual satisfaction and relaxation (50).

Prolactin is also found in high concentrations in semen and is very important for spermatozoa metabolism, that is, glucose oxidation, fructose utilization, and glycolysis (51, 52).

OTHER SOURCES AND FUNCTIONS OF PRL

PRL is secreted by a broad range of other cells in the body, including mammary glands, immune cells, different brain cells, and the decidua of the pregnant uterus. Still, these tissues are probably modulated rather than strictly dependant on PRL.

Prolactin is produced by the decidual cells during pregnancy in large amounts. It was found that the amniotic fluid level of prolactin is usually 10–100 folds higher than the maternal serum level. The exact function of prolactin during this time is not quite clear, but there is evidence that it might contribute to the osmoregulation of the amniotic fluid, uterine contractility, and immune modulation during pregnancy (53, 54).

In addition to uptaking prolactin from the blood, the mammary epithelial cells of lactating animals also synthesize prolactin. Experimental studies on rats have shown that approximately 20 percent of the prolactin ingested in milk passes to the neonatal circulation and that milk prolactin participates in the maturation of their neuroendocrine and immune systems.

Prolactin is also produced by some immune cells especially lymphocytes, and this probably suggests that prolactin may act as an autocrine or paracrine modulator of immune activity (55–57).

Immunoreactivity studies have shown that prolactin is also produced by different parts of the brain like the hypothalamus, brain stem, cerebellum, spinal cord, caudate putamin, amygdale, hippocampus, and the choroid plexus, though its exact role is not clear yet (58).

It had long been known that PRL, GH, and HPL all have in vivo and in vitro angiogenic effects, but what is more surprising is that the proteolytic fragments of native prolactin have antiangiogenic properties. This antiangiogenic activity is inherent to both the N-terminal 16-kDa fragment and the 14-kDa fragment. These fragments were shown to bind to certain sites on the capillary endothelium and prevent angiogenesis (59–61).

Some studies showed that the number of prolactin receptors are increased in the breast and prostate cancer cells, which might point to the fact that prolactin could play a role in these tumor growth (62–65).

Currently, this 16-k PRL and it protease (cathepsin) are also being extensively investigated especially in breast cancer research (66).

HYPERPROLACTINEMIA AND INFERTILITY

Prolactin excess could have a detrimental effect on the reproductive potential both in men and women through its effect on various points of the hypothalamic-pituitary-gonadal axis. In women, this usually presents with menstrual irregularities, galactorrhea, or simply infertility in the absence of the former two symptoms. In men, it might cause impotence, diminished libido, galactorrhea, or abnormal semen analysis (decreased count and increased abnormal morphology). High levels of prolactin decrease the pulsatile release of GnRH from the hypothalamic neurons by binding to prolactin receptors on these neurons. Consequently, this results in reduced pulsatile LH release from the anterior pituitary. Another direct effect of hyperprolactinemia on the pituitary gonadotropins is that it decreases the numbers of GnRH receptors on these cells along with interfering with the positive estrogen feedback loop (67–69).

On the level of the gonads, the role of prolactin is more obscure. Experimental studies have shown that PRL has a trophic effect on the corpus luteum of rats' ovaries, which does not seem to be the case in humans. Still, it is believed that normal levels of prolactin is essential for estrogen and progesterone synthesis. On the contrary, prolactin excess has a direct suppressive effect on estrogen synthesis through antagonizing the stimulatory effect of FSH on aromatase activity (70–72).

Prolactin is also important for progesterone synthesis. Studies showed that when bromocreptin was given to euprolactinemic women, it resulted in shorter luteal phase with a lower progesterone level than their controls. This seems to be due to the PRL stimulatory effect on progesterone synthesis through the induction of 23β hydroxysteroid dehydrogenase, which is an essential enzyme in the progesterone synthesis pathway. However, many women with hyperprolactinemia were also found to have a short luteal phase (73, 74).

Men with hyperprolactinemia not only show abnormal semen analysis but also abnormal histological structure of the testicles with distorted seminiferous tubules and abnormal sertoli cells (75).

Hyperprolactinemia is also frequently reported in patients with polycystic ovarian syndrome (18–40 percent). The nature of association between the two conditions is not clear, but it is believed that androgens excess in PCOS patients lead to higher free estradiol ratio due to reduced sex hormone–binding globulin (even though the total estradiol is not elevated), which in turn leads to prolactin elevation. Others proposed that insulin resistance might be the association between hyperprolactinemia and PCOS (76–78). However, some studies argue against this association stating that such hyperprolactinemia is usually mild and transient and is probably coincidental rather than a pathogenically related phenomenon (79).

CAUSES OF HYPERPROLACTINEMIA

The upper normal value for serum prolactin in most laboratories is about 20 ng/mL (20 mcg/L SI units). Many physiological and or pathological changes involving lactotroph cells can result in hyperprolactinemia.

Physiological Causes

Basal serum prolactin concentrations parallels the increase in serum estradiol concentrations throughout pregnancy, beginning at around seven to eight weeks of gestation and reaching a peak at delivery. The magnitude of the increase is quite variable, ranging from 35 to 600 ng/mL (80). The mechanism for increased prolactin levels in pregnancy is believed to be the suppression of DA and direct stimulation of gene transcription in the pituitary by the high levels of estrogen (81, 82). Regardless of breast feeding, by six weeks after delivery, estradiol secretion decreases and the basal serum prolactin concentration returns to normal. For this reason, postpartum contraception should begin as early as third postpartum week. Nipple stimulation increases serum prolactin concentrations via a neural pathway. Due to the preexisting lactotroph hyperplasia because of high estrogen levels during pregnancy, the serum prolactin concentration increases up to a few hundred ng/mL above baseline in response to suckling in the first weeks of postpartum phase. Several months after delivery, the increase in prolactin in response to suckling in the breast feeding woman is usually less than 10 ng/mL above baseline due to the resolution of lactotroph hyperplasia (80). Physical or psychological stress can cause smaller increases in the serum prolactin concentration, though values rarely exceed 40 ng/mL.

Women have greater increases than men, presumably due to the effect of their higher serum estradiol concentrations on the lactotroph cells.

Pathological Causes

Tumors of the lactotroph cell (prolactinomas), decreased dopaminergic inhibition of prolactin secretion, and decreased clearance of prolactin will all cause pathological hyperprolactinemia. Serum prolactin concentrations in patients who have lactotroph adenomas can range from minimal elevation to 50,000 ng/mL; in hyperprolactinemia due to other causes, the concentrations rarely exceed 200 ng/mL (83).

Prolactinomas

Lactotroph adenomas or else called prolactinomas are true neoplasms of the anterior pituitary arising from monoclonal expansion of a single cell that has undergone a somatic mutation (84, 85). The pituitary tumor-transforming gene is overexpressed in most lactotroph adenomas (86) and appears to play a role in tumor invasiveness since its expression is increased in tumors that invade the sphenoid bone. A truncated form of the receptor for fibroblast growth factor-4 has been identified in human pituitary adenomas. Transgenic mice that express this mutation develop lactotroph adenomas (87). The majority of prolactinomas contain only lactotroph cells and produce prolactin in excess. About 10 percent of prolactinomas are made of both lactotroph and either somatotroph or somatomammotroph cells and secrete growth hormone as well (88).

Lactotroph adenomas are relatively common, accounting for approximately 30–40 percent of all clinically recognized pituitary adenomas and 10 percent of all intracranial neoplasms. The diagnosis is made more frequently in women than in men, especially in reproductive age women (89) because of menstrual irregularities. However, the adenomas that occur in men are usually larger at the time of diagnosis, in part due to the lack of symptoms or delay in seeking medical attention for symptoms such as erectile dysfunction (90). Most lactotroph adenomas are sporadic, but they can rarely occur as part of the multiple endocrine neoplasia type 1 syndrome (91). Almost all lactotroph tumors are benign but a rare tumor can be malignant and metastasize (92). Prolactin secretion by lactotroph adenomas vary with the adenoma size. Adenomas less than 1 cm in diameter are typically associated with serum prolactin values below 200 ng/mL; 1.0–2.0 cm in diameter with values between 200 and 1,000 ng/mL; and those greater than 2.0 cm in diameter with values above 1,000 ng/mL. In less well-differentiated and largely cystic lactotroph adenomas, the size of the adenoma may not correlate well with the level of prolactin. Also due to an artifact in the immunoradiometric assay for prolactin, the reported serum prolactin concentration may be disproportionately low to the large size of the adenoma. This artifact, called the "hook effect," can be obviated by dilution of the sera, which will allow a true assessment of the prolactin concentration (93–95).

CNS Causes

As pointed out earlier, PIF is normally released from the hypothalamic nuclei and inhibits prolactin secretion. Any disease in or near the hypothalamus or pituitary that interferes with the secretion of DA or its delivery to the pituitary gland can cause hyperprolactinemia (83). These include tumors of the hypothalamus, both benign (e.g., craniopharyngiomas) and malignant (e.g., metastatic breast carcinoma), infiltrative diseases of the hypothalamus (e.g., sarcoidosis), section of the hypothalamic-pituitary stalk (e.g., due to head trauma or surgery), and adenomas of the pituitary other than lactotroph adenomas.

Table 29.1: Drugs to Cause Hyperprolactinemia and/or Galactorrhea

Typical antipsychotics	Gastrointestinal drugs
Phenothiazine drugs [e.g., chlorpromazine (Thorazine),	Cimetidine (Tagamet)
clomipramine (Anafranil),	Metoclopramide (Reglan)
fluphenazine (Prolixin),	
prochlorperazine (Compazine),	**Antihypertensive agents**
thioridazine (Mellaril)]	Methyldopa (Aldomet)
Haloperidol (Haldol)	Reserpine (Hydromox, Serpasil, others)
Pimozide (Orap)	Verapamil (Calan, Isoptin)
Atypical antipychotics	**Opiates**
Risperidone (Risperdal)	Codeine
Molindone (Moban)	Morphine
Olanzapine (Zyprexa)	
Antidepressant agents	
Clomipramine (Anafranil)	
Desipramine (Norpramin)	

Medications

A number of drugs may cause hyperprolactinemia (Table 29.1). Many of these drugs are DA D2 receptor antagonists and raise serum prolactin by that mechanism. These include antipsychotic drugs such as risperidone, phenothiazines, haloperidol (96), butyrophenones (97), metoclopramide (98), sulpiride (99), and domperidone (100). Serum prolactin concentrations increase within hours after acute administration of these drugs and return to normal within two to four days after cessation of chronic therapy (97). The magnitude of the elevation varies according to the administered drug, that is, 17 ng/mL with the use of haloperidol compared to 80 ng/mL with risperidone (96).

Antihypertensive drugs like methyldopa and reserpine increase prolactin secretion by a similar mechanism. Methyldopa inhibits DA synthesis (101), while reserpine depletes dopamine stores (102). Verapamil may raise serum prolactin concentrations (103), but other calcium channel blockers do not (104). The mechanism of this verapamil-induced increase is not known. The elevated serum prolactin concentration returns to normal in allpatients after the drug is stopped.

Selective serotonin reuptake inhibitors cause little if any increase in the serum prolactin concentration. In one study (105), 20 mg of paroxetine a day caused no increase in the serum prolactin concentration after one week but did cause a slight increase – only to high normal – after three weeks. In another study, in patients receiving fluoxetine chronically (106), the mean basal serum prolactin concentration was no different from that in untreated patients with similar diseases. These drugs, in short, do not appear to cause clinically significant hyperprolactinemia.

Other Causes

TRH is a potent stimulant of PRL and could be labeled as PRF. Hypothyroidism predisposes to hyperprolactinemia due to elevated levels of TRH. However, basal serum prolactin concentrations are normal in most hypothyroid patients (107), and only the serum prolactin response to stimuli, such as TRH, is increased (108). In the few hypothyroid patients who have elevated basal serum prolactin concentrations, the values return to normal when the hypothyroidism is corrected (109, 110). It is important to recognize hypothyroidism as a potential cause of an enlarged pituitary gland (due to thyrotroph hyperplasia, lactotroph hyperplasia, or both) and hyperprolactinemia and not to confuse this entity with a lactotroph adenoma.

Chest wall injuries, such as severe burns, increase prolactin secretion, presumably due to a neural mechanism similar to that of suckling (111). The serum prolactin concentration is high in patients who have chronic renal failure and returns to normal after renal transplantation (112). The major mechanism is a three fold increase in prolactin secretion, and a one-third decrease in metabolic clearance rate (113).

Occasionally, serum prolactin concentration in some patients would range between 20 and 100 ng/mL, with no identifiable cause. Some studies showed that these patients may have microadenomas not visible on imaging studies and that in most of them the serum prolactin concentrations change little during follow-up for several years (114–116) or even spontaneously decline during follow-up (in about 20 percent) (116).

Approximately, 10 percent of elevated prolactin levels are caused by macroprolactinemia due to decreased clearance of prolactin. The elevated serum prolactin concentration in these patients can be distinguished from hyperprolactinemia of other causes by gel filtration or polyethylene glycol precipitation (117–119).

Macroprolactinemia rarely has any effect on the reproductive potential of the patient. In one study done on fifty-five macroprolactinemic patients, none of them experienced amenorrhea, eight had oligomenorrhea before the age of forty, and one experienced galactorrhea. Also in the same study, no macroadenomas and four microadenomas were seen in these women (120). Similar results were seen in a second study of fifty-one patients (121). Thus, macroprolactinemia appears to be a benign clinical condition, and the only clinical significance of macroprolactinemina is when it is misdiagnosed and treated as ordinary hyperprolactinemia (122). This can be avoided by asking the laboratory to pretreat the serum with polyethylene glycol to precipitate the macroprolactin before the immunoassay for prolactin.

CLINICAL MANIFESTATIONS AND DIAGNOSIS OF HYPERPROLACTINEMIA

Infertility, oligomenorrhea, amenorrhea, galactorrhea, hot flashes, vaginal dryness, headaches, and visual changes are the clinical manifestations of hyperprolactinemia in premenopausal women. Hyperprolactinemia accounts for approximately 10–20 percent of cases of amenorrhea in nonpregnant women (123, 124).

Hypogonadism

The release of GnRH is inhibited in hyperprolactinemia, causing decreased luteinizing hormone (LH) and follicle-stimulating hormone (FSH) secretion, resulting in low serum gonadotropin concentrations and secondary hypogonadism.

The symptoms of hypogonadism due to hyperprolactinemia in premenopausal women directly correlate with the level of the prolactin. A serum prolactin level above 15–20 ng/mL in most laboratories is considered high in women of reproductive age.

Levels above 100 ng/mL are typically associated with overt hypogonadism, causing amenorrhea, hot flashes, and vaginal dryness. Serum prolactin levels of 50–100 ng/mL cause either amenorrhea or oligomenorrhea. Serum prolactin levels of 20–50 ng/mL may cause only insufficient progesterone secretion, and therefore, a short luteal phase of the menstrual cycle (125, 126). About 20 percent of those evaluated for infertility have luteal phase defect caused by subtle elevations of prolactin, causing infertility even when there is no abnormality of the menstrual cycle.

Long-term negative health effects of hyperprolactinemia in women with amenorrhea includes osteopenia and osteoporosis (127, 128). Decreased bone mass has to be diagnosed and managed properly especially in adolescents with prolactinomas. Improvement in bone density after dopamine agonist therapy may not be enough alone (129) and needs close monitoring of bone density with appropriate supplementation of calcium, vitamin D, and rarely bisphoshonates.

Galactorrhea

Hyperprolactinemia in premenopausal women can cause galactorrhea, but most premenopausal women who have hyperprolactinemia do not have galactorrhea. In contrast, many women who have galactorrhea have normal serum prolactin concentrations (130).

Elevated prolactin levels are relatively difficult to diagnose in men and in postmenopausal women due to lack of clear and specific symptoms associated with hyperprolactinemia. Headaches or impaired vision due to the large size of lactotroph adenoma usually leads to the diagnosis of hyperprolactinemia in postmenopausal women. Because these women are markedly hypoestrogenemic, galactorrhea is rare.

Hyperprolactinemia in Men

Decreased libido, impotence, infertility, gynecomastia, or rarely galactorrhea (131, 132) are the signs and symptoms of hyperprolactinemia in men caused by hypogonadotropic hypogonadism. As in women, there is a rough correlation between the presence of any of these symptoms and the degree of hyperprolactinemia. Hyperprolactinemia causes decreased testosterone secretion and low serum testosterone concentrations that are not associated with an increase in LH secretion (131). As in women, the effect of prolactin is on the hypothalamic-pituitary centers. The consequences of the hypogonadism include, in the short term, decreased energy and libido, and in the long term, decreased muscle mass, body hair, and osteoporosis (133).

Hyperprolactinemia also causes erectile dysfunction in some men by a mechanism unrelated to hypogonadism because correcting the hyperprolactinemia with a dopamine agonist drug corrects the impotence, while correcting the hypogonadism by the administration of testosterone does not (131). Hyperprolactinemia can infrequently cause infertility in men by decreasing LH and FSH secretions (132). Men with hyperprolactinemia may develop galactorrhea although less often than in women. This is because the glandular breast tissue in men has not been made sensitive to prolactin by precedent stimulation of estrogen and progesterone.

EVALUATION

Oligomenorrhea, amenorrhea, infertility, or galactorrhea in women and hypogonadism, impotence, or infertility in men calls for serum prolactin determination. The evaluation is aimed at exclusion of pharmacological or extrapituitary causes of hyperprolactinemia and neuroradiological evaluation of the hypothalamic-pituitary region (134). The usual normal range for serum prolactin is 5–20 ng/mL (5–20 mcg/L). The measurement can be performed at any time, but it is preferred to be done early in the morning since prolactin concentrations may increase slightly during sleep, strenuous exercise, and occasionally as a result of emotional or physical stress, intense breast stimulation, and high-protein meals. A slightly high value (21–40 ng/mL) should be confirmed before the patient is considered to have hyperprolactinemia. A persistently elevated serum prolactin value of any magnitude needs proper evaluation for etiology.

Serum prolactin values between 20 and 200 ng/mL can be found in patients with any cause of hyperprolactinemia. Serum prolactin values above 200 ng/mL usually indicate the presence of a lactotroph adenoma.

When there is a macroadenoma and the reported prolactin levels are between 20 and 200 ng/mL, the assay should be repeated using a 1:100 dilution of serum. This is due to the fact that very high serum levels of prolactin, for example, 5,000 ng/mL produced by the large tumor saturates both the capture and signal antibodies used in immunoradiometric and chemiluminescent assays, preventing the binding of the two in a "sandwich." The result is an artifactually low values of prolactin concentration due to this "hook effect" (135–137).

History

Pregnancy (physiologic hyperprolactinemia), medications that can cause hyperprolactinemia (such as estrogen, neuroleptic drugs, metoclopramide, antidepressant drugs, cimetidine, methyldopa, reserpine, verapamil, and risperidone), headache, visual symptoms, symptoms of hypothyroidism, and a history of renal disease should be included in the history.

Physical Examination

Visual field examination to test for a chiasmal syndrome (e.g., bitemporal field loss), chest wall injury, and signs of hypothyroidism or hypogonadism should be evaluated.

Laboratory/Imaging Tests

TSH, BUN, creatinin, and creatinin clearance should be checked to test for hypothyroidism and renal insufficiency. Magnetic resonance imaging (MRI) of the head should be performed in patients with significant hyperprolactinemia to diagnose pituitary adenomas, except if the patient is taking a medication known to cause hyperprolactinemia, such as an antipsychotic drug, which typically causes the magnitude of the prolactin elevation. There are no stimulatory or suppressive endocrine tests that distinguish among the causes of hyperprolactinemia.

If a mass lesion is found in the region of the sella tursica, secretion of other pituitary hormones should also be evaluated. Only a pituitary adenoma can cause hypersecretion of other pituitary hormones, but any mass lesion in the area of the sella can cause hyposecretion of one or more pituitary hormones.

If the MRI shows normal hypothalamic-pituitary anatomy and there is no other identifiable secondary cause of hyperprolactinemia, the diagnosis of idiopathic hyperprolactinemia is made. This syndrome may, in some patients, be due to microadenomas, which are too small to be seen on imaging.

GALACTORRHEA WITHOUT HYPERPROLACTINEMIA

In almost half of the women who present with galactorrhea, the serum prolactin concentration is going to be normal (130). These women will have regular menses. Galactorrhea in the absence of hyperprolactinemia is not the result of any ongoing disease. Often it represents persistent milk secretion following correction of elevated prolactin, most commonly after nursing or drug-induced hyperprolactinemia.

The first step in diagnosis is to be sure the breast secretion is clear or milky. If so, the next step is to measure the serum prolactin concentration. If the prolactin is elevated, the cause should be sought. If the prolactin is not elevated, and there is no ongoing disease, then no further tests are needed. Green or black or bloody fluid is a reason for referral for evaluation of a breast tumor.

Galactorrhea in the absence of hyperprolactinemia does not need treatment. If galactorrhea occurs spontaneously and to a degree that causes staining of the clothes, treatment with a low dose of dopamine agonist, such as 0.25 mg of cabergoline twice a week, will reduce the prolactin concentration to below normal and reduce or eliminate the galactorrhea.

TREATMENT OF HYPERPROLACTINEMIA

DA agonists usually decrease both the secretion and size of lactotroph adenomas and, therefore, are the treatment of choice to achieve fertility, to relieve breast discomfort, reduce galactorrhea, and to restore ovarian function (139). Surgery is recommended when a tumor continues to grow and cause visual impairment, after treatment with DA agonists.

Lactotroph adenoma is called a microadenoma when it is less than 1 cm in diameter. Treatment of asymptomatic microadenomas is not necessary because they rarely grow during pregnancy, very rarely progress to macroadenoma, recur significantly if operated upon, and maintain a natural course even if treated (139, 140). Unsuspected adenomas are found in almost 30 percent of pituitary glands in autopsy specimens (141–143). If microadenoma size remains unchanged at one, two, and five years upon MRI assessments, no further studies are necessary but approximately 5 percent do enlarge during follow-up and these patients should be treated.

A lactotroph adenoma greater than 1 cm is called a macroadenoma. Once macroadenoma is diagnosed, a follow-up MRI should be ordered at six months, one, two, and five years. When the adenoma extends outside of the sella and compresses the optic chiasm or invades the cavernous or sphenoid sinuses or the clivus, treatment is needed. These patients will have neurological symptoms, such as visual impairment or headache. Lesions of this size are likely to continue to grow and eventually cause neurological symptoms.

Treatment of hyperprolactinemia is also indicated when it causes hypogonadism.

Medical Treatment

A dopamine agonist drug should usually be the first line of treatment for patients with hyperprolactinemia of any cause including lactotroph adenomas of all sizes (144). Following are the available DA agonists to treat hyperprolactinemia.

Bromocriptine

Bromocriptine mesylate is marketed under the trade name Parlodel®, which comes in 5-mg capsule and 2.5-mg tablet forms. It belongs to the class of antiparkinsonian and DA agonist drugs and has been used for approximately two decades for treatment of hyperprolactinemia. Bromocriptine mesylate is a DA receptor agonist that activates the postsynaptic DA receptors to inhibit prolactin secretions. It also stimulates DA receptors in the corpus striatum to improve motor functions. It is 90–96 percent protein bound and is completely metabolized. It is excreted 84.6 percent in the feces and 2.5–5.5 percent in urine. The drug is considered as a category B during pregnancy and is excreted in small amounts in milk. The drug is contraindicated in postpartum women with coronary artery disease or other severe cardiovascular conditions and in patients with uncontrollable hypertension. Patients taking bromocriptine should be monitored for blood pressure and renal, liver, and hematopoietic functions. In peptic ulcer patients, signs and symptoms for gastrointestinal bleeding must be watched. Dosing is twice a day, and the initial dose must be one-fourth of the maintenance dose to decrease unpleasant side effects (hypotension, constipation, nausea, vomiting, dizziness, headache, and fatigue), which tends to occur at the beginning of treatment (143).

Cabergoline

It is marketed under the trade name Dostinex® and comes in 0.5-mg oral tablets. It is a long-acting selective DA receptor agonist, exhibiting high affinity for D2 receptors and low affinity for D1, alpha1 and alpha2 adrenergic, and serotonin receptors. It inhibits the synthesis and release of prolactin from the anterior pituitary by directly stimulating the D2 receptors of the pituitary lactotrophs in a dose-related fashion. The elimination half-life is sixty three–sixty nine hours, and it is metabolized mainly by the liver and its excretion is 60 percent fecal, 22 percent renal, and 4 percent unchanged. The drug is considered as a category B during pregnancy and is secreted in milk in small amounts. The drug is contraindicated in patients with uncontrolled hypertension. Patients on cabergoline need to be monitored by checking serum prolactin level, blood pressure measurements, and assessment of liver function. Dose adjustment is needed in liver failure. It is administered once or twice a week and has much less tendency to cause nausea than bromocriptine and pergolide (145, 146). It may be effective in patients resistant to bromocriptine (147). Recently, researchers used cabergoline for prevention of ovarian hyperstimulation syndrome due to its effect in blocking vascular permeability, which is probably due to its ability to block vascular endothelial growth factor receptor 2 phosphorylation. (see chapter 27 for the details of clinical trials) (148).

Pergolide

Pergolide mesylate is marketed under trade name Permax® and comes as 0.05-mg, 0.25-mg, and 1-mg oral tablets. It has been approved by the FDA for the treatment of Parkinson's disease but not for hyperprolactinemia (149). It belongs to the antiparkinsonian and DA agonist class of drugs. Pergolide mesylate is an ergot derivative and a D1 and D2 receptor agonist, exerting direct stimulation on the postsynaptic DA receptors in the nigrostriatal system in patients with Parkinson's disease. It also acts as an inhibitor to prolactin secretion and usually results in a transient elevation in GH concentration and reduced LH concentration. It is 90 percent protein bound and excreted 55 percent by the kidneys. The usual dosing for treatment of hyperprolactinemia is 0.025–0.6 mg PO once daily. Its advantage over bromocriptine is that it can be given once a day, and its advantage over cabergoline is that it costs about one-sixth as much (a one-month supply of a starting dose of pergolide costs about $35 compared to $235 for cabergoline and $85 for bromocriptine).

Recently, the use of the dopamine agonists including pergolide and cabergoline was associated with an increased risk of newly diagnosed cardiac-valve regurgitation. The frequency of valve regurgitation was significantly higher in patients taking pergolide or cabergoline when compared to control subjects (150, 151). Such increased risk was not reported in patients taking non-ergot-derived dopamine agonists (152). It is believed that because of the high affinity for the 5-HT (2B) serotonin receptors, which are expressed in heart valves, ergot-derived dopamine agonists can mediate mitogenesis leading to proliferation of fibroblasts. This ultimately causes fibrotic changes, thickening, retraction, and stiffening of valves, which result in incomplete leaflet coaptation and clinically significant regurgitation (153). Further studies are needed to reveal whether these changes are reversible and whether they are dose or duration dependent.

Other side-effects common to all dopamine agonist drugs include nausea, postural hypotension, mental fogginess, nasal stuffiness, depression, Raynaud phenomenon, alcohol intolerance, and constipation. Side-effects are more likely to occur once treatment is initiated or when the dose is increased. They can be avoided in most patients by starting with a small dose (one-half of the lowest strength pill of bromocriptine) once a day or half a pill of cabergoline twice a week and by giving it with food or at bedtime. The dose can then be increased gradually. Some patients will have side-effects even at the lowest doses. In women, nausea can be avoided by intravaginal administration (154, 155). Nausea is less encountered with the use of cabergoline. CSF rhinorrhea may occur during dopamine agonist treatment for very large lactotroph adenomas that extend inferiorly and invade the floor of the sella (156).

Other drugs that have been studied but are not yet approved in the United States include Quinoglide (CV 205-502), a nonergot DA agonist that is given once a day (157), and a long-acting form of bromocriptine that is administered by injection once a month (158).

Therapeutic Efficacy

DA agonists decrease prolactin secretion (figure 29.5) and reduce the size of the lactotroph adenoma in more than 90 percent of patients. Both effects are mediated by binding of the drug to cell surface dopamine receptors, leading to reductions in the synthesis and secretion of prolactin and in adenoma cell size. Cabergoline is better than bromocriptine in decreasing the serum prolactin concentration (145, 147). If bromocriptine fails to normalize prolactin levels, then the medication should be switched to cabergoline. At a median dose of 1 mg cabergoline weekly, 70 percent of the patients with visual field abnormalities returned to normal, and pituitary tumor size decreased in 67 percent of the 190 patients who had macroadenomas or microadenomas before treatment. The dose was later reduced to 0.5 mg weekly in 25 percent of patients with no increase in serum prolactin concentrations. Quinagolide appears to have equivalent therapeutic effects in reducing serum prolactin and adenoma size (159, 160). The effect on adenoma size is most apparent in patients with lactotroph macroadenomas. The fall in serum prolactin occurs within the first two to three weeks of therapy with a DA agonist (145). The decrease in adenoma size, however, may take six weeks to six months (161). Overall, the greater the decrease in serum prolactin concentration, the greater the decrease in adenoma size, although there is considerable variation from patient to patient. Vision usually begins to improve within days after the initiation of treatment (161, 162). There is recovery of menses and fertility in women, and of testosterone secretion, sperm count, and erectile function in men (144, 145, 163–165). Patients with macroadenomas who are hypothyroid and/or hypoadrenal may also have a return of these functions to normal (166). The therapeutic efficacy of dopamine agonists may be blunted by the concurrent use of drugs known to raise serum prolactin concentrations, including neuroleptic drugs, metoclopramide, sulpiride, domperidone, methyldopa, reserpine, verapamil, and cimetidine.

Cabergoline is very useful in most circumstances because it is most likely to be effective and least likely to cause side effects. The initial dose should be 0.25 mg twice a week

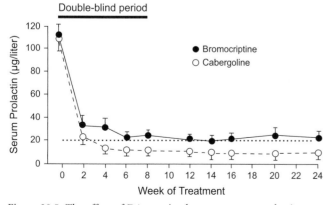

Figure 29.5. The effect of DA agonist drugs on serum prolactin concentration.

(the FDA-approved dose) or 0.5 mg once a week (a dose also reported to be effective). For the treatment of infertility, bromocriptine has a long track record (167), although data to date suggest that cabergoline is also safe in early pregnancy (168, 169). Bromocriptine is 30 percent cheaper than cabergoline to use, and the starting dose is 1.25 mg after dinner or at bedtime for one week, to be increased to 1.25 mg twice a day.

If the serum prolactin concentration has not decreased to normal and no side effects have occurred, the DA agonist dose is further increased gradually up to 1.5 mg of cabergoline two or three times a week or 5 mg of bromocriptine twice a day. If the patient cannot tolerate the first DA agonist administered, another can be tried. If none of these approaches is effective, transsphenoidal surgery or ovulation induction with clomiphene citrate or gonadotropins can be considered. If fertility is not desired, estrogen and progesterone replacement can be considered.

Duration of Treatment

In cases of microadenoma, if the patient tolerates the DA agonist and the serum prolactin eventually returns to normal, the drug should be continued until the patient becomes pregnant. After approximately one year, the dose can often be decreased. If the prolactin has been normal for two or more years and no adenoma is seen on MRI, discontinuation of the drug can be considered and prolactin monitored.

After menopause, the drug can be discontinued. Imaging should be performed if the value rises above 200 ng/mL to determine if the adenoma has enlarged. If so, drug therapy should be resumed.

In macroadenomas, visual field exam should be reassessed within one month of onset of therapy if vision was abnormal. Improvement may occur within a few days. An MRI should be repeated in six–twelve months to determine if the size of the adenoma has decreased. If the serum prolactin concentration has been normal for at least one year and the adenoma has decreased markedly in size, the dose of the dopamine agonist can be decreased gradually, as long as the serum prolactin remains normal (170). In patients with an initial size of macroadenomas less than 1.5 cm, whose serum prolactin concentrations have been normal for more than two years, and whose adenomas can no longer be visualized by MRI, treatment could be stopped. In contrast, discontinuation should not be considered if the adenoma was initially greater than 2 cm, or if it can still be visualized by MRI during treatment, or if the prolactin has not become normal during treatment. The DA agonist should not be discontinued entirely, even after menopause because hyperprolactinemia will probably recur and the adenoma may increase in size (171–173).

Withdrawal of Therapy

The risk of recurrent hyperprolactinemia or adenoma regrowth following discontinuation of the drug is low during two to five years of observation (171–173). After two to five years of observation, hyperprolactinemia recurred in 24, 31, and 36 percent of patients with idiopathic hyperprolactinemia, microadenomas, and macroadenomas, respectively. In patients with adenomas, hyperprolactinemia was more likely to recur if an adenoma remnant was seen on MRI compared to those with no evidence of remnance when treatment was stopped (78 vs. 33 percent for macroadenomas and 42 vs. 26 percent for microadenomas). Giant adenomas (>3 cm) behave more aggressively, growing rapidly within weeks of discontinuation of DA agonist medication (172, 173).

Estrogen

Women who have lactotroph microadenomas causing hyperprolactinemia and hypogonadism and cannot tolerate or do not respond to DA agonists and do not want to become pregnant can be treated with estrogen and progestin. In reproductive age women, oral contraceptive pills, contraceptive patches, or contraceptive rings are possible options. In postreproductive age women, either hormone replacement therapy or nonhormonal bone-building medications should be considered. Estrogen is also a reasonable option for women with hyperprolactinemia and amenorrhea due to antipsychotic agents. Since estrogen treatment might pose a slight risk of increasing the size of the adenoma, the serum prolactin concentration should be measured periodically in these patients. Estrogen should not be used as the sole treatment for lactotroph macroadenomas.

Surgical Treatment

Transsphenoidal surgery is indicated if the patient can not tolerate medical treatment, when DA agonists fail to lower serum prolactin concentration, reduce the size of the adenoma. When a woman with giant lactotroph adenoma (>3 cm) wishes to become pregnant, even if the adenoma responds to a DA agonist, surgery should be considered to prevent aggressive growth of adenoma during pregnancy.

Surgery is usually successful in substantially reducing serum prolactin concentrations in patients with prolactinomas (174–178). It is a safer procedure when performed by an experienced surgeon (179). However, in macroadenomas, only 20–50 percent of patients had normalized prolactin values after surgery, suggesting incomplete excision and removal of adenoma tissue (176). Another shortcoming of surgery is the recurrence of the adenoma (50 percent at four years) and hyperprolactinemia (39 percent at five years) (177, 178). If serum prolactin concentration is 5 ng/mL or less on the first postoperative day, persistent cure is more likely to be expected.

Radiation Therapy

Supervoltage radiation decreases the size and secretion of lactotroph adenomas, but normalization of prolactin levels may take many years after treatment (180, 181). Radiation treatment is primarily used to prevent regrowth of a residual tumor in a patient with a very large macroadenoma after transsphenoidal debulking. Complications of radiation therapy include transient nausea, lassitude, loss of taste and smell, loss of scalp hair, possible damage to the optic nerve, and neurological dysfunction (138). There is also a 50 percent chance of loss of anterior pituitary hormone secretion during the subsequent ten years (182).

Treatment of Hyperprolactinemia due to Other Causes

Treatment of hyperprolactinemia due to an abnormality other than a lactotroph adenoma varies depending on the cause. If hyperprolactinemia is the result of hypothyroidism, treatment of hypothyroidism will correct the problem. If hyperprolactinemia is a result of drug use, and the drug cannot be discontinued because it is essential and no substitute can be found, the resulting hypogonadism can be treated with the appropriate sex steroid. In women where antipsychotic medication use is the cause of hypogonadism, one should use a DA agonist cautiously because it might counteract the DA antagonist property of the antipsychotic drug. Another potential solution is to discuss with the treating psychiatrist the use of an antipsychotic drug that does not raise prolactin, such as quetiapine (Seroquel).

KEY POINTS

- Prolactin is one of the major anterior pituitary hormones but is also released by many other tissues.
- Prolactin secretion is inhibited by dopamine and increased by other hormones as TRH, GAP, PHM, VIP and estrogens.
- Prolactin plays an important part in lactation along with other essential biological activities like immune modulation, osmoregulation, angiogenesis, and sexual gratification.
- Hyperprolactinemia has a detrimental effect on fertility both in women and men, leading to galactorrhea anovulation, amenorrhea, oligomenorrhea, impotence, gynecomastia, and low semen profile.
- The upper normal value for serum prolactin is 20 ng/mL. Slightly high values (21–40 ng/mL) should be confirmed. Values above 200 ng/mL are highly indicative of the presence of a pituitary adenoma.
- Evaluation of the prolactin level should be done early in the morning as there is a diurnal variation in the level of prolactin, which is also influenced by stress and sexual behavior.
- Macroprolactenimia is a common condition where most of the circulating prolactin is in polymeric form with very low biological activity. It is a benign condition that seldom has any effect on the reproductive potential and for which the patient should not be treated.
- Pathological causes of hyperprolactinemia include pituitary and hypothalamic tumors, hypothyrodism, head injury, chest wall lesions, renal failure, and antihypertensive and antipsychotic drug use.
- DA agonist drugs are the first line of treatment for patients with hyperprolactinemia of any cause including lactotroph adenomas of all sizes.
- Although 50 percent of patients with galactorrhea are euprolactinemic, DA agonists still improve their symptoms.
- Cabergoline is a very effective among the DA agonist but is the most expensive. Bromocriptine is still the most widely used drug in infertile patients who want to get pregnant.
- Pergolide is an antiparkinsonian drug, which is not approved by the FDA for treatment of hyperprolactinemia but is currently the most cost-effective drug.
- Intravaginal administration of DA agonists reduces their side effects.
- Transsphenoidal surgery is recommended when symptomatic adenomas continue to grow and cause visual impairment after treatment with DA agonists, for patients who cannot tolerate these drugs and for patients with giant lactotroph adenoma greater than 3 cm who wish to become pregnant.

REFERENCES

1. Davis JR. Prolactin and reproductive medicine. *Curr Opin Obstet Gynecol* 2004;**16**(4):331–7.
2. Bole-Feysot C, Goffin V, Edery M, Binart N, Kelly PA. Prolactin (PRL) and its receptor: actions, signal transduction pathways and phenotypes observed in PRL receptor knockout mice. *Endocr Rev* 1998;**19**:225–68.
3. Rizk B. (Ed.). Ultrasonography in reproductive medicine and infertility. Cambridge: United Kingdom, Cambridge University Press, (in press).
4. Scully KM, Rosenfeld MG. Pituitary development: regulatory codes in mammalian organogenesis. *Science* 22 2002;**295**(5563): 2231–5.
5. Rosenfeld MG, Briate P, Dasen J, Gleiberman AS. Multistep. Signaling and transcriptional requirements for pituitary organogenesis in vivo. *Recent Prog Horm Res* 2000;**55**:1–13.
6. Cohen LE, Wondisford FE, Radovick S. Role of Pit-1 in the gene expression of growth hormone, prolactin, and thyrotropin. *Endocrinol Metab Clin North Am* 1996;**25**:523–40.
7. Gonzalez-Parra S, Chowen JA, Garcia SL, Argente J. Ontogeny of pituitary transcription factor-1 (Pit-1), growth hormone (GH) and prolactin (PRL) mRNA levels in male and female rats and the differential expression of Pit-1 in lactotrophs and somatotrophs. *J Neuroendocr* 1996;**8**:211–25.
8. Sharp ZD. Rat Pit-1 stimulates transcription in vitro by influencing preinitiation complex assembly. *Biochem Biophys Res Commun* 1995;**206**:40–5.
9. Nicoll CS, Mayer GL, Russell SM. Structural features of prolactins and growth hormones that can be related to their biological properties. *Endocr Rev* 1986;**7**:169–203.
10. Goffin V, Shiverick KT, Kelly PA, Martial JA. Sequence-function relationships within the expanding family of prolactin, growth hormone, placental lactogen and related proteins in mammals. *Endocr Rev* 1996;**17**:385–410.
11. Horseman ND, Yu-Lee LY. Transcriptional regulation by the helix bundle peptide hormones: growth hormone, prolactin, and hematopoietic cytokines. *Endocrinol Rev* 1994;**15**:627–49.
12. Bazan JF. Structural design and molecular evolution of a cytokine receptor superfamily. *Proc Natl Acad Sci USA* 1990;**87**: 6934–8.
13. Berwaer M, Monget P, Peers B, Mathy-Hartert M, Bellefroid E, Davis JR, Belayew A, Martial JA. Multihormonal regulation of the human prolactin gene expression from 5000 bp of its upstream sequence. *Mol Cell Endocrinol* 1991;**80**:53–64.
14. Berwaer M, Martial JA, Davis JR. Characterization of an upstream promoter directing extrapituitary expression of the human prolactin gene. *Mol Endocrinol* 1994;**8**:635–42.
15. Peers B, Voz ML, Monget P, Mathy-Hartert M, Berwaer M, et al. Regulatory elements controlling pituitary-specific expression of the human prolactin gene. *Mol Cell Biol* 1990;**10**:4690–700.
16. Truong AT, Duez C, Belayew A, et al. Isolation and characterization of human prolactin gene. *EMBO J* 1984;**3**:429–37.
17. Sinha YN. Structural variants of prolactin: occurrence and physiological significance. *Endocr Rev* 1995;**16**:354–69.
18. Teilum K, Hoch JC, Goffin V, Kinet S, Martial JA, Kragelund BB. Solution structure of human prolactin. *J Mol Biol* 2005; **351**(4):810–23.
19. Keeler C, Dannies PS, Hodsdon ME. The tertiary structure and backbone dynamics of human prolactin. *J Mol Biol* 2003; **328**(5):1105–21.
20. Kasic SV, Ramos IM, Selim A, Gunz G, Morange S, Enjalbert A, Martin PM, Jaquet P, Brue T. Macroprolactinemia revisited: a study on 106 patients. *J Clin Endocrinol Metab* 2002;**87**: 581–8.

21. Hattori N, Ikekubo K, Nakaya Y, Kitagawa K, Inagaki C. Immunoglobulin G subclasses and prolactin (PRL) isoforms in macroprolactinemia due to anti-PRL autoantibodies. *J Clin Endocrinol Metab* 2005;**90**(5):3036–44. Epub 2005 Feb 1.

22. Leanos-Miranda A, Cardenas-Mondragon G, Rivera-Leanos R, Ulloa-Aguirre A, Goffin V. Application of new homologous in vitro bioassays for human lactogens to assess the actual bioactivity of human prolactin isoforms in hyperprolactinaemic patients. *Clin Endocrinol (Oxf)* 2006;**65**(2):146–53.

23. Bazan JF. Haemopoietic receptors and helical cytokines. *Immunol Today* 1990;**11**: 350–54.

24. Rizk B. Genetics of ovarian hyperstimulation syndrome. In Rizk B (Ed.), *Ovarian Hyperstimulation Syndrome*. Cambridge, New York: Cambridge University Press, 2006; Chapter 4, pp. 79–91.

25. Schuler LA, Nagel RM, Gao J, Horseman ND, Kessler MA. Prolactin receptor heterogeneity in fetal and maternal tissues. *Endocrinology* 1997;**138**:3187–94.

26. Bazan JF. Structural design and molecular evolution of a cytokine receptor superfamily. *Proc Natl Acad Sci USA* 1990;**87**: 6934–8.

27. Kline JB, Roehrs H, Clevenger CV. Functional characterization of the intermediate isoform of the human prolactin receptor. *J Biol Chem* 1999;**274**:35461–8.

28. Trott JF, Hovey RC, Koduri S, Vonderhaar BK. Alternative splicing to exon 11 of human prolactin receptor gene results in multiple isoforms including a secreted prolactin-binding protein. *J Mol Endocrinol* 2003;**30**:31–47.

29. Herman A, Bignon C, Daniel N, Grosclaude J, Gertler A, et al. Functional heterodimerization of prolactin and growth hormone receptors by ovine placental lactogen. *J Biol Chem* 2000; **275**:6295–301.

30. Veldhuis JD, Johnson ML. Operating characteristics of the hypothalamo-pituitary-gonadal axis in men: circadian, ultradian, and pulsatile release of prolactin and its temporal coupling with luteinizing hormone. *J Clin Endocrinol Metab* 1988;**67**(1): 116–23.

31. Veldhuis JD, Evans WS, Stumpf PG. Mechanisms that subserve estradiol's induction of increased prolactin concentrations: evidence of amplitude modulation of spontaneous prolactin secretory bursts. *Am J Obstet Gynecol* 1989;**161**(5):1149–58.

32. Freeman ME, Kanyicska B, Lerant A, Nagy G. 2000. Prolactin: structure, function, and regulation of secretion. *Physiol Rev* **80**: 1523–631.

33. Van den Berghe G, de Zegher F, Veldhuis JD, Wouters P, Gouwy S, Stockman W, Weekers F, Schetz M, Lauwers P, Bouillon R, Bowers CY. Thyrotrophin and prolactin release in prolonged critical illness: dynamics of spontaneous secretion and effects of growth hormone-secretagogues. *Clin Endocrinol (Oxf)*. 1997; **47**(5):599–612.

34. Ben-Jonathan N. Dopamine: a prolactin-inhibiting hormone. *Endocr Rev* 1985;**6**:564–589.

35. Lerant A, Freeman ME. Dopaminergic neurons in periventricular and arcuate nuclei of proestrous and ovariectomized rats: endogenous diurnal rhythm of Fos-related antigens expression. *Neuroendocrinology* 1997;**65**:436–445.

36. Binart N, Helloco C, Ormandy CJ, Barra J, Clement-Lacroix P, et al. Rescue of preimplantatory egg development and embryo implantation in prolactin receptor-deficient mice after progesterone administration. *Endocrinology* 2000;**141**:2691–7.

37. Vacher P, Mariot P, Dufy-Barbe L, Nikolics K, Seeburg PH, Kerdelhue B, Dufy B. The gonadotropin-releasing hormone associated peptide reduces calcium entry in prolactin-secreting cells. *Endocrinology* 1991;**128**(1):285–94.

38. Steele MK. The role of brain angiotensin II in the regulation of luteinizing hormone and prolactin secretion. *Trends Endocrinol Metab* 1992;**3**:295–301.

39. Steele MK, McCann SM, Negro-Vilar A. Modulation by dopamine and estradiol of the central effects of angiotensin II on anterior pituitary hormone release. *Endocrinology* 1982;**111**: 722–9.

40. Fessler RG, Deyo SN, Meltzer HY, Miller RJ. Evidence that the medial and dorsal raphe nuclei mediate serotonergically-induced increases in prolactin release from the pituitary. *Brain Res* 1984;**299**:231–7.

41. Dalcik H, Phelps CJ. Median eminence-afferent vasoactive intestinal peptide (VIP) neurons in the hypothalamus: localization by simultaneous tract tracing and immunocytochemistry. *Peptides* 1993;**14**:1059–66.

42. Braund W, Roeger DC, Judd SJ. Synchronous secretion of luteinizing hormone and prolactin in the human luteal phase: neuroendocrine mechanisms. *J Clin Endocrinol Metab* 1984;**58**(2): 293–7.

43. Christiansen E, Veldhuis JD, Rogol AD, Stumpf P, Evans WS. Modulating actions of estradiol on gonadotropin-releasing hormone-stimulated prolactin secretion in postmenopausal individuals. *Am J Obstet Gynecol* 1987;**157**(2):320–5.

44. Van De Kar LD, Bethea CL. Pharmacological evidence that serotonergic stimulation of prolactin secretion is mediated via the dorsal raphe nucleus. *Neuroendocrinology* 1982;**35**: 225–30.

45. Takahashi K, Yoshinoya A, Arihara Z, Murakami O, Totsune K, Sone M, Sasano H, Shibahara S. Regional distribution of immunoreactive prolactin-releasing peptide in the human brain. *Peptides* 2000;**21**(10):1551–5.

46. Barber MC, Clegg RA, Finley E, Vernon RG, Flint DJ. The role of growth hormone, prolactin and insulin-like growth factors in the regulation of rat mammary gland and adipose tissue metabolism during lactation. *J Endocrinol* 1992;**135**:195–202.

47. Tucker HA. Lactation and its hormonal control. In Knobil E, Neill JD (Eds.), *The Physiology of Reproduction*, New York: Raven, 1994; pp. 1065–98.

48. Whitworth NS. Lactation in humans. *Psychoneuroendocrinology* 1988;**13**(1–2):171–88. Review.

49. Speroff L, Glass RH, Kase NG. *Clinical Gynecologic Endocrinology and Infertility*. Sixth edition. Baltimore, MD: Lippincott Williams and Wilkins, 1999. ISNB 0-683-30379-1.

50. Kruger TH, Haake P, Haverkamp J, Kramer M, Exton MS, Saller B, Leygraf N, Hartmann U, Schedlowski M. Effects of acute prolactin manipulation on sexual drive and function in males. *J Endocrinol* 2003;**179**(3):357–65.

51. Sheth AR, Mugatwala PP, Shah GV, et al. Occurrence of prolactin in human semen. *Fertil Steril* 1975;**26**:905–7.

52. Shah GV, Desai RB, Sheth AR. Effect of prolactin on metabolism of human spermatozoa. *Fertil Steril* 1976;**27**:1292–4.

53. Hernandez-Andrade E, Villanueva-Diaz C, Ahued-Ahued JR. Growth hormone and prolactin in maternal plasma and amniotic fluid during normal gestation. *Rev Invest Clin.* 2005; **57**(5):671–5.

54. Shennan DB. Regulation of water and solute transport across mammalian plasma cell membranes by prolactin. *J Dairy Res* 1994;**61**:155–66.

55. Buskila D, Shoenfeld Y. Prolactin, bromocriptine and autoimmune diseases. *Isr J Med Sci* 1996;**32**:23–7.

56. Neidhart M. Prolactin in autoimmune diseases. *Proc Soc Exp Biol Med* 1998;**217**:408–19.

57. Walker SE, Allen SH, McMurray RW. Prolactin and autoimmune disease. *Trends Endocrinol Metab* 1993;**4**:147–51.

58. Roky R, Paut-Pagano L, Goffin V, Kitahama K, Valatx JL, Kelly PA, Jouvet M. Distribution of prolactin receptors in the rat forebrain. Immunohistochemical study. *Neuroendocrinology* 1996;**63**:422–9.

59. Clapp C, Martial JA, Guzman RC, Rentier-Delrue F, Weiner RI. The 16-kilodalton N-terminal fragment of human prolactin is a potent inhibitor of angiogenesis. *Endocrinology* 1993;**133**:1292–9.

60. Clapp C, Torner L, Gutiérrez-Ospina G, Alcántara E, López-Gómez FJ, Nagano M, Kelly PA, Mejía S, Morales MA, Martínez de la Escalera G. The prolactin gene is expressed in the hypothalamic-neurohypophyseal system and the protein is processed into a 14-kDa fragment with activity like 16-kDa prolactin. *Proc Natl Acad Sci USA* 1994;**91**:10384–8.

61. Clapp C, Weiner RI. A specific, high affinity, saturable binding site for the 16-kilodalton fragment of prolactin on capillary endothelial cells. *Endocrinology* 1992;**130**:1380–6.

62. Lissoni P, Mandala M, Rovelli F, Casu M, Rocco F, et al. Paradoxical stimulation of prolactin secretion by L-dopa in metastatic prostate cancer and its possible role in prostate-cancer-related hyperprolactinemia. *Eur Urol* 2000;**37**:569–72.

63. Leav I, Merk FB, Lee KF, Loda M, Mandoki M, et al. Prolactin receptor expression in the developing human prostate and in hyperplastic, dysplastic, and neoplastic lesions. *Am J Pathol* 1999;**154**:863–70.

64. Touraine P, Martini JF, Zafrani B, Durand JC, Labaille F, et al. Increased expression of prolactin receptor gene assessed by quantitative polymerase chain reaction in human breast tumors versus normal breast tissues. *J Clin Endocrinol Metab* 1998; **83**:667–74.

65. Wennbo H, Gebre-Medhin M, Gritli-Linde A, Ohlsson C, Isaksson OG, et al. Activation of the prolactin receptor but not the growth hormone receptor is important for induction of mammary tumors in transgenic mice. *J Clin Invest* 1997;**100**:2744–51.

66. Goffin V, Touraine P, Pichard C, Bernichtein S, Kelly PA. Should prolactin be reconsidered as a therapeutic target in human breast cancer? *Mol Cell Endocrinol* 1999;**151**:79–87.

67. Cheung CY. Prolactin suppresses luteininzing hormone secretion and pituitary responsiveness to luteinizing hormone-releasing hormone by a direct action at the anterior pituitary. *Endocrinology* 1983;**113**:632–638.

68. Milenkovic L, D'Angelo G, Kelly PA, Weiner RI. Inhibition of gonado tropin hormone-releasing hormone release by prolactin from GIT neuronal cell lines through prolactin receptors. *Proc Natl Acad Sci USA* 1994;**91**:1244–7.

69. Glass MR, Shaw RW, Butt WR, et al. An abnormality of estrogen feedback in amenorrhea galactorrhea. *Br Med J* 1975;**3**: 274–5.

70. McNeilly KP, Glasier A, Jonassen J, et al. Evidence for direct inhibition of ovarian function by prolactin. *J Reprod Fert* 1982; **65**:559–69.

71. Dorrington JH, Gore-Langton RE. Antigonadal action of prolactin: further studies on the mechanism of inhibition of follicle stimulating hormone-induced aromatase activity in rat granulosa cell cultures. *Endocrinology* 1982;**110**:1701–7.

72. McNatty KP, Sawers RS, McNeilly AS. A possible role for prolactin in control of steroid secretion by human graffian follicle. *Nature.* 1974 Aug 23;**250**(5468):653–5.

73. Del Pozo E, Wyss H, Tolis G, et al. Prolactin and deficient luteal function. *Obstet Gynecol* 1979;**53**:282–6.

74. Feltus FA, Groner B, Melner MH. Stat5-mediated regulation of the human type II 3α hydroxysteroid dehydrogenase isomerase gene activation by prolactin. *Mol Endocrinol* 1999;**13**: 1084–93.

75. Cameron DF, Murray FT, Drylie DD. Ultrastructural lesions in testes from hyperprolactinemic men. *J Androl* 1984;**5**:283–93.

76. Bahceci M, Tuzcu A, Bahceci S, Tuzcu S. Is hyperprolactinemia associated with insulin resistance in non-obese patients with polycystic ovary syndrome? *J Endocrinol Invest* 2003;**26**(7): 655–9.

77. Isik AZ, Gulekli B, Zorlu CG, Ergin T, Gokmen O. Endocrinological and clinical analysis of hyperprolactinemic patients with and without ultrasonically diagnosed polycystic ovarian changes. *Gynecol Obstet Invest* 1997;**43**(3):183–5.

78. Tanaka T, Fujimoto S. Endocrinological environment of polycystic ovarian disease. *Horm Res* 1990;**33** (Suppl. 2):5–9. Review.

79. Minakami H, Abe N, Oka N, Kimura K, Tamura T, Tamada T. Prolactin release in polycystic ovarian syndrome. *Endocrinol Jpn* 1988;**35**(2):303–10.

80. Tyson JB, Ito P, Guyda H, et al. Studies of prolactin in human pregnancy. *Am J Obstet Gynecol* 1972;**113**:14.

81. Tyson JE, Friesen HG. Factors influencing the secretion of human prolactin and growth hormone in menstrual and gestational women. *Am J Obstet Gynecol* 1973;**116**:377.

82. Barberia JM, Abu-FAdil S, Kletzky OA, Nakamura RM, Mishell DR Jr. Serum prolactin patterns in early human gestation. *Am J Obstet Gynecol* 1975;**121**:1107.

83. Kleinberg DL, Noel GL, Frantz AG. Galactorrhea: a study of 235 cases, including 48 with pituitary tumors. *N Engl J Med* 1977; **296**:589.

84. Alexander JM, Biller BMK, Bikkal H, et al. Clinically nonfunctioning pituitary tumors are monoclonal in origin. *J Clin Invest* 1990;**86**:336.

85. Herman V, Fagin J, Gonsky R, et al. Clonal origin of pituitary adenomas. *J Clin Endocrinol Metab* 1990;**71**:1427.

86. Zhang X, Horwitz GA, Heaney AP, et al. Pituitary tumor transforming gene (PTTG) expression in pituitary adenomas. *J Clin Endocrinol Metab* 1999;**84**:761.

87. Ezzat S, Zheng L, Zhu XF, et al. Targeted expression of a human pituitary tumor-derived isoform of FGF receptor-4 recapitulates pituitary tumorigenesis. *J Clin Invest* 2002;**109**:69.

88. Corenblum B, Sirek AMT, Horvath E, et al. Human mixed somatotrophic and lactotrophic pituitary adenomas. *J Clin Endocrinol Metab* 1976;**42**:857.

89. Mindermann T, Wilson CB. Age-related and gender-related occurrence of pituitary adenomas. *Clin Endocrinol* 1994;**41**:359.

90. Delgrange E, Trouillas J, Maiter D, et al. Sex-related difference in the growth of prolactinomas: a clinical and proliferation marker study. *J Clin Endocrinol Metab* 1997;**82**:2102.

91. Prosser PR, Karam JH, Townsend JJ, et al. Prolactin-secreting pituitary adenomas in multiple endocrine adenomatosis, type 1. *Ann Intern Med* 1979;**91**:41.

92. Walker JD, Grossman A, Anderson JV, et al. Malignant prolactinoma with extracranial metastases: a report of three cases. *Clin Endocrinol* 1993;**38**:411.

93. Petakov MS, Damjanovic SS, Nikolic-Durovic MM, et al. Pituitary adenomas secreting large amounts of prolactin may give false low values in immunoradiometric assays. The hook effect. *J Endocrinol Invest* 1998;**21**:184.

94. St-Jean E, Blain F, Comtois R. High prolactin levels may be missed by immunoradiometric assay in patients with macroprolactinomas. *Clin Endocrinol (Oxf)* 1996;**44**:305.

95. Barkan AL, Chandler WF. Giant pituitary prolactinoma with falsely low serum prolactin: the pitfall of the "high-dose hook effect." *Neurosurgery* 1998;**42**:913.

96. David SR, Taylor CC, Kinon BJ, Breier A. The effects of olanzapine, rispiridone, and haloperiodol on plasma prolactin levels in patients with schizophrenia. *Clin Ther* 2000;**22**:1085.

97. Rivera JL, Lal S, Ettigi P, et al. Effect of acute and chronic neuroleptic therapy on serum prolactin levels in men and women of different age groups. *Clin Endocrinol (Oxf)* 1976;**5**:273.

98. McCallum RW, Sowers JR, Hershman JM, et al. Metoclopramide stimulates prolactin secretion in man. *J Clin Endocrinol Metab* 1976;**42**:1148.

99. Mancini AM, Guitelman A, Vargas CA, et al. Effect of sulpiride on serum prolactin levels in humans. *J Clin Endocrinol Metab* 1976;**42**:181.

100. Sowers JR, Sharp B, McCallum RW. Effect of domperidone, an extracerebral inhibitor of dopamine receptors, on thyrotropin, prolactin, renin, aldosterone, and 181hydroxycorticosterone secretion in man. *J Clin Endocrinol Metab* 1982;**54**:869.

101. Steiner J, Cassar J, Maslliter K, et al. Effect of methyldopa on prolactin and growth hormone. *Br Med J* 1976;**1**:1186.

102. Lee PA, Kelly MR, Wallin JD. Increased prolactin levels during reserpine treatment of hypertensive patients. *JAMA* 1976;**235**: 2316.

103. Fearrington EL, Rand CH, Rose JD. Hyperprolactinemia-galactorrhea induced by verapamil. *Am J Cardiol* 1983;**51**: 1466.

104. Veldhuis JD, Borges JLC, Drake CR. Divergent influences of the structurally dissimilar calcium entry blockers, diltiazem and verapamil, on the thyrotropin- and gonadotropin-releasing hormone-stimulated anterior pituitary hormone secretion in man. *J Clin Endocrinol Metab* 1985;**60**:144.

105. Cowen PJ, Sargent PA. Changes in plasma prolactin during SSRI treatment: evidence for a delayed increase in 5-HT neurotransmission. *J Psychopharmacol* 1997;**11**:345.

106. Meltzer H, Bastani B, Jayathilake K, Maes M. Fluoxetine, but not tricyclic antidepressants, potentiates the 5-hydroxytryptophan-mediated increase in plasma cortisol and prolactin secretion in subjects with major depression or with obsessive compulsive disorder. *Neuropsychopharmacology* 1997;**17**:1.

107. Honbo KS, Van Herle AJ, Kellett KA. Serum prolactin levels in untreated primary hypothyroidism. *Am J Med* 1978;**64**:782.

108. Snyder PJ, Jacobs LS, Utiger RD, Daughaday WH. Thyroid hormone inhibition of the prolactin response to thyrotropin-releasing hormone. *J Clin Invest* 1973;**52**:2324.

109. Groff TR, Shulkin BL, Utiger RD, Talbert LM. Amenorrhea-galactorrhea, hyperprolactinemia, and suprasellar pituitary enlargement as presenting features of primary hypothyroidism. *Obstet Gynecol* 1984;**63**:86S.

110. Grubb MR, Chakeres D, Malarkey WB. Patients with primary hypothyroidism presenting as prolactinomas. *Am J Med* 1987; **83**:765.

111. Morley JE, Hodgkinson DH, Kalk WJ. Galactorrhea and hyperprolactinemia associated with chest wall injury. *J Clin Endocrinol Metab* 1977;**45**:931.

112. Lim VS, Kathpalia SC, Frohman LA. Hyperprolactinemia and impaired pituitary response to suppression and stimulation in chronic renal failure: reversal after transplantation. *J Clin Endocrinol Metab* 1979;**48**:101.

113. Sievertsen GD, Lim VS, Nakawatase C, Frohman LA. Metabolic clearance and secretion rates of human prolactin in normal subjects and patients with chronic renal failure. *J Clin Endocrinol Metab* 1980;**50**:846.

114. Schlechte I, Dolan K, Sherman B, et al. The natural history of untreated hyperprolactinemia: a prospective analysis. *J Clin Endocrinol Metab* 1989;**68**:412.

115. Martin TL, Kim M, Malarkey WB. The natural history of idiopathic hyperprolactinemia. *J Clin Endocrinol Metab* 1985; **60**:855.

116. Sluijmer AV, Lappohn RE. Clinical history and outcome of 59 patients with idiopathic hyperprolactinemia. *Perth Steril* 1992;**58**:72.

117. Carlson HE, Markoff E, Lee DW. On the nature of serum prolactin in two patients with macroprolactinemia. *Perth Steril* 1992; **58**:78.

118. Vallette-Kasic S, Morange-Ramos I, Selim A, et al. Macroprolactinemia revisited: a study on 106 patients. *J Clin Endocrinol Metab* 2002;**87**:581.

119. Olukoga AO, Kane JW. Macroprolactinaemia: validation and application of the polyethylene glycol precipitation test and clinical characterization of the condition. *Clin Endocrinol (Oxf)* 1999;**51**:119.

120. Leslie H, Courtney CH, Bell PM, et al. Laboratory and clinical experience in 55 patients with macroprolactinemia identified by a simple polyethylene glycol precipitation method. *J Clin Endocrinol Metab* 2001;**86**:2743.

121. Strachan MW, Teoh WL, Don-Wauchope AC, et al. Clinical and radiological features of patients with macroprolactinaemia. *Clin Endocrinol (Oxf)* 2003;**59**:339.

122. Gibney J, Smith TP, McKenna TJ. Clinical relevance of macroprolactin. *Clin Endocrinol (Oxf)* 2005;**62**:633.

123. Gomez F, Reyes FI, Faiman C. Nonpuerperal galactorrhea and hyperprolactinemia. Clinical findings, endocrine features and therapeutic responses in 56 cases. *Am J Med* 1977;**62**: 648.

124. Schlechte J, Sherman B, Halmi N, et al. Prolactin-secreting pituitary tumors in amenorrheic women: a comparative study. *Endocr Rev* 1980;**1**:295.

125. Seppala M, Hirvonen E, Ranta T. Hyperprolactinemia and luteal insufficiency. *Lancet* 1976;**1**:229.

126. Corenblum B, Fairaudeau N, Shewchux AB. Prolactin hypersecretion and short luteal phase defects. *Obstet Gynecol* 1976; **47**:486.

127. Biller BMK, Baum HBA, Rosenthal DI, et al. Progressive trabecular osteopenia in women with hyperprolactinemic amenorrhea. *J Clin Endocrinol Metab* 1992;**75**:692.

128. Schlechte J, Walkner L, Kathol M. A longitudinal analysis of premenopausal bone loss in healthy women and women with hyperprolactinemia. *J Clin Endocrinol Metab* 1992;**75**:698.

129. Colao A, Di Somma C, Loche S, et al. Prolactinomas in adolescents: persistent bone loss after 2 years of prolactin normalization. *Clin Endocrinol (Oxf)* 2000;**52**:319.

130. Kleinberg DL, Noel GL, Frantz AG. Galactorrhea: a study of 235 cases, including 48 with pituitary tumors. *N Engl J Med* 1977; **296**:589.

131. Carter JN, Tyson JE, Tolis G, et al. Prolactin-secreting tumors and hypogonadism in 22 men. *N Engl J Med* 1978; **299**:847.

132. Segal S, Yaffe H, Laufer N, Ben-David M. Male hyperprolactinemia: effects on fertility. *Fertil Steril* 1979;**32**:556.

133. Di Somma C, Colao A, Di Sarno A, et al. Bone marker and bone density responses to dopamine agonist therapy in hyperprolactinemic males. *J Clin Endocrinol Metab* 1998;**83**:807.

134. Casanueva FF, Molitch ME, Schlechte JA, et al. Guidelines of the Pituitary Society for the diagnosis and management of prolactinomas. *Clin Endocrinol (Oxf)* 2006;**65**:265.

135. St-Jean E, Blain F, Comtois R. High prolactin levels may be missed by immunoradiometric assay in patients with macroprolactinomas. *Clin Endocrinol (Oxf)* 1996;**44**:305.

136. Petakov MS, Damjanovic SS, Nikolic-Durovic MM, et al. Pituitary adenomas secreting large amounts of prolactin may give false low values in immunoradiometric assays. The hook effect. *J Endocrinol Invest* 1998;**21**:184.

137. Barkan AL, Chandler WF. Giant pituitary prolactinoma with falsely low serum prolactin: the pitfall of the "high-dosehook effect": case report. *Neurosurgery* 1998;**42**:913.

138. Casanueva FF, Molitch ME, Schlechte JA, et al. Guidelines of the Pituitary Society for the diagnosis and management of prolactinomas. *Clin Endocrinol (Oxf)* 2006;**65**:265.

139. Schlechte J, Dolan K, Sherman B, et al. The natural history of untreated hyperprolactinemia: a prospective analysis. *J Clin Endocrinol Metab* 1989;**68**:412.

140. Sisam DA, Sheehan JP, Sheeler LR. The natural history of untreated microprolactinoma. *Fertil Steril* 1987;**48**:67.

141. Costello RT. Subclinical adenoma of the pituitary gland. *Am J Pathol* 1936;**12**:191.

142. Kraus HE. Neoplastic diseases of the human hypophysis. *Arch Pathol* 1945;**39**:343.

143. Burrow GN, Wortzman G, Rewcastle NB, Holgate RC, Kovacs K. Microadenomas of the pituitary and abnormal sellar tomograms in an unselected autopsy series. *New Eng J Med* 1981; **304**:156.

144. Vance ML, Evans WS, Thorner MO. Drugs five years later. *Bromocriptine. Ann Intern Med* 1984;**100**:78.

145. Webster J, Piscitelli MD, Polli A, et al. A comparison of cabergoline and bromocriptine in the treatment of hyperprolactinemic amenorrhea. *N Engl J Med* 1994;**331**:904.

146. Biller BMK, Molitch ME, Vance ML, et al. Treatment of prolactin-secreting macroadenomas with the once-weekly dopamine agonist cabergoline. *J Clin Endocrinol Metab* 1996;**81**: 2338.

147. Verhelst J, Abs R, Maiter D, et al. Cabergoline in the treatment of hyperprolactinemia. *J Clin Endocrinol Metab* 1999;**84**:2518.

148. Rizk B. Treatment of ovarian hyperstimulation syndrome. In Rizk B (Ed.), *Ovarian Hyperstimulation Syndrome.* Cambridge, New York: Cambridge University Press, 2006; Chapter 8, pp. 200–26.

149. Kleinberg DL, Boyd AE 3rd., Wardlaw S, et al. Pergolide for the treatment of pituitary tumors secreting prolactin or growth hormone. *N Engl J Med* 1983;**309**:704.

150. Schade R, Andersohn F, Suissa S, Haverkamp W, Garbe E. Dopamine agonists and the risk of cardiac-valve regurgitation. *N Engl J Med.* 2007 Jan 4;**356**(1):29–38.

151. Zanettini R, Antonini A, Gatto G, Gentile R, Tesei S, Pezzoli G. Valvular heart disease and the use of dopamine agonists for Parkinson's disease. *N Engl J Med.* 2007 Jan 4;**356**(1):39–46.

152. Simonis G, Fuhrmann JT, Strasser RH. Meta-analysis of heart valve abnormalities in Parkinson's disease patients treated with dopamine agonists. *Mov Disord.* 2007 Oct 15;**22**(13):1936–42.

153. Antonini A, Poewe W. Fibrotic heart-valve reactions to dopamine-agonist treatment in Parkinson's disease. *Lancet Neurol.* 2007 Sep;**6**(9):826–9.

154. Kletzky OA, Vermesh M. Effectiveness of vaginal bromocriptine in treating women with hyperprolactinemia. *Fertil Steril.* 1989;**51**:269.

155. Motta T, de Vincentiis S, Marchini M, et al. Vaginal cabergoline in the treatment of hyperprolactinemic patients intolerant to oral dopaminergics. *Fertil Steril.* 1996;**65**:440.

156. Leong KS, Foy PM, Swift AC, et al. CSF rhinorrhoea following treatment with dopamine agonists for massive invasive prolactinomas. *Clin Endocrinol (Oxf)* 2000;**52**:43.

157. Vance ML, Lipper M, Klibanski A, et al. Treatment of prolactin secreting pituitary macroadenomas with the long acting nonergot dopamine agonist CV 205502. *Ann Intern Med.* 1990;**112**:668.

158. Beckers A, Petrossians P, Abs R, et al. Treatment of macroprolactinomas with the long-acting and repeatable form of bromo-

criptine: a report on 29 cases. *J Clin Endocrinol Metab.* 1992;**75**:275.

159. Van der, Lely AL, Brownell J, Lamberts SW. The efficacy and tolerability of CV 205-502 (a nonergot dopaminergic drug) in macroprolactinoma patients and in prolactinoma patients intolerant to bromocriptine. *J Clin Endocrinol Metab.* 1991; **72**:1136.

160. Molitch ME. Macroprolactinoma size reduction with dopamine agonists. *Endocrinologist.* 1997;**7**:390.

161. Molitch ME, Elton RL, Blackwell RE, et al. Bromocriptine as primary therapy for prolactin secreting macroadenomas: results of a prospective multicenter study. *J Clin Endocrinol Metab.* 1985;**60**:698.

162. Moster ML, Savino PJ, Schatz NJ, et al. Visual function in prolactinoma patients treated with bromocriptine. *Ophthalmology.* 1985;**92**:1332.

163. De Rosa M, Colao A, Di Sarno A, et al. Cabergoline treatment rapidly improves gonadal function in hyperprolactinemic males: a comparison with bromocriptine. *Eur J Endocrinol.* 1998;**138**:286.

164. De Rosa M, Zarrilli S, Vitale G, et al. Six months of treatment with cabergoline restores sexual potency in hyperprolactinemic males: an open longitudinal study monitoring nocturnal penile tumescence. *J Clin Endocrinol Metab.* 2004;**89**:621.

165. Colao A, Vitale G, Cappabianca P, et al. Outcome of cabergoline treatment in men with prolactinoma: effects of a 24-month treatment on prolactin levels, tumor mass, recovery of pituitary function, and semen analysis. *J Clin Endocrinol Metab.* 2004;**89**:1704.

166. Warfield A, Finkel DM, Schatz NJ, et al. Bromocriptine treatment of prolactin-secreting pituitary adenomas may restore pituitary function. *Ann Intern Med.* 1984;**101**:783.

167. Turkalj I, Braun P, Krupp P, et al. Surveillance of bromocriptine in pregnancy. *JAMA.* 1982;**247**:1589.

168. Robert E, Musatti L, Piscitelli G, et al. Pregnancy outcome after treatment with the ergot derivative, cabergoline. *Reprod Toxicol* 1996;**10**:333.

169. Ricci E, Parazzini F, Motta T, et al. Pregnancy outcome after cabergoline treatment in early weeks of gestation. *Reprod Toxicol* 2002;**16**:791.

170. Liuzzi A, Dallabonzana D, Oppizzi G, et al. Low doses of dopamine agonists in the long-term treatment of macroprolactinomas. *N Engl J Med* 1985;**313**:656.

171. Colao A, Di Sarno A, Cappabianca P, et al. Withdrawal of long-term cabergoline therapy for tumoral and nontumoral hyperprolactinemia. *N Engl J Med* 2003;**349**:2023.

172. Thorner MO, Perryman RL, Rogol AD, et al. Rapid changes of prolactinoma volume after withdrawal and reinstitution of bromocriptine. *J Clin Endocrinol Metab* 1981;**53**:480.

173. Van't Verlaat JW, Croughs RJ. Withdrawal of bromocriptine after long term therapy for macroprolactinomas: effect on plasma prolactin and tumor size. *Clin Endocrinol* 1991;**34**:175.

174. Passos VQ, Souza JJ, Musolino NR, Bronstein MD. Long-term follow-up of prolactinomas: normoprolactinemia after bromocriptine withdrawal. *J Clin Endocrinol Metab* 2002; **87**:3578.

175. Feigenbaum SL, Downey DE, Wilson CB, et al. Transsphenoidal pituitary resection for preoperative diagnosis of prolactin-secreting pituitary adenoma in women: long term follow-up. *J Clin Endocrinol Metab* 1996;**81**:1711.

176. Randall RV, Laws ER Jr., Abboud CF, et al. Transsphenoidal microsurgical treatment of prolactin-producing pituitary adenomas: results in 100 patients. *Mayo Clin Proc* 1983;**58**: 108.

177. Serri O, Rasio E, Beauregard H, et al. Recurrence of hyperpro-lactinemia after selective transsphenoidal adenomectomy in women with prolactinoma. *N Engl J Med* 1983;**309**:280.

178. Schlechte JA, Sherman BM, Chapler FK, et al. Long-term follow-up of women with surgically treated prolactin-secreting pituitary tumors. *J Clin Endocrinol Metab* 1986;**62**:1296.

179. Ciric I, Ragin A, Baumgartner C, Pierce D. Complications of transsphenoidal surgery: results of a national survey, review of the literature, and personal experience. *Neurosurgery* 1997;**40**:225.

180. Littley MD, Shalet SM, Reid H, et al. The effect of external pituitary irradiation on elevated serum prolactin levels in patients with pituitary macroadenomas. *Q J Med* 1991;**81**:985.

181. Tsagarakis S, Grossman A, Plowman PN, et al. Megavoltage pituitary irradiation in the management of prolactinomas: long-term follow-up. *Clin Endocrinol* 1991;**34**:399.

182. Snyder PJ, Fowble BF, Schatz NJ, et al. Hypopituitarism fol-lowing radiation therapy of pituitary adenomas. *Am J Med* 1986;**81**:457.

30

MEDICAL MANAGEMENT OF POLYCYSTIC OVARY SYNDROME

Nadia Kabli, Togas Tulandi

Polycystic ovary syndrome (PCOS) is the most common endocrine disorder in women. Its prevalence among infertile women is 15–20 percent. The etiology of PCOS remains unclear; however, several studies have suggested that PCOS is an X-linked dominant condition (1). The clinical manifestation of PCOS varies from a mild menstrual disorder to severe disturbance of reproductive and metabolic functions. Women with PCOS are predisposed to type 2 diabetes or develop cardiovascular disease (2).

DEFINITION OF PCOS

In a workshop sponsored by ESHRE (European Society for Human Reproduction and Embryology) and ASRM (American Society for Reproductive Medicine) in Rotterdam in 2003, a new definition of PCOS was proposed (3). This consensus defined PCOS as a syndrome with two out of three of the following features: oligo- or anovulation, clinical and/or biochemical sign of hyperandrogenism, and/or sonographic finding of polycystic ovaries (after exclusion of other etiologies such as congenital adrenal hyperplasia, androgen-secreting tumors, or Cushing's syndrome) (Table 30.1).

Sonographic features of polycystic ovaries (PCO) include the presence of twelve or more follicles in each ovary measuring 2–9 mm in diameter and/or increased ovarian volume (>10 mL). This is regardless of follicle distribution, ovarian stromal echogenicity, or ovarian volume. One ovary fulfilling this definition is sufficient to define PCO (2, 4). It is recognized that some women with sonographic findings of PCO may have regular cycles without clinical or biochemical signs of hyperandrogenism.

DIFFERENTIAL DIAGNOSIS

Other conditions with a similar clinical presentation are congenital adrenal hyperplasia, Cushing's syndrome, and androgen-secreting tumors. Exclusion of nonclassic congenital adrenal hyperplasia (NCAH) secondary to 21-hydroxylase deficiency can be performed using a basal morning 17-hydroxyprogesterone level, with cutoff values ranging between 2 and 3 ng/mL. The diagnosis can also be established by measurement of serum 17-hydroxyprogesterone after ACTH injection (1).

CLINICAL MANIFESTATIONS

- The most common manifestation of PCOS is menstrual disturbances and irregular ovulation. The menstrual pattern in PCOS patients varies from amenorrhea and breakthrough bleeding, to menorrhagia. Due to unopposed estrogen stimulation to the endometrium, women with PCOS are at risk to have endometrial hyperplasia and endometrial cancer. The risk is higher in obese women with PCOS (1, 5).

- Another characteristic of women with PCOS is hyperandrogenis. It is manifested by slowly developing hirsutism (excessive growth of thick, pigmented terminal hair in male pattern). Acne can also be found.

- Acanthosis nigricans in obese patients is a reliable clinical marker of insulin resistance and hyperinsulinemia. Rapidly developing hirsutism and virilization warrant prompt search for underlying ovarian or adrenal neoplasm (1).

ROLE OF INSULIN RESISTANCE

Insulin Resistance, Hyperinsulinemia, and Hyperandrogenisms

Insulin resistance can be encountered in women with PCOS. It is defined as reduced glucose response to a given amount of insulin. This is different from resistance to endogenous insulin, where the serum insulin is high in association with normal or high blood glucose levels. Insulin resistance plays a role in lipoprotein disturbances and body morphology alteration and may predispose to early development of cardiovascular disease.

Several techniques have been proposed to evaluate insulin sensitivity. The gold standard is the glucose clamp technique, but it does not reflect the physiological condition of the patients. A well-accepted alternative is intravenous glucose tolerance test (GTT) (6), fasting insulin and glucose, and oral GTT (OGTT) (7). OGTT provides information about insulin secretion and action, but it is a not a direct measurement of insulin sensitivity.

In any event, insulin resistance is not included in the Rotterdam criteria of PCOS. Diagnosis and treatment are also independent on insulin resistance (Table 30.2).

Criteria have been developed for defining a *metabolic syndrome* (8–10). The metabolic syndrome should include three of the following five parameters:

Hormonal findings in women with PCOS include elevated serum concentration of luteinizing hormone (LH), and ovarian

Hypertension	≥130/85 mmHg
Triglyceride levels	≥150 mg/dL
HDL-cholesterol levels	<50 mg/dL
Abdominal obesity	>35 inches waist circumference
Fasting glucose	≥110 mg/dL or 2 hours glucose >140 mg/dL

Table 30.1: ESHRE/ASRM Definition of PCOS (2)

Presence of two out of the following three criteria

1. Oligo- and/or anovulation

2. Hyperandrogenism (clinical and/or biochemical)

3. PCO by ultrasound (follicular count of ≥12 follicles in each ovary of 2–9 mm in diameter and/or increased ovarian volume of >10 mL)

2003 Rotterdam PCOS concensus reproduced from reference 4.

Table 30.2: Summary of 2003 PCOS Consensus Regarding Screening for Metabolic Disorders

Summary of Rotterdam consensus recommendations

1. Tests for insulin resistance are not necessary to make the diagnosis or to treat PCOS.

2. Obese women with PCOS should be screened for the metabolic syndrome, including glucose intolerance with OGTT.

3. Further studies are necessary in nonobese women with PCOS to determine the utility of these tests, although they may be considered if additional risk factors for insulin resistance, such as family history of diabetes, are present.

2003 Rotterdam PCOS concensus reproduced from reference 4.

androgens [testosterone, androstenedione, dehydroepiandrosterone (DHA)] and, in 50 percent of patients, elevated dehydroepiandrosterone sulfate (DHAS) as adrenal contribution to the system. Estrone level is high mainly due to peripheral conversion of androstendione in the adipose tissues, whereas FSH level is usually low normal.

Sex hormone–binding globulin (SHBG) level is reduced by approximately 50 percent; this is related to increased level of circulating testosterone and hyperinsulinemia (6). The combination of these hormonal changes, peripheral insulin resistance with hyperinsulinemia, and high circulating bioavailable androgens lead to abnormal follicular development (8–10).

MANAGEMENT OF PCOS

Management of women with PCOS depends on the symptoms. These could be ovulatory dysfunction–related infertility, menstrual disorders, or hirsutism.

Weight Reduction

Obesity is observed in 35–60 percent of women with PCOS. The PCOS-related hyperandrogenism causes central obesity with high waist/hip ratio independent on the BMI. Weight loss improves the endocrine profile and increases the likelihood of ovulation and pregnancy. Normalization of the menstrual cycles and ovulation could occur with modest weight loss as little as 5 percent of the initial weight (9).

This could be achieved by diet (high protein, low carbohydrate, and low fat) with adaptation of weight loss programs to meet individual needs and avoidance of "crash diets" and short-term weight loss. In addition, behavior modification, stress reduction, and 150 minutes of regular exercise per week are recommended. It is important to provide long-term observation, monitoring, and encouragements to patients who have managed to lose weight (11, 12).

Treatment of Hirsutism

Oral Contraceptive Pills

In women who have no desire to conceive, they can be treated with oral contraceptive pills (OCPs) (Table 30.3). OCPs reduce hyperandrogenism by promoting direct negative feedback on LH secretion, which results in decreased ovarian synthesis of androgens. Further, it increases liver production of SHBG and subsequently decreases circulating free androgen. Other mechanisms include reduction in adrenal androgen secretion and inhibition of peripheral conversion of testosterone to dihydrotestesterone and binding of dihydrotestosterone to androgen receptors (13).

Most current OCPs contain 30–35 µg of ethinyl estradiol combined with a progestin with minimal androgenic activity (norethindrone, norgestimate, or desogestrel). One of the newest OCPs that might be more effective in reducing the growth of new terminal hair and acne formation is a formula that contains a combination of nonandrogenic progestin, *drospirenone*, and ethinyl estradiol (Yasmin, Berlex Canada, Pointe Claire, Quebec). Drospirenone is a spironolactone analog with mineralocorticoid activity; as a result, it has some diuretic property. However, it should not be prescribed to those predisposed to hyperkalemia. Treatment must be given for at least six to nine months before improvement in hirsutism can be seen (14).

Antiandrogens

Antiandrogens such as spironolactone, cyproterone acetate, or flutamide act by competitive inhibition of androgen-binding receptors or by decreasing androgen production.

Spironolactone (50–100 mg twice daily) can be added after four to six months of unsuccessful treatment with OCP alone (15).

Cyproterone acetate is a progestational antiandrogen. As expected, a combination of ethinyl estradiol and *cyproterone acetate* (Diane 35, Berlex, Montreal, Quebec) is very effective in treating hirsutism and acne. Apart from its antiandrogenic effect, cyproterone acetate has a marked progestational property preventing ovulation (15, 16). Loss of hair, which frequently accompanies seborrhea, also improves.

In moderate to severe forms of androgenization, cyproterone acetate only (Androcur, Berlex) 50–100 mg orally twice per day for two weeks followed by a maintenance dose of 25–50 mg daily can be given. Frequent monitoring of liver and renal function is necessary during therapy with antiandrogens. Similar to

Table 30.3: Medications Used for Hirsutism

Medications	Active ingredient	Oral daily dose	Mode of action	Side effects
Most anti androgenic oral contraceptives *	EE + drospirenone (Yasmin)	Ethinyl estradiol 30 μg + drospirenone 30 μg (one tablet daily)	Suppresses ovarian function and inhibition of androgen receptors	Irregular vaginal bleeding, venous thrombosis.
	EE + cyproterone acetate (Diane-35)	Ethinyl estradiol 30 μg + cyproterone acetate 2 mg (one tablet daily)	Suppresses ovarian function and competitive inhibitor of androgen receptors	Irregular vaginal bleeding, venous thrombosis, difficult loss of weight
Antiandrogens	Spironolactone	50–100 mg twice daily	Competitive inhibitor of androgen receptors	Feminization of male fetus, liver/renal dysfunction
	Cyproterone acetate (Androcur)	Induction 50–100 mg/twice daily for two weeks Maintenance 50 mg/once daily	Competitive inhibitor of androgen receptors	Feminization of male fetus
	Flutamide	125–250 mg, twice daily	Competitive inhibitor of androgen receptors	Feminization of male fetus, hepatotoxicity
	Finasteride	5 mg daily	Type 2, alpha reductase activity inhibitor	
Glucocorticoids	Prednisone	5–7.5 mg once, twice daily	Suppresses adrenal function	Cushing's syndrome
GnRH agonist	Leuprolide acetate (Lupron Depot)	3.75 monthly IM ± add-back estradiol (25–50 μg transdermal)	Suppresses gonadotropins and androgen	Menopausal symptoms and osteopenia

*Besides these two examples, all OCPs are eective in reducing hirsutism.

that of OCP, improvement of hirsutism is expected to be noticeable after six months of treatment. Although there is a considerable variation among individuals, the maximum effect is usually seen after nine to twelve months of antiandrogen treatment (17).

Flutamide is a pure antiandrogen that blocks androgen receptor by competitive inhibition. It is marketed for the treatment of prostate cancer and is very effective in treating hirsutism. However, it is rarely used alone due to its high cost and the risk of hepatocellular toxicity. Recent studies indicated that a combination of flutamide 62.5 mg daily with metformin 850 mg daily was more effective in improving symptoms of PCOS than oral contraceptive alone (18).

Finasteride is a type 2 (5 alpha reductase) activity inhibitor that inhibits the production of dihydrotestosterone. In a randomized trial, the authors compared the efficacy of *finasteride* (5 mg daily) and a combination of cyproterone acetate (25 mg/day on days 5–14) and ethinyl estradiol (20 μm daily on days 5–25) for nine months. Both treatments are equally effective in decreasing hirsutism (19).

Due to the risk of feminization of male fetus, pregnancy must be avoided during treatment with all antiandrogens (19, 20).

Glucocorticoid (5–7.5 mg of prednisone once or twice daily) has been shown to improve hirsutism in women with congenital adrenal hyperplasia. However, its effect on hirsutism due to other causes is unclear (20, 21).

Gonadotropin-releasing hormone agonist (GnRHa) is effective even in women with severe insulin resistance who are unresponsive to OCP (22, 23). GnRHa suppresses pituitary hormones, decreases androgen and estradiol secretion, and improves severe form of hirsutism. To avoid problems asso-

ciated with estrogen deficiency, "add-back" therapy with estrogen-progesterone or low-dose OCP is advisable. However, this method of treatment is expensive, limiting its use to severe forms of ovarian hyperandrogenism with hyperinsulinemia.

Treatment of Menstrual Dysfunction

Menstrual irregularities or dysfunctional uterine bleeding can be controlled with OCP alone. Those who do not need contraception or who have contraindication to estrogen can be treated with cyclic progesterone (medroxyprogesterone acetate 10 mg daily for five days) every two months (13). This will counteract the unopposed estrogen stimulation to the endometrium.

Treatment of Ovulatory Disorder

Clomiphene Citrate

For over four decades, the first line of treatment for ovulatory disorders has been clomiphene citrate (CC). CC is easy to use and results in ovulation in most patients (60–90 percent), but the pregnancy rates are disappointing (10–40 percent). This has been attributed to its peripheral antiestrogenic effects, mainly on the endometrium and the cervical mucus (9, 21–23). The multiple pregnancy rate associated with CC is 10–20 percent (22, 23).

Dexamethazone

In PCOS patients with high adrenal androgen, low-dose dexamethazone (0.25–0.5 mg) at bedtime can be used (22). In a randomized, placebo-controlled study, thirty-eight women with PCOS were randomized to receive either dexamethasone 0.25 mg daily or placebo for twenty-six weeks. All patients were treated with metformin 850 mg three times daily and lifestyle counseling. Compared with placebo, low dose of dexamethazone leads to a lower androgen level (20). In another study of 230 women with PCOS who failed to ovulate with 200 mg of CC for five days, addition of 2 mg of dexamethazone from days 5–14 is associated with a higher ovulation rate and cumulative pregnancy rate (21).

Gonadotropin

Gonadotropin is more effective than CC but is expensive and associated with a higher risk for ovarian hyperstimulation syndrome and multiple gestations. Unlike CC, gonadotropin does not exert peripheral antiestrogenic effect. Conventionally, gonadotropin is administered to patients who failed to respond to CC.

Several treatment protocols have been advocated such as step-up, low-dose step-up, and step-down regimens. Because of high sensitivity of PCO to gonadotropin, small increment of the doses every five to seven days was proposed to avoid the risk of severe ovarian hyperstimulation syndrome and multiple pregnancies (22, 23).

Aromatase Inhibitors

Selective aromatase inhibitors such anastrazole and letrozole are promising new ovulation-inducing agents. They are reversible and highly potent. Unlike CC that has a half-life of five to seven days, the mean half-life of anastrazole and letrozole is approximately forty five hours only (range, thirty–sixty hours). Ovulation regulation with aromatase inhibitors has been suggested to overcome the antiestrogenic effect of clomiphene citrate. Early trials on letrozole either alone or with gonadotropin have been shown to be effective (24–27).

In a small study, twelve PCOS patients with inadequate response to CC were treated with letrozole (24). Nine of the twelve patients ovulated (75 percent) and three conceived; the mean endometrial thickness was 8.1 mm (6.2 mm with CC). The same investigators subsequently evaluated the effects of a single dose of letrozole (20 mg on day 3 of the cycle) in seven patients (nine cycles). The number of follicles, serum estradiol level, and endometrial thickness in women treated with a single dose were similar to those treated with a five-day letrozole regime.

Al-Omari et al. (25) treated clomiphene-resistant PCOS women with 2.5 mg of letrozole (twenty-two patients) or 1 mg of anastrazole daily from days 3 to 7 of the cycle (eighteen patients). Endometrial thickness was thicker in the letrozole group (8.2 mm) than in the anastrazole group (6.5 mm). The ovulation rate in the letrozole group was 84.4 percent and in the anastrazole group was 60 percent. The pregnancy rates were also statistically higher in the letrozole than in the anastrazole group (18.8 vs. 9.7 percent per cycle, respectively). Although, the ideal dose of anastrazole is still unknown, it appears that the dose of 1 mg daily is much too low.

In a nonrandomized study, women with PCOS and those with other causes of infertility (unexplained infertility, male factor infertility, and endometriosis) were treated with either FSH alone or a combination of letrozole/FSH (27). In women with PCOS ($n = 26$), the pregnancy rate in letrozole/FSH group was 26.5 percent per cycle and in the FSH-only group ($n = 46$) was 18.5 percent per cycle. There was no significant difference

in the pregnancy rates among non-PCOS women treated either with letrozole/FSH ($n = 63$) or FSH alone ($n = 308$). The overall pregnancy rate was 11 percent per cycle. However, the additional letrozole to FSH treatment led to a lower FSH requirement without a significant difference in number of follicles of greater than 16 mm. These studies suggest that the addition of letrozole to gonadotropins decreases gonadotropin requirements, increases the number of preovulatory follicles, and decreases endometrial thickness without a negative effect on the pregnancy rates (27).

To date, letrozole has been studied much more extensively than anastrazole. The data on letrozole suggest that it can be used to replace CC as the first-line treatment for women with ovulatory disorders. For superovulation, there is a trend of higher pregnancy rate than that of CC. The ideal dose of letrozole is unknown; however, it seems that the dose of 5 mg daily for five days is the most effective (28).

GnRH Agonist and Antagonist

GnRH agonists play a major role in IVF treatment as well as in superovulation. To reduce LH concentrations throughout the follicular phase and to prevent a premature LH surge, downregulation with GnRHa followed by superovulation with gonadotropin has been advocated (29).

Bahceci et al. used a stimulation protocol incorporating Diane-35 and GnRH antagonist in patients with PCOS who were treated with IVF (30). The fertilization, pregnancy, and implantation rates were similar to those treated with GnRH agonist long protocol, with lower amounts of gonadotropin used and lower serum E_2 levels on the day of HCG injection (30). In a randomized study among women with PCOS undergoing IVF treatment, a combination of Diane and GnRH antagonist, cetrorelix, resulted in a similar pregnancy rate compared to the GnRH agonist long protocol (31).

Insulin-Sensitizing Agents

There are several pharmacological agents available to reduce insulin levels, and the most commonly used for women with PCOS is metformin (32).

Metformin

Metformin is biguanide antihyperglycemic agent. The precise mode of action of metformin is unclear but is believed to act directly at the level of the liver to suppress hepatic glucose output. It also improves peripheral insulin sensitivity, improves the utilization of glucose by skeletal muscles, and decreases intestinal glucose absorption. Metformin also improves the action of insulin at the cellular level by enhancing glucose uptake by fat and muscle cells and by increasing insulin receptor binding. Metformin exerts its beneficial effects on serum androgen in part by its effect on SHBG production by the liver, resulting in decreased free circulating testosterone. It also modulates adrenal androgen production and decreases intraovarian androgens production (32–34) (Table 30.4).

DOSE
Several doses regimen have been proposed (33–36). In order to increase patient tolerance, metformin is started at 500 mg daily with food. After one week, the dose is increased to 1,000 mg for another week and then to 1,500 mg daily. The target dose is 1,500–2,550 mg/day (500 mg or 850 mg three

Table 30.4: Effects of Metformin on the Clinical and Endocrine Parameter of PCOS

Clinical and endocrine parameters	Features of PCOS	Effect of metformin
GnRH pulse	High/frequent	No studies
Estrone	↑	↓
Free testosterone	↑	↓
Other ovarian androgen	↑	↓
DHAS	↑	↓
SHBG	↑	↓
LH	Steadily ↑	Normalize
FSH	↓	Normalize
Insulin	↑	↓
Clinical parameters		
Obesity	Waist circumference 35 inches	No effect
Hirsutism	Variable signs	Improve
Ovulation	Irregular	Improve
Menstruation	Irregular	Normalize
Sleep apnea	At risk	No studies
Epilepsy	More prevalent	No studies
Cardiovascular disease risk	At risk	Risk reduced
Type 2 diabetes	At risk	Control hyperglycemia

Table 30.5: Results of Metformin Treatment in Women with PCOS (Adapted from Ref. 50)

Ovulation rate	82 percent after sixteen weeks of treatment
Pregnancy rate	55 percent with metformin/clomiphene for six months
Miscarriage rate	8.8 percent compared to 41.9 percent in the control group
Hirsutism	Conflicting results
In vitro fertilization	Decreased cancellation, decreased risks of hyperstimulation

Fertil Steril 2003 Aug; 80(2):241–51. Permission to reproduce from the American Society of Reproductive Medicine should be obtained by the publisher.

8 percent ongoing pregnancy of more than thirteen weeks gestation (37) (Table 30.5).

PREGNANCY AND OFFSPRING

Traditionally, oral hypoglycemic agent has been regarded as teratogenic and its use is contraindicated in pregnancy. However, an increasing amount of data support its safety when used throughout the pregnancy. Glueck et al. reported no major birth defects and no effect on motor or social development of infants at three and six months of age (38). Compared with the control group of women who did not receive metformin, the incidence of gestational diabetes in the treated group was significantly lower (4 percent) (38, 39).

EFFECTS OF METFORMIN IN OBESE AND NONOBESE PCOS WOMEN

Tang et al. studied the effect of metformin versus placebo on weight reduction and menstrual frequency in 143 patients (11). They found that metformin did not improve weight loss or menstrual irregularities among obese women with PCO. However, weight loss alone improves menstrual cyclicity, ovulation, and hyperandrogenism in some women. Other studies showed that metformin treatment led to a significant improvement in total testosterone, free testosterone, and androstenedione concentrations in nonobese women but only in free testosterone in obese women (39–42).

Troglitazone, Rosiglitazone, and Pioglitazone

Troglitazone is another insulin-sensitizing drug that has been shown to improve ovulation and increases pregnancy rates. However, due to its hepatotoxic effect, it has been withdrawn from the market (43). Another drug in the same category, *rosiglitazone* (8 mg/day), has been shown to enhance both spontaneous and clomiphene-induced ovulation in women with PCOS with mean BMI of 35.5–38.5 kg/m². *Pioglitazone* appears to be effective as well; however, the study is still limited.

Both rosiglitazone and pioglitazone are classified as category C drugs where they should be given if the potential benefit justifies the potential risk to the fetus. Metformin, on the other

times daily). Clinical response is usually seen at the dose of 1,000 mg daily. It appears that some PCOS patients who did not respond to metformin at a dose of 1,500 mg daily will respond favorably to 2,000 mg daily (33).

SIDE EFFECTS

The most common side effects of metformin are nausea and diarrhea. In order to decrease these side effects, metformin can be ingested with food. Other untoward effects are bloating, flatulence, or vomiting. These side effects are dose dependent and could be mitigated by an incremental dosing protocol. Lactic acidosis has been described mainly in patients with renal impairment, congestive heart failure, and sepsis.

OVULATION AND BMI

A recent meta-analysis demonstrated that metformin is effective in achieving ovulation in women with PCOS with odds ratio of 3.88 (CI 2.25–6.69) for metformin alone and 4.41 (CI 2.37–8.22) for metformin in combination with clomiphene. No beneficial effect of metformin on BMI or waist/hip ratio was found; however, it was associated with a reduction in blood pressure and a slight decrease in LDL-cholesterol (33). In a study evaluating the pregnancy outcomes among seventy-two oligomenorrheic women with PCOS treated with metformin, the authors reported 81 percent spontaneous pregnancy, 75 percent live birth rate, 17 percent spontaneous abortion, and

Table 30.6: Medical Management of PCOS

Clinical problem	Management options
Obesity	■ Lifestyle modification
	■ Weight reduction
	■ Exercise
	■ Diet modification (low fat, low calorie)
Menstrual irregularity	OCPs
Contraception desired	Medroxy progesterone acetate 5–10 mg (up to 30 mg), q.d. for five to ten days/month or every two months
No contraception desired	
Hyperandrogenism	■ OCPs with antiandrogens
	☐ EE + drospirenone (Yasmin)
	☐ EE + cyproterone acetate (Diane-35)
	■ Antiandrogens: spironolactone, cyproterone acetate, flutamide, finasteride
	■ Glucocorticoid
	■ GnRH agonist and antagonists
Insulin resistance	Insulin-sensitizing agents
	1. Metformin
	2. Troglitazone, rosiglitazone, and pioglitazone
	3. Acarbose
Ovulatory disorder	■ Metformin
	■ CC
	■ Aromatase inhibitor
	■ FSH
	■ Assisted reproductive technology (IVF/IVM)

hand, is a category B drug that appears to be safe during pregnancy for the mother and fetus (38, 43).

Administration of D-chiro-inositol as a putative insulin-sensitizing drug in patients with PCOS has also been investigated. It reduces circulating insulin, decreases serum androgens in lean women with PCOS, and ameliorates some of the metabolic abnormalities (increased blood pressure and hypertriglyceridemia) of syndrome X (44).

Acarbose

Acarbose is a pseudotetrasaccharide glucosidase inhibitor, an antidiabetic drug that reduces hydrolysis and absorption of the polysaccharides (45, 46). Penna et al. (45) conducted a double-blind placebo-controlled study in thirty obese hyper-

insulinemic women with PCOS. Women were treated with 150 mg/day acarbose or placebo for six months. The treatment is associated with a reduction in free androgen index and BMI. Hirsutism and menstrual irregularities improved. It appears that acarbose is a good alternative for obese women with PCOS. However, the safety of this drug in pregnancy is still unclear.

LAPAROSCOPIC TREATMENT OF PCO

In 2000, we reported that laparoscopic treatment of PCO with insulated unipolar cautery (ovarian drilling) in 112 clomiphene-resistant women with PCOS-related anovulatory infertility resulted in a cumulative pregnancy of 36, 54, 68, and 82 percent at six, twelve, eighteen, and twenty-four months of follow-up, respectively (47). However, treatment with metformin is equally efficacious in correcting the clinical, endocrine, and metabolic abnormalities associated with PCOS (48–50). As a result, this procedure is rarely performed in our institution.

Our first line of management is advocating weight reduction followed by a trial of treatment with metformin alone and in combination with ovulation-inducing agents for up to three cycles. LOD is used sparingly. (see chapter 31 for clinical details and different approach.)

CONCLUSIONS

Management of women with PCOS should be started with lifestyle modifications and weight reduction (Table 30.6). Menstrual and ovulatory dysfunction should be managed as a part of the syndrome. The type of treatment including OCP, antiandrogen, or ovarian stimulation is dependent on the reproductive need of the patients.

Metformin has replaced the surgical treatment of PCOS with ovarian drilling. Metformin improves insulin resistance and hyperandrogenism, decreases serum lipids, and improves glucose homeostasis. The effects of unopposed estrogen stimulation on the endometrium could be reversed with OCP or oral progestins.

REFERENCES

1. Speroff l, Fritz M. Anovulation and polycystic ovary. In: Clinical Gynecologic Endocrinology and Infertility, 7th edn. Lippincott Williams and Wilkins, Baltimore, MA, 2005; pp. 470–83.
2. Azziz R. Diagnostic criteria for polycystic ovary syndrome: a reappraisal. *Fertil Steril* 2005;83:1343–6.
3a. The Rotterdam ESHRE/ASRM Sponsored PCOS concensus workshop group. Revised 2003 consensus on diagnostic criteria and long-term health risks related to polycystic ovary syndrome (PCOS). *Hum Reprod* 2004;19:41–7.
3b. The Rotterdam ESHRE/ASRM Sponsored PCOS concensus workshop group. Revised 2003 consensus on diagnostic criteria and long-term health risks related to polycystic ovary syndrome (PCOS). *Fertil Steril* 2004;19–25.
4. Bucket WM, Bouzayen R, Watkin KL, Tulandi T, Tan SL. Ovarian stromal echogenicity in women with normal and polycystic ovaries. *Hum Reprod* 2003;18:598–603.
5. Hardiman P, Pillay OC, Atiomo W. Polycystic ovary syndrome and endometrial carcinoma. *Lancet* 2003;361:1810.
6. Ducluzeau PH, Cousin P, Malyoisin E, Bornet H, Vidal H, Laville M, Pugeat M. Glucose-to-insulin ratio rather than sex

hormone-binding globulin and adiponectin levels is the best predictor of insulin resistance in nonobese women with polycystic ovary syndrome. *J Clin Endocrinol Metab* 2003;88:3626–31.

7. Ciampelli M, Leoni F, Cucinelli F, Mancuso S, Panunzi S, De Gaetano A, Lanzone A. Assessment of insulin sensitivity from measurements in the fasting state and during an oral glucose tolerance test in polycystic ovary syndrome and menopausal patients. *J Clin Endocrinol Metab* 2005;90:1398–406.

8. Apridonidze T, Essah PA, Iuorno MJ, Nestler JE. Prevalence and characteristics of the metabolic syndrome in women with polycystic ovary syndrome. *J Clin Endocrinol Metab* 2005;90:1929–35.

9. Patel SM, Nestler JE. Fertility in polycystic ovary syndrome. *Endocrinol Metab Clin North Am* 2006;35:137–55.

10. Lakhani K, Prelevic GM, Seifalian AM, Atiomo WU, Hardiman P. Polycystic ovary syndrome, diabetes and cardiovascular disease: risks and risk factors. *J Obstet Gynaecol* 2004;24:613–21.

11. Tang T, Glanville J, Hayden CJ, White D, Barth JH, Balen AH. Combined life style modification and metformin in obese patients with polycystic ovary syndrome a randomized placebo-controlled, double-blinded multicentre study. *Hum Reprod* 2006;21:80–9.

12. Moran LJ, Noakes M, Clifton PM, et al. Dietary composition in restoring reproductive and metabolic physiology in overweight women with polycystic ovary syndrome. *J Clin Endocrinol Metab* 2003;88:812–19.

13. Aziz R. Use of combination oral contraceptives in the treatment of hyperandrogenism and hirsutism. UpToDate, Clinical Reference Library 2006. www.uptodate.com

14. Falsetti L, Gambera A, Tisi G. Efficacy of the combination ethinyl estradiol and cyproterone acetate on endocrine, clinical and ultrasonographic profile in polycystic ovarian syndrome. *Hum Reprod* 2001;16:36–42.

15. Falsetti L, Gambra A, Platto C, Legrenzi L. Management of hirsutism. *Am J Clin Dermatol* 2000;1:89–99.

16. Rosenfield RL. Clinical practice, hirsutism. *N Engl J Med* 2005;15;353:2578–88.

17. Barbieri R. Treatment of hirsutism. UpToDate, Clinical Reference Library 2006. www.uptodate.com

18. Ibáñez L, De Zegher F. Low-dose flutamide-metformin therapy for hyperinsulinemic hyperandrogenism in non-obese adolescents and women. *Hum Reprod Update* 2006;10.1093.

19. Beigi A, Sobhi A, Zarrinkoub F. Finasteride versus cyproterone acetate-estrogen regimens in the treatment of hirsutism. *Int J Gynaecol Obstet* 2004;87:29–33.

20. Vanky E, Salvesen KA, Carlsen SM. Six-month treatment with low-dose dexamethasone further reduces androgen levels in PCOS women treated with diet and lifestyle advice, and metformin. *Hum Reprod* 2004;19:529–33.

21. Parsanezhad ME, Alborzi S, Motazedian S, Omrani G. Use of dexamethasone and clomiphene citrate in the treatment of clomiphene citrate-resistant patients with polycystic ovary syndrome and normal dehydroepiandrosterone sulfate levels: a prospective, double-blind, placebo-controlled trial. *Fertil Steril* 2002;5:1001–4.

22. Nugent D, Vandekerckhove P, Hughes E, Arnot M, Lilford R. Gonadotropin therapy for ovulation induction in sub fertility associated with polycystic ovary syndrome (Cochrane Review). The Cochrane Library, (4):, CD000410. 2000. Oxford: update Software

23. Cristello F, Cela V, Artini PG, Genazzani AR. Therapeutic strategies for ovulation induction in infertile women with polycystic ovary syndrome. *Gynecol Endocrinol* 2005;21:340–352.

24. Mitwally MF, Casper RF. Aromatase inhibition improves ovarian response to follicle-stimulating hormone in poor responders. *Fertil Steril* 2002;77:776–80.

25. Al-Omari WR, Suliman WR, Al-Hadithi N. Comparison of two aromatase inhibitors in women with clomiphene-resistant polycystic ovary syndrome. *Int J Gynaecol Obstet* 2004;85: 289–91.

26. Al-Fozan H, Al-Khadouri M, Tan SL, Tulandi T. A randomized trial of letrozole versus clomiphene citrate in women undergoing super ovulation. *Fertil Steril* 2004;82:1561–1563.

27. Healy S, Tan SL, Tulandi T, Biljan M. Effects of letrozole on superovulation with gonadotropins in women undergoing intrauterine insemination. *Fertil Steril* 2003;80:1325–9.

28. Al-Fadhli R, Sylvestre C, Buckett W, Tan SL, Tulandi T. A randomized trial of superovulation with two different doses of letrozole. *Fertil Steril* 2006;85:161–4.

29. Grana-Barcia M, Liz-Leston J, Lado-Abeal J. Subcutaneous administration of pulsatile gonadotropin-releasing hormone decreases serum follicle-stimulating hormone and luteinizing hormone levels in women with polycystic ovary syndrome: a preliminary study. *Fertil Steril* 2005;83:1466–72.

30. Bahceci M, Ulug U, Ben-Shalomo I, Erden HF, Akman MA. Use of a GnRH antagonist in controlled ovarian hyperstimulation for assisted conception in women with polycystic ovary disease: a randomized, prospective, pilot study. *J Reprod Med* 2005; 50:84–90.

31. Hwang JL, Seow KM, Lin YH, Huang LW, Hsieh BC, Tsai YL, Wu GJ, Huang SC, Chen CY, Chen PH, Tzeng CR. Ovarian stimulation by concomitant administration of cetrorelix acetate and HMG following Diane-35 pre-treatment for patients with polycystic ovary syndrome: a prospective randomized study. *Hum Reprod* 2004;19:1993–2000.

32. Cheang KI, Nestler JE. Should insulin-sensitizing drugs be used in the treatment of polycystic ovary syndrome? *Reprod Biomed Online* 2004;8:440–7.

33. Harborne LR, Sattar N, Norman JE, Fleming R. Metformin and weight loss in obese women with polycystic ovary syndrome: comparison of doses. *J Am Assoc Gynecol Laparosc* 2005;90(8): 4593–8.

34. Lord JM, Flight IHK, Norman RJ. Insulin-sensitizing drugs (metformin, troglitazone, rosiglitazone, pioglitazone, D-chiro-inositol) for polycystic ovary syndrome. *Cochrane Database Syst Rev* 2003;(2), Art. No: CD003053. DOI:10.1002/14651858.CD003053.

35. Yilmaz M, Karakoc A, Toruner FB, Cakir N, Tiras B, Ayvaz G, Arslan M. The effects of rosiglitazone and metformin on menstrual cyclicity and hirsutism in polycystic ovary syndrome. *Gynecol Endocrinol* 2005;21:154–60.

36. Moghetti P, Castello R, Negri C, Tosi F, Perrone F, Caputo M, et al. Metformin effects on clinical features, endocrine and metabolic profiles, and insulin sensitivity in polycystic ovary syndrome: a randomized, double blinded, placebo controlled 6 month trial, followed by open, long term clinical evaluation. *J Clin Endocrinol Metab* 2000;85:139–46.

37. Eisenhardt S, Schwarzmann N, Henschel V, Germeyer A, von Wolff M, Hamann A, Strowitzki T. Early effects of metformin in women with polycystic ovary syndrome (PCOS): a prospective randomized double blind placebo controlled trial. *J Clin Endocrinol Metab* 2005;10:1210.

38. Glueck CJ, Wang P, Goldenberg N, Sieve-Smith L. Pregnancy outcomes among women with polycystic ovary syndrome treated with metformin. *Hum Reprod* 2002;17:2858–64.

39. Glueck CJ, Goldenberg N, Wang P, Loftspring M, Sherman A. Metformin during pregnancy reduces insulin, insulin resistance, insulin secretion, weight, testosterone and the development of gestational diabetes: prospective longitudinal assessment of women with polycystic ovary syndrome from preconception throughout pregnancy. *Hum Reprod* 2004;19:510–21.

40. Baillargeon JP, Jakubowicz DJ, Iuorno MJ, Jakubowicz S, Nestler JE: Effects of metformin and rosiglitazone, alone and in combination, in nonobese women with polycystic ovary syndrome and normal indices of insulin sensitivity. *Fertil Steril* 2004;82:893–902.

41. Glueck CJ, Moreira A, Goldenberg N, Sieve-Smith L, Wang P. Pioglitazone and metformin in obese women with polycystic ovary syndrome not primarily responsive to metformin. *Hum Reprod* 2003;18:1618–25.

42. Maciel GA, Junior JM, deMaotta EL, Abi Haidar M, deLima GR, Baracat E. Nonobese women with polycystic ovary syndrome respond better than obese women to treatment with metformin. *Fertil Steril* 2004;81:355–60.

43. Azziz R, Ehrmann D, Legro RS, Whitcomb RW, Hanley R, Fereshetian AG. PCOS/Troglitazone Study Group. Troglitazone improves ovulation and hirsutism in the polycystic ovary syndrome: a multicenter, double blind, placebo-controlled trial. *J Clin Endocrinol Metab* 2001;86:1626–32.

44. Iuorno MJ, Jakubowicz DJ, Baillargeon JP, Dillon P, Gunn RD, Allan G, Nestler JE. Effects of d-chiro-inositol in lean women with the polycystic ovary syndrome. *Endocrinol Pract* 2002;8:417–23.

45. Penna IA, Canella PR, Reis RM, Silva de Sa MF, Ferriani RA. Acarbose in obese patients with polycystic ovarian syndrome: a double-blind, randomized, placebo-controlled study. *Hum Reprod* 2005;20:2396–401.

46. Ciotta L, Calogero AE, Farina M, De Leo V, La Marca A, Cianci A. Clinical, endocrine and metabolic effects of acarbose, an α-glucosidase inhibitor, in PCOS patients with increased insulin response and normal glucose tolerance. *Hum Reprod* 2001;16:2066–72.

47. Felemban A, Tan SL, Tulandi T. Laparoscopic treatment of polycystic ovaries with insulated needle cautery: a reappraisal. *Fertil Steril* 2000;73:266–9.

48. Palomba S, Orio FJr., Falbo A, Russo T, Caterina G, Manguso F, Tolinos A, Colao A, Zullo F. Metformin administration and laparoscopic ovarian drilling improve ovarian response to clomiphene citrate in oligo-anovulatory clomiphene citrate resistant women with polycystic ovary syndrome. *Clin Endocrinol* 2005;63:631–5.

49. Al-Fadhli R, Tulandi T. Laparoscopic treatment of polycystic ovaries: is its place diminishing? *Curr Opin Obstet Gynecol* 2004;16:295–8.

50. Pirwany I, Tulandi T. Laparoscopic treatment of polycystic ovaries: is it time to relinquish the procedure. *Fertil Steril* 2003;80:241–51.

31

Surgical Management of Polycystic Ovary Syndrome

Hakan Yarali, Gurkan Bozdag, Ibrahim Esinler

INTRODUCTION

Polycystic ovarian syndrome (PCOS) is a common and ill-understood endocrine disorder with multisystem sequelae. Clinical presentation is variable. It is characterized clinically by oligoamenorrhoea, signs of androgen excess such as hirsutism, acne, alopecia, obesity, and infertility, biochemically by elevation of serum androgens, luteinizing hormone (LH), and LH/follicular-stimulating hormone (FSH) ratio and not infrequently by insulin resistance (1). Morphologically, the ovaries are enlarged and have thick shiny capsules with peripherally placed multiple intermediate sized (2–8 mm in diameter) follicles. However, not all patients with clinically or endocrinologically defined PCOS demonstrate polycystic ovaries, nor do all women with polycystic ovaries have PCOS. Among 257 "normal volunteers," 23 percent were found to have polycystic ovaries, and of the patients with polycystic ovaries, only about 50 percent had PCOS (2). Alternatively, of those women with PCOS, approximately, 70 percent have polycystic ovaries on ultrasonographic examination (3).

The diagnostic criteria of PCOS have been recently revised after a joint meeting of the European Society for Human Reproduction (ESHRE) and American Society for Reproductive Medicine (ASRM) in Rotterdam in May 2003 (4). It was agreed that the diagnosis of PCOS required the presence of at least two of the following three criteria: 1) oligo- and/or anovulation, 2) hyperandrogenism (clinical and/or biochemical), and 3) ultrasonographic appearance of polycystic ovaries, after the exclusion of other etiological factors (4).

Furthermore, the diagnosis of polycystic ovaries has been revised to include at least one of the following: either twelve or more follicles measuring 2–9 mm in diameter, or increased ovarian volume (>10 cm^3) (5). If there is a follicle larger than 10 mm in diameter, the scan should be repeated at a time of ovarian quiescence in order to calculate volume and area. The distribution of follicles and a description of the stroma are no longer required in the diagnosis. However, there is still room for improvement of the Rotterdam Criteria, which may carry the risk of misinterpretation and under- and overestimation of symptoms, as well as of overlooking other hyperandrogenic states (6).

HISTORY OF SURGICAL TREATMENT

Surgical treatment of PCOS associated with infertility, wedge resection of the ovaries, was first reported by Stein and Leventhal (7). They observed restoration of regular menstruation in approximately 80 percent and spontaneous conception in about 50 percent of the patients so treated (8). Stein (9) and others (10) subsequently reported similar results. However, the procedure, whether performed by laparotomy or laparoscopy, is associated with a high percentage of ovarian and periadnexal adhesions (11) that may even lead to infertility in some of the subjects. Ovarian resection, whether performed by laparoscopy or laparotomy, is associated with substantial tissue loss. Furthermore, it may lead to premature ovarian failure if the vascular supply to the ovary is compromised (12). For these reasons, the procedure has largely been abandoned after initial experiences for a period of time.

The introduction of laparoscopic ovarian drilling (LOD) has reawakened interest in surgical treatment of PCOS in patients unresponsive to clomiphene citrate (CC) treatment (13). The procedure is performed in an endeavor to induce ovulation and pregnancy in those women who are resistant to clomiphene citrate.

The alternative strategies in the presence of resistance to CC in patients with PCOS also consist of exogenous gonadotrophins. Exogenous gonadotrophin treatment is commonly employed in infertile PCOS patients who do not respond to CC treatment. Alternative therapeutic options also include glucocorticoids, insulin sensitizers, aromatase inhibitors, and LOD. Although initial studies are promising for the new alternative treatment options, including first-line treatment with insulin sensitizers (14) or aromatase inhibitors (15), their place in routine clinical practice remains uncertain until data from randomized controlled trials employing large series of well-defined patient groups are available.

TECHNIQUE OF OVARIAN DRILLING

Ovarian drilling, or "ovarian electrocautery," is the creation of multiple openings through the ovarian capsule using laparoscopy, laparotomy, or hydrolaparoscopy for surgical access. This can be accomplished electrosurgically using a pointed monopolar or bipolar electrode or with laser energy (CO_2, argon, Nd:YAG, and KTP). In the technique of laparoscopy, instruments should be introduced through two auxiliary portals and each ovary should be immobilized in turn out of harm's way. Each of these craters should be approximately 3 mm in diameter and 4–5 mm in depth. This can be achieved using an insulated monopolar electrode of 1.5–2 mm in diameter with a conical tip. The denuded tip of the electrode should be inserted perpendicular to the ovary for about 3–4 mm, applying 30 W of coagulating current for about four seconds. Depending on the size of the ovary, five to twelve openings are drilled through the capsule. The procedure is concluded by ensuring presence of appropriate hemostasis and by performing a pelvic lavage (16).

There is paucity of data on the optimal energy modality to be used during LOD. Saleh and Khalil (17) reviewed ten studies in which cumulative ovulation and pregnancy rates at twelve months after LOD with electrocoagulation were assessed. They noted that cumulative spontaneous ovulation and pregnancy rates were 82.7 and 64.8 percent at twelve months, respectively, in LOD with electrocoagulation. In the same review, ten studies in which cumulative ovulation and pregnancy rates at twelve months after LOD with laser (6 Nd:YAG, 2 CO_2, 1 CO_2 + KPT, and 1 argon) were reviewed. The respective figures for LOD with laser were 77.5 and 54.5 percent. Although there was no statistically significant difference in ovulation rates following LOD with electrocoagulation or laser (OR 1.4; 95 percent CI 0.9–2.1), a significantly higher cumulative pregnancy rate at twelve months with electrocoagulation was noted (OR 1.5; 95 percent CI 1.1–2.1). The authors hypothesized that the discrepancy between ovulation and pregnancy rates might be due to a greater rate extent of adhesion formation with laser compared to electrocoagulation (17). In concordance this hypothesis, Felemban and Tulandi (18) in their review reported that LOD with laser produced more adhesions than with electrocautery (41.5 vs. 31 percent, respectively; $p < 0.05$). There are limited data on the impact of using different types of laser during LOD on postoperative adhesion formation. CO_2 laser may be associated with a greater extent of adhesion formation than the Nd:YAG laser (19).

Recently, Malkawi and Qublan (20) evaluated the impact of the number of punctures per ovary on the outcome. Five punctures per ovary were compared with ten per ovary in sixty-three clomiphene citrate–resistant women with PCOS. Five punctures per ovary, instead of ten, were sufficient to ameliorate the hyperandrogenic status. Comparable ovulation, pregnancy, multiple pregnancy, and ovarian hyperstimulation syndrome (OHSS) rates were noted in the two groups. However, the study population was too small to make definite conclusions. In another study, Amer et al. (21) showed that four punctures per ovary using a power setting of 30 W for a duration of five seconds per puncture (i.e., 600 J per ovary) appeared to be sufficient to produce an optimal response. They reported that the chance of spontaneous ovulation and conception may be reduced with less than four punctures per ovary. Dabirashrafi (22) reported a case of severe ovarian failure in which eight punctures were created at 400 W. Further studies are warranted to establish the optimum number of punctures to be made to achieve the best ovulation and pregnancy rates, while minimizing the risk of periadnexal adhesions and ovarian failure.

Although surgical access is traditionally via laparoscopy, the procedure may be also carried out by transvaginal hydrolaparoscopy (THL) (23). With hydrolaparoscopy, the surgical principles remain the same. Hydrolaparoscopy is carried out first. A Veress needle is used to enter the peritoneal cavity through the pouch of Douglas. Approximately, 300 mL of normal saline solution is instilled into the peritoneal cavity. Thereafter, a special introducer with a 5-French caliber operative channel is inserted into the distended pouch of Douglas, which permits the introduction of a 2.9-mm scope with a 30-degree lens. After appropriate examination of the pelvic organs, a special bipolar electrode is introduced through the operating channel to carry out the ovarian drilling (23).

Fernandez et al. (23) evaluated the feasibility, ovulation, and pregnancy rates of drilling with bipolar electrocautery via THL in thirteen CC-resistant anovulatory women with PCOS. Mean ($\pm$SD) duration of follow-up time was 6.3 $\pm$ 3.3 months. Six patients recovered to have regular ovulatory cycles. Six pregnancies occurred; three were spontaneous, two occurred with ovarian stimulation and intrauterine insemination, and one occurred after in vitro fertilization (IVF). The cumulative pregnancy rates at three and six months were 33 and 71 percent, respectively. There was no miscarriage. No surgical complication occurred. The authors concluded that ovarian drilling via THL may be an alternative, minimally invasive procedure in patients with PCOS who are resistant to clomiphene therapy.

Branigan et al. (24) evaluated the impact of sonographic oocyte retrieval procedure on subsequent spontaneous ovulation and pregnancy rates in CC-resistant PCOS failing to conceive with IVF. Sixty-four patients failing to conceive with IVF were randomly assigned into two groups. Group I ($n = 34$) had a "thorough" (all follicles including those <10 mm in diameter), and group II ($n = 30$) had a routine (follicles >10 mm in diameter) sonographic oocyte retrieval during IVF. Following failure of IVF, the patients were monitored for steroid hormone levels, evidence of spontaneous ovulation and pregnancy. Cumulative ovulation and pregnancy rates of 53 percent (18/34) and 44 percent (8/18) at six months, respectively, were observed in group I, whereas no ovulation was noted in group II. Significant decreases in LH/FSH ratio (4.1–1.7) and serum testosterone (1.2–0.7 ng/mL) levels were documented in group I, with no significant change in group II. The authors concluded that thorough sonographic oocyte retrieval during in IVF cycle may improve the endocrine status and achieve ovulation and pregnancy rates comparable with those of ovarian wedge resection (24).

MECHANISM OF ACTION OF LOD

The mechanism of action of LOD is unclear. Its beneficial effect is apparently due to destruction of the androgen-producing stroma. This results in a reduction in intraovarian androgen production and decreased circulating androgen concentrations (25, 26). The reduction in total and free testosterone is approximately 50 percent below preoperative concentrations. After LOD, the ovarian volume increases transiently, followed by a reduction.

The serum LH concentration increases immediately after the procedure (27) and then decreases (25, 28). The LH pulse amplitudes are markedly reduced, but the LH pulse frequencies do not change. Pituitary responsiveness to GnRH stimulation also decreases concomitantly with a decline in serum testosterone concentration (29), suggesting that the procedure has an indirect modulating effect on the pituitary-ovarian axis (25).

The effect of LOD on FSH is variable and less pronounced (28). The FSH concentration generally increases rapidly and, thereafter, demonstrates a cyclical rise in keeping with restoration of ovulation. Normal inhibin pulsatility is restored, in association with the onset of regular ovulatory cycles, reflecting the resumption of normal intraovarian paracrine signaling (30). These endocrine changes occur rapidly (25, 31) and are sustained for several years (32, 33) and result in recruitment of new cohort of follicles and restoration of ovulation in most of the subjects.

OVULATION AND CONCEPTION AFTER OVARIAN DRILLING

Numerous published case studies (13, 18, 34–37) have demonstrated that the majority of the PCOS patients who are clomiphene resistant ovulated after drilling (56–94 percent) and that at least half of them obtain a pregnancy (43–84 percent) (Table 31.1).

Considerable variation exists in the reported outcomes of LOD. This is not only the result of the variations of technique but to a large extent the heterogeneity of the patient sample. Although the diagnostic criteria were recently revised (Rotterdam ESHRE/ASRM Sponsored PCOS Consensus Workshop Group, 2004), the criteria that have been used to diagnose the syndrome varied from continent to continent. Whereas in Europe and England the diagnosis was primarily based on ovarian morphology as assessed by transvaginal ultrasound scan, in North America it was based on biochemical features especially that of hyperandrogenemia and chronic anovulation.

Using life-table analysis, Heylen et al. (38) reported cumulative pregnancy rates of 68, 73, and 73 percent, respectively, at 12, 18, and 24 months after LOD with argon laser. In their series, not all patients were previously treated with CC. Li et al. (39), in a series of 111 patients, reported cumulative pregnancy rates of 54, 62, and 68 percent, respectively, at 12, 18, and 24 months follow-up. Felemban et al. (18), following LOD, with an insulated needle electrode, in 112 CC-resistant women reported cumulative pregnancy rates of 36, 54, 68, and 82 percent, respectively, at 6, 12, 18, and 24 months following the procedure. Predictive factors for pregnancy following LOD are younger age and lower body mass index (40, 41).

There are additional advantages provided by LOD. Patients who were resistant to CC may respond to this medication after the procedure (31). Sensitivity to exogenous gonadotrophin treatment is increased (13, 42, 43). Gonadotrophin treatment following LOD is associated with a lower duration of stimulation, lower total dose of gonadotrophins, and higher pregnancy rates. In women undergoing IVF, LOD improves reproductive outcome (44). There is more orderly growth of follicles, serum estradiol concentrations are lower, and the rate of cycle cancellation is reduced, as is the incidence of ovarian hyperstimulation (44–47).

LOD may, therefore, be useful in patients who have previously developed OHSS. LOD has been reported to decrease serum concentrations of vascular endothelial growth factor (VEGF) and insulin-like growth factor-1 (IGF-1), which are typically increased in patients with PCOS (48). The ovarian stromal blood flow, which is significantly lower in PCOS patients, is also increased after the procedure. These changes may contribute to a decreased risk of OHSS following LOD.

Ovarian drilling appears to decrease the spontaneous abortion rate associated with PCOS (32, 49). In a prospective randomized trial, the miscarriage rate following LOD was 21

Table 31.1: Ovulation and Pregnancy Rates following LOD

Author	Year	N	Ovulation (%)	Pregnancy (%)
Aakvaag and Gjonnaess[a] (34)	1985	58	72	NA
Daniell and Miller[b] (72)	1989	85	71	56
Utsunomiya et al.[c] (35)	1990	16	94	50
Campo et al.[c] (36)	1993	23	56	43
Gjonnaess[a] (56)	1994	252	92	84
Kriplani et al.[a] (37)	2001	66	82	55
Felemban et al.[a] (18)	2000	112	73	58

Performed with [a]electrosurgery, [b]laser, and [c]biopsy.

percent less than that of control women with PCOS (49). Amer et al., in a long-term follow-up study, reported a reduction in the miscarriage rate from 54 to 17 percent following LOD (32). In contrast, pretreatment with LOD was noted not to decrease the miscarriage rate after IVF (45). A systematic review of published studies also failed to reveal a difference in the miscarriage rates between women undergoing LOD and those taking gonadotrophins (50).

REPEAT LOD

Amer et al. (21) assessed the effectiveness of a second LOD in twenty women with PCOS and infertility. All twenty had drilling procedures one to six years before. Twelve of these responded positively to the first procedure, but their anovulatory status recurred; in the remaining eight women, the procedure did not yield any response. Following the second drilling procedure, twelve out of twenty (60 percent) started to ovulate and ten out of nineteen (53 percent) became pregnant. It is interesting to note that among the twelve women who had responded to the first procedure, ten (83 percent) became ovulatory, and eight became (67 percent) pregnant. However, of the eight who did not respond to the initial drilling, only two (25 percent) ovulated and were successful at achieving a pregnancy. Furthermore, statistically significant hormonal changes after repeat drilling, including reduction in serum LH, testosterone, and free androgen index, were only observed in the previous responder group. The authors concluded that repeat LOD is highly effective in women who previously responded to the first procedure.

COMPARISON WITH EXOGENOUS GONADOTROPHIN TREATMENT

Ovulation induction with gonadotrophins is commonly used in patients failing to ovulate with CC. Extensive monitoring is necessary because of the high sensitivity of polycystic ovaries to exogenous gonadotrophins, with the risk of multiple follicle development leading to termination of the cycle, OHSS, or multiple pregnancies. To reduce these complications, low-dose regimens are recommended (51).

The choice between the use of gonadotrophins or ovarian drilling in the treatment of CC-resistant PCOS patients continues to be a subject of debate. Four published trials and two abstracts compared surgical treatment with gonadotrophins in patients with CC-resistant PCOS (49, 50, 52, 53). The majority of the studies found no differences in rates for ovulation, pregnancy, and miscarriage (49, 52–54). Farquhar et al. (54) carried out a randomized controlled trial to compare LOD with gonadotrophin treatment. All of the patients were younger than thirty-nine years of age, had a BMI of less than 35 kg/m^2, and twelve months of infertility with no other causes and failed to ovulate with CC (up to 150 mg per day for five days). The gonadotrophin treatment was carried out for three cycles. There were twenty-nine patients in the LOD group and twenty-one patients in the gonadotrophin group. In the LOD group, eight of the twenty-nine patients became pregnant. Fetal heart activity was noted on ultrasound in five of the patients. There were four live births and four spontaneous abortions; three of these patients achieved a second pregnancy. In the gonadotrophin group, of twenty-one women, seven became pregnant, five demonstrating fetal heart activity; there were four live births and three spontaneous abortions.

Bayram et al. (52), in a newly published randomized trial, compared the effectiveness of using recombinant FSH (rFSH) treatment in a low-dose step-up protocol versus laparoscopic "ovarian electrocautery" in 168 PCOS patients who failed to ovulate with CC (52). Of the total group, eighty-three were allocated to laparoscopic ovarian electrocautery and eighty-five to rFSH. In the laparoscopic ovarian electrocautery group, if anovulation persisted for eight weeks after the procedure or if the patient became anovulatory again, CC and rFSH treatment was employed to induce ovulation. The main outcome measure was ongoing pregnancy within twelve months. The cumulative rate of ongoing pregnancy in the rFSH-only arm was 67 percent. With only ovarian electrocautery, it was 34 percent, which increased to 49 percent after CC was given. Subsequent rFSH increased the rate to 67 percent at twelve months. No complications occurred from electrocautery with or without CC. Patients allocated to electrocautery had a significantly lower risk of multiple pregnancy (1/63 pregnancies; 1.6 percent) compared with the rFSH-only arm (9/64 pregnancies; 14 percent) (RR = 0.11; 95 percent CI: 0.01–0.86). It is interesting that the only multiple pregnancy in the ovarian electrocautery arm was quintuplets after rFSH treatment; this finding and the more than expected multiple pregnancy rate in the rFSH-only arm [expected approximately 7 percent (51), observed 14 percent] raises the suspicion whether the low-dose step-up protocol was employed properly.

Farquhar et al. (50) conducted a meta-analysis in which six RCTs were included to compare LOD and gonadotropin treatment. The ongoing and live birth rates were comparable; odds ratios (OR) were 1.04 (95 percent CI 0.74–1.99) and 1.08 (95 percent CI 0.67–1.75), respectively. The multiple pregnancy rates were lower with ovarian drilling than with gonadotrophins (1 vs. 16 percent, OR = 0.13, 95 percent CI: 0.03–0.59). Miscarriage rates were comparable among the two groups (OR = 0.81, 95 percent 0.36–1.86). The authors concluded "There is insufficient evidence among women with CC-resistant PCOS, that either ovarian drilling or ovulation induction with gonadotrophins is superior for the outcomes of ovulation and pregnancy, excepting multiple pregnancy which is rare with ovarian drilling."

The beneficial improvement in menstrual regularity, reproductive performance, and endocrine effects of LOD may continue for years (32, 55). Gjonnaess (56) reported that the late endocrine effects were sustained for eighteen to twenty years following ovarian electrocautery. Besides, subsequent medical induction of ovulation might become easier following ovarian surgery. Gonadotropin use with pretreatment LOD may be associated with lower duration of stimulation, total dose of gonadotropin used, and higher pregnancy rates (57). LOD has been proposed to be employed prior to IVF to minimize the risk of OHSS. Rimington et al. (45) prospectively randomized fifty PCOS patients who underwent IVF into two groups. The patients in group I ($n = 25$) underwent IVF without prior LOD, while the patients in group II ($n = 25$) had LOD before undergoing IVF. A significantly higher rate of cycle cancellation due to OHSS was noted in group I when compared to group II. Furthermore, the incidence of the moderate or severe OHSS was higher in group I compared to group II.

The cost-effectiveness of LOD and gonadotropin treatment has been compared. Obviously, for such a comparison, several issues, including the cost of laparoscopy, IVF cycle, exogenous gonadotropins, and coverage by social security systems should be taken into account. Nevertheless, van Wely et al. (58) conducted a multicenter randomized clinical trial in the Netherlands comparing rFSH treatment and LOD in 168 women with clomiphene citrate–resistant PCOS. In the LOD arm, CC and rFSH was used postoperatively if anovulation persisted. Chronic low-dose step-up protocol was used for rFSH treatment. The ongoing pregnancy rates at twelve months were 67 percent for both the electrocautery and the rFSH arms. The mean total costs per woman were €5308 for the electrocautery arm and €5925 for treatment with rFSH, resulting in a mean difference of €617 (95 percent CI: −€382 to €1614). However, the cost of delivery and neonatal care were not included into these costs. Due to the risk of multiple pregnancies with rFSH treatment, the electrocautery strategy can be expected to result in lower delivery costs and therefore lower total costs (58).

COMPARISON WITH METFORMIN

Pirwany and Tulandi (57), in a recent review article, compared the effectiveness and safety of LOD and metformin. (see chapter 30 for clinical details) LOD and metformin therapy improve menstrual disturbances and ovulatory dysfunction to a similar extent. The pregnancy rates after both treatments are also similar, but the safety of metformin in pregnancy is unproven. Nevertheless, its safety profile in pregnant women with type 2 diabetes is encouraging. Metformin is relatively inexpensive, and unlike LOD, it may decrease the risk for future coronary heart disease. The authors conclude that "Given the availability of treatment with metformin and the fact that it is as efficacious as laparoscopic ovarian drilling in correcting the myriad clinical, endocrine, and metabolic abnormalities associated with PCOS, the role of laparoscopic ovarian drilling in the management of patients with PCOS should be reexamined in the context of a randomized controlled trial."

Recently, a few randomized double-blind placebo-controlled studies have been published comparing LOD and metformin treatment in CC-resistant PCOS patients. Malkawi et al. (59) did not note any significant difference in crude ovulation (79.7 vs. 83.5 percent) and pregnancy rates (64.1 vs. 59.8 percent) in LOD and metformin groups, respectively. Palomba et al. (60) evaluated the effect of LOD and metformin on reproductive outcome in CC-resistant women with PCOS. The first group was prescribed metformin for six months (850 mg twice daily) following diagnostic laparoscopy. The second group underwent LOD and received placebo for six months. After six months of metformin or placebo treatment in women who did not achieve ovulation, CC was administered by the authors at a dose of 150 mg daily from day 3 to day 7 of cycles. At the end of the study, although there were no statistically significant differences between the groups according to the total ovulation rates (54.8 percent compared with 53.2 percent, respectively), the pregnancy rate per cycle was found to be significantly higher in the metformin group (21.8 percent compared with 13.4 percent, $p < 0.05$). The abortion rate was also found to be lower in the metformin group than in the LOD group (9.3 percent compared with 29.0 percent, respectively). After six cycles of treatment, the cumulative pregnancy rate was found to be 72.2 percent (thirty-nine of fifty-four) in the metformin group, whereas it was 56.4 percent (thirty-one of fifty-five) in the LOD group. The authors also evaluated the cost-benefit analysis of the two groups; metformin treatment was approximately twentyfold less expensive than LOD for the first six months if the cost of diagnostic laparoscopy was ignored (60).

Kocak and Ustun (61) randomly and equally divided forty-two PCOS patients into two groups. Patients in group I ($n = 21$) were treated with LOD, and patients in group II ($n = 21$) underwent LOD and subsequently received 1,700 mg per day of metformin for six months. The mean serum androgen levels and insulin response to oral glucose tolerance test decreased significantly in group II, while there was no significant change in group I. The mean serum progesterone level and endometrial thickness at the midluteal phase were found to be significantly higher in group II (34.6 ± 25.4 ng/mL, 8.4 ± 1.1 mm) compared to group I (26.2 ± 24.7 ng/mL, 7.9 ± 2.8 mm) ($p < 0.05$). The ovulation (fifty-six of sixty-five cycles, 86.1 percent, vs. twenty-nine of sixty-five cycles, 44.6 percent) and pregnancy rates (nine of twenty-one women, 47.6 percent, vs. four of twenty-one women, 19.1 percent) were significantly higher in group II than in group I. The authors concluded that metformin improved insulin resistance, reduced androgen levels, and significantly increased the ovulation and pregnancy rates following LOD (61).

HYPERANDROGENISM AND METABOLIC FACTORS

A marked reduction in circulating testosterone concentrations is noted after LOD. However, the data on dehydroepiandrosterone sulfate are conflicting; LOD appears to have a minimal effect on adrenal function, even in hyperinsulinemic women (62). The improvement in hyperandrogenism is thought to be secondary to the reduction in LH concentrations and the decreased androgen production by the ovarian stroma. Insulin sensitivity, however, remains unchanged.

Approximately, 50–70 percent of women with PCOS have insulin resistance (63, 64). Insulin resistance is believed to be secondary to a defect in insulin receptor transduction that is independent of obesity (64). There is a paucity of data on the effect of LOD on insulin sensitivity. Saleh et al. (62) examined the effects of LOD on insulin responses to an oral glucose tolerance test and noted that the effects of surgery on insulin sensitivity differed depending on the patient's preoperative

insulin status. Hyperinsulinemic women tended to have a greater reduction in area under the insulin curve after surgery (62). However, using the hyperglycemic clamp technique, Tiitinen et al. (65) have been unable to demonstrate any change in insulin sensitivity after LOD. One small study (66) found no improvement in insulin sensitivity or a favorable effect on the lipoprotein profile after LOD. In summary, LOD appears to have little or no effect on insulin sensitivity and lipoprotein profile.

PREDICTION OF RESPONSE TO LOD

Although high ovulation and pregnancy rates following LOD in patients with CC-resistant PCOS have been widely documented, 20–30 percent of such cases may fail to respond to surgical therapy (55). In a recent study, Amer et al. (21) evaluated the clinical response to LOD in 200 PCOS patients. They noted that women with BMI greater than 35 kg/m^2, serum testosterone concentration higher than 4.5 nmol/L, free androgen index (testosterone $\times$ 100/sex hormone binding globulin) more than 15, and/or with duration of infertility more than three years associated with poor responders to LOD. The authors concluded that the presence or absence of acne, the menstrual pattern, LH/FSH ratio, and ovarian volume did not influence the outcome of LOD. Of interest, pretreatment LH levels appeared to be associated with the pregnancy but not ovulation rates.

Recently, van Wely et al. (58) performed a study to determine the predictors of failure following LOD in eighty-three CC-resistant PCOS patients. The failure was defined as the persistence of anovulation within eight weeks after electrocautery and failure to reach an ongoing pregnancy after electrocautery with or without CC. Logistic regression analysis revealed that early menarche, low LH/FSH ratio, and low serum glucose levels before the operation were associated with failure of LOD. The LH/FSH level was found to be the strongest predictor of ovarian response after electrocautery.

LONG-TERM EFFECTS OF OVARIAN DRILLING

The endocrine changes resulting from ovarian drilling last for an extended period of time. Gjonnaess reported that over 50 percent of those who had the procedure continued to ovulate more than ten years later (56).

Two recently published studies reported the long-term effects of LOD in 116 women with anovulatory infertility of more than one year duration, who failed to ovulate ($n = 104$) or conceive six to nine cycles of CC up to 150 mg/day for five days and human chorionic gonadotrophin (32, 67). Seven of these women failed to conceive with human menopausal gonadotrophins. During the first postoperative year, 67 percent of the women were having regular menstruations; 50 percent of the total group continued to have regular menstruations seven years later. Of the 116 women, 67 (58 percent) conceived and had a total of 120 pregnancies. The spontaneous abortion rate was 17 percent. Endocrinologically, the serum LH and the LH/FSH ratio demonstrated a statistically significant decline, compared with preoperative concentrations ($p < 0.01$ and $p < 0.001$, respectively). Similarly, the serum testosterone, androstenedione, and the free androgen index were also lower ($p < 0.05$, $p < 0.01$, and $p < 0.001$, respectively). The serum FSH concentrations remained unchanged. These changes in the endocrine profile were still the same three years later.

In a relatively recent report, Lunde et al. (68) presented a follow-up study on fertility and menstrual pattern in 149 patients, fifteen to twenty five years after ovarian wedge resection. The 149 patients were operated on between 1970 and 1980, and the final follow-up was carried out in 1995 using a detailed questionnaire. Responses were obtained from 136 (91 percent) of the 149 women. Of the 129 who attempted a pregnancy, 70 (54 percent) had one or more live births resulting from spontaneous pregnancies. When those who had ovarian stimulation after the procedure are included in the analysis, the number of those who had one or more live births rises to ninety-six (74 percent). These are impressive numbers considering the potential for postoperative adhesions associated with ovarian wedge resection. With regard to menstrual function, the outcome is also very impressive and demonstrates the long-term effect of the procedure; 82 of the 103 premenopausal women were menstruating regularly for more than fifteen years after the operation.

COMPLICATIONS

Complications associated with ovarian drilling may be associated with anesthesia, establishment of the surgical access (laparoscopy or transvaginal hydrolaparoscopy), and/or with the drilling procedure itself, which includes the use of energy, electrical or laser. Related to the drilling itself, the patient may experience bleeding from the drilling sites, laceration of the utero-ovarian ligament, which is frequently grasped to immobilize the ovary. The use of excessive amounts of energy will destroy large numbers of follicles, resulting in decreased ovarian reserve. The use of energy with an electrode introduced too deeply into the ovary may cause desiccation of the hilar vessels, resulting in premature ovarian failure due to necrosis of the ovary (42).

Another important complication is the occurrence of postoperative adhesions. There is a great degree of variation in the reported rates of adhesions, from 0 to 70 percent (Table 31.2) (11, 18, 19, 33, 69–74). Felemban et al. (18) reported a rate of postoperative adhesions of 27 percent in seventeen patients. These were "minimal, filmy adhesions located on the ovarian surface and probably of not great functional significance." The great diversity of the rate of adhesion formation may be partly due to variations in technique and partly on the interpretation of the findings at second look. Adhesion formation seems to be more frequent with laser treatment than with electrocoagulation (33), and use of adhesion barriers do not reduce its incidence. Abdominal lavage and use of insulated needle electrocautery may help to reduce its occurrence (18, 33). Undoubtedly, the procedure must be carried out using a meticulous, atraumatic technique with proper respect to tissues (73, 74).

KEY POINTS

■ Ovarian drilling is a relatively simple procedure performed via minimal access and usually on an outpatient basis. It provides an alternative treatment option for CC-resistant PCOS patient.

■ Ovarian drilling offers several advantages compared with gonadotrophin treatment. They include the following: 1) over 70 percent of patients ovulate spontaneously, 2) more than 50 percent conceive without the need of intensive cycle monitoring as required when gonadotrophins are used, 3) the procedure provides long-term effects, 4) it eliminates the risk of a high incidence of multiple pregnancy and OHSS associated with gonadotrophins, and 5) it creates a favorable response to stimulation with clomiphene citrate or gonadotrophins, if their use becomes necessary to achieve pregnancy.

■ Despite these advantages, ovarian drilling is a surgical procedure and may be associated with minor to major complications. It is essential to use a proper and meticulous technique to avoid such complications.

■ Lifestyle modification (diet and exercise) and/or metformin, which are currently investigated, may well reduce the need for ovarian drilling.

■ Ovarian drilling retains a place in the current treatment of PCOS in well-selected cases. Progress in understanding of this complex syndrome and introduction of effective new treatment option(s) may further diminish the need for surgery in patients with PCOS in the future.

Table 31.2: Postoperative Adhesions following LOD

Author	Year	n	Adhesions (percent of patients)
Weise et al.[a] (69)	1991	10	70
Gurgan et al.[b] (19)	1992	20	68
Corson and Grochmal[b] (70)	1990	30	3
Portuondo et al.[c] (11)	1984	24	0
Naether et al.[a] (33)	1994	62	19
Felemban et al.[a] (18)	2000	15	27

Performed with [a]electrosurgery, [b]laser, and [c]biopsy.

REFERENCES

1. Yildiz BO, Yarali H, Oguz H, Bayraktar M. Glucose intolerance, insulin resistance, and hyperandrogenemia in first degree relatives of women with polycystic ovary syndrome. *J Clin Endocrinol Metab* 2003;**88**:2031–6.
2. Polson DW, Adams J, Wadsworth J, Franks S. Polycystic ovaries—a common finding in normal women. *Lancet* 1988;**1**:870–2.
3. Carmina E, Ditkoff EC, Malizia G, Vijod AG, Janni A, Lobo RA. Increased circulating levels of immunoreactive beta-endorphin in polycystic ovary syndrome is not caused by increased pituitary secretion. *Am J Obstet Gynecol* 1992;**167**:1819–24.
4. The Rotterdam ESHRE/ASRM-Sponsored PCOS consensus workshop group. Revised 2003 consensus on diagnostic criteria and long-term health risks related to polycystic ovary syndrome (PCOS). *Hum Reprod* 2004;**19**:41–7.
5. Balen AH, Laven JS, Tan SL, Dewailly D. Ultrasound assessment of the polycystic ovary: international consensus definitions. *Hum Reprod Update* 2003;**9**:505–14.
6. Geisthovel F. A comment on the European Society of Human Reproduction and Embryology/American Society for Reproductive Medicine consensus of the polycystic ovarian syndrome. *Reprod Biomed Online* 2003;**7**:602–5.
7. Leventhal ML. The Stein-Leventhal syndrome. *Am J Obstet Gynecol* 1958;**76**:825–38.
8. Stein IF, Cohen MR. Surgical treatment of bilateral polycystic ovaries. *Am J Obstet Gynecol* 1939;**38**:465–73.

9. Stein IF. Duration of fertility following ovarian wedge resection—Stein-Leventhal syndrome. *Obstet Gynecol Surv* 1965;**20**:124–7.

10. Adashi EY, Rock JA, Guzick D, Wentz AC, Jones GS, Jones HW, Jr. Fertility following bilateral ovarian wedge resection: a critical analysis of 90 consecutive cases of the polycystic ovary syndrome. *Fertil Steril* 1981;**36**:320–5.

11. Portuondo JA, Melchor JC, Neyro JL, Alegre A. Periovarian adhesions following ovarian wedge resection or laparoscopic biopsy. *Endoscopy* 1984;**16**:143–5.

12. Gomel V. [Reasons for surgical treatment of polycystic ovary syndrome]. *J Gynecol Obstet Biol Reprod (Paris)* 2003;**32**:S46–9.

13. Gjonnaess H. Polycystic ovarian syndrome treated by ovarian electrocautery through the laparoscope. *Fertil Steril* 1984;**41**:20–5.

14. Lord JM, Flight IH, Norman RJ. Insulin-sensitising drugs (metformin, troglitazone, rosiglitazone, pioglitazone, D-chiro-inositol) for polycystic ovary syndrome. *Cochrane Database Syst Rev* 2003;CD003053.

15. Mitwally MF, Casper RF. Aromatase inhibitors for the treatment of infertility. *Expert Opin Investig Drugs* 2003;**12**:353–71.

16. Gomel V, Taylor PJ. Diagnostic and operative gynecologic laparoscopy. Vol. 198. 1995, St. Louis: Mosby.

17. Saleh AM, Khalil HS. Review of nonsurgical and surgical treatment and the role of insulin-sensitizing agents in the management of infertile women with polycystic ovary syndrome. *Acta Obstet Gynecol Scand* 2004;**83**:614–21.

18. Felemban A, Tan SL, Tulandi T. Laparoscopic treatment of polycystic ovaries with insulated needle cautery: a reappraisal. *Fertil Steril* 2000;**73**:266–9.

19. Gurgan T, Urman B, Aksu T, Yarali H, Develioglu O, Kisnisci HA. The effect of short-interval laparoscopic lysis of adhesions on pregnancy rates following Nd-YAG laser photocoagulation of polycystic ovaries. *Obstet Gynecol* 1992;**80**:45–7.

20. Malkawi HY, Qublan HS. Laparoscopic ovarian drilling in the treatment of polycystic ovary syndrome: how many punctures per ovary are needed to improve the reproductive outcome? *J Obstet Gynaecol Res* 2005;**31**:115–9.

21. Amer SA, Li TC, Cooke ID. A prospective dose-finding study of the amount of thermal energy required for laparoscopic ovarian diathermy. *Hum Reprod* 2003;**18**:1693–8.

22. Dabirashrafi H. Complications of laparoscopic ovarian cauterization. *Fertil Steril* 1989;**52**:878–9.

23. Fernandez H, Alby JD, Gervaise A, de Tayrac R, Frydman R. Operative transvaginal hydrolaparoscopy for treatment of polycystic ovary syndrome: a new minimally invasive surgery. *Fertil Steril* 2001;**75**:607–11.

24. Branigan EF, Estes A, Walker K, Rothgeb J. Thorough sonographic oocyte retrieval during in vitro fertilization produces results similar to ovarian wedge resection in patients with clomiphene citrate-resistant polycystic ovarian syndrome. *Am J Obstet Gynecol* 2006;**194**:1696–700; discussion 1700–1.

25. Rossmanith WG, Keckstein J, Spatzier Klauritzen C. The impact of ovarian laser surgery on the gonadotrophin secretion in women with polycystic ovarian disease. *Clin Endocrinol (Oxf)* 1991;**34**:223–30.

26. Keckstein J. Laparoscopic treatment of polycystic ovarian syndrome. *Baillieres Clin Obstet Gynaecol* 1989;**3**:563–81.

27. Liguori G, Tolino A, Moccia G, Scognamiglio G, Nappi C. Laparoscopic ovarian treatment in infertile patients with polycystic ovarian syndrome (PCOS): endocrine changes and clinical outcome. *Gynecol Endocrinol* 1996;**10**:257–64.

28. Alborzi S, Khodaee R, Parsanejad ME. Ovarian size and response to laparoscopic ovarian electro-cauterization in polycystic ovarian disease. *Int J Gynaecol Obstet* 2001;**74**:269–74.

29. Sumioki H, Utsunomiyia T, Matsuoka K, Korenaga M, Kadota T. The effect of laparoscopic multiple punch resection of the ovary on hypothalamo-pituitary axis in polycystic ovary syndrome. *Fertil Steril* 1988;**50**:567–72.

30. Lockwood GM, Muttukrishna S, Groome NP, Matthews DR, Ledger WL. Mid-follicular phase pulses of inhibin B are absent in polycystic ovarian syndrome and are initiated by successful laparoscopic ovarian diathermy: a possible mechanism regulating emergence of the dominant follicle. *J Clin Endocrinol Metab* 1998;**83**:1730–5.

31. Armar NA, McGarrigle HH, Honour J, Holownia P, Jacobs HS, Lachelin GC. Laparoscopic ovarian diathermy in the management of anovulatory infertility in women with polycystic ovaries: endocrine changes and clinical outcome. *Fertil Steril* 1990;**53**:45–9.

32. Amer SA, Gopalan V, Li TC, Ledger WL, Cooke ID. Long term follow-up of patients with polycystic ovarian syndrome after laparoscopic ovarian drilling: clinical outcome. *Hum Reprod* 2002;**17**:2035–42.

33. Naether OG, Baukloh V, Fischer R, Kowalczyk T. Long-term follow-up in 206 infertility patients with polycystic ovarian syndrome after laparoscopic electrocautery of the ovarian surface. *Hum Reprod* 1994;**9**:2342–9.

34. Aakvaag A, Gjonnaess H. Hormonal response to electrocautery of the ovary in patients with polycystic ovarian disease. *Br J Obstet Gynaecol* 1985;**92**:1258–64.

35. Utsunomiya T, Sumioki H, Taniguchi I. Hormonal and clinical effects of multifollicular puncture and resection on the ovaries of polycystic ovary syndrome. *Horm Res* 1990;**33** Suppl. 2:35–9.

36. Campo S, Felli A, Lamanna MA, Barini A, Garcea N. Endocrine changes and clinical outcome after laparoscopic ovarian resection in women with polycystic ovaries. *Hum Reprod* 1993;**8**:359–63.

37. Kriplani A, Manchanda R, Agarwal N, Nayar B. Laparoscopic ovarian drilling in clomiphene citrate-resistant women with polycystic ovary syndrome. *J Am Assoc Gynecol Laparosc* 2001;**8**:511–8.

38. Heylen SM, Puttemans PJ, Brosens IA. Polycystic ovarian disease treated by laparoscopic argon laser capsule drilling: comparison of vaporization versus perforation technique. *Hum Reprod* 1994;**9**:1038–42.

39. Li TC, Saravelos H, Chow MS, Chisabingo R, Cooke ID. Factors affecting the outcome of laparoscopic ovarian drilling for polycystic ovarian syndrome in women with anovulatory infertility. *Br J Obstet Gynaecol* 1998;**105**:338–44.

40. Stegmann BJ, Craig HR, Bay RC, Coonrod DV, Brady MJ, Garbaciak JA Jr. Characteristics predictive of response to ovarian diathermy in women with polycystic ovarian syndrome. *Am J Obstet Gynecol* 2003;**188**:1171–3.

41. Duleba AJ, Banaszewska B, Spaczynski RZ, Pawelczyk L. Success of laparoscopic ovarian wedge resection is related to obesity, lipid profile, and insulin levels. *Fertil Steril* 2003;**79**:1008–14.

42. Gomel V, Yarali H. Surgical treatment of polycystic ovary syndrome associated with infertility. *Reprod Biomed Online* 2004;**9**:35–42.

43. Gjonnaess H. Ovarian electrocautery in the treatment of women with polycystic ovary syndrome (PCOS). Factors affecting the results. *Acta Obstet Gynecol Scand* 1994;**73**:407–12.

44. Tozer AJ, Al-Shawaf T, Zosmer A, et al. Does laparoscopic ovarian diathermy affect the outcome of IVF-embryo transfer in women with polycystic ovarian syndrome? A retrospective comparative study. *Hum Reprod* 2001;**16**:91–5.

45. Rimington MR, Walker SM, Shaw RW. The use of laparoscopic ovarian electrocautery in preventing cancellation of in-vitro

fertilization treatment cycles due to risk of ovarian hyperstimulation syndrome in women with polycystic ovaries. *Hum Reprod* 1997;**12**:1443–7.

46. Farhi J, Soule S, Jacobs HS. Effect of laparoscopic ovarian electrocautery on ovarian response and outcome of treatment with gonadotropins in clomiphene citrate-resistant patients with polycystic ovary syndrome. *Fertil Steril* 1995;**64**:930–5.

47. Colacurci N, Zullo F, De Franciscis P, Mollo A, De Placido G. In vitro fertilization following laparoscopic ovarian diathermy in patients with polycystic ovarian syndrome. *Acta Obstet Gynecol Scand* 1997;**76**:555–8.

48. Amin AF, Abd el-Aal DE, Darwish AM, Meki AR. Evaluation of the impact of laparoscopic ovarian drilling on Doppler indices of ovarian stromal blood flow, serum vascular endothelial growth factor, and insulin-like growth factor-1 in women with polycystic ovary syndrome. *Fertil Steril* 2003;**79**:938–41.

49. Abdel Gadir A, Mowafi RS, Alnaser HM, Alrashid AH, Alonezi OM, Shaw RW. Ovarian electrocautery versus human menopausal gonadotrophins and pure follicle stimulating hormone therapy in the treatment of patients with polycystic ovarian disease. *Clin Endocrinol (Oxf)* 1990;**33**:585–92.

50. Farquhar C, Vandekerckhove P, Lilford R. Laparoscopic "drilling" by diathermy or laser for ovulation induction in anovulatory polycystic ovary syndrome. *The Cochrane Library*, 2002.

51. Homburg R, Howles CM. Low-dose FSH therapy for anovulatory infertility associated with polycystic ovary syndrome: rationale, results, reflections and refinements. *Hum Reprod Update* 1999;**5**:493–9.

52. Bayram N, van Wely M, Kaaijk EM, Bossuyt PM, van der Veen F. Using an electrocautery strategy or recombinant follicle stimulating hormone to induce ovulation in polycystic ovary syndrome: randomised controlled trial. *BMJ* 2004;**328**:192.

53. Vicino M, Loverro G, Bettocchi S, Simonetti S, Mei L, Selvaggi L. Predictive value of serum androstenedione basal levels on the choice of gonadotropin or laparoscopic ovarian electrocautery as ovulation induction in clomiphene citrate-resistant patients with polycystic ovary syndrome. *Gynecol Endocrinol* 2000;**14**:42–9.

54. Farquhar CM, Williamson K, Gudex G, Johnson NP, Garland J, Sadler L. A randomized controlled trial of laparoscopic ovarian diathermy versus gonadotropin therapy for women with clomiphene citrate-resistant polycystic ovary syndrome. *Fertil Steril* 2002;**78**:404–11.

55. Farquhar CM, Williamson K, Brown PM, Garland J. An economic evaluation of laparoscopic ovarian diathermy versus gonadotrophin therapy for women with clomiphene citrate resistant polycystic ovary syndrome. *Hum Reprod* 2004;**19**:1110–5.

56. Gjonnaess H. Late endocrine effects of ovarian electrocautery in women with polycystic ovary syndrome. *Fertil Steril* 1998;**69**:697–701.

57. Pirwany I, Tulandi T. Laparoscopic treatment of polycystic ovaries: is it time to relinquish the procedure? *Fertil Steril* 2003;**80**:241–51.

58. van Wely M, Bayram N, van der Veen F, Bossuyt PM. An economic comparison of a laparoscopic electrocautery strategy and ovulation induction with recombinant FSH in women with clomiphene citrate-resistant polycystic ovary syndrome. *Hum Reprod* 2004;**19**:1741–5.

59. Malkawi HY, Qublan HS, Hamaideh AH. Medical vs. surgical treatment for clomiphene citrate-resistant women with polycystic ovary syndrome. *J Obstet Gynaecol* 2003;**23**:289–93.

60. Palomba S, Orio F, Jr. Falbo A, et al. Metformin administration and laparoscopic ovarian drilling improve ovarian response to clomiphene citrate (CC) in oligo-anovulatory CC-resistant women with polycystic ovary syndrome. *Clin Endocrinol (Oxf)* 2005;**63**:631–5.

61. Kocak I, Ustun C. Effects of metformin on insulin resistance, androgen concentration, ovulation and pregnancy rates in women with polycystic ovary syndrome following laparoscopic ovarian drilling. *J Obstet Gynaecol Res* 2006;**32**:292–8.

62. Saleh A, Morris D, Tan SL, Tulandi T. Effects of laparoscopic ovarian drilling on adrenal steroids in polycystic ovary syndrome patients with and without hyperinsulinemia. *Fertil Steril* 2001;**75**:501–4.

63. Legro RS, Finegood D, Dunaif A. A fasting glucose to insulin ratio is a useful measure of insulin sensitivity in women with polycystic ovary syndrome. *J Clin Endocrinol Metab* 1998;**83**:2694–8.

64. Dunaif A, Segal KR, Futterweit W, Dobrjansky A. Profound peripheral insulin resistance, independent of obesity, in polycystic ovary syndrome. *Diabetes* 1989;**38**:1165–74.

65. Tiitinen A, Tenhunen A, Seppala M. Ovarian electrocauterization causes LH-regulated but not insulin-regulated endocrine changes. *Clin Endocrinol (Oxf)* 1993;**39**:181–4.

66. Lemieux S, Lewis GF, Ben-Chetrit A, Steiner G, Greenblatt EM. Correction of hyperandrogenemia by laparoscopic ovarian cautery in women with polycystic ovarian syndrome is not accompanied by improved insulin sensitivity or lipid-lipoprotein levels. *J Clin Endocrinol Metab* 1999;**84**:4278–82.

67. Amer SA, Banu Z, Li TC, Cooke ID. Long-term follow-up of patients with polycystic ovary syndrome after laparoscopic ovarian drilling: endocrine and ultrasonographic outcomes. *Hum Reprod* 2002;**17**:2851–7.

68. Lunde O, Djoseland O, Grottum P. Polycystic ovarian syndrome: a follow-up study on fertility and menstrual pattern in 149 patients 15-25 years after ovarian wedge resection. *Hum Reprod* 2001;**16**:1479–85.

69. Weise HC, Naether O, Fischer R, Berger-Bispink S, Delfs T. Results of treatment with surface cauterization of polycystic ovaries in sterility patients. *Geburtshilfe Frauenheilkd* 1991;**51**:920–4.

70. Corson SL, Grochmal SA. Contact laser laparoscopy has distinct advantages over alternatives. *Clin Laser Mon* 1990;**8**:7–9.

71. Campo S., Ovulatory cycles, pregnancy outcome and complications after surgical treatment of polycystic ovary syndrome. *Obstet Gynecol Surv* 1998;**53**:297–308.

72. Daniell JF, Miller W. Polycystic ovaries treated by laparoscopic laser vaporization. *Fertil Steril* 1989;**51**:232–6.

73. Rizk B, Nawar MG. Laparoscopic ovarian drilling for surgical induction of ovulation in polycystic ovary syndrome. In Allahbadia G (Ed.) Mumbai: India, Rotunda Medical Technologies (2001), chapter 18, 140–4.

74. Rizk B. Prevention of Ovarian Hyperstimulation Syndrome. In Rizk B (Ed.). Ovarian Hyperstimulation Syndrome. Cambridge: United Kingdom. Cambridge University Press, chapter 7, 130–99.

■ 32 ■

ENDOMETRIOSIS-ASSOCIATED INFERTILITY

Cem S. Atabekoglu, Aydin Arici

INTRODUCTION

Endometriosis is a common pathological process that mostly occurs in the female pelvis. Despite a long history of clinical experience and experimental research, the pathogenesis and management of endometriosis still have a lot of uncertainty. Endometriosis is one of the most common gynecologic diseases affecting fertility potential of women. The prevalence of endometriosis in infertile women ranges from 20 to 55 percent, as compared with 2–5 percent of women undergoing tubal ligation (1, 2). This correlation has led many investigators and clinicians to the assumption that there is a causal relationship between these two entities. There is still no definite answer to the question concerning why patients with endometriosis have subfertility. Several explanations have been proposed for the etiology of infertility of patients with endometriosis. The most straightforward one is anatomical distortion present in advanced disease. However, affected women who have functional, patent tubes, with no anatomic distortion, may also be associated with infertility. Several others possibilities have been suggested, related to immunologic defects and altered characteristics of peritoneal fluid involving cytokines and macrophages, which may affect fertility by means of altered folliculogenesis, ovulatory dysfunction, reduced preovulatory steroidogenesis of granulosa cells, sperm phagocytosis, and impaired fertilization (3).

We do not expect to clarify these enigmas completely in this chapter, but we will try to illustrate different opinions regarding the pathophysiology and management of endometriosis-associated infertility according to the current knowledge.

ENDOMETRIOSIS AND SUBFERTILITY

The prevalence of endometriosis in the general population is not exactly known. There is a wide range of difference in the reported prevalence of endometriosis (3–43 percent) among fertile patients undergoing sterilization, which may be due to the different diagnostic methods used in these studies (4). The interest of the surgeons is very important; as known, some surgeons more eagerly look for minimal or mild endometriosis in a symptomatic patient. Nevertheless, in a recent review, the prevalence of endometriosis among infertile patients was reported to be higher (33 vs. 4 percent among fertile patients). Moreover, prevalence of moderate and severe endometriosis was also found higher in patients with infertility, compared to fertile women undergoing laparoscopic sterilization (32 vs. 9 percent) (4).

Studies carried out on baboons have shown a normal monthly fecundity rate (MFR) with spontaneous minimal endometriosis (18 percent) compared with baboons with a normal pelvis (24 percent) (5, 6). In one of these studies, the authors also demonstrated that the MFR was significantly lower in baboons with mild, moderate, or severe endometriosis than in baboons with minimal endometriosis or a normal pelvis (6). It is now also well established that both the MFR and overall pregnancy rate are reduced in patients with moderate and severe endometriosis who refuse surgery. Olive and co-workers demonstrated an MFR of 3.1 percent in infertile patients with mild to severe endometriosis managed expectantly for an interval of one to twenty-five months. They also found that the MFR and overall pregnancy rate was 0 percent in patients with severe endometriosis. For moderate endometriosis, they reported a 3.2 percent MFR and a 25 percent overall pregnancy rate (7). In a review, it was reported that the average cumulative pregnancy rate with expectant management of minimal or mild endometriosis was approximately 45 percent. In contrast, this rate was reported approximately 58 percent following surgical treatment (8). Unfortunately, the majority of studies are uncontrolled or retrospective, making them prone to selection bias. To date, we have only two randomized controlled trials (RCT) that have evaluated the effect of surgical treatment on fertility in patients with minimal or mild endometriosis. While one study concluded that surgical approach improves fertilization in such patients, the other study did not find any differences (9, 10).

However, when the studies were combined in a meta-analysis, surgical treatment of early-stage endometriosis appeared to provide a significant improvement in pregnancy rates (11). This issue will be discussed in more detail in the following section.

MECHANISM OF ENDOMETRIOSIS-ASSOCIATED INFERTILITY

As previously mentioned, distorted pelvic anatomy is one of the most important mechanisms causing infertility, especially for advanced disease. In this context, pelvic inflammation due to endometriosis may cause adhesion formation and scarring, which leads to a disruption and decrease in fertility, presumably through hampering oocyte release and impairing ovum pickup or transport by the fallopian tube. In contrast, many women with endometriosis ovulate and have functional patent tubes, with no adhesions or anatomic distortions that might be

rate after surgi
et al. suggested
triosis have lo
minimal-mild
28 percent) (2

Deep recta
endometriosis
moval of endoi
of evidence sh
improves fecur
decreases poste
speculate that e
such as segme
rectum slicing,
has very prom
III–IV. Recentl
was 45.5 perce
segmental colo
a history of ur
after surgery i
in mind that t
plications. Du
complications
rates of 3.8 pe
ficial and segn

The prese
1 cm in diame
Conservative
in volume. So
may produce
and reduce o
and number c
has been sug
patients with
Although dat
of operative l
triomas are li
copy represei
endometrioti
scopic proce
removal of th
rate of recurr
Regardless o
approximatel
triomas may
(31, 32).

ART in the
Infertility

Controlled

It has be
ment triples
as compared
cally correcte
of Peterson e
ovulation in
in patients v
with stage I
study, Fedel
was signific
went three

associated with infertility. Several studies have demonstrated increased volume of peritoneal fluid with augmented concentration of many types of cells, especially activated macrophages. Peritoneal macrophages show greater activity, resulting in enhanced phagocytosis and secretion of several soluble substances, such as proteolytic enzymes, cytokines, prostaglandins, and growth factors. It has also been demonstrated that peritoneal macrophages phagocytize sperm and that macrophages from women with endometriosis are more active than those from women without the disease (12). Several investigators have shown that the levels of many cytokines are increased in the peritoneal fluid of women with endometriosis, such as interleukin-1 (IL-1), IL-6, IL-8, IL-17, IL-18, and tumor necrosis factor-α (TNF-α) (13, 14). Since the ovaries and fallopian tubes are bathed in the peritoneal fluid, these alterations may have adverse effects on folliculogenesis, oocyte function and quality, ovulation, sperm, fallopian tube function, embryo quality, or implantation (15).

Diaz et al. showed that, when oocytes from a disease-free donor were transferred, pregnancy, implantation, and live birth rates were similar in patients with either no endometriosis or stage III–IV endometriosis. Therefore, the authors concluded that the reduced fecundity in patients with endometriosis might be related to poor oocyte quality rather than implantation failure (13). Data concerning follicular fluid show that the levels of IL-1, IL-6, IL-8, TNF-α, monocyte chemotactic protein–1 (MCP-1), endothelin-1, and several natural killer cells, B lymphocytes, and monocytes were elevated, but the level of vascular endothelial growth factor was decreased, in women with endometriosis (14). These cytokines and growth factors may also impair folliculogenesis and ovulation. In IVF cycles, some investigators reported reduced fertilization rates in women with endometriosis, but others could not confirm that. A large retrospective study of 980 ICSI cycles for male infertility did not report an adverse outcome in women with endometriosis. No difference was found in fertilization rates, implantation rates, and pregnancy rates between 101 cycles in women with endometriosis and 879 cycles in women with other infertility factors. This finding suggests that ICSI may be a useful tool to overcome fertilization defects in women with endometriosis (15).

A hostile peritoneal environment may cause impaired early embryo development. Although there are conflicting reports, a considerable body of evidence suggests that serum and peritoneal fluid from infertile women with endometriosis are embryotoxic to two-cell mouse embryos (14).

Successful implantation requires a functionally normal embryo at the blastocyst stage and a receptive endometrium. Various genes such as integrins (e.g., $\alpha V\beta 3$), matrix metalloproteinases (e.g., MMP-7 and -11), transcription factors (e.g., hepatocyte nuclear factor), endometrial bleeding factor (ebaf), enzymes involved in steroid hormone metabolism (e.g., aromatase,17β-hydroxysteroid dehydrogenase), leukemia inhibitory factor (LIF), Hox genes, and progesterone receptor isoforms are aberrantly expressed during the window of implantation and at other times of the cycle in women with versus those without endometriosis (16). Recently, Dimitriadis et al. showed that IL-11 and IL-11R-α staining was absent and LIF-staining intensity was significantly lower in the glandular epithelium of the eutrophic endometrium of infertile women with endometriosis when compared with the endometrium of fertile patients during the implantation window (17). Our group showed that the peritoneal fluid of women with endometriosis

has significantly elevated levels of MCP-1 and IL-8 (14). Although some of the evidence supports the hypothesis of impaired implantation, there are now several lines of evidence suggesting that implantation is not impaired in women with endometriosis. For example, as stated earlier, Diaz et al. reported that women with stage III–IV endometriosis had implantation rates similar to those of recipients without endometriosis who received oocytes from the same donor (13). Garcia–Velasco et al. also illustrated that severe endometriosis does not seem to affect the expression of pinopodes, a morphological marker of uterine receptivity (18).

SHOULD LAPAROSCOPY BE MANDATORY FOR DIAGNOSIS OF ENDOMETRIOSIS IN PATIENTS WITH UNEXPLAINED INFERTILITY?

So far, laparoscopy is considered as the gold standard for the definitive diagnosis of endometriosis. In contrast, the precise place of laparoscopy in the line of investigation of infertile patients continues to be a matter of debate. It was shown that laparoscopy reveals tubal pathology or endometriosis in 35–68 percent of cases, even after a normal hysterosalpingography (HSG). There are now several lines of evidence that suggest that laparoscopy may not affect the prognosis of patients with unexplained infertility who have patent tubes. Only a minority of these cases would reveal peritubal adhesions or early endometriosis that can be treated laparoscopically. Nevertheless, as mentioned earlier, there is an ongoing discussion in the literature concerning the role of laparoscopic treatment in the treatment of infertility in patients with minimal and mild endometriosis. Some authors advocate bypassing diagnostic laparoscopy when normal tubal patency is demonstrated on HSG and when there is no sonographic evidence of endometriomas in infertile patients. According to Tanahatoe et al., laparoscopy has considerable value, and laparoscopic findings have altered treatment decisions in 25 percent of patients before the intrauterine insemination (IUI). They found that only 4 percent of patients had severe abnormalities that resulted in a change of treatment to IVF or open surgery, and 21 percent of patients who had endometriosis (stages I and II) or adhesions were directly treated by laparoscopic intervention, followed by IUI treatment (19). More recently, the same authors performed an RCT and compared the value of diagnostic laparoscopy prior to IUI with the value of laparoscopy performed after six cycles of IUI. They could not find any difference between the two groups in regard to the cumulative pregnancy rate (44 percent compared with 49 percent, respectively). The authors also proposed that the prevalence of endometriosis and adhesions at laparoscopy requiring intervention was not significantly higher than when laparoscopy was performed after six cycles of IUI. After this RCT, Tanahatoe and co-workers changed their recommendation and suggested that the impact of detection and treatment of observed pelvic pathology prior to IUI seems negligible in terms of IUI outcome (20). It is still a matter of debate whether the treatment of minimal/mild endometriosis results in higher pregnancy rates of IUI. If diagnostic laparoscopy is performed routinely, it should be recognized that it is an invasive and costly procedure and is not without complications. Furthermore, if surgery to remove minimal and mild endometriosis does not improve pregnancy rates, the additional value of diagnostic laparoscopy after a normal HSG would be very low. If surgical treatment were to

enhance pr
(ART) cycle
to date, the
with stage
viously un
who have
patients wi
with a grea
with mini
with unexp
cess and o
proposed t
on the suc
vere endoi
ples with
irrespectiv
(21). Mor
presenting
likely reve
plaining o
percent) (
patients w
may need
from ider
such pati
for the di
to 2005 I
endometi
ing of lap
it should
hormona

MANAC
ASSOC

Expecta

As woul
nancy in
stages of
taneous
several
ment b
therapie
nancy r
imately
endom
not sig
fertility
suggest
ment o
lignanc
fluid cc
gressio
have e
and wi
expect

Medic

To dat
ical tr

oocyte number because the mean number of mature oocytes that were aspirated from the affected ovary was similar to that from the contralateral ovary (41).

Some authors have declared that surgery might impair ovarian function. Surgery may influence the ovarian reserve or ovarian response to subsequent gonadotropin treatment. The improper use of electrocoagulation during ovarian tissue hemostasis might lead to a reduction in the ovarian reserve, and surgery might be more detrimental than endometriosis itself on the patient's reproductive potential. Pabuccu et al. documented a reduced number of retrieved oocytes as well as a reduced pregnancy rate (42). Garcia-Velasco et al. documented lower peak E2 levels and higher gonadotropin requirements in operated patients when compared to nonoperated patients who had current endometriomas (39). Nevertheless, there are now several studies that failed to observe a reduced ovarian response in patients who previously underwent laparoscopic excision of endometriomas (37). Further supporting this concept, Wong et al. recently showed that the levels of day 3 FSH were similar when patients with previous endometrioma resection were compared with the levels of patients with current endometriomas but no previous resection. The numbers of mature oocytes that were aspirated from the ipsilateral and contralateral ovary (relative to the site of unilateral ovarian cystectomy) were similar (41). These conflicting results may stem from different surgical techniques such as drainage, laser vaporization of the internal wall of the cyst, or removal of the cyst wall. The obtained results support the view that enucleation of endometriomas is associated with significant damage to ovarian reserve. There is the possibility that drainage and laser vaporization of the internal layer may be less detrimental. Dicker et al. documented a significant improvement in number of oocytes and embryos obtained in a cohort of women with ovarian endometriomas who failed to conceive during a previous IVF cycle and who subsequently underwent transvaginal ultrasound-guided aspiration (43). Takuma et al. revealed that the pregnancy rate after complete cystectomy of endometriomas was significantly lower than that after fenestration with electrocoagulation of the cyst wall. The pregnancy rate was also found to be better among patients who underwent aspiration of the cyst followed by ethanol fixation, than with aspiration alone (44). Donnez et al. have shown similar responses to gonadotropins between the affected ovary, operated with CO_2 laser vaporization of the internal cystic wall without cystectomy and the noninvolved ovary (38). Fish and Sher recently reported promising results in a case series of thirty-two women treated with transvaginal-guided aspiration and successive intracystic sclerotherapy with 5 percent tetracycline (45). Randomized studies are required to confirm these interesting preliminary results. In most cases, only one gonad is involved and the contralateral intact gonad may adequately compensate for the reduced function of the affected ovary. Therefore, patients with a single affected ovary do not in general have a reduced fertility potential to conceive through IVF treatment. Women with bilateral endometriotic ovarian cysts may be at elevated risk of ovarian function impairment. Ultrasound-guided aspiration, with or without concomitant local or systemic therapy, may be taken into consideration especially in this circumstance.

It is important to note that, at present, there are no definitive data to clarify whether damage is related to the surgical procedure and/or to the previous presence of the cyst. Indeed, it cannot be excluded that the cyst per se may damage the surrounding ovarian tissue. Using pathological sections of the ovarian cortex surrounding ovarian endometriomas, Maneschi et al. found a reduced number of follicles antecedent to surgery, suggesting that the disease by itself may be detrimental to the ovary (46). Apart from the potential injury related to the presence of the cyst in and of itself, there is some evidence supporting the idea that surgery may negatively affect ovarian reserve. A potential deleterious mechanism is the accidental removal of a significant amount of ovarian tissue during cystectomy. In a histological study performed on pathological specimens, Muzii et al. observed the presence of healthy ovarian tissue adjacent to the cyst wall in fourteen out of twenty-six endometriomas (54 percent), as compared to one case out of sixteen nonendometriotic benign ovarian cysts (6 percent) ($P = 0.002$) (47). The presence of recognizable ovarian tissue adjacent to the wall of enucleated endometriotic cysts has also been documented in a substantial number of cases by Hachisuga and Kawarabayashi (48). A further mechanism potentially responsible for the reduced ovarian reserve is the damage that may be inflicted to the ovarian stroma and vascularization by both surgery-related local inflammation and electrosurgical coagulation during hemostasis. Although the relevance of these pathogenetic mechanisms still needs to be determined, we believe that bipolar coagulation should be performed with caution. This procedure should be selective, directed at the bleeding vessels and not broadly grasping the entire ovarian tissue with the bipolar coagulator. Of note, it has been suggested that laparoscopic ovarian suture may be a less detrimental hemostatic procedure. Removal of the whole capsule wall is very important, especially to prevent recurrence. However, extreme care should be taken during the process of endometrioma cystectomy. It has been speculated that even with experienced hands and extreme care, an unanticipated deleterious effect from cystectomy may remain unavoidable. The cortex must be preserved as much as possible and excessive electrocoagulation during hemostasis must be avoided.

Most investigators believe that reoperation for recurrent endometriotic cysts have deleterious effects on ovarian reserve and reproductive outcome. However, this opinion is based on several earlier studies, where treatment was performed by laparotomy or where the outcome of some studies reported pregnancy rates after conservative laparoscopic treatment of ovarian endometriomas. In contrast, several authors believe that even patients who have undergone previous ovarian surgery might benefit from a second intervention. Paradigas and et al. reported the cumulative pregnancy rate after reoperation for stages III–IV endometriosis-related infertility after three, seven, and nine months to be 6, 18, and 24 percent, respectively (49). It should be kept in mind that if laparoscopic treatment enhances fertility, this effect is more profound within six months after surgery, and only approximately 10 percent additional women become pregnant after two years. Recently, Fedele et al. compared the outcome of reoperation for recurrent endometriomas with the outcome of primary surgery. This study is currently the only clinical trial related to this issue. The authors could not find any significant difference related to reproductive outcome between the two groups and advocated that laparoscopic conservative surgery has a role in the treatment of patients with recurrent ovarian endometriotic cysts. However, it is important to underline that although outcomes were not statistically significant, there was a trend in favor of primary surgery. Lower cumulative pregnancy rates (40.8 vs. 32.4 percent), a higher rate of patients who underwent ART (50 vs. 32.2 percent), and a higher rate of patients with irregular menstrual cycles and FSH higher than 14 IU/mL in the early follicular phase (5.5 vs. 1.3 percent) were demonstrated, especially in patients with bilateral endometriomas (50). It should be noted that many patients with endometriosis selected for IVF had advanced-stage disease and had multiple previous surgeries. Most had pelvic adhesions and were thus at increased risk of complications from further surgery (51).

KEY POINTS

■ There is no single optimal treatment for endometriosis, and physicians should pursue a comprehensive and personalized approach in decision making to identify the best option for the couple.

■ Young patients without significant anatomic distortion and with a short duration of infertility who have endometriosis may be initially managed expectantly.

■ There is no place of medical treatment in patients with endometriosis-associated infertility apart from gonadotropin analog treatment prior to IVF or ICSI.

■ When moderate or severe endometriosis causes pelvic anatomic distortion in women who wish to maintain or restore fertility, surgery may be the treatment of choice.

■ There is still no definite answer to the question concerning the benefit of surgical ablation of minimal to mild endometriosis at the time of diagnostic laparoscopy. However, because of progressive nature of disease, ablation or resection of all visible lesions at the time of laparoscopy is recommended since it may improve future fertility in patients with minimal and mild endometriosis.

■ There is some evidence that excisional surgery for endometriomas provides a more favorable outcome than drainage and ablation, with regard to the recurrence of the endometrioma and subsequent spontaneous pregnancy in women who were previously subfertile.

■ There is insufficient evidence to support a strategy of systematic surgical treatment of endometriomas before IVF-ICSI cycles. Furthermore, there are now several lines of evidence that suggests that laparoscopic cystectomy for endometriomas before commencing an IVF cycle does not improve fertility outcomes and may be hazardous on the ovarian reserve.

■ If laparoscopic surgery will be performed before IVF-ICSI cycles, a less invasive and conservative technique should be used during the operation such as cyst aspiration or fenestration.

REFERENCES

1. Strathy J, Molgaard C, Coulam C, Melton LJ. Endometriosis and infertility: a laparoscopic study of endometriosis among fertile and infertile women. *Fertil Steril* 1982;**38**: 667–72.
2. Suzuki T, Izumi S, Matsubayashi H, Awaji H, Yoshikata K, Makino T. Impact of ovarian endometrioma on oocytes and pregnancy outcome in in vitro fertilization. *Fertil Steril* 2005;**83**:908–13.
3. Buyalos RP, Agarwal SK. Endometriosis-associated infertility. *Curr Opin Obstet Gynecol* 2000;**12**:377–81.
4. D'Hooghe TM, Debrock S, Hill JA, Meuleman C., Endometriosis and subfertility: is the relationship resolved? *Semin Reprod Med* 2003;**21**:243–54.
5. D'Hooghe TM, Bambra CS, Koninckx PR. Cycle fecundity in baboons of proven fertility with minimal endometriosis. *Gynecol Obstet Invest* 1994;**37**:63–5.
6. D'Hooghe TM, Bambra CS, Raeymaekers BM, et al. A prospective controlled study over 2 years shows a normal monthly fertility rate (MFR) in baboons with stage I endometriosis and a decreased MFR in primates with stage II–IV disease. *Fertil Steril* 1996;**66**:809–13.
7. Olive DL, Stohs GF, Metzger DA, Franklin RR. Expectant management and hydrotubations in the treatment of endometriosis-associated infertility. *Fertil Steril* 1985;**44**:35–42.
8. Adamson D. Surgical management of endometriosis. *Semin Reprod Med* 2003;**21**:224–33.
9. Marcoux S, Maheux R, Berube S. Laparoscopic surgery in infertile women with minimal or mild endometriosis. Canadian Collaborative Group on Endometriosis. *N Engl J Med* 1997;**337**:217–22.
10. Parazzini F. Ablation of lesions or no treatment in minimal-mild endometriosis in infertile women: a randomized trial. Gruppo Italiano per lo Studio dell'Endometriosi. *Hum Reprod* 1999;**14**:1332–4.
11. Olive DL. Endometriosis: does surgery make a difference? *OBG Management* 2002;**14**:56–70.
12. Muscato JJ, Haney AF, Weinberg JB. Sperm phagocytosis by human peritoneal macrophages: a possible cause of infertility in endometriosis. *Am J Obstet Gynecol* 1982;**144**:503–10.
13. Diaz I, Navarro J, Blasco L, Simon C, Pellicer A, Remohi J. Impact of stage III–IV endometriosis on recipients of sibling oocytes: matched case-control study. *Fertil Steril* 2000;**74**:31–4.
14. Halis G, Arici A. Endometriosis and inflammation in infertility. *Ann N Y Acad Sci* 2004;**1034**:300–15.
15. Minguez Y, Rubio C, Bernal A, et al. The impact of endometriosis in couples undergoing intracytoplasmic sperm injection because of male infertility. *Hum Reprod* 1997;**12**:2282–5.
16. Giudice LC, Telles TL, Lobo S, Kao L. The molecular basis for implantation failure in endometriosis: on the road to discovery. *Ann N Y Acad Sci* 2002;**955**:252–64.
17. Dimitriadis E, Stoikos C, Stafford-Bell M, et al. Interleukin-11, IL-11 receptor alpha and leukemia inhibitory factor are dysregulated in endometrium of infertile women with endometriosis during the implantation window. *J Reprod Immunol* 2006;**69**:53–64.
18. Garcia-Velasco JA, Nikas G, Remohi J, Pellicer A, Simon C. Endometrial receptivity in terms of pinopode expression is not impaired in women with endometriosis in artificially prepared cycles. *Fertil Steril* 2001;**75**:1231–3.
19. Tanahatoe SJ, Hompes PGA, Lambalk CB. Accuracy of diagnostic laparoscopy in the infertility work-up before intrauterine insemination. *Fertil Steril* 2003;**79**:361–6.
20. Tanahatoe SJ, Lambalk CB, Hompes PG. The role of laparoscopy in intrauterine insemination: a prospective randomized reallocation study. *Hum Reprod* 2005;**20**:3225–30.
21. Calhaz-Jorge C, Chaveiro E, Nunes J, Costa AP. Implications of the diagnosis of endometriosis on the success of infertility treatment. *Clin Exp Obstet Gynecol* 2004;**31**:25–30.
22. Milingos S, Protopapas A, Kallipolitis G, et al. Laparoscopic evaluation of infertile patients with chronic pelvic pain. *Reprod Biomed Online* 2006;**12**:347–53.
23. Kennedy S, Bergqvist A, Chapron C, et al.; on behalf of the ESHRE Special Interest Group for Endometriosis and Endometrium Guideline Development Group. ESHRE guideline for the diagnosis and treatment of endometriosis. *Hum Reprod* 2005;**20**(10):2698–704.
24. Berube S, Marcoux S, Langevin M, Maheux R. Canadian Collaborative Group on Endometriosis. Fecundity of infertile

women with minimal or mild endometriosis and women with unexplained infertility. *Fertil Steril* 1998;**69**:1034–41.

25. Sallam HN, Garcia-Velasco JA, Dias S, Arici A. Long-term pituitary down-regulation before in vitro fertilization (IVF) for women with endometriosis. *Cochrane Database Syst Rev* 2006; 25(1):CD004635.

26. Adamson GD, Pasta DJ. Surgical treatment of endometriosis-associated infertility: meta-analysis compared with survival analysis. *Am J Obstet Gynecol* 1994;**171**:1488–505.

27. Osuga Y, Koga K, Tsutsumi O, et al. Role of laparoscopy in the treatment of endometriosis-associated infertility. *Gynecol Obstet Invest* 2002;**53**:33–9.

28. Darai E, Marpeau O, Thomassin I, et al. Fertility after laparoscopic colorectal resection for endometriosis: preliminary results. *Fertil Steril* 2005;**84**(4):945–50.

29. Duepree HJ, Senagore AJ, Delaney CP, Marcello PW, Brady KM, Falcone T. Laparoscopic resection of deep pelvic endometriosis with rectosigmoid involvement. *J M Coll Surg* 2002;**195**:754–8.

30. Hart RJ, Hickey M, Maouris P, Buckett W, Garry R. Excisional surgery versus ablative surgery for ovarian endometriomata. *Cochrane Database Syst Rev* 2005;**3**:CD004992.

31. Alborzi S, Momtahan M, Parsanezhad ME, Dehbashi S, Zolghadri J, Alborzi SA. Prospective, randomized study comparing laparoscopic ovarian cystectomy versus fenestration and coagulation in patients with endometriomas. *Fertil Steril* 2004;**82**:1633–7.

32. Jones KD, Sutton CJ. Pregnancy rates following ablative laparoscopic surgery for endometriomas. *Hum Reprod* 2002;**17**: 782–5.

33. Deaton JI, Gibson M, Blackmer KM, et al. A randomized, controlled trial of clomiphene citrate and intrauterine insemination in couples with unexplained infertility or surgically corrected endometriosis. *Fertil Steril* 1990;**54**:1083–8.

34. Peterson CM, Hatasaka HH, Jones KP, Pouson AM, Carrell DT, Urry RL. Ovulation induction with gonadotropins and intra-uterine insemination compared with in vitro fertilization and no therapy: a prospective, non-randomized, cohort study and meta-analysis. *Fertil Steril* 1994;**62**:535–44.

35. Fedele L, Bianchi S, Marchini M, Villa L, Brioschi D, Parazzini F. Superovulation with human menopausal gonadotropins in the treatment of infertility associated with minimal or mild endometriosis: a controlled randomized study. *Fertil Steril* 1992; **58**(1):28–31.

36. Al-Azemi M, Bernal AL, Steele J, Gramsbergen I, Barlow D, Kennedy S. Ovarian response to repeated controlled stimulation in in-vitro fertilization cycles in patients with ovarian endometriosis. *Hum Reprod* 2000;**15**(1):72–5.

37. Aboulghar MA, Mansour RT, Serour GI, Al-Inany HG, Aboulghar MM. The outcome of in vitro fertilization in advanced endometriosis with previous surgery: a case-controlled study. *Am J Obstet Gynecol* 2003;**188**(2):371–5.

38. Donnez J, Wyns C, Nisolle M. Does ovarian surgery for endometriomas impair the ovarian response to gonadotropin? *Fertil Steril* 2001;**76**:662–5.

39. Garcia-Velasco JA, Mahutte NG, Corona J, et al. Removal of endometriomas before in vitro fertilization does not improve fertility outcomes: a matched, case-control study. *Fertil Steril* 2004;**81**:1194–7.

40. Suganuma N, Wakahara Y, Ishida D, et al. Pretreatment for ovarian endometrial cyst before in vitro fertilization. *Gynecol Obstet Invest* 2002;**54**:36–40.

41. Wong BC, Gillman NC, Oehninger S, Gibbons WE, Stadtmauer LA. Results of in vitro fertilization in patients with endometriomas: is surgical removal beneficial? *Am J Obstet Gynecol* 2004;**191**:597–606.

42. Pabuccu R, Onalan G, Goktolga U, Kucuk T, Orhon E, Ceyhan T. Aspiration of ovarian endometriomas before intracytoplasmic sperm injection. *Fertil Steril* 2004;**82**(3):705–11.

43. Dicker D, Goldman JA, Feldberg D, Ashkenazi J, Levy T. Transvaginal ultrasonic needle-guided aspiration of endometriotic cysts before ovulation induction for in vitro fertilization. *J In Vitro Fert Embryo Trans* 1991;**8**(5):286–9.

44. Takuma N, Sengoku K, Pan B, Wada K, Tamauchi T, Miyamoto T, et al. Laparoscopic treatment of endometrioma-associated infertility and pregnancy outcome. *Gynecol Obstet Invest* 2002;**54**:30–5.

45. Fisch JD, Sher G. Sclerotherapy with 5% tetracycline is a simple alternative to potentially complex surgical treatment of ovarian endometriomas before in vitro fertilization. *Fertil Steril* 2004; **82**(2):437–41.

46. Maneschi F, Marasa L, Incandela S, Mazzarese M, Zupi E. Ovarian cortex surrounding benign neoplasms: a histologic study. *Am J Obstet Gynecol* 1993;**169**(2):388–93.

47. Muzii L, Bianchi A, Croce C, Manci N, Panici PB. Laparoscopic excision of ovarian cysts: is the stripping technique a tissue-sparing procedure? *Fertil Steril* 2002;**77**(3):609–14.

48. Hachisuga T, Kawarabayashi T. Histopathological analysis of laparoscopically treated ovarian endometriotic cysts with special reference to loss of follicles. *Hum Reprod* 2002;**17**(2):432–5.

49. Pagidas K, Falcone T, Hemmings R, Miron P. Comparison of reoperation for moderate (stage III) and severe (stage IV) endometriosis-related infertility with in vitro fertilization-embryo transfer. *Fertil Steril* 1996;**65**(4):791–5.

50. Fedele L, Bianchi S, Zanconato G, Berlanda N, Raffaelli R, Fontana E. Laparoscopic excision of recurrent endometriomas: long-term outcome and comparison with primary surgery. *Fertil Steril* 2006;**85**(3):694–9.

51. Rizk B and Abdalla H. Surgery for Endometriosis. In: Rizk B and Abdalla H (Eds.) Endometriosis. Second edition. Oxford: United Kingdom, Health Press, 2003; chapter 6, 84–86.

■ 33 ■

MEDICAL MANAGEMENT OF ENDOMETRIOSIS

Botros R. M. B. Rizk, Mary George Nawar, Christine B. Rizk, David B. Rizk

The successful treatment of endometriosis-associated symptoms typically requires surgical as well as medical intervention. Although medical therapies are not curative per se, the medical management of endometriosis remains to be the cornerstone of the treatment of endometriosis-associated pelvic pain (1). However, medical treatment has no place in the management of infertility associated with endometriosis, with the exception of downregulation prior to in vitro fertilization in advanced disease. Historically, the treatment for endometriosis has been high-dose androgens and progestins. These options have been discontinued because of their significant side effects. The modern era for hormonal therapy began with Danazol in 1971. This has been replaced by GnRH agonists two decades ago (2); more recently, the treatment of endometriosis shifted to decreasing the local estrogen production by aromatase inhibitors. Clinical trials are awaited with interest for selective progesterone modulators, angiostatic agents, and matrix metalloproteinase inhibitors (Table 33.1).

Successful treatment of endometriosis depends on the understanding of the effect of hormones and therapeutics on the in situ endometrium. However, there is a significant difference between the in situ endometrium and the ectopic endometrium "endometriosis." Significant aberrant gene expression has been demonstrated in the endometriotic tissue (3). These changes explain excessive local production and decrease inactivation of estrogen in the endometriotic tissue. These include inactivation of 17β-hydroxysteroid dehydrogenase (4), progesterone receptor isoform B (5), and HOXA10 (6) to the upregulation of matrix metalloproteinases (7) and P450 aromatase (8) and to massive gene expression aberration uncovered by the microarray technology (9–12).

PSEUDOPREGNANCY AND ORAL CONTRACEPTIVES

In 1959, Kistner working at Boston Free Hospital (now Brigham and Women's Hospital) reported the use of Enovid (norethynodrel and mestranol) in fifty-eight women with pelvic endometriosis (13). This was a landmark in the history of pharmacological treatment of endometriosis. However, it lost its popularity because of significant side effects.

PROGESTOGENS AND ANTIPROGESTERONES

Progestogens

Progestogen is a hormone that binds to progesterone receptors and results in a progesterone-like action. There are two major forms of progesterone receptors, A and B, that are expressed by a single gene. However, two isotypes exist because of transcription from different promoters. Progesterone receptor agonist induces confirmation of changes that overcomes an inhibitory effect on transcription. Progestogen antagonists permit this inhibitory action to exist. Progesterone receptor A inhibits the activity of the B receptor. Predominant expression of the progesterone receptor A in the endometriotic tissue may play a role in the pathogenesis of endometriosis (5).

Medical treatment of endometriosis by progestogens has been widely used for several decades (Table 33.2). Several randomized controlled trials evaluated the efficacy of progestogen therapy. In 1987, Telimaa et al. performed a trial comparing medroxyprogesterone acetate, 100 mg orally to Danazol 200 mg orally three times daily (14). Fifty-nine patients with mild-to-moderate endometriosis were included in the trial. Electrocoagulation of endometriotic implants was performed in 27 percent of patients. Nine participants were lost to follow-up. The medroxyprogesterone acetate significantly reduced pelvic pain when compared to placebo. There was no significant difference between MPA and Danazol regarding the pelvic pain score at the six-month follow-up. There was also no difference between the two medications regarding the AFS scores.

In 1994, Overton et al. published a double-blind randomized multicenter study comparing progestogen to placebo (15). Sixty-two patients, British, with minimal to mild endometriosis, were investigated. The first group received dydrogesterone (Duphaston) for twelve days starting two days after luteinizing hormone surge, the second group received 40 mg dydrogesterone, and the third received placebo treatment. At twelve months, the second-look laparoscopy was performed. The pelvic pain and AFS scores were not significantly improved.

In 1996, Vercellini performed a randomized trial comparing depot MPA 150 mg every ninety days to a combination of Danazol 50 mg daily for twenty-one to twenty-eight days and oral contraceptives (16).

Danazol

Danazol is an isoxezol derivative of 17α-ethynyl testosterone. It remained the primary medication for the treatment of symptomatic endometriosis until it was replaced by GnRH agonists. Danazol works by altering the endocrinological state of the patients and the immunologic state that is associated with endometriosis. It suppresses gonadotropin surges and lowers circulating estradiol and progesterone by steroidogenic enzyme

Table 33.1: Medical Therapy for Endometriosis-Associated Pelvic Pain

Past Treatment

Methyl testosterone

Danazol

Gestrinone

Mifepristone

Oral contraceptives – high dose

Current therapy

GnRH agonists

Modern oral contraceptives

Progestogens

Future therapy

GnRH antagonist

Aromatase inhibitors

Progesterone receptor modulators

Estrogen receptor modulators

Experimental

Angiogenesis inhibitors

Cytokine inhibitors

Immunomodulators

Metalloproteinases

inhibition (17). Danazol interacts with androgen and progesterone receptors to induce endometrial atrophy. Danazol has an immunomodulatory effect on T-cell function and immunocompetent cells in eutopic endometrium (18).

Danazol is typically administered in doses that ranged from 200 to 800 mg/day to induce amenorrhea. Metzger and Luciano (17) reported an 88 percent symptomatic improvement and 77 percent clinical improvement in sixteen clinical trial involving 1,035 patients (17). Dmowski et al. (19) conducted a six-month double-blind trial comparing the effects of daily doses ranging from 100 to 600 mg of Danazol (19). Clinical symptoms improved in 56 percent of patients receiving 100 mg in daily doses and 83 percent in patients receiving 600 mg of Danazol per day.

Danazol is a synthetic byproduct of testosterone with a half-life of 4.5 hours after oral ingestion and peak levels are reached by two hours, and it is no longer detectable after eight hours (1). Danazol is metabolized in the liver, and methylethisterone, the principal metabolite, exhibits androgenic as well as mild progestational activity.

Danazol has the direct effect on steroidogenesis including cholesterol cleavage enzymes. It has an indirect action by decreasing GnRH pulse frequency.

Side effects

The most common side effects are hyperandrogenism including oily skin and hair, acne, hirsutism, and weight gain. Hot flashes and muscle cramps may also occur. Deepening of the voice, though uncommon, is irreversible. Danazol also has metabolic side effects as it increases LDL and decreases HDL and should be used with caution in women with liver disease.

Cochrane Database Review of Danazol

This meta-analysis was designed to determine the effectiveness of Danazol compared to placebo or no treatment in the management of symptoms or signs other than infertility in women of reproductive age (20). Only four trials were identified. Treatment with Danazol was effective in relieving painful symptoms associated with endometriosis. Side effects were commonly reported in patients taking Danazol rather than placebo.

Antiprogesterones

Gestrinone

Gestrinone is an antiprogestational steroid that has been used in Europe for treatment of endometriosis but is unavailable in the United States (1). Gestrinone is a 19-norsteroid derivative that was originally designed as a weekly oral contraceptive. Gestrinone acts both centrally and peripherally and causes reduction in sex hormone–binding globulin and serum estradiol levels. Gestrinone reduces both progesterone and estrogen receptor concentrations in target tissues.

Gestrinone has a long half-life allowing for administration two to three times weekly. Gestrinone has similar androgenic and metabolic side effects to Danazol but fewer hypoestrogenic side effects.

In randomized clinical trials, Gestrinone was as effective as Danazol in reducing endometriosis-associated pain. Fedele et al. treated thirty-nine patients with endometriosis diagnosed at laparoscopy using gestrinone 2.5 mg twice weekly or Danazol 600–800 mg daily (21). The doses of both drugs were adjusted so as to induce amenorrhea. The primary end-point was infertility, but pain was also evaluated. There was no significant difference in dysmenorrhea or dyspareunia. The AFS scores were similar in the sixteen patients who underwent follow-up laparoscopy.

In a British study that involved 269 women with endometriosis, the patients were randomized to either gestrinone 2.5 mg twice weekly or Danazol 200 mg twice daily for six months (22). The outcome measures were pain scores and AFS scores during therapy as well as twelve months later. There was no difference in the dysmenorrhea or dyspareunia between the two groups (22).

Gestrinone was compared to GnRH agonist, leuprorelin, in a randomized double-blind multicenter Italian study that included fifty-five women aged eighteen to forty with chronic pelvic pain and a laparoscopic diagnosis of endometriosis (23). Gestrinone was administered orally 2.5 mg twice weekly, and leuprorelin was administered intramuscularly 3.75 mg once a month. GnRH agonists had a small advantage in the improvement of dysmenorrheal, but by the end of the follow-up, the advantage was in favor of the gestrinone. Both treatment arms benefited from significant reduction in pain. In 1990, Hornstein et al. compared two doses of gestrinone, 2.5 mg and 1.25 mg, twice weekly (24). There was no difference in pain, and the lower dose had lower side effects. Gestrinone appears to be as effective as GnRH agonists in the treatment of endometriosis.

Mifepristone

Mifepristone, RU486, has been widely used worldwide for pregnancy termination and other medical indications. Mifepristone inhibits ovulation and disrupts endometrial integrity. It has been investigated in patients with symptomatic endometriosis to induce chronic anovulation.

In two pilot studies (25, 26), mifepristone 100 mg per day was given for three months with significant improvement in pelvic pain. Interestingly, at laparoscopy, there was no visible regression of pelvic endometriosis (25, 26). In a follow-up study, treatment was extended six months and the dose was decreased to 50 mg per day. There was a significant decrease in pelvic pain within four weeks. These pilot studies indicate a potential role for antiprogesterone in the treatment of pelvic endometriosis.

Cochrane Database Review of Progestogens in Endometriosis

This review was designed to determine the effectiveness of both the progestogens and antiprogestogens in the treatment of painful symptoms associated with endometriosis (27). Seven studies were identified, and of these, only three studies compared progestogens with placebo, Danazol, and oral contraceptive plus Danazol combination. All other studies compared the antiprogestogen, gestrinone, with other medical therapies. The limited available data suggested that both continuous progestogens and antiprogestogens are effective therapies in the treatment of pain associated with endometriosis. Progestogens given in the luteal phase are not effective.

GONADOTROPHIN-RELEASING HORMONE AGONIST

The native GnRH is a short-acting decapeptide that is secreted episodically into the pituitary circulation to control the formation and release of follicle-stimulating hormone and luteinizing hormone (Figure 33.1). The synthetic GnRH agonist down-regulates the pituitary function, thereby suppressing ovarian steroid production and inducing reversible pseudomenopause. The GnRH agonist must be given parenterally and are available as a nasal spray (nafarelin and buserelin) subcutaneous pellet (goserelin or depo injection) leuprolide/leuprorelin.

GnRH agonists have been extensively used and investigated over the past two decades (2); prospective randomized studies have confirmed GnRH agonist to be as effective as Danazol in endometriosis-associated pain (28–30). The side effect profile is very different. GnRH agonists produce menopausal symptoms such as hot flashes as a result of the hypoestrogenic state that they create.

GnRH Agonist Add-Back Therapy

The estrogen threshold hypothesis was proposed by Barbieri in 1992 (31). Decreased estradiol levels produce changes in different tissues, depending on the sensitivity of the tissues. The most sensitive target is the liver for the manufacture of proteins followed by lipids, vaginal epithelium, vasomotor symptoms, and finally the bone mineral density (BMD). There is no significant loss in the BMD until the serum estradiol level drops to 20 pg/mL. Vasomotor symptoms begin at about 20 pg/mL, and vaginal epithelium starts to become atrophic at 60 pg/mL. In contrast, the treatments for pathological estrogen-dependent disease also have different threshold estradiol levels. Symptomatic endometriosis respond at serum estradiol levels between 30 and 50 pg/mL, and for breast cancer the levels are lower (Figure 33.2).

A variety of medications have been used as add-back therapy in addition to GnRH agonist for treatment of endometriosis in the United States and the UK (32, 33). These include progestogen alone, progestogen and estrogen combination, or progestogen and bisphosphonates (Figure 33.3).

GnRH Agonist Dose Titration

In patients who suffer from pain associated with endometriosis, suppression of estradiol production produces significant pain relief. The price of significant estrogen suppression is vasomotor symptoms and bone loss. This has been the basis of adding low doses of estrogen/progestogen or progestogen only to GnRH agonist. Another successful approach is decreasing the

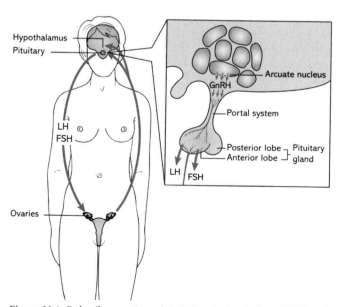

Figure 33.1. Pulsatile secretion of GnRH and stimulation of FSH and LH from the ovary. Reproduced with permission from Rizk and Abdalla (1) and Health Press, Oxford, UK.

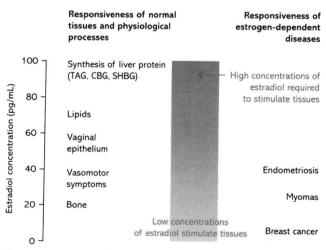

Figure 33.2. Estrogen threshold hypothesis. Reproduced with permission from Barbieri (31).

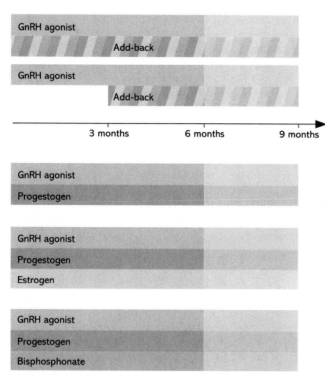

Figure 33.3. Add-back therapy for bone protection for conventional bone loss during GnRh treatment. Reproduced with permission from Rizk and Abdalla (1) and Health Press, Oxford, UK.

dose of GnRH agonist to reduce the suppression of FSH and LH and therefore allow ovarian estrogen production (34).

In practice, this has been performed in a variety of ways. Initiation of therapy was commenced using a standard dose of GnRH agonist such as nafarelin at a dose of 200 mcg bid and then the dose was decreased after one to three months to two nasal sprays on the even calendar days and one nasal spray on the odd calendar days. This will reduce the dose by approximately 25 percent. Further reduction of the dose is possible until pain recurs, and the dose can be increased to achieve more separation of FSH and LH (35–37).

Increasing the time interval between depot injections of RH agonist could be helpful (38). A randomized study, comparing triptorelin depot 3.75 mg i.m. every four weeks to every six weeks found that similar pain improvement occurred in both groups. Body mass index (BMI) was an important issue in predicting whether the extended dose would be effective as patients whose BMI is greater than 30 kg/m^2 and are less likely to achieve amenorrhea with reduced doses of GnRH agonists.

Cochrane Database Review of GnRH Agonist in the Treatment of Endometriosis

The objective of this systematic review was to determine the effectiveness of GnRH agonists in the treatment of the painful symptoms of endometriosis by comparing them with no treatment, placebo, other recognized medical treatments, and surgical interventions (39). Twenty-six studies were identified as appropriate for inclusion in the meta-analysis of the Cochrane Database. The largest group consisted of fifteen studies that compared GnRH agonist with Danazol. There are five studies comparing GnRH agonist with GnRH agonist – add-back

therapy. Three compared GnRH agonist with a different form or dose of GnRH agonist. One with gestrinone, one with the combined oral contraceptive pill, and one with placebo. There was no difference between GnRH agonist in any of the other active comparators with respect to pain relief or reduction in endometriotic deposits. The side effect profiles of the different treatment modalities were very different. With Danazol and gestrinone having more androgenic side effects, while GnRH agonists seem to produce more hypoestrogenic symptoms. The reviewers concluded that GnRH agonist is an effective treatment for endometriosis. The side effects of GnRH agonists could be eliminated by add-back therapy (39).

GnRH ANTAGONISTS

GnRH antagonists' main mechanism of action is competitive receptor occupancy, which results in the blockade of GnRH receptor dimerization, a process that is required for receptor activation. Native GnRH elicits a response when only 1–10 percent of gonadotroph GnRH receptors are occupied. An effective GnRH antagonist must therefore possess high affinity for the receptor, have a prolonged duration of action, and also are given in doses large enough to block the majority of the pituitary GnRH receptors (34).

GnRH antagonists have been used for the treatment of pelvic endometriosis; however, they have not been as widely accepted as GnRH agonists. The serum estradiol levels remain at a mean of 50 pg/mL. At this level, the estrogen production during the course of treatment does not influence the regression of pelvic endometriosis but does not cause the major hypoestrogenic side effect that are experienced when GnRH are given alone without add-back therapy.

In a preliminary study, women with endometriosis and pelvic pain were treated with the GnRH antagonist, cetrorelix 3 mg subcutaneous injection once a week (40). The circulating estradiol levels were suppressed to a mean of 50 pg/mL. Pelvic pain decreased and endometriotic lesions regressed as demonstrated by pretreatment and post-treatment laparoscopy (Figure 33.4).

Another GnRH antagonist, abarelix has been demonstrated to be effective in the treatment of pelvic pain caused by endometriosis (41). It is possible that the use of GnRH antagonist in the future treatment of endometriosis will be more developed once larger clinical trials have been accomplished.

SELECTIVE PROGESTERONE RECEPTOR MODULATORS (SPRMS)

Selective progesterone receptor modulators introduce a new dimension in the medical treatment of endometriosis (1). The concept that hormone receptors exist in a variety of forms within the same tissue has stimulated the design of new compounds with specific actions and side effect profiles. Selective progesterone receptor modulators are a new class of progesterone receptor ligands that have both agonistic and antiagonistic actions (42, 43). There is a variety of progesterone receptor ligands with pure agonistic action similar to progesterone and pure antagonists as onapristone and ZK230211. Many of the selective progesterone receptor modulators are in the middle of the spectrum.

The best known progesterone receptor modulators are J867, J956, J912, and J1042. SPRMs act as weak progestins in the absence of progesterone. In the presence of progesterone,

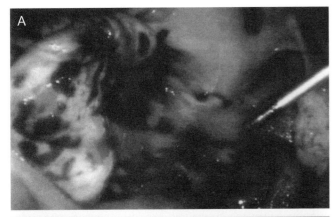

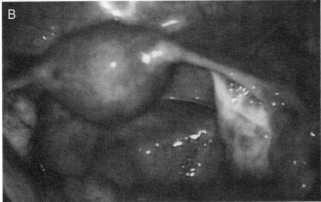

Figure 33.4. Pelvic endometriosis before and after treatment with GnRH antagonist. Reproduced with permission from Kupker (40).

SPRMs have weak progesterone antagonist actions particularly in the endometrium. SPRMs have a reduced glucocorticoid receptor–binding affinity when compared to RU486. SPRMS have minimal binding to estrogen receptors and only in rodents may display a mixed androgenic and antiandrogenic activity.

SPRMs suppress estrogen-dependent endometrial growth and induce reversible amenorrhea (44). Progesterone treatment commonly causes breakthrough bleeding by inducing fragility of the endometrial blood vessels. SPRMs have the spiral arterioles as the target and causing stabilization of the endometrial blood vessels.

SELECTIVE ESTROGEN RECEPTOR MODULATORS (SERMS)

Raloxifene is an SERM developed primarily to prevent and treat postmenopausal osteoporosis. It is the most widely used SERM to date. Raloxifene acts as an estrogen agonist in the bone and liver and as an estrogen antagonist in the uterus and breast.

In experimental animal models, raloxifene have produced encouraging results in two trials (45). In healthy women of reproductive age, the sonographic appearance and progesterone values were particularly ovulatory; therefore, in this age group, Raloxifene does not prevent ovulation, but increases estrogen concentration and produces a minimal antiestrogenic effect on the endometrium. On this basis, Raloxifene would not be effective for treatment of endometriosis.

AROMATASE INHIBITORS

The development and growth of endometriosis is estrogen dependent. Endometriotic tissues have molecular aberration that favor increased local production and decreased inactivation of 17β-estradiol. A positive feedback mechanism for prostaglandin E_2 and 17β-estradiol through upregulation of aromatase and cyclooxygenase-2 (Cox2) in endometriotic stromal cells has been identified. At the same time, there is deficiency of 17β-hydroxysteroid dehydrogenase type II expression in endometriotic epithelial cells. These findings are the molecular basis for the treatment of endometriosis by using aromatase inhibitors (Figure 33.5).

Aromatase enzyme is a target for selective inhibition of estrogen synthesis (see chapter 24 by Mitwally and Casper). Several compounds have been developed over the past decades, with the third generation of aromatase inhibitors currently used for breast cancer patients during the past decade. Letrozole and anastrozole are potent and selective third-generation, nonsteroidal aromatase inhibitors.

The inhibition of local estrogen production in endometriotic implants is an attractive option for the management of endometriosis.

Side Effects

Most of our knowledge about side effects associated with the use of aromatase inhibitors are based upon clinical trials involving postmenopausal women with breast cancer. Generally, third-generation aromatase inhibitors are well tolerated. The main side effects are hot flashes and gastrointestinal side effects such as nausea and leg cramps. Letrozole and anastrozole are associated with less weight gain, fewer thromboembolic events, and less vaginal bleeding than progesterones. It is possible that younger women with endometriosis could tolerate these symptoms better than breast cancer patients. Interestingly, most of the infertility patients who have used clomiphene citrate in the past found that treatment with aromatase inhibitors was better tolerated and was associated with less side effects.

Aromatase Expression in Endometriotic Stromal Cells

Prostaglandin E_2 (PGE_2) is the most potent inducer of aromatase activity in endometriotic stromal cells by increasing cAMP

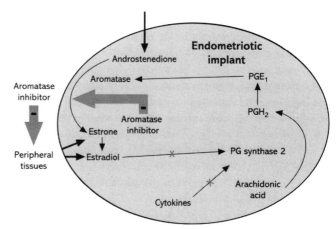

Figure 33.5. The molecular basis of treatment of endometriosis using an aromatase inhibitor. Reproduced with permission from Rizk and Abdalla (1) and Health Press, Oxford, UK.

(46). At the same time, neither PGE_2 nor cAMP analogs were capable of stimulating aromatase activity in eutopic endometrial stromal cells in culture. The molecular alterations leading to local aromatase expression in endometriosis, but not in normal endometrium, is the abnormal production of a stimulatory transcription factor, SF-1 in endometriotic stromal cells, which in turn overrides the protective inhibition that is normally maintained by other transcription factors in the eutopic endometrium (47).

Inactivation of Estradiol in Endometriosis

The primary substrate for aromatase activity in endometriosis is androstenedione of adrenal and ovarian origins in premenopausal women and adrenal androstenedione in postmenopausal women (47). The enzyme 17β-hydroxysteroid dehydrogenase type 1 that catalyzes the conversion of estrone to estradiol is expressed in endometriosis. However, the enzyme 17β-hydroxysteroid dehydrogenase type 2 that inactivates estrodiol to estrone is absent from endometriotic glandular cells. The aberrant expression of aromatase, the presence of 17β-HSD type 1, in the absence of 17β-HSD type 2 from endometriosis results in elevated estradiol levels in comparison with eutopic endometrium. Furthermore, the 17β-HSD type 2 deficiency may also be viewed as defective action of progesterone, which fails to induce this enzyme in endometriotic tissue.

Clinical Basis for Treatment of Endometriosis Using Aromatase Inhibitors

Endometriosis is successfully treated by surgery that includes removal of the ovaries or medications such as GnRH agonist that cause estrogen deprivation. GnRH agonist is usually highly successful during and immediately after the treatment. However, pain invariably returns in up to 75 percent of the patients treated. One of the plausible explanations for this treatment is the estradiol production that continues in the skin adipose tissue and endometriotic implants during the GnRH agonist treatment. Blockage of aromatase activity may possibly keep a larger number of patients in remission for longer periods (47).

The evidence for the significance of extraovarian estrogen is the recurrence of endometriosis after a hysterectomy and bilateral salpingo-oophorectomy in some women. A clinical case of a fifty-seven-year-old overweight woman who had recurrence of severe endometriosis after hysterectomy and bilateral salpingo-oophorectomy has been reported (48). Two additional laparotomies were performed because of bilateral ureteral obstruction leading to left renal atropy and right hydronephrosis. A large 3-cm vaginal endometriotic lesion had unusually high levels of aromatase mRNA. The patient was treated with aromatase inhibitor, anastrozole, for nine months. Dramatic relief of pain and regression of the vaginal endometriotic lesion were observed within the first month of therapy. Circulating estradiol levels were reduced to 50 percent of the baseline value. Aromatase mRNA pretreatment levels became undetectable in a repeat biopsy, six months later. The lesion disappeared after nine months of therapy.

ANTIANGIOGENESIS THERAPY

VEGF is a major mediator in the pathogenesis of endometriosis by promoting angiogenesis. VEGF is produced by activated macrophages in the menstrual effluent and peritoneal cavity. Menstrual blood in the peritoneal cavity could facilitate neoangiogenesis and adhesion of endometrial cells.

Antiangiogenesis therapy has been investigated in rodents, and Nap et al. (2005) demonstrated that angiostatic agents prevent the development of endometriosis-like lesions in the chicken chorioallantoic membrane (49, 50). The future challenge is to successfully utilize it in women suffering from pelvic endometriosis.

IMMUNOMODULATORS

Vignali et al. reviewed the role of immunomodulators in the treatment of endometriosis (51). Four compounds with immune-enhancing properties have been investigated cytokines, interleukin-12 and interferon α-2b, and two synthetic immunomodulators, the guanosine analog loxoribine and the acetyl-choline nicotinic receptor agonist levamisole.

Badawy et al. (51) demonstrated that interferon α-2b inhibits endometrioma cell growth in culture (52). D'Hooghe et al. (52) demonstrated that recombinant tumor necrosis factor–binding protein 1 inhibited the development of experimentally induced endometriosis in the baboon model (53).

Keenan et al. (53) demonstrated the regression of experimentally induced endometriosis in rats using intraperitoneal loxoribine (54).

ANTI-INFLAMMATORY AGENTS

The pain associated with endometriosis is typical of the pain in inflammatory diseases. Nonsteroidal inflammatory drugs are very helpful in pelvic pain and dysmenorrhea associated with endometriosis.

Herbal Medicines in the Treatment of Endometriosis

A significant increase in the lifetime use of herbs and natural products from 12.1 to 18.6 percent was seen between 1998 and 2002 in the United States (54, 55). The WHO, on May 16, 2002, released its global strategy on traditional medicines and announced that it will increase its research in nonallopathic therapies. It also has to be remembered that several important drugs are derived from natural products as aspirin, penicillin, and taxol. Weiser et al. (55) recently reviewed the evidence on the efficacy and safety of herbal medicines in the management of endometriosis-associated pain (56). Although clinical studies on herbs in the literature show promising effects, conclusive clinical evidence of the efficacy of medicinal herbs in the treatment of endometriosis-associated pain is lacking (55).

MEDICAL MANAGEMENT OF ENDOMETRIOSIS-RELATED INFERTILITY

It has been clear over the past three decades that the medical treatment of endometriosis has been very effective in the suppression of the pain associated with this disease. In contrast, medical treatment has never improved the pregnancy chances in patients with endometriosis-associated infertility. Hughes et al. (56) evaluated data from nine trials comparing ovulation suppression with either Danazol, gestrinone, or medroxyprogesterone acetate to no treatment or placebo, which all failed to

Table 33.2: Progestogens Used for Treatment of Endometriosis

Progestogens alone	Dose
Oral medroxyprogesterone acetate	2.5–60 mg daily
Injectable medroxyprogesterone acetate i.m.	50 mg/month or 150 mg every three months
Norethindrone (norethisterone)	2.5–20 mg/day
Megestrol acetate (rarely used in United States)	10–50 mg/day
Dydrogesterone (rarely used in United States)	10 mg, two to three times daily
Progestogens in combination with estrogens	
Desogestrel + ethinyl estradiol	0.15 mg/day and 0.02 mg/day respectively p.o. for twenty-one days of each twenty-eight-day cycle over six months
Cyproterone acetate	12.5 mg/day for six months

show any beneficial effect on enhancing pregnancy rates (OR 0.85; 95% CI 0.95–1.22). In the same study, an additional six randomized trials comparing a GnRH agonist, gestrinone, or an oral contraceptive to Danazol also failed to demonstrate improvement (OR 1.07; 95% CI 0.71–1.61). In a series of well-designed meta-analyses by Adamson and Pasta, it was confirmed that medical treatment of endometriosis did not improve the fertility chances (57).

Surrey (58) proposed several possible explanations of these findings. Minimal and mild endometriosis may have no impact on fertility at all, given the proven efficacy of these agents in treating the underlying disease, but lack of efficacy in improving conception. A second explanation is that the mechanism of infertility associated with endometriosis is different from that associated with pelvic pain and is unaffected by these medications. Surrey states that neither of these explanations are supported by data. A third and perhaps more plausible explanation is that by the time a patient resumes normal ovulatory patterns, which may be months after completion of therapy, the deleterious effects of the disease process on fertility that were initially suppressed by medications reoccur even if the patient remains asymptomatic (58).

Thus, if a patient could attempt conception when the disease process is maximally suppressed, pregnancy rates would be heightened. This could only occur with the use of the assisted reproductive technologies. In a prospective randomized trial, Surrey et al. have recently evaluated the effect of a three-month course of a GnRH agonist administered immediately before in vitro fertilization (IVF) in patients with surgically confirmed endometriosis (59). Significantly higher rates were appreciated in this group of twenty-five patients in comparison to twenty-six controls with endometriosis treated with standard controlled ovarian hyperstimulation techniques before oocyte aspiration in the absence of prolonged GnRH agonist. These findings have been confirmed by other investigators (60–64). This effect may be a result of a beneficial effect of these agents on either peritoneal cytokine levels or endometrial markers of implantations.

KEY POINTS: MEDICAL MANAGEMENT OF ENDOMETRIOSIS

- Medical management is a key component of the management of endometriosis-associated pelvic pain.
- Progestogens are efficacious and inexpensive treatment of pelvic endometriosis.
- Oral contraceptives are widely used for the medical management of endometriosis; there is paucity of data for prospective randomized studies.
- GnRH agonist has been the most efficacious medical option for the past two decades.
- Repeated short courses of GnRH agonist are very helpful in the management of endometriosis pain.
- Add-back therapy with GnRH agonist avoids the menopausal side effects, bone loss, without causing the recurrence of pelvic pain.
- Postoperative GnRH treatment may prolong the time interval to the next treatment modality.
- GnRH agonist downregulation before IVF may improve IVF outcome in patients with advanced endometriosis, provided they have good ovarian reserve.
- Aromatase inhibitors have been successfully used in the treatment of postmenopausal patients and could be the future treatment for premenopausal women.
- Nonsteroidal inflammatory drugs alleviate dysmenorrhea and pelvic pain associated with endometriosis.
- Antiangiogensis therapy and matrix metalloproteinese inhibitors may possibly be useful in the future in the treatment of pelvic endometriosis.
- Selective progesterone receptor modulators could potentially suppress estrogen-dependent endometrial growth and induce reversible amenorrhea.

REFERENCES

1. Rizk B, Abdalla H. (2003). Medical treatment of endometriosis. In: Rizk B, Abdalla H (Eds.). *Endometriosis*, Oxford, England; Health Press, Chapter 4, pp. 55–70.
2. Lemay A, Maheux R, Faure N, et al. (1984). Reversible hypogonadism induced by a luteinizing hormone-releasing hormone (LHRH) agonist (Buserelin) as a new therapeutic approach for endometriosis. *Fertil Steril* **41**:863–71.
3. Wu Y, Strawn E, Basir Z, Halverson G, Guo S-W. (2007). Aberrant expression of deoxyribonucleic acid methyltransferases DNMT1, DNMT3A, and DNMT3B in women with endometriosis. *Fertil Steril* **87**:24–32.
4. Zeitoun K, Takayama K, Sasano H, Suzuki T, Moghrabi N, Andersson S, et al. (1998). Deficient 17beta-hydroxysteriod dehydrogenase type 2 expression in endometriosis: failure to metabolize 17 beta-estradiol. *J Clin Endocrinol Metab* **83**:4474–80.
5. Attia GR, Zeitoun K, Edwards D, Johns A, Carr BR, Bulun SE. (2000). Progesterone receptor isoform A but not B is expressed in endometriosis. *J Clin Endocrinol Metab* **85**:2897–902.
6. Taylor HS, Bagot C, Kardana A, Olive D, Arici A. (1999). HOX gene expression is altered in the endometrium of women with endometriosis. *Hum Reprod* **14**:1328–31.
7. Osteen KG, Yeaman GR, Bruner-Tran KL. (2003). Matrix metalloproteinases and endometriosis. *Semin Reprod Med* **21**:155–64.
8. Noble LS, Simpson ER, Johns A, Bulun SE. (1996). Aromatase expression in endometriosis. *J Clin Endocrinol Metab* **81**:174–9.

9. Kao LC, Germeyer A, Tulax S, Lobo S, Yang JP, Taylor RN, et al. (2003). Expression profiling of endometrium from women with endometriosis reveals candidate genes for disease-based implantation failure and infertility: *Endocrinology* **144**:2870–81.

10. Matsuzaki S, Canis M, Vaurs-Barriere C, Bosespflug-Tanguy O, Penault-Llorca F, et al. (2004). DNA microarray analysis of gene expression profiles in deep endometriosis using laser capture microdissection: *Mol Hum Reprod* **10**:719–28.

11. Matsuzaki S, Canis M, Vaurs-Barriere C, Boespflug-Tanguy O, Dastugue B, Mage G. (2005). DNA microarray analysis of gene expression in eutopic endometrium from patients with deep endometriosis using laser capture microdissection: *Fertil Steril* **84**(Suppl. 2):1180–90.

12. Wu K, Kajdacsy-Balla A, Strawn E, Basir Z, Halverson G, Jailwala P, et al. (2006). Transcriptional characterizations of differences between eutopic and ectopic endometrium. *Endocrinology* **147**:232–46.

13. Kistner RW. (1958). The use of progestins in the treatment of endometriosis. *Am J Obstet Gynecol* **75**:264–78.

14. Telimaa S, Ronnberg L, Kauppila A. (1987). Placebo-controlled comparison of Danazol and high dose medroxyprogesterone acetate in the treatment of endometriosis after conservative surgery. *Gynecol Endocrinol* **1**:363–71.

15. Overton CE, Lindsay PC, Johal B. (1994). A randomized, double blind, placebo controlled study of luteal phase dydrogesterone (Duphasone) in women with minimal to mild endometriosis. *Fertil Steril* **62**:701–7.

16. Vercellini P, De Giorgi O, Oldani S, Cortesti I, Panazza S, Crosignnani PG. (1996). Depot medroxyprogesterone acetate versus an oral contraceptive combined with very-low-dose Danazol for long-term treatment of pelvic pain associated with endometriosis. *Am J Obstet Gynecol* **175**:396–401.

17. Metzger D, Luciano A. (1989). Hormonal therapy of endometriosis. *Obstet Gynecol Clin (N.A.)* **16**:105–22.

18. Ota H, Igarashi S, Hayakawa M, et al. (1996). Effect of danazol on the immunocompetent cell in the eutopic endometrium in patients with endometriosis: a multicenter cooperative study. *Fertil Steril* **65**:545–51.

19. Dmowski W, Kapetanakis E, Scommegna A. (1982). Variable effects of danazol on endometriosis at 4 low-dose levels. *Obstet Gynecol* **59**:408–15.

20. Selak V, Farquhar C, Prentice A, Singla A. (2001). Danazol for pelvic pain associated with endometriosis. *Cochrane Database Syst Rev* (4):CD000068.

21. Fedele L, Bianchi S, Viezzoli T, Arcaini L, Candiani GB. (1989). Gestrinone versus danazol in the treatment of endometriosis. *Fertil Steril* **51**:781–5.

22. Bromham DR, Booker MW, Rose GL, Wardle PG, Newton JR. (1995). A multicentre comparative study of gestrinone and danazol in the treatment of endometriosis. *Am J Obstet Gynecol* **15**:188–94.

23. The Gestrinone Italian Study Group. (1996). Gestrinone versus gonadotropin releasing hormone agonist for the treatment of pelvic pain associated with endometriosis: a multicenter, randomized, double-blind study. *Fertil Steril* **66**:911–19.

24. Hornstein MD, Glaeson RE, Barbieri RI. (1990). A randomized, double-blind prospective trial of two doses of gestrinone in the treatment of endometriosis. *Fertil Steril* **53**:237–41.

25. Kettel LM, Murphy AA, Morales AJ, et al. (1996). Treatment of endometriosis with the antiprogesterone mifepristone (RU486). *Fertil Steril* **65**:23.

26. Kettel LM, Murphy AA, Mortola JF, et al. (1991). Endocrine responses to long-term administration of the antiprogesterone RU486 in patients with pelvic endometriosis. *Fertil Steril* **56**:402.

27. Prentice A, Deary AJ, Bland E. (2000). Progestogens and antiprogestogens for pain associated with endometriosis. *Cochrane Database Syst Rev* (2):CD002122.

28. Henzl MR, Corson SL, Moghissi K, et al. (1988). Administration of nasal nafarelin as compared multicenter double-blind comparative clinical trial with oral danazol for endometriosis. *N Engl J Med* **318**:485–9.

29. Dlugi AM, Miller JD, Knittle J. (1990). Lupron depot (leuprolide acetate for depot suspension) in the treatment of endometriosis: a randomized, placebo-controlled, double-blind study. Lupron Study Group. *Fertil Steril* **54**:419–27.

30. Bergqvist A. (1998). Effects of triptorelin versus placebo on the symptoms of endometriosis. *Fertil Steril* **69**:702–8.

31. Barbieri RL. (1992). Hormone treatment of endometriosis: the oestrogen threshold hypothesis. *Am J Obstet Gynecol* **166**:740–5.

32. Moghissi KS. (1996). Add-back therapy in the treatment of endometriosis: the North American experience. *Br J Obstet Gynecol* **103**:14.

33. Edmonds DK. (1996). Add-back therapy in the treatment of endometriosis: the European experience. *Br J Obstet Gynecol* **103**:10–13.

34. Barbieri RL. (2004). Gonadotropin releasing hormone agonist and antagonist for endometriosis. In: Tulandi T, Redwine D, (Eds.) *Endometriosis: Advances and Controversies*. New York: Marcel Dekker, Chapter 13, pp. 219–43.

35. Hull ME, Barbieri RL. (1994). Nafarelin in the treatment of endometriosis: dose management. *Gynecol Obstet Invest* **37**:263–4.

36. Tahara M, Matsouka T, Yodoi T, Tasaka K, Kurachi H, Murata Y. (2000). Treatment of endometriosis with a decreasing dosage of a gonadotropin releasing hormone agonist (nafarelin): a pilot study with low-dose agonist therapy. *Fertil Steril* **73**:799–804.

37. Uemura T, Shirasu K, Datagiri N, Asukai K, Suzuki T, Suzuki N. (1999). Low-dose GnRH agonist therapy for the management of endometriosis. *J Obstet Gynecol Res* **25**:295–301.

38. Tse CY, Chow AM, Chan SC. (2000). Effects of extended-interval dosing regimen of triptorelin depot on the hormonal profile of patients with endometriosis: prospective observational study. *Hong Kong Med J* **6**:260–4.

39. Prentice A, Deary AJ, Goldbeck-Wood S, Farquhar C, Smith SK. Gonadotropin releasing hormone analogues for pain associated with endometriosis. *Cochrane Database Syst Rev* CD00346.

40. Kupker W, Felberbaum RE, Krapp M, et al. (2002). Use of GnRH antagonists in the treatment of endometriosis. *Reprod BioMed Online* **5**:12–16.

41. Martha P, Gray M, Campion M, Kuca B, Garnick M. (1999). Prolonged suppression of circulating estrogen levels without an initial hormonal flare using abarelix-depot, a pure GnRH antagonist, in women with endometriosis. *Fertil Steril* **72**:S210–11.

42. Chwalisz K, Garg R, Brenner RM, Schubert G, Elger W. (2002). Selective progesterone receptor modulators (SPRMs)—a novel therapeutic concept in endometriosis. *Ann N Y Acad Sci* **955**:373–88.

43. Chwalisz K, Brenner RM, Fuhrmann U, Hess-Stumpp Elger W. (2000). Antiproliferative effects of progesterone antagonists and progesterone receptor modulators on the endometrium. *Steroids* **65**:741–51.

44. Elger W, Bartley J. Schneider B, Kaufmann G, Schubert G, Chwalisz K. (2000). Endocrine pharmacological characterization of progesterone antagonists and progesterone receptor modulators (PRMs) with respect to PR-agonistic and antagonistic activity. *Steroids* **65**:713–23

45. Fanning P, Kuehl T, Lee R, Pearson S, et al. (1997). Video mapping to assess efficacy of an antiestrogen (raloxifene) on spontaneous endometriosis in the rhesus monkey. *Fertil Steril* **68**:S38–9.

46. Noble LS, Takayama K, Zeitoun KM, et al. (1997). Prostaglandin E$_2$ stimulates aromatase expression in endometriosis-derived stromal cells. *J Clin Endocrinol Metab* **82**:600–6.

47. Bulun SE, Gurates B, Fang Z, et al. (2004). Treatment with aromatase inhibitors. In: Tulandi T, Redwine D, (Eds.) *Endometriosis: Advances and Controversies*. New York: Marcel Dekker, Chapter 11, pp. 189–202.

48. Takayama K, Zeitoun K, Gunby RT, et al. (1998). Treatment of severe postmenopausal endometriosis with an aromatase inhibitor. *Fertil Steril* **69**:709–713.

49. Scarpellini F, Sbracia M, Lecchini S, Scarpellini L. (2002). Anti-angiogenesis treatment with thalidomide in endometriosis: a pilot study. *Fertil Steril* **78**:S87.

50. Vignali M, Infantino M, Matrone R, et al. (2002). Endometriosis: novel etiopathogenetic concepts and clinical perspectives. *Fertil Steril* **78**:665–78.

51. Badawy S, Etman A, Cuenca V, et al. (2001). Effect of interferon α-2b on endometrial cells in vitro. *Obstet Gynecol* **98**:417–20.

52. D'Hooghe T, Cuneo S, Nugent N, et al. (2001). Recombinant human TNF binding protein-1 (r-hTBP-1) inhibits the development of endometriosis in baboons: a prospective, randomized, placebo- and drug controlled study. *Fertil Steril* **76**:S1.

53. Keenan J, Williams-Boyle P, Massey P, Chen T, et al. (1999). Regression of endometrial explants in a rat model of endometriosis treated with the immune modulators loxoribine and levamisole. *Fertil Steril* **721**:135–41.

54. Tindle HA, Davis RB, Phillips RS, Eisenberg DM. (2005). Trends in use of complementary and alternative medicine by US adults: 1997-2002. *Altern Ther Health Med* **11**:42–9.

55. Weiser F, Cohen M, Gaeddert A, et al. (2007). Evolution of medical treatment for endometriosis: back to the roots? *Hum Reprod Update* **13**(5):487–99.

56. Hughes EG, Fedorkow DM, Collins JA. (1993). A quantitative overview of controlled trials in endometriosis-associated infertility. *Fertil Steril* **59**:963–70.

57. Adamson GD, Pasta D. (1994). Surgical treatment of endometriosis-associated infertility: meta-analysis compared with survival analysis. *Am J Obstet Gynecol* **171**:1488–505.

58. Surrey ES. (2004). Medical therapy for endometriosis: an overview. In: Tulandi T, Redwine D, (Eds.) *Endometriosis: Advances and Controversies*. New York: Marcel Dekker, Chapter 10, pp. 167–88.

59. Surrey ES, Silverberg K, Surrey MW, Schoolcraft WB. (2002). The effect of prolonged GnRH agonist therapy on in vitro fertilization-embryo transfer cycle outcome in endometriosis patients: a multicenter randomized trial. *Fert Steril* **78**:699–704.

60. Dicker D, Goldman GA, Ashkenazi J, Feldbert D, et al. (1990). The value of pretreatment with long-term gonadotropin-releasing hormone (GnRH) analogue in IVF-ET therapy of severe endometriosis. *Hum Reprod* **5**:418–20.

61. Marcus SF, Edwards RG. (1994). High rates of pregnancy after long-term downregulation of women with severe endometriosis. *Am J Obstet Gynecol* **171**:812–17.

62. Nakamura K, Oosawa M, Kondou I, Inagaki S, et al. (1992). Menotropin stimulation after prolonged gonadotropin releasing hormone agonist pretreatment of in vitro fertilization in patients with endometriosis. *J Assist Reprod Genet* **9**:113–17.

63. Curtis P, Jackson A, Bernard A, Shaw RW. (1993). Pretreatment with gonadotrophin releasing hormone (GnRH) analogue prior to in vitro fertilization for patients with endometriosis. *Eur J Obstet Gynecol Reprod Biol* **52**:211–16.

64. Rizk B, Abdalla H. (2003). Treatment of infertility associated with endometriosis. In: Rizk B, Abdalla H, (Eds.) *Endometriosis*. Oxford: United Kingdom, Health press, Chapter 6, pp. 85–6.

34

REPRODUCTIVE SURGERY FOR
ENDOMETRIOSIS-ASSOCIATED INFERTILITY

Alexis H. Kim, G. David Adamson

In the reproductive-age female, estimates of the general prevalence of endometriosis range from 6 to 11 percent (1–4). Among infertile women, the prevalence of endometriosis has been estimated to be about 20 percent (5). This is in contrast to asymptomatic women undergoing tubal ligation who have a prevalence of 4 percent. Although endometriosis may not be the primary cause of infertility in many of these patients, evidence from several studies support that fecundity is reduced, even in patients with minimal to mild endometriosis (6–8). Having to sort through the diverse therapeutic approaches to endometriosis-associated infertility, to come to a decision regarding the treatment plan often can be a challenging process for even an experienced clinician.

The diversity of choices from expectant management to combined medical/surgical treatment reflects, to some extent, the complex nature of this disease and the explanations for the mechanisms of morbidity. Management decisions are further complicated by coexisting fertility factors, variability of endometriosis presentation, surgical outcome, and, until recently, relatively few good studies to guide us to the best treatment course. Endometriosis may interfere with reproductive outcome by disrupting the hormonal, anatomical, and immunologic milieu of the pelvis. Generally, as the severity of disease increases, alterations within the pelvis become more pronounced, making the timely diagnosis and treatment important to minimize the clinical sequelae.

In patients whose reproductive goals are to maintain or restore fertility, the treatment objectives involve removing or destroying endometrial implants, restoring normal anatomy, and preventing or delaying disease recurrence. Surgery is typically the treatment of choice to accomplish these objectives, especially when moderate or severe endometriosis is involved. In minimal or mild endometriosis where endometrial implants are present typically in the absence of anatomic distortion, the optimal approach to treatment is less obvious. Consideration must be given to other treatment options and their effectiveness relative to surgery to optimize patient care. The increasing availability of basic science and evidence-based data will help us to gain better insight into endometriosis and develop a comprehensive management plan tailored to each patient's reproductive goals.

MECHANISM OF INFERTILITY

Various mechanisms have been proposed to explain the impairment in fertility associated with endometriosis. Except in the case of obvious anatomical distortion by adhesions or tubal occlusion, the exact mechanism by which endometriosis causes subfertility has yet to be determined, but is likely to be a consequence of local inflammation and an altered immune response in the pelvis mediated by cytokines (9). Cytokines promote the growth and spread of endometriosis (10, 11) and propagate chronic inflammatory changes that result in increased peritoneal fluid volume and macrophage number, concentration, and activity (12–15). Within the peritoneal fluid milieu, activated leukocytes are thought to contribute to the impairment of fertility by exerting direct cytotoxic effects or by releasing proteolytic enzymes that affect gamete function or embryo growth. The increase in concentration of activated peritoneal macrophages resulting in sperm phagocytosis is a possible factor in reducing fertility potential (16). The observed changes in the peritoneal environment are also believed to play a role in altered folliculogenesis, ovulatory dysfunction, impaired sperm motility, decreased acrosome reaction rate, disruption of sperm-endosalpingeal interactions, inhibition of oocyte capture, altered gamete interaction, inhibition of early embryo development, defective implantation, and luteal phase defect (17–27). These observations suggest that endometriosis can create abnormalities capable of interfering with normal reproductive function.

The results of other studies have suggested that endometriosis implants alone may not be a cause of infertility. Animal studies have shown that transplanted endometrium reduces fertility only in the presence of adhesions (28–30). In the absence of pelvic distortion, no detrimental effect on fertility was observed (31). In women undergoing donor insemination, no difference in monthly fecundity between women with and without endometriosis was observed (32). A multivariate study of potential infertility factors in a large cohort of infertile women revealed no change in the cumulative conception rate from endometriosis in the absence of adhesions (33). Thus, the association between the presence of endometriosis implants alone and subfertility is still debated.

In a retrospective study, poorer in vitro fertilization (IVF) outcomes were observed in patients with endometriosis compared to patients with tubal factor infertility (34). Pregnancy and implantation rates were similar in recipients with or without endometriosis when oocytes were from donors without endometriosis. However, oocytes from donors with endometriosis (extensive disease inclusive of endometriomas) resulted in lower implantation rates in disease-free recipients compared to oocytes from donors without endometriosis. Moreover, oocytes from women with endometriosis produced embryos with fewer blastomeres and a higher incidence of arrested and abnormal development than women without endometriosis (35, 36). The observations from these studies support, but do not prove, the possibility of endometriosis causing alterations in oocyte quality and subsequent embryo development that result in diminished implantation capacity.

TREATMENT OPTIONS

The optimal management approach to the infertile patient with endometriosis requires an evaluation of the extent of disease and the reproductive goals of the patient. Treatment recommendations typically focus on directly addressing the pelvic implants, improving fecundity through the use of fertility treatments such as IVF, or a combination of both. When attention is primarily focused on treating pelvic implants, restoration of the hormonal, anatomic, or immunologic alterations in the pelvis for future reproduction forms the basis for selection of therapeutic interventions.

The treatment approaches to endometriosis implants can be classified as no treatment, medical treatment, surgical treatment, and combined medical/surgical treatment. For endometriosis-associated infertility, medical therapy alone or in combination with surgery does not improve pregnancy rates (37, 38). In addition to the failure to improve fertility, the ovarian suppression encountered during medical treatment may prolong the duration of infertility for several months. When considering the side effects, additional costs, and the requisite contraceptive period while undergoing treatment, there does not appear to be a role for medical treatment in patients whose only symptom is infertility.

In light of the shortcomings of medical treatment for endometriosis-associated infertility, no treatment has been considered as an alternative in women with minimal or mild disease. This stems from data indicating that no treatment is as effective as surgical treatment for women with minimal or mild endometriosis (38, 39). However, the conclusions from a prospective randomized study suggest that surgical treatment of minimal/mild endometriosis is superior to no treatment (7). The pelvic pathology and anatomic distortion typically associated with moderate or severe endometriosis would likely render the no-treatment approach ineffective. In this situation, surgery is considered the treatment of choice.

The surgical approaches to endometriosis treatment are accomplished by laparotomy or laparoscopy. With the advent of advanced laparoscopic and imaging equipment and operative techniques, laparoscopy has been used more commonly to perform the increasingly complex operations that endometriosis often requires. In general, laparoscopy is the preferred surgical approach, given the advantages of improved visualization, reduced foreign body exposure and possibly reduced adhesion formation, less tissue trauma, a lower incidence of complications, and quicker recovery due to smaller, less painful incisions (40–44). In most situations, these advantages outweigh the disadvantages of laparoscopy such as the inability to palpate structures, the lack of a three-dimensional perspective, and a greater possibility of operator fatigue. However, laparotomy may be more appropriate for performing bowel resection, extensive enterolysis, or removing large endometriomas (45, 46).

The primary laparoscopic techniques used to remove or destroy endometriosis implants involve the laser, electrosurgery, or sharp resection. The preferred method is primarily dependent upon the familiarity and skills of the surgeon with a certain technique and what is considered to yield the best possible outcome. Different types of lasers may be chosen based upon the desired characteristic for a particular clinical situation. For example, the CO_2 laser is used when excellent precision is desired that will allow the creation of a well-defined area of tissue destruction. However, this precision comes at the expense of poor coagulating ability. The argon and KTP532 lasers have better coagulating ability than the CO_2 laser but are less precise. The Nd:YAG laser has the least precision but good coagulating properties that make it more susceptible to unnoticed large-volume thermal injury. Unipolar electrosurgery is effective at removing implants but has a risk of deeper tissue damage. Bipolar electrosurgery is used to desiccate endometriosis implants. However, inadequate treatment is a risk due to the inability to determine the precise extent of tissue destruction. In contrast, sharp resection is effective at removing disease with a low risk of inadequate treatment but is more likely to be affected by bleeding.

SURGICAL PRINCIPLES

Surgical treatment for endometriosis-associated infertility employs techniques that are designed to minimize trauma, maintain hemostasis, and reduce operating time while facilitating the removal of all disease. In order to accomplish these goals, the surgical approach and instruments selected for each case should reflect the skill level and best judgment of the surgeon. Copious irrigation with physiological fluids during the operation assists with the maintenance of a clean surgical field and the reduction in tissue desiccation, allowing for good visualization and the preservation of serosal integrity. These factors in combination with attention to meticulous surgical techniques decrease the risk of de novo adhesion formation (47). The likelihood of operative success will be further enhanced by adhering to surgical principles (Table 34.1).

A detailed description of the status of the pelvis following surgery is an important component of any surgical procedure, especially in the evaluation of fertility potential. In addition to the operative report, an objective recording of the findings and results of surgery through standardized forms such as those from the American Society of Reproductive Medicine (48), photographs, and/or videos will provide a comprehensive document from which future recommendations can be made with respect to fertility. Most importantly, an honest and thorough assessment of the surgical outcome obtained will enable a realistic estimation of the probability of pregnancy to be made.

EVALUATION OF TREATMENT OUTCOME

An association between endometriosis and subfertility has been supported by numerous studies. In the presence of significant pelvic distortion, the role that endometriosis has in disrupting the normal reproductive processes and causing infertility is obvious. Adhesions interfere with normal anatomic relationships and restrict the mobility and distensibility of organs. In the absence of anatomic distortion, however, a causation relationship between endometriosis and subfertility becomes less clear. Although it is logical and reasonable to suggest that

Table 34.1: Surgical Principles in the Treatment of Endometriosis

Principles of surgical management

Knowledge of disease and treatment modalities

Experienced surgeon

Adequate facilities, personnel, and equipment

Appropriate patient selection

Informed consent

Proper patient position

Careful pelvic evaluation

Maximum exposure

Use of magnification

Minimum tissue trauma

Excellent hemostasis

Removal of all diseased tissue

Avoidance of foreign body material

Confirmation of tissue pathology

Follow-up of surgical results (outcome)

From Adamson (47), with permission.

endometriosis implants are responsible for a decline in fecundity, we have to consider the possibility of endometriosis coexisting as a marker for an underlying pathological process that interferes with fertility. This may be problematic when evaluating treatments for endometriosis-associated infertility because the basis for current treatment paradigms relies on the premise that endometriosis causes infertility.

Results from outcomes assessment will be the primary data of interest to the patient. Several studies have attempted to evaluate the effectiveness of infertility treatments in increasing the monthly chance of conceiving or shortening the interval to conception. Although the use of pregnancy as an outcome measure for clinical response seems obvious, it is important to understand the method of data reporting and analysis and to consider that multiple factors often have an effect on fertility. A commonly used outcome measure that is easy to calculate has been crude or simple pregnancy rates. However, pregnancy rates increase with longer patient follow-up, which limits the value of crude pregnancy rates. In order to account for the time-dependent nature of pregnancy, life-table analyses or fecundity rates have been frequently used. Although these calculations are often preferred in studies of infertility treatment, they cannot correct for selection bias. Another useful method for analyzing data is meta-analysis. Since the data from several studies are pooled together, a more robust analysis may be obtained that is less subject to the limitations of a small study. However, a meta-analysis does not correct for the variable lengths of follow-up among the studies, is subject to limitations in study design, and may lose the subtleties of the data from each study during the process of analysis.

Another factor to consider in infertility studies is the background rate of conception. In many situations, endometriosis does not result in an absolute inability to conceive but rather a relative decrease in fertility. Without any intervention, pregnancies will occur at a certain background rate in these women. Thus, this pregnancy rate in the untreated woman must be determined and used as a source of comparison to assess the efficacy of a treatment.

Studies addressing stage-specific treatment comparisons are hindered further by the use of an endometriosis classification system that has focused on the observed extent of disease involvement and is limited in its ability to correlate disease stage with the degree of infertility (49, 50). The ideal classification system should facilitate accurate assessment of the extent and location of disease, be useful in predicting outcome based upon the stage of disease, allow predictable outcomes from similar stages of disease in response to treatment, and provide guidance in selecting the appropriate treatment (51). Unfortunately, attempts to develop a classification scheme for endometriosis that fulfill these criteria have been unsuccessful. For example, deeply invasive nodules of endometriosis may be categorized as mild disease according to the American Society of Reproductive Medicine classification scheme but yet may have significant adverse effects on fertility. Nonetheless, despite a lack of correlation with fertility prognosis, a framework for classifying disease is necessary to enable comparisons to be made regarding the effectiveness of treatments.

In light of the various factors related to outcome variables, data analysis, and disease classification, carefully designed studies that are ideally prospective, randomized, and controlled are required to yield meaningful information as to the most effective treatment approach. These studies should have sufficient sample size, appropriate follow-up, and proper statistical analysis. However, many studies are uncontrolled or retrospective, making them prone to selection bias. As a result, conclusions from these studies are more likely to indicate that a treatment is efficacious when in reality it is not.

OTHER FACTORS

The probability of conception may potentially be affected by other factors in addition to the outcome of surgery. This complicates the ability to develop a system that predicts pregnancy following surgery for endometriosis (52). In addition to the pelvic status after surgery, consideration of the age of the patient, duration of infertility, and prior gravidity is helpful in evaluating postsurgical fertility potential (53). Other fertility factors such as ovulatory disorders and male factor problems usually reduce the fecundity in patients following surgery compared to those who have endometriosis alone. In these patients, further assistance with ovulation induction or assisted reproductive technologies (ART) after surgery may be beneficial.

Management decisions before and after surgical treatment are also influenced by factors that are unrelated to the primary medical condition. These factors include the availability of health insurance coverage for infertility treatment, religious and moral perspectives on various treatment options, timeliness of treatments, emotional status, and personal preferences of the patient. Formulating a plan of treatment requires the integration of these factors along with the anticipated surgical outcome. In some situations, the best approach for the patient may be to forgo surgery in favor of fertility treatments. Communicating treatment recommendations effectively is necessary for patient understanding, appropriate participation in decision making, and implementation of the treatment plan (54).

RESULTS OF SURGICAL TREATMENT

Stage-Specific Outcome

Generally, a pregnancy rate of about 65 percent can be expected within one to two years after surgery for endometriosis. A meta-analysis of studies comparing surgery to nonsurgical treatment for all stages of endometriosis-associated infertility showed that the surgical approach was superior with crude pregnancy rates, estimated to be 38 percent higher than the nonsurgical approach (95 percent confidence interval 28 to 48 percent higher) (Figure 34.1) (55). The time lost due to the required period of contraception while taking medications accounts primarily for the pregnancy rate differences between surgical and medical treatment of endometriosis. This is an important consideration when recommending treatment, especially among older infertility patients, since a delay of up to six months in attempting to conceive may significantly reduce fertility potential.

In patients with moderate to severe endometriosis, sufficient anatomic distortion is usually present to cause impaired fertility through mechanical interference of gamete interaction (Figure 34.2). Surgery is the commonly accepted approach to correcting this pelvic distortion caused by invasive, adhesive, endometriotic disease. Besides restoring anatomy, removing rather than dividing adhesions is considered to be important due to the possible presence of endometriosis within adhesions. Nonsurgical treatments are not effective at restoring normal anatomy and treating adhesions, which are the primary obstacles for oocyte pickup and transport. Support for the surgical approach to moderate or severe endometriosis-associated infertility arises from the observation of an extremely low background pregnancy rate and studies showing that pregnancies occur following corrective surgery. Repeated surgical intervention for infertility patients has not been supported by any large randomized studies. Instead, these patients are more likely to benefit from IVF if pregnancy does not occur after the initial surgery (56). Despite the paucity of prospective, randomized, controlled trials, it is reasonable to favor surgery over no treatment or medical treatment in moderate to severe endometriosis (55).

More uncertainty exists regarding the benefits of surgical treatment for infertility in patients with early-stage (minimal or mild) endometriosis (Figure 34.3). Often, treatment has been opportunistic and easily accomplished simultaneously during diagnostic laparoscopy. However, one of the concerns is that the risk of adhesion formation following the removal or ablation of endometriosis implants may be increased and potentially interfere with fertility to a greater degree than was present prior to surgery. Although an association between early-stage endometriosis and reproductive dysfunction has been recognized, whether a cause-effect relationship exists between minimal/mild endometriosis and infertility is not clear (57, 58). Data from earlier studies evaluating surgical treatment of minimal/mild endometriosis revealed an average pregnancy rate of 58 percent compared to 45 percent for expectant management (38, 59–74). Based on these studies, it would appear that surgery is a more effective approach than expectant management. However, the average monthly fecundity calculated for expectant management of 6.8 percent was not clearly different than the monthly fecundity for surgery (61, 75–77). In light of the heterogeneity and variable lengths of follow-up with these studies, the superiority of surgery over expectant management in early-stage endometriosis has been difficult to demonstrate.

More recently, published studies have supported the surgical approach to infertile patients with minimal or mild endometriosis. In a prospective, multicenter, double-blinded, controlled study by the Canadian collaborative trial (ENDO-CAN), 41 infertile women with minimal or mild endometriosis

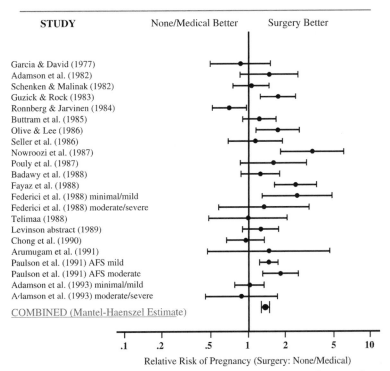

Figure 34.1. Meta-analysis of data comparing the surgical to nonsurgical approaches to endometriosis-associated infertility treatment. From Adamson and Pasta (55), with permission.

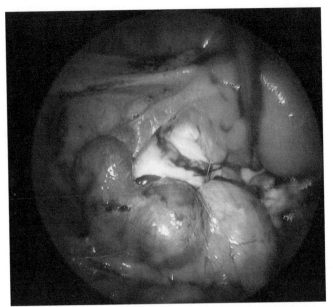

Figure 34.2. Severe endometriosis with adnexal and cul-de-sac adhesions.

were randomized to either diagnostic laparoscopy or laparoscopic treatment of the disease (7). Surgical treatment resulted in a significantly higher pregnancy rate after nine months compared to no treatment (37.5 vs. 22.5 percent). This large, well-designed study provided the first convincing evidence that surgery for minimal or mild endometriosis-associated infertility was beneficial. However, a second, similarly designed multicenter, randomized, controlled study of 101 women with minimal or mild endometriosis did not demonstrate a difference in the live birth rate between surgery and no treatment (19.6 vs. 22.2 percent, respectively) within one year following the excision or ablation of endometriosis implants (78). This study had a smaller sample size than the ENDOCAN trial with patients that had a longer duration of infertility and more advanced disease. When the results of these two trials are

combined into a meta-analysis, surgical treatment is still favored over no treatment (odds ratio for pregnancy 1.7; 95 percent confidence limits, 1.1–2.5), although to a lesser extent than seen in the ENDOCAN trial alone (79). Based on the ENDOCAN trial, the number needed to treat to obtain one additional pregnancy is approximately 7.7 women. This relatively small benefit of surgery needs to be balanced against the costs, risks, and alternative options such as controlled ovarian stimulation when recommending treatment for early-stage endometriosis.

Laparoscopy versus Laparotomy

One of the major concerns with surgery for endometriosis-associated infertility is the risk of post surgical adhesion formation that interferes with fertility. It would appear that laparoscopy would be more advantageous than laparotomy due to the possibility of less adhesion formation from reduced foreign body exposure and tissue trauma (80). In a life-table analysis of patients without other infertility factors, laparoscopy does not appear to confer any advantage over laparotomy for minimal or mild endometriosis (38). However, for moderate or severe endometriosis, laparoscopy resulted in higher pregnancy rates than laparotomy. A survival analysis with multiple fixed covariates also showed higher pregnancy rates with laparoscopy compared to laparotomy in the endometriosis-only group (87 percent higher pregnancy rate).

In contrast, a meta-analysis of studies comparing laparoscopy to laparotomy revealed no significant difference in pregnancy rates (55). A plausible explanation for the observed discrepancy between the meta-analysis and survival analysis is that the meta-analysis only accounts for the final pregnancy rate, not the duration of time to pregnancy. Furthermore, patients treated by laparotomy generally had longer follow-up, thus allowing for more time to conceive. In most cases of endometriosis-associated infertility, laparoscopy would appear to be the preferred approach given the evidence supporting the same or better pregnancy outcome with laparoscopy compared to laparotomy.

Endometriomas

Ovarian endometriomas are typically treated utilizing various techniques such as cyst stripping or ablation, drainage, and wide excision. Improvements in technology have facilitated the advanced treatment of endometriomas by the laparoscopic approach. Among the various techniques utilized, resection of the cyst wall is preferable in order to minimize thermal injury to the ovary, have greater assurance of complete removal, and obtain a specimen for pathological examination (Figure 34.4). In a prospective cohort study of endometrioma treatment by laparoscopy or laparotomy, the estimated cumulative pregnancy rate at three years was approximately 50 percent (Figure 34.5) (81). The pregnancy outcome was not dependent on the number or size of endometriomas. Following the resection, stripping, or ablation of endometriomas, a less than 10 percent rate of recurrence has been reported with a 20 percent incidence of de novo adhesion formation and approximately 80 percent incidence of partial or complete dense adhesion recurrence (82). With regard to the laparoscopic technique used, a prospective, randomized, clinical trial reported a higher pregnancy rate (59 vs. 23 percent) and lower reoperation rate (6 vs.

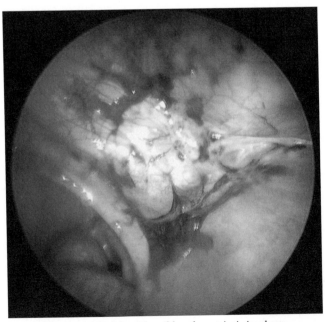

Figure 34.3. Pelvis with mild endometriosis implants.

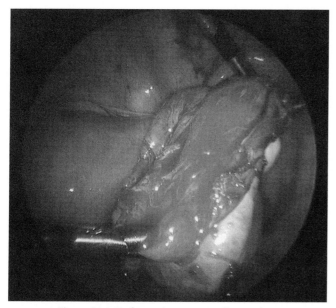

Figure 34.4. Endometrioma cyst wall resection.

23 percent) with ovarian cystectomy compared to fenestration and coagulation (83).

The value of operating on ovarian endometriomas for endometriosis-associated infertility has been questioned over the concern of reduced ovarian function, especially prior to IVF treatment. Retention of normal ovarian function following surgery has been reported in some patients but not in others (84–89). Controversy also exists regarding the best tissue-sparing technique for minimization of follicle loss (89–92). A meta-analysis of pregnancy outcome after IVF in patients with ovarian endometriomas did not demonstrate an adverse effect on the pregnancy rates in the presence of an endometrioma (93). In a prospective, randomized study of the effect on pregnancy outcome of endometrioma cystectomy prior to IVF treatment versus

IVF alone, patients undergoing ovarian surgery had diminished ovarian responsiveness but no difference in pregnancy (34 vs. 38 percent) and implantation rates (16.5 vs. 18.5 percent) (94). Thus, the benefit of surgery for endometriomas prior to IVF is questionable, although most clinicians recommend the removal of endometriomas larger than 3 or 4 cm in size (95–97).

Posterior Cul-De-Sac

The posterior cul-de-sac and rectovaginal septum are locations where deeply invasive endometriosis can sometimes be found. These areas also can be some of the most difficult to dissect. Access to endometriosis implants can be challenging and difficult to treat completely. In one study of infertile patients with partial or complete cul-de-sac obliteration, laparoscopic treatment resulted in 74 percent (thirty-four of forty-six) of the patients conceiving of which 38 percent (thirteen of thirty-four) required more than one laparoscopy (98). In another study, life-table analysis of twenty-seven infertility patients with complete cul-de-sac obliteration resulted in a pregnancy rate of 29.6 percent at one and two years for eleven patients following laparoscopic treatment and 0 percent at one year and 23.7 percent at two years for the remaining patients treated by laparotomy (99).

CONCLUSIONS

Surgery is an important treatment option for endometriosis-associated infertility. Although our knowledge is somewhat limited with respect to the optimal treatment approach, the current evidence generally supports the surgical approach for all stages of endometriosis. While laparoscopy is a commonly chosen treatment approach for many situations, the outcome is dependent on appropriate patient selection and the skill level of the surgeon.

Current studies on endometriosis-associated infertility rely on a classification scheme that does not allow an entirely predictable outcome based on stage-specific treatment plans. The development of an endometriosis scoring system that has good correlation with the severity of reproductive impairment would contribute significantly to future studies. Better understanding of the immunologic, hormonal, genetic, and environmental aspects of endometriosis may lead to new insights for treatment that might be complimentary to surgery. As our knowledge about this complex disease increases, it will allow more refined conclusions to be made regarding the optimal treatment approach to endometriosis-associated infertility and enable patients to benefit from better outcomes.

KEY POINTS

■ The prevalence of endometriosis among infertile women has been estimated to be about 20 percent.

■ Significant anatomic distortion from adhesions that interferes with fertility may be caused by moderate/severe endometriosis.

■ Minimal/mild endometriosis may also create abnormalities capable of impairing fertility. The exact mechanism for subfertility has yet to be determined but is likely associated with local inflammation and an altered immune response in the pelvis mediated by cytokines.

■ The optimal management approach for endometriosis-associated infertility requires an evaluation of the extent of disease and the reproductive goals of the patient.

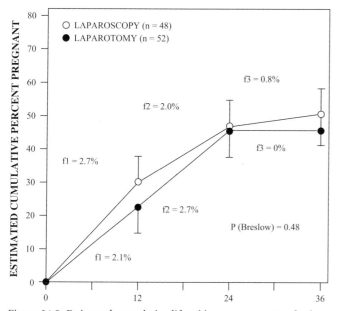

Figure 34.5. Estimated cumulative life-table pregnancy rates for laparoscopy and laparotomy for treatment of endometriomas. From Adamson et al. (81), with permission.

- Treatment typically focuses on eliminating endometriosis implants through surgery, improving fecundity with fertility treatments, or a combination of both.
- Surgical treatment for endometriosis-associated infertility should employ techniques that reduce tissue injury by preserving serosal integrity, maintaining hemostasis, and reducing operating time. These techniques help to reduce adhesion formation.
- Laparoscopy in conjunction with the laser, electrosurgery, or sharp resection is commonly used to treat most cases of endometriosis. Laparotomy may be more appropriate for performing bowel resection, extensive enterolysis, or removing large endometriomas, although even these procedures can be treated effectively through the laparoscope by highly skilled surgeons.
- Ovarian suppression, which forms the basis of medical treatment of pain associated with endometriosis, prolongs the duration of infertility, with no improvement in fertility status, and is not indicated for endometriosis-associated infertility. The only exception is the use of ovarian suppression prior to IVF.
- Studies of stage-specific treatments are hindered by a classification system for endometriosis that has focused on the observed extent of disease involvement and is limited in its ability to correlate disease stage with the degree of infertility.
- Other fertility factors may influence the outcome of surgery for endometriosis-associated infertility. These factors need to be considered prior to surgery in order to formulate a comprehensive management plan.
- Surgery is the commonly accepted approach to correcting pelvic distortion caused by moderate to severe endometriosis.
- For minimal to mild endometriosis, the data favor surgical treatment over no treatment. However, approximately 7.7 women need to be treated to obtain one additional pregnancy. This relatively small benefit of surgery needs to be balanced against the cost, risks, and alternative options such as fertility treatments.
- Cyst wall resection is the preferred approach to treating endometriomas.
- The benefit of endometrioma surgery prior to IVF treatment is questionable, although many clinicians recommend removal of endometriomas greater than 3 or 4 cm.

REFERENCES

1. Boling RO, Abbasi R, Ackerman G, et al. Disability from endometriosis in the United States Army. *J Reprod Med* 1988;33: 49–52.
2. Wheeler JM. Epidemiology of endometriosis-associated infertility. *J Reprod Med* 1989;34:41–46.
3. Velebil P, Wingo PH, Xia Z, et al. Rate of hospitalization for gynecologic disorders among reproductive-age women in the United States. *Obstet Gynecol* 1995;86:764–769.
4. Houston DE, Noller KL, Melton LJ, et al. Incidence of pelvic endometriosis in Rochester, Minnesota, 1970-1979. *Am J Epidemiol* 1987;125:959–969.
5. Eskenazi B, Warner ML. Epidemiology of endometriosis. *Obstet Gynecol Clin North Am* 1997;24:235–258.
6. Hammond MG, Jordan S, Sloan CS. Factors affecting pregnancy rates in a donor insemination program using frozen semen. *Am J Obstet Gynecol* 1986;155:480–485.
7. Marcoux S, Maheux R, Berube S. Laparoscopic surgery in infertile women with minimal or mild endometriosis: Canadian Collaborative Group in Endometriosis. *N Engl J Med* 1997;337: 217–222.
8. Toma SK, Stovall DW, Hammond MG. The effect of laparoscopic ablation or danocrine on pregnancy rate in patients with stage I or II endometriosis undergoing donor insemination. *Obstet Gynecol* 1992;80:253–256.
9. Harada T, Iwabe T, Terakawa N. Role of cytokines in endometriosis. *Fertil Steril* 2001;76:1–10.
10. Arici A, Seli E, Zeyneloglu HB, et al. Interleukin-8 induces proliferation of endometrial stromal cells: a potential autocrine growth factor. *J Clin Endocrinol Metab* 1998;83:1201–1205.
11. Iwabe T, Harada T, Tsudo T, et al. Pathogenetic significance of increased levels of interleukin-8 in peritoneal fluid of patients with endometriosis. *Fertil Steril* 1998;69:924–930.
12. Dunselman G, Hendrix M, Bouckaert P, Evers J. Functional aspects of peritoneal macrophages in endometriosis of women. *J Reprod Fertil* 1988;82:707–710.
13. Haney A, Muscato J, Weinberg J. Peritoneal fluid cell populations in infertility patients. *Fertil Steril* 1981;35:696–698.
14. Olive DL, Weinberg JB, Haney AF. Peritoneal macrophages and infertility: the association between cell number and pelvic pathology. *Fertil Steril* 1985;44:772–777.
15. Halme J, Becker S, Hammond MG, et al. Increased activation of pelvic macrophages in infertile women with mild endometriosis. *Am J Obstet Gynecol* 1983;145:333–337.
16. Muscato JJ, Haney AF, Weinberg JB. Sperm phagocytosis by human peritoneal macrophages: a possible cause of infertility in endometriosis. *Am J Obstet Gynecol* 1982;144:503–510.
17. Harlow CR, Cahill DJ, Maile LA, et al. Reduced preovulatory granulosa cell steroidogenesis in women with endometriosis. *J Clin Endocrinol Metab* 1996;81:426–429.
18. Tummon IS, Maclin VM, Radwanska E, et al. Occult ovulatory dysfunction in women with minimal endometriosis or unexplained infertility. *Fertil Steril* 1988;50:716–720.
19. Curtis P, Lindsay P, Jackson AE, Shaw RW. Adverse effects on sperm movement characteristics in women with minimal and mild endometriosis. *Br J Obstet Gynecol* 1993;100:165–169.
20. Oral E, Arici A, Olive DL, Huszar G. Peritoneal fluid from women with moderate or severe endometriosis inhibits sperm motility: the role of seminal fluid components. *Fertil Steril* 1996;66:787–792.
21. Arumugam K. Endometriosis and infertility: raised iron concentration in the peritoneal fluid and its effect on the acrosome reaction. *Hum Reprod* 1994;9:1153–1157.
22. Reeve L, Lashen H, Pacey AA. Endometriosis affects sperm-endosalpingeal interactions. *Hum Reprod* 2005;20:448–451.
23. Suginami H, Yano K. An ovum capture inhibitor (OCI) in endometriosis peritoneal flUID:an OCI-related membrane responsible for fimbrial failure of ovum capture. *Fertil Steril* 1988;50:648–653.
24. Coddington CC, Oehninger S, Cunningham DS, et al. Peritoneal fluid from patients with endometriosis decreases sperm binding to the zona pellucida in the hemizona assay: a preliminary report. *Fertil Steril* 1992;57:783–786.
25. Morcos RN, Gibbons WE, Findley WE. Effect of peritoneal fluid on in vitro cleavage of 2-cell mouse embryos: possible role in infertility associated with endometriosis. *Fertil Steril* 1985;44: 678–683.
26. Arici A, Oral E, Bukulmez O, et al. The effect of endometriosis on implantation: results from the Yale University in vitro fertilization and embryo transfer program. *Fertil Steril* 1996;65:603–607.
27. Pittaway DE, Maxson W, Daniell J, et al. Luteal phase defects in infertility patients with endometriosis. *Fertil Steril* 1983;39: 712–713.

28. Schenken RS, Asch RH, Williams RF, Hodgen GD. Etiology of infertility in monkeys with endometriosis: luteinized unruptured follicles, luteal phase defects, pelvic adhesions, and spontaneous abortions. *Fertil Steril* 1984;41:122–130.

29. Schenken RS, Asch RH. Surgical induction of endometriosis in the rabbit: effects on fertility and concentrations of peritoneal fluid prostaglandins. *Fertil Steril* 1980;34:581–587.

30. Kaplan CR, Eddy CA, Olive DL, Schenken RS. Effects of ovarian endometriosis on ovulation in rabbits. *Am J Obstet Gynecol* 1989;160:40–44.

31. Dunselman GA, Dumoulin JC, Land JA, Evers JL. Lack of effect of peritoneal endometriosis on fertility in the rabbit model. *Fertil Steril* 1991;56:340–342.

32. Chauhan M, Barratt CL, Cooke SM, Cooke ID. Differences in the fertility of donor insemination recipients – a study to provide prognostic guidelines as to its success and outcome. *Fertil Steril* 1989;51:815–819.

33. Dunphy BC, Kay R, Barratt CL, Cooke ID. Female age, the length of involuntary infertility prior to investigation and fertility outcome. *Hum Reprod* 1989;4:527–530.

34. Símon C, Gutiérrez A, Vidal A, et al. Outcome of patients with endometriosis in assisted reproduction: results from in-vitro fertilization and oocyte donation. *Hum Reprod* 1994;9:725–729.

35. Pellicer A, Oliveira N, Ruiz A, et al. Exploring the mechanism(s) of endometriosis-related infertility: an analysis of embryo development and implantation in assisted reproduction. *Hum Reprod* 1995;10(Suppl. 2):91–97.

36. Brizek CL, Schlaff S, Pellegrini VA, et al. Increased incidence of aberrant morphological phenotypes in human embryogenesis – an association with endometriosis. *J Assist Reprod Genet* 1995;12:106–112.

37. Hughes EG, Fedorkow DM, Collins JA. A quantitative overview of controlled trials in endometriosis-associated infertility. *Fertil Steril* 1993;59:963–970.

38. Adamson GD, Hurd SJ, Pasta DJ, Rodriguez BD. Laparoscopic endometriosis treatment: is it better? *Fertil Steril* 1993;59:35–44.

39. Gruppo Italiano per lo Studio dell' Endometriosi. Ablation of lesions or no treatment in minimal-mild endometriosis in infertile womena randomized trial. *Hum Reprod* 1999;14:1332–1334.

40. Bruhat MA, Mage C, Chapron C, et al. Present-day endoscopic surgery in gynecology. *Eur J Obstet Gynecol Reprod Biol* 1991;41:4–13.

41. Operative Laparoscopy Study Group. Postoperative adhesion development following operative laparoscopy: evaluation at early second-look procedures. *Fertil Steril* 1991;55:700–704.

42. Carbon Dioxide Laser Laparoscopy Study Group. Initial report of the carbon dioxide laser laparoscopy study group: complications. *J Gynecol surg* 1989;5:269–272.

43. Azziz R, Steinkampf MP, Murphy A. Post-operative recuperation: relation to the extent of endoscopic surgery. *Fertil Steril* 1989;51:1061–1064.

44. Peterson HB, Hulka JF, Phillips JM. American Association of Gynecologic Laparoscopists 1988 membership survey on operative laparoscopy. *J Reprod Med* 1990;35:587–589.

45. Luciano AA, Manzi D. Treatment options for endometriosis: surgical therapies. *Infertil Reprod Med Clin N Am* 1992;3:657–682.

46. Redwine DB. Treatment of endometriosis-associated pain. *Infertil Reprod Med Clin N Am* 1992;3:683–695.

47. Adamson GD. Laparoscopic treatment of endometriosis. In: Adamson GD, Martin DC, eds. Endoscopic Management of Gynecologic Disease. Philadelphia: Lippincott-Raven;1996:147–187.

48. American Society for Reproductive Medicine. Revised American Society for Reproductive Medicine classification of endometriosis: 1996. *Fertil Steril* 1997;67:817–821.

49. Adamson GD, Frison L, Lamb EJ. Endometriosis: studies of a method for design of a surgical staging system. *Fertil Steril* 1982;38:659–666.

50. Fedele L, Parozzini F, Bianchi S, et al. Stage and localization of pelvic endometriosis and pain. *Fertil Steril* 1990;53:155–158.

51. Hoeger KM, Guzick DS. Classification of endometriosis. *Obstet Gynecol Clin North Am* 1997;24:347–359.

52. Guzick DS, Silliman NP, Adamson GD, et al. Prediction of pregnancy in infertile women based on the American Society for Reproductive Medicine's revised classification of endometriosis. *Fertil Steril* 1997;67:822–829.

53. Adamson GD, Pasta DJ. Pregnancy rates can be predicted by validated endometriosis fertility index (EFI). *Fertil Steril* 2002;77(Suppl. 1):S48.

54. Epstein RM, Alper BS, Quill TE. Communicating evidence for participatory decision making. *JAMA* 2004;291(19):2359–2366.

55. Adamson GD, Pasta DJ. Surgical treatment of endometriosis-associated infertility: meta-analysis compared with survival analysis. *Am J Obstet Gynecol* 1994;171:1488–1505.

56. The Practice Committee of the American Society for Reproductive Medicine. Endometriosis and infertility. *Fertil Steril* 2004;81:1441–1446.

57. Akande VA, Hunt LP, Cahill DJ, Jenkins JM. Differences in time to natural conception between women with unexplained infertility and infertile women with minor endometriosis. *Hum Reprod* 2004;19:96–103.

58. D'Hooghe TM, Debrock S, Hill JA, Meuleman C. Endometriosis and subfertility: is the relationship resolved? *Semin Reprod Med* 2003; 21(2):243–254.

59. Garcia CD, David SS. Pelvic endometriosis: infertility and pelvic pain. *Am J Obstet Gynecol* 1977;129:740–747.

60. Schenken RS, Malinak LR. Conservative surgery versus expectant management for the infertile patient with mild endometriosis. *Fertil Steril* 1982;37:183–186.

61. Seibel MM, Berger MJ, Weinstein FG, Taymor ML. The effectiveness of danazol on subsequent fertility in minimal endometriosis. *Fertil Steril* 1982;38:534–537.

62. Portuondo JA, Echanojauregui AD, Herran C, Alijarte I. Early conception in patients with untreated mild endometriosis. *Fertil Steril* 1983;39:22–25.

63. Olive DL, Stohs GF, Metzger DA, Franklin RR. Expectant management and hydrotubations in the treatment of endometriosis-associated infertility. *Fertil Steril* 1985;44:351–352.

64. Hull ME, Moghissi KS, Magyar DM, Hayes MF. Comparison of different modalities of endometriosis in infertile women. *Fertil Steril* 1987;47:40–44.

65. Thomas EJ, Cooke ID. Successful treatment of asymptomatic endometriosis: does it benefit infertile women? *Br Med J* 1987;294:1117–1119.

66. Bayer SR, Seibel MM, Saffan DS, et al. Efficacy of danazol treatment for minimal endometriosis in infertile women. A prospective randomized study. *J Reprod Med* 1988;33:179–183.

67. Rodriguez-Escudero FJ, Neyro JL, Corcostegui B, Benito JA. Does minimal endometriosis reduce fecundity? *Fertil Steril* 1988;50:522–524.

68. Badawy SZA, El Bakry MM, Samuel F, Dizer M. Cumulative pregnancy rates in infertile women with endometriosis. *J Reprod Med* 1988;33:757–760.

69. Paulson JD, Asmar P, Saffan DS. Mild and moderate endometriosis: comparison of treatment modalities for infertile couples. *J Reprod Med* 1991;36:151–155.

70. Inoue M, Kobayashi Y, Honda I, et al. The impact of endometriosis on the reproductive outcome of infertile patients. *Am J Obstet Gynecol* 1992;167:278–282.

71. Schenken RS, Malinak LR. Reoperation after initial treatment of endometriosis with conservative surgery. *Am J Obstet Gynecol* 1978;131:416–424.

72. Buttram VC. Conservative surgery for endometriosis in the infertile female: a study of 206 patients with implications for both medical and surgical therapy. *Fertil Steril* 1979;31:117–123.

73. Rantala ML, Kahanpaa KV, Koskimies AI, Widholm O. Fertility prognosis after surgical treatment of pelvic endometriosis. *Acta Obstet Gynaecol Scand* 1983;62:11–14.

74. Gordts S, Boeckx W, Brosens IA. Microsurgery of endometriosis in infertile patients. *Fertil Steril* 1984;42:520–525.

75. Rock JA, Guzick DS, Sengol C, et al. The conservative surgical treatment of endometriosis: evaluation of pregnancy success with respect to the extent of disease as categorized using contemporary classification system. *Fertil Steril* 1981;35:131–137.

76. Olive DL, Martin DC. Treatment of endometriosis-associated infertility with CO_2 laser laparoscopy: the use of one- and two-parameter exponential models. *Fertil Steril* 1987;48:18–23.

77. Nezhat C, Crowgey R, Nezhat F. Videolaseroscopy for the treatment of endometriosis associated with infertility. *Fertil Steril* 1989;51:237–240.

78. Gruppo Italiano per lo Studio dell'Endometriosi. Ablation of lesions or no treatment in minimal-mild endometriosis in infertile womena randomized trial. *Hum Reprod* 1999;14:1332–1334.

79. Olive DL. Endometriosis: does surgery make a difference? *OBG Management* 2002;Jul:56–70.

80. Diamond MP, Daniell JF, Feste J, et al. Adhesion reformation and de novo adhesion formation following reproductive pelvic surgery. *Fertil Steril* 1987;47:864–866.

81. Adamson GD, Subak LL, Pasta DJ, et al. Comparison of CO_2 laser laparoscopy with laparotomy for treatment of endometriomata. *Fertil Steril* 1992;57:965–973.

82. Canis M, Mage G, Wattiez A, et al. Second-look laparoscopy after laparoscopic cystectomy of large ovarian endometriomas. *Fertil Steril* 1992;58:617–619.

83. Alborzi S, Momtahan M, Parsanezhad ME, et al. A prospective, randomized study comparing laparoscopic ovarian cystectomy versus fenestration and coagulation in patients with endometriomas. *Fertil Steril* 2004;82:1633–1637.

84. Sayegh R, Garcia CR. Ovarian function after conservational ovarian surgery: a long-term follow-up study. *Int J Gynaecol Obstet* 1992;39:303–309.

85. Marconi G, Vilela M, Quintana R, Sueldo C. Laparoscopic ovarian cystectomy of endometriomas does not affect the ovarian response to gonadotropin stimulation. *Fertil Steril* 2002;78:876–878.

86. Hemmings R, Bissonnette F, Bouzayen R. Results of laparoscopic treatments of ovarian endometriomas: laparoscopic ovarian fenestration and coagulation. *Fertil Steril* 1998;70:527–529.

87. Loh F-H, Tan AT, Kumar J, Ng S-C. Ovarian response after laparoscopic ovarian cystectomy for endometriotic cysts in 132 monitored cycles. *Fertil Steril* 1999;72:316–321.

88. Donnez J, Wyns C, Nisolle M. Does ovarian surgery for endometriomas impair the ovarian response to gonadotropin? *Fertil Steril* 2001;76:662–665.

89. Canis M, Pouly JL, Tamburro S, et al. Ovarian response during IVF-embryo transfer cycles after laparoscopic ovarian cystectomy for endometriotic cysts of >3 cm in diameter. *Hum Reprod* 2001;16:2583–2586.

90. Muzii L, Bianchi A, Croce C, et al. Laparoscopic excision of ovarian cysts: is the stripping technique a tissue-sparing procedure? *Fertil Steril* 2002;77:609–614.

91. Jones KD, Sutton CJG. Pregnancy rates following ablative laparoscopic surgery for endometriomas. *Hum Reprod* 2002;17:782–785.

92. Garry R. The effectiveness of laparoscopic excision of endometriosis. *Curr Opin Obstet Gynecol* 2004;16:299–303.

93. Gupta S, Agarwal A, Agarwal R, Loret de Mola JR. Impact of ovarian endometriomas on assisted reproduction outcomes. *Reprod Biomed Online* 2006;13:349–360.

94. Demirol A, Guven S, Baykal C, Gurgan T. Effect of endometriomas cystectomy on IVF outcome: a prospective randomized study. *Reprod Biomed Online* 2006;12:639–643.

95. Canis M, Pouly JL, Tamburro S, Mage G, Wattiez A, Bruhat MA. Ovarian response during IVF–embryo transfer cycles after laparoscopic ovarian cystectomy for endometriotic cysts of >3 cm in diameter. *Hum Reprod* 2001;16:2583–2586.

96. Kennedy S, Bergqvist A, Chapron C, D'Hooghe T, Dunselman G, Greb R, Hummelshoj L, Prentice A, Saridogan E on behalf of the ESHRE Special Interest Group for Endometriosis and Endometrium Guideline Development Group. *Hum Reprod* 2005;10:2698–2704.

97. Rizk B. Treatment of Infertility associated with endometriosis. In: Rizk B, and Abdalla H, eds. Endometriosis. Oxford: UK, Health Press, 2003: chapter 6; 85–86.

98. Reich H, McGlynn F, Salvat J. Laparoscopic treatment of cul-de-sac obliteration secondary to retrocervical deep fibrotic endometriosis. *J Reprod Med* 1991;36:516–522.

99. Adamson GD, Hurd SJ, Rodriguez BD.Laparoscopy versus laparotomy for treatment of posterior cul-de-sac obliteration. Presented at the American Association of Gynecologic Laparoscopists; September 24–27, 1992; Chicago. Abstract.

35

Congenital Uterine Malformations and Reproduction

Theodore A. Baramki

The genital tract in the female arises from two embryonic sources, the Mullerian ducts (mesodermal in origin) and the urogenital sinus (endodermal in origin). Abnormal Mullerian differentiation is frequently associated with urologic malformations.

EMBRYOLOGY

The Mullerian (paramesonephric) ducts appear in the 10-mm crown-rump length embryo (about five weeks) by an invagination of the coelomic epithelium into the underlying mesenchyme lateral to the cranial extremity of the Wolffian ducts (Figure 35.1).

In the female, the site of invagination becomes the future abdominal opening of the Fallopian tube. At the caudal tip of this invagination, a solid bud is formed, which burrows in the mesenchyme lateral to and parallel with the Wolffian ducts. At the caudal extremity of the mesonephros, the Mullerian duct crosses ventrally and medially and grows mediocaudally to meet and fuse with the duct of the opposite side (Figure 35.2). Fusion of the Mullerian ducts is at first incomplete, so that for a short while a septum separates their two cavities. In embryos about 56 mm long (about twelve weeks), the septum degenerates and gives a single cavity, the uterovaginal (genital) canal. The caudal tip of this canal comes in contact with the dorsal wall of the urogenital sinus, producing an elevation, the Mullerian tubercle (Figure 35.3). Proliferation of the tip of the uterovaginal canal results in the formation of a solid vaginal cord.

At around ten weeks, two sinovaginal bulbs appear in the form of bilateral posterior endodermal evaginations from the urogenital sinus close to the attachment of the Wolffian ducts. These fuse with the caudal end of the vaginal cord to form the vaginal plate. The part of the urogenital sinus immediately cranial to the bulbs forms the female urethra, while the bulbs move caudally to form the vestibule. Later in fetal life, the uterovaginal canal extends caudally and canalizes the vaginal plate, while the epithelium of the sinovaginal bulb breaks. A communication is thus established between the urogenital sinus and the uterovaginal canal.

The hymen is formed of the partition, which persists to varying degrees between the urogenital sinus and the canalized fused sinovaginal bulbs. It has two layers of epithelium of endodermal origin enclosing an intermediate layer of mesoderm; the internal layer is derived from the sinovaginal bulbs and the external layer from the urogenital sinus.

The musculature of the female genital tract arises from the mesenchyme surrounding the Mullerian ducts.

CLASSIFICATION

1. Congenital absence of the vagina (Mayer-Rokitansky–Kuster-Hauser Syndrome)
2. Anomalous vertical fusion
   - ■ Obstructive
     - □ imperforate hymen
     - □ transverse vaginal septum
   - ■ Nonobstructive
     - □ incomplete transverse vaginal septum
3. Anomalous lateral fusion
   - ■ Obstructive
     - □ unicornuate uterus with a noncommunicating rudimentary horn
     - □ unilateral obstruction of a cavity of double uterus
     - □ unilateral vaginal obstruction associated with uterus didelphys
   - ■ Nonobstructive
     - □ unicornuate uterus
     - □ septate uterus
     - □ bicornuate uterus
     - □ uterus didelphys
     - □ DES exposure in utero

CONGENITAL ABSENCE OF THE VAGINA

Patients with congenital absence of the vagina usually lack the uterus as well (1). Therefore, a more accurate term might be aplasia or dysplasia of the Mullerian ducts. However, by common usage, the term congenital absence of the vagina is used to describe this entity.

The patient usually presents as a phenotypic female with normal secondary sex characters and primary amenorrhea. On examination, the external genitalia are female and the vagina is short and blind. The uterus is represented by solid fibromuscular anlagen attached to the proximal ends of the tubes. Ovarian development is normal and the karyotype is 46, XX. Urinary (15 percent) and skeletal (5 percent) anomalies may be encountered in this syndrome.

Management of this condition depends on when the patient is interested in having a functional vaginal. Dilators have been used successfully (2, 3), and if no progress is made,

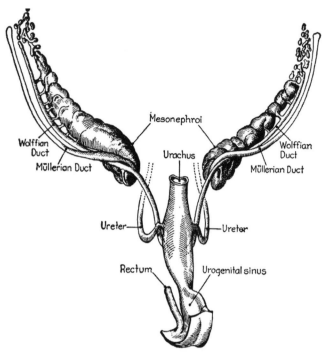

Figure 35.1. Wax plate reconstruction of the urogenital system in a human embryo of 23-mm C-R length (about six weeks ovulation age). (Courtesy of Carnegie Institution of Washington.)

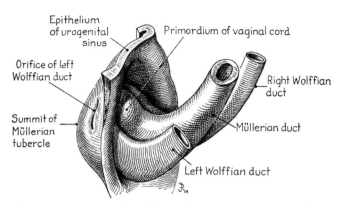

Figure 35.3. Reconstruction of the epithelial elements of the Mullerian tubercle region of a 48-mm C-R length embryo (about nine weeks). (Courtesy of Carnegie Institution of Washington.)

guidance, in vitro fertilization with husband's sperm, and embryo transfer in the uterus of a surrogate mother.

ANOMALOUS VERTICAL FUSION

Imperforate Hymen

The patient usually presents with normal sexual development, no periods (cryptomenorrhea), cyclic pelvic pain, a pelvic mass, and a bulging hymen. Ultrasonography can confirm the presence of hematocolpos, hematometra, or hematosalpinx. When the diagnosis is established, a cruciate incision is made in the hymen and the angles are cut. The more the delay in establishing egress of the menstrual flow, the more the chances that retrograde menstruation will occur with its chemical irritation to the peritoneum and the induction of endometriosis.

Transverse Vaginal Septum

A transverse vaginal septum occurs when the junction of the vaginal (Mullerian) cord and urogenital sinus does not canalize. The clinical picture is similar to that of an imperforate hymen, except that the obstruction occurs higher up. The septum may be in the upper, middle, or lower third of the vagina (Figure 35.4). Here ultrasonography can give an idea about the thickness of the vaginal septum. Excision of this septum should be done as soon as the diagnosis is established. Retrograde menstruation through the uterus and tubes may occur earlier in patients with a higher transverse vaginal septum, thus giving them a poorer fertility prognosis.

ANOMALOUS LATERAL FUSION (OBSTRUCTIVE)

A noncommunicating rudimentary horn presents as a case of a unicornuate uterus with no symptoms. However, if one functional horn does not communicate with the uterus, the patient presents with cyclic pelvic pain and an adnexal mass representing a hematometra. Excision of the noncommunicating horn is advisable.

In case of a uterus didelphys, where one of the vaginas does not communicate with the outside, the patient presents with cyclic pelvic pain and a hematometra and hematosalpinx may occur (Figure 35.5). Excision of the vaginal septum should be

surgery using the split-thickness graft (McIndoe procedure) (4) may be resorted to. It should be emphasized that surgery should not be done as soon as the diagnosis is made, but until such time that the patient is interested in becoming sexually active.

Pregnancy in patients with Mayer-Rokitansky–Kuster–Hauser syndrome is possible with IVF and surrogate motherhood. The oocytes can be retrieved vaginally by ultrasound

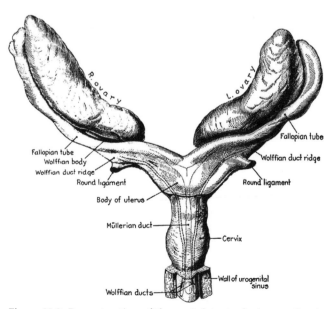

Figure 35.2. Reconstruction of the genital tract of a human female embryo of 48-mm C-R length (about nine weeks). Wolffian ducts are no longer present (Courtesy of Carnegie Institution of Washington.)

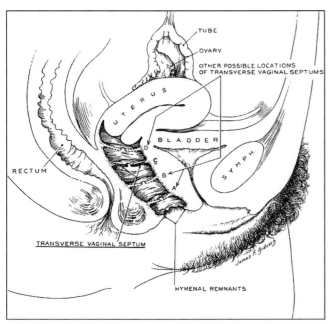

Figure 35.4. Different locations where a transverse vaginal septum may be found.

done. Renal anomalies occur, especially congenital absence of a kidney usually on the side of the abnormal Mullerian duct.

Unicornuate Uterus

The unicornuate uterus results from normal differentiation of only one Mullerian duct. The chances of having a live birth is 37 percent (5). Abortion rates (38 percent), especially early miscarriages (37.5 percent) are high (6). The rate of preterm

delivery is 25 percent, and only 31 percent of all pregnancies go to term.

It is common to find an absent kidney on the side of the absent Mullerian duct.

Double Uterus

If the partition between the two Mullerian ducts does not break down, varying degrees of double uterus will result. Complete duplication is uterus didelphys, where we have two uterine horns, two cervices, and two vaginas. If the cranial part of the partition does not break down, the result will be a septate uterus, where there is no depression in the fundus, or a bicornuate uterus, where there is a depression in the fundus at the junction of the two Mullerian ducts (Figure 35.6).

Unlike asymmetrical obstructive maldevelopment of the uterus, only a small percentage of patients with symmetrical double uterus have anomalies of the urinary tract.

Septate Uterus

This represents 66 percent of the Mullerian malformations. It results from failure of resorption of the medial segments of the Mullerain ducts. It is usually associated with the poorest reproductive prognosis with fetal survival of 6–28 percent and a high rate of spontaneous abortion (>60 percent) (7–10).

Pregnancy losses associated with septate uterus classically occur between eight and sixteen weeks of gestation. Spontaneous

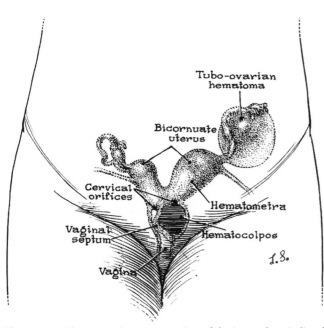

Figure 35.5. Diagrammatic representation of the internal genitalia of a patient with uterus didelphys with an obstructive left side. The patient menstruated regularly but had excruciating pelvic pain with each menstrual period.

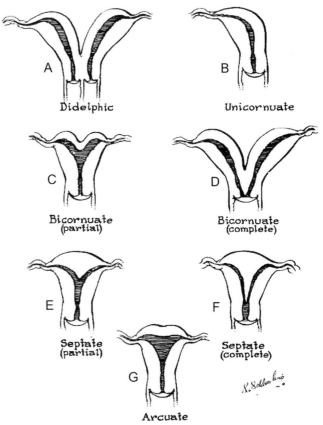

Figure 35.6. Nonobstructive maldevelopment of the uterus. (A) Uterus didelphys, (B) unicornuate uterus, (C) partial bicornuate uterus, (D) complete bicornuate uterus, (E) and (F) septate uterus showing normal external configuration the uterus, and (G) arcuate uterus.

abortion may be the result of poor blood supply to the septum leading to poor implantation (11). Premature delivery may be caused by increased intrauterine pressure and relative cervical incompetence (12).

Any patient with a double uterus who has repeated pregnancy wastage should be evaluated thoroughly before considering surgical unification of the two cavities. It should be kept in mind that although there may be a septum in the uterus, there may be other causes of repeated fetal wastage as incompetent cervical os, corpus luteum inadequacy, genital infection, immunologic factors, or chromosome abnormalities.

UNIFICATION OPERATIONS

Strassman Procedure (13)

In this operation, a transverse fundal incision is made in case of a bicornuate uterus and the two uterine cavities are unified.

Tompkins Procedure (14)

This is a procedure for septate uteri. A median bivalve is made and no tissue is excised. The two cavities are opened and unified.

Jones Procedure (15)

In this operation, which is usually reserved for the wide septum, a wedge resection of the septum is done and the uterine cavities are unified.

With the above procedures, it would be advisable to deliver the patient by cesarean section at thirty-eight weeks pregnancy because of the scar in the uterus.

Hysteroscopic incision of the septum is preferred over abdominal metroplasty. The septum may be cut by scissors, laser, or resectoscope.

Advantages of hysteroscopic metroplasty over abdominal metroplasty.

    no risk of sequelae of laparotomy.
    shorter convalescence
    no reduction in volume of the uterine cavity.
    shorter interval to conception after the operation
    no fundal uterine scar to compromise the safety of vaginal delivery
    significant cost saving.

The reproductive performance was not adversely affected by a residual septum up to 1 cm.

Regardless of the unification operation, the literature shows that properly selected patients can anticipate 70–80 percent chance of delivering a live child (16).

Bicornuate Uterus

The bicornuate uterus results when two normally differentiated Mullerian ducts partially fuse in the region of the fundus. The chances of having a term pregnancy are >60 percent.

The diagnostic accuracy of differentiating between septate and bicornuate uterus using a hysterogram (Figures 35.7 and 35.8) is only 55 percent. Three-dimensional ultrasound, however, gives 91.6 percent accuracy (17). MRI appears to be confined to the research setting or dedicated referral centers.

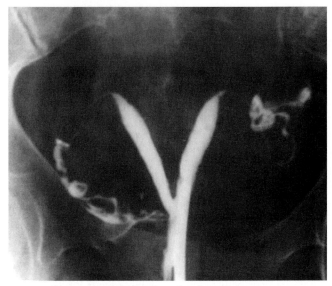

Figure 35.7. Hysterogram showing septate uterus.

Uterus Didelphys

In this abnormality, there is duplication of the uterus, cervix, and vagina. The incidence of this abnormality is about 10 percent of all uterine anomalies.

An obstructed hemivaginia was found in 18 percent of cases of uterus didelphys. Ipsilateral renal agenesis was the rule in case of obstruction. Where no obstruction is found, kidney abnormalities were found in 23 percent of uterus didelphys cases.

Fertility of women with didelphic uterus was comparatively good. Thirty-four (94 percent) out of thirty-six women who wanted to conceive had at least one pregnancy, and thirty-two (89 percent) had at least one living infant. Ten women had fifteen (25 percent) spontaneous abortions (8). There is a high frequency of breech presentation (51 percent) favoring cesarean section as a mode of delivery.

With blind hemivagina, hematometra and hemosalpinx occur, with endometriosis resulting in 38 percent of cases (18).

Arcuate Uterus

This represents a simple change in the uterine cavity shape with no external dimpling. It has no impact on reproduction.

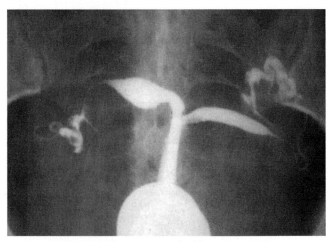

Figure 35.8. Hysterogram of a biocornuate uterus.

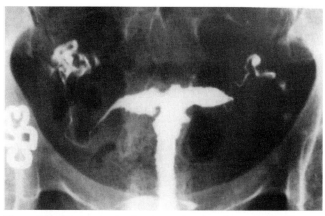

Figure 35.9. Hysterogram of a uterus showing changes of DES exposure in utero.

DES Exposure in Utero

The effect of DES exposure in utero is seen in the vagina, cervix, uterus, and the fallopian tubes. The typical hysterographic picture is that of a T-shaped uterus (Figure 35.9). Patients with DES exposure in utero tend to have an increased incidence of tubal pregnancy, first-trimester spontaneous abortions, and second-trimester spontaneous abortions due to an incompetent cervical os. The clinician should be aware of these possibilities whenever he or she is managing a patient with DES exposure in utero.

GENERAL REMARKS

The general frequency of uterine malformations is 4 percent. Infertility patients (6.3 percent) had a higher incidence of Mullerian anomalies in comparison with fertile women (3.8 percent) (6). Patients with congenital uterine malformations undergoing IVF have a good pregnancy rate (19).

REFERENCES

1. Hauser GA, Schreiner WE. Das Mayer-Rokitansky-Kuster-Hauser Syndrome. *Separatabdruck aus der Sweizerischen Medizinschen Wochenschrift* 1961;12:381.
2. Frank RT. The formation of an artificial vagina without operation. *Am J Obstet Gynecol* 1955;35:1057.
3. Ingram JM. The bicycle seat-stool in the treatment of vaginal agenesis and stenosis. A preliminary report. *Am J Obstet Gynecol* 1989;140:867.
4. McIndoe A. Treatment of congenital absence or obliterative condition of the vagina. *Brit J Plast Surg* 1950;2:254.
5. Raga F, Bauset C, Remohi J, Bonilla-Musoles F, Simon C, Pellicer A. Reproductive impact of congenital Mullerian anomalies. *Hum Reprod* 1997;12:2277.
6. Acien P. Reproductive performance of women with uterine malformations. *Hum Reprod* 1993;8:122.
7. Golan A, Langer R, Bukovsky R, Caspi E. Congenital anomalies of the Mullerian system. *Fertil Steril* 1989;51:747.
8. Heinonen PK, Saarikoski S, Pyskynen P. Reproductive performance of women with uterine anomalies. *Acta Obstet Gynecol Scand* 1982;61:157.
9. Harger JH, Archer DF, Marchese SG, Muracca-Clemens M, Garver KL. Etiology of recurrent pregnancy losses and outcome of subsequent pregnancies. *Obstet Gynecol* 1983;62:547.
10. Green LK, Harris RE. Uterine anomalies. Frequency of diagnosis and associated obstetrical complications. *Obstet Gynecol* 1976;47:427.
11. Burchell RC, Creed F, Rasoulpour M, Whitcomb M. Vascular anatomy of the human uterus and pregnancy wastage. *Brit J Obstet Gynaecol* 1978;85:698.
12. Rock JA, Murphy AA. Anatomic abnormalities. *Clin Obstet Gynecol* 1986;29:886.
13. Strassman P. Die operative Vereinigung eines droppelten Uterus. *Zbl Gynaek* 1907;31:1322.
14. Tompkins P. Comments on bicornuate uterus and twinning. *Surg Clin North Am* 1962;42:1049.
15. Jones HW Jr., Delfs E, Jones GES. Reproductive difficulties in double uterus. The place of plastic reconstruction. *Am J Obstet Gynecol* 1956;72:865.
16. Ayhan A, Yucel I, Tuncer Z, Kisnichi H. Reproductive performance after conventional metroplasty: an evaluation of 102 cases. *Fertil Steril* 1992;57:1194.
17. Raga F, Bonilla-Musoles F, Blaner J, Osborne NG. Congenital Mullerian anomalies: diagnostic accuracy of three-dimensional ultrasound. *Fertil Steril* 1996;65:523.18.
18. Candiani GB, Fedele L, Zamberletti D, De Virgilis D, Carinelli S. Endometrial patterns in malformed uteri. *Acta Eur Fertil* 1983;14:35.
19. Marcus S, Al-Shawaf T, Brinsden P. The obstetric outcome of in vitro fertilization and embryo transfer in women with congenital uterine malformations. *Am J Obstet Gynecol* 1996;75:89.

36

UNEXPLAINED INFERTILITY

Juan Balasch

INTRODUCTION

Human beings are not very fertile mammals, with an average monthly fecundity rate of only 20 percent. Formal evaluation of infertility is generally indicated in women attempting pregnancy who fail to conceive after a year or more of regular, unprotected intercourse; 85 percent of couples who will achieve pregnancy without assistance succeed within this interval of time (1,2). However, most couples seeking therapy for infertility are not truly sterile but have some degree of subfertility (i.e., the couples have conditions associated with a relative decrease in the monthly likelihood of conception) and can achieve pregnancy without treatment (1,3,4). Thus, in contrast to the treatment of sterility, it cannot be assumed that the pregnancy that occurs after treatment for subfertility is attributable solely to the treatment because it could have occurred by chance. Such treatment-independent pregnancies are more likely in couples designated as having unexplained infertility.

Despite advances in the diagnosis of causes of subfertility, inability to conceive remains unexplained in 15–30 percent of fully investigated couples (1,5). In these couples, the delay in conception may represent a chance delay or may be, in many cases, the result of an as yet undetected abnormality in the reproductive process. Cumulative pregnancy rates of 60 percent may be achieved within two years; however, for infertility of greater than three years duration, monthly fecundity rates in untreated couples are 1–2 percent (6,7).

The incidence of unexplained infertility varies with the population studied and with the criteria used. Different potential factors may contribute to unexplained infertility, including age of the partners, duration of infertility, coital frequency, and professional status (5). Among all of the potential contributing factors, female age over thirty years is the only significant predictor. A couple in which the female partner is aged thirty years or more is 1.7-fold more likely (95 percent confidence interval 1.3–1.9) to have unexplained infertility. In fact, the distribution of the age of female partners with this condition is significantly more advanced than the age distribution with other diagnoses (4,5).

Therefore, unexplained infertility seems to arise mainly from undetectable reproductive defects, some of which may be associated with an age-related decline in fertility (4,5,8). However, another scenario could be present: unexplained infertility represents in fact our lack of knowledge or missing information about reproductive processes because in addition to the recognized causes of infertility, numerous undetectable defects in the reproductive process might prevent conception among infertile couples (9). Thus, the relationships between semen quality and biological fertility remain controversial, direct diagnostic tests do not exist that can allow an assessment of ovulation and oocyte quality, tests of tubal assessment are mainly descriptive (appearance) but they do not assess function (conditions that foster oocyte pick up, fertilization and embryo development), and the exact mechanisms leading to successful embryo implantation are still largely unknown (9). On this basis, it has been recently claimed that the so-called unexplained infertility appears not only didactically but also clinically unsustainable as an independent diagnosis (10).

In summary, unexplained infertility may be considered as a misfortune due to the laws of chance or a limitation in our knowledge because numerous reproductive defects cannot be detected with current diagnostic methods (11,12).

DIAGNOSTIC CRITERIA OF UNEXPLAINED INFERTILITY

Unexplained infertility is a diagnosis made by exclusion after a complete infertility evaluation (13). However, the establishment of this diagnosis is complicated by the existence of different diagnostic protocols, various definitions of a normal test result, and the limited scope of the diagnostic assessment (5).

Traditionally, the cornerstones of assessing an infertile couple have been grouped into five standard testing categories. These include semen analysis, assessment of ovulation (usually by endometrial biopsy), evaluation of uterine architecture and tubal patency, the postcoital test (PCT), and laparoscopy (14,15). Despite the basic workup outlined by the American Fertility Society (14) and the World Health Organization (WHO) guidelines (15), a lack of agreement exists among trained fertility subspecialists with regard to the diagnostic tests to be performed and their prognostic utility as well as criteria for normality. Thus, a questionnaire survey among the teaching departments of obstetrics and gynecology in Western Europe revealed only weak adherence to the WHO recommendations for the standard investigation of the infertile couple with large differences among countries in the preferred standard testing methods. From this study, it was concluded that fertility investigations are based more on tradition and personal preference, than on the demonstrated usefulness of its components (16).

This agrees with the findings of similar studies performed among the U.S. board–certified reproductive endocrinologists, which demonstrated that, although most trained specialists agree on the major areas of the performance of infertility testing as outlined by the American Fertility Society (14), there was significant variability in details of the performance of most testing (including both criteria for normality and the interpretation of results), especially with respect to physician sex, age, type of practice, and geographic location. There was even less agreement with regard to additional modes of testing (e.g., hormonal testing, use of pelvic ultrasounds, hysteroscopy, cervical cultures, and antisperm antibody) besides those five "traditional" infertility tests (17,18). It can be argued that performing comprehensive investigations may explain or define causes of otherwise unexplained infertility; but when many tests are carried out that are independent or partially independent, then the chances of encountering a false-positive result increases exponentially (19,20).

Finally, the definition of unexplained infertility also is affected by the inclusion criteria for studies. If a couple conceives prior to having a test such as laparoscopy, to what category should they be allocated? The choice here is a trade-off between uncertainty and overselection (5). Requiring laparoscopy increases the certainty of being correct about the unexplained diagnosis, but any infertile group that includes only couples who have had a laparoscopy no longer represents typical infertile couples (5).

On the above evidence is therefore important to seek agreement on which diagnostic tests are required to be done prior to concluding that a couple have unexplained infertility. Such agreement is not readily obtained because of different views about the evidence and the variety of clinical experience. Although some believe that any abnormal diagnostic test result define a cause of infertility, there is now general agreement that abnormal tests' results define a cause of infertility only if treatment of this cause enhances fecundability as compared with no treatment (9,12,13,19,21,22). In other words, the current focus of diagnostic testing is on the use of a limited panel of specific investigations that correlate with the likelihood of live birth, rather than a broad range of screening tests (12).

Based on the latter view, diagnostic tests for infertility have been sorted into three categories (13,21,22):

1. Abnormal test results that have an established correlation with impaired fecundability: semen analysis, tubal patency by hysterosalpingogram or laparoscopy, and laboratory assessment of ovulation. In each case, when the test result is unequivocally abnormal (azoospermia, bilateral tubal occlusion, or anovulation), fertility is unarguably impaired without therapy.
2. Abnormal test results that are not consistently correlated with pregnancy: PCT, laparoscopic finding of mild endometriosis, cervical mucus penetration test, hysteroscopy, antisperm antibody assays, and the zona-free hamster egg penetration test. For these diagnostic tests, abnormal results frequently are associated with subsequent fertility without therapy.
3. Abnormal test results that do not appear to be correlated with impaired fecundability: endometrial dating, varicocele assessment, and falloscopy. For these diagnostic tests, either there are data that confirm the lack of a correlation with pregnancy or such follow-up studies do not exist.

Therefore, standard testing should include semen analysis (evaluated according to the WHO criteria), assessment of ovulation (serum progesterone determination in the midluteal phase), and an evaluation of tubal patency (hysterosalpingography is considered as the standard method to assess tubal patency as well as size and shape of the uterine cavity) (5,12,13,19,21,22). At present, other additional investigations contribute relatively little to effective diagnosis of unexplained infertility.

Laparoscopy is required to make a diagnosis of endometriosis or adnexal adhesions, but in the presence of tubal patency, these lesions seems to be of lesser significance. The medical treatment of endometriosis does not improve pregnancy rates, and intraoperative destruction of the lesions has only a small and short-lived beneficial effect (5,9). In fact, The Canadian Collaborative Group on Endometriosis (23) reported that the fecundity of infertile women with minimal or mild endometriosis is not significantly lower than that of women with unexplained infertility. In addition, if a *Chlamydia trachomatis* antibody titer is not elevated and pelvic sonography does not demonstrate the presence of an endometrioma, the incidence of major pelvic abnormalities is found in less than 5 percent of the patients (9,22). Therefore, as previously stressed by Collins (5), in these circumstances, having a laparoscopy should be determined by patient preference rather than the clinician's wish to define unexplained infertility in a more precise manner.

TREATMENT STRATEGIES

The efficacy of treatment for infertility disorders may be assessed easily and objectively by the resulting pregnancy rates. Cycle fecundity after in vitro fertilization (IVF) and embryo transfer in women who have had their fallopian tubes surgically removed provides a good indication of the efficacy of IVF for that condition. Similarly, in partners of azoospermic males undergoing artificial insemination with donor semen, the cycle fecundity is a good indicator of the suitability of this therapeutic approach.

The underlying assumption in the analysis of efficacy for any infertility treatment is that the likelihood of pregnancy without treatment is negligible. Therefore, designing and assessing the efficacy (or lack thereof) of treatment of unexplained infertility is rather challenging for several reasons (1,6,21,24):

1. There is a lack of consistency in the literature in defining the condition, and couples with only mild endometriosis are frequently considered to have unexplained infertility.
2. Therapy of unexplained infertility does not fit standard practice for medical decision making. Such standard practice requires a specific pathophysiological rationale that allows the correction of a biological defect. Because no such defect is known in unexplained infertility, treatment approaches are usually empiric.
3. Given the high probability for conception in such couples with observation alone, especially with infertility lasting less than three years and when the female partner is older than thirty years of age, a decrease in the time to conception may be seen rather than an increase in the absolute number of couples conceiving. However, this situation, where expectant management could be offered, is unusual in the current days when women are delaying childbearing to an age where they are more likely to encounter problems having a child (20).
4. There is a paucity of prospective, randomized, controlled trials evaluating pregnancy rates in treated and untreated patients with unexplained infertility.

During the past two decades, there has been a marked increase in the use of two treatments (used alone or in combination) for unexplained infertility: induction of super-ovulation, in which the ovaries are stimulated mainly with exogenous gonadotropins to develop several dominant follicles, and intrauterine insemination (IUI), in which motile sperm are suspended in culture medium and injected transcervically into the uterine cavity. IVF techniques are used as a final therapeutic step in couples who have tried IUI and ovarian stimulation without success. Other treatment modalities have been proposed or attempted for the treatment of unexplained infertility, but the majority have insufficient evidence to show efficacy.

Ovulation Induction and/or IUI

Taking into account the above considerations, what might be the rationale for administering gonadotropins to stimulate follicular development in patients with unexplained infertility, who by definition have regular ovulatory menstrual cycles? Why introduce washed sperm into the uterine cavity in situations in which the semen analysis is normal and there is no cervical factor present? With respect to ovarian stimulation, two explanations have been offered (25–27): 1) it may overcome a subtle defect in ovulatory function not uncovered by conventional testing and 2) it may enhance the likelihood of pregnancy by increasing the number of eggs available for fertilization.

According to the latter rationale, ovarian stimulation might improve the monthly pregnancy rate by simply increasing the number of oocytes available for fertilization and implantation. In fact, superovulation therapy was developed as a result of a fortuitous clinical observation. Some patients who received gonadotropins in preparation for an IVF or gamete intrafallopian transfer (GIFT) cycle had their oocyte retrieval procedure canceled (owing to inadequate numbers of follicles or endogenous LH surge) but became pregnant anyway (28,29). This observation suggested that multiple follicular recruitment and egg release might be the most critical element contributing to pregnancy. The direct relationship found between the intensity of stimulation protocols used for superovulation and IUI and the multiple pregnancy rates further supports this contention (30,31).

Along similar lines of thinking, increasing the density of motile sperm with a high proportion of normal forms available to these oocytes by IUI might further increase the monthly probability of pregnancy. In addition, timing the insemination as close to ovulation as possible optimizes the likelihood for gamete interaction (27). Thus, by increasing the numbers of gametes at the site of fertilization, the probability of conception can be increased. In fact, this is also the rationale behind IUI in couples with moderate male factor subfertility where sperm morphology using strict criteria and the inseminating motile sperm count after sperm preparation are the two most important sperm parameters related to IUI success (32).

IUI can be carried out during the natural ovarian cycle or following ovarian stimulation. IUI has gained increased clinical use in conjunction with ovarian stimulation using CC alone or in combination with gonadotropins, or, more commonly, gonadotropins alone. The use of CC, however, in women with unexplained infertility is associated with a small absolute effect on treatment per cycle (33) and pregnancy rates obtained are lower than with gonadotropin treatment, mainly when ovarian stimulation is associated with IUI (21,34–38).

To allow firm conclusions to be drawn on whether superovulation, with or without IUI, significantly improves the probability of conception in cases of subfertility compared with timed intercourse (TI) and to identify the independent effects of gonadotropins and IUI, four comparisons should be performed in randomized clinical trials (39,40). First, IUI should be compared with TI in natural cycles (comparison 1) and in superovulated cycles (comparison 2). Whether superovulation in combination with TI improves the probability of conception should be investigated in a trial comparing TI in stimulated cycles with TI in natural cycles (comparison 3). Whether superovulation in combination with IUI improves the probability of conception should be investigated in a trial comparing IUI in stimulated cycles with IUI in natural cycles (comparison 4). The best clinical scenario to perform these comparisons is unexplained infertility where there is absence of an apparent correctable abnormality.

We have recently analyzed the literature in this regard to determine, after performing the four above-mentioned comparisons, whether for unexplained infertility, superovulation improves the probability of conception compared with TI and whether IUI improves the results any further (41). For the analysis, four meta-analyses (21,35,36,42), two analyses of combined data from the literature (26,43), and three published, large, randomized clinical trials (two multicenter trials) (44–46) were considered relevant. Despite clinical heterogeneity and different methodological qualities of the trials, the following recommendation can be made based on the evidence found in the analyzed data (Table 36.1). In couples with unexplained infertility, superovulation with gonadotropins significantly improves the probability of conception, particularly when associated with IUI. This is in agreement with results from a recent Cochrane review (47).

The use of IUI together with ovulation induction in normally ovulating women carries a risk of ovarian hyperstimulation syndrome and multiple pregnancy. Both risks are proportional to the treatment protocol and dosages used. The use of current chronic low-dose (≤75 IU per day) protocols of FSH administration, careful ovarian response monitoring to determine the size and number of follicles (and estradiol serum levels if necessary), as well as strict cancellation criteria minimize those complications. Cases of moderate or severe ovarian hyperstimulation syndrome were observed neither in two large studies (48,49) nor in our own series of 1,360 IUI cycles. According to a recent review of studies with cancellation criteria reporting the results of ovarian stimulation-IUI cycles using low doses of gonadotropins and including 681 pregnancies among 6,670 IUI cycles initiated, the mean rate of high-order multiple pregnancy rate was 0.3 percent (being 0 percent in most of the studies included), with a mean success rate of 10 percent pregnancies per treatment cycle (49).

Most couples (>90 percent) who get pregnant using IUI in association with ovarian stimulation do so within the first three to four cycles of treatment, and there is a significant decline in cycle fecundity afterward. Therefore, it is not advisable to continue treatment with IUI after this number of attempts and it is reasonable to switch from IUI to IVF after a maximum of three to four IUI cycles (50–54). This is our decision-making process in most infertile couples.

IVF and Related Assisted Reproductive Technologies (ART)

Although IVF and embryo transfer was first used to bypass the fallopian tubes in women with inoperable tubal disease, it is

Table 36.1: Summary of Reported Results of Treatment with IUI and/or Gonadotropin Ovarian Stimulation for Unexplained Infertility*

Study, year (references)	IUI versus TI	FSH + IUI versus FSH + TI	FSH + TI versus TI	FSH + IUI versus IUI
Cohlen, 1998 (36)	No difference	FSH + IUI better	FSH + TI better	FSH + IUI better
Zeyneloglu et al., 1998 (42)	—	FSH + IUI better	—	—
Hughes, 1997 (35)	IUI better	FSH + IUI better	FSH + TI better	FSH + IUI better
ESHRE Capri Workshop Group, 1996 (21)	IUI better	FSH + IUI better	FSH + TI better	FSH + IUI better
Guzick et al., 1998 (26)	No difference	FSH + IUI better	FSH + TI better	FSH + IUI better
Crosignani et al., 1991 (44)	—	FSH + IUI better	—	—
Guzick et al., 1999 (45)	IUI better	FSH + IUI better	FSH + TI better	FSH + IUI better
Goverde et al., 2000 (46)	—	FSH + IUI better	—	FSH + IUI better
Aboulghar et al., 2003 (43)	—	FSH + IUI better	—	FSH + IUI better

*Adapted from reference 41.
FSH is used as synonymous with ovarian stimulation with gonadotropins, that is, HMG or FSH.

now performed in couples with a variety of infertility causes as a method to enhance conception. In fact, IVF is considered the last resort in the treatment of almost all infertile patients, and it is widely accepted as treatment for unexplained infertility despite that very few studies have compared the live birth rates achieved with assisted reproduction with placebo in this condition (55,56).

IVF is advocated by most clinicians for couples with unexplained infertility based on evidence from retrospective and/or uncontrolled trials. Thus, in the Centers for Disease Control and Prevention, the American Society for Reproductive Medicine, and the Society for Assisted Reproductive Technology report on ART results for 2003, a total of 35,785 pregnancies resulting from 122,872 ART procedures were reported (57). Unexplained infertility involved 11.6 percent of the treatment cycles, and while the national average success rate was slightly more than 28 percent, the live birth rate among women with unexplained infertility was 30.4 percent. In that report, it was concluded that, in general, couples diagnosed with tubal factor, ovulatory dysfunction, endometriosis, male factor, or unexplained infertility had above-average success rates (57). Also, in the 2004 Fertility Clinical Guidance, the National Institute of Clinical Excellence (NICE) (58) stressed that in cases of tubal, endocrinological, and unexplained infertility, the success rate of IVF was comparable with the probability of natural conception for young and fertile couples. A recent Cochrane review (59), however, concluded that IVF might result in more pregnancies than other options for unexplained infertility; but this is still uncertain and more research is needed on birth rates, adverse outcomes, and costs. Thus, IVF may not be the preferred first line of treatment for these couples.

Interestingly enough, on the other side, it has recently been suggested that IVF should be offered as first-line therapy as opposed to IUI and superovulation with gonadotropins for the treatment of unexplained infertility because of the high risk of high-order multiple pregnancy when using IUI and ovula-

tion induction (31,60). In response to this argument, others (61,62) regretted the lack of good-quality, large, prospective randomized trials to settle the argument. Notably, Homburg (63,64) has critically and thoughtfully analyzed this subject using the results of randomized controlled trials wherever possible, live birth rates rather than pregnancy rates and taking into account efficacy; complications, especially multiple pregnancy rates; patient compliance; and cost efficiency. The efficiency of the IVF is still limited; although less efficient per cycle in terms of basis, findings are consistent in concluding that IUI and superovulation are nevertheless capable of producing a pregnancy and delivery within a reasonable time. There is little doubt that IVF is a much more invasive procedure than IUI and that superovulation and IUI are unequivocally less complicated and safer compared with IVF. In fact, the cumulative drop-out rate in an IVF programme is significantly higher than that for IUI. Ovulation induction coupled with IUI is more cost effective than IVF (63,64). The cost of an IVF cycle is approximately four times higher than the cost of a cycle of gonadotropin/IUI treatment (61). Cost-effectiveness, which is the ratio of cost to success, tends to decrease when success is better and increase when costs go up. Thus, given the fourfold higher cost of IVF, the live birth rate with a cycle of IVF would have to be fourfold greater than the live birth rate with a cycle of gonadotropin/IUI to achieve a similar level of cost-effectiveness (61). In contrast, because gonadotropin/IUI is more tolerable and less expensive than IVF, repeated cycles are possible, further increasing the absolute number of pregnancies associated with these treatments (62).

Despite being empirical, expensive, and invasive, IVF is considered to be an effective treatment option because it can circumvent most of the putative causes of unexplained infertility. These include ovarian dysfunction, cervical factors, sperm and egg transport, and problems with sperm-egg interaction. IVF may also have a diagnostic role in identifying couples with fertilization failure (59). Unsuspected sperm abnormalities or oocyte dysfunction may result in fertilization failure even after IVF and may be responsible for unexplained infertility. Although intracytoplasmic sperm injection (ICSI) does not overcome oocyte defects, it may be a good solution for undetected sperm abnormalities. ICSI appears to be a better choice of treatment, at least for a subgroup of patients, if not all (65). Couples with unexplained infertility treated with IVF usually have the same oocyte recovery rate as other subgroups, but they have been shown to have reduced fertilization and cleavage rates, and a complete failure of fertilization has been reported in 5–30 percent of the cycles (66). If no fertilization has occurred in previous IVF attempt, ICSI is the treatment of choice, as it is also in cases of low fertilization percentage with conventional IVF. Studies comparing IVF and ICSI on sibling oocytes from couples with unexplained infertility showed no difference regarding overall fertilization rates between the two groups, but cases with total fertilization failure were significantly higher in the IVF group (65). This is also our experience, and thus, we agree with those authors who suggest that performing ICSI in some of the oocytes from the first attempt may help in eliminating fertilization failures in couples with supposedly unexplained infertility (65–67).

GIFT and zygote intrafallopian transfer (ZIFT) were used in the 1980s and 1990s to treat unexplained infertility. As both these treatments were more invasive and expensive and offered no advantages compared with IVF and, in addition, fertilization cannot be observed and assessed after GIFT, they have largely been abandoned (66). In fact, in the 2004 Fertility Clinical Guidance, the NICE (58) clearly stresses that GIFT and ZIFT are not recommended for treatment of unexplained infertility.

Alternative Therapies

Other treatment modalities have been proposed or attempted for the treatment of unexplained infertility. Clomiphene citrate is a common treatment for this condition, although it has been suggested that the empiric use of this drug in ovulatory women can cause alterations in the normal endocrinology of ovulation (56). A Cochrane review concluded that clomiphene citrate appears to modestly improve pregnancy rates in women with unexplained subfertility, but adverse effects include a possible ovarian cancer risk and risk of multiple pregnancy (33). Although it seems logical that clomiphene citrate in combination with IUI would have greater value than clomiphene citrate alone, the data in this respect are contradictory and the reported effects are compromised by crossover designs and unequal loss to follow-up (56). In addition, pregnancy rates obtained are lower in comparison with gonadotropin and IUI treatment (21,34–38). Bromocriptine and danazol have distinct size effects and both are a poor choice as an empiric therapy for unexplained infertility (5,68,69). Finally, although there exists a strong motivation to find answers to what is otherwise unexplained, the use of widespread immune testing in clinical practice cannot be supported by existing data. Thus, the implementation of therapies to correct presumed immunologic defects that are proposed to lead to reproductive failure in the form of unexplained infertility cannot be recommended and may cause harm (70,71). Similarly, although psychological factors have been considered to play a part in unexplained infertility, there is no evidence that such factors are causative, and there are no controlled trials showing that psychological or educational counselling is effective (21).

KEY POINTS FOR CLINICAL PRACTICE

■ Despite advances in the diagnosis of causes of subfertility, inability to conceive remains unexplained in 15–30 percent of fully investigated couples.

■ The incidence of unexplained infertility varies with the population studied and with the criteria used being female age, the most significant contributing factor.

■ The diagnosis of unexplained infertility is one of exclusion.

■ The dilemma of unexplained infertility is double: 1) an agreement on which diagnostic tests are required to be done prior to concluding that a couple have unexplained infertility is not readily obtained and 2) although there have been numerous advances in the diagnostic assessment of infertility, undetectable defects in the reproductive process might still prevent conception among infertile couples.

■ The treatment of unexplained infertility is hampered primarily, by definition, by the lack of a specific abnormality the practitioner can attempt to correct. Thus, treatment approaches are usually empiric.

■ Based on the available information, it is reasonable to recommend an escalating course of gonadotropin ovarian stimulation with IUI and then IVF/ICSI.

REFERENCES

1. Evers JLH. Female subfertility. *Lancet* 2002; 360:151–159.
2. The Practice Committee of the American Society for Reproductive Medicine. Optimal evaluation of the infertile female. *Fertil Steril* 2004; 82 (Suppl. 1):S169–S172.
3. Collins JA, Wrixon W, Janes LB, Wilson EH. Treatment-independent pregnancy among infertile couples. *N Engl J Med* 1983; 309:1201–1206.
4. Collins JA, Crosignani PG. Unexplained infertility: a review of diagnosis, prognosis, treatment efficacy and management. *Int J Gynecol Obstet* 1992; 39:267–275.
5. Collins J. An overview of medical care issues in unexplained infertility. In: Filicori M, Flamigni C, (eds.) Treatment of Infertility: The New Frontiers. New Jersey: Communications Media for Education, 1998: 15–27.
6. Hull MGR. Infertility treatment: relative effectiveness of conventional and assisted conception methods. *Hum Reprod* 1992; 7:785–796.
7. Collins JA, Burrows EA, Willan AR. The prognosis for live birth among untreated infertile couples. *Fertil Steril* 1995; 64:22–28.
8. The ESHRE Capri Workshop Group. Fertility and ageing. *Hum Reprod Update* 2005; 11:261–276.
9. The ESHRE Capri Workshop Group. Diagnosis and management of the infertile couple: missing information. *Hum Reprod Update* 2004; 10:295–307.
10. Gleicher N, Barad D. Unexplained infertility: does it really exist? *Hum Reprod* 2006; 21:1951–1955.
11. Southam AL. What to do with the "normal" infertile couple? *Fertil Steril* 1960; 11:543–549.
12. Collins JA. Evidence-based infertility: evaluation of the female partner. In: Daya S, Harrison RF, Kempers RD, (eds.) Advances in Fertility and Reproductive Medicine. Amsterdam, The Netherlands: Elsevier, 2004:57–62.
13. Crosignani PG, Collins J, Cooke ID, Diczfalusy E, Rubin B. Unexplained infertility. *Hum Reprod* 1993; 8:977–980.
14. American Fertility Society. Investigation of the Infertile Couple. Birmingham, AL: American Fertility Society, 1992.

15. Rowe PJ, Comhaire FH, Hargreave TB et al. WHO Manual for the Standardized Investigation of the Infertile Couple. Cambridge, UK: Cambridge University Press, 1993.

16. Helmerhorst FM, Oei SG, Bloemenkamp KWM et al. Consistency and variation in fertility investigations in Europe. *Hum Reprod* 1995; 10:2027–2030.

17. Glatstein IZ, Harlow BL, Hornstein MD. Practice patterns among reproductive endocrinologists: the infertility evaluation. *Fertil Steril* 1997; 67:443–451.

18. Glatstein IZ, Harlow BL, Hornstein MD. Practice patterns among reproductive endocrinologists: further aspects of the infertility evaluation. *Fertil Steril* 1998; 70:263–269.

19. Zayed F, Abu-Heija A. The management of unexplained infertility. *Obstet Gynecol Survey* 1999; 54:121–130.

20. Balasch J. Investigation of the infertile couple in the era of assisted reproductive technology: a time for reappraisal. *Hum Reprod* 2000; 15:2251–2257.

21. The ESHRE Capri Workshop Group. Guidelines to the prevalence, diagnosis, treatment and management of infertility, 1996. *Hum Reprod* 1996; 11:1775–1807.

22. The ESHRE Capri Workshop Group. Optimal use of infertility diagnostic tests and treatments. *Hum Reprod* 2000; 15:723–732.

23. Bérubé S, Marcoux S, Langevin RN et al. Fecundity of infertile women with minimal or mild endometriosis and women with unexplained infertility. *Fertil Steril* 1998; 69:1034–1041.

24. Hull MGR, Glazener CMA, Kelly NJ et al. Population study of causes, treatment, and outcome of infertility. *Br Med J* 1985; 291:1693–1697.

25. Collins JA. Superovulation in the treatment of unexplained infertility. *Sem Reprod Endocrinol* 1990; 8:165–173.

26. Guzick DS, Sullivan MW, Adamson GD et al. Efficacy of treatment for unexplained infertility. *Fertil Steril* 1998; 70:207–213.

27. Stewart JA. Stimulated intra-uterine insemination is not a natural choice for the treatment of unexplained subfertility. Should the guidelines be changed? *Hum Reprod* 2003; 18:903–907.

28. Haney AF, Hughes CL, Whitesides DB, Dodson WC. Treatment-independent, treatment-associated and pregnancies after additional therapy in a program of in vitro fertilization and embryo transfer. *Fertil Steril* 1987; 47:634–638.

29. Curole DN, Dickey RP, Taylor SN, Rye PH, Olar TT. Pregnancies in canceled gamete intrafallopian transfer cycles. *Fertil Steril* 1989; 51:363–364.

30. Nan PM, Cohlen BJ, te Velde ER et al. Intra-uterine insemination or timed intercourse after ovarian stimulation for male subfertility? A controlled study. *Hum Reprod* 1994; 9:2022–2026.

31. Gleicher N, Oleske DM, Tur-Kaspa I, Vidali A, Karande V. Reducing the risk of high-order multiple pregnancy after ovarian stimulation with gonadotropins. *N Engl J Med* 2000; 343:2–7.

32. Ombelet W. Semen quality and intrauterine insemination. *Reprod BioMed Online* 2003; 7:485–492.

33. Hughes EG, Collins J, Vandekerckhove P. Clomiphene citrate for unexplained subfertility in women. Cochrane Review, In: The Cochrane Library, Issue 2, 2001. Oxford: Update Software.

34. Balasch J, Ballescá JL, Pimentel C et al. Late low-dose pure follicle stimulating hormone for ovarian stimulation in intrauterine insemination cycles. *Hum Reprod* 1994; 9:1863–1866.

35. Hughes EG. The effectiveness of ovulation induction and intra-uterine insemination in the treatment of persistent infertility: a meta-analysis. *Hum Reprod* 1997; 12:1865–1872.

36. Cohlen BJ. Intrauterine insemination and controlled ovarian hyperstimulation. In: Templeton A, Cooke I and O'Brien PMS (eds.). Evidence-Based Fertility Treatment. London, UK: RCOG Press, 1998: 205–216.

37. Matorras R, Díaz T, Corcostegui B et al. Ovarian stimulation in intrauterine insemination with donor sperm: a randomized study comparing clomiphene citrate in fixed protocol versus highly purified urinary FSH. *Hum Reprod* 2002; 17:2107–2111.

38. Costello MF. Systematic review of the treatment of ovulatory infertility with clomiphene citrate and intrauterine insemination. *Aust NZ J Obstet Gynecol* 2004; 44:93–102.

39. Cohlen BJ, te Velde ER, van Kooij RJ. Is there still a place for intra-uterine insemination as a treatment for male subfertility? *Intern J Androl* 1995; 18 (Suppl. 2):72–75.

40. Cohlen BJ, Hughes E, te Velde ER. Intra-uterine insemination for unexplained infertility (Protocol for a Cochrane Review). In: The Cochrane Library, Issue 3, 2004. Chichester, UK: John Wiley & Sons, Ltd.

41. Balasch J. Gonadotrophin ovarian stimulation and intrauterine insemination for unexplained infertility. *Reprod BioMed Online* 2004; 9:664–672.

42. Zeyneloglu HB, Arici A, Olive DL et al. Comparison of intrauterine insemination with timed intercourse in superovulated cycles with gonadotropins: a meta-analysis. *Fertil Steril* 1998; 69:486–491.

43. Aboulghar MA, Mansour RT, Serour GI et al. Diagnosis and management of unexplained infertility: an update. *Arch Gynecol Obstet* 2003; 267:177–188.

44. Crosignani PG, Walters DE, Soliani A. The ESHRE multicentre trial on the treatment of unexplained infertility: a preliminary report. *Hum Reprod* 1991; 6:953–958.

45. Guzick DS, Carson SA, Coutifaris C et al. Efficacy of superovulation and intrauterine insemination in the treatment of infertility. *N Engl J Med* 1999; 340:177–183.

46. Goverde AJ, McDonnell J, Vermeiden JPW et al. Intrauterine insemination or in-vitro fertilisation in idiopathic subfertility and male subfertility: a randomised trial and cost-effectiveness analysis. *Lancet* 2000; 355:13–18.

47. Verhulst SM, Cohlen BJ, Hughes E, Te Velde E, Heineman MJ. Intra-uterine insemination for unexplained subfertility. *Cochrane Database of Systematic Reviews* 2006, Issue 4. Art. No.: CD001838. DOI: 10.1002/14651858.CD001838.pub3.

48. Papageorgiou TC, Guibert J, Savale M et al. Low dose recombinant FSH treatment may reduce multiple gestations caused by controlled ovarian hyperstimulation and intrauterine insemination. *BJOG* 2004; 111:1277–1282.

49. Ragni G, Caliari I, Nicolosi AE, Arnoldi M, Somigliana E, Crosignani PG. Preventing high-order multiple pregnancies during controlled ovarian hyperstimulation and intrauterine insemination: 3 years' experience using low-dose recombinant follicle-stimulating hormone and gonadotropin-releasing hormone antagonists. *Fertil Steril* 2006; 85:619–624.

50. Ombelet W, Puttemans P, Bosmans E. Intrauterine insemination: a first-step procedure in the algorithm of male subfertility treatment. *Hum Reprod* 1995; 10 (Suppl. 1):90–102.

51. Dodson WC, Haney AF. Superovulation and intrauterine insemination. In Adashi EY et al. (eds.), Reproductive Endocrinology, Surgery, and Technology, vol. 2. Philadelphia: Lippincott-Raven, 1996:2234–2243.

52. Aboulghar MA, Mansour RT, Serour GI et al. Controlled ovarian hyperstimulation and intrauterine insemination for treatment of unexplained infertility should be limited to a maximum of three trials. *Fertil Steril* 2001; 75:88–91.

53. Meniru GI. Cambridge Guide to Infertility Management and Assisted Reproduction. Cambridge, UK: Cambridge University Press, 2001.

54. Ludwig AK, Diedrich K, Ludwig M. The process of decision making in reproductive medicine. *Sem Reprod Med* 2005; 23: 348–353.

55. RCOG Infertility Guideline Group. The Management of Infertility in Secondary Care. London, UK: RCOG, 1998.

56. The Practice Committee of the American Society for Reproductive Medicine. Effectiveness and treatment for unexplained infertility. *Fertil Steril* 2006; 86 (Suppl. 4):S111–S114.

57. Centers for Disease Control and Prevention. 2003 Assisted Reproductive Technology (ART) Report. USA, 2006.

58. NICE. National Collaborating Centre for Women's and Children's Health. Fertility: Assessment and Treatment for People with Fertility Problems. Clinical Guideline. London, UK: RCOG Press, 2004.

59. Pandian Z, Bhattacharya S, Vale L, Templeton A. In vitro fertilisation for unexplained subfertility. *Cochrane Database of Systematic Reviews* 2005, Issue 2. Art. No.: CD003357. DOI: 10.1002/14651858.CD003357.pub2.

60. Gleicher N, Karande V. Forget about ovulation induction! Proceed directly to IVF. In Proceedings of the 2nd World Congress on Controversies in Obstetrics and Gynecology, edited by Ben-Rafael Z, Shoham Z, Frydman R. Monduzzi Editore, Bologna: 2001:211–215.

61. Collins J. Stimulated intra-uterine insemination is not a natural choice for the treatment of unexplained subfertility. Current best evidence for the advanced treatment of unexplained subfertility. *Hum Reprod* 2003; 18:907–912.

62. Hughes EG. Stimulated intra-uterine insemination is not a natural choice for the treatment of unexplained subfertility.

'Effective treatment' or 'not a natural choice'? *Hum Reprod* 2003; 18:912–914.

63. Homburg R. The case for initial treatment with intrauterine insemination as opposed to in vitro fertilization for idiopathic infertility. *Hum Fertil (Cambridge)* 2003; 6:122–124.

64. Homburg R, Insler V. Ovulation induction in perspective. *Hum Reprod Update* 2002; 8:449–462.

65. Mercan R, Sertac A, Urman B. Role of assisted reproductive technologies in the treatment of unexplained infertility. *Reprod Technol* 2001;10:288–294.

66. Isaksson R, Tiitinen A. Present concept of unexplained infertility. *Gynecol Endocrinol* 2004;18:278–290.

67. Aboulghar MA, Mansour RT, Serour GI et al. Management of long-standing unexplained infertility: a prospective study. *Am J Obstet Gynecol* 1999; 181:371–375.

68. Hughes EG, Collins J, Vandekerckhove P. Bromocriptine for unexplained subfertility in women. *Cochrane Database Syst Rev* 2000;(2):CD000044.

69. Hughes EG, Tiffin G, Vandekerckhove P. Danazol for unexplained infertility. *Cochrane Database Syst Rev* 2000;(2): CD000069.

70. Stovall DW, Van Voorhis BJ. Immunologic tests and treatments in patients with unexplained infertility, IVF-ET, and recurrent pregnancy loss. *Clin Obstet Gynecol* 1999; 42:979–1000.

71. Kallen CB, Arici A. Immune testing in fertility practice: truth or deception? *Curr Opin Obstet Gynecol* 2003; 15:225–231.

37

"Premature Ovarian Failure": Characteristics, Diagnosis, and Management

Robert W. Rebar

"Premature ovarian failure" (POF), sometimes termed premature menopause, is an enigmatic disorder. Although generally defined as consisting of the triad of amenorrhea (primary or secondary), hypergonadotropinism, and hypoestrogenism in women younger than forty years, it is now apparent that many affected women will ovulate and even conceive after the diagnosis is established. Thus, the name itself, implying permanent ovarian dysfunction, is actually inappropriate. In this regard, suggestions that the disorder be referred to as (primary) ovarian insufficiency, hypergonadotropic hypogonadism, or hypogonadotropic amenorrhea may be more accurate.

Definitive criteria for diagnosis have not been established. However, several groups have suggested that at least four months of amenorrhea in association with menopausal levels of gonadotropins on two or more occasions should qualify as an operational definition for the disorder (1, 2).

It has become clear that clinicians who provide reproductive care for women are likely to identify individuals with POF. Estimates of the prevalence of the disorder have varied. In one study, 7 of 300 consecutive women presenting with amenorrhea had POF (3). An estimate based on several studies concluded that 0.3 percent of reproductive-aged women (or approximately 200,000 in the United States) have POF (4). The risk of experiencing menopause prior to age forty was calculated as 0.9 percent in Rochester, Minnesota, based on 1950 data (5).

THE CLINICAL SPECTRUM OF PREMATURE OVARIAN FAILURE

We compiled data from 115 consecutive women with hypergonadotropic amenorrhea seen over a ten-year period in order to characterize the clinical presentation of affected individuals (1). These data have been confirmed by the more than 300 additional women with POF we have seen since that report (unpublished) and by series published by other groups of clinicians as well. Most apparent are striking differences between women who present with secondary as opposed to primary amenorrhea (Table 37.1).

About 85 percent of women with secondary amenorrhea complained of symptoms of estrogen deficiency, principally hot flashes and dyspareunia, whereas these complaints were present in only 20 percent of women with primary amenorrhea. Moreover, only those women with primary amenorrhea who had been given exogenous estrogen and then stopped taking it complained of these symptoms. On physical examination, about 90 percent of women with secondary amenorrhea had Tanner stage 5 breast and pubic hair development, whereas only 10 percent of women with primary amenorrhea were completely developed. Karyotypic abnormalities were present in a little more than 10 percent of women with secondary amenorrhea but were found in over half the women with primary hypergonadotropic amenorrhea. Moreover, the kinds of abnormalities found differed in the two groups of amenorrheic women: women with secondary amenorrhea often had an additional X chromosome, whereas those with primary amenorrhea were more apt to have all or a portion of an X chromosome missing. Bone density in comparison to age-matched controls was diminished in at least half the women in each group. About half the women with secondary amenorrhea had withdrawal bleeding in response to administration of exogenous progestin, whereas only 20 percent of those with primary amenorrhea withdrew to progestin. In any case, the fact that so many women in each group withdrew was surprising and provides strong evidence that administration of progestin is not a reliable test of estrogen status and of the possibility of responding to exogenous clomiphene citrate. More than one-third of women with second amenorrhea had been pregnant at least once before diagnosis, about 25 percent had evidence of ovulation after the diagnosis was established, and 8 percent became pregnant without assistance after diagnosis. Pregnancies occurred in none of the women with primary hypergonadotropic amenorrhea.

Four of the women with secondary amenorrhea and normal karyotypes gave a family history of early menopause prior to age forty. More recently, other investigators have documented the importance of family history. Premutations of the FMR1 gene are present in as many as 14 percent of women with familial POF, as well as about 2 percent of women with isolated POF (6).

Immune disorders have been identified in about 20 percent of affected women, regardless of whether they present with primary or secondary amenorrhea. In our series, thyroid abnormalities were most frequent, with five women developing Hashimoto thyroiditis, two developing primary hypothyroidism, one developing subacute thyroiditis, and one presenting with Graves disease. One of the women had vitiligo and hypoparathyroidism, one developed Addison disease, and one developed insulin-dependent diabetes mellitus. Because the prevalence of autoimmune diseases is also common in normal women, it is not clear if the incidence of these disorders is any higher in women with POF than it is in the general population.

Table 37.1: Features of Women with Primary and Secondary Amenorrhea

Characteristic	1° Amenorrhea (%)*	2° Amenorrhea (%)*
Symptoms of estrogen deficiency	20	85
Incomplete sexual development	90	8
Karyotypic abnormalities	55	13
Immune abnormalities	20	20
Decreased spinal bone density +	50	60
Progestin-induced withdrawal bleeding	20	50
Pregnancies before diagnosis	0	35
Evidence of ovulation after diagnosis	0	25
Pregnancies after diagnosis	0	8

*Approximate percentages of affected individuals based on data from Rebar and Connolly, 1990. + Compared to age-matched normal controls.

In this series, twenty-five women with secondary amenorrhea were treated with clomiphene citrate in an effort to induce ovulation, but only four (16 percent) ovulated as determined by serial ultrasound examinations and serum progesterone levels. Because each of the four women who ovulated had evidence of spontaneous episodic ovulation before therapy, it is not clear if the clomiphene actually induced ovulation or ovulation just occurred by chance alone. Nineteen of the women had gonadotropin secretion suppressed either with exogenous estrogen and progestin ($n = 14$) or with gonadotropin-releasing hormone agonist ($n = 5$) for one to three months. Then, ovulation induction with exogenous gonadotropins was attempted. Only two of the patients ovulated and one conceived. These data are consistent with the spontaneous ovulation and pregnancy rates in these women and with a later controlled trial documenting that ovulation induction is unlikely to be successful (7).

A total of twelve women with secondary amenorrhea had ovarian biopsies, and apparently viable oocytes were identified in tissue from seven of the women. Yet, two of the eight pregnancies occurring subsequently in this series occurred in women with biopsies containing no follicles. Moreover, about seven of the eight pregnancies occurred while the women were taking exogenous estrogens – in some case, combination oral contraceptive agents. Five of these eight pregnancies resulted in normal-term live births, two ended in miscarriage, and one was terminated by elective abortion. Only three women with primary amenorrhea underwent biopsy of gonadal tissue; the two with 46,XY karyotypes had dysgerminomas. The third patient had only fibrous streaks present.

ETIOLOGY OF PREMATURE OVARIAN FAILURE

The characteristics of series of patients with POF make it very clear that this disorder has several etiologies. In considering possible etiologies, the largest category is still idiopathic, but each year more and more genetic causes are being identified. It is likely that gene mutations ultimately will be identified in the majority of women who present with POF. Among the various causes of POF that now have been identified, it is clear that some are present only in those who have no oocytes remaining, whereas others may be associated with remaining follicles and offer the potential for ovulation and spontaneous pregnancy. Given current knowledge, it is impossible to develop a classification scheme for POF that does not include some overlap, but one possible classification is suggested in Table 37.2.

Cytogenetic Abnormalities Involving the X chromosome

Individuals who have any of the various forms of gonadal dysgenesis, with or without the stigmata of Turner syndrome, typically present with hypergonadotropic amenorrhea, whether or not they have pubertal development. Cytogenetic abnormalities of the X chromosome clearly impair ovarian development and function. Studies of 45,X individuals and those with various deletions of one of their two X chromosomes have confirmed that two intact X chromosomes are necessary for maintenance of the normal complement of oocytes and normal ovarian function (8). The gonads of fetuses who are 45,X contain normal numbers of oocytes at twenty to twenty-four weeks of fetal age, but there is rapid atresia such that virtually none are present at birth (9); thus, individuals with classic Turner syndrome really can be considered as having POF and virtually always have primary amenorrhea. Individuals with deletions in either the short or the long arm of the X chromosome commonly present with primary or secondary amenorrhea. Structural abnormalities of the X chromosome also can lead to hypergonadotropic amenorrhea. The association of submicroscopic deletions of the X chromosome with POF indicates that even very subtle molecular defects can affect ovarian function (10, 11). Extra X chromosomes also may be found in some women with POF (12). Women with 47,XXX karyotypes typically develop normally and only later develop POF.

Perhaps one of the most important associations with POF is with abnormalities of the familial mental retardation-1 (FMR1) gene. A constellation of disorders is now known to be associated with a dynamic triple-repeat sequence mutation (cytosine-guanine-guanine, CGG) in the FMR1 gene located on the end of the long arm of the X chromosome at Xq27 (13). In normal individuals, the CGG repeat typically numbers fewer than 45. In the so-called premutation, from 50 to 200 CGG repeats are present, and individuals with the full mutation have more than 200 CGG repeats. In its fully expanded form, the mutation inactivates the gene and leads to the fragile X syndrome, the most common cause of inherited mental retardation and the leading single-gene defect associated with autism. It has been estimated that the premutation is present in 1 of every 129 females and in 1 of every 800 males in the United States.

The premutation is now known to be associated with two disorders that are distinct from the fragile X syndrome. The first, affecting primarily males, is a neurological disorder now termed the fragile X–associated tremor/ataxia syndrome (FXTAS). The second, affecting approximately 15 percent of those women carrying the premutation, is premature ovarian

Table 37.2: Causes of Premature Ovarian Failure

I. Cytogenetic abnormalities involving the X chromosome

A. Structural alterations or absence of an X chromosome

B. Premutations of the FMR1 gene (fragile X; 6 percent of cases) at Xq27

C. Trisomy X with or without mosaicism

II. Enzymatic defects

A. Steroidogenic enzyme defects

1. 17α-hydroxylase or 17, 20-lyase deficiency

2. 20, 22-desmolase deficiency

3. Aromatase deficiency

B. Galactosemia

III. Other known genetic alterations of specific genes

A. FSHR (the FSH receptor)

B. INHA (inhibin alpha)

C. FOXL2 (a forkhead transcription factor associated with the blepharophimosis/ptosis/epicanthus inversus syndrome)

D. EIF2B (a family of genes associated with CNS leukodystrophy and ovarian failure)

E. BMP15 (bone morphogenetic factor 15, involved with folliculogenesis)

F. PMM2 (phosphomannomutase)

G. AIRE (autoimmune polyendocrinopathy-candidiasis-ectodermal dystrophy syndrome)

IV. Defective gonadotropin secretion or action

A. Receptor or postreceptor defects

1. FSH receptor mutations

2. LH receptor mutations

3. G-protein alterations

B. Secretion of biologically inactive gonadotropin

V. Environmental insults

A. Chemotherapeutic agents

B. Ionizing radiation

C. Viral infection

D. Surgical injury or extirpation

VI. Autoimmune disorders

A. In association with other autoimmune disturbances (15–20 percent of cases; 4 percent with steroidogenic cell autoimmunity)

B. Isolated

C. In association with congenital thymic aplasia

VII. Idiopathic

---

failure. Individuals with the premutation also may present with emotional features including anxiety, excessive outbursts, impulsivity, short attention span, hyperactivity, and even autism. Current estimates suggest that about 6 percent of women with POF have the fragile X premutation (14).

Enzymatic Defects

Three enzymatic defects in the steroidogenic pathway – 17α-hydroxylase (also known as 17,20-lyase) deficiency, 20,22-lyase deficiency, and aromatase deficiency – also may result in hypergonadotropic amenorrhea. 17α-Hydroxylase deficiency is identified easily because affected individuals present with primary amenorrhea, failure to develop secondary sexual characteristics, hypergonadotropinism, hypertension, hypokalemic alkalosis, and increased circulating concentrations of deoxycorticosterone and progesterone (15).

Several individuals have now been described with documented mutations in the CYP19 (aromatase P450) gene (16). Estrogen biosynthesis is virtually absent in all affected individuals. Regardless of the specific mutation present in the gene, aromatase deficiency in 46,XX individuals is characterized by female pseudohermaphroditism with clitoromegaly and posterior labioscrotal fusion at birth; enlarged cystic ovaries with elevated FSH levels during childhood; further enlargement of the clitoris, normal development of pubic and axillary hair, and continued existence of enlarged cystic ovaries during the teenage years; and severe estrogen deficiency, virilization, and enlarged multicystic ovaries in association with markedly elevated levels of gonadotropins in adulthood. Follicles are abundant early in life, but there appears to be accelerated atresia. Affected 46,XY individuals appear normal at birth and during childhood but develop eunuchoid proportions and osteoporosis as they continue to grow during childhood because estrogen is required for epiphyseal closure. Because of the absence of aromatase enzyme in the placenta to convert fetal androgens to estrogens, mothers of affected children develop reversible virilization during the second half of pregnancy.

It has been recognized for several years now that women with galactosemia may develop hypergonadotropic amenorrhea even when treated with a galactose-restricted diet from an early age (17). Although the etiology of the ovarian failure in this disorder has not been determined, pregnant rats fed a 50 percent galactose diet deliver pups with significantly reduced numbers of oocytes, apparently because of decreased germ cell migration to the genital ridges (18). Galactose also inhibits follicular development in the rat ovary (19).

Other Known Genetic Alterations of Specific Genes

Mutations to any of an increasing number of genes can result in POF. In addition to the gene mutations discussed thus far, mutations involving *FSHR* (the FSH receptor gene), *FOXL2* (a forkhead transcription factor associated with the blepharophimosis/ptosis/epicanthus inversus syndrome), *INHA* (the inhibin alpha gene), *EIF2B* (a family of genes associated with central nervous system leukodystrophy and ovarian failure), *BMP15* (the gene for bone morphogenetic protein 15), *PMM2* (the gene for phosphosmannomutase), and *AIRE* (leading to the autoimmune polyendocrinopathy-candidiasis-ectodermal dystrophy syndrome) have been reported to cause POF (20–24).

Defective Gonadotropin Secretion or Action

There are now data indicating that abnormal gonadotropin structure, secretion, metabolism, or action can lead to POF in some women. We have reported altered forms of immunoreactive LH and FSH in urinary extracts from women with POF (25), suggesting that altered metabolism and/or excretion of gonadotropins exists in some cases. As noted previously, genetic mutations in the FSH receptor may manifest as POF (20). It also appears that there may be some individuals with a low–molecular-weight peptide that binds to the FSH receptor, antagonizes normal FSH binding, and leads to POF with only intermittent follicular activity (26).

Environmental Insults

A variety of environmental insults, including ionizing radiation, various chemotherapeutic agents, certain viral infections, and even cigarette smoking, can accelerate follicular atresia (27).

About half of the women who receive 400–500 rads to the ovaries over four to six weeks, as may occur in treatment for lymphomas such as Hodgkins disease, will develop POF (28). For any given dose of radiation, the older the woman, the greater the likelihood of her developing hypergonadotropic amenorrhea. It appears that 800 rads is sufficient to result in permanent sterility in virtually all women.

It is also known that the hypergonadotropic amenorrhea following radiation therapy is not always permanent, suggesting that some follicles are damaged but not destroyed by relatively low doses of radiation. This information has led to the practice of transposing the ovaries to the pelvic sidewall before radiation therapy begins in an effort to reduce the radiation to the ovaries; one review has reported that transposition in women younger than forty results in preservation of ovarian function in almost 90 percent of women (29).

It has also been known for several years that chemotherapeutic agents, particularly alkylating agents, may produce either temporary or permanent ovarian failure (28). As is true for radiation therapy, the older the woman at the time of therapy, the more likely is it that ovarian function will be compromised. There is now evidence that the frequency of congenital anomalies is not increased in the children of women previously treated with chemotherapeutic agents (30).

There is the possibility, however, that dactinomycin may be associated with an increased risk of congenital heart disease, and further studies are clearly indicated.

Suggestions that viruses can affect ovarian follicles are difficult to confirm. The best documented series includes three presumptive cases of "mumps oophoritis" preceding onset of ovarian failure, including cases in a mother and her daughter in which the mother had documented mumps parotiditis and abdominal pain during pregnancy just prior to the delivery of a daughter who later suffered from hypergonadotropic amenorrhea (31).

Although there is no evidence that cigarette smoking will lead to POF, data exist documenting that cigarette smokers experience menopause on average several months earlier than nonsmokers (32).

Autoimmune Disorders

Several autoimmune disorders appear to be associated with POF. It appears that 15–20 percent of women with POF con-

currently also have an autoimmune disorder (33). Because these series were not controlled and because autoimmune disorders are also common in women who do not have ovarian failure, it is not clear that autoimmune disorders are actually increased in POF. However, evidence that some cases of POF may have an autoimmune etiology is provided by sporadic case reports documenting return of ovarian function following either immunosuppressive therapy or recovery from an associated autoimmune disease (34–36). In a few cases, lymphocytic infiltrates suggesting autoimmune dysfunction have been observed in ovarian biopsy specimens (36).

In fact, it has become clear that women with POF who have steroidogenic cell autoimmunity have lymphocytic oophoritis as the mechanism for the ovarian failure.

In one review, all patients with histologically confirmed lymphocytic autoimmune oophoritis had adrenal antibodies when tested using an indirect immunofluorescence assay (37). Either testing for adrenal antibodies by indirect immunofluorescence or for antibodies to the 21-hydroxylase enzyme by an immunoprecipitation assay will identify the 4 percent of women with spontaneous POF who have steroidogenic cell autoimmunity and are at risk for potentially fatal adrenal insufficiency (38–40). When adrenal insufficiency occurs in association with POF, the ovarian failure presents first about 90 percent of the time (41). Because adrenal crisis can occur even in those women with occult adrenal insufficiency, it is important to identify women with adrenal antibodies who may have unrecognized adrenal insufficiency or who are at risk of developing adrenal insufficiency in the future (42).

Indirect immunofluorescence of ovarian biopsy specimens from a few women with POF has revealed antibodies reacting with various ovarian components (43). Circulating immunoglobulins to ovarian proteins have been detected by immunochemical techniques by several different groups (33). We utilized a solid-phase, enzyme-linked immunosorbent assay to detect antibodies to ovarian tissue in 22 percent of women with spontaneous POF, but nonspecific positive findings in normal women preclude routine use of this test (44). The most well-documented evidence of autoantibodies to ovarian tissue comes from a study of two women with myasthenia gravis and POF who had circulating immunoglobulin G that blocked binding of FSH to ovarian cell surface receptors (45). However, to the present time, there is no test to detect ovarian tissue-specific antibodies that is of any proven clinical utility.

Abundant data indicate links between the immune and reproductive systems. Congenitally athymic girls dying before puberty have been found to have ovaries that are devoid of oocytes on autopsy (46). Congenitally athymic mice, known to develop premature ovarian failure, have lower gonadotropin concentrations prepubertally than do their normal littermates (47). These hormonal alterations, as well as the accelerated loss of oocytes, can be prevented by thymic transplantation into the athymic mice at birth (48). Ovarian development occurring during the first few weeks of life in mice occurs in utero in humans and in nonhuman primates. Thus, thymic ablation in fetal rhesus monkeys in late gestation is associated with a marked reduction in oocyte number at birth (49). One possible explanation for the association of thymic aplasia and ovarian failure may be found in our observation that peptides produced by the thymus gland can stimulate release of gonadotropin-releasing hormone (GnRH) and consequently luteinizing hormone (LH) (50). The fact that fetal hypophysectomy in rhesus monkeys leads to the newborns having no oocytes in their ovaries suggests that gonadotropins are required for normal ovarian development (51).

Because ovarian activity appears to wax and wane in women with autoimmune POF, it may be important to identify those with an autoimmune disorder so that they might be treated effectively in the future to prevent final loss of all viable oocytes.

Idiopathic

The diagnosis of "idiopathic" POF should be one of exclusion, even if most patients today are not found to have a definitive etiology for the POF. No doubt additional causes of POF will be identified as investigation of the human genome continues.

The "Resistant Ovary Syndrome": An Outdated Term

The resistant ovary or "Savage" syndrome was originally defined as present in young amenorrheic women who had (1) elevated peripheral gonadotropin levels, (2) normal but immature follicles in the ovaries, (3) a 46,XX karyotype, (4) mature secondary sex characteristics, and (5) decreased sensitivity to stimulation with exogenous gonadotropin (52). However, it is now clear that these criteria might be the result of several differing etiologies. In addition, these criteria might apply to all or most women with incipient POF. Thus, the term "resistant ovary syndrome" is outdated and should no longer be used.

EVALUATION OF WOMEN WITH HYPERGONADOTROPIC AMENORRHEA

The objectives of the evaluation of young women with hypergonadotropic amenorrhea are to identify any treatable causes and any potentially dangerous associated disorders. It is important to make the diagnosis in a timely fashion. One series noted that over half the women who presented with secondary amenorrhea saw three or more clinicians before laboratory testing established the diagnosis (53).

In general, young women who miss three or more consecutive menstrual periods warrant evaluation (Table 37.3). Clinical evaluation may rule out pregnancy and may help determine if endogenous estrogen is present. At a minimum, laboratory evaluation of any amenorrheic woman should include measurement of basal levels of prolactin, FSH, and TSH (after pregnancy is ruled out). FSH levels are typically greater than 30 mIU/mL in women who do not have functioning gonads. If the FSH level is greater than 15 mIU/mL in the initial measurement and the woman is less than forty years of age, then the measurement of FSH should be repeated and serum estradiol should also be measured to confirm hypogonadism. FSH levels may be persistently increased or increased only in the early follicular phase in regularly menstruating women who have so-called "diminished ovarian reserve." Diminished reserve may be an early harbinger of POF, although this remains to be established. The additional measurement of basal LH levels may aid in determining if any functional follicles are present. In general, if the estradiol concentration is greater than 50 pg/mL or if the LH concentration is greater than the FSH concentration (in terms of mIU/mL) on any occasion, then at least a few viable follicles must be present. This is true because most estradiol is produced by granulosa cells in functional follicles and

Table 37.3. Evaluation for Suspected POF

Rule out pregnancy

Measurement of basal serum prolactin and TSH

Measurement of basal serum FSH and estradiol on at least two occasions

Karyotype in women with primary amenorrhea, those younger than thirty-five, and those with children

Careful family history

Evaluation for premutations in FMR1

Testing for adrenal antibodies using indirect immunofluorescence

Thyroid-stimulating immunoglobulins

because estradiol is more effective in suppressing FSH relative to LH than are other estrogens. Irregular uterine bleeding, indicative of continuing estradiol production, also suggests the presence of remaining functional oocytes. The presence of identifiable follicles on transvaginal ultrasonography also can be used to identify women with remaining oocytes. Because about one-half of the women with POF will experience withdrawal bleeding in response to a progestin challenge (1), this test should not be used as a substitute for measuring basal FSH levels.

Although our series suggests that less than 15 percent of women developing secondary hypergonadotropic amenorrhea prior to age thirty have karyotypic abnormalities, compared to the 50 percent incidence in women with primary hypergonadotropic amenorrhea, it seems reasonable to obtain a karyotype in women with the onset of hypergonadotropic amenorrhea prior to age thirty-five to identify those with various forms of gonadal dysgenesis, individuals with mosaicism, those with trisomy X, and those with a portion of a Y chromosome. Gonadal extirpation is warranted in women with a portion of a Y chromosome present because of the increased risk of gonadal malignancy (54). Karyotypes also are justified to rule out familial transmission of a sex chromosomal disorder in women who develop POF after delivery of children. Given recent data indicating the presence of molecular cytogenetic defects in Xq as detected by fluorescent in situ hybridization (FISH), this technique may have increasing value in establishing the cause in affected individuals (11).

Because approximately 6 percent of women with 46,XX spontaneous POF have premutations of the FMR1 gene, testing for this abnormality is warranted in all such women. Testing for adrenal antibodies by indirect immunofluorescence is also warranted. If antibodies are detected, a corticotropin stimulation test is indicated to identify individuals with adrenal insufficiency. Because of the frequency of autoimmune thyroid disease in women with POF, serum TSH and thyroid-stimulating immunoglobulins also should be measured in women with POF.

Evaluation of bone density appears warranted in women with POF because of the high incidence of osteopenia (1). In fact, periodic assessment may be indicated, regardless of therapy, to assess the rate of bone loss. Similarly, monitoring patients for development of autoimmune endocrinopathies seems warranted even if all the tests are normal when the patient is first evaluated. Development of other disorders after diagnosis of POF is known to occur (1), and little is known about the natural history of the development of associated autoimmune disorders.

In distinct contrast, ovarian biopsy is not indicated in women with POF and a normal karyotype. The results are not sufficiently definitive so as to alter any proposed therapy. In one series, one of two women who eventually conceived had no oocytes present on biopsy (4). In another series, two of eight subsequent pregnancies among ninety-seven women with POF occurred in women with no oocytes present in specimens obtained by ovarian biopsy at laparotomy (1). These findings are not surprising given calculations suggesting that oocytes are sought in tissue representing only 0.15 percent of an ovary 2 × 3 × 4 cm in size (55).

TREATMENT

The very first, and perhaps most important, challenge in providing appropriate treatment to women with POF is informing the patient of the diagnosis in a sensitive and caring fashion. The manner in which the diagnosis is provided can affect the magnitude of emotional trauma experienced, especially if the patient originally sought assistance because of infertility or is likely to desire children in the future. It is often best to schedule a separate visit to review the findings and discuss treatment options. Members of the International POF Association (IPOFA) indicate that they were not infrequently informed of the diagnosis over the telephone (personal communication)! It is important to explain that remissions and spontaneous pregnancies can occur; moreover, POF differs from normal menopause in several important ways. Because the diagnosis can be so devastating emotionally, it is important to provide appropriate psychological support. Referral to an organization such as IPOFA (www.pofsupport.org) also should be considered.

Hormone *replacement* therapy with exogenous estrogen and progestogen is warranted in women with POF. The accelerated bone loss frequently accompanying this disorder may be prevented by the administration of exogenous estrogens (56). Moreover, hormone therapy has been shown to restore the impaired cardiovascular endothelial function noted in young women with POF to normal within six months of initiation of therapy (57). Whether women with POF are at increased risk of cardiovascular disease if not treated with estrogen, however, is not known at this time.

It is important to counsel patients that spontaneous pregnancies can occur whether or not they are taking exogenous estrogens – even in the form of combined oral contraceptive agents (1). However, even though about 25 percent of women actually ovulate again after the diagnosis is established, the likelihood of pregnancy is less than 10 percent, regardless of therapy (1). Women who do not desire pregnancy and are sexually active should be advised to use barrier contraception even if they are taking oral contraceptives. Women also should be advised to contact their physician if they develop any signs or symptoms consistent with pregnancy or if they do not have withdrawal bleeding while taking exogenous estrogen and progestogen. It is not at all clear why women with this disorder can ovulate and conceive while taking high-dose steroids as are found in oral contraceptive agents.

There are no controlled trials to guide clinicians in how best to provide exogenous estrogen to women with POF. Thus, these comments represent the opinions of this author only, and other clinicians may arrive at different recommendations and conclusions. Data documenting significant risks of exogenous estrogen when administered to postmenopausal women do not apply to patients with POF. At present, there are no data suggesting risk – or absence of risk – in these young women. Although exogenous estrogen can be provided in the form of oral contraceptive agents, it would appear that exogenous estrogen with addition of periodic progestogen is more physiological. Generally speaking, these young women may require twice as much estrogen as do postmenopausal women to alleviate signs and symptoms of hypoestrogenism. Although different clinicians suggest different therapeutic regimens for women with POF, I prefer to administer the estrogen continuously, most commonly in the form of transdermal estradiol-17β skin patches (generally beginning with 0.1 mg). I then add a progestogen, most commonly micronized progesterone (100 mg daily), for fourteen days the first two weeks of every other month. Some clinicians believe that a progestogen should be provided for twelve to fourteen days every month in order to eliminate any increased risk of endometrial hyperplasia, but I prefer to reduce the number of episodes of uterine bleeding even in the absence of much data documenting reduced risk of endometrial hyperplasia when progestogen is provided less frequently than monthly. There is no evidence that any one form of estrogen or of progestogen is safer or more efficacious than any other.

Trials have established that ovulation induction, even after gonadotropin suppression, is no more successful in women with POF than is the likelihood of spontaneous ovulation and pregnancy (1, 7, 58). Thus, there is no point in attempting to induce ovulation in these patients; rather, adoption and in vitro fertilization utilizing donor oocytes should be discussed with women with POF desiring children.

The first successful case of oocyte donation in humans was reported in 1984 (59). A young woman with POF was given estradiol valerate and progesterone pessaries to prepare the endometrium for transfer of a single donated oocyte following fertilization with her husband's sperm. Use of oocyte donation is now widespread, and success rates are generally greater than those observed with traditional in vitro fertilization (60–62). Thus, oocyte donation offers the possibility of pregnancy to all women with POF who have a normal uterus.

Recent information, however, indicates the need for special caution in two particular circumstances. First, women with Turner syndrome have an increased risk of aortic rupture during pregnancy (63, 64). An echocardiogram to exclude dilatation of the aortic root is indicated in women with Turner syndrome contemplating pregnancy; but even if the findings are normal, the risk of aortic rupture may be increased because the structure of the aortic wall is abnormal. Thus, these women must be counseled very carefully before oocyte donation is contemplated, and adoption is clearly the more prudent course of action. If the patient still chooses to become pregnant, careful cardiac monitoring is warranted throughout the course of the pregnancy. Second, premutation carriers for the FMR1 gene need to be counseled carefully regarding the possibility of transmitting the premutation and of expansion to the full mutation. Affected women and their partners need to understand all of the medical ramifications associated with the FMR1 gene; careful genetic counseling is clearly warranted. Preimplantation genetic diagnosis to test for the presence of the FMR1 premutation and mutation should be discussed as well.

KEY POINTS FOR CLINICAL PRACTICE

■ POF is sufficiently common that clinicians can expect to see some patients with this disorder.

■ Evaluation is warranted to exclude treatable causes and associated health concerns.

■ It is particularly important to exclude thyroid dysfunction, adrenal insufficiency, and the fragile X premutation.

■ Affected patients should be provided with sensitive care and extensive counseling as needed.

■ Pregnancy occurs spontaneously in a small percentage of women affected with POF.

■ In vitro fertilization with donor oocytes is the most effective way of providing a pregnancy for any affected woman – but should be used with caution in women with Turner syndrome and the fragile X premutation.

REFERENCES

1. Rebar RW, Connolly HV. Clinical features of young women with hypergonadotropic amenorrhea. *Fertil Steril* 1990;**53**:804–10.

2. Nelson LM, Anasti JN, Kimzey LM, et al. Development of luteinized graafian follicles in patients with karyotypically normal spontaneous premature ovarian failure. *J Clin Endocrinol Metab* 1994;**79**:1470–5.

3. de Moraes-Ruehsen M, Jones GS. Premature ovarian failure. *Fertil Steril* 1967;**18**:440–61.

4. Aiman J, Smentek C. Premature ovarian failure. *Obstet Gynecol* 1985;**66**:9–14.

5. Coulam CB, Adamson SC, Annegers JF. Incidence of premature ovarian failure. *Obstet Gynecol* 1986;**67**:604–6.

6. Sherman SL. Premature ovarian failure in the fragile X syndrome. *Am J Med Genet* 2000;**97**:189–94.

7. Nelson LM, Kimzey LM, White BJ, Merriam GR. Gonadotropin suppression for the treatment of karyotypically normal spontaneous premature ovarian failure: a controlled trial. *Fertil Steril* 1992;**57**:50–5.

8. Simpson JL, Rajkovic A. Ovarian differentiation and gonadal failure. *Am J Med Genet* 1999;**89**:186–200.

9. Singh RP, Carr DH. The anatomy and histology of XO human embryos and fetuses. *Anat Rec* 1966;**155**:369–83.

10. Krauss CM, Turksoy RN, Atkins L, et al. Familial premature ovarian failure due to an interstitial deletion of the long arm of the X chromosome. *N Engl J Med* 1987;**317**:125–31.

11. Portnoi MF, Aboura A, Tachdjian G, Bouchard P, Dewailly D, Bourcigaux N, Frydman R, et al. Molecular cytogenetic studies of Xq critical regions in premature ovarian failure patients. *Hum Reprod* 2006;2329–34.

12. Villanueva AL, Rebar RW. Triple-X syndrome and premature ovarian failure. *Obstet Gynecol* 1983;**62**(3 Suppl.):70–3s.

13. Wittenberger MD, Hagerman RJ, Sherman SL, McConkie-Rosell A, Welt CK, Rebar RW, Corrigan EC, et al. The FMR1 premutation and reproduction. *Fertil Steril* 2006. DOI: 10.1016/j.fertnstert.2006.09.004

14. Sullivan AK, Marcus M, Epstein MP, Allen EG, Anido AE, Paquin JJ, Yadav-Shah M, et al. Association of *FMR1* repeat size with ovarian dysfunction. *Hum Reprod* 2005;**20**:402–12.

15. Biglieri EG, Herron MA, Brust N. 17-hydroxylation deficiency in man. *J Clin Invest* 1966;**45**:1946–54.

16. Morishima A, Grumbach MM, Simpson ER, Fisher C, Qin K. Aromatase deficiency in male and female siblings caused by a novel mutation and the physiological role of estrogens. *J Clin Endocrinol Metab* 1995;**80**:3689–98.

17. Kaufman FR, Kogut MD, Donnell GN, et al. Hypergonadotropic hypogonadism in female patients with galactosemia. *N Engl J Med* 1981;**304**:994–8.

18. Chen YT, Mattison DR, Feigenbaum L, Fukui H, Schulman JD. Reduction in oocyte number following prenatal exposure to a diet high in galactose. *Science* 1981;**214**:1145–7.

19. Liu G, Shif F, Blas-Machado U, et al. Dietary galactose inhibits GDF-9 mediated follicular development in the rat ovary. *Reprod Toxicol* 2006;**21**:26–33.

20. Aittomaki K, Herva R, Stenman UH, et al. Clinical features of primary ovarian failure caused by a point mutation in the follicle-stimulating hormone receptor gene. *J Clin Endocrinol Metab* 1996;**81**:3722–6.

21. De Baere E, Dixon MJ, Small KW, et al. Spectrum of FOXL2 gene mutations in blepharophimosis-ptosis-epicanthus inversus (BPES) families demonstrates a genotype–phenotype correlation. *Hum Mol Genet* 2001;**10**:1591–600.

22. Fogli A, Rodriguez D, Eymard-Pierre E, et al. Ovarian failure related to eukaryotic initiation factor 2B mutations. *Am J Hum Genet* 2003;**72**:1544–50.

23. Di Pasquale E, Beck-Peccoz P, Persani L. Hypergonadotropic ovarian failure associated with an inherited mutation of human bone morphogenetic protein-15 (BMP15) gene. *Am J Hum Genet* 2004;**75**:106–11.

24. Ahonen P, Myllarniemi S, Sipila I, Perheentupa J. Clinical variation of autoimmune polyendocrinopathy-candidiasis-ectodermal dystrophy (APECED) in a series of 68 patients. *N Engl J Med* 1990;**322**:1829–36.

25. Silva de Sa MF, Matthews MJ, Rebar RW. Altered forms of immunoreactive urinary FSH and LH in premature ovarian failure. *Infertility* 1988;**11**:1–11.

26. Sluss PM, Schneyer AL. Low molecular weight follicle-stimulating hormone receptor binding inhibitor in sera from premature ovarian failure patients. *J Clin Endocrinol Metab* 1992;**74**:1242–6.

27. Verp M. Environmental causes of ovarian failure. *Semin Reprod Endocrinol* 1983;**1**:101–11.

28. Damewood MD, Grochow LB. Prospects for fertility after chemotherapy or radiation for neoplastic disease. *Fertil Steril* 1986;**45**:443–59.

29. Bisharah M, Tulandi T. Laparoscopic preservation of ovarian function: an underused procedure. *Am J Obstet Gynecol* 2003;**188**:367–70.

30. Green DM, Zevon MA, Lowrie G, Seigelstein N, Hall B., Congenital anomalies in children of patients who received chemotherapy for cancer in childhood and adolescence. *N Engl J Med* 1991;**325**:141–6.

31. Morrison JC, Givens JR, Wiser WL, Fish SA. Mumps oophoritis: a cause of premature menopause. *Fertil Steril* 1975;**26**:655–9.

32. Jick H, Porter J. Relation between smoking and age of natural menopause. Report from the Boston Collaborative Drug Surveillance Program, Boston University Medical Center. *Lancet* 1977;**1**:1354–5.

33. LaBarbera AR, Miller MM, Ober C, Rebar RW. Autoimmune etiology in premature ovarian failure. *Am J Reprod Immunol Microbiol* 1988;**16**:115–22.

34. Lucky AW, Rebar RW, Blizzard RM, Goren EM. Pubertal progression in the presence of elevated serum gonadotropins in girls with multiple endocrine deficiencies. *J Clin Endocrinol Metab* 1977;**45**:673–8.

35. Bateman BG, Nunley WC Jr., Kitchin JD, 3rd. Reversal of apparent premature ovarian failure in a patient with myasthenia gravis. *Fertil Steril* 1983;**39**:108–10.

36. Rabinowe SL, Berger MJ, Welch WR, Dluhy RG. Lymphocyte dysfunction in autoimmune oophoritis. Resumption of menses with corticosteroids. *Am J Med* 1986;**81**:347–50.

37. Hoek A, Schoemaker J, Drexhage HA. Premature ovarian failure and ovarian autoimmunity. *Endocr Rev* 1997;**18**:107–34.

38. Chen S, Sawicka J, Betterle C, et al. Autoantibodies to steroidogenic enzymes in autoimmune polyglandular syndrome, Addison's disease, and premature ovarian failure. *J Clin Endocrinol Metab* 1996;**81**:1871–6.

39. Bakalov VK, Vanderhoof VH, Bondy CA, Nelson LM. Adrenal antibodies detect asymptomatic auto-immune adrenal insufficiency in young women with spontaneous premature ovarian failure. *Hum Reprod* 2002;**17**:2096–100.

40. Falorni A, Laureti S, Candeloro P, et al. Steroid-cell autoantibodies are preferentially expressed in women with premature ovarian failure who have adrenal autoimmunity. *Fertil Steril* 2002;**78**:270–9.

41. Turkington RW, Lebovitz HE. Extra-adrenal endocrine deficiencies in Addison's disease. *Am J Med* 1967;**43**:499–507.

42. Betterle C, Volpato M, Rees Smith B, et al. I. Adrenal cortex and steroid 21-hydroxylase autoantibodies in adult patients with organ-specific autoimmune diseases: markers of low progression to clinical Addison's disease. *J Clin Endocrinol Metab* 1997; **82**:932–8.

43. Muechler EK, Huang KE, Schenk E., Autoimmunity in premature ovarian failure. *Int J Fertil* 1991;**36**:99–103.

44. Kim JG, Anderson BE, Rebar RW, LaBarbera AR. A biotin-streptavidin enzyme immunoassay for detection of antibodies to porcine granulosa cell antigens. *J Immunoassay* 1991;**12**:447–64.

45. Chiauzzi V, Cigorraga S, Escobar ME, Rivarola MA, Charreau EH. Inhibition of follicle-stimulating hormone receptor binding by circulating immunoglobulins. *J Clin Endocrinol Metab* 1982; **54**:1221–8.

46. Miller ME, Chatten J. Ovarian changes in ataxia telangiectasia. *Acta Paediatr Scand* 1967;**56**:559–61.

47. Rebar RW, Morandini IC, Erickson GF, Petze JE. The hormonal basis of reproductive defects in athymic mice: diminished gonadotropin concentrations in prepubertal females. *Endocrinology* 1981;**108**:120–6.

48. Rebar RW, Morandini IC, Benirschke K, Petze JE. Reduced gonadotropins in athymic mice: prevention by thymic transplantation. *Endocrinology* 1980;**107**:2130–2.

49. Healy DL, Bacher J, Hodgen GD. Thymic regulation of primate fetal ovarian-adrenal differentiation. *Biol Reprod* 1985;**32**:1127–33.

50. Rebar RW, Miyake A, Low TL, Goldstein AL. Thymosin stimulates secretion of luteinizing hormone-releasing factor. *Science* 1981;**214**:669–71.

51. Gulyas BJ, Hodgen GD, Tullner WW, Ross GT. Effects of fetal or maternal hypophysectomy on endocrine organs and body weight in infant rhesus monkeys (Macaca mulatta): with particular emphasis on oogenesis. *Biol Reprod* 1977;**16**(2):216–27.

52. Jones GS, De Moraes-Ruehsen M. A new syndrome of amenorrhea in association with hypergonadotropism and apparently normal ovarian follicular apparatus. *Am J Obstet Gynecol* 1969;**104**:597–600.

53. Alzubaidi NH, Chapin HL, Vanderhoof VH, Calis KA, Nelson LM. Meeting the needs of young women with secondary amenorrhea and spontaneous premature ovarian failure. *Obstet Gynecol* 2002;**99**:720–5.

54. Manuel M, Katayama PK, Jones HW Jr. The age of occurrence of gonadal tumors in intersex patients with a Y chromosome. *Am J Obstet Gynecol* 1976;**124**:293–300.

55. Alper MM, Garner PR, Seibel MM. Premature ovarian failure. Current concepts. *J Reprod Med* 1986;**31**:699–708.

56. Metka M, Holzer G, Heytmanek G, Huber J. Hypergonadotropic hypogonadic amenorrhea (World Health Organization III) and osteoporosis. *Fertil Steril* 1992;**57**:37–41.

57. Kalantaridou SN, Naka KK, Papanikolaou E, Kazakos N, Kravariti M, Calis KA, Paraskevaidis EA, et al. Impaired endothelial function in young women with premature ovarian failure: normalization with hormone therapy. *J Clin Endocrinol Metab* 2004;**89**:3907–13.

58. Ledger WL, Thomas EJ, Browning D, Lenton EA, Cooke ID. Suppression of gonadotrophin secretion does not reverse premature ovarian failure. *Br J Obstet Gynaecol* 1989;**96**:196–9.

59. Lutjen P, Trounson A, Leeton J, et al. The establishment and maintenance of pregnancy using in vitro fertilization and embryo donation in a patient with primary ovarian failure. *Nature* 1984;**307**:174–5.

60. Chan CL, Cameron IT, Findlay JK, et al. Oocyte donation and in vitro fertilization for hypergonadotropic hypogonadism: clinical state of the art. *Obstet Gynecol Surv* 1987;**42**:350–62.

61. Sauer MV, Paulson R. Oocyte donation for women who have ovarian failure. *Contemp Obstet Gynecol* 1989:125–35.

62. Rebar RW, Cedars MI. Hypergonadotropic forms of amenorrhea in young women. *Endocrinol Metab Clin North Am* 1992; **21**:173–91.

63. Karnis MF, Zimon AE, Lalwani SI, et al. Risk of death in pregnancy achieved through oocyte donation in patients with Turner syndrome: a national survey. *Fertil Steril* 2003;**80**:498–501.

64. Practice Committee of the American Society for Reproductive Medicine. Increased maternal cardiovascular mortality associated with pregnancy in women with Turner syndrome. *Fertil Steril* 2005;**83**:1074–5.

PART III

ASSISTED REPRODUCTION

38

MEDICAL STRATEGIES TO IMPROVE ART
OUTCOME: CURRENT EVIDENCE

C. M. Boomsma, N. S. Macklon

INTRODUCTION

In recent years, much progress has been made in improving embryo quality and selection for transfer after in vitro fertilization (IVF). These include technical improvements in oocyte and embryo culture conditions, assisted hatching, the use of sequential media, and the use of embryo-endometrial coculture for selected patients. Moreover, preimplantation genetic screening (PGS) has been introduced with the aim of improving embryo selection on the basis of chromosomal compliment. However, despite these advances, even when embryos are considered to be of high quality using morphological and chromosomal criteria, implantation rates remain around 25–35 percent per embryo transfer procedure (The European IVF-monitoring program, 2005).

High rates of implantation failure and early pregnancy loss in IVF continue to be a considerable cause of frustration to both patients and clinicians. The practice of transferring multiple embryos to increase the chance of implantation continues in contemporary practice. However, this approach is now being seen less as the "solution" to low implantation rates but rather more as the cause of the most important problem arising from IVF treatment: that of multiple pregnancy (Fauser et al., 2005). The widespread adoption of single-embryo transfer (SET) is recognized to be necessary if the morbidity associated with IVF multiple pregnancies is to be reduced (Fauser et al., 2005). In order to improve implantation rates in the age of SET, medical strategies designed to increase the chance of successful implantation are sought and applied in practice, often before they have been subject to appropriate clinical assessment in the context of randomized controlled trials (RCTs) (Boomsma and Macklon, 2006). In this chapter, five sequential medical "steps" to successful implantation are described, and the evidence supporting their efficacy and safety are reviewed.

STEP ONE: SELECT AND PREPARE THE PATIENT

The most important determinant of IVF outcome is the patient herself. A number of studies have addressed the patient-related factors predictive of successful IVF treatment, and it is becoming clear that prognostic factors other than the underlying "diagnosis" of infertility cause are the prime determinants of success (Macklon et al., 2004). Therefore, when counseling patients regarding their chances of achieving successful pregnancy with IVF treatment, a number of factors should be addressed.

Age and Duration of Infertility

One of the most important determinants of IVF outcome is the individual ovarian response to stimulation. Poor response, which is highly correlated with chronological aging, is highly resistant to therapeutic intervention (Tarlatzis et al., 2003). A multiple regression analysis of factors influencing IVF outcome has revealed a decline in live birth rate of 17 percent in women at the age of thirty to 7 percent in women at the age of forty (Templeton et al., 1996). Chronological age is, however, poorly correlated with ovarian aging. Moreover, studies have shown that young women with a poor response demonstrate higher implantation rates compared to women older than forty years with normal basal FSH levels (van Rooij et al., 2003). In recent years, much attention has been given to the identification of markers of ovarian aging, which may predict the success of IVF. A meta-analysis revealed basal FSH levels to have only a moderate predictive performance for poor response, and a low predictive performance for nonpregnancy was observed (Bancsi et al., 2003). The issue of poor response and markers of ovarian reserve are addressed more fully in Chapter 47.

While duration of infertility has been shown to be associated with the chance of a spontaneous pregnancy, its impact on the chance of success in IVF is less clear (Collins, 1995). However, a large retrospective analysis of factors affecting outcomes in IVF showed a significant decrease in age-adjusted live birth rates with increasing duration of infertility. A previous pregnancy had a significantly positive impact on the chance of success with IVF, with the effect being stronger after a live birth, in particular resulting from a previous IVF treatment (Templeton et al., 1996).

Cause of Infertility

The extent to which the underlying pathology itself can impact on the chance of success has been the subject of considerable study. The largest study yet published on factors determining IVF outcome, carried out in the United Kingdom between 1991 and 1994, including 36,961 cycles, showed no significant effect of the indication for IVF treatment (Templeton et al., 1996) (Table 38.1). However, a meta-analysis studying the effect of endometriosis on the success rate of IVF versus tubal factor controls did show significantly lower fertilization, implantation, and pregnancy rates in women with endometriosis. Stronger negative associations consistently were noted in women

Table 38.1: Impact of Cause of Infertility on Live Birth Rate from IVF

Cause of infertility	Number of cycles	Live birth rate (percent) (95 percent CI)		
		Per treatment cycle	Per egg collection	Per embryo transfer
Tubal disease	19,096	13.6 (13.0–14.0)	15.0 (14.5–15.6)	16.5 (15.9–17.1)
Endometriosis	4,117	14.2 (13.2–15.3)	15.9 (14.7–17.0)	17.9 (16.6–19.3)
Unexplained	12,340	13.4 (12.9–14.1)	15.2 (14.6–15.9)	19.7 (18.8–20.5)
Cervical	4,232	14.2 (13.2–15.3)	16.2 (15.1–17.4)	18.8 (17.5–20.2)

Reprinted from Templeton et al. (1996), with permission from Elsevier.

with severe disease. When directly compared, women with severe endometriosis were noted to have a decrease in pregnancy rate and implantation rates than women with mild endometriosis (Barnhart et al., 2002).

The impact of tubal dysfunction on IVF outcome is controversial, although there is now convincing evidence that distal tubal disease associated with hydrosalpinx has a detrimental effect on the chances from IVF treatment. A meta-analysis, evaluating differences in pregnancy rates after IVF in tubal infertility with or without hydrosalpinx, showed an odds ratio (OR) 0.64, 95 percent confidence interval (CI) 0.56–0.74 (Aboulghar et al., 1998). Current evidence indicates that laparoscopic salpingectomy before IVF treatment should be advised for women with hydrosalpinges: a meta-analysis of three RCTs comparing surgical intervention versus no intervention showed an OR 1.8, 95 percent CI 1.1–2.9 (Johnson et al., 2002). The major study addressed in this meta-analysis demonstrated that this effect was entirely due to the positive effect among those with a hydrosalpinx visible on ultrasound (Strandell et al., 2001; Strandell, 2005). A recent RCT compared the clinical impact of proximal tubal occlusion and salpingectomy prior to IVF in patients with hydrosalpinges. Proximal tubal occlusion was shown to be as effective as salpingectomy in improving implantation rates compared to no intervention (Kontoravdis, in press). Furthermore, anovulation is a common cause of infertility, but cumulative live birth rates of up to 71 percent can be achieved in two years by ovulation induction among women with polycystic ovary syndrome (PCOS). Those women who may benefit from IVF as first-line therapy can be identified by older age, longer duration of infertility, and a higher insulin to glucose ratio (Eijkemans et al., 2003). A recent meta-analysis of outcomes in IVF in women with PCOS versus controls showed no significant differences in pregnancy rates per embryo transfer (Heijnen et al., 2005).

Lifestyle Factors and Concurrent Medical Conditions

There is now a substantial amount of evidence showing that environmental and life style factors influence the success rates of ART (Lintsen et al., 2005; Younglai et al., 2005), and it is therefore important that serious attempts are made to provide adequate preconceptional screening, counseling, and interventions in order to optimize health prior to starting IVF. The importance of full medical assessment prior to IVF treatment is increasing as the average age of our patients continues to rise.

A greater proportion of infertility patients may now also present with concurrent medical conditions, which may impact on the safety and management of the IVF treatment as well as pregnancy. The appropriate management of the medically complicated patient presenting for IVF can be complex and often requires an interdisciplinary approach. For further information in this field, the reader is referred to Macklon (2005).

The most important lifestyle factor impacting on fertility outcomes is tobacco smoking. Smoking during pregnancy has long been known to increase the risk of a number of adverse obstetric and fetal outcomes such as miscarriage, placenta previa, preterm birth, and low birth weight (Younglai et al., 2005). In recent years, the association between smoking and infertility in women has become clear. Chemicals present in cigarette smoke can reach the developing egg in vivo, as both cotinine, the metabolite of nicotine, and cadmium and heavy metal in cigarette smoke are increased in the follicular fluid surrounding the egg (Zenzes et al., 1995a). It has also been demonstrated that active smoking increases oxidative stress in the growing follicle and cytotoxicity in the egg and surrounding granulosa cells (Paszkowski et al., 2002). Reports have appeared linking smoking to damage of the meiotic spindle in oocytes, increasing the risk of chromosomal errors (Zenzes et al., 1995b). In men who smoke, all parameters of sperm quality are reduced (Younglai et al., 2005). Smoking in men and passive and active smoking in women has been associated with a longer time to achieve a pregnancy (Younglai et al., 2005).

The effects of smoking on live birth rate among women who undergo IVF is similar in magnitude to the effect of an increase in female age of more than ten years (Lintsen et al., 2005). As a result, smokers require twice as many IVF cycles to become pregnant as nonsmokers (Lintsen et al., 2005). A recent ASRM practice committee published on smoking and infertility has highlighted the considerable contribution of smoking to infertility and treatment outcomes and the need for a more proactive approach to stop smoking prior to fertility treatment (The Practice Committee of the American Society for Reproduction, 2006). Epidemiological evidence clearly shows that being overweight contributes to menstrual disorders, infertility, miscarriage, poor pregnancy outcome, impaired fetal well-being, and diabetes mellitus (Norman and Clark, 1998). Overweight women (BMI > 27 kg/m^2) have been shown to have a 33 percent reduced chance of a live birth after their first IVF cycle compared to women with a BMI 20–27 kg/m^2. The association was strongest in women with unexplained infertility (Lintsen et al., 2005). In men, a BMI less than 20 or greater than 25 kg/m^2 is associated with reduced sperm quality (Younglai et al., 2005).

A number of studies have shown that weight loss can improve fecundity in overweight women, and many centers include weight loss programs as part of their fertility treatment. However, little data are available regarding the impact of the type of diet on IVF outcomes. Recent studies have highlighted the importance of certain nutritional factors. Folic acid supplementation was shown to alter the vitamin microenvironment of the oocyte (Boxmeer et al., 2005), while seminal plasma cobalamin levels were demonstrated to effect sperm concentration (Boxmeer et al., 2006). Moreover, the intake of alcohol and caffeine are associated with the success rate of IVF. A high intake of caffeine has been linked to an increase risk of spontaneous abortions and lower live birth rates after IVF treatment. Similarly, female alcohol consumption was associated with a decrease in pregnancy rates and an increase of spontaneous miscarriages. Male alcohol consumption up to one week before sperm collection may increase the risk of miscarriage (Younglai et al., 2005).

STEP TWO: OPTIMIZE THE OVARIAN STIMULATION PROTOCOL

The contemporary approach to ovarian stimulation in IVF treatment is based on the perceived need to maximize the number of oocytes available for fertilization, in order to generate multiple embryos for selection and transfer. Ovaries are stimulated with exogenous FSH in order to obtain multiple oocytes during IVF treatment. However, ovarian hyperstimulation and the resultant elevated estradiol levels have been shown to impact negatively on endometrial receptivity (Simon et al., 1995; Macklon and Fauser, 2000; Macklon et al., 2006). Endometrial receptivity may be declined due to advanced postovulatory endometrial maturation and defective induction of progesterone receptors. Supraphysiological estrogen concentrations may increase sensitivity to progesterone action and lead to secretory advancement. Studies of the impact of ovarian stimulation on endometrial maturation several days after ovulation have shown either no effect or endometrial delay. Additionally, a study on endometrial histology has shown that advancement on the day of oocyte retrieval exceeding three days was associated with no subsequent pregnancies (Devroey et al., 2004). Moreover, the magnitude of estrogen dose to which the endometrium is exposed has been shown to affect the duration of the receptive phase (Ma et al., 2003). Kolibianakis et al. have demonstrated the effect of prolongation of the follicular phase by delaying human chorionic gonadotropin (hCG) administration by two days in a randomized controlled trial. They showed endometrial advancement on the day of oocyte retrieval of two to three days in all women when hCG was delayed versus no secretory changes in the control group (Kolibianakis et al., 2005).

Increasing awareness of the possible detrimental effects of standard ovarian stimulation regimens and their burdens on the patient have stimulated a reassessment of the optimal approach to ovarian stimulation for IVF (Fauser et al., 1999; Macklon and Fauser, 2000). Increasing knowledge regarding the physiology of ovarian follicle development, together with the clinical availability of GnRH antagonists, which allows ovarian stimulation to be commenced in the undisturbed menstrual cycle, has presented the opportunity to develop novel,

milder approaches for ovarian stimulation for IVF (Fauser and Macklon, 2004; Macklon et al., 2006). In an RCT, it has been shown that the initiation of exogenous FSH (fixed dose, 150 IU/day, GnRH antagonist cotreatment) as late as cycle day 5 results in a comparable clinical IVF outcome, despite a reduced duration of stimulation (and total dose of FSH given) and increased cancellation rates (Hohmann et al., 2003). The quality of embryos obtained after mild stimulation was significantly greater compared to the conventional long protocol. Moreover, almost all the pregnancies after minimal stimulation were observed in patients with a relatively low oocyte yield, whereas no pregnancies were observed when a similar yield was obtained after conventional IVF.

The optimal number of growing follicles or oocytes retrieved in order to maximize IVF outcome following conventional ovarian stimulation regimens in combination with a GnRH agonist in a long protocol has been shown to be around thirteen (Gaast van der et al., 2006). The optimal number is likely to be lower following mild ovarian stimulation. The stimulation of large numbers of follicles may result in the generation of poorer quality oocytes and hence lower quality embryos. In a recent randomized study, PGS was employed to investigate the chromosomal constitution of embryos obtained after conventional ovarian stimulation compared to embryos obtained after mild ovarian stimulation (Baart et al., 2006). Although more oocytes were obtained in the conventional ovarian stimulation group, the mild group demonstrated an increased percentage of euploid embryos per number of oocytes retrieved. These observations support the concept of a "natural" selection of oocytes during follicular development, which may be overridden by conventional "maximal" stimulation protocols. Employing mild stimulation regimens may aid embryo selection by increasing the chance that the transferred embryo is euploid.

Although current mild stimulation regimens employ fixed doses of FSH (usually 150 IU/day), it is likely that outcomes could further be improved by individualizing the FSH dose. However, individualized ovarian stimulation regimens are difficult to design due to the variable ovarian response between patients and indeed from cycle to cycle. Prognostic models have been developed, which enable the response dose to FSH to be determined on the basis of initial screening parameters. A model developed by Popovic-Todorovic et al. included the number of antral follicles, ovarian volume, age, and smoking habits (Popovic-Todorovic et al., 2003b). Application of such a model promises greater individualization of treatment, lower risk of OHSS, and shorter, more successful treatment cycles. A subsequent prospective RCT comparing an individualized dose of recFSH with a standard starting dose of 150 IU/day suggested indeed that this approach could improve outcomes (Popovic-Todorovic et al., 2003a). This concept is illustrated graphically in Figure 38.1, which shows the relationship between oocyte numbers, benefits (pregnancies), and risks. Currently, other studies are in progress prospectively testing alternative models. Developments and applications of these normograms in practice may benefit from fill-by mass preparations, which enable more reliable dose administration. Recently, the field of pharmacogenetics has emerged and may offer a route toward further individualization of FSH dosing. Clinical studies are required to investigate the usefulness of genotyping for certain FSH mutations as a routine diagnostic test before ovarian stimulation (Greb et al., 2005).

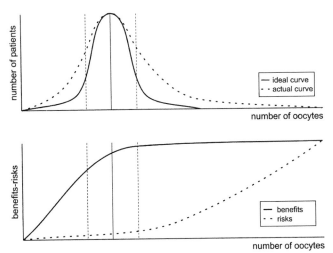

Figure 38.1. Distribution of oocytes, benefits, and risks: the present and the ideal situation. Reprinted from Popovic-Todorovic et al. (2003). ©European Society of Human Reproduction and Embryology. Reproduced by permission of Oxford University Press/Human Reproduction.

STEP THREE: ADJUVANT MEDICAL THERAPIES?

Adjuvant medical therapies to those required for ovarian hyperstimulation are frequently applied in an empirical manner with the aim of improving embryo implantation (Tables 38.2 and 38.3). However, the evidence for their efficacy and safety does not always justify the enthusiasm with which they are prescribed (Rizk and Abdalla, 2008).

Aspirin

The rationale for the use of aspirin as an adjuvant drug in IVF is based on its vasodilatation and anticoagulant properties. The main method of action of aspirin is the inhibition of cyclooxygenase (the rate-limiting enzyme in the prostaglandin synthesis pathway) and subsequent reduction of platelet aggregation. As a result, blood perfusion to the ovaries and the endometrium are both presumed to be improved. Indeed, a significant improvement in the uterine blood perfusion (reduction of the pulsatility index of the uterine artery) in the peri-implantation period after aspirin supplementation has been shown (Kuo et al., 1997).

Aspirin has been shown to be effective in combination with heparin, in the treatment of recurrent miscarriage in women with antiphospholipid antibody syndrome (APS) (Empson et al., 2005). However, efficacy in recurrent miscarriage in women without APS has not been proven (Di Nisio et al., 2005). In the context of IVF treatment, an RCT was performed comparing aspirin plus heparin treatment with placebo from embryo transfer onward in 143 women with antiphospholipid or antinuclear antibodies with a history of embryo implantation failure (Stern et al., 2003). No significant differences in implantation or pregnancy rates were observed.

RCTs investigating the use of aspirin in a nonselected IVF population as an empirical therapy have shown conflicting results (Tables 38.2 and 38.3). One study showed significantly improved ovarian response and implantation rates (Rubinstein et al., 1999); all other studies showed no significant differences

(Urman et al., 2000; Waldenstrom et al., 2004; Pakkila et al., 2005; Duvan et al., 2006). A meta-analysis of ten RCTs showed no statistically significant improvement in clinical pregnancy rates with aspirin versus no, or placebo, treatment (OR 1.18, 95 percent CI 0.86–1.61) (Daya, 2006). At present, there is insufficient evidence to support the use of aspirin outwith the context of RCTs.

Nitric Oxide Donors

NO acts as a relaxant of arterial and smooth muscle and inhibits platelet aggregation. On the day of either hCG administration or embryo transfer, a high resistance to uterine blood flow is reported to be correlated with a poor clinical outcome for patients undergoing IVF (Coulam et al., 1995). These observations suggested that uterine vasodilatation induced by an NO donor might improve endometrial receptivity. However, while initial studies suggested beneficial effects on ovarian response and implantation (Battaglia et al., 1999), more recent studies suggested a detrimental effect of NO on implantation (Battaglia et al., 2002). In addition, a recent prospective study on women undergoing IVF reported an association between high follicular NO levels and advanced embryo fragmentation and implantation failure (Lee et al., 2004). Although subgroups of women may be identified who benefit from NO donor therapy, at present, the available data demand caution in its use, which at present should be restricted to well-designed studies.

Aromatase Inhibitors

The conversion of androstenedione and testosterone to estriol and estradiol, respectively, is blocked by aromatase inhibitors (Cole and Robinson, 1990). This approach reduces the amount of estrogens synthesized, rather than antagonizing estrogen feedback activity at the hypothalamic-pituitary axis as with clomiphene citrate. As a result, gonadotropin secretion is increased and follicular growth is stimulated. Moreover, by preventing excessive estradiol synthesis, it has been hypothesized that adjuvant treatment with aromatase inhibitors during ovarian stimulation may result in less disruption of endometrial receptivity. One RCT has been performed on women with a poor ovarian response (defined by Goswami et al. as less than two dominant follicles). Women using aromatase inhibitors required a significantly lower total dose of FSH; however, the pregnancy rates were comparable (Goswami et al., 2004). These results are in line with three nonrandomized trials investigating aromatase inhibitors as an adjunct treatment in normal responders (Healey et al., 2003; Mitwally and Casper, 2003; Mitwally and Casper, 2004). Only a subgroup of women with PCOS showed significantly higher pregnancy rates after addition of an aromatase inhibitor (Mitwally and Casper, 2004). While of considerable potential value, further studies are required to confirm the value and safety of aromatase inhibitors in IVF.

Ascorbic Acid

Ascorbic acid (AA) appears to be involved in normal folliculogenesis (Luck et al., 1995) and luteal formation and regression (Luck and Zhao, 1993). Moreover, transient high plasma levels can be achieved by high dose intake of AA, which can exert anti-inflammatory and immunostimulant effects. These effects

Table 38.3: Summary Table "What Can the Clinician Do to Improve Embryo Implantation?"

What can the clinician do to improve implantation?	(Presumed) Method of action	Empirical use in nonselected IVF population
Careful ET technique	Minimize trauma and cervical manipulation	Soft ET catheter: significantly higher pregnancy rates
Adjuvant pharmaceutical therapies		
Aspirin	Vasodilatation and anticoagulant properties	No significant beneficial effect on pregnancy rates in a nonselected IVF population
Nitric oxide donors	Uterine vasodilatation	No significant beneficial effect on pregnancy rates. Possible detrimental effect on the embryo
Aromatase inhibitors	Reduction estrogen synthesis: improving endometrial receptivity	No significant beneficial effect on pregnancy rates in a nonselected IVF population
Ascorbic acid	Anti-inflammatory and immunostimulant effects	No significant beneficial effect on pregnancy rates in a nonselected IVF population
Prolonged progesterone	Luteal phase supplementation in a downregulated cycle	No significant beneficial effect on pregnancy rates in a nonselected IVF population
Luteal E2 supplementation	Luteal phase supplementation in a downregulated cycle	Application of luteal E2 supplementation remains controversial
Glucocorticoids	Immunomodulatory effect reduction number NK cells	No significant beneficial effect on pregnancy rates in a nonselected IVF population
Insulin-sensitizing drugs	Minimizing insulin resistance	No significant beneficial effect on pregnancy rates, may reduce miscarriage/OHSS rate in PCOS; empirical use in a nonselected IVF population has not been investigated
GnRH agonist	LH-releasing properties	Can possibly be exploited as luteal support: no beneficial effect on implantation rates described
Ovarian stimulation		
Mild stimulation regimens	Improvement of endometrial receptivity and embryo quality	Comparable IVF outcomes, despite fewer oocytes
Prediction of optimal starting dose FSH in the patient	Optimal stimulation level	Prediction models may have a role. In the future, pharmacogenetics is likely to become important
Selecting optimal embryo, endometrium, and patient		
Preimplantation genetic screening	Selection of euploid embryos	No RCTs in a nonselected IVF population have been published yet
Marker for endometrial receptivity	Correcting and optimizing receptivity prior to ET	A reliable test remains elusive
Selecting patients for SET	Identification of patients in which SET does not reduce the pregnancy rate	No prospective analysis of prediction models has yet been performed
Optimize lifestyle and nutrition	Optimizing oocyte and semen quality and implantation rates. Decrease rate pregnancy complications	Significant higher pregnancy rates among women with a lower BMI, nonsmokers. Higher miscarriage rate in women using caffeine or alcohol

Adapted from Boomsma et al. (2006).

KEY POINTS FOR CLINICAL PRACTICE

■ Many clinical interventions aimed at increasing the chance of implantation in IVF have been proposed, but few have been shown to be effective in well-designed studies. Significant improvements in clinical pregnancy rates can be achieved by giving due attention to ET technique. However, the empirical use of adjuvant medical therapies during IVF treatment have not been shown to be effective and may in some cases be detrimental. Subgroups of patients who may benefit from such therapies still need to be identified. Recently, it has been shown that milder stimulation protocols may improve embryo and endometrial quality. In addition greater attention to optimizing preconceptional care is likely to be beneficial (Table 38.3).

REFERENCES

Aboulghar MA, Mansour RT, Serour GI. 1998. Controversies in the modern management of hydrosalpinx. *Human Reproduction Update* 4 882–890.

Ando T, Suganuma N, Furuhashi M, Asada Y, Kondo I, Tomoda Y. 1996. Successful glucocorticoid treatment for patients with abnormal autoimmunity on in vitro fertilization and embryo transfer. *Journal of Assisted Reproduction and Genetics* 13 776–781.

Baart EB, Martini E, Eijkemans MJC, Van Opstal D, Beckers NG, Verhoeff A, Macklon NS, Fauser BC. 2006. Milder ovarian stimulation for in vitro fertilization reduces aneuploidy in the human preimplantation embryo: a randomized controlled trial. *Human Reproduction* (in press).

Bancsi La, Broekmans FJM, Mol BWJ, Habbema JD, te Velde ER. 2003. Performance of basal follicle-stimulating hormone in the prediction of poor ovarian response and failure to become pregnant after in vitro fertilization: a meta-analysis. *Fertility and Sterility* 79 1091–1100.

Barker DJ. 1994. Maternal and fetal origins of coronary heart disease. *Journal of the Royal College of Physicians of London* 28 544–551.

Barnhart K, Dunsmoor-Su R, Coutifaris C. 2002. Effect of endometriosis on in vitro fertilization. *Fertility and Sterility* 77 1148–1155.

Battaglia C, Regnani G, Marsella T, Facchinetti F, Volpe A, Venturoli S, Flamigni C. 2002. Adjuvant L-arginine treatment in controlled ovarian hyperstimulation: a double-blind, randomized study. *Human Reproduction* 17 659–665.

Battaglia C, Salvatori M, Maxia N, Petraglia F, Facchinetti F, Volpe A. 1999. Adjuvant L-arginine treatment for in-vitro fertilization in poor responder patients. *Human Reproduction* 14 1690–1697.

Beckers NG, Macklon NS, Eijkemans MJ, Ludwig M, Felberbaum RE, Diedrich K, Bustion S, Loumaye E, Fauser BC. 2003. Nonsupplemented luteal phase characteristics after the administration of recombinant human chorionic gonadotropin, recombinant luteinizing hormone, or gonadotropin-releasing hormone (GnRH) agonist to induce final oocyte maturation in in vitro fertilization patients after ovarian stimulation with recombinant follicle-stimulating hormone and GnRH antagonist cotreatment. *Journal of Clinical Endocrinology Metabolism* 88 4186–4192.

Blois SM, Joachim R, Kandil J, Margni R, Tometten M, Klapp BF, Arck PC. 2004. Depletion of CD8+ Cells abolishes the pregnancy protective effect of progesterone substitution with dydrogesterone in mice by altering the Th1/Th2 cytokine profile. *The Journal of Immunology* 172 5893–5899.

Boomsma CM, Eijkemans MJ, Keay SD, Macklon NS. 2006. Periimplantation glucocorticoid administration for assisted reproductive technology cycles. *Cochrane Database of Systematic Reviews* (in press).

Boomsma CM, Macklon NS. 2006. What can the clinician do to improve implantation? *Reproductive Biomedicine Online* 13 845–855.

Boxmeer JC, Brouns MM, Lindemans J, Martini E, Macklon NS, Steegers-Teunissen RPM. 2005. Folic acid treatment affects oocyte environment. *Journal of Social Gynecological Investigation* 12 24A.

Boxmeer JC, Smit M, Weber RFA, Lindemans J, Romijn JC, Eijkemans MJC, Macklon NS, Steegers-Teunissen RPM. 2006. Seminal plasma cobalamin significantly correlates with sperm concentration. *Journal of Social Gynecological Investigation* (in press).

Buckett WM. 2003. A meta-analysis of ultrasound-guided versus clinical touch embryo transfer. *Fertility and Sterility* 80 1037–1041.

Buckett WM. 2006. A review and meta-analysis of prospective trials comparing different catheters used for embryo transfer. *Fertility and Sterility* 85 728–734.

Checa MA, Requena A, Salvador C, Tur R, Callejo J, Espinos JJ, Fabregues F, Herrero J; Reproductive Endocrinology Interest Group of the Spanish Society of Fertility. 2005. Insulin-sensitizing agents: use in pregnancy and as therapy in polycystic ovary syndrome. *Human Reproduction Update* 11 375–390.

Cole PA, Robinson CH. 1990. Mechanism and inhibition of cytochrome P-450 aromatase. *Journal of Medicinal Chemistry* 33 2933–2942.

Collins JA BEWAR. 1995. The prognosis for live birth among untreated infertile couples. *Fertility and Sterility* 64 22–28.

Coroleu B, Barri PN, Carreras O, Martinez F, Parriego M, Hereter L, Parera N, Veiga A, Balasch J. 2002. The influence of the depth of embryo replacement into the uterine cavity on implantation rates after IVF: a controlled, ultrasound-guided study. *Human Reproduction* 17 341–346.

Costea DM, Gunn LK, Hargreaves C, Howell RJ, Chard T. 2000. Delayed luteo-placental shift of progesterone production in IVF pregnancy. *International Journal of Gynaecology and Obstetrics* 68 123–129.

Costello MF, Chapman M, Conway U. 2006. A systematic review and meta-analysis of randomized controlled trials on metformin co-administration during gonadotrophin ovulation induction or IVF in women with polycystic ovary syndrome. *Human Reproduction* 21 1387–1399.

Coulam CB, Stern JJ, Soenksen DM, Britten S, Bustillo M. 1995. Comparison of pulsatility indices on the day of oocyte retrieval and embryo transfer. *Human Reproduction* 10 82–84.

Daya S, Gunby J. 2004. Luteal phase support in assisted reproduction cycles. *Cochrane Database of Systematic Review* CD004830.

Daya S. 2006. Is there a benefit of low-dose aspirin in assisted reproduction? *Current Opinions in Obstetrics and Gynecology* 18 313–318.

de Jong-Potjer LC, Elsinga J. 2006. Preconception counselling in general practice. *Doctoral thesis.*

Devroey P, Bourgain C, Macklon NS, Fauser BC. 2004. Reproductive biology and IVF: ovarian stimulation and endometrial receptivity. *Trends in Endocrinology and Metabolism* 15 84–90.

Dey SK, Lim H, Das SK, Reese J, Paria BC, Daikoku T, Wang H. 2004. Molecular cues to implantation. *Endocrine Reviews* 25 341–373.

Di Nisio M, Peters L, Middeldorp S. 2005. Anticoagulants for the treatment of recurrent pregnancy loss in women without antiphospholipid syndrome. *Cochrane Database of Systematic Reviews* CD004734.

Donderwinkel PF, Schoot DC, Pache TD, de Jong FH, Hop WC, Fauser BC. 1993. Luteal function following ovulation induction in polycystic ovary syndrome patients using exogenous gonadotrophins in combination with a gonadotrophin-releasing hormone agonist. *Human Reproduction* 8 2027–2032.

Duvan CI, Ozmen B, Satiroglu H, Atabekoglu CS, Berker B. 2006. Does addition of low-dose aspirin and/or steroid as a standard treatment in nonselected intracytoplasmic sperm injection cycles improve in vitro fertilization success? A randomized, prospective, placebo-controlled study. *Journal of Assisted Reproductive Genetics* 23 15–21.

Eijkemans MJC, Imani B, Mulders AGMG, Habbema JD, Fauser BCJM. 2003. High singleton live birth rate following classical ovulation induction in normogonadotrophic anovulatory infertility (WHO 2). *Human Reproduction* 18 2357–2362.

Empson M, Lassere M, Craig J, Scott J. 2005. Prevention of recurrent miscarriage for women with antiphospholipid antibody or lupus anticoagulant. *Cochrane Database of Systematic Reviews* CD002859.

Empson M, Lassere M, Craig JC, Scott JR. 2002. Recurrent pregnancy loss with antiphospholipid antibody: a systematic review of therapeutic trials. *Obstetrics Gynecology* 99 135–144.

The European IVF-monitoring program. 2005. Assisted reproductive technology in Europe, 2001. Results generated from European registers by ESHRE. *Human Reproduction* **20** 1158–1176.

Fanchin R, Righini C, de Ziegler D, Olivennes F, Ledee N, Frydman R. 2001. Effects of vaginal progesterone administration on uterine contractility at the time of embryo transfer. *Fertility and Sterility* **75** 1136–1140.

Fanchin R, Righini C, Olivennes F, Taylor S, de Ziegler D, Frydman R. 1998. Uterine contractions at the time of embryo transfer alter pregnancy rates after in-vitro fertilization. *Human Reproduction* **13** 1968–1974.

Fauser BC, Devroey P, Macklon NS. 2005. Multiple birth resulting from ovarian stimulation for subfertility treatment. *Lancet* **365** 1807–1816.

Fauser BC, Devroey P, Yen SS, Gosden R, Crowley WF Jr., Baird DT, Bouchard P. 1999. Minimal ovarian stimulation for IVF: appraisal of potential benefits and drawbacks. *Human Reproduction* **14** 2681–2686.

Fauser BC, Macklon NS. 2004. Medical approaches to ovarian stimulation for infertility. In *Yen and Jaffe's Reproductive Endocrinology*, Strauss BRJF, Ed. Elsevier Saunders: Philadelphia.

Fauser BCJM, Devroey P. 2003. Reproductive biology and IVF: ovarian stimulation and luteal phase consequences. *Trends in Endocrinology and Metabolism* **14** 236–242.

Gaast van der MH, Eijkemans MJC, Net van der JB, Boer de EJ, Burger CW, Leeuwen van FE, Fauser BC, Macklon NS. 2006. The optimum number of oocytes for a successful first IVF treatment cycle. *Reproductive Biomedicine Online* (in press).

Garcia J, Jones GS, Acosta AA, Wright GL Jr. 1981. Corpus luteum function after follicle aspiration for oocyte retrieval. *Fertility and Sterility* **36** 565–572.

Geva E, Amit A, Lerner-Geva L, Yaron Y, Daniel Y, Schwartz T, Azem F, Yovel I, Lessing JB. 2000. Prednisone and aspirin improve pregnancy rate in patients with reproductive failure and autoimmune antibodies: a prospective study. *American Journal of Reproductive Immunology* **43** 36–40.

Goswami SK, Das T, Chattopadhyay R, Sawhney V, Kumar J, Chaudhury K, Chakravarty BN, Kabir SN. 2004. A randomized single-blind controlled trial of letrozole as a low-cost IVF protocol in women with poor ovarian response: a preliminary report. *Human Reproduction* **19** 2031–2035.

Greb RR, Behre HM, Simoni M. 2005. Pharmacogenetics in ovarian stimulation—current concepts and future options. *Reproductive Biomedicine Online* **11** 589.

Griesinger G, Franke K, Kinast C, Kutzelnigg A, Riedinger S, Kulin S, Kaali SG, Feichtinger W. 2002. Ascorbic acid supplement during luteal phase in IVF. *Journal of Assisted Reproduction and Genetics* **19** 164–168.

Guimond MJ, Wang B, Croy BA. 1998. Engraftment of bone marrow from severe combined immunodeficient (SCID) mice reverses the reproductive deficits in natural killer cell-deficient tg epsilon 26 mice. *Journal of Experimental Medicine* **187** 217–223.

Healey S, Tan SL, Tulandi T, Biljan MM. 2003. Effects of letrozole on superovulation with gonadotropins in women undergoing intrauterine insemination. *Fertility and Sterility* **80** 1325–1329.

Heijnen EM, Eijkemans MJ, Hughes EG, Laven JS, Macklon NS, Fauser BC. 2005. A meta-analysis of outcomes of conventional IVF in women with polycystic ovary syndrome. *Human Reproduction Update*.

Heijnen EM, Macklon NS, Fauser BC. 2004. What is the most relevant standard of success in assisted reproduction? The next step to improving outcomes of IVF: consider the whole treatment. *Human Reproduction* **19** 1936–1938.

Hohmann FP, Macklon NS, Fauser BC. 2003. A randomized comparison of two ovarian stimulation protocols with gonadotropin-releasing hormone (GnRH) antagonist cotreatment for in vitro fertilization commencing recombinant follicle-stimulating hormone on cycle day 2 or 5 with the standard long GnRH agonist protocol. *Journal of Clinical Endocrinology Metabolism* **88** 166–173.

Johnson NP, Mak W, Sowter MC. 2002. Laparoscopic salpingectomy for women with hydrosalpinges enhances the success of IVF: a Cochrane review. *Human Reproduction* **17** 543.

Jones HW Jr. 1996. What has happened? Where are we? *Human Reproduction* **11** 7.

Kolibianakis EM, Bourgain C, Papanikolaou EG, Camus M, Tournaye H, Van Steirteghem AC, Devroey P. 2005. Prolongation of follicular phase by delaying hCG administration results in a higher incidence of endometrial advancement on the day of oocyte retrieval in GnRH antagonist cycles. *Human Reproduction* **20** 2453–2456.

Kontoravdis A, Makrakis E, Pantos K, Botsis D, Deligeoroglou E, Creatsas G. Proximal tubal occlusion and salpingectomy result in similar improvement in in vitro fertilization outcome in patients with hydrosalpinx. *Fertility and Sterility* (in press).

Korn AP, Bolan G, Padian N, Ohm-Smith M, Schachter J, Landers DV. 1995. Plasma cell endometritis in women with symptomatic bacterial vaginosis. *Obstetrics and Gynecology* **85** 387–390.

Kuo HC, Hsu CC, Wang ST, Huang KE. 1997. Aspirin improves uterine blood flow in the peri-implantation period. *Journal of the Formosan Medical Association* **96** 253–257.

Ledee-Bataille N, Bonnet-Chea K, Hosny G, Dubanchet S, Frydman R, Chaouat G. 2005. Role of the endometrial tripod interleukin-18, -15, and -12 in inadequate uterine receptivity in patients with a history of repeated in vitro fertilization-embryo transfer failure. *Fertility and Sterility* **83** 598–605.

Lee TH, Wu MY, Chen MJ, Chao KH, Ho HN, Yang YS. 2004. Nitric oxide is associated with poor embryo quality and pregnancy outcome in in vitro fertilization cycles. *Fertility and Sterility* **82** 126–131.

Lintsen AM, Pasker-de Jong PC, de Boer EJ, Burger CW, Jansen CA, Braat DD, van Leeuwen FE. 2005. Effects of subfertility cause, smoking and body weight on the success rate of IVF. *Human Reproduction* **20** 1867–1875.

Liversedge NH, Turner A, Horner PJ, Keay SD, Jenkins JM, Hull MG. 1999. The influence of bacterial vaginosis on in-vitro fertilization and embryo implantation during assisted reproduction treatment. *Human Reproduction* **14** 2411–2415.

Lord JM, Flight IH, Norman RJ. 2003. Insulin-sensitising drugs (metformin, troglitazone, rosiglitazone, pioglitazone, D-chiro-inositol) for polycystic ovary syndrome. *Cochrane Database of Systematic Reviews*. Issue 2. Art.No.: CD003053.

Luck MR, Jeyaseelan I, Scholes RA. 1995. Ascorbic acid and fertility. *Biology of Reproduction* **52** 262–266.

Luck MR, Zhao Y. 1993. Identification and measurement of collagen in the bovine corpus luteum and its relationship with ascorbic acid and tissue development. *Journal of Reproduction and Fertility* **99** 647–652.

Ma Wg, Song H, Das SK, Paria BC, Dey SK. 2003. Estrogen is a critical determinant that specifies the duration of the window of uterine receptivity for implantation. *Proceedings of the National Academy of Sciences* **100** 2963–2968.

Macklon NS, Fauser BC. 2000. Impact of ovarian hyperstimulation on the luteal phase. *Journal of Reproduction and Fertility* **55** 101–108.

Macklon NS, Pieters MHEC, Fauser BCJM. 2004. Indications for IVF treatment: from diagnosis to prognosis. In *Textbook of Assisted Reproductive Techniques: Laboratory and Clinical Perspectives*, edn 2, Gardner DK, Weissman A, Howles CM, Shoham Z, Eds. London: Taylor and Francis.

Macklon NS, Stouffer RL, Giudice LC, Fauser BC. 2006. The science behind 25 years of ovarian stimulation for in vitro fertilization. *Endocrine Reviews* **27** 170–207.

Mitwally MF, Casper RF. 2003. Aromatase inhibition reduces gonadotrophin dose required for controlled ovarian stimulation in women with unexplained infertility. *Human Reproduction* **18** 1588–1597.

Mitwally MF, Casper RF. 2004. Aromatase inhibition reduces the dose of gonadotropin required for controlled ovarian hyperstimulation. *Journal of Social Gynecological Investigation* **11** 406–415.

Miyazaki S, Tanebe K, Sakai M, Michimata T, Tsuda H, Fujimura M, Nakamura M, Kiso Y, Saito S. 2002. Interleukin 2 receptor gamma chain (gamma(c)) knockout mice show less regularity in estrous cycle but achieve normal pregnancy without fetal compromise. *American Journal of Reproductive Immunology* **47** 222–230.

Nestler JE. 2002. Should patients with polycystic ovarian syndrome be treated with metformin?: an enthusiastic endorsement. *Human Reproduction* **17** 1950–1953.

Norman RJ, Clark AM. 1998. Obesity and reproductive disorders: a review. *Reproduction, Fertility and Development* **10** 55–63.

Nyboe AA, Popovic-Todorovic B, Schmidt KT, Loft A, Lindhard A, Hojgaard A, Ziebe S, Hald F, Hauge B, Toft B. 2002. Progesterone supplementation during early gestations after IVF or ICSI has no effect on the delivery rates: a randomized controlled trial. *Human Reproduction* **17** 357–361.

Oliveira JB, Martins AM, Baruffi RL, Mauri AL, Petersen CG, Felipe V, Contart P, Pontes A, Franco JG Jr. 2004. Increased implantation and pregnancy rates obtained by placing the tip of the transfer catheter in the central area of the endometrial cavity. *Reproductive Biomedicine Online* **9** 435–441.

Pakkila M, Rasanen J, Heinonen S, Tinkanen H, Tuomivaara L, Makikallio K, Hippelainen M, Tapanainen JS, Martikainen H. 2005. Low-dose aspirin does not improve ovarian responsiveness or pregnancy rate in IVF and ICSI patients: a randomized, placebo-controlled double-blind study. *Human Reproduction* **20** 2211–2214.

Paszkowski T, Clarke RN, Hornstein MD. 2002. Smoking induces oxidative stress inside the Graafian follicle. *Human Reproduction* **17** 921–925.

Popovic-Todorovic B, Loft A, Bredkjaeer HE, Bangsboll S, Nielsen IK, Andersen AN. 2003a. A prospective randomized clinical trial comparing an individual dose of recombinant FSH based on predictive factors versus a 'standard' dose of 150 IU/day in 'standard' patients undergoing IVF/ICSI treatment. *Human Reproduction* **18** 2275–2282.

Popovic-Todorovic B, Loft A, Lindhard A, Bangsboll S, Andersson AM, Andersen AN. 2003b. A prospective study of predictive factors of ovarian response in 'standard' IVF/ICSI patients treated with recombinant FSH. A suggestion for a recombinant FSH dosage normogram. *Human Reproduction* **18** 781–787.

The Practice Committee of the American Society for Reproductive M. 2006. Smoking and infertility. *Fertility and Sterility* **86** S172–S177.

Quenby S, Kalumbi C, Bates M, Farquharson R, Vince G. 2005. Prednisolone reduces preconceptual endometrial natural killer cells in women with recurrent miscarriage. *Fertility and Sterility* **84** 980–984.

Rizk B, Abdalla H. 2008. In Vitro fertilization. In: Rizk B, Abdalla H (Eds.), Infertility and Assisted Reproductive Technology. Oxford: United Kingdom. Cambridge University Press, chapter 7, pp. 112–114.

Romundstad LB, Romundstad PR, Sunde A, During Vv, Skjarven R, Vatten LJ. 2006. Increased risk of placenta previa in pregnancies following IVF/ICSI; a comparison of ART and non-ART pregnancies in the same mother. *Human Reproduction* **21** 1532–4.

Rubinstein M, Marazzi A, Polak dF. 1999. Low-dose aspirin treatment improves ovarian responsiveness, uterine and ovarian blood flow velocity, implantation, and pregnancy rates in patients undergoing in vitro fertilization: a prospective, randomized, double-blind placebo-controlled assay. *Fertility and Sterility* **71** 825–829.

Salim R, Ben Shlomo I, Colodner R, Keness Y, Shalev E. 2002. Bacterial colonization of the uterine cervix and success rate in assisted reproduction: results of a prospective survey. *Human Reproduction* **17** 337–340.

Simon C, Cano F, Valbuena D, Remohi J, Pellicer A. 1995. Clinical evidence for a detrimental effect on uterine receptivity of high serum oestradiol concentrations in high and normal responder patients. *Human Reproduction* **10** 2432–2437.

Stern C, Chamley L, Norris H, Hale L, Baker HW. 2003. A randomized, double-blind, placebo-controlled trial of heparin and aspirin for women with in vitro fertilization implantation failure and antiphospholipid or antinuclear antibodies. *Fertility and Sterility* **80** 376–383.

Strandell A, Lindhard A, Waldenstrom U, Thorburn J. 2001. Hydrosalpinx and IVF outcome: cumulative results after salpingectomy in a randomized controlled trial. *Human Reproduction* **16** 2403–2410.

Strandell A. 2005. The patient with hydrosalpinx. In *IVF in the Medically Complicated Patient: A Guide to Management*, Macklon NS, Ed. Abingdon: Taylor and Francis.

Tang T, Glanville J, Orsi N, Barth JH, Balen AH. 2006. The use of metformin for women with PCOS undergoing IVF treatment. *Human Reproduction* **21** 1416–1425.

Tarlatzis BC, Zepiridis L, Grimbizis G, Bontis J. 2003. Clinical management of low ovarian response to stimulation for IVF: a systematic review. *Human Reproduction Update* **9** 61–76.

Templeton A, Morris JK, Parslow W. 1996. Factors that affect outcome of in-vitro fertilisation treatment. *Lancet* **348** 1402–1406.

Urman B, Mercan R, Alatas C, Balaban B, Isiklar A, Nuhoglu A. 2000. Low-dose aspirin does not increase implantation rates in patients undergoing intracytoplasmic sperm injection: a prospective randomized study. *Journal of Assisted Reproduction and Genetics* **17** 586–590.

van Rooij IAJ, Bancsi LFJM, Broekmans FJM, Looman CWN, Habbema JD, te Velde ER. 2003. Women older than 40 years of age and those with elevated follicle-stimulating hormone levels differ in poor response rate and embryo quality in in vitro fertilization. *Fertility and Sterility* **79** 482–488.

Waldenstrom U, Hellberg D, Nilsson S. 2004. Low-dose aspirin in a short regimen as standard treatment in in vitro fertilization: a randomized, prospective study. *Fertility and Sterility* **81** 1560–1564.

Wegmann TG, Lin H, Guilbert L, Mosmann TR. 1993. Bidirectional cytokine interactions in the maternal-fetal relationship: is successful pregnancy a TH2 phenomenon? *Immunology Today* **14** 353–356.

Younglai EV, Holloway AC, Foster WG. 2005. Environmental and occupational factors affecting fertility and IVF success. *Human Reproduction Update* **11** 43–57.

Zenzes MT, Krishnan S, Krishnan B, Zhang H, Casper RF. 1995a. Cadmium accumulation in follicular fluid of women in in vitro fertilization-embryo transfer is higher in smokers. *Fertility and Sterility* **64** 599–603.

Zenzes MT, Wang P, Casper RF. 1995b. Cigarette smoking may affect meiotic maturation of human oocytes. *Hum Reprod* **10** 3213–3217.

39

Surgical Preparation of the Patient for In Vitro Fertilization

Eric S. Surrey

Surgical management of tubal abnormalities, endometriosis, and uterine fibroids has traditionally been employed to enhance fertility in the absence of the assisted reproductive technologies as has been reviewed elsewhere in this text. Can these procedures be employed not only as alternatives to the assisted reproductive technologies but also as adjuncts? In this chapter, we will review the evidence surrounding the effect of reproductive surgery for these conditions on in vitro fertilization (IVF) cycle outcome.

DISTAL TUBAL DISEASE

IVF was originally designed to overcome infertility due to irreversible tubal disease or for those who did not wish to undergo surgical repair. A large body of literature has reported that either unilateral or bilateral hydrosalpinges may exert deleterious effects on IVF cycle outcome (1–10) (Table 39.1). Camus et al. performed a meta-analysis of nine retrospective controlled series and five published abstracts encompassing 1,004 patients with hydrosalpinges and 4,588 control patients with tubal factor infertility but without hydrosalpinges (11). Significant decreases in pregnancy, implantation, and delivery rates were appreciated in the hydrosalpinx groups (odds ratios 0.64, 0.63, and 0.58, respectively). Only one investigation included in the meta-analysis noted no difference in pregnancy or implantation rates in hydrosalpinx patients as opposed to controls (12). One confounding variable in that particular trial may be the low implantation and ongoing pregnancy rates in the control group.

Several potential causes for this general decline in pregnancy and implantation rates have been proposed. The accumulation of fluid of any source within the endometrial cavity has been shown to impair embryonic implantation (13). Employing a murine model, several investigative teams have shown that hydrosalpinx fluid may have a direct embryotoxic effect (14–16). Using a similar model, Arrighi et al. demonstrated a deleterious effect of hydrosalpinx fluid on fertilization when preincubated with sperm during capacitation but not when preincubated with oocytes alone (17). This effect on sperm function has been confirmed by others (18). Inflammatory cytokines present within hydrosalpinx fluid may also play an inhibitory role on implantation (19–22). Meyer et al. have demonstrated that women with hydrosalpinges expressed significantly less $\alpha_v\beta_3$ integrin, a presumptive marker of endometrial receptivity, than fertile controls (23). This finding has been reported by others (24). Daftary and Taylor reported that endometrial expression of HOXA-10, purported to be a regulator of endometrial receptivity, is diminished in the presence of hydrosalpinx fluid (25). Blastocyst attachment and trophoblast proliferation may also be inhibited in the presence of this fluid (26). Others have suggested that the deleterious effect of hydrosalpinges may be due in part to a decrease in endometrial and subendometrial blood flow (27).

Prophylactic salpingectomy has been performed in hydrosalpinx patients prior to IVF-ET in an effort to eliminate the retrograde flow of potentially embryotoxic substances. Strandell et al. randomized 204 patients with hydrosalpinges to either salpingectomy or no intervention prior to IVF-ET of which 192 began an actual treatment cycle (28). This group reported significantly increased delivery rates with a trend toward increased clinical pregnancy rates in patients randomized to salpingectomy. In a smaller trial of sixty patients performed by Dechaud et al., a trend toward increased pregnancy and implantation rates, which did not reach statistical significance, was reported after salpingectomy (29). Johnson et al. recently reported the results of a Cochrane review of these two studies as well as one additional unpublished trial (30). They calculated that the likelihood of live birth was significantly higher after salpingectomy (OR = 2.13, 95 percent CI 1.25–3.65). However, there were no significant differences regarding implantation, ectopic pregnancy, or miscarriage rates. It is interesting to note that one trial demonstrated that women who underwent surgical resection of a unilateral hydrosalpinx experienced an 88 percent spontaneous intrauterine pregnancy rate within a mean of 5.6 months postoperatively (31).

It has not been conclusively demonstrated that all hydrosalpinges exert a deleterious effect on IVF outcome. Csemiczky et al. noted that pregnancy rates were compromised only in those patients with a high degree of tubal damage (32). Others have reported that only large hydrosalpinges, visible on ultrasound, resulted in reduced implantation and pregnancy rates (33). Strandell et al. also noted that implantation, clinical pregnancy, and delivery rates were all significantly decreased only in this subgroup (28).

The mechanism of action by which salpingectomy may enhance IVF outcome has not been clearly demonstrated. It has been proposed that salpingectomy may improve endometrial receptivity by enhancing $\alpha_v\beta_3$ integrin expression (34). Ito et al. have demonstrated a significant reduction of lymphocyte clusters within the endometrium after salpingectomy, suggesting suppression of natural killer cell activation (35). Others have

Table 39.1: Effect of Hydrosalpinx on IVF Pregnancy (PR) and Implantation Rates (IR)

First author	References	PR/transfer (%)		IR/transfer (%)	
		Hydrosalpinx	Control	Hydrosalpinx	Control
Anderson	2	27.0 (20/91)	35.6 (265/744)	2.9 (8/273)	10.3 (221/2152)
Strandell	3	13.2 (12/91)	26.0 (74/285)	NR	NR
Kasabji	4	18.4 (43/234)	31.4 (70/223)	7.7 (59/796)	11.7 (83/710)
Vandromme	5	11.3 (7/62)	31.6 (30/95)	4.2 (8/190)	13.4 (36/269)
Katz	6	16.8 (16/95)	36.8 (467/1268)	3.9 (17/434)	11.5 (643/5577)
Blazar	7	39.0 (26/67)	45.0 (81/180)	NR	NR
Sharara	8	24.5 (25/101)	33.7 (30/89)	9.8 (43/437)	12.6 (50/396)
Murray	9	8.5 (4/47)	38.6 (56/146)	2.8 (5/167)	15.8 (189/565)
Akman	10	7.1 (1/14)	24.5 (24/98)	5.0 (2/40)	10.4 (30/289)

All differences statistically significant. NR = not reported.

shown that endometrial leukemia inhibitory factor expression, which is thought to serve as a potential marker for endometrial receptivity, is suppressed in hydrosalpinx patients but increased after surgery (36).

However, there are potential disadvantages to the performance of salpingectomy. This procedure is clearly invasive and may become technically difficult in the face of extensive pelvic adhesions, with an increased potential for injury to surrounding structures. In addition, transection of the tube too close to the cornua may also increase the risk of an interstitial pregnancy after embryo transfer, a devastating complication (37).

Salpingectomy could also theoretically result in a decrease in ovarian perfusion given that a portion of the blood supply to the ovary is derived from the branches of the uterine artery and the mesosalpingeal vascular arcade (38). McComb and Relbeke noted fewer corpora lutea after fimbriectomy in the rabbit (39). Clinically, Lass et al. reported development of fewer follicles and retrieved fewer oocytes from the ipsilateral ovary in women who had undergone unilateral salpingectomy (40). More recently, Chan et al. reported that ovarian blood flow and antral follicle counts were reduced on the ipsilateral side of women who had undergone unilateral salpingectomy at laparoscopy or laparotomy (41). Others have demonstrated compromise in ovarian response to gonadotropins without an effect on pregnancy rates in patients who had undergone prior salpingectomy (42). In contrast, Dar et al. assessed ovarian response in assisted reproductive technology cycles performed before and after laparoscopic salpingectomy for ectopic pregnancy and noted no ill effect of surgery (43). These findings have been confirmed by others (44, 45).

Proximal tubal occlusion represents a significantly less invasive approach, which requires less surgical dissection and operating time while still eliminating retrograde flow of hydrosalpingeal fluid into the endometrial cavity. Surrey and Schoolcraft demonstrated that laparoscopic proximal occlusion and transection of the affected fallopian tube resulted in similar ovarian response and cycle outcome as control groups with nonocclusive tubal disease or those who had undergone bilateral tubal ligation for sterilizations or those who have undergone

laparoscopic salpingectomy (46). The extent of peritubal adhesions, size of hydrosalpinges, and extent of tubal mucosal damage was similar between the two study groups. The slightly lower implantation and pregnancy rates in patients undergoing proximal tubal occlusion did not reach statistical significance and may have been a function of sample size (Table 39.2).

These findings were confirmed by two other series. Murray et al. reported the outcome of fifteen embryo transfers performed in women with hydrosalpinges who had undergone proximal tubal occlusion (9). Implantation and ongoing pregnancy rates were similar to those of twenty-three women who had undergone salpingectomy and seven who had undergone proximal tubal occlusion. Ovarian response was not addressed in this trial. Stadtmauer et al. reported that proximal occlusion yielded significantly improved outcomes in comparison to patients with hydrosalpinges, which were not treated surgically (47). Interestingly, a trend toward higher pregnancy and implantation rates were noted in thirty patients treated with proximal tubal cautery in comparison to fifteen treated with salpingectomy.

Other less invasive approaches have also been attempted. A single published series describes the hysteroscopic placement of an occlusive microinsert into the proximal portion of the fallopian tube prior to IVF in two patients (48). Two of three of IVF cycles were successful. Although this approach is clearly less invasive, it is an off-label use of the device and more clinical data are clearly required.

Sharara et al. reported a trend toward reduced implantation and pregnancy rates, which did not reach statistical significance in women with hydrosalpinges in whom antibiotic therapy was administered prior to an IVF cycle (49). Hurst et al. have shown that such therapy resulted in similar implantation and live birth rates as several groups of untreated controls (50). This approach, which has not been addressed in a randomized trial, should theoretically only have an impact on acutely or chronically infected tubal fluid but might not address the embryotoxic effects of hydrosalpingeal fluid derived from a noninfectious etiology.

Others have attempted to drain hydrosalpinges surgically prior to cycle initiation or under ultrasound guidance at the

Table 39.2: IVF Cycle Outcome in Hydrosalpinx Patients: Salpingectomy versus Proximal Tubal Occlusion

Group	I (salpingectomy)	II (proximal tubal occlusion)	III (tubal disease without hydrosalpinx)	IV (bilateral tubal ligation for sterilization)
Parameter				
Cycles	35	17	37	15
Age	35.1 ± 0.7^c	$35.4 \pm 1.0^{a,b}$	35.6 ± 0.7	38.2 ± 1.0
E_2 day of hCG (pg/mL)	$2555 \pm 219^{a,b}$	$2366 \pm 282^{a,b}$	2925 ± 259	2479 ± 281
Fertilization (%)	61.8 ± 2.8^a	$63.6 \pm 3.5^{a,b}$	57.7 ± 2.9	65.5 ± 5.5
Embryos transferred/cycle	2.79 ± 0.2^a	$3.5 \pm 0.4^{a,b}$	3.2 ± 0.2	3.0 ± 0.3
Clinical pregnancy/embryo transfer (%)	$16/28 (57.1)^a$	$7/15 (46.7)^{a,b}$	18/34 (52.9)	7/12 (58.3)
Group implantation (%)	$21/78 (26.9)^a$	$8/49 (16.3)^{a,b}$	23/108 (21.3)	12/36 (33.3)
Individual implantation rate/embryo transfer procedure (%)	29.2 ± 5.9^a	$19.4 \pm 6.1^{a,b}$	25.4 ± 5.6	36.1 ± 11.3

Results expressed as mean ± SEM unless otherwise indicated. Modified from Surrey and Schoolcraft (46).
[a] P = not significant (vs. group III or IV).
[b] P = not significant (vs. group I).
[c] $P < 0.05$ versus group IV.

time of oocyte aspiration with mixed results (51–54). Although this technique would reduce the overall volume of hydrosalpingeal fluid, drainage would neither eliminate its source nor its ability to flow into the endometrial cavity even in reduced amounts. In addition, Bloechle et al. have demonstrated reaccumulation of hydrosalpingeal fluid within three days of aspiration performed at oocyte retrieval, which would precede the time of embryo implantation (55). This would theoretically obviate the benefit of drainage alone. Similarly, aspiration of uterine fluid resulting from hydrosalpinges before planned embryo transfer is not beneficial due to its rapid reaccumulation (56).

From an economic standpoint, Strandell et al. have shown that the incremental cost required to perform salpingectomies was outweighed by an overall decreased cost per live birth due to increased pregnancy rates and resulting need for patients to undergo fewer IVF cycles (57).

Thus, the phenomenon of distal tubal obstruction represents an ideal circumstance in which reproductive surgery might serve not only as an alternative but also as an adjunct to enhance IVF cycle outcome.

UTERINE FIBROIDS

It is critical that the uterine cavity is appropriately evaluated and clinically significant abnormalities managed prior to initiation of an IVF cycle. The majority of investigators have relied upon hysterosalpingography or standard transvaginal sonography to assess cavitary distortion and confirm the location of lesions. The lack of a strong correlation between either of these techniques and hysteroscopic findings has previously been described. Wang et al. reported that the sensitivity and specificity of hysterosalpingography in revealing intrauterine abnormalities were 80.3 and 70.1 percent, respectively (58). Similarly, transvaginal ultrasonography may not clearly demonstrate the presence of intracavitary lesions (59, 60). Shamma et al. have reported that 43 percent of patients with a normal hysterosal-

pingogram preparing for IVF were noted to have abnormal hysteroscopic findings (61). These patients had a significantly lower pregnancy rate than those with hysteroscopically normal endometrial cavities. More recently, Oliveira et al. performed hysteroscopy on patients who had a normal hysterosalpingogram and had failed two prior IVF cycles despite transfer of good-quality embryos (62). Forty-eight percent were noted to have abnormal findings at hysteroscopy, including leiomyoma, polyps, or adhesions, which were subsequently treated. These patients then underwent a third IVF cycle with 50 percent clinical pregnancy rate. Evaluation of the cavity by sonohysterography has been shown to correlate well with hysteroscopy and may be even more accurate for preoperative measurement of lesions (63).

The effect of leiomyomata in general on fertility has not been definitively demonstrated. Since these tumors are extremely common in reproductive-age women, it is difficult to truly determine a causal relationship with infertility. Although the effect on implantation of submucosal leiomyomas that distort the endometrial cavity is readily understandable, the mechanism by which intramural lesions in an infertile patient with a normal uterine cavity might exert a deleterious effect is less than clear. A variety of hypotheses have been proposed, including potential effects on implantation and sperm transport as well as on uterine contractility and perfusion (64, 65). Others have shown that the uterine artery pulsatility index is significantly lower in patients with fibroids than in those without (66, 67). Abnormal local expression of growth factors involved with angiogenesis as well as other regulatory processes and aberrant gene expression may play a role (68, 69).

In a review of the literature, Pritts reported that women with submucosal lesions experienced lower pregnancy (RR 0.3, 95 percent CI 0.13–0.7) and implantation (RR 0.28, 95 percent CI 0.1–0.72) rates than fertile controls (70). In this analysis, no other types of fibroids appeared to have an effect on fertility.

The impact of uterine leiomyomata specifically on the outcome of assisted reproductive technologies has been evaluated by others with conflicting results. Farhi et al. compared the outcome of 141 IVF cycles performed on patients with leiomyomata to age-matched controls and reported a deleterious effect on both pregnancy and implantation rates only in the group of patients with endometrial cavitary distortion (71). Stovall et al. reported that patients with intramural and subserosal myomas undergoing assisted reproductive technologies experienced a significant reduction in the likelihood of achieving a live birth (RR = 0.68, 95 percent CI = 0.47–0.98) (72). ElderGeva et al. stratified patients by leiomyoma location and noted that the presence of either intramural or submucosal leiomyomas greatly reduced both implantation and pregnancy rates in comparison to matched controls, whereas subserosal lesions alone exerted no impact (73). In a prospective trial, Hart et al. evaluated 106 women with intramural fibroids diagnosed by ultrasound, hysteroscopy, or sonohysterography (74). The presence of fibroids produced significantly negative effects on clinical pregnancy, implantation, and ongoing pregnancy rates. In an analysis of six previously published trials, Donnez and Jadoul emphasized that only fibroids that induced cavitary distortion exerted a deleterious effect (75).

Surrey et al. noted a significant decrease in implantation rates in women with intramural leiomyomata and hysteroscopically normal endometrial cavities younger than forty years of age undergoing IVF in comparison to age-matched controls (76). Trends toward lower clinical pregnancy and live birth rates, which failed to reach statistical significance, were also appreciated. Regression analyses revealed that neither leiomyoma size nor volume per se correlated with implantation. Similarly, no correlation between mean uterine artery Doppler flow and implantation was appreciated when controlled for age.

Oliveira et al. recently evaluated 245 IVF-ICSI patients with subserosal and/or intramural fibroids, which did not distort the endometrial cavity (77). They also noted that location and number had no correlation with cycle outcome. However, patients with intramural lesions larger than 4 cm had lower pregnancy rates than those with smaller tumors.

Not all investigators have shown that intramural fibroids exert a deleterious effect. One study evaluated seventy-three women with intramural fibroids and thirty-five women with subserosal fibroids in a case-controlled design of patients undergoing IVF and ICSI and noted no adverse effect on either clinical pregnancy or implantation rates (78). These findings have been reported by others (79, 80).

One possible explanation for the discrepancy in outcomes among the various studies described may rest with a difference in patient selection technique. Mean sizes and numbers of leiomyomata vary among the studies. The method of evaluating the uterus is not consistent among investigators. The extent of normal intervening myometrium between the fibroid and degree of distortion of the endometrial cavity is not universally defined. Similarly, differences in outcomes among various IVF laboratories make comparing trials difficult.

The implied benefit of excising fibroids in patients with clinically significant lesions prior to IVF has not been extensively evaluated. In the aforementioned meta-analysis, Pritts reported that when submucosal lesions were resected, delivery rates were equivalent to those of infertile women without fibroids (RR 0.98, 95 percent CI 0.45–2.41) (70). However, this analysis did not solely address patients who were undergoing IVF. In a retrospective series, Seoud et al. reported that ongoing pregnancy rates were similar in forty-seven patients who had undergone precycle myomectomies (16.9 percent) in comparison with controls without fibroids (19.0 percent) (81). Unfortunately, the majority of these patients were noted to have subserosal lesions and only ten were described as having abnormal cavities prior to surgery.

More recently, Surrey et al. evaluated the effect of myomectomy on IVF outcomes in patients with leiomyomata considered to be clinically significant: submucosal or intramural lesions exhibiting evidence of cavitary distortion or direct impingement (82). In this retrospective series, patients who underwent precycle myomectomy for uterine leiomyomata felt to be clinically significant had ongoing pregnancy, implantation, and biochemical cycle pregnancy loss rates, which were similar to controls. The outcome for patients with smaller submucosal lesions resected hysteroscopically was the same as for those with large submucosal lesions with a significant intramural component or those intramural lesions, which directly impinged upon or distorted the endometrial cavity resected at laparotomy. In an effort to control for the variables of oocyte quality and endometrial receptivity, oocyte donor recipients were evaluated independently from patients using their own oocytes. Yet, the net effect of surgical resection was similar (Figure 39.1). The inherent weakness of this investigation is its retrospective nature, although a degree of control was achieved by creating strict criteria for the indications for myomectomy, that is, only those fibroids that were clearly distorting or impinging upon the endometrial cavity were removed and a normal endometrial cavity was achieved prior to cycle initiation. An appropriately designed prospective randomized trial would clearly provide definitive answers, although recruitment would be challenging.

In summary, evaluation of the uterine cavity should be a routine part of the precycle evaluation. It appears that leiomyomata that distort the endometrial cavity have an impact on cycle outcome. The effect of intramural lesions has not been uniformly demonstrated due to the heterogeneous nature of the investigations. Consideration should be given to resection of submucosal fibroids and intramural lesions that distort directly impinge upon the endometrial cavity prior to IVF. In

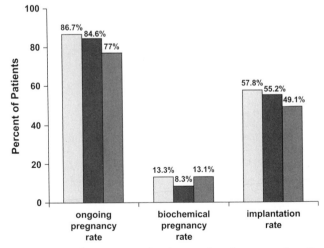

Figure 39.1. Cycle outcomes of patients undergoing oocyte donation (Surrey et al., 82). Reprinted with permission from the American Society for Reproductive Medicine. (□) Group A: hysteroscopic myomectomy; (▤) Group B: myomectomy at laparotomy; (■) Group C: recipient controls.

contrast, the benefit of resecting other asymptomatic intramural or subserosal lesions with a normal uterine cavity has not been demonstrated.

ENDOMETRIOSIS

The relationship between endometriosis and infertility and the roles of both surgical and medical therapies have been reviewed in this text in chapter 42. Pregnancy rates achieved with ART have increased progressively in recent years, and in endometriosis, patients achieve levels of success that are significantly higher than those obtained with alternative therapies.

A controversial issue is whether endometriosis per se exerts a deleterious effect on ART outcomes. Several early studies implied that fertilization, implantation, and pregnancy rates in endometriosis patients were significantly compromised in comparison to controls (83–86). In contrast, Olivennes et al. reported a delivery rate per embryo transfer of 30 percent in 360 IVF cycles performed on 214 endometriosis patients in contrast to a rate of 37.5 percent in 166 cycles performed on 111 tubal factor controls, a difference that was not statistically significant (87). Geber et al. confirmed these findings reporting a 40 percent overall pregnancy rate in 140 endometriosis patients that was not significantly different when compared to three control groups (88).

In an effort to resolve these issues, Barnhart et al. performed a meta-analysis that included twenty-seven trials published from 1983 to 1998 (89). After performing bivariate and multivariate logistic regression analyses, the authors concluded that the chance of conceiving from IVF was significantly lower for endometriosis patients than for tubal factor controls (OR 0.56, 95 percent CI 0.44–0.70). These authors also reported that endometriosis patients experienced significantly lower fertilization and implantation rates as well as number of oocytes obtained. Needless to say, these pregnancy rates still remain higher than those achieved with other forms of therapy as has been reviewed elsewhere in this text.

The effect of disease severity on cycle outcome has also been evaluated. Several large investigations have demonstrated no relationship between disease severity and ongoing pregnancy or miscarriage rates (87, 88). More recently, Azem et al. reported significantly reduced fertilization, pregnancy, and live birth rates per cycle in fifty-eight patients with stage III and IV endometriosis in comparison to sixty controls with tubal factor infertility (90). No comparisons were made to patients with less extensive disease, however. Interestingly, delivery rates were low in both of the groups (6.7 vs. 16.6 percent, respectively). Pal et al. reported that although fertilization rates were significantly lower in patients with stages III and IV in comparison to stages I and II, endometriosis, implantation, clinical pregnancy, and miscarriage rates were similar between the groups (91). As part of the aforementioned meta-analysis, Barnhart et al. compared outcomes in patients previously diagnosed with stage I–II endometriosis to those with stage III–IV disease (89). Women with severe disease were noted to have significantly lower peak estradiol levels, number of oocytes retrieved, implantation, and pregnancy rates than those with less extensive disease.

The presence of ovarian endometriotic cysts (endometriomas) should perhaps be addressed separately from patients with stage IV disease in the absence of these lesions. However, the effect of endometrioma size has not been evaluated as an independent variable in any trial. It is also extremely difficult to assess the effect of the endometrioma per se on cycle outcome given that the majority of patients with these lesions are likely to have peritoneal disease as well, which could have an independent effect.

Uniformly poor outcomes in patients with endometriomas with regard to ovarian response, number of embryos available for transfer, as well as fertilization and pregnancy rates in comparison to controls with hydrosalpinges were reported in an earlier study (92). Yanushpolsky et al. reported a higher incidence of pregnancy loss and an adverse effect on number of oocytes retrieved and embryo quality in endometriosis patients (93). Others have described a decrease in ovarian response requiring the use of higher gonadotropin doses with no effect on cumulative pregnancy and live birth rates in patients with such lesions (94). However, Olivennes et al. demonstrated no effect of persistent endometriomas on any outcome parameter of either controlled ovarian hyperstimulation or IVF (87). Despite traditional teaching, at least one group of investigators reported that limited inadvertent exposure of oocytes to endometrioma fluid does not appear to have a significant impact on fertilization rates or early embryo development (95). However, it is only logical to make every effort to avoid placing the aspirating needle through an endometrioma during oocyte retrieval procedures to prevent rupture and inadvertent exposure of oocytes to cyst contents if at all possible.

The benefit of surgical management of endometriosis on achieving spontaneous conception has been reviewed elsewhere. The question of whether surgical management would benefit outcome of the assisted reproductive technologies has not been extensively addressed. One prospective randomized trial reported that although laparoscopic laser ablation of endometriosis at the time of GIFT (gamete intrafallopian transfer) had no effect on cycle outcome, pregnancy rates in subsequent cycles of patients who failed to conceive from GIFT were significantly higher than in controls with endometriosis who underwent GIFT alone (96). More recently, Surrey and Schoolcraft reported that controlled ovarian hyperstimulation and IVF cycle outcomes were similar between two groups of endometriosis patients without ovarian endometriomata, one of which had undergone surgical resection of disease within six months and the other had undergone surgical resection greater than six months to five years prior to oocyte aspiration (ongoing pregnancy rates 63.6 vs. 60.6 percent, respectively) (97) (Figure 39.2). Regression analyses revealed no effect of the time interval between surgery and oocyte aspiration or stage of disease on implantation rates. In contrast, Aboulghar et al. reported that stage IV endometriosis patients who had undergone surgery prior to IVF experienced significantly higher cancellation rates due to poor response (29.7 vs. 1.1 percent) and lower clinical pregnancy rates (15.3 vs. 52.5 percent) in comparison to similarly stimulated age-matched controls with tubal factor infertility (98).

The question of whether endometriomas should be resected prior to initiation of an IVF cycle has not been resolved. Canis et al. described a series of forty-one patients who had undergone precycle laparoscopic resection of large (>3 cm in diameter) ovarian endometriotic cysts (unilateral in thirty patients and bilateral in eleven patients) in comparison to 139 controls with endometriosis but without endometriomata and 59 additional controls with tubal infertility (99). No differences with regard to number of oocytes retrieved or available embryos for

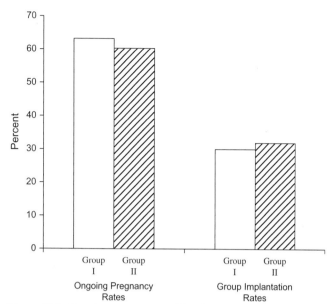

Figure 39.2. Ongoing pregnancy and implantation rates in endometriosis patients undergoing surgical resection less than six months (Group I) or six months to five years (Group II) prior to oocyte aspiration. Surrey and Schoolcraft (97). Reprinted with permission.

transfer were noted despite extensive ovarian surgery. Donnez et al. reported upon 187 cycles (eighty-five patients) who underwent laparoscopic cyst wall vaporization of ovarian endometriomas prior to IVF and compared responses to 633 cycles (289 patients) with tubal factor infertility (100). Response to stimulation and clinical pregnancy rates were also similar between the groups. Others have reported similar cycle outcomes although higher gonadotropin doses were required to achieve adequate ovarian response (101). It is important to note that in these studies there were no controls with endometriomas left in situ and no analyses of the relative effects of cyst size.

The aforementioned studies suggest that precycle resection of endometriomas is not harmful but do not address the question of whether this procedure is advantageous. In an interesting trial, Ho et al. compared relative ovarian responses between ovaries of patients who had undergone unilateral cystectomy for an endometrioma prior to IVF (102). The number of dominant follicles and oocytes retrieved was significantly lower in the ovary that had been previously operated upon. This suggests that aggressive ovarian surgery could compromise ovarian blood supply or result in the destruction of normal ovarian tissue. In a retrospective series, Garcia-Velasco et al. compared the outcomes of fifty patients who had at least one endometrioma larger than 3 cm in mean diameter at the time of oocyte aspiration to those of eighty-seven patients who had undergone laparoscopic resection of endometriomas within three months of an IVF cycle (103). There were no differences in ovarian response, fertilization rates, number of embryos available for transfer, or pregnancy rates between the groups. However, the relative sizes of lesions in the two groups were not described, which may have been a confounding variable. The authors concluded that although laparoscopic resection of ovarian endometriomata does not have a deleterious effect on IVF cycle outcome, it does not appear to offer any specific benefit.

A summary of studies addressing the resection of these lesions is presented in Table 39.3. Resection of large lesions will clearly enhance access to follicles within underlying normal ovarian tissue and eliminate the potential for rupture during oocyte aspiration. However, meticulous surgical technique with an eye toward carefully avoiding compromise of ovarian blood supply and destroying healthy ovarian tissue is clearly mandatory.

Traditional medical therapies for symptomatic endometriosis, such as progestins, danazol, and GnRH agonists have been shown to have little impact on enhancing spontaneous pregnancy rates as has been reviewed previously. However, if the negative effect of this disease process on fertility returns rapidly after discontinuation of medication, then one could hypothesize that any benefits of medical suppression on enhancing fertility would be most evident if pregnancy could be achieved during a time of maximal suppression. This could only occur with the use of the assisted reproductive technologies.

In a prospective randomized multicenter trial, Surrey et al. evaluated the effect of a three-month course of a GnRH agonist administered to patients with surgically confirmed endometriosis immediately prior to controlled ovarian hyperstimulation and IVF (104). Significantly higher ongoing pregnancy rates (78.3 vs. 56.5 percent; $P < 0.03$) with a trend toward higher implantation rates were appreciated in this group of twenty-five patients in comparison to twenty-six controls with endometriosis treated with standard controlled ovarian hyperstimulation techniques in the absence of prolonged GnRH agonist therapy. These findings have been demonstrated by others. Seven previous studies of varying design have assessed the effect of suppression with a GnRH agonist before IVF or GIFT (105–111). The length of suppression varied from six weeks to seven months. Some studies lacked control groups, but a beneficial effect of pretreatment was suggested by all. In a recent Cochrane database review, Sallam analyzed three of the aforementioned trials that were prospective and randomized including 163 patients with endometriosis undergoing three to six months of precycle GnRH agonist therapy (112). A significant improvement in live birth rates (OR 9.19, 95 percent CI 1.08–78.22) was noted.

The mechanism of action for this effect has not been established. Investigators have suggested that GnRH agonists may have been a positive input on natural killer cell activity, metalloproteinase tissue inhibitor concentrations, peritoneal cytokine levels, and endometrial cell apoptosis (113–116). Alternatively, suppressive therapy with danazol and GnRH agonists has been suggested to have a beneficial effect on restoring aberrant endometrial $\alpha_v\beta_3$ integrin expression, which may enhance implantation (117, 118).

In summary, the effects of endometriosis in general and disease stage in specific on IVF outcome have not been definitively demonstrated. Although it would be logical to resect larger endometriomas (>3 cm) prior to initiation of an IVF cycle, the data supporting this approach are inconclusive. Needless to say, great care should be taken to preserve ovarian blood supply when these lesions are resected. However, there is no evidence to suggest that resection of nonovarian endometriosis has any effect on the outcome of a subsequent IVF cycle. Prolonged pretreatment of selected endometriosis patients with a GnRH agonist may enhance IVF cycle outcome. Whether this approach is uniformly beneficial or of value only in a subset of patients has not, as yet, been established (119, 120).

Table 39.3: Resection of Ovarian Endometriomas and IVF Outcome: Summary

First author (reference)	Cycles	Patients	Controls			COH			
			Endometrioma (unoperated)	Endometriosis, No endometrioma	Other	Days	Dose	CPR	SAb
Camus (99)	41	Postresection	No	Yes (139)	Tubal (59)	NS	NS	NS	NR
Donnez (100)	633	Postresection	No	No	Tubal (633)	NS	NS	NS	NR
Marconi (101)	39	Postresection	No	No	Tubal (39)	↑	↑	NS	NR
Garcia-Velasco (103)	147	Postresection	Yes (63)	No	No	NS (↓ peak estradiol)	NS	NS	NS

COH, controlled ovarian hyperstimulation; CPR, clinical pregnancy rate; NR, not reported; NS, no significant difference; SAb, spontaneous abortion.

KEY POINTS FOR CLINICAL PRACTICE

- Hydrosalpinges should either be removed or occluded proximally prior to an IVF cycle in order to maximize outcome.
- The uterine cavity should be evaluated prior to initiating an IVF cycle. Consideration for resection of submucosal and intramural leiomyomata that impinge upon or distort the endometrial cavity prior to an IVF cycle is vital. The benefit of resection of other fibroids, which do not impinge upon the endometrial cavity, has not been demonstrated.
- The surgical management of nonovarian endometriosis, prior to initiation of an IVF cycle does not improve outcomes.
- The benefit of resection of large ovarian endometriotic cysts before undertaking an IVF cycle is controversial. Great care should be taken to preserve ovarian blood supply when such procedures are performed.
- The prolonged use of a GnRH agonist, in at least a subset of endometriosis patients, appears to improve IVF cycle outcome.

REFERENCES

1. Wainer R, Camus E, Camier B, Martin C, Vasseur C, Merlet F. Does hydrosalpinx reduce the pregnancy rate after in vitro fertilization? *Fertil Steril* 1997;68:1022–6.
2. Andersen AN, Yue Z, Meng FJ, Petersen K. Low implantation rate after in-vitro fertilization in patients with hydrosalpinges diagnosed by ultrasonography. *Hum Reprod* 1994;9:1935–8.
3. Strandell A, Waldenstrom U, Nilsson L, Hamberger L. Hydrosalpinx reduces in-vitro fertilization/embryo transfer pregnancy rates. *Hum Reprod* 1994;9:861–3.
4. Kasebji M, Sims J, Butler L, Muashe S. Reduced pregnancy rate with unilateral or bilateral hydrosalpinx after in vitro fertilization. *Eur J Obstet Gynecol Reprod Biol* 1994;56:129–32.
5. Vandromme J, Chasse E, Lejeune B, van Rysselborge M, Delvigne A, Leroy F. Hydrosalpinges in in-vitro fertilization: an unfavorable prognostic feature. *Hum Reprod* 1995;10:579–9.
6. Katz E, Akman M, Damewood M, Garcia J. Deleterious effect of the presence of hydrosalpinx on implantation and pregnancy rates with in vitro fertilization. *Fertil Steril* 1996;66:122–5.
7. Blazar AS, Hogan JW, Seifer DB, Frishman GF, Wheeler CA, Haning RV. The impact of hydrosalpinx on successful pregnancy in tubal factor infertility treated by in vitro fertilization. *Fertil Steril* 1997;67:517–20.
8. Sharara F, Scott R, Marut E, Queenan J. In vitro fertilization outcomes in women with hydrosalpinx. *Hum Reprod* 1996;11:526–30.
9. Murray DL, Sagoskin AW, Widra EA, Levy MJ. The adverse effect of hydrosalpinges on in vitro fertilization pregnancy rate and the benefit of surgical correction. *Fertil Steril* 1998;69:41–5.
10. Akman M, Garcia S, Damewood M, Watts L, Katz E. Hydrosalpinx affects the implantation of previously cryopreserved embryos. *Hum Reprod* 1996;11:1013–14.
11. Camus E, Poncelet C, Goffinet F, et al. Pregnancy rates after in vitro fertilization in cases of tubal infertility with and without hydrosalpinx: a meta-analysis of published comparative studies. *Hum Reprod* 1999;14:1243–9.
12. Ng EH, Yeung WS, Ho PC. The presence of hydrosalpinx may not adversely affect the implantation and pregnancy rates in in vitro fertilization. *J Reprod Genet* 1997;14:508–12.
13. Mansour RT, Aboulghar MA, Serour GI, Raafat R. Fluid accumulation of the uterine cavity before embryo transfer: a possible hindrance for implantation. *J In Vitro Fert Embryo Transf* 1991;8:157–9.
14. Mukherjee T, Copperman AB, McCaffrey C, Cook CA, Bustillo M, Obasaju MF. Hydrosalpinx fluid has embryotoxic effects on murine embryogenesis: a case for prophylactic salpingectomy. *Fertil Steril* 1996;66:851–3.
15. Beyler SA, James KP, Fritz MA, Meyer WR. Hydrosalpingeal fluid inhibits in-vitro embryonic development in a murine model. *Hum Reprod* 1997;12:2724–8.
16. Rawe VJ, Liu J, Shaffer S, Compton MG, Garcia JE, Katz E. Effect of human hydrosalpinx fluid on murine embryo development and implantation. *Fertil Steril* 1997;68:668–70.
17. Arrighi C, Lucas H, El-Mowafi D, Campana A, Chardonnens D. Effects of human hydrosalpinx fluid on in-vitro murine fertilization. *Hum Reprod* 2001;16:676–82.
18. Ajonuma L, Chan L, Ng E, et al. Characterization of epithelial cell culture from human hydrosalpinges and effects of its conditioned medium on embryo development and sperm motility. *Hum Reprod* 2003;18:291–8.
19. Toth M, Jeremias J, Ledger WJ, Witkin SS. In vivo tumor necrosis factor production in women with salpingitis. *Surg Gynecol Obstet* 1992;174:359–62.
20. Barmat L, Nasti K, Yang X, Spandorfer S, Kowalik A, El-Roiey A. Are cytokines and growth factors responsible for the detrimental effects of hydrosalpingeal fluid on pregnancy rates after in vitro fertilization-embryo transfer. *Fertil Steril* 1999;72:1110–12.
21. Lam P, Briton-Jones C, Cheung C, Po L, Cheung L, Hames F. Increased mRNA expression of vascular endothelial growth

factor and its receptor (flt-1) in the hydrosalpinx. *Hum Reprod* 2003;18:2264–9

22. Strandell A, Twinburn J, Wallin A. The presence of cytokines and growth factors in hydrosalpingeal fluid. *J Assist Reprod Genet* 2004;21:241–7.

23. Meyer WR, Castelbaum AJ, Somkuti S, et al. Hydrosalpinges adversely affect markers of endometrial receptivity. *Hum Reprod* 1997;12:1393–8.

24. Savains R, Pedrini J, Flores R, Fabris G, Zettler C. Expression of alpha 1 and beta 3 integrins subunits in the endometrium of patients with tubal phimosis or hydrosalpinx. *Fertil Steril* 2006; 85:188–92.

25. Daftary G, Taylor H. Hydrosalpinx fluid diminishes endometrial HOXA 10 expression. *Fertil Steril* 2002;78:577–80.

26. Choi B, Koong M, Lee J, et al. Hydrosalpinx fluid inhibits trophoblast cell proliferation in vitro culture system: implication for early implantation failure in women with hydrosalpinx fluid. Abstr O-197. *Fertil Steril* 1999;72:S76.

27. Ng E, Chan C, Tang O, Ho P. Comparison of endometrial and subendometrial blood flows among patients with and without hydrosalpinx shown on scanning during in vitro fertilization treatment. *Fertil Steril* 2006;85:333–8.

28. Strandell A, Lindhard A, Waldenstrom U, Thorburn J, Janson P, Hamberger L. Hydrosalpinx and IVF outcome: a prospective randomized multicentre trial in Scandinavia on salpingectomy prior to IVF. *Hum Reprod* 1999;14:2762–9.

29. Dechaud H, Daures JP, Arnal F, Humeau C, Hedon B. Does previous salpingectomy improve implantation and pregnancy rates in patients with severe tubal factor infertility who are undergoing in vitro fertilization? A pilot prospective randomized study. *Fertil Steril* 1998;69:1020–5.

30. Johnson N, Mak W, Sowter M. Laparoscopic salpingectomy for women with hydrosalpinges enhances the success of IVF: a Cochrane review. *Hum Reprod* 2002;17:543–8.

31. Sagoskin A, Lessey B, Mottla G, et al. Salpingectomy of proximal tubal occlusion of unilateral hydrosalpinx increases the potential for spontaneous pregnancy. *Hum Reprod* 2003;18:2634–7.

32. Czemiczky G, Landgren BM, Fried G, Wramsby H. High tubal damage grade is associated with low pregnancy rate in women undergoing in-vitro fertilization treatment. *Hum Reprod* 1996;11:2438–40.

33. deWit W, Gowrising CJ, Kuik DJ, Lens JW, Schats R. Only hydrosalpinges visible on ultrasound are associated with reduced implantation and pregnancy rates after in-vitro fertilization. *Hum Reprod* 1998;13:1696–701.

34. Bildirci I, Bukulmez O, Ensari A, Yarali H, Guregan T. A prospective evaluation of the effect of salpingectomy on endometrial receptivity in cases of women with communicating hydrosalpinges. *Hum Reprod* 2001;96:2422–6.

35. Ito C, Ito M, Itakura A, Hsai M, Ninta O, Mizutani S. A prospective evaluation of the effect of salpingectomy on endometrial lymphocyte clusters in patients with hydrosalpinges. *Fertil Steril* 2004;80:149–53.

36. Seli E, Kagiski U, Lakniak H, et al. Removal of hydrosalpinges increases endometrial leukemia inhibitory factor (LIF) expression at the time of the implantation window. *Hum Reprod* 2005; 20:3012–17.

37. Sharif K, Kaufmann M, Sharma V. Heterotopic pregnancy obtained after in-vitro fertilization and embryo transfer following bilateral total salpingectomy: case report. *Hum Reprod* 1994;9:1966–7.

38. San Filippo JS, Lincoln SR. Surgical treatment of diseases of the ovary. In: Keye W, Chang R, Rebar R, Soules M, eds. *Infertility: Evaluation and Treatment*. Philadelphia, PA: WB Saunders, 1995:539–51.

39. McComb P, Relbeke L. Decreasing the number of ovulations in the rabbit with surgical division of the blood vessels between the fallopian tube and ovary. *J Reprod Med* 1984;29:827–9.

40. Lass A, Ellenbogen A, Croucher C, et al. Effect of salpingectomy on ovarian response to superovulation in an in vitro fertilization-embryo transfer program. *Fertil Steril* 1998;70:1035–8.

41. Chan C, Ng E, Li C, Ho P. Impaired ovarian blood flow and reduced antral follicle count following laparoscopic salpingectomy for ectopic pregnancy. *Hum Reprod* 2003;18: 2175–80.

42. Gelbaya T, Navio L, Fitzgerald C, Horne G, Bason D, Veherman B. Ovarian response to gonadotropins after laparoscopic salpingectomy or the division of fallopian tubes for hydrosalpinges. *Fertil Steril* 2006;85:1464–8.

43. Dar P, Sachs AS, Strassburger D, Bukovsky I, Arieli S. Ovarian function before and after salpingectomy in artificial reproductive technology patients. *Hum Reprod* 2000;15:142–4.

44. Tal J, Paltieli Y, Korobotchka R, Ziskind G, Eibschitz I, Ohel G. Ovarian response to gonadotropin stimulation in repeated IVF cycles after unilateral salpingectomy. *J Assist Reprod Genet* 2002; 18:451–5.

45. Strandell A, Lindhard A, Waldenstrom U, Thorburn J. Prophylactic salpingectomy does not impair the ovarian response of IVF treatment. *Hum Reprod* 2001;16:1135–9.

46. Surrey E Schoolcraft W. Laparoscopic management of hydrosalpinges prior to in-vitro fertilization-embryo transfer (IVF-ET): salpingectomy vs. proximal tubal occlusion. *Fertil Steril* 2001;75:612–17.

47. Stadtmauer L, Riehl R, Toma S, Talbert L. Cauterization of hydrosalpinges before in vitro fertilization is an effective surgical treatment associated with improved pregnancy rates. *Am J Obstet Gynecol* 2000;183:367–71.

48. Kerin J and Cattanach S. Successful pregnancy outcome with the use of in vitro fertilization after essure hysteroscopic sterilization. *Fertil Steril* 2007;87:1212.

49. Sharara F, Scott R Jr., Marut E, Queenan J Jr. In-vitro fertilization outcome in women with hydrosalpinx. *Hum Reprod* 1996;11: 526–30.

50. Hurst B, Tucker K, Awoniyi C, Schlaff W. Hydrosalpinx treated with extended doxycycline does not compromise the success of in vitro fertilization. *Fertil Steril* 2001;75:1017–19.

51. Hammadieh N, Afnan M, Khaldoun S, Evans J, Amso N. The effect of hydrosalpinx on IVF outcome: a prospective randomized controlled trial of ultrasound guided hydrosalpinx aspiration during egg collection. Abstr P-35. *Fertil Steril* 2003;80: S131.

52. Van Voorhis B, Sparks A, Syrop C, Stovall D. Ultrasound-guided aspiration of hydrosalpinges is associated with improved pregnancy and implantation rates after in-vitro fertilization cycles. *Hum Reprod* 1998;13:736–9.

53. Aboulghar M, Mansour R, Serour G, Settar M, Awad M, Amin Y. Transvaginal ultrasonic guided aspiration of pelvic inflammatory cystic masses before ovulation induction for in vitro fertilization. *Fertil Steril* 1990:53;311–14.

54. Sowter M, Akande V, Williams J, Hull M. Is the outcome of in-vitro fertilization and embryo transfer treatment improved by spontaneous or surgical drainage of a hydrosalpinx? *Hum Reprod* 1997;10:2147–50.

55. Bloeche M, Schreiner T, Lisse K. Recurrence of hydrosalpinges after transvaginal aspiration of tubal fluid in an IVF cycle with development of a serometra. *Hum Reprod* 1997;12:266–71.

56. Hinkley M, Milki A. Rapid reaccumulation of hydrometra after drainage at embryo transfer in patients with hydrosalpinx. *Fertil Steril* 2003;80:1268–71.

57. Strandell A, Lindhard A, Eckerlind I. Cost effectiveness analysis of salpingectomy prior to IVF based on a randomized controlled trial. *Hum Reprod* 2005;20:3289–92.

58. Wang C, Lee C, Lai Y, Tsai C, Chang M, Soong Y. Comparison of hysterosalpingography and hysteroscopy in female infertility. *J Am Assoc Gynecol Laparosc* 1996;3:581–4.

59. Kerin J, Surrey E. Transvaginal imaging and the infertility patient. *Obstet Gynecol Clin (NA)*. 1991;18:749–77.

60. Battarowich O, Kurtz A, Pennell R, et al. Pitfalls in the sonographic diagnosis of uterine fibroids. *Am J Roentgenol* 1988;151:725–8.

61. Shamma F, Lee G, Gutmann J, Lavy G. The role of office hysteroscopy in in vitro fertilization. *Fertil Steril* 1992;58:1237–9.

62. Oliveira F, Abdelmassih V, Diamond M. Uterine cavity findings and hysteroscopic intervention in patients undergoing in vitro fertilization-embryo transfer who repeatedly cannot conceive. *Fertil Steril* 2003;80:1371–5.

63. de Kroon C, Jansen F, Louwe L, Dieben S, Van Houwelingen H, Trimbos J. Technology assessment of saline contrast hysterosonography. *Am J Obstet Gynecol* 2003;188:945–9.

64. Coutinko V, Maie H. The contractile response of the human uterus, fallopian tubes and ovary to prostaglandins in vivo. *Fertil Steril* 1971;22:539–43.

65. Deligdish L, Lowenthal M. Endometrial changes associated with myomata of the uterus. *J Clin Pathol* 1970;23:676–80.

66. Ng E, Ho P. Doppler ultrasound examination of uterine arteries on the day of oocyte retrieval in patients with uterine fibroids undergoing IVF. *Hum Reprod* 2002;17:765–70.

67. Sladkevicius P, Valentin L, Marsal K. Transvaginal Doppler examination of uteri with myoma. *J Clin Ultrasound* 1996;24:135–40.

68. Rein M, Powell W, Walter F, et al. Cytogenetic abnormalities in uterine myomas are associated with myoma size. *Mol Hum Reprod* 1998;4:83–6.

69. Lepper P, Catherino W, Segars J. A new hypothesis about the origin of uterine fibroids based on gene expression profiling with microarrays. *Am J Obstet Gynecol* 2006;195:415–20.

70. Pritts E. Fibroids and infertility: a systematic review of the evidence. *Obstet Gynecol Surv* 2001;56:483–91.

71. Fahri J, Ashkenazi J, Feldberg D, Dicker D, Orvieto R, Ben Rafael Z. Effect of uterine leiomyomata on the results of in vitro fertilization treatment. *Hum Reprod* 1995;10:2576–8.

72. Stovall D, Parrish S, Van Voorhis B, Hahn S, Sparks A, Syrop C. Uterine leiomyomas reduce the efficacy of assisted reproduction cycles. *Hum Reprod* 1998;13:192–7.

73. Eldar-Geva T, Meagher S, Healy D, MacLachlan V, Breheny S, Wood C. Effect of intramural, subserosal, and submucosal uterine fibroids on the outcome of assisted reproductive technology treatment. *Fertil Steril* 1998;70:687–91.

74. Hart R, Khalaf Y, Yeong C-T, Seed P, Taylor A, Braude P. A prospective controlled study of the effect of intramural fibroids on the outcome of assisted conception. *Hum Reprod* 2001;16:2411–17.

75. Donnez J, Jadoul P. What are the implications of myomas on fertility? *Hum Reprod* 2002;17:1424–30.

76. Surrey E, Lietz A, Schoolcraft W. Impact of intramural leiomyomata in patients with normal endometrial cavity on in vitro fertilization-embryo transfer cycle outcome. *Fertil Steril* 2001;75:405–10.

77. Olivera F, Abdelmassih V, Diamond M, Dozortseo D, Melo N, Abdelmassih R. Impact of subserosal and intramural uterine fibroids that do not distort the endometrial cavity on the outcome of in vitro fertilization-intracytoplasmic sperm injection. *Fertil Steril* 2004;81:582–7.

78. Yarali H, Bukulmez O. The effect of intramural and subserous uterine fibroids on implantation and clinical pregnancy rates in patients having intracytoplasmic sperm injection. *Arch Gynecol Obstet* 2002;266:30–3.

79. Jun S, Ginsburg E, Racowsky C, Wise L, Hornstein M. Uterine leiomyomas and their effect on in vitro fertilization outcome: a retrospective study. *J Assist Reprod Genet* 2001;13:139–43.

80. Check J, Choe J, Lee G, Dieterich C. The effect on IVF outcome of small intramural fibroids not compressing the uterine cavity as determined by a prospective matched control study. *Hum Reprod* 2002;17:1244–8.

81. Seoud M, Patterson R, Muasher S, Coddington C. Effect of myomas on prior myomectomy or in vitro fertilization (IVF) performance. *J Assist Reprod Genet* 1992;9:655–8.

82. Surrey E, Minjarez D, Stevens J, Schoolcraft W. Effect of myomectomy on the outcome of the assisted reproductive technologies. *Fertil Steril* 2005;83:1473–9.

83. Bergendal A, Naffah S, Nagy C, et al. Outcome of IVF in patients with endometriosis in comparison with tubal-factor infertility. *J Assist Reprod Genet* 1998;15:530–4.

84. Simon C, Gutierrez A, Vidal A, et al. Outcome of patients with endometriosis in assisted reproduction: results from in-vitro fertilization and oocyte donation. *Hum Reprod* 1994;9:725–9.

85. Wardle PG, Mitchell JD, McLaughlin EA, et al. Endometriosis and ovulatory disorder: reduced fertilization in vitro compared with tubal and unexplained infertility. *Lancet* 1985;2:236–9.

86. Arici A, Oral E, Bukulmez O, et al. The effect of endometriosis on implantation: results from the Yale University in vitro fertilization and embryo transfer program. *Fertil Steril* 1996;65:603–7.

87. Olivennes F, Feldberg D, Liu HC, et al. Endometriosis: a stage by stage analysis in the role of in vitro fertilization. *Fertil Steril* 1995;64:392–8.

88. Geber S, Paraschos T, Atkinson G, et al. Results of IVF in patients with endometriosis: the severity of the disease does not affect outcome, or the incidence of miscarriage. *Hum Reprod* 1995;10:1507–11.

89. Barnhart K, Dunsmoor-Su R, Coutifaris C. Effect of endometriosis on in vitro fertilization. *Fertil Steril* 2002;77:1148–55.

90. Azem F, Lessing JB, Geva E, et al. Patients with stages III and IV endometriosis have a poorer outcome of in vitro fertilization-embryo transfer than patients with tubal infertility. *Fertil Steril* 1999;72:1107–9.

91. Pal L, Shifren JL, Isaacson K, et al. Impact of varying stages of endometriosis on the outcome of in vitro fertilization-embryo transfer. *J Assist Reprod Genet* 1998;15:27–31.

92. Dlugi A, Loy R, Dieterle S, et al. The effect of endometriomas on in vitro fertilization outcome. *J In Vitro Fertil Emb Transf* 1989;6:338–41.

93. Yanushpolsky E, Best C, Jackson K, et al. Effects of endometriomas on oocyte quality and pregnancy rates in in vitro fertilization cycles; a prospective case-controlled study. *J Assist Reprod Genet* 1998;15:193–7.

94. Al-Azemi M, Lopez Bernal A, Steele J, et al. Ovarian response to repeated controlled stimulation in in vitro cycles in patients with ovarian endometriosis. *Hum Reprod* 2000;15:72–5.

95. Khamsi F, Yavas Y, Lacanna IC, et al. Exposure of human oocytes to endometrioma fluid does not alter fertilization or early embryo development. *J Assist Reprod Genet* 2001;18:106–9.

96. Surrey M, Hill D. Treatment of endometriosis by carbon dioxide laser during gamete intrafallopian transfer. *J Am Coll Surg* 1994;79:440–2.

97. Surrey E, Schoolcraft W. Does surgical management of endometriosis within 6 months of an in vitro fertilization-embryo transfer cycle improve outcome? *J Assist Reprod Genet* 2003;20:365–70.

98. Aboulghar M, Mansour R, Serour G, et al. The outcome of in vitro fertilization in advanced endometriosis with previous surgery: a case-controlled study. *Am J Obstet Gynecol* 2003;188:371–5.

99. Canis M, Pouly S, Tamburro S,et al. Ovarian response during embryo transfer cycles after laparoscopic ovarian cystectomy for endometriotic cysts of >3 cm diameter. *Hum Reprod* 2001;12:2583–6.

100. Donnez J, Wyns C, Nisolle M. Does ovarian surgery for endometriomas impair the ovarian response to gonadotropin? *Fertil Steril* 2001;76:662–5.

101. Marconi G, Vilela M, Quintana R, et al. Laparoscopic ovarian cystectomy of endometriomas does not affect ovarian response to gonadotropin stimulation. *Fertil Steril* 2002;78:876–8.

102. Ho H-Y, Lee R, Hwu Y-M, et al. Poor response of ovaries with endometrioma previously treated with cystectomy to controlled ovarian hyperstimulation. *J Assist Reprod Genet* 2002;19:507–11.

103. Garcia-Velasco J, Corona J, Requena A, Remohi J, Simon C, Pellicer A. Should we operate on ovarian endometriomas prior to IVF? *Fertil Steril* 2002;78:S203.

104. Surrey E, Silverberg K, Surrey M, Schoolcraft W. The effect of prolonged GnRH agonist therapy on in vitro fertilization-embryo transfer cycle outcome in endometriosis patients: a multicenter randomized trial. *Fertil Steril* 2002;78:699–704.

105. Chedid S, Camus W, Smitz J, et al. Comparison among different ovarian stimulation regimens for assisted procreation procedures in patients with endometriosis. *Hum Reprod* 1995;10:2406–10.

106. Wardle P, Foster P, Mitchel J, et al. Endometriosis and IVF: effect of prior therapy. *Lancet* 1986;8475(1):276–7.

107. Dicker D, Goldman GA, Ashkenazi J, et al. The value of pretreatment with long-term gonadotropin-releasing hormone (GnRH) analogue in IVF-ET therapy of severe endometriosis. *Hum Reprod* 1990;5:418–20.

108. Marcus S, Edwards R. High rates of pregnancy after long-term down-regulation of women with severe endometriosis. *Am J Obstet Gynecol* 1994;171:812–17.

109. Curtis P, Jackson A, Bernard A, Shaw R. Pretreatment with gonadotrophin releasing hormone (GnRH) analogue prior to in vitro fertilization for patients with endometriosis. *Eur J Obstet Gynecol Reprod Biol* 1993;52:211–16.

110. Nakamura K, Oosawa M, Kondou I, et al. Menotropin stimulation after prolonged gonadotropin releasing hormone agonist pretreatment for in vitro fertilization in patients with endometriosis. *J Assist Reprod Genet* 1992;9:113–17.

111. Remorgida V, Anserini P, Croce S, et al. Comparison of different ovarian stimulation protocols for gamete intrafallopian transfer in patients with minimal and mild endometriosis. *Fertil Steril* 1990;53:1060–3.

112. Sallam H, Garcia-Velasco J, Dias S, Arici A. Long-term pituitary down-regulation before in vitro fertilization (IVF) for women with endometriosis. *The Cochrane Database for Systemic Reviews* 2006, Iss. No. 1 Art No.: CD004635. pub 2.

113. Imai A, Takagi A, Tamaya T. Gonadotropin-releasing hormone analog repairs reduced endometrial cell apoptosis in endometriosis in vitro. *Am J Obstet Gynecol* 2000;182:1142–6.

114. Taketani Y, Kuo T-M, Mizuno M. Comparison of cytokine levels and embryo toxicity in peritoneal fluid in infertile women with untreated or treated endometriosis. *Am J Obstet Gynecol* 1992;167:265–70.

115. Sharpe-Timms K, Keisler L, McIntush E, et al. Tissue inhibitors of metalloproteinase-1 concentrations are attenuated in peritoneal fluid and sera of women with endometriosis and restored in sera by gonadotropin-releasing hormone agonist therapy. *Fertil Steril* 1998;69:1128–34.

116. Garzetti GG, Ciavattini A, Provinciali M, et al. Natural cytoxicity and GnRH agonist administration in advanced endometriosis: positive modulation on natural killer cell activity. *Obstet Gynecol* 1996;88:234–40.

117. Lessey BA. Medical management of endometriosis and infertility. *Fertil Steril* 2000;73:1089–96.

118. Tei C, Maruyama T, Kuji N, et al. Reduced expression of $\alpha_v\beta_3$ integrin in the endometrium of unexplained infertility patients with recurrent IVF-ET failures: improvement by danazol treatment. *J Assist Reprod Genet* 2003;20:13–20.

119. Rizk B, Abdalla H. Assisted Reproductive Technology in Endometriosis. In: Rizk B, Abdalla H (Eds.), *Endometriosis. Second Ed.* Oxford: United Kingdom, Health Press, 2003, chapter 6, pp. 74–76.

120. Rizk B, Abdalla H. In Vitro fertilization. In: Rizk B, Abdalla H (Eds.), *Infertility and Assisted Reproductive Technology*. Cambridge: United Kingdom, Cambridge University Press, 2008, chapter 10, pp. 112–114.

40

IVF in the Medically Complicated Patient

Botros R. M. B. Rizk, Christopher B. Rizk, Sameh Mikhail, Christine B. Rizk, Hany F. Moustafa, James Hole, Sheri Owens, Susan Baker, Kathy B. Porter

The majority of women undergoing assisted reproduction are healthy and relatively young. However, the tendency to delay pregnancy to later on in life may mean that some of the patients may present with a concurrent condition that may have implications for in vitro fertilization (IVF), pregnancy, and its outcome. Preparing the couple for pregnancy is an important task, which the infertility specialist has to undertake.

Some of the important issues that may be challenging to the clinician are medical problems that affect a variety of systems. With the increasing survival of cancer patients, many patients are not only satisfied with their cure but are also eager to fulfill their reproductive potential. The patient with endocrine problems such as hyperprolactinemia and hypopituitarism, Cushing's syndrome, and diabetes mellitus have to be addressed prior to assisted conception couples that are discordant for human immunodeficiency virus (HIV) present their own challenge regarding infertility treatment. Couples with sexual dysfunction may also present for assisted conception. Finally, patients at risk for thrombosis could pose tremendous challenges during assisted reproduction treatment and a subsequent pregnancy as discussed in the chapter 45.

Some patients present with gynecologic problems that are either challenging or that impact the IVF outcome. Patients with endometriosis exemplify this scenario as discussed in the chapter 42. Patients with fibroids and hydrosalpynx require surgical treatment prior to IVF as discussed in the chapter 39. Patients with congenital uterine abnormalities can also impact the outcome of assisted reproduction or result in miscarriage as discussed in the chapter 35.

PRECONCEPTION COUNSELING

Despite tremendous advances in prenatal care, certain adverse pregnancy outcomes such as preterm delivery and birth defects have not changed. A confounding factor for IVF pregnancies is the increased number of multiple pregnancies and the relatively increased number of high-risk pregnancies among women with chronic medical problems.

The principal goal of preconception counseling is to maximize the quality of fetal and newborn life through primary prevention. We believe that even low-risk populations should be offered preconception care; however, there is no consensus in offering preconception care to this group of patients, and practically speaking, most of these patients do not seek the advice of a specialist.

In contrast, patients with diabetes, hypertension, and those taking potentially teratogenic drugs and patients with previous deep vein thromboses (DVTs) are typically offered preconception care.

The components of preconception care have been summarized by Steegers and Wildschut (1). The four main components are risk assessment, health promotion, intervention to eliminate risk factors, and adequate counseling.

Medical Risk Assessment

Risk assessment includes screening for medical risk factors by the evaluation of the couple's obstetric and medical history, family history, medication use, teratogen exposure, and dietary habits. Assessment of the partner's history is crucial, particularly regarding genetic abnormalities. Additional evaluation often includes laboratory tests and imaging including blood typing and antibody screen, hemoglobinopathies, sickle cell anemia, Tay-Sachs disease, and infectious disease such as hepatitis and sexually transmitted disease such as HIV.

Health Promotion

Health promotion should focus on the stoppage of alcohol use, smoking, and substance abuse. It also addresses the prevention of infection of toxoplasmosis and listeria. Preconception health promotion should encourage the use of folic acid. In healthy women, 400 µg per day is advised and in patients with a previous child with a neural tube defect, 4 mg per day is advised.

Alcohol

Alcohol is the most common human teratogen used. Heavy drinking during pregnancy could possibly result in serious adverse outcomes.

Tobacco

Cigarette smoking could possibly increase pregnancy complications including spontaneous abortion, low birth weight, premature delivery, and placental abruption. Unfortunately, it is estimated that 20–30 percent of pregnant women smoked.

Vaccines

Appropriate administration of vaccines that are safe during pregnancy should be encouraged. In contrast, use of live vaccines should be discouraged. The World Health Organization (WHO) recommends that active vaccination with live attenuated measles, mumps, rubella, bacillus calmette Guerin; and yellow fever virus vaccines should be avoided in pregnancy.

Counseling

Counseling prior to IVF should focus on specific issues such as genetics or previous complications.

CANCER PATIENTS

Cancer patients present particular challenges to the IVF unit. In the United States, cancer is diagnosed in approximately 650,000 women each year. As many of these women are of reproductive age, the effect of their cancer treatment on their fertility has to be considered.

The Impact of Cancer and Its Treatment on IVF

Patients with malignant disease may have reduced fertility as a result of their disease. Men with Hodgkin's disease have impaired semen quality (2, 3). Cancer may also influence female fertility by reducing the oocyte quality and fertility (4).

The Impact of IVF on Malignant Disease

The main concerns about IVF and malignant disease relate to the issue of the potential delay in the starting of the patient's chemotherapy or of any possible effect of hormonal changes on the cancer. The impact and the magnitude of the delay should always be discussed with the patient and the patient's oncologist. Other factors such as the patient's normal menstrual cycle might also influence the time until the treatment is started. Oral contraceptives are frequently used to regulate the menstrual cycle prior to IVF. Gonadotropin-releasing hormone antagonists have also been used to shorten the IVF cycle (5).

Breast cancer is the most common cancer in women of reproductive age. Approximately, 15 percent of breast cancers are diagnosed in women younger than forty years (2). Potentially, there may be time to perform IVF with cryopreservation. This may not be recommended because of preexisting metastases in the ovary. Controlled superovulation exposes the patients to very high estradiol concentrations but only for a few days. The use of antiestrogens, used for the treatment of breast cancer, for ovarian stimulation has been successfully demonstrated (6).

It is of utmost importance for the patient to have the time to consider IVF. Independent counseling is valuable in some circumstances. Measurement of early-cycle FSH is paramount before the patient receives any form of chemotherapy. In addition, antral follicle count and ovarian volume is tremendously useful and is part of the preparation. The effects of radiation on uterine artery blood flow and endometrial development is important to consider. The use of GnRH antagonists is attractive to shorten the IVF cycle. It is usually started in the early follicular phase of the cycle. If the patient is in luteal phase at the time of presentation, a small dose of GnRH antagonist can be used to cause follicular regression or luteolysis, allowing gonadotropin administration to begin a few days later (2). Antiestrogen medication such as tamoxifen has been demonstrated to result in a modest increase in oocytes and embryos recovered in breast cancer patients. The use of aromatase inhibitors has also been advocated (7).

COUPLES DISCORDANT FOR HIV

HIV affects fifty million people worldwide. It affects men and women equally, although in the United States, the majority of cases are in reproductive-age males.

Despite statements made by the American Society for Reproductive Medicine (8), the American College of Obstetrics and Gynecology (9), and the European Society of Human Reproduction and Embryology (10) encouraging physicians to provide fertility services to HIV-seropositive men and women, few programs are known to be openly compliant (11). It is almost a decade ago that we participated in a debate about IVF treatment in couples with HIV, and we have to admit that at that time, we were opposed to offer treatment to these couples (12). Our main concern had been that the infected parent or parents might not survive long enough to offer their children the care and support that children need to reach adulthood. At this point in time, we feel that this position has to be changed because of the significant improvement in the length and quality of life of these patients. One issue that we feel very strongly about is that close collaboration with infectious disease specialists remains to be a prior requisite for us before initiating the infertility treatment. Since then, we encourage active treatment of couples discordant for HIV, keeping in mind that their personal health and their children's health come first. Our limited experience has been rewarded by successful IVF outcome, and the children continue to remain HIV negative.

Preparing the Couple for IVF

HIV-infected patients are usually under close medical surveillance by infectious disease specialists. Plasma HIV-RNA viral counts and CD4 status should be repeated before their IVF cycle. Other infections should be screened for including hepatitis A, B, and C and syphilis (RPR). Liver functions and renal functions should be recently performed. We emphasize that the couples should be evaluated and obtain medical clearance by a maternal-fetal and infectious disease specialist before they embark on assisted reproduction. Genetic testing that could be offered include cystic fibrosis, hemoglobin electrophoresis, and Tay-Sachs disease if deemed necessary.

Their partners should be HIV tested and be seronegative. The couples should comply with safe-sex practices and agree to use condoms. HIV-seropositive women should receive antibiotics prior to hysterosalpingography or sonohysterography and medications may be continued for seven to ten days. Ultrasonographers should avoid performing sonograms during the menstrual cycle to avoid blood contamination of the ultrasound equipment and a thorough cleaning with a mild bleach solution to eliminate the presence of live virus (11, 13).

Managing the IVF Cycle in HIV Discordant Couples

Standard IVF protocols are used for controlled ovarian hyperstimulation: aspiration of oocytes is performed thirty-five to thirty-six hours following the injection of human chorionic gonadotropin injection, a fresh semen sample is requested for ICSI, and sperm-washing techniques have been recommended to reduce the likelihood of horizontal transmission of HIV (11, 14) reviewed the pregnancy rates in more than 3,600 published attempts and no seroconversions occurred in women or children. Embryo transfers are scheduled on the third or fifth day and assisted hatching is not performed on the embryos of HIV patients.

Post-IVF Follow-up

Serial blood testing is done every trimester during the pregnancy. Newborns are tested at birth and three months of age. Mothers are tested at delivery and three months postpartum using sensitive assays to detect a level of less than fifty copies per ml of blood.

The Special Needs of HIV-Seropositive Women

There has been a significant improvement in the outcome of pregnant women who are seropositive. The risk of vertical transmission of HIV to the fetus is significantly reduced from 25 percent to less than 2 percent with the use of appropriate therapy.

OBESITY AND ASSISTED REPRODUCTIVE TECHNOLOGY

Obesity results from a combination of genetic and environmental factors. Several methods have been used to estimate obesity including body mass index (BMI), waist to hip ratio, abdominal volume index, abdominal-visceral adiposity, and body fat content (15). The most widely used index is BMI. It is defined as the weight in kilograms divided by the square of the height in meters. The WHO defines "overweight" as having a BMI of 25–29.9 and "obese" as greater than or equal to a BMI of 30. A BMI of more than twenty-five is associated with a risk of type 2 diabetes mellitus, essential hypertension, hypercholesterolemia, coronary artery disease, gall bladder disease, asthma, and osteoarthritis.

Impact of Obesity on IVF Outcome

Pregnancy rates after IVF among obese (BMI = 30–35) and very obese (BMI = 35) is reduced compared with normal-weight women (15, 16). Android body fat distribution in females may impair the pregnancy rate after IVF-ET (17).

Obesity may impact ART through a variety of mechanisms. Obese patients are more likely to have menstrual and ovulatory disorders, making it more difficult to plan the start of their treatment. An increased cancellation rate may result from the failure to downregulate the pituitary-ovarian axis. An association between obesity and FSH requirements for IVF has been suggested. Obesity may increased lead to complications at oocyte retrieval.

Pregnancy Outcome in Obese Patients

Obese patients are more prone to several adverse pregnancy outcomes. Obesity is associated with an increased risk in first-trimester miscarriages in IVF pregnancies. Obesity also predisposes to hypertension, glucose intolerance, and gestational diabetes and venous thrombolic disorders. Obesity is also associated with fetal macrosomia and shoulder dystocia. They are more likely to require a cesarean section for failure to progress and a higher rate of postnatal thromboembolic complications. Compared with normal-weight women, obese mothers are more likely to have infants with neural tube defects, heart defects, omphaloceles, and multiple anomalies. This could possibly be related to hyperglycemia, hyperinsulinemia, and dietary vitamin deficiencies.

Ola and Ledger (15) proposed the question whether a cutoff BMI should be imposed for withholding IVF treatment in obese patients. They noted that some reports link obesity with reproductive disorders and reduced fecundity. Others have not found a significant negative effect on IVF pregnancy outcome. In the United Kingdom, clinical guidelines or the evaluation and treatment of infertility problems were commissioned by the National Institute for Clinical Excellence and published in 2004. They recommended that BMI outside the range of ninteen–thirty is likely to reduce the success of ART procedures, based on evidence of four retrospective studies. However, they concluded that withholding assisted conception treatment for moderate to obese patients based on reduced pregnancy rates is still open to question.

In summary, obesity might affect the outcome of IVF and pregnancy, but with careful management, a good outcome can be achieved. Provided that obese patients are carefully advised about the problems that may be encountered during IVF and the pregnancy that follows and that they give informed consent that they wish to proceed, the refusal of treatment may be unethical. Adequate advice must always be given about healthy lifestyle, exercise, and weight loss.

PATIENTS WITH SYSTEMIC LUPUS ERYTHEMATOSUS (SLE)

Fertility is thought to be almost normal in patients with SLE except for amenorrhea during flare-ups and ovarian failure secondary to cyclophosphamide therapy. Preservation of ovarian function during and after chemotherapy has attracted both scientific researchers and clinicians to contribute significant research. Blumenfeld (18) described the preliminary encouraging experience in women with lymphoma and in with temporary induction of prepubertal hormonal milieu during chemotherapy resulted in a decreased risk of premature ovarian failure. These preliminary studies suggest that a monthly injection of gonadotropin-releasing hormone agonist in eighteen patients with SLE undergoing chemotherapy. Their results demonstrated that none of the eighteen women receiving GnRH agonist at the same time as an alkylating agent chemotherapy or chlorambucil suffered from premature ovarian failure. Five of nine patients that did not receive GnRH experienced premature ovarian failure.

Effect of IVF on SLE

The exponential rise of serum estradiol in controlled ovarian hyperstimulation in ART may cause an SLE flare-up. The risks of controlled ovarian hyperstimulation in SLE patients have been reported by Gubbala (21). In nineteen women with SLE and APS who have undergone sixty-eight IVF cycles, four IVF cycles (25 percent) have resulted in SLE flare-up and two cycles (13 percent) in OHSS.

Impact of SLE on IVF

It has been suggested that SLE may reduce the success of IVF-ET. The presence of antinuclear antibodies may reduce the implantation rate in IVF patients. The exact mechanism remains to be elucidated. Patients with long-standing SLE may have poor pregnancy outcomes. Active renal disease and maternal hypertension may increase the chances of premature birth and fetal loss. Routine screening for SLE and other immunologic conditions always creates a stimulating discussion. It is estimated that one to two percent of undiagnosed SLE may be present in a cohort of infertile women. Their results demonstrated that none of the eighteen women receiving GnRH agonist at the same time as an alkylating agent chemotherapy or chlorambucil suffered from premature ovarian failure. Five of nine patients that did not receive GnRH experienced premature ovarian failure (19,20).

CONCLUSIONS

In the majority of cases women undergoing ART are healthy. As a result of delay in child bearing there may be a higher preponderance of medical problems in this group. Multiple pregnancies might complicate the pregnancy. Prepregnancy counseling physical, psychological and ethical is of paramount importance. It is argued that it should be offered to every couple. Alcohol and smoking cessation is a priority. Weight loss and physical fitness are useful. Control of hypertension and diabetes is usually attended to well. Pregnancy in cancer survivors is ever increasing. Optimizing IVF outcome requires detailed attention to medical, surgical and psychological preparation. The influence of religious and ethical views should be respected.

KEY POINTS

■ The majority of women undergoing assisted reproduction are healthy and relatively young.

■ Despite tremendous advances in prenatal care, certain adverse pregnancy outcomes such as preterm delivery and birth defects have not changed.

■ A confounding factor for IVF pregnancies is the increased number of multiple pregnancies and the relatively increased number of high risk pregnancies among women with chronic medical problems.

■ The four main components of preconception care are risk assessment, health promotion, intervention to eliminate risk factors, and adequate counseling.

■ Breast cancer is the most common cancer in women of reproductive age.

■ Aromatase inhibitors, tamoxifen, and GnRH antagonists are useful for controlled ovarian hyperstimulation in breast cancer patients.

■ The main concerns about IVF and malignant disease relate to the issue of the potential delay in the starting of the patient's chemotherapy or of any possible effect of hormonal changes on the cancer.

■ Couples discordant for HIV should be treated with respect, fair consideration, and in close communication with their infectious disease specialist.

■ Pregnancy rates after IVF among obese and very obese patients is reduced compared to women of normal weight.

■ Fertility is thought to be almost normal in patients with SLE except for amenorrhea during flare-ups and ovarian failure secondary to cyclophosphamide therapy.

■ Preservation of ovarian function during and after chemotherapy has attracted both scientific researchers and clinicians to contribute significant research.

REFERENCES

1. Steegers EAP and Wildschut HIJ. Preparing for pregnancy: preconception care. In: Macklon NS (ed.), *IVF in the Medically Complicated Patient: A Guide to Management*. Taylor and Francis, London: 2005, Chapter 12, pp. 181–203.

2. Anderson RA. The patient with malignant disease. In: Macklon NS (ed.), *IVF in the Medically Complicated Patient: A Guide to Management*. Taylor and Francis, London: 2005, Chapter 3, pp. 41–50.

3. Rueffer U, Breuer K, Josting A, et al. Male gonadal dysfunction in patients with Hodgkin's disease prior to treatment. *Ann Oncol* 2001; 12:1307–1311.

4. Pal L, Leykin L, Schifren JL, et al. Malignancy may adversely influence the quality and behaviour of oocytes. *Hum Reprod* 1998; 13:1837–1840.

5. Andersen RA, Kinniburgh D, Baird DT. Preliminary evidence of the use of gonadotrophin releasing-hormone antagonist in superovulation/IVF prior to cancer treatment. *Hum Reprod* 1999; 14:2665–2668.

6. Oktay K, Buyuk E, Davis O, et al. Fertility preservation in breast cancer patients: IVF and embryo cryopreservation after ovarian stimulation with tamoxifen. *Hum Reprod* 2003; 18:90–95.

7. Sonmezer M, Oktay K. Fertility preservation in female patients. *Hum Reprod Update* 2004; 10:251–266.

8. Ethics Committee of the ASRM. HIV and infertility treatment. *Fertil Steril* 2002; 77: 218–222.

9. American College of Obstetrics and Gynecologists. HIV: Ethical Guidelines for Obstetricians and Gynecologists, April 2001. ACOG Committee Opinion 255, Washington DC; ACOG, 2001.

10. The ESHRE Ethics and Law Task Force. Task Force 8: Ethics of medically assisted fertility treatment for HIV positive men and women. *Hum Reprod* 2004; 19: 2454–6.

11. Sauer MV. The couple discordant for human immunodeficiency virus. In: Macklon NS (ed.), *IVF in the Medically Complicated Patient: A Guide to Management*. Taylor and Francis, London: 2005, Chapter 5, pp. 61–71.

12. Rizk B, Dill R. Counseling HIV patients pursuing infertility investigation and treatment. *Hum Reprod* 1997;12(3):415–416.

13. Sauer MV. Sperm washing techniques address the fertility needs of HIV-seropositive men: a clinical review. *Reprod Biomed Online* 2005; 10:135–140.

14. Semprini AE, Levi-Seti P, Bozzo M, et al. Insemination of HIV-negative women with processed semen of HIV-positive partners. *Lancet* 1992; 340:1317–1319.

15. Ola B, Ledger L. The obese patient. In: Macklon NS (ed.), *IVF in the Medically Complicated Patient: A Guide To Management*. Taylor and Francis, London: 2005, Chapter 7, pp. 87–100.

16. Wang JX, Davies M, Norman RJ. Body mass and probability of pregnancy during assisted reproduction treatment: retrospective study. *BMJ* 2000; 321:1320–1321.

17. Wass P, Waldenstrom U, Rossner S, Hellberg D. An android body fat distribution in females impairs the pregnancy rate of in-vitro fertilization-embryo transfer. *Hum Reprod* 1997; 12:2057–2060.

18. Blumenfeld Z. The patient with systemic lupus erythematosus. In: Macklon, Nick S (ed.), *IVF in the Medically Complicated Patient: A Guide To Management*. Taylor and Francis, London: 2005, Chapter 4, pp. 51–60.

19. Blumenfeld Z, Shapiro D, Shteinberg M, et al. Preservation of fertility and ovarian function and minimizing gonadotoxicity in young women with systemic erythematosus treated by chemotherapy. *Lupus* 2000; 9:1–5.

20. Blumenfeld Z. Ovarian cryopreservation versus ovarian suppression by GnRH analogues: primum non nocere. *Hum Reprod* 2004; 19:1924–1925.

21. Guballa N, Sammaritano L, Schwartzman S, et al. Ovulation induction and in vitro fertilization in systemic lupus erythematosus and antiphospholipid syndrome. *Arthritis Rheum* 2000; 43:550–556.

22. Rizk B, Abdalla H. In vitro fertilization. In Rizk B, Abdalla H (Eds.) Infertility and assisted reproductive technology. Oxford: United Kingdom, Health Press, 2008, Chapter 7, pp. 112–114.

41

Polycystic Ovary Syndrome and IVF

Timur Gurgan, Aygul Demirol

INTRODUCTION

Polycystic ovary syndrome (PCOS), characterized by ovulatory dysfunction and hyperandrogenism, is the most common cause of infertility in women. Although prevalence data are limited, PCOS is thought to be one of the most common endocrinopathies in women (1). The prevalence of PCOS in women of reproductive age is changed in between 4.7 and 6.8 percent (2–4).

The classic syndrome originally was described by Stein and Leventhal as the association of amenorrhea with polycystic ovaries and, variably, hirsutism and obesity (5). It is now recognized that PCOS represents a spectrum of disease characterized primarily by the following features: hyperandrogenism, menstrual irregularity, polycystic ovaries (PCO), and central adiposity.

Two diagnostic criteria have been developed to identify and diagnose all patients with PCOS (6). In 1990, the National Institutes of Health Conference on PCOS defined PCOS as chronic, unexplained hyperandrogenism and menstrual dysfunction. Hyperandrogenism could be defined by either clinical or biochemical findings. In 2003, the European Society of Human Reproduction and Embryology/American Society of Reproductive Medicine consensus workshop group added polycystic ovaries as an alternative finding (7). The Rotterdam criteria define PCOS when two of the three primary features are present: PCO, oligoanovulation, and/or clinical or biochemical signs of unexplained hyperandrogenism.

The woman with PCOS usually presents to the gynecologist with menstrual dysfunction and complaints secondary to hyperandrogenism or unsuccessful reproduction. The reproductive problems relate both to subfertility, secondary to anovulation, and to early pregnancy loss.

THE PATHOGENESIS OF PCOS-ASSOCIATED INFERTILITY

Epidemiological studies have demonstrated PCO in about 20 percent of apparently normal women (8). Considering the subfertile population, PCOS is diagnosed in about 75 percent of patients with anovulatory infertility and high prevalence rates of PCOS have been reported among women with recurrent miscarriages (9).

Ovarian function in infertile women with PCOS is characterized by disordered folliculogenesis and abnormal steroidogenesis. The phase of early follicular development up to an average follicular diameter of 5 mm is normal in PCOS. Thereafter, follicular maturation is disturbed, resulting in premature arrest of follicular growth. Many factors implicated in chronic anovulation in PCOS have been reported: relative FSH deficiency (results in inadequate follicle stimulation), LH hypersecretion (results in hyperandrogenemia and follicle growth arrest), insulin hypersecretion (results in hyperandrogenemia and follicle growth arrest), androgen hypersecretion (results in abnormal gonadotrophin secretion and follicle growth arrest), estrogens hypersecretion [results in suppression of FSH secretion and increased (tonic) LH secretion], inhibin B hypersecretion (results in suppression of FSH secretion), attenuated apoptosis (results in increased cohort of small follicles active in steroidogenesis), and aberrant growth factors expression (results in abnormal apoptosis, follicle growth arrest, and suppression of estrogen synthesis) (10).

Closely linked to abnormal folliculogenesis are the abnormalities in ovarian steroid production. Hyperandrogenemia and abnormality in estrogen and progesterone production are the biochemical and clinical features of PCOS. The theca cells of women with ovulatory and anovulatory PCOS hypersecrete androgens secondary to increased activity of P450c17, the key regulatory enzyme of androgen biosynthesis, which is modulated by serine phosphorylation (11). The granulosa cells of women with PCOS and anovulation show evidence of increased aromatase activity response to both FSH and LH stimulation, resulting in enhanced estrogen and progesterone synthesis (12). The increased levels of circulating estrogen induce a tonic effect on LH production and give negative feedback to FSH secretion, thus perpetuating the cycles of abnormal folliculogenesis, abnormal steroidogenesis, and abnormal gonadotrophin secretion (13).

The other factors modulating ovarian functions are obesity, high vascular endothelial growth factor expression (may be related to chronic anovulation and the risk of ovarian hyperstimulation with ovulation-inducing agents in this group of women), and increased plasminogen activator inhibitor-1 activity in the serum of women with PCOS (it may contribute to abnormal follicle maturation and rupture) (10).

INFERTILITY MANAGEMENT FOR PCOS

For obese women with PCOS, the first line of therapy is comprehensive attention to weight reduction. Clomiphene citrate is then the first-line active medical treatment. If clomiphene fails to induce ovulation and pregnancy, several therapeutic paths are open, depending on the individual case: low-dose FSH therapy, metformin alone or in cotreatment with clomiphene or FSH, and laparoscopic ovarian drilling. If all else fails for the infertile PCOS patient, then in vitro fertilization is a last resort providing excellent results. Although a smaller percentage of recovered oocytes are fertilized, the larger number of oocytes recovered from PCOS patients balances out the pregnancy rate in comparison with, for example, women with a mechanical factor (14). Alternative possibilities for treatment in the near future include aromatase inhibitors and in vitro maturation of oocytes. Aromatase inhibitors do not possess the adverse antiestrogenic effects of clomiphene by suppressing estrogen production and mimic the central reduction of negative feedback through which clomiphene acts. Although some encouragement can be taken from the solidity of the working hypothesis and the success of the preliminary results, hard evidence on efficacy and safety are awaited from larger trials (15, 16).

The recovery of immature oocytes followed by in vitro maturation (IVM) and in vitro fertilization has many advantages to conventional in vitro fertilization treatment in selected cases with an experienced team. Many advances have been reported in IVM procedures. In comparison with conventional IVF, the major advantages of IVM treatment include avoidance of the risk of OHSS, reduced cost, and simplified treatment. Approximately 300 healthy infants have been born following immature oocyte retrieval and IVM. In general, the clinical pregnancy and implantation rates have reached 30–35 percent and 10–15 percent, respectively, in women with polycystic ovaries or PCOS. Therefore, as an option, IVM treatment can be offered to women whose infertility is due to polycystic ovaries or PCOS (17).

Assisted reproduction technologies (ART) like intrauterine insemination (IUI) or IVF are increasingly applied (18), although well-designed studies documenting efficacy and safety in PCOS are lacking in this patient group. Certainly, with improved outcome and the more frequent use of single embryo transfer, eliminating chances for multiple pregnancies, IVF has become a serious alternative to ovulation induction (19).

IVF FOR PCOS

Favorable IVF outcomes have been reported; however, uncertainty remains with regard to risk of ovarian hyperstimulation syndrome, cycle cancellation rate, oocyte quality, and fertilization rates in PCOS women undergoing IVF and also whether pregnancy rates differ between PCOS and non-PCOS or PCO women is still uncertain.

In one retrospective study, the results of sixteen patients with PCO treated by IVF were compared with thirty normoovulatory women with tubal disease. Although more oocytes were recovered per cycle from the PCO group than from the control group, the pregnancy rate was comparable in both groups (30.7 versus 29.7 percent, respectively). The authors suggested that these may be because of the lower fertilization and cleavage rates in PCO patients (20).

In another retrospective, well-designed and large sample – size study, the IVF results of patients with PCOS were compared with controls who had normal ovaries and who were matched for the main determinants of success in IVF-ET. Reduced fertilization rate, and increased pregnancy and miscarriage rates were observed in patients with PCOS, although statistically significant values were not obtained (21).

In contrast, Kodama et al. also compared the outcome of IVF-ET in patients with PCOS with control group. It was

reported that the pregnancy rate per transfer was not different in the two groups of patients (25 versus 34 percent, PCOS versus control group); however, the PCOS group had a significantly lower pregnancy rate per follicle aspiration (19 versus 31 percent) (22).

The recent meta-analysis was conducted to compare outcomes of conventional IVF in women presenting with PCOS and non-PCOS patients. Studies in which PCOS patients undergoing IVF were compared with a matched – no male factor – control group were considered for that review. Nine out of 290 identified studies reporting data on 458 PCOS patients (793 cycles) compared with 694 matched controls (1,116 cycles). It was reported that PCOS patients demonstrated a significantly reduced chance of oocyte retrieval per started cycle. Although significantly more oocytes per retrieval were obtained in PCOS patients compared with controls, the number of oocytes fertilized did not differ significantly between groups. No significant difference was also reported in the clinical pregnancy rates per started cycle. It was concluded that PCOS patients had the risks of an increased cycle cancellation rate, increased oocytes retrieved per retrieval, and a decreased fertilization rate and similar pregnancy and live birth rates per cycle (19).

The other controversial subject in PCOS patients is that "Do IVF results in PCOS patients differ from PCO ones?" In a recent retrospective study, it was reported that patients with the full-blown picture of PCOS or isolated PCO-only morphology behave exactly in the same manner during all stages of assisted reproduction. Owing to the availability of more fertilized oocytes and grade 1 embryos, patients with PCOS or PCO-only morphology are associated with higher clinical pregnancy rates per ET compared to patients with isolated male factor infertility (23). Another recent study also supported these findings, and in that study, it was concluded that the response to follicular stimulation in PCO women was better than that for women with normal ovaries; however, the outcome of pregnancy in IVF was similar (24).

WHICH GONADOTROPIN FOR PCOS?

There are sufficient data in the literature derived from ovulation induction from ovulation induction cycles using gonadotrophins in women with clomiphene citrate – resistant PCOS. Information gained from these data suggests that for induction of ovulation in the PCOS patient, human menopausal gonadotrophin (hMG), urinary-derived FSH (uFSH), and recombinant FSH (r-FSH) appear to be equally effective for achieving pregnancy (25, 26). The inter- and intraindividual differences in the daily amount of FSH required to induce ongoing follicle growth (the FSH "response" dose) can be indicated as the major complicating factor in FSH ovulation induction. This variation may result in complications such as multifollicular growth, ovarian hyperstimulation, and multiple pregnancy (27).

There has been a long-standing debate regarding the gonadotrophin of choice for ovarian stimulation in women with PCOS. Elevated LH concentrations commonly associated with the syndrome have been blamed for increased incidence of OHSS and spontaneous abortions. Due to such concerns, gonadotrophin preparations devoid of LH were advocated.

Daya et al. reviewed the controlled trials comparing rFSH and uFSH for ovarian stimulation in ART. It was concluded that rFSH produced higher pregnancy rates per cycle than uFSH when follitropin alpha was used in IVF and the total gonadotropin dose required was lower (28).

Recent meta-analysis comparing the effectiveness of hMG and FSH after downregulation for ovulation stimulation in assisted reproductive cycles revealed that the group of women treated with hMG had higher pregnancy rates. However, there was no evidence of a difference in rates of ongoing pregnancy or live birth per woman between hMG recipients and FSH recipients and no differences were found in gonadotropin dose used, oocytes retrieved, miscarriage rate, or multiple pregnancy rate. It was concluded that use of hMG resulted in higher clinical pregnancy rates than did use of recombinant FSH in IVF/ICSI cycles after GnRH agonist downregulation in a long protocol (29).

Another recent meta-analysis reported the comparison of rFSH preparations (devoid of LH) and hMG in terms of clinical efficacy. Pooling the results of these RCTs showed no significant difference between rFSH and hMG regarding the different outcomes: ongoing pregnancy/live birth, clinical pregnancy, miscarriage, multiple pregnancy rate, and incidence of moderate/severe OHSS. However, there was significant reduction in the amount of gonadotrophins in favor of hMG over rFSH. It was also concluded that there is no clinically significant difference between hMG and rFSH IVF/ICSI cycles (30).

Although there are no clear comparative data regarding the outcome of IVF in PCOS patients stimulated with different gonadotrophin preparations, data for ovulation induction cycles suggest that there are no outcome differences in the gonadotrophin preparation studied (25, 29).

THE USE OF GnRH AGONIST

The ability of GnRH agonists (GnRH-a) to suppress LH concentrations before and during ovarian stimulation has earned them an undisputed place in IVF treatment protocols. They confer the advantage of eliminating, almost completely, the annoying occurrence of premature luteinization. Their possible application during ovulation induction should therefore be particularly relevant in the presence of the chronic, tonic, high serum concentrations of LH observed in a high proportion of women with PCOS. Theoretically, by suppressing LH concentrations, GnRH-a should eliminate premature luteinization and alleviate the relatively low pregnancy rates and the high miscarriage rates witnessed in this group of patients (16).

Dor et al. investigated the effect of GnRH-a on pituitary suppression, subsequent ovarian response, and results of IVF treatments in PCOS. The pituitary responsiveness was abolished in all patients fourteen days after GnRH-a administration, and early luteinization was prevented. They also reported that administration of GnRH-a in patients with PCOS decreased progesterone and androstenedione production by the granulosa cells and prevents early luteinization. However, it does not affect the IVF results (31).

In a retrospective study, the effect of treatment with GnRH-a in cumulative live birth and miscarriage rate of pregnancies achieved in women with PCOS was compared. Miscarriage rates after treatment in ovulation induction with (16.7 percent) and without GnRH-a (39.4 percent) and in IVF with (18.2 percent) and without GnRH-a (38.5 percent) were almost identical. However, of pregnancies achieved with GnRH-a, 17.6 percent miscarried compared with 39.1 percent of those achieved with gonadotrophins alone. Cumulative live birth rate

after four cycles for GnRH-a was 64 percent compared with 26 percent for gonadotropins only. This suggested the idea that the cotreatment with GnRH-a/hMG for anovulatory women with PCOS reduces the miscarriage rate and improves the live birth rate compared with treatment with gonadotrophins alone (32).

Cochrane database systematic review also revealed a reduction in the incidence of OHSS with FSH compared to hMG in stimulation cycles without the concomitant use of a GnRH-a, a higher OHSS rate when a GnRH-a is added to gonadotrophins. It was concluded that there was a trend toward better pregnancy rates with the addition of a GnRH-a to gonadotrophin stimulation, and these interventions warrant further study. The only demonstrable benefit was a reduced risk of OHSS in cycles when administered without the concomitant use of a GnRH-a (25).

In summary, there are conflicting results in the literature with regard to the effect of GnRH-a on IVF success for PCOS patients, and the current results from meta-analysis may suggest the beneficial effect of GnRH-a on pregnancy and miscarriage rates in IVF cycles although statistical significant values were not obtained. In another point of view, the combination of a GnRH agonist with gonadotrophin either hMG or r-FSH may probably be reserved for women with high serum concentrations of LH who have repeated premature luteinization, stubbornly do not conceive on gonadotrophin therapy alone, or have conceived and had early miscarriages on more than one occasion (16).

THE USE OF GnRH ANTAGONISTS

GnRH antagonists have several theoretical advantages over the agonists because they act by the mechanism of competitive binding and this allows a modulation of the degree of hormonal suppression by adjustment of the dose. Further, antagonists suppress gonadotrophin release within a few hours and have no flare-up effect, and gonadal function resumes without a lag effect following their discontinuation. Considering the PCOS patient, GnRH antagonist in combination with low-dose FSH administration, the antagonist could be given in single or repeated doses when a leading follicle of 13–14 mm is produced. This would theoretically prevent premature luteinization, protect the oocyte from the deleterious effects of high LH concentrations, and still allow the follicle to grow unhindered to ovulatory size. Compared to agonist-treated cycles, this would confer the advantages of a much shorter cycle of treatment, promise more conceptions and fewer miscarriages, reduce the amount of gonadotrophin required, and increase the incidence of monofollicular ovulation with a consequent reduction in the prevalence of OHSS and multiple pregnancies (16).

Recent meta-analysis assessing the effect of GnRH antagonists in ART concluded that GnRH antagonist protocol is a short and simple protocol with good clinical outcome with significant reduction in incidence of severe OHSS and amount of gonadotrophins, but the lower pregnancy rate compared to the GnRH-a-long protocol necessitates counseling subfertile couples before recommending change from GnRH-a to antagonist (33).

A recent prospective study assessed the reproductive outcome of 110 patients with PCOS treated by IVF/ICSI with rFSH and GnRH antagonists. A significantly lower ongoing pregnancy rate per oocyte retrieval (25.6 versus 46.7 percent) and a higher occurrence of OHSS (16.3 versus 3.0 percent) was observed in the group of patients with BMI greater than 29 kg/m^2 as compared with the group of patients with BMI lesser than or equal to 29 kg/m^2, respectively. It was concluded that in GnRH antagonist cycles, a worse reproductive outcome is expected in PCOS patients with BMI greater than 29 kg/m^2 in whom stimulation is initiated with 200 IU of rFSH as compared with PCOS patients with BMI lesser than or equal to 29 kg/m^2 in whom stimulation is initiated with 100 IU of rFSH (34).

Bahceci et al. compared the outcome of using GnRH antagonists versus agonists in women with PCOS who underwent controlled ovarian hyperstimulation for ART. It was found that there was no significant difference between the antagonist and agonist arms in the number of gonadotrophin ampules consumed per cycle. However, in the antagonist arm, a shorter duration of ovarian stimulation and a lower quality of the oocytes was recorded as compared to the agonist arm. Pregnancy rates were 57.6 and 58.5 percent in the antagonist and agonist arms, respectively. Implantation rates and the frequency of OHSS were not different between the treatment groups. Although the size of their study, on a specific subgroup of patients, does not allow a reliable conclusion regarding ART outcome following the use of a GnRH antagonist versus agonist, the protocol with the antagonist gave results that were as good as those of the protocol with the agonist in this PCOS patient population (35).

In a recent study, whether elevated LH levels in PCOS might be suppressed to normal range values by the administration of different low doses of GnRH antagonist was investigated. Twenty-four PCOS patients with elevated endogenous LH concentrations were randomized into three different dose groups, receiving 0.125, 0.250, or 0.500 mg ganirelix sc daily for seven subsequent days. Six hours after ganirelix administration, endogenous LH was suppressed by 49, 69, and 75 percent and endogenous FSH was suppressed by 23, 19, and 25 percent, respectively. The decrease in serum LH and FSH levels was transient and lasted for twelve hours, after which serum levels returned to baseline levels at twenty-four hours after drug administration. They concluded that the GnRH antagonist ganirelix is capable of normalizing elevated LH levels in PCOS patients, in doses similar to the ones previously shown to prevent a premature LH rise during ovarian hyperstimulation for IVF. In addition, the transient suppression of elevated endogenous LH levels per se does not reestablish normal follicle development in PCOS. However, follicle development may be insufficiently supported by the accompanied subtle suppression of endogenous FSH. Similarly, a transient decline in E2 levels does not effectively restore normal pituitary ovarian feedback. Moreover, these results support the contention of a limited role of LH in the pathogenesis of PCOS (36).

Patients with PCOS may need a longer period of pituitary downregulation to suppress the elevated serum LH and androgen levels effectively during IVF treatment using the GnRH-a long protocol. Recently, it was proposed a stimulation protocol incorporating Diane-35 and GnRH antagonist and this protocol was compared with the GnRH-a long protocol for PCOS patients. The clinical results for both protocols were comparable, with significantly fewer days of injection, lower amounts of gonadotrophin used, and lower estradiol levels on the day of HCG injection following the Diane/cetrorelix protocol. Furthermore, there was no significant difference in clinical pregnancy outcome between the two stimulation protocols. This study suggested the similar outcome with the Diane/cetrorelix protocol and the GnRH-a long protocol for women with PCOS undergoing IVF treatment (37).

The combination of GnRH antagonist and gonadotrophin represents a valid alternative to the classical protocol with GnRH-a for ovulation induction in patients with PCOS. The use of metformin may be of benefit to women with PCOS. In one recent study, the stimulation characteristics and IVF-ET outcomes of the standard short GnRH antagonist protocol for ovarian stimulation with or without metformin were compared. In metformin-used group, a statistically significant decrease in the number of ampules of rFSH and estradiol levels, fewer canceled cycles, and lower incidence of OHSS were observed. However, the mean number of mature oocytes was increased with metformin treatment. These findings may suggest the improvement in the outcome of ovarian stimulation in IVF-ET cycles in PCOS patients by using of metformin with GnRH antagonist (38).

Although GnRH antagonists seem to be as effective as established therapy, but with shorter treatment times, less use of gonadotropic hormones, improved patient acceptance, and fewer follicles and oocytes in ART (39), there are no peer-reviewed data regarding the application of these medications specifically for patients with PCOS, so large multicenter studies comparing the effect of agonists and antagonists should have been conducted.

THE COADMINISTRATION OF METFORMIN

The strong association between hyperinsulinemia and anovulation suggests that a reduction of insulin concentrations could be of great importance. For those who fail to achieve this by losing weight, or are of normal weight but hyperinsulinemic, an insulin-sensitizing agent such as metformin might be indicated (16).

In a prospective RCT on women with PCOS undergoing IVF, overall, metformin had no effect on the results of IVF, dose of FSH required, estradiol levels on the day of human chorionic gonadotrophin, oocytes retrieved, or fertilization rate. The only positive effect of metformin was seen in the lean (but not obese) subgroup, in whom it improved implantation and pregnancy rates (40).

Another recent prospective randomized study investigated the impact of metformin therapy on IVF/ICSI outcomes in patients with PCOS. They found that metformin does not lead to any improvement in IVF/ICSI outcomes among patients with PCOS (41).

A systematic review of randomized controlled trials comparing whether metformin coadministration with gonadotrophins for IVF improves outcome in women with PCOS revealed that metformin coadministration to IVF treatment does not improve pregnancy rates but reduces the risk of ovarian hyperstimulation syndrome (42).

Metformin appears to improve reproductive function in some women with PCOS. Recently, Tang et al. investigated the effect of metformin in women with PCOS undergoing IVF in a randomized, placebo-controlled, double-blind study. No differences in the total dose of rFSH required, the median number of oocytes retrieved per cycle, and the overall fertilization rates in both group were observed. However, both the clinical pregnancy rates beyond twelve weeks gestation per cycle and per embryo transfer were significantly higher in those treated with metformin. Furthermore, a significant decrease in the incidence of severe OHSS was also observed. Based on this study findings, it may be concluded that short-term cotreatment with metformin for patients with PCOS undergoing IVF/ICSI cycles does not improve the response to stimulation but significantly improves the pregnancy outcome and reduces the risk of OHSS (43).

In conclusion, current data on the use of metformin in IVF treatment settings are encouraging. Further RCTs are necessary to definitively clarify whether metformin coadministration during IVF will improve the efficacy of these treatments in PCOS women.

CONCLUSIONS

Unsuccessful reproduction is a common problem for woman with PCOS, and the reproductive problems relate both to subfertility, secondary to anovulation, and to early pregnancy loss.

IVF seems an appropriate treatment option for PCOS patients. It is not easy to conclude that PCOS patients undergoing IVF have reduced chances for success and increased complication rates. The woman with PCOS has a similar chance for pregnancy or live birth per started IVF cycle as a non-PCOS or PCO woman. More research is necessary to define the optimal place of IVF, the best ovulation induction protocol, the choice of gonadotropin, the use of GnRH analog, antagonist, and the impact of coadministration of metformin for anovulatory infertile PCOS patients subjected to IVF.

KEY NOTES

- PCOS, characterized by ovulatory dysfunction and hyperandrogenism, is the most common cause of infertility in women.
- The factors implicated in chronic anovulation in PCOS have been reported: relative FSH deficiency, LH hypersecretion, insulin hypersecretion, androgens hypersecretion, estrogens hypersecretion, inhibin B hypersecretion, attenuated apoptosis, and aberrant growth factors expression.
- Clomiphene citrate is the first-line active medical treatment. If clomiphene fails to induce ovulation and pregnancy, several therapeutic paths are open, depending on the individual case: low-dose FSH therapy, metformin alone or in cotreatment with clomiphene or FSH, and laparoscopic ovarian drilling.
- Favorable IVF outcomes have been reported; however, uncertainty remains with regard to risk of ovarian hyperstimulation syndrome, cycle cancellation rate, oocyte quality, and fertilization rates.
- There are no outcome differences in the gonadotrophin preparation studied for patients with PCOS.
- The GnRH-a may have beneficial effect on pregnancy and miscarriage rates in IVF cycles.
- GnRH antagonists seem to be as effective as established therapy, but with shorter treatment times, less use of gonadotropic hormones, improved patient acceptance, and fewer follicles and oocytes in ART.
- The use and the beneficial effect of metformin in IVF treatment settings are not clear.

REFERENCES

1. Azziz R, Woods KS, Reyna R, Key TJ, Knochenhauer ES, Yildiz BO. The prevalence and features of the polycystic ovary syndrome in an unselected population. *J Clin Endocrinol Metab* 2004;89:2745–9.

2. Asuncion M, Calvo RM, San Millan JL, Sancho J, Avila S, Escobar-Morreale HF. A prospective study of the prevalence of the polycystic ovary syndrome in unselected Caucasian women from Spain. *J Clin Endocrinol Metab* 2000;85:2434–8.

3. Diamanti-Kandarakis E, Kouli CR, Bergiele AT, Filandra FA, Tsianateli TC, Spina GG, et al. A survey of the polycystic ovary syndrome in the Greek island of Lesbos: hormonal and metabolic profile. *J Clin Endocrinol Metab* 1999;84:4006–11.

4. Knochenhauer ES, Key TJ, Kahsar-Miller M, Waggoner W, Boots LR, Azziz R. Prevalence of the polycystic ovary syndrome in unselected black and white women of the southeastern United States: a prospective study. *J Clin Endocrinol Metab* 1998;83:3078–82.

5. Stein I. Amenorrhea associated with bilateral polycystic ovaries. *Am J Obstet Gynecol* 1935;29:181.

6. Azziz R. PCOS: a diagnostic challenge. *Reprod Biomed Online* 2004;8:644–8.

7. Revised 2003 consensus on diagnostic criteria and long-term health risks related to polycystic ovary syndrome (PCOS). *Hum Reprod* 2004;19:41–7.

8. Polson DW, Adams J, Wadsworth J, Franks S. Polycystic ovaries—a common finding in normal women. *Lancet* 1988;1: 870–2.

9. Kousta E, White DM, Cela E, McCarthy MI, Franks S. The prevalence of polycystic ovaries in women with infertility. *Hum Reprod* 1999;14:2720–3.

10. van der Spuy ZM, Dyer SJ. The pathogenesis of infertility and early pregnancy loss in polycystic ovary syndrome. *Best Pract Res Clin Obstet Gynaecol* 2004;18:755–71.

11. Dunaif A, Xia J, Book CB, Schenker E, Tang Z. Excessive insulin receptor serine phosphorylation in cultured fibroblasts and in skeletal muscle. A potential mechanism for insulin resistance in the polycystic ovary syndrome. *J Clin Invest* 1995;96:801–10.

12. Barnes RB. The pathogenesis of polycystic ovary syndrome: lessons from ovarian stimulation studies. *J Endocrinol Invest* 1998;21:567–79.

13. Marx TL, Mehta AE. Polycystic ovary syndrome: pathogenesis and treatment over the short and long term. *Cleve Clin J Med* 2003;70:31–3, 36–41, 45.

14. Homburg R. Management of infertility and prevention of ovarian hyperstimulation in women with polycystic ovary syndrome. *Best Pract Res Clin Obstet Gynaecol* 2004;18:773–88.

15. Mitwally MF, Casper RF. Use of an aromatase inhibitor for induction of ovulation in patients with an inadequate response to clomiphene citrate. *Fertil Steril* 2001;75:305–9.

16. Homburg R. The management of infertility associated with polycystic ovary syndrome. *Reprod Biol Endocrinol* 2003;1:109.

17. Chian RC, Lim JH, Tan SL. State of the art in in-vitro oocyte maturation. *Curr Opin Obstet Gynecol* 2004;16:211–19.

18. Fauser BC, Devroey P, Macklon NS. Multiple birth resulting from ovarian stimulation for subfertility treatment. *Lancet* 2005; 365:1807–16.

19. Heijnen EM, Eijkemans MJ, Hughes EG, Laven JS, Macklon NS, Fauser BC. A meta-analysis of outcomes of conventional IVF in women with polycystic ovary syndrome. *Hum Reprod Update* 2006;12:13–21.

20. Dor J, Shulman A, Levran D, Ben-Rafael Z, Rudak E, Mashiach S. The treatment of patients with polycystic ovarian syndrome by in-vitro fertilization and embryo transfer: a comparison of results with those of patients with tubal infertility. *Hum Reprod* 1990;5:816–18.

21. Doldi N, Marsiglio E, Destefani A, Gessi A, Merati G, Ferrari A. Elevated serum progesterone on the day of HCG administration in IVF is associated with a higher pregnancy rate in polycystic ovary syndrome. *Hum Reprod* 1999;14:601–5.

22. Kodama H, Fukuda J, Karube H, Matsui T, Shimizu Y, Tanaka T. High incidence of embryo transfer cancellations in patients with polycystic ovarian syndrome. *Hum Reprod* 1995;10:1962–7.

23. Esinler I, Bayar U, Bozdag G, Yarali H. Outcome of intracytoplasmic sperm injection in patients with polycystic ovary syndrome or isolated polycystic ovaries. *Fertil Steril* 2005;84:932–7.

24. Esmailzadeh S, Faramarzi M, Jorsarai G. Comparison of in vitro fertilization outcome in women with and without sonographic evidence of polycystic ovarian morphology. *Eur J Obstet Gynecol Reprod Biol* 2005;121:67–70.

25. Nugent D, Vandekerckhove P, Hughes E, Arnot M, Lilford R. Gonadotrophin therapy for ovulation induction in subfertility associated with polycystic ovary syndrome. *Cochrane Database Syst Rev* 2000:CD000410.

26. van Wely M, Bayram N, van der Veen F. Recombinant FSH in alternative doses or versus urinary gonadotrophins for ovulation induction in subfertility associated with polycystic ovary syndrome: a systematic review based on a Cochrane review. *Hum Reprod* 2003;18:1143–9.

27. Fauser BC, Van Heusden AM. Manipulation of human ovarian function: physiological concepts and clinical consequences. *Endocr Rev* 1997;18:71–106.

28. Daya S. Updated meta-analysis of recombinant follicle-stimulating hormone (FSH) versus urinary FSH for ovarian stimulation in assisted reproduction. *Fertil Steril* 2002;77:711–14.

29. van Wely M, Westergaard LG, Bossuyt PM, van der Veen F. Effectiveness of human menopausal gonadotropin versus recombinant follicle-stimulating hormone for controlled ovarian hyperstimulation in assisted reproductive cycles: a meta-analysis. *Fertil Steril* 2003;80:1086–93.

30. Al-Inany H, Aboulghar MA, Mansour RT, Serour GI. Ovulation induction in the new millennium: recombinant follicle-stimulating hormone versus human menopausal gonadotropin. *Gynecol Endocrinol* 2005;20:161–9.

31. Dor J, Shulman A, Pariente C, Levran D, Bider D, Menashe Y, et al. The effect of gonadotropin-releasing hormone agonist on the ovarian response and in vitro fertilization results in polycystic ovarian syndrome: a prospective study. *Fertil Steril* 1992;57:366–71.

32. Homburg R, Levy T, Berkovitz D, Farchi J, Feldberg D, Ashkenazi J, et al. Gonadotropin-releasing hormone agonist reduces the miscarriage rate for pregnancies achieved in women with polycystic ovarian syndrome. *Fertil Steril* 1993;59:527–31.

33. Al-Inany HG, Abou-Setta AM, Aboulghar M. Gonadotrophin-releasing hormone antagonists for assisted conception. *Cochrane Database Syst Rev* 2006;3:CD001750.

34. Kolibianakis E, Zikopoulos K, Albano C, Camus M, Tournaye H, Van Steirteghem A, et al. Reproductive outcome of polycystic ovary syndrome patients treated with GnRH antagonists and recombinant FSH for IVF/ICSI. *Reprod Biomed Online* 2003;7: 313–18.

35. Bahceci M, Ulug U, Ben-Shlomo I, Erden HF, Akman MA. Use of a GnRH antagonist in controlled ovarian hyperstimulation for assisted conception in women with polycystic ovary disease: a randomized, prospective, pilot study. *J Reprod Med* 2005;50: 84–90.

36. Hohmann FP, Laven JS, Mulders AG, Oberye JJ, Mannaerts BM, de Jong FH, et al. LH suppression following different low doses of the GnRH antagonist ganirelix in polycystic ovary syndrome. *J Endocrinol Invest* 2005;28:990–7.

37. Hwang JL, Seow KM, Lin YH, Huang LW, Hsieh BC, Tsai YL, et al. Ovarian stimulation by concomitant administration of cetrorelix acetate and HMG following Diane-35 pre-treatment for patients with polycystic ovary syndrome: a prospective randomized study. *Hum Reprod* 2004;19:1993–2000.

38. Doldi N, Persico P, Di Sebastiano F, Marsiglio E, Ferrari A. Gonadotropin-releasing hormone antagonist and metformin for treatment of polycystic ovary syndrome patients undergoing in vitro fertilization-embryo transfer. *Gynecol Endocrinol* 2006; 22:235–8.

39. Schultze-Mosgau A, Griesinger G, Altgassen C, von Otte S, Hornung D, Diedrich K. New developments in the use of peptide gonadotropin-releasing hormone antagonists versus agonists. *Expert Opin Investig Drugs* 2005;14:1085–97.

40. Kjotrod SB, von During V, Carlsen SM. Metformin treatment before IVF/ICSI in women with polycystic ovary syndrome; a prospective, randomized, double blind study. *Hum Reprod* 2004;19:1315–22.

41. Onalan G, Pabuccu R, Goktolga U, Ceyhan T, Bagis T, Cincik M. Metformin treatment in patients with polycystic ovary syndrome undergoing in vitro fertilization: a prospective randomized trial. *Fertil Steril* 2005;84:798–801.

42. Costello MF, Chapman M, Conway U. A systematic review and meta-analysis of randomized controlled trials on metformin co-administration during gonadotrophin ovulation induction or IVF in women with polycystic ovary syndrome. *Hum Reprod* 2006;21:1387–99.

43. Tang T, Glanville J, Orsi N, Barth JH, Balen AH. The use of metformin for women with PCOS undergoing IVF treatment. *Hum Reprod* 2006; 21:1416–25.

42

ENDOMETRIOSIS AND ASSISTED REPRODUCTIVE TECHNOLOGY

Juan A. Garcia-Velasco, Alfredo Guillén, Guillermo Quea, Antonio Requena

WHY WOMEN WITH ENDOMETRIOSIS NEED ART?

Endometriosis, the disease characterized by the presence of both functional endometrial glands and stroma outside of the uterine cavity, is usually related to infertility, even though the relationship is still being debated (1). As this disease is most likely observed in women of reproductive ages – although few cases have been described in adolescents and/or postmenopausal women – there is a strong interest in solving the problem on whether endometriosis and infertility are causally related, and if so, how can we help these women.

Although the prevalence of the disease is difficult to evaluate, it seems reasonable to state that there is an increased prevalence in subfertile women when compared with fertile women. But obviously, this does not mean that all women with endometriosis are infertile or need assisted reproduction (ART). In fact, there are women with endometriosis and with proven fertility. However, their fecundability or chances of achieving a pregnancy per month seems to be reduced.

The ideal study, comparing the fecundability of women with endometriosis (diagnosed by biopsy) with women without endometriosis (laparoscopically confirmed) would be unethical to perform. But from the baboon model, we have learned that their monthly fecundity rate (MFR) drops from 24 percent in baboons with normal pelvis to 18 percent if minimal endometriosis developed, and even lower if mild, moderate, or severe forms of the disease were present (2).

In women, we can only have access to data from women with endometriosis and expectant management. A low MFR – around 8 percent – has been described in these women (3, 4). In a study from Spain (5), women with minimal endometriosis had a 6 percent MFR, with a cumulative pregnancy rate of 47 percent at twelve months, confirming that not all women with endometriosis require treatment. From the Canadian study that evaluated the benefit of laparoscopic intervention in women with minimal/mild endometriosis (ENDOCAN), an even lower MFR was observed (2.5 percent) (6). A close correlation can be observed with MFR and severity of the disease, as MFR was 8.7, 3.2, and 0 percent in women with mild, moderate, or severe endometriosis, respectively (3).

Thus, an infertile woman who has been diagnosed with endometriosis may be considered for treatment after a reasonable time of expectant management, as she can conceive if no other concomitant factors limit her chances. The "reasonable time" period will depend basically on her age, but less than thirty-five years old from one to two years would be correct if ovarian reserve is not diminished and over thirty-five probably from six months to one year would be reasonable.

WHERE CAN ART ACT TO IMPROVE ENDOMETRIOSIS SUBFERTILITY?

In a previous chapter of this book, the different mechanisms of endometriosis-associated infertility are reviewed, so we will not go over them again. Just to mention that although endometriosis may be affecting the reproductive process at various stages (Table 42.1), ART may bypass these difficulties as data from large registries from women with endometriosis are similar to other ART indications (7). However, this is not in accordance with data from smaller studies pulled together in meta-analysis (8).

WHAT ARE THE RESULTS?

Intrauterine Insemination

According to ESHRE 2005 Guidelines for the Diagnosis and Treatment of Endometriosis, treatment with intrauterine insemination (IUI) improves fertility in minimal-mild endometriosis: IUI with ovarian stimulation is effective but the role of unstimulated IUI is uncertain – evidence level 1b (9).

The efficacy of controlled ovarian hyperstimulation (COH) and IUI versus no treatment for infertility associated with minimal or mild endometriosis was reported by Tummon (10) in a randomized controlled trial. Ovarian stimulation was performed with FSH, and live birth rate was the main outcome measure. Three hundred eleven cycles in 103 couples (female age twenty to thirty-nine years) with minimal or mild endometriosis (laparoscopy procedure in the twelve months before enrolment) was the only identified subfertility factor. The odds ratio (OR) was 5.6 [95 percent confidence interval (CI) 1.8–17.4] in favor of COH and IUI. Live birth occurred in 14 of 127 (11 percent) treatments cycles compared with 4 of 184 (2 percent) control cycles.

A previous meta-analysis by Peterson (11) on using gonadotrophins for ovulation induction and IUI reported a pooled total pregnancy rate per cycle of 8 percent in endometriosis stages III and IV (three studies – 15 pregnancies/179 cycles) and 13 percent (five studies – 100 pregnancies/783 cycles) in endometriosis stages I and II.

Table 42.1: Where Endometriosis May Affect Human Reproduction

Defective folliculogenesis

Poor oocyte quality

Luteinized unruptured follicle

Altered tubal permeability and functionality

Diminished sperm motility in the uterus

Reduced oocyte fertilization

Slower embryo cleavage

Reduced embryo implantation

Meta-analyses suggest that COH in combination with IUI has a significant improvement in success rates (12, 13) for unexplained infertility, but a significant lower pregnancy rate (10, 14, 15) has been found in patients with endometriosis when compared to women with unexplained infertility (6.5–16 percent).

Hughes published a meta-analysis (13) where it is showed that endometriosis reduced the effectiveness of ovarian stimulation/IUI by approximately half in the treatment of endometriosis (adjusted OR for the likelihood of conception per cycle).

Nevertheless, a recent retrospective controlled cohort study (16) confirmed another interesting hypothesis. Clinical pregnancy rate (PR) and clinical live birth rate were similar in women with recently surgically treated minimal to mild endometriosis and in women with unexplained infertility after COH (23 cycles with clomiphene citrate and 236 cycles with gonadotrophins) and IUI. Minimal or mild endometriosis lesions had been removed by laparoscopy within seven months before the treatment. In 107 patients during 259 cycles, the clinical PR for minimal (21 percent) or mild (18.9 percent) endometriosis was comparable to women with unexplained infertility (20.5 percent).

In Vitro Fertilization

According to ESHRE 2005 Guidelines for the Diagnosis and Treatment of Endometriosis, in vitro fertilization (IVF) is an appropriate treatment especially if tubal function is compromised, if there is also male factor infertility, and/or when other treatments have failed – evidence level 2b. IVF pregnancy rates are lower in patients with endometriosis than in those with tubal infertility (9) – evidence level 1a.

A meta-analysis by Barnhart (8) in 2002 pooled data from twenty-two studies, for a total of 2,377 IVF cycles in patients with endometriosis and 4,383 cycles in women without endometriosis. The results after adjusting the confounding variables showed a 35 percent decrease in the chance of achieving a pregnancy with IVF for women with endometriosis compared with women undergoing IVF without endometriosis (OR, 0.63; 95 percent; CI, 0.51–0.77). ORs were also significantly lower for fertilization rate (FR), implantation rate (IR), and peak serum estradiol (E2) concentrations in women with endometriosis. The adjusted analysis also demonstrated a significant lower number of oocytes retrieved in women with endometriosis (OR, 0.92; CI, 0.85–0.99).

After the independent evaluation of variables according to endometriosis stages compared with tubal factor infertility, significant differences were demonstrated. The comparing of women with stage III or IV endometriosis to women with tubal infertility confirm a diminished pregnancy rate (OR, 0.46; CI, 0.28–0.74). Comparing results of mild endometriosis to patients with tubal factor showed significant differences in all variables except for pregnancy rate, where the strength of association was similar to other comparisons, but results did not achieve statistical significance.

The different outcomes of IVF according to the stage of endometriosis were also studied in this meta-analysis and a poorer success was observed in IVF with increase in severity of the disease. Lower pregnancy and implantation rates have been documented in women with severe (stage III or IV) endometriosis when compared to mild (stage I or II) endometriosis. A smaller number of oocytes and a lower peak of serum estradiol concentration, but no significant difference in fertilization rate, were reported. Overall, there was a 36 percent reduction in pregnancy rate for women with severe endometriosis compared with those with mild disease (OR, 0.64; CI, 0.35–1.17).

All these data suggest that endometriosis affects developing follicles, oocyte, and embryo quality and not only by distorting normal anatomy. The AFS classification is useful in predicting the outcome of infertility treatment and can be used for counseling couples.

A more recent observational study (17) on ninety-eight consecutive women with endometriosis who underwent IVF or ICSI compared to eighty-seven women with tubal infertility showed a significantly lower pregnancy rate after pooled cycles (1–4) in stage III or IV endometriosis (22.6 percent) compared to stage I or II disease group (40.0 percent) or tubal infertility (36.6 percent).

So again, ART may bypass some of the mechanisms of endometriosis-associated infertility, but the disease may have an impact on cycle outcome.

Oocyte Donation

Oocyte donation appears as an alternative in patients with endometriosis with low response, poor embryo quality, or repeated ART failures. Implantation is not affected in this group of patients according to this particular therapeutic modality. Moreover, oocyte donation provides an excellent scenario to obtain relevant data about reproductive outcome in patients with endometriosis.

An appropriate set up to address how endometriosis affects fertility was postulated by Diaz (18) by allocating sibling oocytes to recipients with or without endometriosis. Twenty-five recipients with documented stage III or IV endometriosis and thirty-three without the disease were compared. There were no differences between number of donated oocytes, fertilization rate, number of transferred embryos, or mean number of good-quality embryos between groups. Pregnancy, implantation, and miscarriage rates were not affected by stage III–IV endometriosis when compared with the control group.

Another previous article by our group (19) showed that patients with endometriosis had the same chances of implantation and pregnancy as other recipients when the oocytes came from donors without known endometriosis. Same results were published by Sung (20): 18 recipients with mild endometriosis and 37 with moderate to severe disease were compared to 184 recipients without endometriosis. Pregnancy and implantation rates were comparable between groups reaching the same conclusion that the adverse effect of endometriosis is not related to implantation or uterine receptivity.

DOES COH AFFECT ENDOMETRIOSIS?

Does Repeated COH Affect Ovarian Reserve?

The first question to be solved is whether repeated cycles of COH will compromise ovarian reserve, specially in these women with already a lower amount of healthy ovarian tissue present, as not all women achieve a pregnancy in their first cycle and may require more than one cycle. According to ovarian physiology, there is no rationale to speculate that repeated COH will diminish ovarian function in any women (21). Oocytes retrieved in one specific cycle come from the antral follicle pool that otherwise would become atretic due to dominant follicle selection (22). Apart from anecdotal reports (23), ovarian response persists with subsequent cycles of COH. The number of oocytes retrieved may diminish with subsequent cycles, but this seems to be more related to the advancing maternal age with repeated cycles. So we may confirm that repeated COH is not detrimental for ovarian function.

When we specifically look at this not in the general IVF population but in women with endometriosis, it seems that they require – each subsequent cycle – a larger dose of FSH to adequately respond and that the number of eggs retrieved was lower each time. However, this did not decrease the chances of successful IVF treatment in terms of cumulative pregnancy rate and live birth rate (24).

Does COH Affect Endometriosis Stage?

Another issue that worries clinicians when stimulating the ovaries of women with endometriosis is whether the elevated estradiol levels to which these women are exposed during COH may be harmful, stimulating the growth of endometriotic lesions, and hypothetically increasing the recurrence rate. In fact, there is not much evidence of the effect of temporary but repeated exposure to high estradiol levels in women with endometriosis undergoing COH that have had previous endometriosis surgery.

In a recent study, D'Hooghe et al. (25) recently reviewed with life-table analysis with their experience of eleven years investigating the cumulative endometriosis recurrence rate after fertility surgery for stages III and IV of the disease in women undergoing fertility treatment. The overall Cumulative Endometriosis Recurrence Rate (CERR) at twenty-one months after the start of ovulation induction was 31 percent, which is in accordance with the recurrence rate of other groups (26). Interestingly, it was significantly lower in women undergoing IVF (7 percent), much lower than expected as COH in IVF will expose women to higher E2 levels that in IUI, as higher doses are usually administered. Women treated with both IVF and IUI showed a CERR of 43 percent, which was even higher in women that were treated just with IUI (70 percent). Thus, COH for IVF is not a major risk factor of the recurrence of endometriosis, as it might be expected. Whether this was a protective effect of the GnRH analog exposure in IVF cycles or if the fact that women undergoing IUI – with a much higher CERR – had open tubes and were exposed to recurrent retrograde menstruation that may increase the risk of developing new endometriosis lesions remains open to speculation.

Does Surgery for Ovarian Endometriosis Affect ART?

The Presence of Ovarian Endometriomas has an Impact on ART

Until recently, most clinicians would remove any ovarian cyst if diagnosed by ultrasound, and especially if it was likely to be an endometrioma, with the idea to prepare the ovary and leave it in a better condition prior to COH. The risk of damaging ovarian reserve has challenged this unproven gold-standard approach, and many publications have appeared in the past few years evaluating this issue (27, 28).

Considering that ovarian surgery may affect ovarian reserve and that the contralateral ovary may compensate the altered function of the affected ovary, the ideal model to study the impact of the presence of ovarian endometriomas would be women with unilateral disease who had not undergone previous surgery. Somigliana et al. (29) evaluated fifty-six IVF cycles performed in thirty-six women with these conditions and confirmed that the presence of ovarian endometriomas is associated with a reduced responsiveness to gonadotrophins, which is estimated to be around 25 percent less. This effect was more pronounced with larger cysts or with if more than one lesion was present.

Surgical Removal of Endometriomas and the Effect on ART

It has been classically admitted that endometriomas in infertile women require surgery to improve their fertility status, an unproven dogma. The fact that most (24, 30–32) but not all (33–35) studies suggested the ovarian response to gonadotrophins may be impaired after cystectomy led us to investigate if there was any benefit from removing the cyst prior to ART. In a retrospective analysis of 189 women with ovarian endometriomas undergoing IVF, we compared fifty-six women that proceeded directly to IVF with 133 that first underwent conservative ovarian surgery (36). Women with operated ovarian endometrioma had a lower peak estradiol level and required a larger dose of gonadotrophins, but no other differences were observed between the two groups. Thus, laparoscopic cystectomy does not offer any benefit in terms of fertility outcome. If the patient is asymptomatic, proceeding directly to COH might reduce the time to pregnancy, diminish patient costs, and avoid the potential complications of surgery. In contrast, symptomatic women may be advised that careful, conservative ovarian surgery does not impair their chances of a successful IVF cycle.

Risk of Damaging the Ovary and Premature Ovarian Failure

Although a consensus exists that laparoscopy is the first-line approach in women with endometriotic ovarian cysts (37), we have to balance the benefit of this surgery to the patient versus the potential damage to ovarian reserve (Table 42.2). The fact that healthy ovarian tissue has been described in 54 to 68 percent of the endometriotic cysts that have been removed by stripping the capsule reminds us to be extremely careful with the indication as well as with the technique itself (38, 39).

Candiani et al. have provided evidence that three months after laparoscopic surgical excision of endometriotic cysts, a significant reduction in ovarian volume occurs (40). No other changes were described in the number of antral follicles or Doppler analysis of ovarian blood flow. Being as it is the size

Table 42.2: Pros and Cons of Operating Ovarian Endometriomas Prior to ART

Pros	Cons
Eliminate risk of malignancy	Damage ovarian reserve
Facilitate oocyte retrieval	Surgical risks
Diminish disease progression	Delayed pregnancy
Reduce risk of cyst rupture	Costs of surgery

of the ovary a prognostic marker of ovarian reserve, it seems clear that laparoscopic excision of these cysts is associated with damage to this reserve.

When the endometriotic cyst removal is bilateral, the risk of damaging ovarian function is even higher. Busacca et al. recently confirmed this in a retrospective analysis (41). They followed, for a mean time of 4.6 years, 126 patients who underwent bilateral laparoscopic removal of endometriomas and found that 2.4 percent (CI 0.5–6.8 percent) had postsurgical ovarian failure, which in all cases occurred immediately after surgery.

So, we have to take into consideration when indicating surgery in these patients the significant benefits of relieving pain and improving fertility by surgical intervention, without forgetting the low but definitive risk of POF (42, 43).

KEY POINTS FOR CLINICAL PRACTICE

■ Most of the available evidence supports the hypothesis that endometriosis compromises fertility.

■ Advanced stages of the disease compromise further the monthly fecundity rate.

■ ART is able to bypass most of the endometriosis-altered mechanisms to achieve a pregnancy.

■ The only ART outcome that is not affected by endometriosis is oocyte donation.

■ Surgery for endometriomas in women undergoing ART is indicated in symptomatic women; otherwise, it does not add any benefit to cycle outcome. However, careful surgery does not compromise ovarian reserve.

REFERENCES

1. D'Hooghe T, Debrock S, Hill J, Meuleman C. Endometriosis and subfertility: is the relationship resolved? *Sem Reprod Med* 2003; 21: 243–53.

2. D'Hooghe T, Bambra C, Koninckx P. Cycle fecundity in baboons of proven fertility with minimal endometriosis. *Gynecol Obstet Invest* 1994; 37: 63–5.

3. Olive D, Stohs F, Metzger D, Franklin R. Expectant management and hydrotubations in the treatment of endometriosis-associated infertility. *Fertil Steril* 1985; 44: 35–42.

4. Portuondo JA, Echanojauregui A, Herran C, Alijarte I. Early conception in patients with untreated mild endometriosis. *Fertil Steril* 1983; 39: 22–5.

5. Rodriguez-Escudero F, Negro J, Corcostegui B, Benito J. Does minimal endometriosis reduce fecundity? *Fertil Steril* 1988; 50: 522–4.

6. Berube S, Marcoux S, Langevin M, Maeux R, and the Canadian Collaborative Group on Endometriosis. Fecundity of infertile women with minimal or mild endometriosis and women with unexplained infertility. *Fertil Steril* 1998; 69: 1034–41.

7. Centers for Disease Control: 2004 Assisted Reproductive Technology (ART) Report (accessed January 15, 2007, at http://www.cdc.gov/ART/ART2004/index.htm).

8. Barnhart K, Dunsmoor-Su R, Coutifaris C. Effect of endometriosis on in vitro fertilization. *Fertil Steril* 2000; 77: 1148–55.

9. Kennedy S, Bergqvist A, Chapron C, D'Hooghe T, Dunselman G, Greb R, Hummelshoj L, Prentice A, Saridogan E; on behalf of the ESHRE Special Interest Group for Endometriosis and Endometrium Guideline Development Group. ESHRE guideline for the diagnosis and treatment of endometriosis. *Hum Reprod* 2005; 20: 2698–704.

10. Tummon IS, Asher LJ, Martin JS, Tulandi T. Randomized controlled trial of superovulation and insemination for infertility associated with minimal or mild endometriosis. *Fertil Steril* 1997; 68: 8–12.

11. Peterson CM, Hatasaka HH, Jones KP, Poulson AM Jr., Carrell DT, Urry RL. Ovulation induction with gonadotropins and intrauterine insemination compared with in vitro fertilization and no therapy: a prospective, nonrandomized, cohort study and meta-analysis. *Fertil Steril* 1994; 62: 535–44.

12. Infertility revisited: the state of the art today and tomorrow. The ESHRE Capri Workshop. European Society for Human Reproduction and Embryology. *Hum Reprod* 1996; 11: 1779–807.

13. Hughes EG. The effectiveness of ovulation induction and intrauterine insemination in the treatment of persistent infertility: a meta-analysis. *Hum Reprod* 1997; 12: 1865–72.

14. Nuojua-Huttunen S, Tomas C, Bloigu R, Tuomivaara L, Martikainen H. Intrauterine insemination treatment in subfertility: an analysis of factors affecting outcome. *Hum Reprod* 1999; 14: 698–703.

15. Chaffkin LM, Nulsen JC, Luciano AA, Metzger DA. A comparative analysis of the cycle fecundity rates associated with combined human menopausal gonadotropin (hMG) and intrauterine insemination (IUI) versus either hMG or IUI alone. *Fertil Steril* 1991; 55: 252–7.

16. Werbrouck E, Spiessens C, Meuleman C, D'Hooghe T. No difference in cycle pregnancy rate and in cumulative live-birth rate between women with surgically treated minimal to mild endometriosis and women with unexplained infertility after controlled ovarian hyperstimulation and intrauterine insemination. *Fertil Steril* 2006; 86: 566–71.

17. Kuivasaari P, Hippelainen M, Anttila M, Heinonen S. Effect of endometriosis on IVF/ICSI outcome: stage III/IV endometriosis worsens cumulative pregnancy and live-born rates. *Hum Reprod* 2005; 20: 3130–5.

18. Diaz I, Navarro J, Blasco L, Simon C, Pellicer A, Remohi J. Impact of stage III-IV endometriosis on recipients of sibling oocytes: matched case-control study. *Fertil Steril* 2000; 74: 31–4.

19. Pellicer A, Oliveira N, Gutierrez A, Remohí J, Simón C. Implantation in endometriosis: lessons learned from IVF and oocyte donation. In Spinola PY, Coutinho EM (eds.), *Progress in endometriosis*, Parthenon Publishing Group, Casterton-Hill, 1994, 177–83.

20. Sung L, Mukherjee T, Takeshige T, Bustillo M, Copperman AB. Endometriosis is not detrimental to embryo implantation in oocyte recipients. *J Assist Reprod Genet* 1997; 14: 152–156.

21. Messinis I. Ovulation induction: a mini-review. *Hum Reprod* 2005; 20: 2688–97.

22. Serna J, Garcia-Velasco J. Effect of repeated assisted reproduction techniques on the ovarian response. *Curr Opin Obstet Gynecol* 2005; 17: 233–6.

23. Isikoglu M, Ozgur K. Rapid decline in ovarian reserve after ART cycles in a 22-year old IVF patient. *Arch Gynecol Obstet* 2003; 268: 206–8.

24. Al-Hazemy M, Bernal A, Steele J, Gramsbergen I, Barlow D, Kennedy S. Ovarian response to repeated controlled stimulation in in-vitro fertilization cycles in patients with ovarian endometriosis. *Hum Reprod* 2000; 15: 72–5.

25. D'Hooghe T, Denys B, Spiessens C, Meuleman C, Debrock S. Is the endometriosis recurrence rate increased after ovarian hyperstimulation? *Fertil Steril* 2006; 86: 283–90.

26. Koga K, Takemura Y, Osuga Y, et al. Recurrence of ovarian endometrioma alter laparoscopic excision. *Hum Reprod* 2006; 21: 2171–4.

27. Somigliana E, Vercellini P, Vigano P, Ragni G, Crosignani P. Should endometriomas be treated before IVF-ICSI cycles? *Hum Reprod Update* 2006; 12: 57–64.

28. Gupta S, Agarwal A, Agarwal R, Loret de Mola R. Impact of ovarian endometrioma on assisted reproductive outcomes. *Reprod Biomed Online* 2006; 13: 349–60.

29. Somigliana E, Infantino M, Benedetti F, Arnoldi M, Calanna G, Ragni G. The presence of ovarian endometriomas is associated with a reduced responsiveness to gonadotropins. *Fertil Steril* 2006; 86: 192–6.

30. Pagidas K, Falcone T, Hemmings R, Miron P. Comparison of reoperation for moderate (stage III) and severe (stage IV) endometriosis-related infertility with in vitro fertilization-embryo transfer. *Fertil Steril* 1996; 65: 791–5.

31. Loh FH, Tan AT, Kumar J, Ng SC. Ovarian response after laparoscopic ovarian cystectomy for endometriotic cysts in 132 monitored cycles. *Fertil Steril* 1999; 72: 316–21.

32. Tinkanen H, Kujansuu E. In vitro fertilization in patients with ovarian endometriomas. *Acta Obstet Gynecol Scand* 2000; 79: 119–22.

33. Donnez J, Wyns C, Nisolle M. Does ovarian surgery for endometriomas impair the ovarian response to gonadotropin? *Fertil Steril* 2001; 76: 662–5.

34. Canis M, Pouly JL, Tamburro S, Mage G, Wattiez A, Bruhat MA. Ovarian response during IVF-embryo transfer cycles after laparoscopic ovarian cystectomy for endometriotic cysts of >3cm in diameter. *Hum Reprod* 2001; 16: 2583–6.

35. Marconi G, Vilela M, Quintana R, Sueldo C. Laparoscopic ovarian cystectomy of endometriomas does not affect the ovarian response to gonadotropin stimulation. *Fertil Steril* 2002; 78: 876–8.

36. Garcia-Velasco JA, Mahutte N, Corona J, et al. Renoval of endometriomas before in vitro fertilization does not improve fertility outcomes: a matched, case-control study. *Fertil Steril* 2004; 81: 1194–97.

37. Chapron C, Vercellini P, Barakat H, Vieira M, Dubuisson J. Management of ovarian endometriomas. *Hum Reprod Update* 2002; 8: 591–597.

38. Muzii L, Bianchi A, Croce C, Manci N, Panici P. Laparoscopic excision of ovarian cysts: is the stripping technique a tissue-sparing procedure? *Fertil Steril* 2002; 77: 609–14.

39. Hachisuga T, Kawarabayashi T. Histopathological analysis of laparoscopically treated ovarian endometriotic cysts with special reference to loss of follicles. *Hum Reprod* 2002; 17: 432–5.

40. Candiani M, Barbieri M Bottani B et al. Ovarian recovery after laparoscopic enucleation of ovarian cysts: insights from echographic short-term postsurgical follow-up. *J Minim Invasive Gynecol* 2005; 12: 409–14.

41. Busacca M, Riparini J, Somigliana E et al. Postsurgical ovarian failure after laparoscopic excision of bilateral endometriomas. *Am J Obstet Gynecol* 2006; 195: 421–5.

43

EVIDENCE-BASED MEDICINE COMPARING hMG/FSH AND AGONIST/ANTAGONIST AND REC/URINARY hCG/LH/GnRH TO TRIGGER OVULATION

Mohamed Aboulghar, Hesham Al Inany

INTRODUCTION

The first in vitro fertilization (IVF) baby was born after a natural IVF cycle. In the early days of IVF, clomiphene citrate was used for ovarian stimulation, and later urinary gonadotrophins were used for controlled ovarian hyperstimulation. A decade later, recombinant follicle-stimulating harmone (FSH) was produced (2), and since then, there is an ongoing debate between using urinary versus recombinant gonadotrophins (3).

From the mid-1980s, ovarian stimulation protocols combined the use of gonadotrophins with gonadotrophin-releasing hormone agonist (GnRHa) in order to increase oocyte number and to avoid premature luteinizing hormone (LH) surge (4). In the twenty-first century, GnRH antagonist became available as an alternative to GnRHa (5).

With the recent interest in evidence-based medicine, it would be logical to search for the optimum protocol of ovarian stimulation, decreasing rate of OHSS, and yet achieving at least the same success rate to provide our patients with the best possible care. Randomized controlled trials and systematic reviews are considered the source of the top-quality evidence. One big advantage of systematic reviews is pooling the results of studies with similar methodology and addressing the same topic, hence achieving large sample size and tightening the confidence in the results obtained (Al-Inany et al., 2003).

COH PROTOCOLS: WHAT CHALLENGED THE GOLDEN RULE?

Pharmaceutical preparations of human gonadotrophins play an important role to achieve multifollicular development (6). In the late 1970s, human menopausal gonadotrophin (hMG) containing FSH and LH in a 1:1 ratio with urinary proteins was the most widely used gonadotrophin for ovarian stimulation in assisted reproduction. However, the often concurrent problem of premature LH surges and premature luteinizations resulted in cancellations of many cycles (7). This was efficiently overcome by reversible medical "hypophysectomy," performed by GnRHa, introduced in 1982 (5).

According to time of initiation and duration of administration, GnRHa use was divided into three protocols: the long, most widely used, protocol, which was the most efficient for suppression of endogenous, high tonic LH levels, especially in polycystic ovary syndrome and normogonadotropic patients;

and the short and ultrashort protocols, which are mainly used in poor responders or older or hypergonadotropic patients with elevated FSH because of the well-known flare-up phenomenon (8).

With the use of GnRHa, human chorionic gonadotrophin (hCG) was necessary to induce final follicular maturation and triggering of ovulation. Accordingly, in the 1980s, the use of gonadotrophins, GnRHa, and hCG became a standard successful protocol for ovulation induction in assisted conception cycles. However, this standard protocol was challenged by the introduction of recombinant gonadotrophins and GnRH antagonists.

The manufacture of human FSH by recombinant DNA technology made production independent of urine collection and guaranteed the availability of an almost pure FSH preparation (>99 percent free from urinary protein contaminants) with minimal batch-to-batch variation. The high purity and low immunogeneity allowed SC administration (9). Despite proven efficacy of recombinant FSH (rFSH), its wide-spread use was hampered by its relatively high cost as compared with hMG (10). Both effectiveness and cost are important to decide whether to prefer one drug over the other. The decision to adopt a more expensive treatment could result in a lower number of couples receiving IVF treatment, especially in societies with decreasing health resources where financial implications should always be considered.

SELECTION OF THE TYPE OF GONADOTROPHINS

All types of the urinary-derived gonadotrophins contain FSH, the only difference lies in the content of LH and urinary proteins. hMG contains FSH and LH in a 1:1 ratio with urinary proteins, and recently, urinary hMG free of urinary proteins was manufactured (11).

Several randomized trials compared urinary FSH products with rFSH. Daya and Gunby published the first meta-analysis comparing urinary FSH with rFSH (12). Daya updated the meta-analysis and he showed that rFSH produced higher pregnancy rates per cycle than urinary FSH (OR 1.21; 95 percent CI 1.04–1.42), with a 3.7 percent absolute increase in pregnancy rate with rFSH. He included both randomized and quasirandomized trials ($n = 18$) including 3,421 cycles (13).

Al-Inany et al. published a meta-analysis comparing urinary FSH with rFSH. They included twenty truly randomized studies (4,610 IVF/ICSI cycles using long GnRH downregulation protocol) showing no statistically significant difference in the pregnancy rate per started cycle between rFSH and urinary-derived FSH gonadotrophins (OR 1.07; 95 percent CI 0.94–1.22). Subgroup analysis showed no significant difference in the pregnancy rate per started cycle between recombinant FSH and hMG (OR 0.81; 95 percent CI 0.63–1.05). The conclusion was that there is no evidence for superiority in terms of clinical pregnancy rate between rFSH and urinary FSH (14).

van Wely et al. (15) compared the effectiveness of hMG versus rFSH in a meta-analysis including six studies with 2,030 IVF/ICSI cycles. They concluded that hMG resulted in a higher clinical pregnancy rate than rFSH in IVF/ICSI cycles downregulated by the long protocol. However, one of the studies included was a quasirandomized, and if the data of this study were excluded, there will be no significant difference in clinical pregnancy rate between hMG and rFSH (15).

AL-Inany et al. updated their meta-analysis focusing only on comparison between rFSH and hMG demonstrating no significant difference between rFSH and hMG regarding, different outcomes (ongoing pregnancy/live birth rate OR 1.18, 95 percent CI 0.93–1.50; clinical pregnancy rate OR 1.2, 95 percent CI 0.99–1.47; miscarriage rate OR 1.2, 95 percent CI 0.70–2.16; multiple pregnancy rate OR 1.35, 95 percent CI 0.96–1.90; and incidence of moderate/severe OHSS OR 1.79, 95 percent CI 0.74–4.33). However, there was significant reduction in the amount of gonadotrophins in favor of hMG over rFSH (OR −317.8; 95 percent CI −346.6, −289.0) (6a).

Finally, by 2008, The Egyptian group updated their meta-analysis focusing mainly upon live birth rate, which is a patient-oriented outcome, and showed it to be significantly higher with hMG (OR 1.20; 95% CI 1.01–1.42) than with rFSH (6b). The findings of our meta-analysis were further supported by another recently published systematic review (6c), which ultimately strengthens the take-home message derived from our meta-analysis showing that hMG could achieve better live birth rate than rFSH.

Several points should be discussed within the frame of the comparison between the two gonadotrophin preparations:

First, do some patients require LH supplementation during stimulation with rFSH? It is theoretically possible that GnRHa may result in profound suppression of LH concentration, subsequently there will be a need for LH supplementation during ovarian stimulation (16). Until recently, there was no evidence in the literature that this actually happens; moreover, women who would require additional LH during ovarian stimulation could not be identified. Several recent studies identified subgroup of patients who require LH supplementation (17, 18).

Further documentation that LH activity may influence treatment response and outcome in IVF cycles came from the MERIT trial. Pharmacodynamic differences in follicular development, oocyte/embryo quality, endocrine response, and endometrial echogenicity exist between HP-hMG and rFSH preparations, which may be relevant for treatment outcome (19).

Second, there is a general trend in the field of medicine to move away from drugs extracted from biological material for safety reasons. It has been recently found that a prion protein

isoform is present in the urine of animals and affected humans with transmissible spongiform encephalopathies (20). This prion protein was also found in the urine of hamsters inoculated with prions. However, the urinary prion protein failed to cause prion disease in hamsters when inoculated intracerebrally (21). Urinary preparations of gonadotrophins have been used widely for more than forty years, and no infections have been associated with their use, even in the past when urinary products were crude (22). The current advice from the World Health Organization is that urine has zero infectivity for prion disease (23).

However, the cell culture medium for rFSH requires the presence of fetal calf serum, which theoretically can be risky. However, this serum is obtained from countries where prion disease is absent and the serum is prepared via a validated purification process.

Both urinary and recombinant gonadotropin preparations require purification, including a number of filtration, ionic exchange, chromatography, and precipitation steps, and thus bacteria, viruses, and prions may be physically removed from the final gonadotropin preparations. It is also reassuring to note that similar fractionation procedures are used in the production of human plasma. These steps are capable of removing prion proteins (24). In conclusion, concerning efficacy and safety, the available evidence showed that there is no significant difference between urinary and recombinant FSH and both products are safe and effective.

LH IN OVULATION INDUCTION

According to the "two-cells two-gonadotrophins" model (25, 26), LH exerts its activity in theca cells and expresses enzymatic pathways of androgen synthesis. The granulosa cells' activities and proliferation are directly regulated by FSH. LH induces the expression of the aromatase enzyme, which in turn converts theca-deriving androgens into estradiol. This theory reinforced the notion that granulosa and theca cells are distinct compartments regulated by FSH and LH, respectively. However, it was subsequently found that LH receptors are detectable on the granulosa compartment at the intermediate follicular phase (26, 27) at a time when blood concentrations of LH increase. Therefore, it appears that LH regulates both granulosa and theca cells. The optimal ratio of FSH-to-LH activity during ovarian stimulation has been a matter of controversy since the very early days of gonadotrophin therapy (28).

The use of GnRHa and antagonist, which prevents the rise of LH, together with the development of recombinant FSH devoid of LH activity made it possible to study in depth the role of LH in controlled ovarian hyperstimualtion for IVF.

The treatment of profoundly hypogonadotrophic women with FSH alone induces multiple follicle development but is associated with ovarian endocrine abnormalities and low oocyte fertilization rates (29). These findings indicate that, in spite of apparently normal follicular development induced by FSH, some exogenous LH is strictly necessary to optimize ovulation induction.

Recombinant FSH (r-hFSH), which is free of LH activity, is used in many cases of COH after downregulation with long protocol. The degree of pituitary suppression also depends on the GnRHa formulation, dose, and mode of administration (30). Although the postsuppression decline of LH concentrations is variable, concentrations ranging between 0.5 and 2.5 IU/L are usually observed. These concentrations often fall to less than 0.5 IU/L during the intermediate late stages of stimulation. Thus, multiple follicular growth is induced without exogenous LH and in a low endogenous LH environment. Nevertheless, an adequate ovarian response is achieved in almost all patients (31).

In a large multicenter, randomized trial using GnRHa long protocol, patients were randomized to receive either 225 IU/day of r-hFSH or the same dose of r-hFSH plus r-hLH (150 IU/day, from day S6). No significant difference in the number of metaphase II oocytes retrieved or in the cumulative pregnancy rate was found (32). It was also shown that rLH supplementation does not improve IVF outcome in GnRH antagonist cycles (33).

In a double-blind study using long GnRHa protocol, patients were randomized when the lead follicle reached a diameter of 14 mm to receive r-hFSH in addition to r-hLH, 75 IU, or placebo daily for a maximum of ten days prior to oocyte retrieval and IVF. Serum estradiol concentrations on the day of hCG administration were significantly higher in the group receiving r-hLH plus r-hFSH ($P = 0.0001$), but there were no significant differences between the groups in dose and duration of r-hFSH treatment required, oocyte maturation, fertilization rate, pregnancy rate, and live birth rate (34). Although the study was underpowered, it was very well designed and executed. The results of the study were supported by other trials (17a).

There is a Cochrane systematic review (17b) showing that LH supplementation may be of value for older women and poor responders.

Kolibianakis et al. performed a systematic review including four retrospective and two prospective studies to assess among women with normal ovulation or WHO Group II patients undergoing ovarian stimulation in GnRH analog IVF cycles, whether endogenous LH levels predict ongoing pregnancy beyond twelve weeks. Their conclusion was that there was no adverse effect of low LH level on probability of ongoing pregnancy beyond twelve weeks (35).

Some observational trials with r-hFSH have examined the relationship between LH serum concentrations and ovarian/IVF outcome in normogonadotrophic women undergoing ovarian stimulation in a GnRHa long protocol (36, 37). No LH cutoff value able to identify women requiring LH activity supplementation could be found by any of those authors. Differences in patient selection criteria, clinical end points, serum LH assays, and LH cutoff value may account for discrepancies among results. Hence, there is a need for adequately sized, prospective observational trials (38).

STEADY RESPONSE DURING COH AND LH

De Placido et al. found that in about 10–12 percent of normogonadotrophic patients, an initial response (i.e., at least five 2- to 9-mm follicles in each ovary) during the first days of stimulation is followed by a plateau in which there is no significant increase in follicular size or estradiol production in the next 3–4 days of stimulation (39). This profile of initial ovarian response to r-hFSH is referred to as "steady response" and usually leads physicians to increase the r-hFSH dose. In a prospective randomized trial, women who had no follicle with a mean diameter greater than 10 mm and estradiol serum concentrations 180 pg/mL or less on day S8 were randomized to receive LH activity supplementation ($n = 20$) in the form of hMG (150 IU/day) or an increase in the r-hFSH daily dose (maximum daily dose of 375 IU; $n = 23$). In order not to modify the daily FSH administration, the r-hFSH dose was reduced to 150 IU in women of

the hMG group. Forty matched women with an initial adequate response to r-hFSH (i.e., a tripling of serum estradiol concentration between days S5 and S8 in association with more than four follicles >10 mm on day S8) served as a nonrandomized control population. The mean number of oocytes retrieved was significantly higher in women treated with hMG supplementation than in those who received r-hFSH "step-up." Moreover, the ovarian outcome of the hMG group was comparable with that observed in "normal responders," suggesting that LH activity supplementation was able to "rescue" this apparently abnormal response to r-hFSH. Interestingly, when serum LH concentrations were measured on day S8, there was no statistically significant difference between women whose ovarian outcome improved with hMG and normal responders to r-hFSH. These findings revealed the existence of a subgroup of hyporesponders who benefit more from LH activity supplementation than from an increase in the daily r-hFSH dose (39).

In a preliminary dose-finding design, De Placido et al. (40) evaluated the efficacy of r-hLH supplementation in women displaying an initial steady response to r-hFSH. Women displaying a steady response were randomized on day 8 to receive a daily r-hLH dose of 75 ($n = 23$) or 150 IU ($n = 23$). The control population consisted of "normal" responders to r-hFSH ($n = 46$). The mean number of oocytes retrieved (primary end point) and the percentage of mature oocytes in women treated with 150 IU of r-hLH (9.65 ± 2.16, 79.0 percent) were similar to those observed in "normal responders" (10.65 ± 2.8, 82.5 percent) and were significantly higher than those of subjects receiving 75 IU [6.39 ± 1.53, 65.7 percent ($P < 0.001$ and $P < 0.05$ respectively)] (40).

The effectiveness of r-hLH in steady responders was then evaluated in a larger multicenter randomized trial (41). A total of 229 IVF/ICSI cycles of long GnRHa protocol performed in seven Italian units were analyzed. Steady responders were identified on day 8 and randomized to receive either r-hLH supplementation of 150 IU/day ($n = 59$) or an increase of 150 IU in the daily r-hFSH dose ($n = 58$; r-hFSH step-up protocol). Also a matched normal responders group was selected as a control group ($n = 112$). The number of cumulus-oocyte complexes (primary end point) and mature oocytes retrieved was significantly higher in women receiving r-hLH than in those treated with the r-hFSH step-up protocol. Moreover, the mean number of mature oocytes of r-hLH group was similar to that observed in normal responders. Also in this study, endogenous LH serum concentrations on day S8 (before randomization) did not differ between steady responders undergoing r-hLH supplementation and normal responders (41).

Ferraretti et al. conducted an RCT (42) on 184 patients and reached similar conclusion to that of previous studies (39–41), and it should be noted that in all these studies women treated with r-hLH had a significantly lower consumption of r-hFSH.

Thus, there is a subset of normogonadotrophic women who cannot be classified as either "poor responders," or "normal responders." These patients have a suboptimal IVF outcome and seem to benefit from r-hLH administration. Thus, a clinical history of high r-hFSH consumption during ovarian stimulation should suggest the use of r-hLH-containing drugs for restimulation. In case of a first ovarian stimulation cycle, early identification of women who require a high r-hFSH dose may result in timely integration with r-hLH, which, in turn, may rescue the ovarian response and improve the ovarian IVF outcome.

Recent publications (41, 43) suggested that the direction and extent of change of LH serum concentration during ovarian stimulation might be predictive of outcome (41, 43). From this, the suggestions were derived to add recombinant LH or switch from recombinant FSH only to partly hMG in GnRH antagonist–based ovarian stimulation protocols in all first cycle patients, as soon as GnRH antagonist administration starts (44).

ENDOGENOUS LH LEVELS

Kol suggests that the need for exogenous LH could possibly be predicted by the dynamics of endogenous LH levels during stimulation. Generally, this appears to be a difficult task, as the concentration of immunoreactive LH seems not to be related to the concentration of bioactive LH (44).

Clinical response to r-hFSH more than basal LH concentration seems to be predictive of exogenous LH requirement during ovarian stimulation (39–41), supporting the idea that a discrepancy between immunoreactive and bioactive LH may exist (45). The hypothesis that carriers of a less bioactive LH may require higher gonadotrophin doses and/or benefit from LH activity supplementation during ovarian stimulation is supported by other lines of evidence.

In this context, an association between ovarian resistance to r-FSH monotherapy and presence of an LH polymorphism (V-beta LH) in normogonadotrophic women undergoing GnRHa long protocol has been recently suggested (38).

There is growing evidence showing that circulating LH measurements do not accurately reflect LH administration (39–43, 46). Serum LH concentrations assayed by immunoassay do not necessarily reflect circulating LH bioactively (47, 48). This may be explained in various ways. First, LH circulating concentrations may not be representative of local hormonal activity, which is also related to receptor status and paracrine networks. During critical phases of folliculogenesis, LH concentrations may fall below the threshold of single follicles: this phenomenon could be counteracted by FSH-dependent mechanisms in almost all patients. Conversely, in some women, local variables may interfere with adaptive mechanisms and render the lack of LH critical. Alternatively, incongruence between LH serum concentration and exogenous LH requirement may be related to genetic variables (41, 42). Some polymorphic variants of the FSH receptor are associated with a poor ovarian response to exogenous FSH (49). In such cases, an initial suboptimal response to r-hFSH would be rescued by LH, which is able to substitute FSH activity during the intermediate-late stages of folliculogenesis (27). Filicori et al. tried in an RCT low-dose hCG (200 IU/day) alone to replace FSH-containing gonadotropins in the final few days of COH (50). Interestingly, both duration and dose of gonadotrophins administration were reduced; small but not large preovulatory follicles were reduced; fertilization rates were higher, but no difference in pregnancy rate. These data may point to low-dose hCG, which can support the growth and stimulate the maturation of larger ovarian follicles as a result of specific granulosa cell receptors that develop after a few days of FSH priming. Finally, it is possible that LH is less biologically active in women who benefit from exogenous LH. In other words, serum concentrations of the "immunoreactive" molecule may be not representative of the bioactivity of the hormone (51–54).

GnRHa VERSUS ANTAGONIST IN COH FOR IVF

The GnRH antagonists emerged as an alternative to GnRHa in preventing premature LH surges. In comparison with the GnRHa, the pharmacological mechanism by which GnRH antagonists suppress the release of gonadotrophins is completely different (55). While the agonists act on chronic administration through downregulation of receptors and desensitization of the gonadotrophic cells, the antagonists bind competitively to the receptors and thereby prevent the endogenous GnRH from exerting its stimulatory effects on the pituitary cells. The competitive blockade of the receptors leads to an immediate arrest of gonadotrophin secretion (56). This mechanism of action is dependent on the equilibrium between endogenous GnRH and the applied antagonist. Because of this, the antagonistic effect is highly dose dependent in contrast with the GnRHa. The efficacy and safety of GnRH antagonists was demonstrated in a number of studies (57–59).

In addition, GnRH antagonists for COH in assisted conception reduced the amount of gonadotrophin needed for stimulation and avoided estrogen deprivation symptoms (e.g., hot flushes, sleep disturbances, and headache) as frequently observed in the prestimulation phase of a long GnRHa protocol (60). Whether the benefits mentioned above justify a change in routine treatment from the standard long GnRHa protocol to the newly designed GnRH antagonist regimen depends on whether the clinical outcome using these protocols is equivalent. Although multicenter RCTs showed that there was no statistically significant difference between GnRHa and antagonist in prevention of premature LH surge, there was a consistent trend toward lower pregnancy rate with the antagonist (61).

A Cochrane systematic review was published comparing the long protocol of GnRHa to the antagonist, the overall OR for the prevention of premature LH surges was 1.76 (95 percent CI 0.75–4.16), which is not statistically significant. There were significantly fewer clinical pregnancies in those treated with GnRH antagonists (OR 0.79, 95 percent CI 0.62–0.97). The absolute treatment effect was calculated to be 5 percent. The number needed to treat was 20. There was no statistically significant reduction in incidence of severe ovarian hyperstimulation syndrome between the two regimens (RR 0.51, 95 percent CI 0.22–1.18) (62).

An update of this Cochrane review, which included twenty-nine RCTs (4,424 subjects), including only long GnRH protocol versus GnRH antagonist showed that clinical pregnancy rate was significantly lower in the antagonist group (OR 0.79, 95 percent CI 0.68–0.9) as was the ongoing pregnancy/live birth rate (OR 0.79, 95 percent CI 0.68–0.9). There was statistically significant reduction in the incidence of severe OHSS with the antagonist protocol (OR 0.60, 95 percent CI 0.41–0.89). The authors concluded that GnRH antagonist protocol is associated with a lower pregnancy rate compared with GnRHa long protocol but with a significant reduction in severe OHSS (63).

A recent systematic review that included twenty-two RCTs that involved 3,176 patients compared GnRHa versus antagonist, and they found no significant difference in live birth rate between the two groups studied (OR 0.86, 95 percent 0.72–1.02) (64). This meta-analysis was criticized in several points: first, it mixed both long and short GnRHa protocols. It is well known that short protocol is associated with significant lower pregnancy rate (65). The inclusion of short protocol will dilute the data extracted from the long GnRH protocol studies, and this may affect the outcome of the meta-analysis. Second, the authors calculated the probability of live birth rate in several studies in which the only clinical pregnancy rate was published (66), so the real birth rate was not compared in the meta-analysis. Third, the studies published as abstracts in major scientific meetings were excluded. Although it is a prerequisite to include these studies in Cochrane reviews, it may be difficult to extract detailed information from abstracts particularly when contact with the authors fails.

In an attempt to tailor the GnRH antagonist to individual patients, flexible protocol was used. The day of the onset of GnRH antagonist was adjusted according to the response of the patient. A meta-analysis of four RCTs compared GnRH antagonist administration on a fixed day versus starting it according to follicular size. There was statistically no significant difference in pregnancy rate per woman randomized, although there was a trend toward a lower pregnancy rate in favor of the fixed protocol (OR 0.7, 95 percent CI 0.47–1.05). However, there was a statistically significant reduction both in number of antagonist ampoules and amount of gonadotrophins used in the flexible protocol (OR −1.2, 95 percent CI −1.26 to −1.15) (67).

With GnRHa, the pituitary is downregulated and secretion of endogenous gonadotrophins is extremely low during stimulation and follicular growth will depend only on exogenous gonadotrophins, whereas in antagonist cycles, follicular growth depends on both exogenous and endogenous FSH and LH. However, both endogenous FSH and LH secretion will fall when antagonist is started. The hypothesis is that on the day of starting GnRH antagonist, the endogenous FSH will suddenly stop and this will reduce the total FSH available for the growing follicles until the day of hCG.

An RCT included 151 patients where couples were randomly allocated on the day of starting the antagonist into two groups: no increase in hMG dose or an increase of 75 U of hMG on the day of antagonist administration, and continued till the day of hCG administration. There was no statistically significant difference between both groups regarding number of oocytes retrieved, embryos obtained, implantation rate, clinical pregnancy rate, and multiple pregnancy rate. Clinical pregnancy rate was 32.1 percent in group A versus 36.2 percent in group B (OR 1.3, 95 percent CI 0.63–2.6). The multiple pregnancy rate was 41.2 versus 38.9 percent. In summary, there was no evidence of clinical value for increasing the dose of hMG on day of antagonist administration (68a).

However, GnRH antagonist was proved to be effective in mild stimulation protocols, which may change the trend in IVF programs. In an RCT by the Dutch group, cumulative rates of term live births and patients' discomfort are much the same for mild ovarian stimulation with single embryos transferred and for standard stimulation with two embryos transferred. However, a mild IVF treatment protocol can substantially reduce multiple pregnancy rates and overall costs (68b). In such trial, GnRH antagonist was the cornerstone to prevent premature LH surge.

Another new option for GnRH antagonist comes from our group that conducted an RCT to compare coasting versus the use of GnRH antagonist for prevention of severe ovarian hyperstimulation syndrome in cycles downregulated by GnRHa and it proved to be effective (68c) GnRH antagonist was superior to coasting in producing significantly more high-quality embryos and more oocytes as well as reducing the time until

hCG administration. There was no significant difference in pregnancy rate between the two groups.

GONADOTROPHINS FOR TRIGGERING OF OVULATION

LH surge is essential in the final stages of follicular maturation for triggering follicle rupture, expelling the oocyte from the follicle, and leading to its capture by the fallopian tube. In addition, the LH surge promotes luteinization forming an active corpus luteum. These effects of LH are essential for conception to occur (69).

In assisted conception, urinary hCG has been used for many years to mimic the endogenous LH surge as there are considerable structural similarities between hCG and human LH and hence both hormones stimulate the same receptor (70). Preparations of hCG are easy and cheap as hCG is readily available in the urine of pregnant women, whereas only low concentrations of LH are found in the urine of postmenopausal women.

Recombinant hCG (rhCG) and r-LH preparations are derived from genetically engineered Chinese hamster ovary cell through recombinant DNA technology. Thus, it is necessary to assess the efficacy of recombinant hCG and r-LH compared to urinary hCG (used for more than twenty-five years) for induction of final follicular maturation and luteinization in women undergoing assisted conception. One systematic review included seven RCTs, four comparing rhCG and uhCG, and three RCTs comparing r-hLH and uhCG were published. There was no statistically significant difference between rhCG versus uhCG regarding the ongoing pregnancy/live birth rate (OR 0.98, 95 percent CI 0.69–1.39), pregnancy rate, miscarriage rate, or incidence of OHSS, but rhCG was associated with a reduction in the incidence of local site reactions and other minor adverse effects (OR 0.47, 95 percent CI 0.32–0.70) (71).

Results of one trial showed that increasing the dose of recombinant hCG (single 500-μg dose of rhCG) may lead to a higher rate of ovarian hyperstimulation syndrome compared with a 250-μg dose (this difference was not statistically significant), with no significant improvement in pregnancy rate. As both safety and efficacy are required for any medication, the dose of 250 μg seems the dose of choice for triggering ovulation. Pooling the data from the trials comparing recombinant r-hLH versus urinary hCG demonstrated that clinical pregnancy rates were significantly lower in the r-hLH group than in the uhCG group ($P = 0.018$ and $P = 0.023$, respectively) (71).

GnRHa was used for triggering final oocyte maturation in the GnRH antagonist protocols. However, a systematic review of three randomized studies comparing triggering ovulation with a bolus of GnRHa versus hCG showed that GnRHa is associated with a significantly reduced likelihood of achieving clinical pregnancy (0.21, 95 percent CI 0.05–0.84, $P = 0.03$) (72).

ECONOMIC EVALUATION

The cost of ovulation induction drugs is one of the main limiting factors in assisted reproduction. There are few studies that examined the cost difference of recombinant FSH versus hMG in ART (10, 73, 74). These studies were based on meta-analysis of Daya, which showed superiority of rFSH, but as recent publications (6, 14) showed no significant difference in the pregnancy rate between recFSH and hMG then, the results of these studies are not valid anymore.

For any drug, the optimum position of an experimental treatment would be both to save costs and have greater effectiveness relative to a comparator. In a recently published guidelines for the management of infertility (75), the cost of antagonists for a five-day treatment schedule is around £120 and the cost of agonists for a much longer schedule (24–31 days) is £111. However, the cost of agonists increases with longer schedules of treatment (from around £88 for a shorter schedule to around £111 for a longer schedule). This could be an underestimate if a woman requires a few more doses of agonists, which may only be available in thirty-dose or sixty-dose units (75).

The total cost of gonadotrophins (using the British National Formulary prices) is around £544 for a low-dose schedule for women who are expected to respond well to ovulation induction and around £1,050 for a high-dose schedule. The overall cost of a schedule of ovulation induction with antagonists is between £645 and £1,170 per cycle of treatment. The cost of agonists is between £623 and £1,138 per cycle of treatment. In practice, the cost of the antagonist schedule is likely to be toward the lower end of the cost range as the patient uses fewer doses of gonadotrophins. The agonist schedule of treatment is likely to cost toward the higher end of the range since women tend to use the agonist for longer periods of time before starting gonadotrophins.

CONCLUSIONS

In general, there is no clinical significant difference in the effectiveness between urinary hMG and rFSH. A small subgroup of patients may require extra LH in the form of hMG or rLH. It seems that there is no significant difference in the cost of the cycle between agonist and antagonist protocols. GnRHa protocol as compared to GnRH antagonists results in a small but significantly higher pregnancy rate; however, it is also associated with a higher incidence of ovarian hyperstimulation syndrome. It is up to the clinician to decide the clinical relevance of these data and choose the type of Analogue.

KEY POINTS FOR CLINICAL PRACTICE

■ With the use of GnRHa, hCG was necessary to induce final follicular maturation and triggering of ovulation. Accordingly, in the 1980s, the use of gonadotrophins, GnRHa, and hCG became a standard successful protocol for ovulation induction in assisted conception cycles. However, this standard protocol was challenged by the introduction of recombinant gonadotrophins and GnRH antagonists.

■ The most up-to-date meta-analysis (Al-Inany 2005) focused only on comparison between rFSH and hMG, demonstrating no significant difference between rFSH and hMG regarding different outcomes (ongoing pregnancy/live birth rate OR 1.18, 95 percent CI 0.93–1.50), clinical pregnancy rate OR 1.2 (95 percent CI 0.99–1.47), miscarriage rate OR 1.2 (95 percent CI 0.70–2.16), multiple pregnancy rate OR 1.35 (95 percent CI 0.96–1.90), and incidence of moderate/severe OHSS OR 1.79 (95 percent CI 0.74–4.33). However, there was significant reduction in the amount of gonadotrophins in favor of hMG over rFSH (OR −317.8, 95 percent CI −346.6 to −289.0).

■ The conclusions of the above meta-analyses were that there is no advantage for either rFSH or urinary FSH concerning the clinical pregnancy rate, miscarriage rate, or OHSS rate.

■ The GnRH antagonists emerged as an alternative to GnRHa in preventing premature LH surges. While the agonists act on chronic administration through downregulation of receptors and desensitization of the gonadotrophic cells, the antagonists bind competitively to the receptors and thereby prevent the endogenous GnRH from exerting its stimulatory effects on the pituitary cells. The competitive blockade of the receptors leads to an immediate arrest of gonadotrophin secretion.

■ A Cochrane systematic review was published comparing the long protocol of GnRHa to the antagonist; the overall OR for the prevention of premature LH surges was 1.76 (95 percent CI 0.75–4.16), which is not statistically significant. There were significantly fewer clinical pregnancies in those treated with GnRH antagonists (OR 0.79, 95 percent CI 0.62–0.97). The absolute treatment effect was calculated to be 5 percent. The number needed to treat was 20. There was no statistically significant reduction in incidence of severe ovarian hyperstimulation syndrome between the two regimens (RR 0.51, 95 percent CI 0.22, 1.18) (62).

■ An update of this Cochrane review showed that clinical pregnancy rate was significantly lower in the antagonist group and there was statistically significant reduction in the incidence of severe OHSS with the antagonist protocol (OR 0.60, 95 percent CI 0.41–0.89).

REFERENCES

1. International Committee for Monitoring Assisted Reproductive Technology; Adamson GD, de Mouzon J, Lancaster P, Nygren KG, Sullivan E, Zegers-Hochschild F. World collaborative report on in vitro fertilization, 2000. *Fertil Steril*. 2006;85(6):1586–622.

2. Coelingh Bennink HJ, Fauser BC, Out HJ. Recombinant follicle-stimulating hormone (FSH; Puregon) is more efficient than urinary FSH (Metrodin) in women with clomiphene citrate-resistant, normogonadotropic, chronic anovulation: a prospective, multicenter, assessor-blind, randomized, clinical trial. European Puregon Collaborative Anovulation Study Group. *Fertil Steril*. 1998;69(1):19–25.

3. van Wely M, Yding Andersen C, Bayram N, van der Veen F. Urofollitropin and ovulation induction. *Treat Endocrinol*. 2005; 4(3):155–65.

4. Albano C, Felberbaum RE, Smitz J, Riethmuller-Winzen H, Engel J, Diedrich K, Devroey P. Ovarian stimulation with HMG: results of a prospective randomized phase III European study comparing the luteinizing hormone-releasing hormone (LHRH)-antagonist cetrorelix and the LHRH-agonist buserelin. European Cetrorelix Study Group. *Hum Reprod*. 2000;15(3):526–31.

5. Macklon NS, Stouffer RL, Giudice LC, Fauser BC. The science behind 25 years of ovarian stimulation for in vitro fertilization. *Endocr Rev*. 2006;27(2):170–207.

6a. Al-Inany H, Aboulghar MA, Mansour RT, Serour GI. Ovulation induction in the new millennium: recombinant follicle-stimulating hormone versus human menopausal gonadotropin. *Gynecol Endocrinol*. 2005;20(3):161–9.

6b. Al-Inany HG, Abou-Setta AM, Aboulghar MA et al. Efficacy and safety of human menopausal gonadotrophins versus recombinant FSH: a meta-analysis. *Reprod BioMed Online*. 2008;16:81–88.

6c. Coomarasamy A, Afnan M, Cheema D et al. Urinary hMG versus recombinant FSH for controlled ovarian hyperstimulation following an agonist long down-regulation protocol in IVF or ICSI treatment: a systematic review and meta-analysis. *Hum Reprod*. 2008;23:310–315.

7. Zafeiriou S, Loutradis D, Michalas S. The role of gonadotropins in follicular development and their use in ovulation induction protocols for assisted reproduction. *Eur J Contracept Reprod Health Care* 2000;5(2):157–67.

8. Albuquerque LE, Saconato H, Maciel MC, Baracat EC, Freitas V. Depot versus daily administration of GnRH agonist protocols for pituitary desensitization in assisted reproduction cycles: a Cochrane Review. *Hum Reprod.* 2003;18(10):2008–17.

9. Bergh C. Recombinant follicle stimulating hormone. *Hum Reprod.* 1999;14:1418–20.

10. Sykes D, Out HJ, Palmer SJ, Loon Jv J. The cost-effectiveness of IVF in the UK: a comparison of three gonadotrophin treatments. *Hum Reprod.* 2001; 16(12):2557–62.

11. Platteau P, Andersen AN, Balen A, Devroey P, Sorensen P, Helmgaard L, Arce JC. Menopur Ovulation Induction (MOI) Study Group. Similar ovulation rates, but different follicular development with highly purified menotrophin compared with recombinant FSH in WHO Group II anovulatory infertility: a randomized controlled study. *Hum Reprod.* 2006;21(7):1798–804.

12. Daya S, Gunby J. Recombinant versus urinary follicle stimulating hormone for ovarian stimulation in assisted reproduction cycles. *Cochrane Database Syst Rev.* 2000;(4):CD002810.

13. Daya S. Updated meta-analysis of recombinant follicle-stimulating hormone (FSH) versus urinary FSH for ovarian stimulation in assisted reproduction. *Fertil Steril.* 2002;77(4):711–14.

14. Al-Inany H, Aboulghar M, Mansour R, Serour G. Meta-analysis of recombinant versus urinary-derived FSH: an update. *Hum Reprod.* 2003;18(2):305–13.

15. van Wely M, Westergaard LG, Bossuyt PM, van der Veen F. Human menopausal gonadotropin and recombinant follicle-stimulating hormone for controlled ovarian hyperstimulation in assisted reproductive cycles. *Fertil Steril.* 2003;80(5):1121–2.

16. Fleming R, Rehka P, Deshpande N, Jamieson ME, Yates RW, Lyall H. Suppression of LH during ovarian stimulation: effects differ in cycles stimulated with purified urinary FSH and recombinant FSH. *Hum Reprod.* 2000;15:1440–5.

17a. Lisi F, Rinaldi L, Fishel S, Lisi R, Pepe GP, Picconeri MG, Campbell A. Use of recombinant LH in a group of unselected IVF patients. *Reprod Biomed Online* 2002;5(2):104–8.

17b. Mochtar MH, Van der Veen, Ziech M, van Wely M. Recombinant Luteinizing Hormone (rLH) for controlled ovarian hyperstimulation in assisted reproductive cycles. Cochrane Database Syst Rev. 2007 Apr 18;(2):CD005070.

18. Humaidan P, Bungum M, Bungum L, Yding Andersen C. Effects of recombinant LH supplementation in women undergoing assisted reproduction with GnRH agonist down-regulation and stimulation with recombinant FSH: an opening study. *Reprod Biomed Online* 2004;8(6):635–43.

19. Andersen AN, Devroey P, Arce JC. Clinical outcome following stimulation with highly purified hMG or recombinant FSH in patients undergoing IVF: a randomized assessor-blind controlled trial. *Hum Reprod.* 2006;21(12):3217–27.

20. Zygmunt M, Herr F, Keller-Schoenwetter S, Kunzi-Rapp K, Munstedt K, Rao CV, Lang U, Preissner KT. Characterization of human chorionic gonadotropin as a novel angiogenic factor. *J Clin Endocrinol Metab.* 2002;87:5290–6.

21. Matorras R, Rodriguez-Escudero FJ. The use of urinary gonadotrophins should be discouraged. *Hum Reprod.* 2002;17:1675.

22. Shaked GM, Shaked Y, Kariv-Inbal Z, Halimi M, Avraham I, Gabizon R. A protease-resistant prion protein isoform is present in urine of animals and humans affected with prion diseases. *J Biol Chem.* 2001;276:31479–82.

23. Crosignani PG. Risk of infection is not the main problem. *Hum Reprod.* 2002;17:1676.

24. Reichl H, Balen A, Jansen CA. Prion transmission in blood and urine: what are the implications for recombinant and urinary-derived gonadotrophins? *Hum Reprod.* 2002;17:2501–8

25. Fevold H. Synergism of follicle stimulating and luteinizing hormones in producing estrogen secretion. *Endocrinology* 1941;28:33–6.

26. Hillier SG, Whitelaw PF, Smyth CD. Follicular oestrogen synthesis: the 'two-cell, two-gonadotrophin' model revisited. *Mol Cell Endocrinol.* 1994;100:51–4.

27. Filicori M, Cognigni GE, Pocognoli P et al. Current concepts and novel applications of LH activity in ovarian stimulation. *Trends Endocrinol Metab.* 2003;14:267–73.

28. Jacobson A, Marshall JR. Ovulatory response rate with human menopausal gonadotropins of varying FSH-LH ratios. *Fertil Steril.* 1969;20:171–5.

29. Balasch J. The role of FSH and LH in ovulation induction: current concepts and the contribution of recombinant gonadotropins. In: Gardner DK, Weissman A, Howles CM, Shoham Z (Eds.). *Textbook of Assisted Reproductive Techniques: Laboratory and Clinical Perspectives, 2nd edn.* Taylor and Francis, London, 2004; pp. 541–65.

30. Westergaard LG, Erb K, Laursen SB et al. Human menopausal gonadotropin versus recombinant follicle-stimulating hormone in normogonadotropic women down-regulated with a gonadotropin-releasing hormone agonist who were undergoing in vitro fertilization and intracytoplasmic sperm injection: a prospective randomized study. *Fertil Steril.* 2001;76:543–9.

31. Chappel SC, Howles C. Reevaluation of the roles of luteinizing hormone and follicle-stimulating hormone in the ovulatory process. *Hum Reprod.* 1991;6(9):1206–12.

32. Marrs R, Meldrum D, Muasher S, Schoolcraft W, Werlin L, Kelly E. Randomized trial to compare the effect of recombinant human FSH (follitropin alfa) with or without recombinant human LH in women undergoing assisted reproduction treatment. *Reprod Biomed Online* 2004;8(2):175–82.

33. Griesinger G, Schultze-Mosgau A, Dafopoulos K, Schroeder A, Schroer A, von Otte S, Hornung D, Diedrich K, Felberbaum R. Recombinant luteinizing hormone supplementation to recombinant follicle-stimulating hormone induced ovarian hyperstimulation in the GnRH-antagonist multiple-dose protocol. *Hum Reprod.* 2005;20(5):1200–6.

34. Tarlatzis B, Tavmergen E, Szamatowicz M, Barash A, Amit A, Levitas E, Shoham Z. The use of recombinant human LH (lutropin alfa) in the late stimulation phase of assisted reproduction cycles: a double-blind, randomized, prospective study. *Hum Reprod.* 2006;21(1):90–4.

35. Kolibianakis EM, Collins J, Tarlatzis B, Papanikolaou E, Devroey P. Are endogenous LH levels during ovarian stimulation for IVF using GnRH analogues associated with the probability of ongoing pregnancy? A systematic review. *Hum Reprod Update* 2006;12(1):3–12.

36. Westergaard LG, Laursen SB, Andersen CY. Increased risk of early pregnancy loss by profound suppression of luteinizing hormone during ovarian stimulation in normogonadotrophic women undergoing assisted reproduction. *Hum Reprod.* 2000;15:1003–8.

37. Humaidan P, Bungum L, Bungum M, Yding Andersen C. Ovarian response and pregnancy outcome related to mid-follicular LH levels in women undergoing assisted reproduction with GnRH agonist down-regulation and recombinant FSH stimulation. *Hum Reprod.* 2002;17:2016–21.

38. Alviggi C, Pettersson K, Mollo A et al. Impaired multiple follicular development in carriers of Trp8Arg and Ile15 Thr LH-beta variant undergoing controlled ovarian stimulation.

Abstracts of the 21st Annual Meeting of ESHRE. *Hum Reprod.* 2005;20 (Suppl. 1):P-385, i139.

39. De Placido G, Mollo A, Alviggi C et al. Rescue of IVF cycles by HMG in pituitary down-regulated normogonadotrophic young women characterized by a poor initial response to recombinant FSH. *Hum Reprod.* 2001;16:1875–9.

40. De Placido G, Alviggi C, Perino A et al. Recombinant human LH supplementation versus recombinant human FSH (rFSH) step-up protocol during controlled ovarian stimulation in normogonadotrophic women with initial inadequate ovarian response to rFSH. A multicentre, prospective, randomized controlled trial. *Hum Reprod.* 2005;20:390–6.

41. De Placido G, Alviggi C, Mollo A et al. Effects of recombinant LH (rLH) supplementation during controlled ovarian hyperstimulation (COH) in normogonadotrophic women with an initial inadequate response to recombinant FSH (rFSH) after pituitary downregulation. *Clin Endocrinol (Oxf)* 2004;60:637–43.

42. Ferraretti AP, Gianaroli L, Magli MC et al. Exogenous luteinizing hormone in controlled ovarian hyperstimulation for assisted reproduction techniques. *Fertil Steril.* 2004;82:1521–6.

43. Huirne JA, van Loenen AC, Schats R et al. Dose-finding study of daily GnRH antagonist for the prevention of premature LH surges in IVF/ICSI patients: optimal changes in LH and progesterone for clinical pregnancy. *Hum Reprod.* 2005;20:359–67.

44. Kol S. To add or not to add LH: considerations of LH concentration changes in individual patients. *Reprod BioMed Online* 2005;11:664–66.

45. Huhtaniemi I, Jiang M, Nilsson et al. Mutations and polymorphisms in gonadotropin genes. *Mol Cell Endocrinol.* 1999;25:89–94.

46. Fabregues F, Creus M, Penarrubia J, Manau D, Vanrell JA, Balasch J. Effects of recombinant human luteinizing hormone supplementation on ovarian stimulation and the implantation rate in down-regulated women of advanced reproductive age. *Fertil Steril.* 2006;85(4):925–31.

47. Jaakkola T, Ding Y, Valavaara R et al. The ratios of serum bioactive/immunoreactive luteinizing hormone and follicle stimulating hormone in various clinical conditions with an increased and decreased gonadotropin secretion: reevaluation by a highly sensitive immunometric assay. *J Clin Endocrinol Metab.* 1990;70:1496–505.

48. Schroor E, van Weissenbruch M, Engelbert M et al. Bioactivity of luteinizing hormone during normal puberty in girls and boys. *Horm Res.* 1999;51:230–7.

49. Simoni M, Nieschlag E, Gromoll J. Isoforms and single nucleotide polymorphisms of the FSH receptor gene: implications for human reproduction. *Hum Reprod Update* 2002;8:413–21.

50. Filicori M, Cognigni GE, Gamberini E, Parmegiani L, Troilo E, Roset B. Efficacy of low-dose human chorionic gonadotropin alone to complete controlled ovarian stimulation. *Fertil Steril.* 2005;84(2):394–401.

51. Jiang M, Pakarinen P, Zhang FP et al. A common polymorphic allele of the human luteinizing hormone beta-subunit gene: additional mutations and differential function of the promoter sequence. *Hum Mol Gen.* 1999;8:2037–46.

52. Themmen APN, Huhtaniemi IT. Mutations of gonadotropins and gonadotropin receptors: elucidating the physiology and pathophysiology of pituitary-gonadal function. *Endocrine Rev.* 2000;21:551–83.

53. Ropelato MG, Garcia-Rudaz MC, Castro-Fernandez C et al. A preponderance of basic luteinizing hormone (LH) isoforms accompanies inappropriate hypersecretion of both basal and pulsatile LH in adolescents with polycystic ovarian syndrome. *J Clin Endocrinol Metab.* 1999;84:4629–36.

54. Mitchell R, Hollis S, Rothwell C et al. Age related changes in the pituitary-testicular axis in normal men; lower serum testosterone results from decreased bioactive LH drive. *Clin Endocrinol.* 1995;42:501–7.

55. Olivennes F, Alvarez S, Bouchard P, Fanchin R, Salat-Baroux J, Frydman R. The use of GnRH antagonist (Cetrorelix) in a single dose protocol in IVF-embryo transfer: a dose finding study of 3 versus 2mg. *Hum Reprod.* 1998;13(9):2411–14.

56. Felberbaum RE, Reissmann T, Kuper W, Bauer O, al Hasani S, Diedrich C et al. Preserved pituitary response under ovarian stimulation with hMG and GnRH-antagonists (Cetrorelix) in women with tubal infertility. *Euro J Obstet Gynecol Reprod Biol.* 1995;61(2):151–5.

57. Borm G, Mannaerts B. Treatment with the gonadotrophin-releasing hormone antagonist ganirelix in women undergoing ovarian stimulation with recombinant follicle stimulating hormone is effective, safe and convenient: results of a controlled, randomized, multicentre trial. The European Orgalutran Study Group. *Hum Reprod.* 2000;15(7):1490–8.

58. The European Middle East Orgalutran Study Group. Comparable clinical outcome using the GnRH antagonist ganirelix or a long protocol of the GnRH agonist triptorelin for the prevention of premature LH surges in women undergoing ovarian stimulation. *Hum Reprod.* 2001;16:644–51.

59. North American Study. Fluker M, Grifo J, Leader A, Levy M, Meldrum D, Muasher SJ, Rinehart J, Rosenwaks Z, Scott RT Jr., Schoolcraft W, Shapiro DB. Efficacy and safety of ganirelix acetate versus leuprolide acetate in women undergoing controlled ovarian hyperstimulation. *Fertil Steril.* 2001;75(1):38–45.

60. Ortmann O, Weiss JM, Diedrich K. Embryo implantation and GnRH antagonists: ovarian actions of GnRH antagonists. *Hum Reprod.* 2001;16(4):608–11.

61. Rongieres-Bertrand C, Olivennes F, Righini C, Fanchin R, Taieb J, Hamamah S, Bouchard P, Frydman R. Revival of the natural cycles in in-vitro fertilization with the use of a new gonadotrophin-releasing hormone antagonist (Cetrorelix): a pilot study with minimal stimulation. *Hum Reprod.* 1999;14(3):683–8.

62. Al-Inany H, Aboulghar M. GnRH antagonist in assisted reproduction: a Cochrane review. *Hum Reprod.* 2002;17(4):874–85.

63. Al-Inany HG, Abou-Setta AM, Aboulghar M. Gonadotrophin-releasing hormone antagonists for assisted conception. *Cochrane Database Syst Rev.* 2006;3:CD001750.

64. Kolibianakis EM, Collins J, Tarlatzis BC, Devroey P, Diedrich K, Griesinger G. Among patients treated for IVF with gonadotrophins and GnRH analogues, is the probability of live birth dependent on the type of analogue used? A systematic review and meta-analysis. *Hum Reprod Update* 2006;12(6):651–71.

65. Daya S. Gonadotropin releasing hormone agonist protocols for pituitary desensitization in in vitro fertilization and gamete intrafallopian transfer cycles. *Cochrane Database Syst Rev.* 2000;(2):CD001299.

66. Arce JC, Nyboe Andersen A, Collins J. Resolving methodological and clinical issues in the design of efficacy trials in assisted reproductive technologies: a mini-review. *Hum Reprod.* 2005;20(7):1757–71.

67. Al-Inany H, Aboulghar MA, Mansour RT, Serour GI. Optimizing GnRH antagonist administration: meta-analysis of fixed versus flexible protocol. *Reprod Biomed Online* 2005;10(5):567–70.

68a. Aboulghar MA, Mansour RT, Serour GI, Al-Inany HG, Amin YM, Aboulghar MM. Increasing the dose of human menopausal gonadotrophins on day of GnRH antagonist administration: randomized controlled trial. *Reprod Biomed Online* 2004;8(5):524–7.

68b. Heijnen EM, Eijkemans MJ, De Klerk C, Polinder S, Beckers NG, Klinkert ER, Broekmans FJ, Passchier J, Te Velde ER, Macklon NS, Fauser BC. A mild treatment strategy for in-vitro fertilisation: a randomised non-inferiority trial. *Lancet.* 2007 Mar 3;369(9563):743–9.

68c. Aboulghar MA, Mansour RT, Amin YM, Al-Inany HG, Aboulghar MM, Serour GI. A prospective randomized study comparing coasting with GnRH antagonist administration in patients at risk for severe OHSS. *Reprod Biomed Online* 2007 Sep;15(3): 271–9.

69. Loraine JA. Assays of human chorionic gonadotrophin in relation to clinical practice. *J Reprod Fertil.* 1966;12(1):23–31.

70. Chang P, Kenley S, Burns T, Denton G, Currie K, DeVane G et al. Recombinant human chorionic gonadotropin (rhCG) in assisted reproductive technology: results of a clinical trial comparing two doses of rhCG (Ovidrel) to urinary hCG (Profasi) for induction of final follicular maturation in in vitro fertilization-embryo transfer. *Fertil Steril.* 2001;76(1):67–74.

71. Al-Inany HG, Aboulghar M, Mansour R, Proctor M. Recombinant versus urinary human chorionic gonadotrophin for ovulation induction in assisted conception. *Cochrane Database Syst Rev.* 2005;(2):CD003719.

72. Griesinger G, Diedrich K, Devroey P, Kolibianakis EM. GnRH agonist for triggering final oocyte maturation in the GnRH antagonist ovarian hyperstimulation protocol: a systematic review and meta-analysis. *Hum Reprod Update* 2006;12(2):159–68.

73. Silverberg K, Daya S, Auray JP, Duru G, Ledger W, Wikland M, Bouzayen R, O'Brien M, Falk B, Beresniak A. Analysis of the cost effectiveness of recombinant versus urinary follicle-stimulating hormone in in vitro fertilization/intracytoplasmic sperm injection programs in the United States. *Fertil Steril.* 2002;77(1): 107–13.

74. Daya S, Ledger W, Auray JP, Duru G, Silverberg K, Wikland M, Bouzayen R, Howles CM, Beresniak A. Cost-effectiveness modelling of recombinant FSH versus urinary FSH in assisted reproduction techniques in the UK. *Hum Reprod.* 2001;16(12): 2563–9.

75. National Institute of Clinical Excellence. Fertility: assessment and treatment of people with fertility problems, Clinical guidelines No. 11. London: Abba Litho Ltd. UK, 2004.

44

LUTEAL PHASE SUPPORT IN ASSISTED REPRODUCTION

Luciano G. Nardo, Tarek A. Gelbaya

INTRODUCTION

Despite numerous developments in assisted reproduction, the implantation rate of good-quality embryos remains low. Over the years, implantation failure has been questioned for many cases of unsuccessful in vitro fertilization (IVF) with or without intracytoplasmic sperm injection (ICSI).

Implantation is the end result of complex molecular crosstalks between the hormonally primed uterus and the blastocyst. Failure to synchronize the component processes involved in these interactions results in unsuccessful implantation. During the implantation window (day 19 to day 24 of the menstrual cycle), the endometrium undergoes precise morphological changes under the control of the sex steroid hormones – estrogen and progesterone (P). During the secretory phase, the endometrial glands display enhanced secretory activity, the endometrium becomes more vascular and edematous, and pinopodes (bulky pedunculated extrusions of the luminal epithelial cell membrane) develop on the luminal surface of the epithelium. Although these changes are useful predictors of the outcome of pregnancy, the molecular mechanisms underlying them are unknown. Of the many aspects of the synchronization process, the role of steroid hormones is indeed the best understood.

In order to improve implantation rates, a variety of therapeutic strategies have been proposed, including immunologic testing and treatment, blastocyst transfer, assisted hatching, embryo coculture, preimplantation genetic screening for aneuploidy, and embryo donation. Nevertheless, the inadequacy of luteal phase remains a cause of implantation failure in some of the patients undergoing assisted reproductive techniques (ART). The luteal phase is defined as the period from occurrence of ovulation until the establishment of pregnancy or the resumption of menses two weeks later. Numerous studies have confirmed that ovarian stimulation used in IVF cycles is associated with luteal phase deficiency, even when gonadotrophin-releasing hormone (GnRH) antagonists are used. In the context of ART, luteal phase therapy identifies the administration of drugs to support the process of implantation.

In this chapter, we discuss the physiology of the luteal phase both in natural and stimulated cycles, while a lot of emphasis is given to the current evidence-based approaches for luteal phase support in assisted reproduction.

LUTEAL PHASE IN THE NATURAL CYCLE

Progesterone and estrogen are required to prepare the uterus for embryo implantation and to modulate the endometrium during the early stages of pregnancy. In the normal luteal phase of a nonpregnant woman, steroid production peaks four days after ovulation and continues for one week until falling several days before the next menses. If pregnancy occurs, progesterone production is restored by human chorionic gonadotrophin (hCG) stimulation. Once the oocyte is released, the follicle collapses and the remaining granulosa cells, which have acquired receptors for luteinizing hormone (LH), rapidly undergo luteinization under the influence of LH. The formed corpus luteum requires regular stimulation by LH to maintain adequate production of progesterone (Vande Wiele et al., 1970).

A shift from ovarian to placental production of gonadal steroids occurs over a period of weeks. In one study, placental progesterone secretion was detected as early as fifty days of gestational age (thirty-six days after embryo transfer) in oocyte recipients (Scott et al., 1991). The timing accords with the observation that surgical removal of the corpus luteum in early pregnancy leads to miscarriage (Caspo et al., 1972).

LUTEAL PHASE IN ART CYCLE

Luteal Phase and Controlled Ovarian Hyperstimulation

The advent of follicular maturation drugs, like gonadotrophins, showed that serum progesterone increases to supraphysiological levels. Simon et al. (1995) have reported significantly decreased implantation and pregnancy rates per cycle in IVF patients whose serum estradiol (E_2) concentrations were higher than 2,500 pg/mL on the day of hCG (high responders) as compared with normal responders. The authors concluded that elevated E_2 levels on the day of hCG injection, regardless of the number of oocytes retrieved and the serum progesterone measurements, adversely affect uterine receptivity. A matched-control study found higher clinical and ongoing pregnancy rates in oocyte recipients compared to patients undergoing IVF treatments (Paulson et al., 1990). Data from an oocyte-sharing program have demonstrated that pregnancy rates following fresh embryo transfer were twice as high in older recipients as in younger donors. Interestingly, there was no significant difference in pregnancy rate after frozen embryo transfer between the two groups (Check et al., 1995). These findings support the view that controlled ovarian hyperstimulation may have a detrimental effect on the receptivity of the endometrium and indirectly on implantation.

Luteal Phase and GnRH Agonist

Over two decades ago, Edwards and Steptoe (1980) suggested that luteal phase inadequacy due to ovarian stimulation could be the cause of IVF failure. Other researchers have shown that luteal phase support was beneficial in establishing an IVF pregnancy (Smitz et al., 1992; Smitz et al., 1993; Soliman et al., 1994). A meta-analysis of all available quasirandomized trials showed that the use of GnRH agonists increased IVF pregnancy rates by 80–127 percent in women who responded normally to exogenous gonadotrophins (Hughes et al., 1992). Luteal phase deficiency is more pronounced in GnRH agonist long protocols compared with short protocols (Devreker et al., 1996) and is present even if GnRH agonists are ceased early (Beckers et al., 2000).

Endometrial biopsies on the day of oocyte retrieval in agonist-controlled IVF cycles have shown endometrial advancement in more than 90 percent of patients. Of note, there were no pregnancies in cases where the endometrial advancement was exceeded by three days (Ubaldi et al., 1997; Lass et al., 1998). It has been reported that pinopodes appear during the early luteal phase in women undergoing ovarian stimulation (Nikas et al., 1999). In agreement with these studies, Soliman et al. (1994) observed a delay of two to four days in midluteal endometrial biopsies taken in stimulated cycles. When progesterone or hCG was used to support the luteal phase, mid- and late – luteal phase histology, scanning electron microscopy, and immunochemistry showed in-phase endometrium (Balasch et al., 1991).

It is plausible that one or more of the following mechanisms may compromise the luteal phase: 1) suppression of endogenous LH secretion during the luteal phase as a result of persistent pituitary suppression by GnRH agonist; 2) supraphysiological levels of E_2 and P in the early luteal phase, leading to advanced development of the endometrium, hence asynchrony between the embryo and the endometrium; 3) shorter duration of ovarian steroid production in stimulated cycles compared to natural cycles; and 4) aspiration of the granulosa cells that surround the oocyte.

A number of meta-analyses have concurred to document that luteal support improves IVF outcome (Soliman et al., 1994; Pritts and Atwood, 2002; Daya and Gunby, 2004; Nosarka et al., 2005). In their review of fifty-nine randomized controlled trials on luteal support in ART cycles, Daya and Gunby (2004) found that luteal phase support with hCG provided significant benefit as compared to placebo or no treatment, with a significant increase in ongoing pregnancy rate and a decrease in miscarriage rate when GnRH agonist was used. Luteal phase support with progesterone, compared to placebo or no treatment in GnRH agonist and non-GnRH agonist cycles, also resulted in a significant increase in pregnancy rates but without any effect on the early pregnancy loss rate.

Luteal Phase and GnRH Antagonist

Due to the immediate recovery of pituitary gonadotrophin release just after discontinuation of the GnRH antagonists, it has been hypothesized that the luteal phase would be less disturbed in these cycles (Elter and Nelson, 2001; Ragni et al., 2001). Although preliminary observations in intrauterine insemination cycles favored this contention, studies on a limited number of cases undergoing IVF demonstrated that there was a significant reduction in pregnancy rates without luteal phase support (Albano et al., 1998; Albano et al., 1999; Beckers et al., 2002).

The serum LH levels in the early and midluteal phase of GnRH antagonist–treated cycles were low, regardless of the regimen used to induce oocyte maturation (Tavaniotou et al., 2001; Beckers et al., 2003). In the absence of luteal phase support, the area under the curve for P was suboptimal and this was accompanied by premature luteolysis (Penarrubia et al., 1998). In nonsupported cycles, the length of the luteal phase was shortened and early bleeding occurred (Albano et al., 1998). Based on this body of evidence, luteal phase support should be considered in IVF cycles where GnRH antagonists are used.

LUTEAL PHASE DEFECT

Preparation of the endometrium starts in the proliferative phase and extends throughout the luteal phase. A decrease in the amount or the duration of P secretion by the corpus luteum, or the lack of an adequate response by the endometrium, results in luteal phase deficiency (Jones, 1991) and subsequent pregnancy failure (Porter and Scott, 2005). Adequate secretory transformation of the endometrium is therefore essential for embryo implantation (Navot et al., 1991; Dominguez et al., 2003). Normal luteal phase depends on the duration of exposure to adequate P concentration, provided that sufficient estrogen priming has occurred during the follicular phase (De Ziegler et al., 1992). While estrogen controls the endometrial gland secretions that sustain the embryo prior to implantation, P has a prime effect on the stroma (Good and Moyer, 1968). Thus, around the time of implantation, the endometrium is associated with maximal glandular secretory activity and secretion of an extracellular matrix consisting of fibronectin, laminin, heparin sulphate, and type IV collagen from the perivascular stromal cells (Strauss and Gurpide, 1991). Without appropriate stimulation of P and estrogen, endometrial receptivity may be compromised, resulting in low implantation and pregnancy rates (reviewed by Nardo and Sallam, 2006).

Diagnosis of Luteal Phase Defect

Luteal phase defect has been regarded as a cause of poor reproductive performance for more than fifty years (Jones, 1949). The preferred diagnostic method remains the morphological examination of a precisely timed luteal phase endometrial biopsy according to the Noyes' criteria (Noyes et al., 1950). The endometrium is considered "out of phase" when, based on morphological criteria, it lags two days behind the actual ovulation date estimated by counting backward from the date of onset of the next menstrual period. The diagnosis of luteal phase defect is made if two consecutive biopsies are found to be out of phase (Wentz, 1980).

Multiple reports have demonstrated significant inter- and intraobserver variability in the histological evaluation of human endometrium (Li et al., 1989; Myers et al., 2004). Recently, the need and usefulness of histological dating, but not the existence of the diagnosis of luteal phase defect, has been questioned (Coutifaris et al., 2004). Collectively, these observations indicate that the timed endometrial biopsy and histological dating of the endometrium provide no additional clinical benefits to the routine assessment of infertility.

Table 44.1: Summary of Prospective Randomized Studies Comparing Different Routes of P Support in GnRH Agonist IVF Cycles

Author	Stimulation protocol	No. of cycles	Luteal phase support	Pregnancy rate (%) (implantation rate, %)
Buvat et al. (1990)	Triptorelin/HMG (short)	19	Utrogest 400 mg/day orally	5
		20	Utrogest 400 mg/day vaginally	55[a]
	Triptorelin/HMG (long)	41	Utrogest 400 mg/day orally	27
		35	Utrogest 400 mg/day vaginally	40
Smitz et al. (1992)	Buserelin/HMG (long)	131	P 50 mg i.m. + estradiol valerated 6 mg/day	30.5 (11.6)
		131	Utrogest 600 mg vaginally + estradiol valerated 6 mg/day	35.5 (16.3)
Artini et al. (1995)	Buserelin/pFSH or HMG (long)	44	P 50 mg i.m./day	13.6
		44	Micronized P in vaginal cream 100 mg/day	15.6
Pouly et al. (1996)	Decapeptyl/HMG (long)	139	Crinone 90 mg/day vaginally	28.8 (35.3)
		144	Utrogest 300 mg/day orally	25 (29.9)
Licciardi et al. (1999)	GnRH/FSH/HMG (long)	19	P 50 mg i.m	57.9 (40.9)[b]
		24	Micronized P 600 mg/day orally	45.8 (18.1)
Friedler et al. (1999)	Decapeptyl/HMG (long)	30	Utrogest 200 mg ×4/day orally	33 (10.7)
		34	Utrogest 100 mg ×2/day vaginally	47 (30.7)[a]
Abate et al. (1999)	GnRH/(long)	52	P 50 mg/day i.m	34.3[c]
		52	Crinone 90 mg/day vaginally	19.1
Strehler et al. (1999)	GnRH/HMG (short)	48	Utrogest	37.5
		51	Crinone	35.3
Schwartz et al. (2000)	GnRH (long) or multiple doses GnRH antagonist/HMG or rFSH	53	Utrogest 600 mg/day vaginally	18.9
		73	Crinone 90 mg/day vaginally	28.8
Geusa et al. (2001)	GnRH/rFSH (long)	150	Crinone 90 mg/day vaginally	26.6
		150	P i.m. 50 mg daily	28
Ludwig et al. (2002)	GnRH-a (long) or GnRH antagonist (multiple doses)/rFSH or HMG	73	Crinone 90 mg/day vaginally	28.7
		53	Utrogest 600 mg/day vaginally	18.9
Ng et al. (2003)	GnRH (long)	30	Crinone 90 mg/day vaginally	23.3
		30	P vaginal pessaries 400 mg × 2 daily	30
la Saucedo et al. (2003)	GnRH/rFSH	44	Crinone 90 mg/day vaginally	38.6
		42	P i.m. 50 mg daily	31
Sumita and Sofat (2003)	GnRH/FSH (long)	50	Utrogest 600 mg vaginally/day	34
		50	P 50 mg i.m./day	26
Geber et al. (2004)	GnRH (long)	122	Utrogest 600 mg/day	36.1
		122	Crinone 90 mg/day	44.3

Utrogest: natural micronized P capsules; Crinone: natural P in vaginal gel; [a]$P < 0.01$ vs. oral; [b]$P = 0.004$; [c]$P < 0.01$. versus vaginal.

Table 44.2: Summary of Prospective Randomized Studies Comparing hCG Versus P for Luteal Support in GnRH Agonist IVF Cycles

Author	Stimulation protocol	No. of cycles	Luteal phase support	Pregnancy rate (%)
Buvat et al. (1990)	Triptorelin/HMG (short)	32	hCG 1,500 IU ×3	62.5[a]
		19	Utrogest 400 mg/day orally	5
		20	Utrogest 400 mg/day vaginally	55[a]
	Triptorelin/HMG (long)	47	hCG 1,500 IU ×3	40
		41	Utrogest 400 mg/day orally	27
		35	Utrogest 400 mg/day vaginally	40
Claman et al. (1992)	GnRH/HMG (long)	49	P 12.5 mg i.m. daily from the day before retrieval, increased to 25 mg daily from the day of ET	14.3
		72	hCG 1,500 IU on days 1, 4, and 7 after retrieval	18
Golan et al. (1993)	GnRH/HMG (ultra-short)	26	P 100 mg i.m. daily	3.8
		30	hCG 1,000 IU or 2,500 IU every 3 days (4 times)	23.3
Araujo et al. (1994)	GnRH/HMG or FSH (long)	38	hCG 2,000 IU on days 1, 4, 7, and 10 after ET	37.7
		39	50 mg P i.m. daily	35.3
Artini et al. (1995)	Buserelin/pFSH or HMG (long)	44	hCG 2000 IU ×3	13.6
		44	P 50 mg i.m./day	13.6
		44	Micronized P in vaginal cream 100 mg/day	15.6
Martinez et al. (2000)	GnRH/FSH or HMG	168	Vaginal utrogest 100 mg ×3 daily	38.7
		142	hCG 2,500 IU on days 2, 4, and 6 after retrieval.	33.1
Ludwig et al. (2001)	GnRH/HMG or rFSH (long)			
	Low-risk	77	hCG 5,000 IU on day of ET and 3 days after, 2500 IU 6 days after	19.5
		62	hCG 5,000 IU on day of ET + utrogest 600 mg/day	21
		70	Utrogest 600 mg/day	18.6
	High-risk	83	hCG 5,000 IU on day of ET + utrogest 600 mg/day	27.2
		121	Utrogest 600 mg/day	28.1

Crinone, natural P in vaginal gel; ET, embryo transfer; high risk, estradiol >2,500 pg/mL or >12 oocytes retrieved; low risk, P estradiol <2,500 pg/mL and <12 oocytes retrieved; USOR, ultrasound-guided oocyte retrieval; Utrogestan, natural micronized P capsules; [a]$P < 0.01$ versus oral.

LUTEAL PHASE SUPPORT

The ideal luteal phase support regimen in stimulated cycles has been a matter of debate since the early days of IVF. Luteal phase supplementation is crucial between the disappearance of exogenous hCG, administered for final oocyte maturation, and the rise in endogenous hCG during early implantation (Nyboe Andersen et al., 2002).

Progesterone versus hCG for Luteal Support in Assisted Reproduction

It has been suggested that intramuscular hCG might be superior to P alone as luteal support in assisted reproduction cycles. The rationales behind it are 1) hCG administration in the luteal phase will rescue the corpus luteum and allow continuation of secretion of both estrogen and P (Hutchins-Williams et al., 1990) and 2) hCG stimulates other unknown products secreted by the corpus luteum and affects implantation. Enhancement of the corpus luteum function may be more beneficial than just replacing sex steroids in the luteal phase (Mochtar et al., 1996). Although a meta-analysis suggested that hCG could be a better alternative than progesterone for luteal phase support in GnRH agonist cycles (Soliman et al., 1994), these data were not confirmed by more recent studies (Martinez et al., 2000; Ludwig et al., 2001) (Table 44.2). Further, two meta-analyses have failed to show any significant difference in clinical and ongoing pregnancy rates between IVF patients who received P and those who had hCG (Pritts and Atwood, 2002; Daya and Gunby, 2004). Of note, the risk of OHSS was about half when P was given as compared with hCG, hence making P a more attractive option (Daya and Gunby, 2004).

Table 44.3: Summary of Prospective Randomized Studies Comparing Estradiol Plus P versus P Alone for Luteal Support in GnRH Agonist IVF Cycles

Author	Stimulation protocol	No. of cycles	Luteal phase support	Pregnancy rate (%)
Lewin et al. (1994)	GnRH-a/HMG (long)	50	IM P 50 mg/day	28
		50	IM P 50 mg/day + estradiol valerate 2 mg/day	26.5
Smitz et al. (1993)	GnRH-a/HMG (long)	183	Vaginal utrogest 600 mg/day	29.5
		195	Vaginal utrogest 600 mg + estradiol 6 mg/day	35.8
Farhi et al. (2000)	GnRH-a/uFSH/hMG (long or short)	149	IM P 50 mg/day + vaginal 100 mg/day	23.4
		136	IM P 50 mg/day + vaginal 100 mg/day + estradiol valerate 4 mg/day	33.8
Tay and Lenton (2003)	GnRH-a/FSH (long)	35	Vaginal utrogest 400 mg day	20
		28	Vaginal utrogest 400 mg + estradiol valerate 2 mg day	17.9
Gorkemli et al. (2004)	GnRH-a (long)	148	Vaginal utrogest 600 mg/day	13.5
		140	Transdermal estradiol 100 μg/day + utrogest 600 mg/day	38.5
Lukaszuk et al. (2005)	GnRH-a/uFSH (long)	80	Vaginal utrogest 600 mg/day	23.1
		73	Vaginal utrogest 600 mg/day + estradiol valerate 2 mg day	32.8
		78	Vaginal utrogest 600 mg/day + estradiol valerate 6 mg day	51.3

Progesterone and hCG for Luteal Support in Assisted Reproduction

A number of fertility specialists have recommended the combination of P and hCG for luteal support in assisted reproduction (Herman et al., 1996; Mochtar et al., 1996; Ludwig et al., 2001; Fujimoto et al., 2002). In their meta-analysis, Daya and Gunby (2004) found no statistically significant difference in clinical pregnancy, ongoing pregnancy, and miscarriage rates between combined P and hCG versus P alone. The odds ratio of OHSS was more than threefold higher when hCG was added to the luteal phase support regimen, confirming that P alone is a better strategy.

Progesterone and Estrogen for Luteal Support in Assisted Reproduction

The justification of estrogen support in stimulated IVF cycles arose from the observation of an abrupt fall in E_2 levels occurring in the mid- to late stages of the luteal phase. In humans, luteal estrogen depletion does not seem to adversely affect the morphological developmental capacity of the endometrium (Younis et al., 1994). Although some authors suggested that combining E_2 and P for luteal support in ART cycles may increase pregnancy and implantation rates (Smitz et al., 1993; Farhi et al., 2000; Gorkemli et al., 2004; Lukaszuk et al., 2005), others (Lewin et al., 1994; Tay and Lenton, 2003) could not confirm these findings. The meta-analysis by Pritts and Atwood (2002) suggested that P in combination with estrogen is the best luteal support in long and short agonist protocols. In contrast, the Cochrane review by Daya and Gunby (2004) showed no significant difference in clinical

pregnancy, ongoing pregnancy, miscarriage, or live birth rates between luteal support therapy with P and E_2 as compared with P alone.

A beneficial effect of E_2 might be related to the dose in which it is used. In a prospective randomized study, Lukaszuk et al. (2005) investigated the effect of different E_2 supplementation doses on implantation and pregnancy rates in the luteal phase of women undergoing IVF. All subjects received luteal phase support with natural micronized progesterone (600 mg/day vaginally in three divided doses) starting on the day of oocyte retrieval. Women were randomly allocated to daily doses of 0, 2, or 6 mg of estradiol valerate during the whole luteal phase. It was shown that the addition of a high dose of E_2 to daily P supplementation significantly improved the probability of pregnancy in women treated with a long GnRH agonist protocol for controlled ovarian stimulation. A recent RCT (Fatemi et al., 2006) demonstrated that the addition of estradiol valerate (4 mg per day) to micronized P for luteal phase supplementation did not enhance the likelihood of pregnancy. The implantation rate per embryo transfer was 37.8 percent in the P group versus 42.4 percent in the P plus E_2 group. No significant differences in the ongoing pregnancy rates per oocyte retrieval and per embryo transfer between the two groups were found. Table 44.3 summarizes the RCTs comparing E_2 plus P versus P alone for luteal support in GnRH agonist IVF cycles.

GnRH Agonist for Luteal Support in Assisted Reproduction

Many authors have reported independently on the potential use of GnRH agonist for luteal phase support (Tesarik et al.,

2004; Pirard et al., 2005; Hughes et al., 2006; Pirard et al., 2006; Tesarik et al., 2006). In the study by Tesarik et al. (2004), two recipients of oocytes from the same donor received either a single injection of GnRH agonist (triptorelin) six days after ICSI or placebo. Implantation and live birth rates were substantially higher in the GnRH agonist group. Pirard et al. (2005, 2006) reported on the benefits of intranasal GnRH agonist (buserelin) for induction of final oocyte maturation and support of luteal phase in intrauterine insemination and IVF patients. In an RCT involving 600 women undergoing GnRH agonist or antagonist IVF/ICSI with hCG for final oocyte maturation, women were randomized to receive a single injection of 100 µg triptorelin or placebo. The authors reported improved implantation, ongoing pregnancy, and live birth rates per embryo transfer after luteal phase administration of GnRH agonist. It was difficult to explain whether this significant effect had occurred because of improved corpus luteum function or as a result of a direct effect on the endometrium or the embryo.

ROLE OF P

P plays an important role in postovulatory regulation of the menstrual cycle. It has been aptly named the hormone of pregnancy because in preparing the endometrium for embryo implantation and facilitating endometrial development, it is critical to the maintenance of early pregnancy. This key hormone decreases myometrial activity and sensitivity throughout pregnancy. A growing body of evidence suggests that P plays a crucial role in establishing an adequate immune environment for the early stages of pregnancy (Piccinni et al., 1995; Choi et al., 2000; Kalinka and Szekeres-Bartho, 2005; Raghupathy et al., 2005). During pregnancy, the maternal immune system is carefully modulated by P via control of cytokine production (Szekeres-Bartho et al., 1997).

In normal pregnancies, there is a shift in the decidua from cellular immune response (Th1 cytokines) to humoral immunity (Th2 cytokines), which is highly controlled by progesterone-inhibiting blocking factor (Szekeres-Bartho et al., 1996). Some authors postulated that significantly increased Th1 cytokine expression may represent the underlying phenomenon, leading to reproductive failure (Ng et al., 2002). Further, the activation of peripheral blood mononuclear cells with trophoblast antigens confirmed that women with idiopathic recurrent spontaneous pregnancy loss have a Th1-type cytokine profile, characterized by production of IL-2, tumor necrosis factor, and interferon γ (Raghupathy et al., 2000). The possible association between maternal Th1 dominance and recurrent miscarriage provides researchers with the challenge of trying to manipulate the Th1/Th2 cytokine balance to suppress the cell-mediated immunity (reviewed by Nardo and Sallam, 2006). P has been proposed to act as an immunologic suppressant blocking Th1 activity and inducing release of Th2 cytokines (IL-4 and IL-10).

ROUTES OF P ADMINISTRATION

Possible routes of P delivery include transdermal, oral, intramuscular, vaginal, sublingual, nasal, and rectal. Of these, only three – oral, intramuscular, and vaginal – have been widely used. Table 44.1 shows the prospective randomized studies comparing different routes of P supplementation in GnRH agonist IVF cycles.

Oral Route

Since natural P is rapidly metabolized after oral administration, synthetic progestins that resist enzymatic degradation have been designed. The latter have been associated with a number of undesirable effects, and those with androgenic properties have been connected with an increased risk of fetal congenital malformations (Revesz et al., 1960; Wilkins, 1960; Aarskog, 1979). Natural P does not appear to have teratogenic effect (Chez, 1978; Rock et al., 1985; Check et al., 1986), and it is more effective in inducing secretory endometrial changes than P derivatives, like dydrogesterone (Pellicer et al., 1989). The development of the micronization process allowed for much improved absorption of oral P (Maxon and Hargrove, 1985; Kimzey et al., 1991). However, its systemic levels are too low after oral administration to provide adequate endometrial support (Levine and Watson, 2000). The first passage of P through the liver after oral ingestion leads to massive metabolism and at best only 10 percent of the administered dose circulates as active compound (Nahoul et al., 1993). Any effort to increase the oral dose sufficiently to achieve the requisite serum P levels produces a degree of somnolence unacceptable to most patients. Clinical trials that utilized oral P supplementation in IVF cycles confirmed the inadequacy of this route (Table 44.1). Oral P should therefore not be prescribed as luteal support treatment.

Intramuscular Route

Intramuscular P results in high serum P concentrations, adequate endometrial secretory features (Navot et al., 1986; Devroey et al., 1989; Sauer et al., 1991), satisfactory pregnancy rates (Navot et al., 1986; Younis et al., 1992; Smitz et al., 1992; Artini et al., 1995), and delayed menses in most women. Daily injections are uncomfortable, especially for long-term treatments, and may lead to marked inflammation and sterile abscess formation at the injection site.

Intramuscular 17 α-hydroxyprogesterone caproate given twice weekly represents a suitable option. Pregnancy and miscarriage rates were not different when comparing this therapeutic approach with daily intramuscular injections (Costabile et al., 2001).

Six RCTs (Table 44.1) compared intramuscular (50 mg/day) with vaginal P for luteal support in IVF. Only one study showed that intramuscular P was associated with higher pregnancy rates compared with vaginal P (Abate et al., 1999). Daya and Gunby (2004) concluded that intramuscular route is advantageous compared with the vaginal route. This conclusion remains open for debate as the authors did not include a large prospective randomized trial (Smitz et al., 1992) that compared vaginal and intramuscular P administration in IVF. In their trial including 262 patients undergoing IVF using a long GnRH agonist protocol, Smitz et al. (1992) showed similar pregnancy and implantation rates in women who received vaginal or intramuscular P. Of interest, miscarriage rate was lower in women receiving P vaginally. Inclusion of this trial in the meta-analysis might have altered the conclusions in favor of the intramuscular route.

Vaginal Route

Vaginal P results in adequate endometrial secretory transformation, even though serum P levels may be lower than those measured during the luteal phase (Salat-Baroux et al., 1988; Cicinelli et al., 1996; Fanchin et al., 1997). The discrepancies between P concentrations and histological features after vaginal P administration are indicative of the so-called "first uterine pass effect" (Miles et al., 1994; Balasch et al., 1996; Fanchin et al., 1997).

Vaginal P supplementation can cause discharge, irritation, and/or local warmth (Kimzey et al., 1991; Pouly et al., 1996). Formulations used per vagina have included micronized P tablets, pharmacist-formulated suppositories (usually in a paraffin base), Crinone 8 percent (a gel), and Prometrium (a gelatin capsule). All these products have higher patient acceptability than intramuscular injections. Comparison of luteal support with vaginal P gel versus vaginal micronized P tablets demonstrated statistical equivalence in IVF cycles for most clinical end points (Table 44.1). Vaginal supplementation is also possible via P-impregnated rings. Zegers-Hochschild et al. (2000) reported on a ring that releases 10–20 nmol/L P daily for up to ninety days. In their RCT, pregnancy rate was similar after vaginal and intramuscular supplementation therapy.

LUTEAL PHASE SUPPORT IN OOCYTE DONATION CYCLES

The challenge of oocyte donation programs is to prime endometrial receptivity with exogenous steroid hormones. This approach has proved to be successful as shown by implantation and pregnancy rates higher than those following standard IVF (Lutjen et al., 1985; Navot et al., 1986; Rosenwaks et al., 1986). Hormonally controlled cycles have a degree of flexibility in terms of dose of drugs and duration of treatments. The duration of estrogen therapy can vary from 10 days or less to greater than 100 days without impairing endometrial receptivity. A large multicentre oocyte donation program showed that implantation and pregnancy rates were unaffected by estrogen priming lasting up to 100 days, but started to decrease thereafter (Remohi et al., 1995).

Estrogen supplementation in women undergoing oocyte donation and frozen embryo transfers (FET) can be delivered either orally or transdermally (Steingold et al., 1991). The latter route should be preferred in women whose hepatic metabolism is abnormal, for example, those who smoke, ingest neuropsychiatric medications, or have been exposed to chemotherapy in the past. Patients whose endometrial response to oral estrogen is suboptimal should be recommended the transdermal route. Estrogen priming is regarded as inappropriate when the endometrial thickness is less than 7 mm on ultrasound. Ensuring that the endometrial exposure to P coincides with the stage of embryo development is of paramount importance. It has been suggested that four- to eight-cell embryos require three to four days of exogenous P therapy (or cycle days 17–18 when progesterone is started on day 15) (Navot et al., 1986; Rosenwaks et al., 1987; Navot et al., 1991), while blastocysts need a couple of days more. Looking at the outcome of embryo transfers performed outside this optimal window, it is possible to conclude that earlier transfers may result in pregnancies, whereas embryos transferred later fail to implant.

The majority of successful oocyte donation cycles have used P intramuscularly or vaginally. Studies have evaluated the hormonal and histological parameters after P supplementation using various routes and doses. In a study including oocyte recipients with absent ovaries, serum P concentrations were higher after intramuscular as compared to vaginal administration. Classical endometrial secretory morphology was similar in both groups but endometrial maturation was better with the vaginal route (Devroey et al., 1989). Several authors have observed inadequate endometrial secretory transformation in oocyte recipients taking oral P supplementation (Devroey et al., 1989; Dehou et al., 1987; Bourgain et al., 1990; Critchley et al., 1990).

LUTEAL SUPPORT IN FET CYCLES

Frozen-thawed embryo transfer has been equally successful in natural cycles following spontaneous ovulation, in stimulated cycles using clomiphene citrate or gonadotrophins and in cycles in which the endometrium was prepared with exogenous steroids (Al-Shawaf et al., 1993; Loh and Leong, 1999; Simon et al., 1999; El Toukhy et al., 2004; Wright et al., 2006; Gelbaya et al., 2006). In natural-cycle FET, pregnancy rates were similar when comparing women who received vaginal P (800 mg daily) starting on the day of replacement and those who did not receive P (Bjuresten et al., 2005).

Undoubtedly P supplementation is essential in downregulated FET cycles. Protocols using GnRH agonists have been developed mainly on the experience gained from oocyte donation. In such cycles, endometrial preparation is successfully performed using estrogen (oral, transdermal, or vaginal preparations) and P (intramuscular and vaginal preparations). E_2 is given for a minimum of ten days (usually fifteen days), and once the endometrial thickness is 7 mm or larger, P is added.

The regimen of estrogen supplementation varies between IVF centers. It is our current practice to prescribe E_2 in a step-up regimen, starting with a dose of 1 mg/day from day 1 to day 5, then 2 mg/day from day 6 to day 9, followed by 6 mg/day from day 10 onward up to the day of pregnancy test or onset of next spontaneous period. Different doses and preparations have been used for P supplementation in stimulated and down-regulated, hormonally controlled FET cycles. Currently, there are no robust data in the literature to support the use of one preparation over the other. Most centers use either intramuscular or vaginal P in doses similar to those used in oocyte donation programs.

TIMING OF LUTEAL PHASE SUPPORT

In stimulated IVF cycles, the steroid production in the first week after oocyte retrieval is likely to be well timed and more than sufficient, so the start of exogenous support is not apt to be critical within this window. Williams et al. (2001) reported higher pregnancy rates in IVF when P was started three rather than six days after oocyte collection. Vaginal P supplementation before embryo transfer may be useful in quieting uterine contractions and thereby reducing embryo displacement (Fanchin et al., 2001). Sohn et al. (1999) found that starting intramuscular P before oocyte collection negatively affected the implantation rate. More recently, a well-conducted RCT showed no significant differences in the ongoing pregnancy rate when vaginal P was started on the day of hCG administration, the day of oocyte retrieval, or the day of embryo transfer (Mochtar et al., 2006). In programmed cycles, however, the timing is critical as the only source of P is exogenous. Over two decades ago, Navot et al. (1986) showed that day-2 embryos transferred on day 2 to day 4 of P therapy produced pregnancies, while transfers out of that window failed. In a larger study, Prapas et al. (1998) concluded that the highest pregnancy rates occurred when day-2 embryos were transferred on day 4 or day 5 of P supplementation therapy. In the attempt to synchronize endometrial development and embryo stage, P should be commenced on the same day or the day after the oocyte donor is given hCG.

The evidence supporting P supplementation during early pregnancy is conflicting. In an RCT, Prietl et al. (1992) found that patients receiving combined treatment of intramuscular estradiol valerate and 17 alpha-hydroxyprogesterone caproate from the time of a positive pregnancy test until twelve weeks of gestation had higher pregnancy rates compared with controls. Other authors (Stovall et al., 1998) showed that P supplementation could be withdrawn at six weeks of gestation in patients with high serum progesterone concentrations. A retrospective controlled study demonstrated that in women who conceived after ART, withdrawal of vaginal P at the time of a positive pregnancy test had no influence on the miscarriage and delivery rates (Schmidt et al., 2001). These data were in agreement with that of an RCT subsequently published by the same authors (Nyboe Andersen et al., 2002).

CONCLUSIONS

Failed implantation is a major limiting factor in assisted reproduction. A better understanding of the molecular mechanisms responsible for implantation and placentation may improve the clinicians' ability to treat disorders related to these processes, including idiopathic infertility and early pregnancy loss. P and estrogen play central roles in preparation for and establishment of human pregnancy. Until the luteoplacental shift occurs at about seven weeks of gestational age, the ovary production of these hormones is critical to pregnancy maintenance. Beyond seven weeks of gestation, the placenta normally makes enough sex steroids to obviate any dependence on ovarian or exogenously supplied hormones.

In most cases of contemporary ART, P supplementation is common practice. Various routes of administration have been developed, but most have proved to have limitations and to cause untoward effects. While intramuscular delivery of P continues to remain an option, an increasing number of fertility specialists prefer the vaginal route of delivery.

As yet, the role of estrogen supplementation therapy during the luteal phase of IVF cycles lacks enough evidence to be employed in routine practice.

KEY POINTS

- Luteal phase support is necessary to optimize the outcome of ART.
- Luteal phase support with hCG is not superior to luteal phase support with P.
- Supplementary administration of hCG brings no advantage when P is administered.
- Luteal phase support with hCG increases the risk of OHSS as compared with P.
- The administration of estrogen to supplement the luteal phase in standard stimulated IVF cycles needs further clarification and evidence.
- The use of oral P is clearly inferior to intramuscular or vaginal administration and is associated with an increased rate of side effects due to its metabolites.
- At present, there are insufficient data for a direct comparison between intramuscular and vaginal P therapy; therefore, physicians should be guided by their own clinical experience.

REFERENCES

Aarskog D (1979) Maternal progestins as a possible cause of hypospadias. *N Engl J Med* 300:75–8.

Abate A, Perino M, Abate FG, Brigandi A, Costabile L, Manti F (1999) Intramuscular *versus* vaginal administration of progesterone for luteal phase support after *in vitro* fertilization and embryo transfer. A comparative study. *Clin Exp Obstet Gynecol* 26:203–6.

Albano C, Grimbizis G, Smitz J, et al. (1998) The luteal phase of nonsupplemented cycles after ovarian superovulation with human menopausal gonadotropin and the gonadotropin releasing hormone antagonist Cetrorelix. *Fertil Steril* 70:357–9.

Albano C, Smitz J, Tournaye H, et al. (1999) Luteal phase and clinical outcome after human menopausal gonadotrophin/gonadotropin releasing hormone antagonist treatment for ovarian stimulation in in-vitro fertilization/intracytoplasmic sperm injection cycles. *Hum Reprod* 14:1426–30.

Al-Shawaf T, Yang D, Al-Magid Y, Seaton A, Iketubosin F, Craft I (1993) Ultrasonic monitoring during replacement of frozen-thawed embryos in natural and hormone replacement cycles. *Hum Reprod* 8:2068–74.

Araujo E, Bernardini L, Frederick JL, Asch RH, Balmaceda JP (1994) Prospective randomized comparison of human chorionic gonadotropin versus intramuscular progesterone for luteal-phase support in assisted reproduction. *J Assist Reprod Genet* 11: 74–8.

Artini PG, Volpe A, Angioni S, et al. (1995) A comparative, randomized study of three different progesterone support of the luteal phase following IVF/ET program. *J Endocrinol Invest* 18:51–6.

Balasch J, Fabregues F, Ordi J, et al. (1996) Further data favouring the hypothesis of the uterine first-pass effect of the vaginally administered micronized progesterone. *Gynecol Endocrinol* 10:421–6.

Balasch J, Jove I, Marquez M, Vanrell JA (1991) Hormonal and histological evaluation of the luteal phase after combined GnRH agonist/gonadotropin treatment for superovulation in IVF or GIFT. *Hum Reprod* 6:914–17.

Beckers NGM, Laven JS, Eijkemans MJC, Fauser BC (2000) Follicular and luteal phase characteristics following early cessation of gonadotrophin-releasing hormone agonist during ovarian stimulation for in-vitro fertilization. *Hum Reprod* 15:43–9.

Beckers NGM, Macklon NS, Eijkemans MJC, et al. (2002) Comparison of the nonsupplemented luteal phase characteristics after recombinant (r)HCG, rLH or GnRH agonist for oocyte maturation in IVF. *Hum Reprod* 17 (Suppl. 1):55.

Beckers NG, Macklon NS, Eijkemans MJ, et al. (2003) Nonsupplemented luteal phase characteristics after the administration of recombinant human chorionic gonadotropin, recombinant luteinizing hormone, or gonadotropin-releasing hormone (GnRH) agonist to induce final oocyte maturation in in vitro fertilization patients after ovarian stimulation with recombinant follicle-stimulating hormone and GnRH antagonist cotreatment. *J Clin Endocrinol Metab* **88**:4186–92.

Bjuresten K, Hreinsson J, Hovatta O (2005) Can pregnancy rate outcome be improved with vaginal progesterone as luteal phase support in frozen embryo replacement normal cycle. *Acta Obstet Gynecol Scand* **84**:500–13.

Bourgain C, Devroey P, Van waesberghe L, et al. (1990) Effects of natural progesterone on the morphology of the endometrium in patients with primary ovarian failure. *Hum Reprod* **5**: 537–43.

Buvat J, Marcolin G, Guittard C, et al. (1990) Luteal support after luteinizing hormone-releasing hormone agonist for in vitro fertilization: superiority of human chorionic gonadotrophin over oral progesterone. *Fertil Steril* **53**:490–4.

Caspo AI, Pulkkinen MO, Rutter B, et al. (1972) The significance of the human corpus luteum in pregnancy maintenance. *Am J Obstet Gynecol* **112**:1061–7.

Check JH, O'Shaughnessy A, Lurie D, Fisher C, Adelson HG (1995) Evaluation of the mechanisms for higher pregnancy rates in donor oocyte recipients by comparison of fresh with frozen embryo transfer pregnancy rates in a shared oocyte programme. *Hum Reprod* **10**:3022–7.

Check JH, Rankin A, Teichman M (1986) The risk of fetal anomalies as a result of progesterone therapy during pregnancy. *Fertil Steril* **45**:575–7.

Chez RA (1978) Proceedings of the symposium "Progesterone, progestins and fetal development". *Fertil Steril* **30**:16–26.

Choi BC, Polgar K, Xiao L, Hill JA (2000) Progesterone inhibits in-vitro embryotoxic Th1 cytokine production to trophoblast in women with recurrent pregnancy loss. *Hum Reprod* **15**:46–59.

Cicinelli E, Borraccino V, Petruzzi D, et al. (1996) Pharmacokinetics and endometrial effects of the vaginal administration of micronized progesterone in an oil-based solution to postmenopausal women. *Fertil Steril* **65**:860–2.

Claman P, Domingo M, Leader A (1992) Luteal phase support for invitro fertilization using gonadotrophin releasing hormone analogue before ovarian stimulation: a prospective randomized study of human chorionic gonadotrophin versus intramuscular progesterone. *Hum Reprod* **7**:487–9.

Costabile L, Gerli S, Manna C, et al. (2001) A prospective randomized study comparing intramuscular progesterone and 17-alpha-hydroxyprogesterone caproate in patients undergoing in vitro fertilization and embryo transfer cycles. *Fertil Steril* **76**:394–6.

Coutifaris C, Myers ER, Guzick DS, et al. (2004) Histological dating of timed endometrial biopsy tissue is not related to fertility status. *Fertil Steril* **82**:1264–72.

Critchley H, Buckley CH, Anderson D (1990) Experience with 'physiological' steroid replacement regimen for the establishment of a receptive endometrium in women with premature ovarian failure. *BJOG* **97**:804–10.

Daya S, Gunby J (2004) Luteal phase support in assisted reproduction cycles. *Cochrane Database Syst Rev*, CD004830.

De Ziegler D, Bergeron C, Cornel C, et al. (1992) Effects of luteal estradiol on the secretory transformation of human endometrium and plasma gonadotropins. *J Clin Endocrinol Metab* **74**:322–31.

Dehou MF, Lejeune B, Arijs C, et al. (1987) Endometrial morphology in stimulated in vitro fertilization cycles and after steroid replacement therapy in cases of primary ovarian failure. *Fertil Steril* **48**:995–1000.

Devreker F, Govaerts I, Bertrand E, et al. (1996) The long acting gonadotrophin releasing hormone analogues impaired the implantation rate. *Fertil Steril* **65**:122–6.

Devroey P, Palermo G, Bourgain C, et al. (1989) Progesterone administration in patients with absent ovaries. *Int J Fertil* **34**:188–93.

Dominguez F, Galan A, Martin JJ, Remohi J, Pellicer A, Simon C (2003) Hormonal and embryonic regulation of chemokine receptors CXCR1, CXCR4, CCR5 and CCR2B in the human endometrium and the human blastocyst. *Mol Hum Reprod* **9**: 189–98.

Edwards RG, Steptoe P (1980) Establishing full-term human pregnancies using cleavage embryos grown in vitro. *BJOG* **87**:737–56.

Elter K, Nelson LR (2001) Use of third generation gonadotropin releasing hormone antagonists in in vitro fertilization–embryo transfer: a review. *Obstet Gynecol Surv* **56**:576–88.

El-Toukhy T, Taylor A, Khalaf Y, et al. (2004) Pituitary suppression in ultrasound-monitored frozen embryo replacement cycles. A randomized study. *Hum Reprod* **19**:874–9.

Fanchin R, de Ziegler D, Bergeron C, et al. (1997) Transvaginal administration of progesterone. *Obstet Gynecol* **90**:396–401.

Fanchin R, Righini C, de Ziegler D, et al. (2001) Effects of vaginal progesterone administration on uterine contractility at the time of embryo transfer. *Fertil Steril* **75**:1136–40.

Farhi J, Weissman A, Steinfeld Z, Shorer M, Nahum H, Levran D (2000) Estradiol supplementation during the luteal phase may improve the pregnancy rate in patients undergoing in vitro fertilization-embryo transfer cycles. *Fertil Steril* **73**:761–5.

Fatemi HM, Kolibianakis EM, Camus M, et al. (2006) Addition of estradiol to progesterone for luteal supplementation in patients stimulated with GnRH antagonist/rFSH for IVF: a randomized controlled trial. *Hum Reprod* **21**:2628–32.

Friedler S, Raziel A, Schachter M, Strassburger D, Bukovsky I, Ron-El R (1999) Luteal support with micronized progesterone following in-vitro fertilization using a down-regulation protocol with gonadotrophin-releasing hormone agonist: a comparative study between vaginal and oral administration. *Hum Reprod* **14**: 1944–8.

Fujimoto A, Osuga Y, Fujiwara T, et al. (2002) Human chorionic gonadotrophin combined with progesterone for luteal support improves pregnancy rate in patients with low late-midluteal estradiol levels in IVF cycles. *J Assist Reprod Genet* **19**:550–4.

Geber S, Moreira ACF, de Paula S, Veado B, Sampaio MAC (2004) Comparison between two different preparations of vaginal progesterone for luteal phase support in assisted reproduction treatment. *Hum Reprod* **19** (Suppl. 1):i111.

Gelbaya TA, Nardo LG, Hunter HR, et al. (2006) Cryopreserved-thawed embryo transfer in natural or down regulated hormonally controlled cycles: a retrospective study. *Fertil Steril* **85**:603–9.

Geusa S, Causio F, Marinaccio M, Stanziano A, Sarcina E (2001) Luteal phase support with progesterone in IVF/ET cycles: a prospective, randomized study comparing vaginal and intramuscular administration. *Hum Reprod* **16**:145 (P-111).

Golan A, Herman A, Soffer Y, et al. (1993) Human chorionic gonadotrophin is a better luteal support than progesterone in ultrashort gonadotrophin-releasing hormone agonist/menotrophin in vitro fertilization cycles. *Hum Reprod* **8**:1372–5.

Good RG, Moyer DL (1968) Estrogen-progesterone relationships in the development of secretory endometrium. *Fertil Steril* **19**: 37–43.

Gorkemli H, Ak D, Akyurek C, Aktan M, Duman S (2004) Comparison of pregnancy outcomes of progesterone or progesterone + estradiol for luteal phase support in ICSI-ET cycles. *Gynecol Obstet Invest* **58**:140–4.

Herman A, Raziel A, Strassburger D, et al. (1996) The benefits of mid-luteal addition of human chorionic gonadotrophin in in-vitro fertilization using a down-regulation protocol and luteal support with progesterone. *Hum Reprod* **11**:1552–7.

Hughes EG, Fedorkow DM, Daya S, Sagle MA, Van de Koppel P, Collins JA (1992) The routine use of gonadotropin-releasing hormone agonists prior to in vitro fertilization and gamete intrafallopian transfer: a meta-analysis of randomized controlled trials. *Fertil Steril* **58**:888–96.

Hughes JN, Cedrin-Durnerin I, Bstandig B, et al. (2006) Administration of gonadotropin-releasing hormone agonist during the luteal phase of the GnRH-antagonist IVF cycles. *Hum Reprod* **21** (Suppl. 1):O-007.

Hutchins-Williams KA, Decherney AH, Lavy G, et al. (1990) Luteal rescue in in vitro fertilization-embryo transfer. *Fertil Steril* **53**:495–501.

Jones GS (1991) Luteal phase defect: a review of pathophysiology. *Curr Opin Obstet Gynecol* **3**:641–8.

Jones GS (1949) Some newer aspects of the management of infertility. *J Am Med Assoc* **141**:1123–9.

Kalinaka J, Szekeres-Bartho J (2005) The impact of dydrogesterone supplementation on hormonal profile and progesterone-induced blocking factor concentrations in women with threatened abortion. *Am J Reprod Immunol* **53**:166–71.

Kimzey LM, Gumowski J, Merriam GR, et al. (1991) Absorption of micronized progesterone from a nonliquefying vaginal cream. *Fertil Steril* **56**:995–6.

la Saucedo-de Llata E, Batiza V, Arenas L, et al. (2003) Progesterone for luteal support: randomized, prospective trial comparing vaginal and i.m. administration. *Hum Reprod* **18**:130(382).

Lass A, Peat D, Avery S, Brinsden B (1998) Histological evaluation of endometrium on the day of oocyte retrieval after gonadotropin releasing hormone agonist follicle stimulating hormone ovulation induction for in vitro fertilization. *Hum Reprod* **13**:3203–5.

Levine H, Watson N (2000) Comparison of the pharmacokinetics of Crinone 8% administered vaginally versus Prometrium administered orally in postmenopauasal women. *Fertil Steril* **73**:516–21.

Lewin A, Benshushan A, Mezker E, et al. (1994) The role of estrogen support during the luteal phase of in vitro fertilization-embryo transplant cycles: a comparative study between progesterone alone and estrogen and progesterone support. *Fertil Steril* **62**:121–5.

Li TC, Dockery P, Rogers AW, Cooke ID (1989) How precise is histological dating of endometrium using the standard dating criteria? *Fertil Steril* **51**:759–63.

Licciardi FL, Kwiatkowski A, Noyes NL, Berkeley AS, Krey LL, Grifo JA (1999) Oral *versus* intramuscular progesterone for *in vitro* fertilization: a prospective randomized study. *Fertil Steril* **71**:614–18.

Loh SK, Leong NK (1999) Factors affecting success in an embryo cryopreservation program. *Ann Acad Med Singapore* **28**:260–5.

Ludwig M, Finas A, Katalinic A, et al. (2001) Prospective, randomized study to evaluate the success rates using hCG, vaginal progesterone or a combination of both for luteal phase support. *Acta Obstet Gynecol Scand* **80**:574–82.

Ludwig M, Schwartz P, Babahan B, et al. (2002) Luteal phase support using either Crinone 8% or Utrogest: results of a prospective, randomized study. *Eur J Obstet Gynaecol* **103**:48–52.

Lutjen PJ, Leeton JF, Findlay JK (1985) Oocyte and embryo donation in IVF programmes. *Clin Obstet Gynaecol* **12**:799–813.

Lukaszuk K, Liss J, Lukaszuk M, Maj B (2005) Optimization of estradiol supplementation during the luteal phase improves the pregnancy rate in women undergoing in vitro fertilization-embryo transfer cycles. *Fertil Steril* **83**:1372–6.

Martinez F, Coroleu B, Parera N, et al. (2000) Human chorionic gonadotropin and intravaginal natural progesterone are equally effective for luteal phase support in IVF. *Gynecol Endocrinol* **14**:316–20.

Maxon W, Hargrove J (1985) Bioavailability of oral micronized progesterone. *Fertil Steril* **44**:622–6.

Miles R, Paulson R, Lobo R, et al. (1994) Pharmacokinetics and endometrial tissue levels of progesterone after administration by intramuscular and vaginal routes: a comparative study. *Fertil Steril* **62**:485–90.

Mochtar MH, Hogerzeil HV, Mol BW (1996) Progesterone alone versus progesterone combined with HCG as luteal support in GnRHa/HMG induced IVF cycles: a randomized clinical trial. *Hum Reprod* **11**:1602–5.

Mochtar MH, Wely MV, der Veen FV (2006) Timing luteal phase support in GNRH agonist down-regulated IVF/embryo transfer cycles. *Hum Reprod* **21**:905–8.

Myers ER, Silva S, Barnhart K, et al. (2004) Interobserver and intraobserver variability in the histological dating of the endometrium in fertile and infertile women. *Fertil Steril* **82**:1278–82.

Nahoul K, Dehennin L, Jondent M, et al. (1993) Profiles of plasma estrogens, progesterone and their metabolites after oral or vaginal administration of estradiol or progesterone. *Maturitas* **16**:185–202.

Nardo LG, Sallam HN (2006) Progesterone supplementation to prevent recurrent miscarriage and to reduce implantation failure in assisted reproduction cycles. *Reprod Biomed Online* **13**:47–57.

Navot D, Laufer N, Kopolovic J, et al. (1986) Artificially induced endometrial cycles and establishment of pregnancies in the absence of ovaries. *N Engl J Med* **314**:806–11.

Navot D, Scott RT, Droesch K, Veeck LL, Liu HC, Rosenwaks Z (1991) The window of embryo transfer and the efficiency of human conception in vitro. *Fertil Steril* **55**:114–18.

Ng SC, Gilman-Sachs A, Thaker P, et al. (2002) Expression of intracellular Th1 and Th2 cytokines in women with recurrent spontaneous abortion, implantation failure after IVF/ET or normal pregnancy. *Am J Reprod Immunol* **48**:77–86.

Ng EHY, Miao B, Cheung W, Ho PC (2003) A randomised comparison of side effects and patient inconvenience of two vaginal progesterone formulations used for luteal support in in vitro fertilisation cycles. *Eur J Obstet Gynecol Reprod Biol* **111**:50–4.

Nikas G, Develioglu OH, Toner JP, Jones HW Jr (1999) Endometrial pinopode indicate a shift in the window of receptivity in IVF cycles. *Hum Reprod* **14**:787–92.

Nosarka S, Kruger T, Siebert I, et al. (2005) Luteal phase support in in vitro fertilization: metaanalysis of randomized trials. *Gynecol Obstet Invest* **60**:67–74.

Noyes RW, Hertig AT, Rock J (1950) Dating the endometrial biopsy. *Fertil Steril* **1**:3–25.

Nyboe Andersen A, Popovic-Todorovic B, Schmidt KT, et al. (2002) Progesterone supplementation during early gestations after IVF or ICSI has no effect on the delivery rates: a randomized controlled trial. *Hum Reprod* **17**:357–61.

Paulson RJ, Sauer MV, Lobo RA (1990) Embryo implantation after human in vitro fertilization: importance of endometrial receptivity. *Fertil Steril* **53**:870–4.

Pellicer A, Matallin P, Miro F, et al. (1989) Progesterone versus dydrogesterone as replacement therapy in women with premature ovarian failure. *Hum Reprod* **4**:777–81.

Penarrubia J, Balasch J, Fabregues F, et al. (1998) Human chorionic gonadotrophin luteal support overcomes luteal phase inadequacy after gonadotrophin releasing hormone agonist-induced ovulation in gonadotrophin stimulated cycles. *Hum Reprod* **13**:3315–18.

Piccinni MP, Giudizi MG, Biagiotti R, et al. (1995) Progesterone favours the development of human T helper cells producing Th2-type cytokines and promotes both IL-4 production and membrane CD30 expression in established T cell clones. *J Immunol* **155**:128–33.

Pirard C, Donnez J, Loumaye E (2005) GnRH agonist as novel luteal support: results of a randomised, parallel group, feasibility study using intranasal administration of buserelin. *Hum Reprod* **20**:1798–804.

Pirard C, Donnez J, Loumaye E (2006) GnRH agonist as luteal phase support in assisted reproduction technique cycles: results of a pilot study. *Hum Reprod* **21**:1894–900.

Porter TF, Scott JR (2005) Evidence-based care of recurrent miscarriage. *Best Pract Res Clin Obstet Gynaecol* **19**:85–101.

Pouly JL, Bassil S, Frydman R, et al. (1996) Luteal support after in-vitro fertilization: Crinone 8%, a sustained release vaginal progesterone gel, versus Utrogestan, an oral micronized progesterone. *Hum Reprod* **11**:2085–9.

Prapas Y, Parapas N, Jones EE, et al. (1998) The window for embryo transfer in oocyte donation cycles depends on the duration of progesterone therapy. *Hum Reprod* **13**:720–3.

Prietl G, Diedrich K, Van der ven HH, Luckhaus J, Krebs D (1992) The effect of 17 alpha-hydroxyprogesterone caproate/oestradiol valerate on the development and outcome of early pregnancies following in vitro fertilization and embryo transfer: a prospective and randomised controlled trial. *Hum Reprod* **7**:1–5.

Pritts E, Atwood A (2002) Luteal phase support in infertility treatment: a meta-analysis of the randomized trials. *Hum Reprod* **17**:2287–99.

Raghupathy R, Al Mutawa E, Makhseed M, et al. (2005) Modulation of cytokine production by dydrogesterone in lymphocytes from women with recurrent miscarriage. *BJOG* **112**:1096–101.

Raghupathy R, Makhseed M, Azizieh F, et al. (2000) Cytokine production by maternal lymphocytes during normal human pregnancy and in unexplained recurrent spontaneous abortion. *Hum Reprod* **15**:713–18.

Ragni G, Vegetti W, Baroni E, et al. (2001) Comparison of luteal phase profile in gonadotrophin stimulated cycles with or without a gonadotrophin-releasing hormone antagonist. *Hum Reprod* **16**:2258–62.

Remohi J, Gutierrez A, Cano F, et al. (1995) Long oestradiol replacement in an oocyte donation programme. *Hum Reprod* **10**:1387–91.

Revesz C, Chappel CI, Caudry R (1960) Masculinization of female fetuses in the rat by progestational compounds. *Endocrinology* **66**:140–4.

Rock J, Colston Wentz A, Cole K, et al. (1985) Fetal malformation following progesterone therapy during pregnancy: a preliminary report. *Fertil Steril* **44**:17–19.

Rosenwaks Z (1987) Donor eggs: their application in modern reproductive technologies. *Fertil Steril* **47**:895–9.

Rosenwaks Z, Veeck LL, Liu HC (1986) Pregnancy following transfer of in vitro fertilized donated oocytes. *Fertil Steril* **45**:417–20.

Salat-Baroux J, Cornet D, Alvarez S, et al. (1988) Pregnancies after replacement of frozen thawed embryos in a donation program. *Fertil Steril* **49**:817–21.

Sauer MV, Stein AL, Paulson RJ, et al. (1991) Endometrial responses to various hormone replacement regimens in ovarian failure patients preparing for embryo donation. *Int J Gynecol Obstet* **35**:61–8.

Schmidt KT, Ziebe S, Popovic B, Lindhard A, Loft A, Andersen AN (2001) Progesterone supplementation during early gestation after IVF has no effect on the delivery rates. *Fertil Steril* **75**:337–41.

Schwartz P, Ludwig M, Babahan B, et al. (2000) Luteal phase support using either progesterone gel (Crinone 8%®) or progesterone suppositories (Utrogest®): results of a prospective randomized study. *Hum Reprod* **15**:43–4.

Scott R, Navot D, Liu H-C, Rosenwaks Z (1991) A human in vivo model for the luteoplacental shift. *Fertil Steril* **56**:481–4.

Simon A, Hurwitz A, Pharhat M, Revel A, Zentner BS, Laufer N (1999) A flexible protocol for artificial preparation of the endometrium without prior gonadotropin-releasing hormone agonist suppression in women with functioning ovaries undergoing frozen-thawed embryo transfer cycles. *Fertil Steril* **71**:609–13.

Simon C, Cano F, Valbuena D, Remohi J, Pellicer A (1995) Clinical evidence for a detrimental effect on uterine receptivity of high serum oestradiol concentrations in high and normal responder patients. *Hum Reprod* **10**:2432–7.

Smitz J, Bourgain C, Van Waesberghe L, Camus M, Devroey P, Van Steirteghem A (1993) A prospective randomized study on estradiol valerate supplementation in addition to intravaginal micronized progesterone in buserelin and HMG induced superovulation. *Hum Reprod* **8**:40–5.

Smitz J, Devroey P, Faguer B, et al. (1992) A prospective randomized comparison of intramuscular or intravaginal natural progesterone as a luteal phase and early pregnancy supplement. *Hum Reprod* **7**:168–75.

Sohn SH, Penzias AS, Emmi AM, et al. (1999) Administration of progesterone before oocyte retrieval negatively affects the implantation rate. *Fertil Steril* **71**:11–14.

Soliman S, Daya S, Collins J, Hughes EG (1994) The role of luteal support in infertility treatments: a meta-analysis of randomised trials. *Fertil Steril* **61**:1068–76.

Steingold KA, Matt DW, de Ziegler D, et al. (1991) Comparison of transdermal to oral estradiol administration on hormonal and hepatic parameters in women with premature ovarian failure. *J Clin Endocrinol Metab* **73**:275–80.

Stovall DW, Van Voorhis BJ, Sparks AE, Adams LM, Syrop CH (1998) Selective early elimination of luteal support in assisted reproduction cycles using a gonadotrophin releasing hormone agonist during ovarian stimulation. *Fertil Steril* **70**:1056–62.

Strauss JR, Gurpide E (1991) The endometrium: regulation and dysfunction. In: Yen SSC, Jaffe RB, editors. *Reproductive Endocrinology: Physiology, Pathophysiology and Clinical Management*. Philadelphia: WB Saunders Co, 309–56.

Strehler E, Abt M, el-Danasouri I, Sterzik K (1999) Transvaginal administration of micronized progesterone does not differ to progesterone gel application in the efficacy of luteal phase support in IVF cycles. In: *Abstract Book. 11th World Congress on In Vitro Fertilization and Human Reproductive Genetics*, 9–14 May 1999, Sydney, Australia, 287.

Sumita S, Sofat S Sr. (2003) Intramuscular versus intravaginal progesterone as luteal phase and early pregnancy support in patients undergoing IVF-ET. *Fertil Steril* **80**:S134–5 (P-44).

Szekeres-Bartho J, Par G, Dombay GY, et al. (1997) The anti-abortive effect of PIBF in mice is manifested by modulating NK activity. *Cell Immunol* **177**:194–9.

Szekeres-Bartho J, Wegman TG (1996) A progesterone-dependant immunomodulatory protein alters the Th1/Th2 balance. *J Reprod Immunol* **31**:81–95.

Tavaniotou A, Albano C, Smitz J, Devroey P (2001) Comparison of LH concentrations in the early and mid-luteal phase in IVF cycles after treatment with HMG alone or in association with the GnRH antagonist Cetrorelix. *Hum Reprod* **16**:663–7.

Tay PY, Lenton EA (2003) Inhibition of progesterone secretion by oestradiol administered in the luteal phase of assisted conception cycles. *Med J Malaysia* **58**:187–95.

Tesarik J, Hazout A, Mendoza C (2004) Enhancement of embryo developmental potential by a single administration of GnRH agonist at the time of implantation. *Hum Reprod* **19**:1176–80.

Tesarik J, Hazout A, Mendoza-Tesarik R, Mendoza N, Mendoza C (2006) Beneficial effect of luteal-phase GnRH agonist administration on embryo implantation after ICSI in both GnRH agonist- and antagonist-treated ovarian stimulation cycles. *Hum Reprod* **21**: 2572–9.

Ubaldi F, Bourgain C, Tournaye H, et al. (1997) Endometrial evaluation by aspiration biopsy on the day of oocyte retrieval in the embryo transfer cycles in patients with serum progesterone rise during the follicular phase. *Fertil Steril* **67**: 521–6.

Vande Wiele RL, Bogumil J, Dyrenfurth I, et al. (1970) Mechanisms regulating the menstrual cycle in women. *Recent Prog Horm Res* **26**:63–103.

Wentz AC (1980) Endometrial biopsy in the evaluation of infertility. *Fertil Steril* **33**:121–4.

Wilkins L (1960) Masculinization of female fetus due to use of orally given progestins. *JAMA* **172**:1028–30.

Williams SG, Oehninger S, Gibbons WE, et al. (2001) Delaying the initiation of progesterone supplementation results in decreased pregnancy rates after in vitro fertilization: a randomized prospective study. *Fertil Steril* **76**:1140–3.

Wright KP, Guibert J, Weitzen S, Davy C, Fauque P, Olivennes F (2006) Artificial versus stimulated cycles for endometrial preparation prior to frozen-thawed embryo transfer. *Reprod Biomed Online* **13**:321–5.

Younis JS, Mordel N, Lewin A, et al. (1992) Artificial endometrial preparation for oocyte donation: the effects of estrogen stimulation on clinical outcome. *J Assist Reprod Genet* **9**:222–7.

Younis S, Ezra Y, Sherman Y, Simon A, Schencker G, Laufer N (1994) The effect of estradiol depletion during the luteal phase on endometrium development. *Fertil Steril* **62**:103–7.

Zegers-Hochschild F, Balmaceda JP, Fabres C, et al. (2000) Prospective randomized trial to evaluate the efficacy of a vaginal ring releasing progesterone for IVF and oocyte donation. *Hum Reprod* **15**:2093–7.

45

THROMBOPHILIA AND IMPLANTATION FAILURE

Sameh Mikhail, Botros R. M. B. Rizk, Mary George Nawar, Christopher B. Rizk

INTRODUCTION

Human reproduction is an inefficient process. It is estimated that approximately one-fifth of conceptions result in life birth (1, 2). During the past three decades, substantial progress has been achieved in improving stimulation protocols and fertilization procedures. In the same period, however, there was only minimal advancement embryo implantation and pregnancy rate per embryo transfer (3). The average birthrate per complete cycle of in vitro fertilization (IVF) still ranges from 29.9 to 43.7 percent per egg retrieval (4).

It has been estimated that 30 percent of embryos are lost in the preimplantation phase, and 30 percent are lost after the embryo is implanted in the uterus (5). It has been suggested that unsuccessful implantation is attributed to abnormal embryo karyotype (6). Data from genetic studies, however, indicate that the overall prevalence of karyotype abnormalities among preimplantation embryos ranges from 50 to 60 percent (7, 8). Based on these data, the expected implantation rate would be much higher than currently observed (9). This discrepancy suggests that implantation failure could be the result of abnormalities in the mother (6).

Recent evidence suggest that abnormalities such as thyroid anomalies, increased levels of circulating natural killer cells (10, 12), the presence of mouse embryo assay factor (13, 14), and inherited and acquired thrombophilia may contribute to the failure of implantation (15).

Some inherited thrombophilic disorders have been implicated as a possible mechanism for adverse pregnancy outcomes and fetal loss (15). Moreover, it has been suggested that recurrent miscarriage and subfertility may have overlapping pathogenetic mechanisms. This theory is supported by the finding that women with infertility/subfertility have a higher risk of pregnancy failure (16). Additionally, subfertility is an adverse prognostic factor in women with recurrent pregnancy loss (17).

The relation between recurrent miscarriage and inherited thrombophilia is discussed elsewhere. In this chapter, we focus on the association between acquired and inherited thrombophilia and implantation failure (IF).

OVERVIEW OF THROMBOPHILIA

Hypercoagulability can be acquired or inherited (Table 45.1). Acquired and genetic causes of thrombophilia frequently interact (18), which occasionally poses diagnostic and therapeutic challenges when managing patients with hypercoagulability.

Inherited Thrombophilia

Activated Protein C Resistance and Factor V Leiden

Activated protein C resistance (APCR) was described by Dahlback and Hildebrand in 1994 (19). Activated protein C inhibits coagulation by inactivating coagulation factors Va and VIIIa. Ninety percent of patients with APCR have a factor V allele that is resistant to the effect of protein C. This mutation, factor V Leiden (FVL), involves a single amino acid change (Arg 506 to Gln) at the site where activated protein C proteolitically cleaves factor Va (20, 22).

FVL is very common: it is present in 5 percent of healthy individuals of northern European descent, in 10 percent of patients presenting with venous thrombosis, and in 30–50 percent of patients evaluated for hypercoagulability (23–26). FVL is common in Whites but rare in individuals of African or Asian descent (26). Although patients homozygous for FVL do not exhibit severe thrombotic disorders, they are still at higher risk of venous thrombosis than patients heterozygous for FVL (27). Patients with FVL are at a low risk for venous thromboembolism: by the age of sixty-five years, only 6 percent of patients would have developed venous thrombosis, the majority of which occur in the presence of other risk factors, such as surgery (20).

Prothrombin Gene Mutation

The prothrombin gene mutation was first described in 1996 (28). This mutant allele is associated with a gain of function leading to increased levels of functionally normal prothrombin. It is present in about 4 percent of the population, 5–10 percent of patients presenting with venous thrombosis, and 15 percent of patients being evaluated for thrombophilia (25, 29).

The prothrombin gene mutation is common in Whites of northern European descent but rare in individuals of African and Asian descent (29). Patients with this disorder have a low risk of venous thromboembolism, and most individuals with this mutation will not have an episode of venous thrombosis by the age of fifty.

Antithrombin Deficiency

Antithrombin deficiency was first described in 1965 (30). Antithrombin inactivates thrombin (factor IIa) and factors Xa,

Table 45.1: Inherited and Acquired Hypercoagulable States

Inherited

Resistance to activated protein C/factor V Leiden

Prothrombin gene mutation 20210A

Antithrombin III deficiency

Protein C deficiency

Protein S deficiency

Hyperhomocysteinemia

Acquired

Antiphospholipid antibody syndrome

Hypercoagulable state associated with other clinical conditions

Nephrotic syndrome

Hyperviscosity (polycythemia vera, Waldenström macroglobinemia, and multiple myeloma)

Myeloproliferative disorders (polycythemia vera and essential thrombocythemia)

Paroxysmal nocturnal hemoglobinuria

Sickle cell anemia

Rare or not well established

Dysfibrinogenemia

Hypoplasminogenemia, dysplasminogenemia

Abnormal thrombomodulin

Factor XII deficiency

Elevated factor VII, factor VIII, fibrinogen, lipoprotein (a), plasminogen activator inhibitor-1

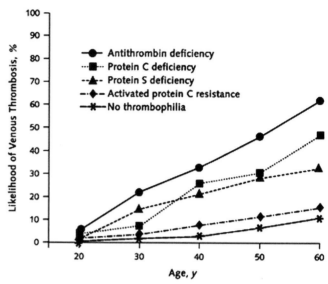

Figure 45.1. Thrombosis-free survival for patients with the major thrombophilic states.

IXa, XIa, and XIIa. Patient with antithrombin deficiency have the highest risk of thrombosis among patients with congenital thrombophilic states (Figure 45.1). Even mild antithrombin deficiency will lead to thrombosis. Approximately 30 percent of patients with antithrombin deficiency will experience an episode of venous thrombosis by the age of forty (31). Antithrombin deficiency is present in about 0.2 percent of the general population and in 0.5–7.5 percent of patient with venous thrombosis (32).

Protein C Deficiency

Protein C deficiency was first described in 1981 (33). Activated protein C exerts its anticoagulant effect through inactivating factors Va and VIIIa. Protein C deficiency is present in about 0.2 percent of the population and in 2.5–6 percent of patients presenting with venous thrombosis (32, 34–37). Approximately 25 percent of patients with protein C deficiency will develop venous thrombosis by the age of forty (31).

Protein S Deficiency

Protein S deficiency was first described in 1984 (38, 39). Protein S exerts its anticoagulant activity by acting as a cofactor

for inactivation of factor Va and VIIIa by activated protein C. The prevalence of protein S deficiency in the general population is unknown. It is found in 1.3–5 percent of patients presenting with venous thromboembolism (37, 40). About 20 percent of individuals with protein S deficiency will develop venous thrombosis by the age of forty (Figure 45.1).

Hyperhomocystenemia

Elevated homocysteine levels can be congenital or acquired. Acquired hyperhomocysteinmia is caused by folate, vitamine B_{12}, or vitamin B_6 deficiency (43). The congenital form is most commonly caused by a mutation in the cystathione B-synthase or the methylenetetrahydrofolate reductase (MTHFR) gene (41, 42). The MTHFR gene mutation is the most common genetic abnormality associated with this disorder. In some groups, 50 percent of patients were heterozygous for the abnormal allele, while 15 percent were homozygous (44). The homozygous mutation is associated with elevated homocysteine levels in the presence of concomitant folate, vitamine B_{12}, or vitamin B_6 deficiency. The heterozygous mutation, however, is not associated with hyperhomocysteinemia. Elevated homocysteine levels may be associated with venous or arterial thrombosis (45, 46).

Acquired Thrombophilia

Antiphospholipid Antibody (APA) Syndrome

The (APA) syndrome is a group of closely related clinical syndromes: 1) the lupus anticoagulant (LA) syndrome, 2) the anticardiolipin antibody syndrome, and 3) syndromes caused by other (APA), such as antiphosphatidylserine, antiphosphatidylethanolamine, antiphosphatidylglycerol, antiphosphatidylcholine, antiphosphatidylinositol anti-annexin B antibody, and antiphosphatidic acid (47). All APA may be associated with arterial and venous thrombosis, fetal wastage, infertility, and thrombocytopenia in descending order of frequency (47). The LA is estimated to account for approximately 6–8 percent of thrombosis in otherwise healthy individuals. Thromboembolism, however, develops in 50 percent of patients with concomitant LA and systemic lupus erythromatosis (48).

Mechanism of IF in Patients with Thrombophilia

Inherited Thrombophilia

Recent data propose an association between thrombophilic gene mutations and IF (15). An accurate balance of coagulation and fibrinolysis is essential for trophobastic invasion, fibrin polymerization, and stabilization of the placental basal plate. This balance also prevents fibrin deposition in forming intervillous spaces and placental blood vessels (49). The main regulator of coagulation and fibrinolysis is thrombin. Thrombin is converted from its proenzyme prothrombin by the prothrombinase complex that includes factor V. Activated protein C is an essential part of the feedback mechanism of the prothrombinase complex. It inactivates factor V, resulting in a decrease in thrombin generation. Moreover, once thrombin is formed it stimulates fibrin formation. Fibrin catalyzes the conversion of plasminogen to plasmin, which in turn stimulates fibrinolysis. This process is tightly regulated, and the balance between coagulation, anticoagulation, and fibrinolysis may be offset by the presence of thrombophilic gene mutations (49).

Some investigators suggest that coagulation factors may also exert nonhemostatic functions during implantation. Thrombophilic genes also encode proteins involved in inflammation and tissue remodeling (50). The pathogenesis of recurrent IF in patients with thrombophilic gene mutation may involve the effect of hypofibrinolysis on trophoblast migration (51, 52). Trophoblastic migration and invasion during implantation involves extracellular matrix degradation, which is facilitated by matrix metalloproteinases (MMP). Expression of MMP is enhanced by plasmin (53, 54). Therefore, it is postulated that trophoblastic implantation depends on the controlled production of plasmin from plasminogen (55). This observation is supported by data showing improved implantation rate in patients with factor V Leiden, a mutatin that leads to increased thrombin generation and consequently increased fibrinolysis (19, 56).

Acquired Thrombophilia

Recently, a variety of pathogenetic mechanisms have been suggested to explain the prothrombotic effect of APA, the main cause of acquired thrombophilia. APA are thought to cause thrombosis through disruption of anticoagulant mechanisms, such as the annexin V network and increased production of tissue factor (57, 58). However, these theories are being challenged now by emerging evidence that thrombosis of the uteroplacental circulation is not the primary mechanism by which APA cause reproductive failure. This is supported by the studies showing that placentae of the majority of women with APA are not severely infarcted (59, 61). During the first few weeks of pregnancy, extravillous trophoblast invades the uterine spiral arteries and form plugs within the lumen of these vessels that prevent the passage of maternal blood to the placenta (62). These plugs do not disappear until the tenth or twelfth week of gestation. Therefore, thrombosis of the maternal arteries cannot explain implantation failure or miscarriages that occur prior to the tenth week of gestation. Since it became clear that thrombosis is unlikely to be the pathogenetic mechanism of IF, a variety of other mechanisms have been proposed to explain this phenomenon. It has been shown that APA can adversely affect proliferation, invasion of trophoblasts, and production hormones such as human chorionic gonadotropin (63, 67). These mechanisms, however, did not fully explain IF in patients with APA. Recently, it has been suggested that APA may negatively impact the transformation of the endometrium into decidua, creating a hostile environment for blastocyst implantation (68). A growing body of evidence suggests that APA exert their effect by interfering with cell membrane vital reactions or by reacting with antigens on cell membrane surface and thus interfering with their activity (69).

Clinical Studies of Thrombophilia and IF

The association between acquired and inherited causes of thrombophilia and IF was the focus of several studies that showed variable results (70, 79).

In 2001, Grandone et al. (71) investigated the prevalence of FVL, prothrombin gene mutation (G20210A), antithrombin III (AT-III), protein C, and protein S deficiencies as well as LA and anticardiolipin (ACL) antibodies in eighteen patients with at least three IVF cycles with subsequent fetal loss (group A). The two control groups included women at the first or second IVF cycle, those with almost one successful pregnancy after an IVF attempt (group B), and parous women who conceived spontaneously with uneventful pregnancies (group C).

Overall, the prevalence of one prothrombotic mutation was 27.7, 0, and 6 percent in groups A, B, and C, respectively. The frequency of FVL and G20210 was not significantly different between groups A and C.

In 2001, Gopel et al. (76) evaluated 102 mother-child pairs with successful IVF/intracytoplasmic sperm injection (ICSI) to determine the effect of the FVL mutation on implantation. Ten of the 102 pairs had the FVL mutation (mother only = 4, child only = 4, and mother and child = 2). Implantation was successful at first attempt in nine out of ten (90 percent) pairs who had the mutation compared to forty-five of ninety-two (49 percent) pairs who did not ($P = 0.018$). Moreover, pairs with the FVL allele had significantly lower median number of unsuccessful transfers than pairs without the allele [0 (range 0–2) vs. 1 (0–8)], respectively ($P = 0.02$). On multivariate analysis, only the FVL mutation status predicted the success of the first embryo transfer.

In 2003, Martinellli et al. (72) conducted a case-control study to determine the frequency of FVL, prothrombin gene G20210A, MTHFR C677T gene mutations, LA, and ACL antibodies in 234 women undergoing either IVF or ICSI. The control group included 234 women who conceived naturally. Among women who underwent IVF or ICSI, seventy-two (31 percent) became pregnant. The study did not find an association between thrombophilia and failure of the assisted reproductive procedures (Table 45.2). Moreover, when women where stratified according to age or total number of embryo transfer procedures performed, no association was observed between thrombophilia and failure of IVF or ICSI.

In 2004, Azem et al. (73) conducted a case-control study comparing the prevalence of hereditary thrombophilia between forty-five women with a history of four or more failed IVF cycles (group A), forty-four apparently healthy women with at least one uneventful pregnancy matched for age and ethnic origin (group B), and fifteen women who conceived in the first IVF cycle. The prevalence of FVL, G20210A, MTHFR, as well as deficiencies of protein C, protein S, and AT-III were assessed in all 104 women. The prevalence of at least one inherited

Table 45.2: Prevalence of Mutations in Factor V, Prothrombin and MTHFR in Women Undergoing Assisted Reproductive Procedures and Control Women

	Women in whom assisted reproductive procedures failed, n = 162 (%)	Women with spontaneous conception, n = 234 (%)	OR (95 percent CI),
Factor V mutation	8 (5)	5 (2)	2.4 (0.7–8.3)
Prothrombin gene mutation	5 (3)	13 (6)	0.5 (0.2–1.6)
MTHFR gene mutation	31 (19)	46 (20)	1.0 (0.5–1.7)

Adapted from Matinelli et al. (72).

Table 45.3: Summary of the Incidence of Inherited Thrombophilias in the Study Population

Thrombophilia	Group A, n = 45 (%)	Group B, n = 44 (%)	Group C, n = 15 (%)
All thrombophilias	20 (44.4)	8 (18.2)[a]	3 (20)
All thrombophilias without MTHFR	12 (26.7)	4 (9.1)[b]	1 (6.7)
MTHFR homozygote	8 (17.8)	4 (9.1)	2 (13.3)
FVL	3 (6.7)	3 (6.8)	0

Adapted from Azem et al. (73).
[a]$P = 0.012$; OR 3.6; 95 percent CI 1.25–10.6.
[b]$P = 0.03$; OR 2.9; 95 percent CI 1.02–8.4.

thrombophilic disorder was 44, 18.2, and 20 percent in groups A, B, and C, respectively. Women who failed IVF had significantly more thrombophilia than women in group B ($P = 0.012$; odds ratio OR) 3.6; 95 percent confidence interval (CI) 1.25–10.6]. The prevalence of MTHFR, protein S deficiency, and G20210A in group A was 17.8, 8.9, and 8.9 percent, respectively. Since folic acid intake was not known in most women, the study results were reanalyzed, without the MTHFR mutation. The frequency of thrombophilia was 26.7 percent in group A compared to 9.1 percent in group B ($P = 0.03$, OR 2.9; 95 percent CI 1.02–8.4) (Table 45.3).

In 2005, Van Dunne et al. (75) evaluated 115 female patients with history of deep venous thrombosis or pulmonary embolism with the FVL mutation and 230 age-matched control subjects who also suffered from venous thromboembolism but did not have the FVL mutation. The aim of the study was to determine the effect of FVL on embryo implantation and human reproduction. Time to first pregnancy, proportion of patients who achieved their first pregnancy within three months, and proportion of patients who reported a time to first pregnancy of more than twelve months was similar between FVL carriers and noncarriers.

In 2006, Qublan et al. (70) evaluated the prevalence of thrombophilia in 90 consecutive women with a history of at least three previously failed IVF embryo transfer cycles (group A), 90 women who have had successful pregnancy after their first IVF cycle (group B), and 100 women who had conceived spontaneously with at least one uneventful pregnancy and no history of miscarriages. All women were investigated for the presence of FVL, MTHFR, G20210A mutations, LA, ACL, as well as deficiency in protein C and S and AT-III. The frequency of at least one thrombophilic defect was 68.9, 25.6, and 25 percent in groups A, B, and C, respectively. This difference was statistically significant ($P < 0.01$). In women with repeated IVF failure, homozygosity for FVL was found in 4.4 percent (4/90) of patients, compared with none in the other two groups. Similarly, 14.4 percent (13/90) patients in group A were homozygous for the MTHFR mutation compared to 3.3 percent (3/90) and 2 percent (2/100) patients in groups B and C, respectively. In women with MTHFR mutation, hyperhomocysteinemia was more prevalent in the study group [60 percent (12/20)] compared with each control group [9.1 percent (1/11)] ($P < 0.001$). Homozygosity for MTHFR mutation with hyperhomocysteinemia was found in 55 percent (11/20) of patients in group A compared with none in the other two groups ($P < 0.042$). The frequency of combined thrombophilia was 35.6, 4.4, and 3 percent in groups A, B, and C, respectively. The prevalence of the G20210A mutation, LA, ACL, as well as deficiency in protein C and S and AT-III was not significantly different between the study group and each of the control groups (Table 45.4).

In 2006, Coulam et al. (74) evaluated the prevalence of FVL, G20210A mutations, factor XIII, B-fibrinogen, plasminogen activator inhibitor-1 (PAI-1), human platelet antigen 1, and MTHFR mutations in forty-two women with a history of recurrent IF. The control group consisted of twenty fertile women who were also evaluated for the thrombophilic gene mutations. PAI-1 was the only specific gene mutation to show significantly higher frequency in women with IF compared with controls [38 percent (16/42) vs. 10 percent (2/20) ($P = 0.03$)]. Women with history of recurrent IF demonstrated significantly more total homozygous mutations than controls [74 percent (31/42)] than control women [20 percent (4/20)] ($P = 0.007$). Similarly, when total number of mutations was calculated by counting a heterozygous mutation as one mutation and a homozygous mutation as two mutations, women experiencing recurrent IF had more total mutations than controls (74 vs. 20 percent, $P = 0.0004$).

The association between APA and IF was the focus of a variety of research studies. In 1998, Stern et al. (70) evaluated the incidence of LA, antinuclear (ANA), antiphospholipid, anticardiolipin, and anti-B_2 glycoprotein (B_2 GPI) I antibodies in 105 patients who have previously had at least ten embryos transferred with no success. Other groups evaluated in this study were 52 newly referred patients for IVF, 97 women with recurrent miscarriage, and 106 women with at least one child born

Table 45.4: Frequency of Thrombophilic Factors in the Study Groups

Thrombophilic factors	Study group	Control group		P-Value	
	Group A (n = 90)	Group B (n = 90)	Group C (n = 100)	A versus B	A versus C
FVL					
Homozygous	4 (4.4)	0	0	0.049	0.294
MTHFR (C677T) mutation					
Homozygous	13 (14.4)	3 (3.3)	2 (2)	0.046[a]	0.012[a]
Combined thrombophilia	32 (35.6)	4 (4.4)	3 (3)	<0.0001[a]	<0.0001[a]

Adapted from Qublan et al. (70).

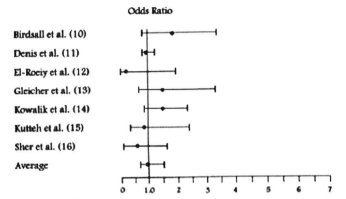

Figure 45.2. The relative likelihood of clinical pregnancy in women undergoing IVF who have antiphospholipid antibodies compared with women lacking such antibodies. Circles represent odds ratios, whereas the bars indicate 95 percent confidence intervals. Adapted from Hornstein. In vitro fertilization success. *Fertil Steril* 2000.

without any major pregnancy complication or any period of subfertility. A significantly higher frequency of ANA and B_2 GPI IgM antibodies was detected in women with recurrent miscarriage and IVF IF than in the fertile controls. B_2 GPI IgM antibodies were present in 8.6 percent (9/105) of patients with IF versus 0 percent of fertile controls. Similarly, ANA was detected in 21 percent (22/105) of patients with IF versus 9.4 percent (10/106) of fertile controls. The study did not find a statistically significant association between other autoantibodies and any specific patient group.

In 2001, Matsubayashi et al. (79) investigated the incidence of anti-annexin V antibodies (aANX) in forty-eight patients with recurrent (two or more) IVF-ET failure, 179 normal nonpregnant women, and 120 pregnant women. The group with recurrent IVF-ET failure had significantly increased number of positive aANX patients compared with normal pregnant and nonpregnant control groups ($P < 0.05$).

In 1999, Hornstein et al. (77) conducted a meta-analysis of seven studies that investigated the association between APA and IVF success. The aggregate clinical pregnancy rate was 57 and 49 percent in APA-positive and APA-negative patients, respectively (OR 0.99; 95 percent CI 0.64–1.53) (Figure 45.2). The studies, however, included, in this review were heteroge-neous and included differing study designs and patient populations, making interpretation of these results difficult (81).

TREATMENT

A small number of studies have explored the therapeutic options in patients with acquired thrombophilia and IF (82–88). The treatment of patients with IF and inherited hypercoagulable states has not been studied to date. The main therapeutic modalities investigated are heparin, aspirin (ASA), corticosteroids, and intravenous immunoglobulin alone or in combinations.

Heparin/ASA

Heparin is to exerts its therapeutic effect by several mechanisms. Heparin has an antithrombotic effect through a 1,000-fold acceleration of the action of antithrombin III, a naturally occurring inhibitor of the coagulation cascade (89). Moreover, in vitro studies (90) have shown that heparin, at therapeutic doses, inhibits the binding of APA binding as measured by ELISA. This, in vivo, may prevent the detrimental effect of APA on the trophoblastic layer. Additionally, heparin and ASA modulate trophoblast apoptosis in vitro, thus providing an additional explanation for their mechanism of action in patients with reproductive failure (91). In 1994, Sher et al. (84) explored the possibility that women with organic pelvic disease and APA might benefit from heparin and ASA administration. The viable pregnancy rate in patients with APA and organic pelvic disease receiving heparin and ASA was much higher compared to the untreated APA seronegative patients (49 vs. 16 percent, respectively) ($P < 0.05$). These results were subsequently challenged by Kutteh et al. (83) and Stern et al. (84) in 1997 and 2002, respectively. Kutteh et al. prospectively tested 191 women with infertility undergoing IVF for the first time for APA. They subsequently evaluated the effect of treating APA-positive women with heparin and ASA. The control population consisted of 200 nonpregnant, reproductive-age women with no history of fertility problems, 200 nonpregnant women with recurrent pregnancy loss (three or more), and 200 nonpregnant women with systemic lupus erythematosus. The implantation rate in women who had a positive APA and received heparin and ASA was 25 percent. In comparison, women with positive APA antibodies and standard treatment had an implantation rate of 19.4 percent. Additionally, the implantation rate of women who tested negative for APA and received standard treatment compared to those who received heparin and ASA were 19.4 and 26.7 percent, respectively. The difference between the groups was not statistically significant.

Stern et al. conducted a double-blind, placebo-controlled trial of heparin and ASA for 143 women with history of IF associated with IVF who tested positive for at least one APA. The intervention group received unfractionated heparin sodium 5,000 units twice daily and ASA 100 oral, once a day. The was no significant difference between intervention and placebo cycles in combined positive pregnancy tests per embryo transfer (14.6 and 17.6 percent, respectively) and fetal heart detection rate per embryo (6.8 and 8.5 percent).

Corticosteroids

The benefit of glucocorticoids in women with implantation failure and APA was the focus of a small number of studies (92–94).

In 1996, Ando et al. (94) investigated the use of low-dose prednisolone in forty-one women with positive APA who underwent fifty-one embryo transfer cycles. The implantation rate of this group was compared to forty-eight cycles without corticosteroid therapy. The implantation rate with corticosteroids was significantly better than without corticosteroids (13.2 and 3.8 percent, respectively).

In 1998, Hasegawa et al. (93) conducted a nonrandomized study to evaluate the effect of prednisolone 10 mg daily and ASA 81 mg daily in women with APA enroled in IVF program. Women positive for ANA and negative for ACL and antiphosphatidylserin (APS) who had received the intervention had a better implantation rate than women who had not received the intervention (20.3 and 6.8 percent, respectively) ($P < 0.01$). There was no significant difference, however, between women positive for ANA, ACL, and APS, who were treated and those who were not treated with the intervention medication.

In 2005, Taniguchi conducted a nonrandomized study to evaluate the effect of five days 15–60 mg of prednisolone on ANA-positive women referred for IVF. The study population consisted of 120 women who underwent 223 IVF embryo transfer cycles. Implantation and clinical pregnancy rates in steroid-nontreated ANA-positive women were significantly lower than in the other groups (0/41 transplanted embryos and 0/15 cycles).

Intravenous Immunoglobulin

Sher et al. (95) conducted a nonrandomized study to investigate the effect of intravenous immunoglobulin (IVIG) in women with positive APA who underwent IVF. Six hundred eighty seven women were initially offered heparin and ASA. Six hundred three of these women agreed to receive the treatment medications. The APA profile of the study population was tested, and 322 patients tested positive to only one APA. IVIG in combination with heparin and ASA was subsequently administered to 121 women who had received only heparin and ASA and did not achieve a viable pregnancy following two consecutive IVF attempts. Women who had an IgM- or IgG-related APA directed specifically toward phosphatidylserin (PS) or phosphatidylethanolamine (PE) had a significant increase in IVF birthrate following addition of IVIG to heparin and

ASA therapy (41 vs. 17 percent, respectively; $P < 0.0001$). Women whose APA were directed toward epitopes other than PS and PE did not experience a significantly improved IVF birthrate after addition of IVIG to heparin and ASA (43 vs. 36 percent; $P > 0.05$).

CONCLUSIONS

Studies have shown conflicting and inconclusive data about the association between thrombophilia and IF (96). The current literature is flawed by using different study and control populations and different methods for detecting and reporting diagnostic tests. At the present time the optimal diagnostic workup and no treatment recommendation have to be individualized for women with recurrent IF.

KEY POINTS

- A significant proportion of embryos is lost in the implantation and pre-implantion phase.
- Acquired and inherited thrombophilia may be associated with IF.
- Thrombophilia is hypothesized to cause IF through hemostatic and non-hemostatic mechanisms.
- Studies evaluating the association between thrombophilia and IF were heterogenous and showed inconsistent results.
- It is premature to recommend anticoagulation for patients with thrombophilia and IF.

REFERENCES

1. Robert CJ, Lowe Cr. Where have all the conceptions gone? *Lancet* 1975; I: 498–9.
2. ZinMn MJ, O'Connor J, Clegg ED et al. Estimates of human fertility and pregnancy loss. *Fertil Steril* 1996; 65: 503–9.
3. Christiansen OB, Nielsen H, Kolte A. Future directions of failed implantation and recurrent miscarriage research.
4. Assisted reproductive technology in the United States: 2000 results generated from the American Society for Reproductive Medicine/Society for Assisted Reproductive Technology Registry. *Fertil Steril* 2004; 81(5): 1207–20.
5. Macklon NS, Geraedts JPM, Fauser BCJM. Conception to ongoing pregnancy: the 'black box' of early pregnancy loss. *Hum Reprod Update* 2002; 8: 333–43.
6. Vaquero E, Lazzrin N, Caserta D et al. Diagnostic evaluation of women experiencing repeated in vitro fertilization failure. *Eur J Obstet Gynecol* 2005.
7. Clark DA, Coulam CB, Daya S et al. Unexplained sporadic and recurrent miscarriage in the new millennium: a critical analysis of immune mechanisms and treatments. *Hum Reprod Update* 2001; 7: 501–11.
8. Gianaroli L, Masgli C, Ferraretti AP et al. Preimplantation diagnosis for aneuploidies in patients undergoing in vitro fertilization with a poor prognosis: identification of the categories for which it should be proposed. *Fertil Steril* 1999; 72: 837–44.
9. Coulam CB, Roussev RG. Correlation of NK cell activation and inhibition markers with NK cytotoxicity among women experiencing immunological implantation failure after in vitro fertilization and embryo transfer. *J Assist Reprod Genet* 2003; 20: 58–62.
10. Ntrivalas EI, Kwak-Kim JYH, Gilman-Sachs A et al. Status of peripheral blood natural killer cells in women with recurrent

spontaneous abortions and infertility of unknown aetiology. *Hum Reprod* 2001; 16: 855–61.

11. Michou VI, Kanavaros P, Athanasssiou V et al. Fraction of the peripheral blood concentration of CD56+/CD16-/CD3- cells in total natural killer cells as an indication of fertility and infertility. *Fertil Steril* 80: 691–7.

12. Roussev FR, Kaider BD, Price DE et al. Laboratory evaluation of women experiencing reproductive failure. *Am J Reprod Immunol* 1996; 35: 415–20.

13. Kaider AS, Kaider BD, Janowicz PB et al. Immunodiagnostic evaluation in women with reproductive failure. *Am J Reprod Immunol* 1999; 42: 335–46.

14. Christiansen O, Nielsen H, Kolte A. Future directions of failed implantation and recurrent miscarriage research. *Reprod Biomed Online* 2006; 13(1): 71–83.

15. Kupferminc MJ, Eldor A, Steinman N et al. Increased frequency of genetic thrombophilia in women with complications of pregnancy. *N Eng J Med* 1999; 340: 9–13.

16. Hakim RB, Gray RH, Zacur H. Infertility and early pregnancy loss. *Am J Obstet Gynecol* 1995; 172(5): 1510–17.

17. Cauchi MN, Coulam CB, Cowchock S et al. Predictive factors in recurrent spontaneous aborters—a multicenter study. *Am J Reprod Immunol* 1995; 33: 165–70.

18. Seligsohn U, Lubetski A. Genetic susceptibility to venous thrombosis. *N Eng J Med* 2001; 344: 1222–30.

19. Dahlback B, Hildebrand B. Inherited resistance to activated protein C is corrected by anticoagulant cofactor activity found to be a property of factor V. *Proc Natl Acad Sci USA* 1994; 91: 1396–400.

20. Rodeghiero F, Tosetto A. Activated protein C resistance and factor V Leiden mutation are independent risk factors for venous thromboembolism. *Ann Intern Med* 1999; 130: 643–50.

21. Kalafatis M, Bertina RM, Rand MD, Mann KG. Characterization of the molecular defect in factor VR506Q. *J Biol Chem* 1995; 270: 4053–7.

22. Camire RM, Kalafatis M, Cushman M, Tracy RP, Mann KG, Tracy PB. The mechanism of inactivation of human platelet factor Va from normal and activated protein C-resistant individuals. *J Biol Chem* 1995; 270: 20794–800.

23. Lee DH, Henderson PA, Blajchman MA. Prevalence of factor V Leiden in a Canadian blood donor population. *CMAJ* 1996; 155: 285–9.

24. Ridker PM, Hennekens CH, Lindpaintner K, Stampfer MJ, Eisenberg PR, Milletich JP. Mutation in the gene coding for coagulation factor V and the risk of myocardial infraction, stroke, and venous thrombosis in apparently healthy men. *N Engl J Med* 1995; 332: 912–17.

25. Salomon O, Steinberg DM, Zivelin A, Gitel S, Dardik R, Rosenberg N et al. Single and combined prothrombotic factors in patients with idiopathic venous thromboembolism: prevalence and risk assessment. *Arterioscler Thromb Vasc Biol* 1999; 19: 511–18.

26. Ridker PM, Miletich JP, Hennekens CH, Buring JE. Ethnic distribution of factor V Leiden in 4047 men and women. Implications for venous thromboembolism screening. *JAMA* 1997; 277: 1305–7.

27. Dulicek P, Maly J, Safarova M. Risk of thrombosis in patients homozygous and heterozygous forfactro V Leiden in the East Bohemian region. *Clin Appl Thromb Hemost* 2000; 6: 87–9.

28. Poort SR, Rosendaal FR, Reitsma PH, Bertina RM. A common genetic variation in the 3'-untranslated region of the prothrombin gene is associated with elevated plasma prothrombin levels and an increase in venous thrombosis. *Blood* 1996; 88: 3698–703.

29. Rosendaal FR, Doggen CJ, Zivelin A, Arruda VR, Aiach M, Siscobick DS et al. Geographic distribution of the 20210 G to A prothrombin variant. *Thromb Haemost* 1998; 79: 706–8.

30. Egberg O. Inherited antithrombin deficiency causing thrombophilia. *Thromb Diath Haemorrh* 1965; 13: 516–30.

31. Martinelli I, Mannucci PM, De Stefano V, Taioli E, Rossi B, Crosti F et al. Different risks of thrombosis in four coagulation defects associated with inherited thrombophilia: a study of 150 families. *Blood* 1998; 92: 2353–8.

32. Mateo J, Oliver A, Borrell M, Sala N, Fontcuberta J. Laboratory evaluation and clinical characteristics of 2.132 consecutive unselected patients with venous thromboembolism—results of the Spanish Multicentric Study on Thrombophilia (EMET-Study). *Thromb Haemost* 1997; 77: 444–51.

33. Griffin JH, Evatt B, Zimmerman TS, Kleiss AJ, Wideman C. Deficiency of protein C in congenital thrombotic disease. *J Clin Invest* 1981; 68: 1370–3.

34. Ben-Tal O, Zivelin A, Seligsohn U. The relative frequency of hereditary thrombotic disorders among 107 patients with thrombophilia in Israel. *Thromb Haemost* 1989; 61: 50–4.

35. Tait RC, Walker ID, Reitsma PH, Islam SI, McCall F, Poort SR et al. Prevalence of protein C deficiency in the healthy population. *Thromb Haemost* 1995; 73: 87–93.

36. Sakata T, Kario K, Katayama Y, Matsuyama T, Kato H, Miyata T. Studies on congenital protein C deficiency in Japanese: prevalence, genetic analysis, and relevance to the onset of arterial occlusive diseases. *Semin Thromb Hemost* 2000; 26: 11–16.

37. Pabinger I, Brucker S, Krle PA, Schneider B, Korninger HC, Neissner H et al. Hereditary deficiency of antithrombin III, protein C and protein S: prevalence in patients with a history of venous thrombosis and criteria for rational patients screening. *Blood Coagul Fibrinolysis* 1992; 3: 547–53.

38. Comp PC, Nixon RR, Cooper MR, Esmon CT. Familial protein S deficiency is associated with recurrent thrombosis. *J Clin Invest* 1984; 74: 2082–8.

39. Comp PC, Esmon Ct. Recurrent venous thromboembolism in patients with a partial deficiency of protein S. *N Engl J Med* 1984; 311: 1525–8.

40. Gladson CL, Sharrer I, Hach V, Beck KH, Griffin JH. The frequency of type I heterozygous protein S and protein C deficiency in 141 unrelated young patients with venous thrombosis. *Thromb Haemost* 1988; 59: 18–22.

41. Goyette P, Frosst P, Rosenblatt DS, Rozen R. Seven novel mutations in the methylenetetrahydrofolate reductase gene and genotype/phenotype correlations in severe methylenetetrahydrofolate reductase deficiency. *Am J Hum Genet* 1995; 56: 1052–9.

42. Mudd SH, Skovby F, Levy HL, Pettigrew KD, Wilcken B, Pyeritz RE et al. The natural history of homocysteinuria due to cystathionine beta-synthase deficiency. *Am J Hum Genet* 1985; 37: 1–31.

43. Jacques PF, Bostom AG, Williams RR, Ellison RC, Eckfeldt JH, Rosenberg IH et al. Relation between folate status, a common mutation in the methylenetetrahydrofolate reductase, and plasma homocysteine concentrations. *Circulation* 1996; 93: 7–9.

44. Kluijtmans LA, van den Heuvel LP, Boers GH, Frosst P, Stevens EM, van Oost BA et al. Molecular genetic analysis in mild hyperhomocysteinemia: a common mutation in the methylenetetrahydrofolate reductase gene is a genetic risk factor for cardiovascular disease. *Am J Hum Genet* 1996; 58: 35–41.

45. Cattaneo M. Hyperhomocysteinemia, atherosclerosis and thrombosis. *Thromb Haemost* 1999; 81: 165–76.

46. Ray JG. Meta-analysis of hyperhomocysteinemia as a risk factor for venous thromboembolic disease. *Arch Intern Med* 1998; 158: 2101–6.

47. Bick RL. Antiphospholipid thrombosis syndromes. *Hematol Oncol Clin North Am* 2003; 17: 115.

48. Bick RL, Baker WF. Antiphospholipid syndrome and thrombosis. *Semin Thromb Hemost* 1999; 25: 333.

49. Coulam DB, Jeyendran RS, Fishel LA, Roussev R. *Reprod Biomed Online* 2006; 12(3): 322–7.

50. Rawlins ND, Barrett AJ et al. Evolutionary families of peptidases. *Biochem J* 1993; 290: 205–18.

51. Axelrod HR. Altered trophoblast functions in implantation-defective mouse embryos. *Dev Biol* 1985; 108: 185–90.

52. Many A, Schrieber L, Rosner S et al. Pathologic features of the placenta in women with severe pregnancy complications and thrombophilia. *Obstet Gynecol* 2001; 1041–4.

53. Chung HW, Wen Y, Ahn JJ et al. Interluekin-1 beta regulates urokinase plasminogen activator (u-PA), u-PA receptor, soluble u-PA receptor, and plasminogen activator inhibitor-1 messenger ribonucleic acid expression in cultured human endometrial stromal cells. *J Clin Endocrinol* 2001; 86: 1332–40.

54. Aflalo ED, Sod-Moriah UA, Patashnik G, Har-Vardi I. Differences in the implantation rates of rat embryos developed in viva and in vitro: possible role from plasminogen activators. *Fertil Steril* 2004; 1: 780–5.

55. Solberg H, Rinkenberger J, Dano K et al. A functional overlap of plasminogen and MMPs regulates vascularization during placental development. *Development* 2003; 130: 4439–50.

56. Gopel W, Ludwig M, Junge A et al. Selection pressure for the factor-V Leiden mutation and embryo implantation. *Lancet* 2001; 358: 1238–9.

57. Rand JH, Wu XX, Quinn AS et al. Human monoclonal antiphospholipid antibodies disrupt the annexin A5 anticoagulant crystal shield on phospholipid bilayers: evidence from atomic force microscopy and functional assay. *Am J Path* 2003; 163: 1193–200.

58. Amengual O, Atsumi T, Khamashta MA. Tissue factor in antiphospholipid syndrome: shifting the focus from coagulation to endothelium. *Rheumatology* 2003; 42: 1029–31.

59. Out HJ, Bruinse HW, Derksen RH. Anti-phospholipid antibodies and pregnancy loss. *Hum Reprod* 1999; 6: 889–97.

60. Salafia CM, Cowchock FS. Placental pathology and antiphospholipid antibodies: a descriptive study. *Am J Perinatol* 1997; 14: 435–41.

61. Van Horn JT, Crave C, Ward K. Features of placentas and abortion specimens from women with antiphospholipid and antiphospholipid-like syndromes. *Placenta* 2004; 25: 642–8.

62. James JL, Stone PR, Chamley LW. The regulation of trophoblast differentiation by oxygen in the first trimester of pregnancy. *Hum Reprod update* 2006; 12: 137–44.

63. Shurtz-Swirski R, Inbar O, Blank M et al. In vitro effect of anti-cardiolipin autoantibodies upon total and pulsatile placental hCG secretion during early pregnancy. *Am J Reprod Immunol* 1993; 29: 206–10.

64. Adler RR, Ng AK, Rote NS. Monoclonal antiphosphatidylserine antibody inhibits intercellular fusion of the choriocarcinoma line, JAR. *Biol Reprod* 1995; 53: 905–10.

65. Di Simone N, De Carolis S, Lanzone A et. In vitro effect of antiphospholipid antibody-containing sera on basal and gonadotrophin releasing hormone-dependent human chorionic gonadotrophin release by cultured trophoblast cells. *Placenta* 1995; 16: 75–83.

66. Di Simone N, Meroni PL, de Papa N et al. Antiphospholipid antibodies affect trophoblast gonadotropin secretion and invasiveness by binding directly and through adhered B2-glycoprotein I. *Arthritis Rheum* 2000; 43: 140–50.

67. Chamley LW, Duncalf A, Mitchell M et al. Action of anticardiolipin and antibodies to B2 glycoprotein I on trophoblast

68. Mak IY, Brosens JJ, Christian M et al. Regulated expression of signal transducer and activator of transcription, Stat5, and its enhancement of PRL expression in human endometrial stromal cells in vitro. *J Clin Endocrinol Metab* 2002; 87: 2581–8.

69. Rouby RA, Hoffman M. From antiphospholipid syndrome to antibody-mediated thrombosis. *Lancet* 1997; 350: 1491–2.

70. Qublan HS, Eid SS, Ababneh HA, Amarin ZO, Al-Khafaji FF, Khader YS. Acquired and inherited thrombophilia: implication in recurrent IVF and embryo transfer failure. *Hum Reprod* 2006; 21(10): 2694–8.

71. Grandone E, Colaizzo D, Lo Bue A, Checola MG, Cittadini E, Margaglione M. Inherited thrombophilia and in vitro fertilization implantation failure. *Fertil Steril* 2001; 76(1): 201–2.

72. Martinelli I, Taioli E, Ragni G, Levi-Setti P, Passomonti SM, Battaglioli T, Lodigiani C, Mannucci PM. Embryo implantation after assisted reproductive procedures and maternal thrombophilia. *Haematologica* 2003; 88(7): 789–93.

73. Azem F, Many F, Yovel I, Amit A, Lessing J, Kuperminc M. Increased rates of thrombophilia in women with repeated IVF failures. *Hum Reprod* 2004; 19(2): 368–74.

74. Coulam C, Jeyendran RS, Fishel L, Roussev R. Multiple thrombophilic gene mutations are risk factors for implantation failure. *Reprod Biomed Online* 2006; 12(3): 322–7.

75. Van Dunne FM, Doggen CJM, Heemskerk M, Rosendall FR, Helmerhorst FM. Factor V Leiden mutation in relation to fecundity and miscarriage in women with venous thrombosis. *Hum Reprod* 2005; 20(3): 802–6.

76. Gopel W, Ludwig M, Junge A, Kohlmann T, Diedrich K, Moller J. Selection pressure for the factor-V-Leiden mutation and embryo implantation. *Lancet* 2001; 358: 1238–9.

77. Hornstein M, Davis O, Massey J, Paulson R, Collins J. Antiphospholipid antibodies and in vitro fertilization success: a meta-analysis. *Fertil Steril* 2000; 73(2): 330–3.

78. McIntyre JA. Antiphospholipid antibodies in implantation failure. *Am J Reprod Immunol* 2003; 49: 221–9.

79. Matsubayashi H, Arai T, Izumi S, Sugi T, McIntyre J, Makino T. Anti-annexin V antibodies in patients with early pregnancy loss or implantation failures. *Fertil Steril* 2001; 76(4): 694–9.

80. Stern C, Chamley L, Hale L, Kloss M, Speirs A, Baker HW. Antibodies to B2 glycoprotein I are associated with in vitro fertilization implantation failure as well as recurrent miscarriage: results of a prevalence study. *Fertil Steril* 1998; 70(5): 938–44.

81. Gleicher N, Vidali A, Karande V. The immunological 'war of the roses': disagreements amongst reproductive immunologists. *Hum Reprod* 2002; 17: 539–42.

82. Stern C, Chamley L, Norris H, Hale L, Baker HW. A randomized, double-blind, placebo controlled trial of heparin and aspirin for women with fertilization implantation failure and antiphospholipid or antinuclear antibodies. *Fertil Steril* 2004; 81(5): 376–83.

83. Kutteh WH, Yetman DL, Chantilis SJ, Crain J. Effect of antiphospholipid antibodies in women undergoing in-vitro fertilization: role of heparin and aspirin. *Hum Reprod* 1997; 12(6): 1171–5.

84. Sher G, Feinman M, Zouves C, Duttner G, Maassarani G, Salem R, Matzner W, Ching W, Chong P. High fecundity rates following in-vitro fertilization and embryo transfer in antiphospholipid antibody seropositive women treated with heparin and aspirin. *Hum Reprod* 1994; 9(12): 2278–83.

85. Fiedler K, Wurfel W. Effectivity of heparin in assisted reproduction. *Eur J Med Res* 2004; 9(4): 207–14.

86. Sher G, Zouves C, Geinman M, Maassarani G, Matzner W, Chong P, Ching W. A rational basis for the use of combined

proliferation as a mechanism for fetal death. *Lancet* 1998; 352: 1037–8.

heparin/aspirin and IVIG immunotherapy in the treatment of recurrent IVF failure associated with antiphospholipid antibodies. *Am J Reprod Immunol* 1998; 39(6): 391–4.

87. Taniguchi F. Results of prednisolone given to improve the outcome of in vitro fertilization-embryo transfer in women with antinuclear antibodies. *J Reprod Med* 2005; 50(6): 383–8.

88. Sher G, Matzner W, Feinman M, Maassarani G, Zouves C, Chong P, Ching W. The selective use of heparin/aspirin therapy, alone or in combination with intravenous immunoglobulin G, in the management of antiphospholipid antibody-positive women undergoing in vitro fertilization. *Am J Reprod Immunol* 1998; 40(2): 74–82.

89. Rosenberg RD, Edelberg J, Zhang L. The heparin/antithrombin system: a natural anticoagulant mechanism. In: Colman RW, Hirsh J, Marder VJ, Clowes AW, George JN, Eds. *Thrombosis and Hemostasis: Basic Principles and Clinical Practice.* 4th ed. Philadelphia: Lippincott Williams & Wilkins; 2001: 711–31.

90. Di Simone N, Ferrazzani S, Castellani R, De Carolis S, Mancuso S, Caruso A. Heparin and low-dose aspirin restore placental human chorionic gonadotrophin secretion abolished by antiphospholipid antibody-containing sera. *Hum Reprod* 1997; 12(9): 2061–5.

91. Bose P, Black S, Dadyrov M, Weissebborn U, Neulen J, Regan L, Huppertz B. Heparin and aspirin attenuate placental apoptosis in vitro: implications for early pregnancy failure. *Am J Obstet Gynecol* 2005; 192(1): 23–30.

92. Hasegawa I, Yamanoto Y, Suzuki M, Murakawa H, Kuraboyashi T, Takakuwa K, Tanaka K. Prednisolone plus low-dose aspirin improves the implantation rate in women with autoimmune conditions who are undergoing in vitro fertilization. *Fertil Steril* 1998; 70(6): 1044–8.

93. Ando T, Suganuma N, Furuhashi M, Asada Y, Kondo I, Tomoda Y. Successful glucocorticoid treatment for patients with abnormal autoimmunity on in vitro fertilization and embryo transfer. *J Assist Reprod Genet* 1996; 13(10): 776–81.

94. Taniguchi F. Results of prednisolone given to improve the outcome of in vitro fertilization-embryo transfer in women with antinuclear antibodies. *J Reprod Med* 2005; 50(6): 383–8.

95. Sher G, Matzner W, Feinman M, Maassarani G, Zouves C, Chong P, Ching W. The selective use of heparin/aspirin therapy, alone or in combination with intravenous immunoglobulin G in the management of antiphospholipid antibody positive women undergoing in vitro fertilization. *Am J Reprod Immunol* 1998; 40(2): 74–82.

96. Rizk B, Abdalla HI. In Vitro fertilization. In: Rizk B, Abdalla HI, Eds. *Infertility and assisted reproductive technology.* 2008; chapter 9, 116–118.

46

INTRAUTERINE INSEMINATION

Norman F. Angell, Hany F. Moustafa, Botros R. M. B. Rizk, Mary George Nawar, Christopher B. Rizk,
Chris A. Huff, Ruth Kennedy, Scherri B. Holland, Julie Hazelton,
Juan A. Garcia-Velasco, Hassan N. Sallam

INTRODUCTION

Intrauterine insemination (IUI) is one of the most commonly performed treatments for infertile or hypofertile couples. Although the technique was first reported by Dickinson in 1921 (1), it was not until the 1980s when IUI started to become popular. Over the past twenty-five years, there has been a substantial amount of research evaluating this method. As in much of infertility, methodological problems preclude clear conclusions. In particular, well-planned randomized controlled trials are rare. However, the data available allow us to scientifically treat our patients even if that science is not perfect.

INDICATIONS FOR IUI

General indications for IUI include cervical factor infertility, male infertility, minimal to mild endometriosis, and unexplained infertility (Table 46.1).

Cervical Factor

An abnormal postcoital test is frequently treated by IUI. However, the test is difficult to standardize and the predictability of the test is low. Inadequate cervical mucus is difficult to quantitate, and whether a threshold amount of cervical mucus is necessary for proper function also is unknown. The epidemic of cervical dysplasia secondary to HPV infection has resulted in a great number of cervical operations via cryotherapy, LEEP and cone biopsy, may result in removing significant amount of cervical glands. The impact of these interventions on subsequent fertility is variable.

An abnormal Spinbarkeit test may show either a low amount of cervical mucus or an increase in viscosity of the mucus. Similar to the above, the prediction of the effect of abnormal Spinbarkeit on fertility is uncertain. Many practitioners prescribe estrogen therapy to improve the amount and viscosity of cervical mucus, particularly while treating with clomiphene citrate despite its limited efficiency (2).

Despite the uncertainty about cervical effects on infertility and the uncertainty about the effects of treatment, IUI seems to be a reasonable treatment option to use for these factors. Conceptually, one may fold these factors into the category of unexplained infertility and once again one would be left with the treatment of ovarian stimulation and IUI.

Male Factor

Male factor infertility is a major indication for IUI. John Hunter was the first to introduce the concept of IUI more than 200 years ago when he injected the semen of one of his patients with hypospadias into his spouse vagina. It is currently estimated that 40–50 percent of infertility causes are due to male factor. Ejaculatory dysfunction, sexual dysfunction, and retrograde ejaculation do not necessarily involve abnormal sperm production but IUI can effectively overcome these mechanical problems.

Most oligozoospermia, asthenozoospermia, and teratozoospermia remain idiopathic, with no clear cause found after investigation. Many studies have shown that men with abnormal semen analysis can still produce spontaneous pregnancies (3).

Investigators have attempted to quantitate a lower limit that predicts the likelihood of success with IUI (see chapter 18 by Kruger and Oehninger). It is important to advise couples about their chances of success with IUI so that time and money are not wasted on IUI rather than advancing directly to IVF.

Ejaculatory dysfunction (see chapter 21 by Fifer, Gurkan and Hellstrom) may prevent the ability to deposit semen into the vagina during intercourse. Retrograde ejaculation is relatively uncommon. In these men, it is possible to recover significant numbers of sperm by alkalinization of urine and subsequent masturbation followed by voiding. Sperm is recovered from the voided urine and concentrated in the usual manner, resulting in a specimen that may be used for IUI (4). Anejaculatory men with spinal cord injury can also be treated effectively (5, 6). If hypospadias is severe enough to prevent deposition of semen in the vagina through intercourse and cannot be treated, then IUI with washed sperm can overcome this problem.

Sexual dysfunction is more common than thought. If the clinician does not specifically ask about sexual dysfunction, this problem may not be identified as a reason for infertility. Erectile dysfunction may occur even in young men (see chapter 21 by Hellstrom). The stress of infertility evaluation and treatment itself may result in difficulty with erections. Effective treatment of erectile dysfunction is now available and may eliminate the need for advanced reproductive technologies. Other disabilities that prevent effective vaginal intercourse may require use of cervical or IUI.

Table 46.1: List of the Possible Mechanisms of Action of IUI

Male	Increase motility of sperm
	Increase concentration of sperm
	Increase concentration of normal sperm
	Improve sperm selection
	Assist sperm migration
Female	Bypass cervical barrier
	Bypass need of cervical mucus
	Increase number of sperm in tube
Ovarian stimulation	Increase number of fertilizable oocytes
	Improve timing for fertilization

Unexplained Infertility and Minimal Endometriosis

Unexplained infertility is a diagnosis of exclusion, (see chapter 36 by Balasch) although some may include minimal endometriosis in this category. Generally, 10 percent of infertile couples end up with this diagnosis after complete infertility workup.

Unexplained infertility is now a major indication for controlled ovarian hyperstimulation + IUI. According to the National Institute of Clinical Excellence (NICE) guidelines, all couples with unexplained infertility should be offered IUI treatment before restoring to other modalities of assisted reproduction, that is, IVF (7).

POSSIBLE MECHANISMS OF ACTION OF IUI

The indications for IUI are related to the possible mechanisms of action (Table 46.2). In general, there are two main mechanisms thought to be responsible for the efficacy of IUI. These include increasing the number of gametes and increasing the probability that the gametes are present in the female reproductive tract at the same time thereby enhancing fertilization.

In Males

Sperm washing results in increasing the number and concentration of motile sperms (8). In addition to improving those factors, IUI eliminates the filter mechanism of the cervix, thereby helping to maintain these concentrations in the female genital tract. Injection of the washed sperm also results in deposition of sperm higher in the genital tract, and this perhaps may do some of the work required by sperms to swim to the ampulla of the Fallopian tube and may result in increasing the number of sperm available for fertilization. IUI has been shown to increase pregnancy rates even if semen parameters are normal (9).

In Females

IUI bypasses the cervix and may overcome cervical factors thought to result in infertility. Immunological infertility resulting from antisperm antibodies in cervical mucus is avoided by injecting sperm directly into the uterine cavity. Widespread screening for precursors of cervical cancer has dramatically decreased the incidence of cervical cancer, but treatments of dysplasia of the cervix may contribute to cervical mucus changes that interfere with conception. Removal of much or all the endocervical glands may decrease the amount of cervical mucus or change its composition. IUI eliminates the need for cervical mucus to serve as the capacitation site for sperm as capacitation occurs in vitro as part of the sperm-washing procedure. Cervical mucus is not required as a medium for sperm migration when IUI is used. However, the loss of the reservoir function of the cervical crypts requires precise timing of the insemination.

Ovarian Stimulation

The use of controlled ovarian hyperstimulation (COH) in conjunction with IUI is designed to increase the number of oocytes available for fertilization in each cycle. Studies have shown

Table 46.2: Indications for IUI

Cervical factor	Immunologic	
	Inadequate cervical mucus	
	Viscous cervical mucus	
Male factor	Idiopathic oligozoospermia	
	Asthenozoospermia	
	Teratozoospermia	
	Ejaculatory dysfunction	Retrograde ejaculation
		Anejaculation
		Hypospadias
	Sexual dysfunction	Erectile dysfunction
		Other disabilities that prevent sexual intercourse
Unexplained Infertility		
Minimal endometriosis		

a positive correlation between the number of mature follicles and the pregnancy rate in IUI (10).

Unexplained Infertility

By definition, unexplained infertility does not allow a specific mechanism for the effectiveness of IUI and COH. It is thought that various factors may result in decreased fecundity in such couples. These factors may include subtle ovulatory disorders, cervical factors, and male factors not identified by the usual workup. All the factors identified above may be involved in improving the outcome of this group of couples when IUI is used.

WORKUP PRIOR TO IUI

The workup for couples prior to IUI does not differ much from that offered to any infertile couples to determine the cause of infertility. This includes semen analysis for the male along with treatment of any reversible condition. For the female, basic evaluation entails a baseline ultrasound, ovarian reserve FSH and estradiol monitoring of ovulatory function, hysterosalpingogram, and, if indicated, laparoscopy with chromotubation. This evaluation is not only essential in determining the type of infertility and whether IUI will be a suitable option for the couple but will also allow screening for subtle pathologies that might decrease the chances of IUI success, like endometrial polyps or ovarian cysts. In fact, studies showed that many of these patients especially those with uterine polyps may even get pregnant spontaneously once polyps are removed before they even start their IUI cycles (11). Other factors that could be treated prior to IUI to increase the chances of success include treatment minor tubal adhesions.

DETERMINANTS OF IUI OUTCOME

The overall success rates of IUI are variable. The mean pregnancy rate per IUI cycle in most of the international literature is around 9 percent. Pregnancy rates range from as low as 5 percent up to 70 percent. This wide range is probably because there are many variables, that is, heterogeneity of patient's population, different IUI and ovarian stimulation protocols, which all could affect the pregnancy rate when using IUI. Unfortunately, most of the published studies are retrospective, with few being prospective and randomized trails.

Knowledge of these variables is very important in order for physicians to have insight of the probable success rates, which helps to provide couples with more objective counseling.

Female Age

By far, age is the most important predictor factor of IUI success among other female factors. This is due to the negative impact of age on ovarian reserve, oocyte quality, and possibly on the endometrial receptivity. In a retrospective statistical analysis of the outcomes of 9,963 consecutive IUI cycles, Stone et al. showed that the pregnancy rates were 18.9, 13.9, 12.4, 11.4, 4.7, and 0.5 percent in the age groups of less than 26, 26–30, 31–35, 36–40, 41–45, and greater than 45, respectively. A significant decline in conception rates was noticed beyond the age of thirty two (12).

Increased male age was also shown to have a negative impact on IUI outcome, although not as evident as female age (13, 14).

Duration of Infertility

The duration of infertility especially in patients with unexplained infertility has been shown to negatively correlate with the conception rate after IUI. The increased duration of infertility reduce probability of conception after IUI (20 percent conception rate if the duration of infertility was less than six years versus 10 percent conception rate if the duration of infertility was more than six years) (15).

Many studies have supported such negative correlation (16). In a study by Iberico et al., it was shown that higher clinical pregnancy rates could be significantly demonstrated in patients with infertility duration less than three years (17).

Type of Infertility

The outcome of IUI cycles in terms of clinical pregnancy rates, cycle fecundity rates, and live birth rates depends on which class of infertility we are dealing with. In general, it seems that the best pregnancy rates after IUI were reported in patients with unexplained infertility and with anovulation (18). Among patients with male subfertility, ejaculatory dysfunction had the highest pregnancy rates.

Other factors that have been shown to negatively affect the pregnancy rates include endometriosis and history of pelvic infection, even if they do not cause obvious tubal damage.

A recent study showed that COH and IUI for patients with minimal to mild endometriosis shortly after laparoscopic excision is as effective as when COH and IUI are used in patients with unexplained subfertility. The clinical PR per cycle was shown to be comparable in both groups (21 and 18.9 percent, respectively) (19, 20).

Follicular Count

Another important factor is the number of the leading follicles in the IUI cycles. It is well documented that increased follicular count is strongly associated with higher pregnancy rates after IUI (e.g., 6.2, 12.9, and 30 percent with one, two, and three follicles) (17, 21, 22).

Also antral follicular count and E2 at the day of hCG administration in IUI cycles were positively correlated with higher CPRs (23).

Unfortunately, this increase in CPRs is also paralleled by another increase in multiple birth rates, as high as 39 percent (24). It was once recommended to cancel the cycle by withholding the hCG injection and advising the couple to abstain from intercourse if the number of the mature follicles was over six or if E2 levels were more than 1,000 pg/mL (25). This high follicular count is no longer accepted in current clinical practice due to the high incidence of high-order multiple pregnancy (HOMP) (triplets or more), (see chapter 28 by RP Dickey) currently, it is generally advised to cancel the cycle if there are more than three mature follicles. A more reliable method to avoid HOMP is to use previously tested prediction models, which are based on a number of variables as age, serum E2 levels, and follicular count (see chapter 28). These models were shown to decrease HOMP by 285 percent, although the price to pay is a reduction in the overall pregnancy rate by 8 percent (26) (see chapter 28).

Some practitioners may restore to aspiration of supernumerary follicles before IUI or even multifetal pregnancy reduction, but these should not be considered as a routine practice and perhaps it is wise to cancel the cycle if the risk of multifetal gestation is high (based on the follicular count and estradiol level). Others may advocate for rescue IVF and embryo transfer (IVF-ET) for those who overresponded to COH (more than three follicles measuring larger than 15 mm in diameter on the planned day of hCG administration). Some studies showed that the clinical pregnancy and live birth rates could be as high as 52 and 48 percent, respectively, in those cycles (27).

The Endometrium

The presence of trilaminar endometrium on the day of IUI in patients with COH provides a favorable prediction of pregnancy (see chapter 15). It seems that neither the endometrial thickness nor the Doppler surveys of the spiral uterine arteries have a good predictive value in COH + IUI.

Sperm Count and Morphology

Determining the semen parameters significantly affect the IUI outcome requires well-designed randomized controlled trials with all possible female factors eliminated (see chapter 18).

Another important variable to consider while interpreting the results of these studies is the lack of standardization of semen analysis criteria and semen-processing techniques.

Some semen parameters were found by some researchers to correlate directly with the clinical pregnancy rates and live birth rates after IUI. These include the total motile sperm (TMS) count per insemination, sperm motility, and sperm morphology (see chapter 18 by TF Kruger and SC Oehninger).

Although there is no threshold count below which pregnancy is impossible, it is extremely difficult to achieve pregnancy if the total motile sperm is $<2 \times (10)6/mL$ (28). Van der Westerlaken et al. showed significant decrease in CPR in couples where TMS was $<2 \times (10)6/mL$ as opposed to $\geq 2 \times (10)6/mL$ per insemination (4.6 vs. 9.2 percent) (29).

In a retrospective analysis of 1,115 cycles by Campana et al., the TMS was also shown to significantly decrease the pregnancy rates (2.1 vs. 6.7 percent), only this time the threshold of significance for TMS was $<1 \times (10)6/mL$ (30). Other studies showed dramatic increase in CPR with motile sperm count (TMS) of more than 10 million/mL when compared with less than 10 million/mL (12.3 vs. 2.8 percent) (21, 31).

Some centers even councel their patients for IVF if the TMS count is less than ten millions based on the fact that although pregnancy could be achieved by IUI, IVF with ICSI will be a more cost-effective alternative (32).

Still, it is very obvious that even though the effect of the TMS on pregnancy rate with IUI has been studied extensively, most of the studies and many meta-analysis failed to show a threshold of total sperm count that should result in discouraging couples from attempting IUI (33).

The degree of sperm motility and percent of fast motile sperm following preparation significantly correlate with positive IUI outcome. Studies showed that patients with original sperm motility more than 30 percent had a four time increase in the cumulative pregnancy rate than patient with motility less than 30 percent (34, 35).

Also, a study by Stone et al. showed that sperm motility less than 20 percent significantly decreases the CPR when compared to sperm motility of 20 percent or more (5.5 vs. 14 percent, respectively) (12).

Some studies even showed that the percentage of post-wash sperm motility could be more strongly correlated to successful IUI outcome when compared to post-wash TMS count (36).

Isolated teratozoospermia (<10 percent normal forms using strict criteria with normal motility and normal count) also affects the clinical birth rate after IUI cycles. In fresh semen, a normal morphology of more than 10 percent by WHO criteria was shown to result in an 18.2 percent pregnancy rate per cycle, while less than 10 percent normal forms showed only a 4.3 percent per cycle pregnancy rate (37). The effect of isolated teratospermia was shown to be as significant as those of TMS count and sperm motility (38). Other studies also showed marked decrease of the CPR when the percentage of normal forms was less than 15.5 percent (39, 40).

Other motion characteristic parameters that were evaluated by studies using computer-aided sperm analysis and were identified as good predictors of pregnancy after IUI include rapid motiliy 25.5 percent or more and VCL (average path velocity) 102.65 µm/second or more after sperm separation. Less importantly were the curvilinear velocity (VCL) and straight-line velocity (39).

DIFFERENT IUI PROTOCOLS

In treating couples with IUI, a number of possible treatment options should be discussed with the couple before starting the cycle. Although there is a large body of literature addressing the efficacy of these various options, the choice of a method for a particular couple remains that of balancing the diagnosis, chances of obtaining pregnancy, and the risk and cost associated with each choice. These include the choice of IUI versus other forms of artificial insemination, the use of natural cycles versus COH, timing of insemination, the number of IUI cycles to be carried, whether the couple will need single or double insemination, the type of catheter used, and the choice of sperm preparation technique.

IUI versus Timed Intercourse (TI)

Most of the recently published studies show that IUI is more effective than TI either in couples with unexplained infertility or with male subfertility. In a review of 3,662 completed cycles by Cohlen et al., IUI was shown to significantly increase the pregnancy rates when compared to TI in natural cycles regardless of the type of infertility [odds ratio (OR) 2.43]. Similarly, cycles where IUI and COH were employed yielded higher pregnancy rates than in TI + COH cycles (OR 2.2). When IUI + COH was compared to TI + natural cycle, the odds of pregnancy was 6.23 (41). In a recent review by Verhulst et al. of six RCTs, IUI was superior to TI, both in natural and stimulated cycles, and was showed to significantly increase the chance of pregnancy, with OR 1.68, (42).

A meta-analysis of 980 cycles by Zeyneloglu et al. also showed that the pregnancy rates after IUI were significantly higher than after TI (20.04 vs. 11.37 percent) in cycles superovulated with gonadotropins (43).

Intrauterine versus Other Forms of Artificial Insemination

The term artificial insemination includes a wide range of techniques including IUI, intracervical insemination (ICI), direct intraperitoneal insemination (DIPI), intrafallopian insemination (IFI), fallopian tube sperm perfusion (FSP), and intrafollicular insemination.

Regardless of the method used, the primary goal is it to deliver a concentrate of highly motile spermatozoa as near as possible to the oocyte (44).

Generally, most of the available studies to date did not show any major difference between these methods in term of CPR, fecundity rates, or LBR (45).

Direct Intraperitoneal Insemination

In DIPI, sperms are deposited intraperitoneally at both tubal fimbria under transvaginal sonographic guidance usually using a seventeen-gauge single-lumen IVF needle. However, most of the published literature did not show any significant differences between pregnancy rates for IUI and DIPI in the different categories of subfertility (46). DIPI could be useful in certain situations as in severe cervical stenosis (47).

Intracervical Insemination

ICI is a cheaper alternative used in some fertility centers for those couples who cannot afford IUI. The reason of being cheaper is that the procedure does not require in vitro sperm processing nor the presence of a medical staff. The semen is simply deposited in the cervical canal, either using a straw or by mean of a cervical cap (48).

Regardless of the various attempts to improve this technique, IUI results remain significantly better than those of ICI. Cycle fecundity rates ranged between 14 and 23 percent for IUI versus 3.9 and 5 percent for ICI (49–52).

The National Cooperative Reproductive Medicine Network published a study in 1999 (53), where 932 couples with unexplained infertility were randomized to one of four groups. 1) ICI alone, 2) IUI alone, 3) COH + ICI, or 4) COH + IUI. The results showed the pregnancy rates of:

- ICI, 10 percent
- IUI, 18 percent
- COH + ICI, 19 percent
- COH + IUI, 33 percent

Fallopian Tube Sperm Perfusion

FSP is based on pressure injection of higher volume of sperm suspension (4 mL as opposed to 0.2–0.5 mL as in regular IUI procedures), with the attempt of keeping the cervix sealed to prevent reflux. The procedure aims at increasing the sperm density in the tubes at the time of ovulation (54–56).

The reported results of FSP vary significantly probably because of the wide heterogeneity of patient studied, differences in techniques, and types of catheters used. It is worth noting here that the lowest FSP results were reported when Foley catheters were employed (57, 58).

Although some studies showed significantly higher pregnancy rates in FSP compared to IUI, more solid evidence needed before this technique is offered in standard clinical practice (57, 59).

Increasing the insemination volume to 10 mL will ensure peritoneal delivery of spermatozoa and should significantly increase the CPR. The procedure in this case is better referred to as intrauterine tuboperitoneal insemination (60).

Natural Cycles versus COH

IUI could be carried out in natural cycles or in combination with COH. The use of IUI in natural cycles has the advantage of lower cost and adds no risk from drug treatment. COH could be achieved by using clomiphene citrate (CC), letrozole and/or gonadotrophins, alone or with gonadotrophin-releasing hormone (GnRH-a, GnRH-ant). Studies showed that during IUI, the use of certain protocols of COH might yield better results than others, according to which type of infertility we are dealing with. In couples with unexplained infertility, IUI combined with COH either by CC, letrozole, or gonadotrophins results in significantly higher conception rates compared to IUI alone (61, 62).

In couples with male subfertility, randomized controlled trials showed that there are no significant differences between the conception rates when IUI alone was compared to IUI + COH using CC. Significant increase of conception rates was only achieved in this group of patients when gonadotrophins were used in COH instead of CC. Further analysis of the subgroups revealed that IUI + COH usually leads to higher conception rates in couples with TMS count $\geq 10 \times 10(6)$ when compared to those with a total $< 10 \times 10(6)$ (21, 63).

In couples with male subfertility, IUI even when used alone without COH, was shown to have more superior results than when COH was done using CC without IUI (64).

In conclusion, RCTs have clearly showed that IUI in cycles with COH generally improves the probability of conception compared with IUI in natural cycles (42, 65, 66).

The efficacy of different gonadotrophins versus CC and letrozole has been extensively investigated. While some studies show that rFSH was better than urinary FSH and HMG in terms of clinical pregnancy rates (25.9, 13.8, and 12.5 percent) (65), other studies showed that there were no significant differences in conception rates when CC + IUI was compared to rFSH + IUI in couples with unexplained infertility nor have there been any differences when letrozol + IUI was compared to CC + IUI or HMG + IUI (67–70).

In light of these controversies, CC seems to be the most cost-effective method of COH with IUI in patients with unexplained infertility, specially that it does not need extensive monitoring and is associated with lower risks of OHSS and multiple pregnancy when compared to gonadotrophins (71).

A recent study by Mitwally and Casper showed that letrozole is as effective as CC in terms of pregnancy rates with the advantage of lower incidence of multiple pregnancy, which might encourage the use of this drug as a first-line ovulation induction agent (72, 73).

Recently, there have been a number of studies that showed that low-dose gonadotrophins (50 IU) reduce the incidence of multiple birth rate without much influencing the clinical pregnancy rates (74).

There is no current evidence to support the use of GnRH agonists and antagonists during IUI cycles. A recent multicentric RCT study reported by Crosignani et al. did not show any significant increase in the pregnancy rates with the use of GnRH antagonists. GnRH antagonists are only useful in women who showed evidence of premature lutinization in previous cycles (75, 76).

GnRH antagonists could be used in IUI cycles with COH to prevent premature lutinization in certain situations, that is, if the patient shows follicles that are 17 mm or more in diameter, just before weekends where IUI is unavailable. In these situations, insemination could be safely delayed till next Monday without any changes in the IUI outcomes, if these women receive GnRH antagonist, for example, Cetrorelix during that weekend until the day of hCG administration (77).

Women using this protocol are expected to have higher E2 levels and increased endometrial thickness on the day of hCG administration due to prolonged ovarian stimulation, but there is no evidence suggesting any increase risk of OHSS (78).

It is very important when considering the use of ovarian stimulation during IUI cycles to counsel the patient with regard to the higher pregnancy rates that has to be balanced against the increased cost and complications as OHSS and the risk of multiple pregnancy (71).

In fact, the NICE guidelines advise against the use of COH during IUI cycles that are offered to couples with unexplained infertility and male subfertility (7).

Once COH is started, monitoring the follicular growth and the endometrial development is crucial during IUI cycles. This is usually achieved through serial pelvic ultrasound scanning and measurement of plasma estradiol (E2) to assess the follicular maturation. This is along with measurement of lutinizing hormone (LH) and progesterone to detect possible premature lutinization. This monitoring serves to decrease the risk of OHSS and multiple pregnancy that commonly occur in patients younger than thirty and especially those known to have PCOS (79).

Timing of Insemination

Timing of insemination is very important regardless of the method of insemination used to make sure that sperms will be present in the female genital tract just about the time of ovulation. There are several methods to time the insemination, perhaps the simplest of which is the basal body temperature measurement or assessment of the cyclical changes in the cervical mucus. Unfortunately, both methods are very insensitive and not reliable. The recently introduced urinary LH kits could also be used to detect the preovulatory LH surge. In a study by Vermesh et al., these dip-stick LH kits had a positive predictive value of 84 percent in predicting ovulation (80).

Ultrasound was shown to be the most precise method to confirm ovulation by scanning for ruptured follicles. During COH, ovulation could be induced by the administration of hCG (10,000 IU) or rLH and ovulation should be expected to occur thirty-four to thirty-six hours after the injection. Recently, there have been controversies about the benefits of hCG in triggering the ovulation versus spontaneous ovulation. A recent meta-analysis of seven studies with 2,623 patients by Kosmas et al. showed that hCG-induced ovulation had no benefit when compared with spontaneous ovulation for IUI timing (81).

Single versus Double Insemination

An important question that is frequently addressed is how many inseminations should be done in each IUI cycle?

Single insemination is usually done thirty-four to thirty-six hours after the LH surge or after the hCG injection. In double-insemination protocols, an additional insemination is done either at twelve hours or sixty hours from the LH surge. Obviously, the rationale behind this is to increase the sperm availability during the periovulatory window.

Although many studies showed no difference between single versus double insemination (82–84), other studies showed that double insemination may result in a significant increase in pregnancy rates specially in couples with low sperm count or male factor infertility (85).

If it is decided that couple should receive double insemination, it is best to perform them at twelve hours and thirty-four hours from the hCG administration (86).

To avoid the cost of a second insemination setting, some fertility specialists may advise the couples to have timed coitus on the day of hCG administration. Again, most of the studies showed that this technique does not increase the pregnancy rates except in couples with lower sperm count ($<40 \times 10(6)$) (87, 88).

Number of Cycles

IUI with or without COH should be offered for four to six cycles to the infertile couples who are eligible for IUI. Evidence from published literature show little benefit if any beyond the sixth cycle (89).

In a study by Khalil et al., the pregnancy rates were highest in the first treatment cycle and the cumulative birth rate rose only slightly after the fourth treatment cycle (18). In fact, most of the CPR (97 percent) reported in most studies were obtained in the first four treatment cycles (15).

Dickey et al. showed that after four cycles, CPRs were 46 percent for ovulatory dysfunction; 38 percent for cervical factor, male factor, and unexplained infertility; 34 percent for endometriosis; and 26 percent for tubal factor. After six cycles, CPRs were 65 percent for ovulation dysfunction, 35 percent for endometriosis, and unchanged for other diagnoses (90).

The NICE fertility guidelines advocate for up to six IUI cycles for patients with unexplained infertility, male subfertility, cervical factor, and minimal to mild endometriosis (7).

If no pregnancy is achieved by the end of the fourth to sixth cycle, patients should be offered IVF. Some centers may even offer this option after the third cycle if pregnancy does not occur. Aboulghar et al. showed that in women who were offered IVF after their third IUI cycles, the cycle fecundity increased to 36.6 percent per cycle compared to 5.6 percent, if they were offered another three IUI cycles (91).

Type of Catheter

Currently, there are different kinds of IUI catheters in the market that vary in price, frequency of sperm regurgitation, or the difficulty in introduction. They are generally classified into hard- and soft-tip catheters. None of the published literature showed any difference in pregnancy rates when IUI was done using a soft-tip catheters compared to hard-tip catheters (92–94).

Sperm Preparation Technique

All the currently employed methods of sperm preparation were originally developed to separate the motile, morphologically normal spermatozoa from other harmful components in the seminal fluid like leucocytes, bacteria, and dead spermatozoa, which produce oxygen radicals that negatively influence the fertilizing capacity of sperms. These techniques for sperm wash and preparation not only increased the pregnancy rate but also decreased other possible complications like infection and uterine cramps (44).

Currently, there is no consensus on sperm-processing methods for IUI patients. Some centers use the swim-up technique, which is the simplest and the cheapest, while others use the density gradient centrifugation (DGC).

Most of the published studies and systematic reviews show no difference in the IUI outcomes with the use of either technique (95–97), although a borderline benefit of DGC over swim-up technique was shown by a meta-analysis by Duran et al. (98).

Currently, there is no evidence that the time duration between the collection of semen and IUI have any significant influence on IUI outcomes as studies showed that the same results could be obtained when IUI was done any time between 30 and 150 minutes after the sample collection.

There had been recently a number of publications about the in vitro use of substances to stimulate the sperm function and protect them from the influence of reactive oxygen species such as xanthines, pentoxifylline and 2-deoxyadenosine, bicarbonate, metal chelators, prostaglandins, kinine-enhancing drugs, and platelet-activating factor (PAF) (99–103). Although many of these substances were shown to improve the sperm function in vitro, more clinical studies are needed to prove their clinical usefulness in IUI setting. In one study, the CPR was significantly increased in couples with unexplained infertility when sperms were treated with PAF (23.07 vs. 7.92 percent) (104). However, it seems that this significant improvement can only be shown to affect men presenting with normal semen parameters (105).

RISKS OF IUI

The risks of IUI are summarized in Table 46.3. In general, the risks of the actual IUI procedure are minimal. While the procedure is mildly uncomfortable, pain rarely results in patients abandoning the procedure. Pain is more intense in those who require more manipulation such as straightening of the cervix with a tenaculum or dilation of the cervix because of stenosis. In these patients, one should consider the use of a local anesthetic such as lidocaine jelly or a cervical block. Anaphylaxis is possible but extremely rare. A report of anaphylaxis may have been secondary to a reaction to penicillin added to the media (106). A vasovagal response can be frightening to the patient but resolves without treatment other than psychological support.

A practice with multiple couples simultaneously in treatment is at greatest risk. Labeling at each step of the procedure is important. All raw specimens and prepared specimens should contain the name of the donor, name of the recipient, and the time in which the specimen was obtained and processed. The donor must label the semen sample, and he must hand the specimen to the person who brings the specimen to the laboratory. Some men are embarrassed by the procedure and wish to leave the specimen in the collection room, but for safety this should not be allowed despite their discomfort.

A "time-out" in the same manner as in the operating room should precede an insemination. The matching of names with

Table 46.3: Risks of IUI

Risks of procedure	Infection
	Pain
	Anaphylaxis
	Vasovagal response
Clerical error in handling of specimens	
Risks of ovarian stimulation	Multiple births
	OHSS

the labeling prior to insemination is necessary. Couples with different last names complicate the problem. Communication with the couple and between the partners in the couple is important. Everyone is busy, including the patients. It is important that the patients know about the scheduling of the procedure for each partner so that the timing can be matched during the time-out. Checking by more than one person at each level of the procedure provides extra safety. These procedures should be documented in the record.

The risk of increasing the rate of birth of abnormal children is present in all advanced reproductive procedures. Theoretically, a deficit in semen may be indicative of a genetic problem in the sperm. By allowing fertilization that otherwise would not occur may increase the risk of abnormalities. The same argument can be made for the female if ovarian stimulation is required. Not to mention that there is growing evidence that exogenous gonadotophins is associated with increased rate of aneuploidies. Developmental toxicity of ovarian stimulation may occur even if the drugs are used only to increase the chances of conception in women who spontaneously ovulate. Fortunately, there is little evidence that this risk is substantial (107). However, given the 3–8 percent background of a birth defect, small differences would be difficult to detect. There may be an increase in preterm birth after COH + IUI treatment even in the absence of multiple pregnancies (108).

The risk of multiple births continues to be the major complication of all advanced reproductive procedures. IUI has inherent problems that even IVF does not have. In IVF, limiting the numbers of embryos can decrease the number of multiple births. The practitioner has even less control in IUI (109). Using soft stimulation protocols, canceling the cycle when there are three or more mature follicles or using prediction models are all means to decrease the incidence of multiple pregnancy.

OHSS can occur in any ovulation induction. It is particularly severe in PCOS patients and gets more severe in cases in which conception occurs (71). The usual diagnosis and treatment of the syndrome is the same as in other settings (110).

DISCORDANT COUPLES WITH VIRAL INFECTIONS

Hepatitis B virus (HBV), hepatitis C virus (HCV), and human immunodeficiency virus (HIV) have been transmitted in donor insemination programs. Because of these risks, strict testing of donors of semen has been implemented. Contamination with viruses has also occurred during use of reproductive technologies. However, there is evidence that use of IUI with washed sperm may decrease the risk of contamination.

Until recently, HIV infection resulted in an early death. Because of the poor prognosis of these patients and the risk of viral transmission, most infertility centers denied treatment to those infected, which was very disappointing especially that most of HIV-infected people are in their reproductive years. However, the existence of effective antivirals has placed HIV infection into the category of a chronic disease. With the likelihood of survival of more than twenty years after diagnosis, the attitude toward those infected with HIV is changing (111).

The ethics committees of both the American College of Obstetrics and Gynecology and the American Society for Reproductive Medicine have suggested that infection with HIV should not result in denying treatment for infertility. The Center for Disease Control and Prevention recommends against insemination with semen from HIV-infected men because safety has not been proven (112).

Male to female transmission of HIV occurs at the rate of between 0.1 and 0.5 percent in a stable couple. There is a low correlation between the circulating viral load and the viral load in semen (112). There is no unanimous agreement about whether sperm itself can act as a vector for HIV, but there is evidence that sperm does not appear to be responsible for the transmission of the virus. Flow cytometry studies showed that spermatozoa did not express significant levels of CD4, CCR5, or CXCR4, suggesting that they are unlikely to be major targets for HIV infection (113).

There are still concerns regarding the ability of an HIV surface glycoprotein (gp120) to bind to galactosyl-alkyl-acylglyerol (GAL AAG) that is present on the surface membrane of spermatozoa (114). Viral binding is mostly limited to other cellular elements of semen (CD4 leukocytes and macrophages) that are removed by sperm washing. Effective sperm washing by density gradient plus swim-up followed by nested polymerase chain reaction of HIV-1 RNA and proviral DNA can result in a sperm preparation that contains an undetectable viral load (115).

It is important to mention that approximately 10 percent of the performed sperm washes remain positive, and in this case another sample must be prepared (116).

In a recent review summarizing the published experience of IUI in 581 HIV-1 serodiscordant couples, the incidence of viral transmission was 0 percent (117).

In another review, 3,019 cycles in 1,111 serodiscordant couples also resulted in zero infections (114). While these data are encouraging, the CDC reported two cases of contamination at the beginning of the 1990s. Although worrisome, these two cases may not be method failures. In one case a method of sperm centrifugation followed by insemination of the cell pellet was used. The pellet contained both sperm and round cells, the latter of which are known to bind HIV. The second case involved a patient with a high viral load and a test of HIV presence in the final preparation was not used (111).

Safety continues to be a concern. While more than 3,000 cases have been reported with no infection, the estimated rate of contamination would require about 30,000 cases to have adequate statistical power to detect a difference.

Practitioners should consider offering IUI or ICSI to discordant couples with HIV to decrease the incidence of viral transmission. These options should be also offered to couples who are both infected with HIV but with different strains (118).

Couples should be advised that HIV infection may decrease the effectiveness of treatment in men (119) and women (120).

It is recommended that patients receive systematic screening before assisted reproductive technologies and that HIV detection in the post-preparation inseminant be utilized in those who are HIV positive. A separate "infected laboratory" should be established to prevent cross-contamination.

Many questions remain. We know much less about other relatively common viruses (HBV and HCV). Optimal sperm preparation and methods of post-preparation are the subject of research.

KEY POINTS FOR CLINICAL PRACTICE

■ IUI is an effective treatment for unexplained infertility, cervical factor, male factor infertility, and sexual dysfunction.

■ IUI is the most effective among other methods of artificial insemination.

■ All patients should receive a baseline ultrasound and hormonal assessment before IUI, especially if COH is to be used.

■ The highest pregnancy rate is obtained by the use of COH with gonadotropins in combination with IUI, but this has to be balanced against the increased cost and possible risk of OHSS and multiple pregnancy. Using this method, one-third or even up to one half of couples are expected to become pregnant.

■ Risks of IUI are minimal except for the risk of multiple births and OHSS. The risk of multiple births is substantial, especially if gonadotropins are utilized. It is advised to cancel the cycle if more than three mature follicles show upon monitoring.

■ There are many variables that affect IUI success, perhaps the most important of which is the female age.

■ Most pregnancies occur with this treatment within three to six cycles. The number of cycles offered must take into account the diagnosis, age of the patient, and the financial situation of the couple.

■ Timing of insemination is important – the highest pregnancy rate is associated with IUI at thirty-six to forty hours after ovulation.

■ "Natural" cycles have a lower follicular count and the difficulty of precise timing of insemination. If natural cycles are used, then daily measurement of LH surge in morning urine should be started a few days prior to predicted ovulation to improve the timing of the insemination and increase the pregnancy rate.

■ A single, well-timed insemination per cycle is effective. Little is gained from multiple inseminations per cycle except in males with low sperm count.

■ Neither the sperm preparation technique nor the type of catheter used for IUI affects the success rate.

■ Consideration should be given to offering IUI to serodiscordant couples with HIV infection and perhaps to those with other chronic viral diseases.

REFERENCES

1. Dickinson RL. Artificial impregnation: essays in tubal insemination. *Am J Obstet Gynecol*. 1921;1:252–61.
2. Gerli S, Gholami H, Manna C, Di Frega AS, Vitiello C, Unfer V. Use of ethinyl estradiol to reverse the antiestrogenic effects of clomiphene citrate in patients undergoing intrauterine

insemination: a comparative, randomized study. *Fertil Steril.* 2000;73(1):85–9.

3. Nallella KP, Sharma RK, Aziz N, Agarwal A. Significance of sperm characteristics in the evaluation of male infertility. *Fertil Steril.* 2006;85(3):629–34.

4. Zhao Y, Garcia J, Jarow JP, Wallach EE. Successful management of infertility due to retrograde ejaculation using assisted reproductive technologies: a report of two cases. *Arch Androl.* 2004;50(6):391–4.

5. Shieh JY, Chen SU, Wang YH, Chang HC, Ho HN, Yang YS. A protocol of electroejaculation and systematic assisted reproductive technology achieved high efficiency and efficacy for pregnancy for anejaculatory men with spinal cord injury. *Arch Phys Med Rehabil.* 2003;84(4):535–40.

6. Ohl DA, Wolf LJ, Menge AC, Christman GM, Hurd WW, Ansbacher R, Smith YR, Randolph JF Jr. Electroejaculation and assisted reproductive technologies in the treatment of anejaculatory infertility. *Fertil Steril.* 2001;76(6):1249–55.

7. National Institute of Clinical Excellence. Fertility: assessment and treatment of people with fertility problems, Clinical guidelines No11. London: Abba Litho Ltd. UK, 2004.

8. Zimmerman ER, Robertson KR, Kim H, Drobnis EZ, Nakajima ST. Semen preparation with the sperm select system versus a washing technique. *Fertil Steril.* 1994;61(2):269–75.

9. Goldberg JM, Mascha E, Falcone T, Attaran M. Comparison of intrauterine and intracervical insemination with frozen donor sperm: a meta-analysis. *Fertil Steril.* 1999;72(5):792–5.

10. Kaplan PF, Katz SL, Thompson AK, Freund RD. Cycle fecundity in controlled ovarian hyperstimulation and intrauterine insemination. Influence of the number of mature follicles at hCG administration. *J Reprod Med.* 2002;47(7):535–9.

11. Perez-Medina T, Bajo-Arenas J, Salazar F, Redondo T, Sanfrutos L, Alvarez P, Engels V. Endometrial polyps and their implication in the pregnancy rates of patients undergoing intrauterine insemination: a prospective, randomized study. *Hum Reprod.* 2005;20(6):1632–5.

12. Stone BA, Vargyas JM, Ringler GE, Stein AL, Marrs RP. Determinants of the outcome of intrauterine insemination: analysis of outcomes of 9963 consecutive cycles. *Am J Obstet Gynecol.* 1999;180(6 Pt. 1):1522–34.

13. Mathieu C, Ecochard R, Bied V, Lornage J, Czyba JC. Cumulative conception rate following intrauterine artificial insemination with husband's spermatozoa: influence of husband's age. *Hum Reprod.* 1995;10(5):1090–7.

14. Brzechffa PR, Buyalos RP. Female and male partner age and menotrophin requirements influence pregnancy rates with human menopausal gonadotrophin therapy in combination with intrauterine insemination. *Hum Reprod.* 1997;12(1):29–33.

15. Nuojua-Huttunen S, Tomas C, Bloigu R, Tuomivaara L, Martikainen H. Intrauterine insemination treatment in subfertility: an analysis of factors affecting outcome. *Hum Reprod.* 1999;14(3):698–703.

16. Steures P, van der Steeg JW, Mol BW, Eijkemans MJ, van der Veen F, Habbema JD, Hompes PG, Bossuyt PM, Verhoeve HR, van Kasteren YM, van Dop PA; CECERM (Collaborative Effort in Clinical Evaluation in Reproductive Medicine). Prediction of an ongoing pregnancy after intrauterine insemination. *Fertil Steril.* 2004;82(1):45–51.

17. Iberico G, Vioque J, Ariza N, Lozano JM, Roca M, Llacer J, Bernabeu R. Analysis of factors influencing pregnancy rates in homologous intrauterine insemination. *Fertil Steril.* 2004;81(5):1308–13.

18. Khalil MR, Rasmussen PE, Erb K, Laursen SB, Rex S, Westergaard LG. Intrauterine insemination with donor semen. An evaluation of prognostic factors based on a review of 1131 cycles. *Acta Obstet Gynecol Scand.* 2001;80(4):342–8.

19. Rizk B. Clinical guidelines for treatment of selected cases of endometriosis by ART or surgery. *American Society For Reproductive Medicine*, 60th Annual Meeting, Postgraduate Course, Endometriosis Treatment: Medical, Surgical and Assisted Reproductive Technology. ASRM Postgraduate course syllabus. October 16, 2004.

20. Werbrouck E, Spiessens C, Meuleman C, D'Hooghe T. No difference in cycle pregnancy rate and in cumulative live-birth rate between women with surgically treated minimal to mild endometriosis and women with unexplained infertility after controlled ovarian hyperstimulation and intrauterine insemination. *Fertil Steril.* 2006;86(3):566–71.

21. Sikandar R, Virk S, Lakhani S, Sahab H, Rizvi J. Intrauterine insemination with controlled ovarian hyperstimulation in the treatment of subfertility. *J Coll Physicians Surg Pak.* 2005;15(12):782–5.

22. Tomlinson MJ, Amissah-Arthur JB, Thompson KA, Kasraie JL, Bentick B. Prognostic indicators for intrauterine insemination (IUI): statistical model for IUI success. *Hum Reprod.* 1996;11(9):1892–6.

23. Chang MY, Chiang CH, Hsieh TT, Soong YK, Hsu KH. Use of the antral follicle count to predict the outcome of assisted reproductive technologies. *Fertil Steril.* 1998;69(3):505–10.

24. van Rumste MM, den Hartog JE, Dumoulin JC, Evers JL, Land JA. Is controlled ovarian stimulation in intrauterine insemination an acceptable therapy in couples with unexplained non-conception in the perspective of multiple pregnancies? *Hum Reprod.* 2006;21(3):701–4. Epub 2005 Oct 27.

25. Valbuena D, Simon C, Romero JL, Remohi J, Pellicer A. Factors responsible for multiple pregnancies after ovarian stimulation and intrauterine insemination with gonadotropins. *J Assist Reprod Genet.* 1996;13(8):663–8.

26. Tur R, Barri PN, Coroleu B, Buxaderas R, Parera N, Balasch J. Use of a prediction model for high-order multiple implantation after ovarian stimulation with gonadotropins. *Fertil Steril.* 2005;83(1):116–21.

27. Olufowobi O, Sharif K, Papaioannou S, Mohamed H, Neelakantan D, Afnan M. Role of rescue IVF-ET treatment in the management of high response in stimulated IUI cycles. *J Obstet Gynaecol.* 2005;25(2):166–8.

28. Dickey RP, Pyrzak R, Lu PY, Taylor SN, Rye PH. Comparison of the sperm quality necessary for successful intrauterine insemination with World Health Organization threshold values for normal sperm. *Fertil Steril.* 1999;71(4):684–9.

29. van der Westerlaken LA, Naaktgeboren N, Helmerhorst FM. Evaluation of pregnancy rates after intrauterine insemination according to indication, age, and sperm parameters. *J Assist Reprod Genet.* 1998;15(6):359–64.

30. Campana A, Sakkas D, Stalberg A, Bianchi PG, Comte I, Pache T, Walker D. Intrauterine insemination: evaluation of the results according to the woman's age, sperm quality, total sperm count per insemination and life table analysis. *Hum Reprod.* 1996;11(4):732–6.

31. Miller DC, Hollenbeck BK, Smith GD, Randolph JF, Christman GM, Smith YR, Lebovic DI, Ohl DA. Processed total motile sperm count correlates with pregnancy outcome after intrauterine insemination. *Urology.* 2002;60(3):497–501.

32. Van Voorhis BJ, Barnett M, Sparks AE, Syrop CH, Rosenthal G, Dawson J. Effect of the total motile sperm count on the efficacy and cost-effectiveness of intrauterine insemination and in vitro fertilization. *Fertil Steril.* 2001;75(4):661–8.

33. van Weert JM, Repping S, Van Voorhis BJ, van der Veen F, Bossuyt PM, Mol BW. Performance of the postwash total motile

sperm count as a predictor of pregnancy at the time of intrauterine insemination: a meta-analysis. *Fertil Steril.* 2004;82(3):612–20.

34. Yalti S, Gurbuz B, Sezer H, Celik S. Effects of semen characteristics on IUI combined with mild ovarian stimulation. *Arch Androl.* 2004;50(4):239–46.

35. Shulman A, Hauser R, Lipitz S, Frenkel Y, Dor J, Bider D, Mashiach S, Yogev L, Yavetz H. Sperm motility is a major determinant of pregnancy outcome following intrauterine insemination. *J Assist Reprod Genet.* 1998;15(6):381–5.

36. Pasqualotto EB, Daitch JA, Hendin BN, Falcone T, Thomas AJ Jr., Nelson DR, Agarwal A. Relationship of total motile sperm count and percentage motile sperm to successful pregnancy rates following intrauterine insemination. *J Assist Reprod Genet.* 1999; 16(9):476–82.

37. Burr RW, Siegberg R, Flaherty SP, Wang XJ, Matthews CD. The influence of sperm morphology and the number of motile sperm inseminated on the outcome of intrauterine insemination combined with mild ovarian stimulation. *Fertil Steril.* 1996;65(1): 127–32.

38. Spiessens C, Vanderschueren D, Meuleman C, D'Hooghe T. Isolated teratozoospermia and intrauterine insemination. *Fertil Steril.* 2003;80(5):1185–9.

39. Shibahara H, Obara H, Ayustawati Hirano Y, Suzuki T, Ohno A, Takamizawa S, Suzuki M. Prediction of pregnancy by intrauterine insemination using CASA estimates and strict criteria in patients with male factor infertility. *Int J Androl.* 2004;27(2):63–8.

40. Grigoriou O, Pantos K, Makrakis E, Hassiakos D, Konidaris S, Creatsas G. Impact of isolated teratozoospermia on the outcome of intrauterine insemination. *Fertil Steril.* 2005;83(3):773–5.

41. Cohlen BJ, Vandekerckhove P, te Velde ER, Habbema JD. Timed intercourse versus intra-uterine insemination with or without ovarian hyperstimulation for subfertility in men. *Cochrane Database Syst Rev.* 2000;(2):CD000360. Review.

42. Verhulst SM, Cohlen BJ, Hughes E, Te Velde E, Heineman MJ. Intra-uterine insemination for unexplained subfertility. *Cochrane Database Syst Rev.* 2006;(4):CD001838.

43. Zeyneloglu HB, Arici A, Olive DL, Duleba AJ. Comparison of intrauterine insemination with timed intercourse in superovulated cycles with gonadotropins: a meta-analysis. *Fertil Steril.* 1998;69(3):486–91.

44. Marcus SF. Intrauterine insemination. In (Brinsden PR Ed.), *Textbook of In Vitro Fertilization and Assisted Reproduction.* Chapter 13. Carnforth, UK: Parthenon Publishing, 2005; pp. 259–69.

45. Noci I, Dabizzi S, Evangelisti P, Cozzi C, Cameron Smith M, Criscuoli L, Fuzzi B, Branconi F. Evaluation of clinical efficacy of three different insemination techniques in couple infertility. A randomized study. *Minerva Ginecol.* 2007;59(1):11–18.

46. Tiemessen CH, Bots RS, Peeters MF, Evers JL. Direct intraperitoneal insemination compared to intrauterine insemination in superovulated cycles: a randomized cross-over study. *Gynecol Obstet Invest.* 1997;44(3):149–52.

47. Sills ES, Palermo GD. Intrauterine pregnancy following low-dose gonadotropin ovulation induction and direct intraperitoneal insemination for severe cervical stenosis. *BMC Pregnancy Childbirth.* 2002; Nov. 26;2(1):9.

48. Flierman PA, Hogerzeil HV, Hemrika DJ. A prospective, randomized, cross-over comparison of two methods of artificial insemination by donor on the incidence of conception: intracervical insemination by straw versus cervical cap. *Hum Reprod.* 1997;12(9):1945–8.

49. Carroll N, Palmer JR. A comparison of intrauterine versus intracervical insemination in fertile single women. *Fertil Steril.* 2001; 75(4):656–60.

50. Patton PE, Burry KA, Thurmond A, Novy MJ, Wolf DP. Intrauterine insemination outperforms intracervical insemination in a randomized, controlled study with frozen, donor semen. *Fertil Steril.* 1992;57(3):559–64.

51. Hurd WW, Randolph JF Jr., Ansbacher R, Menge AC, Ohl DA, Brown AN. Comparison of intracervical, intrauterine, and intratubal techniques for donor insemination. *Fertil Steril.* 1993; 59(2):339–42.

52. Rizk B, Lenton W, Vere M, Martin R, Latarche E. Superovulation and intrauterine insemination in couples with azoospermia after failed intracervical insemination. 7th World Congress on In vitro Fertilization and Assisted Procreation, Paris, June 1991. *Hum Reprod, Abstract book,* p. 171–2.

53. Guzick DS, Carson SA, Coutifaris C, Overstreet JW, Factor-Litvak P, Steinkampf MP, Hill JA, Mastroianni L, Buster JE, Nakajima ST, Vogel DL, Canfield RE. Efficacy of superovulation and intrauterine insemination in the treatment of infertility. National Cooperative Reproductive Medicine Network. *N Engl J Med.* 1999; Jan. 21;340(3):177–83.

54. Trout SW, Kemmann E. Fallopian sperm perfusion versus intrauterine insemination: a randomized controlled trial and meta-analysis of the literature. *Fertil Steril.* 1999;71(5):881–5.

55. Fanchin R, Olivennes F, Righini C, Hazout A, Schwab B, Frydman R. A new system for fallopian tube sperm perfusion leads to pregnancy rates twice as high as standard intrauterine insemination. *Fertil Steril.* 1995;64(3):505–10.

56. Kahn JA, Sunde A, Koskemies A, von During V, Sordal T, Christensen F, Molne K. Fallopian tube sperm perfusion (FSP) versus intra-uterine insemination (IUI) in the treatment of unexplained infertility: a prospective randomized study. *Hum Reprod.* 1993;8(6):890–4.

57. Ricci G, Nucera G, Pozzobon C, Boscolo R, Giolo E, Guaschino S. A simple method for fallopian tube sperm perfusion using a blocking device in the treatment of unexplained infertility. *Fertil Steril.* 2001;76(6):1242–8.

58. Cantineau AE, Cohlen BJ, Al-Inany H, Heineman MJ. Intrauterine insemination versus fallopian tube sperm perfusion for non tubal infertility. *Cochrane Database Syst Rev.* 2004;(3): CD001502. Review.

59. Nuojua-Huttunen S, Tuomivaara L, Juntunen K, Tomas C, Martikainen H. Comparison of fallopian tube sperm perfusion with intrauterine insemination in the treatment of infertility. *Fertil Steril.* 1997;67(5):939–42.

60. Mamas L. Comparison of fallopian tube sperm perfusion and intrauterine tuboperitoneal insemination: a prospective randomized study. *Fertil Steril.* 2006;85(3):735–40.

61. Nulsen JC, Walsh S, Dumez S, Metzger DA. A randomized and longitudinal study of human menopausal gonadotropin with intrauterine insemination in the treatment of infertility. *Obstet Gynecol.* 1993;82(5):780–6.

62. Chaffkin LM, Nulsen JC, Luciano AA, Metzger DA. A comparative analysis of the cycle fecundity rates associated with combined human menopausal gonadotropin (hMG) and intrauterine insemination (IUI) versus either hMG or IUI alone. *Fertil Steril.* 1991;55(2):252–7.

63. Cohlen BJ, te Velde ER, van Kooij RJ, Looman CW, Habbema JD. Controlled ovarian hyperstimulation and intrauterine insemination for treating male subfertility: a controlled study. *Hum Reprod.* 1998;13(6):1553–8.

64. Martinez AR, Bernardus RE, Voorhorst FJ, Vermeiden JP, Schoemaker J. Intrauterine insemination does and clomiphene citrate does not improve fecundity in couples with infertility due to male or idiopathic factors: a prospective, randomized, controlled study. *Fertil Steril.* 1990;53(5):847–53.

65. Arcaini L, Bianchi S, Baglioni A, Marchini M, Tozzi L, Fedele L. Superovulation and intrauterine insemination vs. superovulation alone in the treatment of unexplained infertility. A randomized study. *J Reprod Med.* 1996;41(8):614–18.

66. Mahani IM, Afnan M. The pregnancy rates with intrauterine insemination (IUI) in superovulated cycles employing different protocols (clomiphene citrate (CC), human menopausal gonadotropin (HMG) and HMG + CC) and in natural ovulatory cycle. *J Pak Med Assoc.* 2004;54(10):503–5.

67. Demirol A, Gurgan T. Comparison of different gonadotrophin preparations in intrauterine insemination cycles for the treatment of unexplained infertility: a prospective, randomized study. *Hum Reprod.* 2007;22(1):97–100. Epub 2006 Sep 5.

68. Dankert T, Kremer JA, Cohlen BJ, Hamilton CJ, Pasker-de Jong PC, Straatman H, van Dop PA. A randomized clinical trial of clomiphene citrate versus low dose recombinant FSH for ovarian hyperstimulation in intrauterine insemination cycles for unexplained and male subfertility. *Hum Reprod.* 2007;22(3):792–7. Epub 2006 Nov 16.

69. Baysoy A, Serdaroglu H, Jamal H, Karatekeli E, Ozornek H, Attar E. Letrozole versus human menopausal gonadotrophin in women undergoing intrauterine insemination. *Reprod Biomed Online.* 2006;13(2):208–12.

70. Jee BC, Ku SY, Suh CS, Kim KC, Lee WD, Kim SH. Use of letrozole versus clomiphene citrate combined with gonadotropins in intrauterine insemination cycles: a pilot study. *Fertil Steril.* 2006;85(6):1774–7. Epub 2006 May 4.

71. Rizk B. Epidemiology of ovarian hyperstimulation syndrome: iatrogenic and spontaneous. In Rizk B (Ed.), *Ovarian Hyperstimulation Syndrome.* Chapter 2. Cambridge, New York: Cambridge University Press, 2006; pp. 10–42.

72. Mitwally MF, Biljan MM, Casper RF. Pregnancy outcome after the use of an aromatase inhibitor for ovarian stimulation. *Am J Obstet Gynecol.* 2005;192(2):381–6.

73. Casper RF, Mitwally MF. Review: aromatase inhibitors for ovulation induction. *J Clin Endocrinol Metab.* 2006;91(3):760–71.

74. Dhaliwal LK, Sialy RK, Gopalan S, Majumdar S. Minimal stimulation protocol for use with intrauterine insemination in the treatment of infertility. *Int J Fertil Womens Med.* 2000;45(3):232–5.

75. Crosignani PG, Somigliana E; Intrauterine Insemination Study Group. Effect of GnRH antagonists in FSH mildly stimulated intrauterine insemination cycles: a multicentre randomized trial. *Hum Reprod.* 2007;22(2):500–5. Epub 2006 Oct 24.

76. Allegra A, Marino A, Coffaro F, Scaglione P, Sammartano F, Rizza G, Volpes A. GnRH antagonist-induced inhibition of the premature LH surge increases pregnancy rates in IUI-stimulated cycles. A prospective randomized trial. *Hum Reprod.* 2007;22(1):101–18. Epub 2006 Oct 10.

77. Checa MA, Prat M, Robles A, Carreras R. Use of gonadotropin-releasing hormone antagonists to overcome the drawbacks of intrauterine insemination on weekends. *Fertil Steril.* 2006;85(3):573–7.

78. Matorras R, Ramon O, Exposito A, Corcostegui B, Ocerin I, Gonzalez-Lopera S, Rodriguez-Escudero FJ. Gn-RH antagonists in intrauterine insemination: the weekend-free protocol. *J Assist Reprod Genet.* 2006;23(2):51–4. Epub 2006 Mar 22.

79. Rizk B. Prevention of ovarian hyperstimulation syndrome. In Rizk B (Ed.), *Ovarian Hyperstimulation Syndrome.* Cambridge: United Kingdom, Cambridge University Press, 2006: chapter 7; 130–199.

80. Vermesh M, Kletzky OA, Davajan V, Israel R. Monitoring techniques to predict and detect ovulation. *Fertil Steril.* 1987;47(2):259–64.

81. Kosmas IP, Tatsioni A, Fatemi HM, Kolibianakis EM, Tournaye H, Devroey P. Human chorionic gonadotropin administration vs. luteinizing monitoring for intrauterine insemination timing, after administration of clomiphene citrate: a meta-analysis. *Fertil Steril.* 2007;87(3):607–12. Epub 2006 Dec 14.

82. Alborzi S, Motazedian S, Parsanezhad ME, Jannati S. Comparison of the effectiveness of single intrauterine insemination (IUI) versus double IUI per cycle in infertile patients. *Fertil Steril.* 2003;80(3):595–9.

83. Cantineau AE, Heineman MJ, Cohlen BJ. Single versus double intrauterine insemination (IUI) in stimulated cycles for subfertile couples. *Cochrane Database Syst Rev.* 2003;(1):CD003854. Review.

84. Ng EH, Makkar G, Yeung WS, Ho PC. A randomized comparison of three insemination methods in an artificial insemination program using husbands' semen. *J Reprod Med.* 2003;48(7):542–6.

85. Liu W, Gong F, Luo K, Lu G. Comparing the pregnancy rates of one versus two intrauterine inseminations (IUIs) in male factor and idiopathic infertility. *J Assist Reprod Genet.* 2006;23(2):75–9. Epub 2006 Feb 23.

86. Ragni G, Maggioni P, Guermandi E, Testa A, Baroni E, Colombo M, Crosignani PG. Efficacy of double intrauterine insemination in controlled ovarian hyperstimulation cycles. *Fertil Steril.* 1999;72(4):619–22.

87. Casadei L, Zamaro V, Calcagni M, Ticconi C, Dorrucci M, Piccione E. Homologous intrauterine insemination in controlled ovarian hyperstimulation cycles: a comparison among three different regimens. *Eur J Obstet Gynecol Reprod Biol.* 2006;129(2):155–61. Epub 2006 May 9.

88. Huang FJ, Chang SY, Chang JC, Kung FT, Wu JF, Tsai MY. Timed intercourse after intrauterine insemination for treatment of infertility. *Eur J Obstet Gynecol Reprod Biol.* 1998;80(2):257–61.

89. Crosignani PG, Somigliana E, Colombo M et al. The current role of intrauterine insemination for the treatment of male factor and unexplained infertility. *Middle East Fertil Soc J.* 2005;10:29–42.

90. Dickey RP, Taylor SN, Lu PY, Sartor BM, Rye PH, Pyrzak R. Effect of diagnosis, age, sperm quality, and number of preovulatory follicles on the outcome of multiple cycles of clomiphene citrate-intrauterine insemination. *Fertil Steril.* 2002;78(5):1088–95.

91. Aboulghar M, Mansour R, Serour G, Abdrazek A, Amin Y, Rhodes C. Controlled ovarian hyperstimulation and intrauterine insemination for treatment of unexplained infertility should be limited to a maximum of three trials. *Fertil Steril.* 2001;75(1):88–91.

92. Vermeylen AM, D'Hooghe T, Debrock S, Meeuwis L, Meuleman C, Spiessens C. The type of catheter has no impact on the pregnancy rate after intrauterine insemination: a randomized study. *Hum Reprod.* 2006;21(9):2364–7. Epub 2006 May 16.

93. Fancsovits P, Toth L, Murber A, Szendei G, Papp Z, Urbancsek J. Catheter type does not affect the outcome of intrauterine insemination treatment: a prospective randomized study. *Fertil Steril.* 2005;83(3):699–704.

94. Miller PB, Acres ML, Proctor JG, Higdon HL 3rd, Boone WR. Flexible versus rigid intrauterine insemination catheters: a prospective, randomized, controlled study. *Fertil Steril.* 2005;83(5):1544–6.

95. Boomsma CM, Heineman MJ, Cohlen BJ, Farquhar C. Semen preparation techniques for intrauterine insemination. *Cochrane Database Syst Rev.* 2004;(3):CD004507. Review.

96. Carrell DT, Kuneck PH, Peterson CM, Hatasaka HH, Jones KP, Campbell BF. A randomized, prospective analysis of five sperm preparation techniques before intrauterine insemination of husband sperm. *Fertil Steril.* 1998;69(1):122–6.

97. Dodson WC, Moessner J, Miller J, Legro RS, Gnatuk CL. A randomized comparison of the methods of sperm preparation for intrauterine insemination. *Fertil Steril*. 1998;70(3):574–5.

98. Duran HE, Morshedi M, Kruger T, Oehninger S. Intrauterine insemination: a systematic review on determinants of success. *Hum Reprod Update*. 2002;8(4):373–84.

99. Henkel RR, Schill WB. Sperm preparation for ART. *Reprod Biol Endocrinol*. 2003;1:108. Review.

100. Fountain S, Rizk B, Palmer C, Wada I, Macnamee M, Blayney M, Brinsden P, Smith SK. A prospective randomized controlled trial of pentoxifylline in severe male factor infertility and previous failure of in vitro fertilization. The 49th Annual Meeting of the AFS, Montreal, Canada, October 1993. *Fertil Steril*, ProgramSupplement, 1993, S17–18.

101. Brown SE, Toner JP, Schnorr JA, Williams SC, Gibbons WE, de Ziegler D, Oehninger S. Vaginal misoprostol enhances intrauterine insemination. *Hum Reprod*. 2001;16:96–101.

102. Toner J, de Ziegler D, Brown S, Gibbons WE, Oehninger S, Schnorr JA, Williams SC. High rates of cramping with misoprotol administration for intrauterine insemination. *Hum Reprod*. 2001;16:1051.

103. Vandekerckhove P, Lilford R, Vail A, Hughes E. Kinin enhancing drugs for unexplained subfertility in men (Cochrane Review). In *The Cochrane Library*, Issue 1, 2002. Oxford: Update Software.

104. Grigoriou O, Makrakis E, Konidaris S, Hassiakos D, Papadias K, Baka S, Creatsas G. Effect of sperm treatment with exogenous platelet-activating factor on the outcome of intrauterine insemination. *Fertil Steril*. 2005;83(3):618–21.

105. Roudebush WE, Toledo AA, Kort HI, Mitchell-Leef D, Elsner CW, Massey JB. Platelet-activating factor significantly enhances intrauterine insemination pregnancy rates in non-male factor infertility. *Fertil Steril*. 2004;82(1):52–6. Erratum in: *Fertil Steril*. 2004;82(3):768.

106. Al-Ramahi M, Leader A, Leveille MC. An allergic reaction following intrauterine insemination. *Hum Reprod*. 1998;13(12):3368–70.

107. Nuojua-Huttunen S, Gissler M, Martikainen H, Tuomivaara L. Obstetric and perinatal outcome of pregnancies after intrauterine insemination. *Hum Reprod*. 1999;14(8):2110–15.

108. Wang JX, Norman RJ, Kristiansson P. The effect of various infertility treatments on the risk of preterm birth. *Hum Reprod*. 2002;17(4):945–9.

109. Dickey RP, Taylor SN, Lu PY, Sartor BM, Rye PH, Pyrzak R. Relationship of follicle numbers and estradiol levels to multiple implantation in 3,608 intrauterine insemination cycles. *Fertil Steril*. 2001;75(1):69–78.

110. Rizk B, Dickey RP. In: Dickey RP, Brinsden PR, Pryzak R (Eds.), Intrauterine insemination. Cambridge: United Kingdom, Cambridge University Press, 2009, in press.

111. Rizk B, Dill SR. Counseling HIV patients pursuing infertility investigation and treatment. *Hum Reprod* 1997;12(3):415–16.

112. Englert Y, Lesage B, Van Vooren JP, Liesnard C, Place I, Vannin AS, Emiliani S, Delbaere A. Medically assisted reproduction in the presence of chronic viral diseases. *Hum Reprod Update*. 2004;10(2):149–62. Review.

113. Kim LU, Johnson MR, Barton S, Nelson MR, Sontag G, Smith JR, Gotch FM, Gilmour JW. Evaluation of sperm washing as a potential method of reducing HIV transmission in HIV-discordant couples wishing to have children. *AIDS*. 1999;13(6):645–51.

114. Sauer MV. Sperm washing techniques address the fertility needs of HIV-seropositive men: a clinical review. *Reprod Biomed Online*. 2005;10(1):135–40. Review.

115. Kato S, Hanabusa H, Kaneko S, Takakuwa K, Suzuki M, Kuji N, Jinno M, Tanaka R, Kojima K, Iwashita M, Yoshimura Y, Tanaka K. Complete removal of HIV-1 RNA and proviral DNA from semen by the swim-up method: assisted reproduction technique using spermatozoa free from HIV-1. *AIDS*. 2006;20(7):967–73.

116. Garrido N, Meseguer M, Remohí J, Simón C, Pellicer A. Semen characteristics in human immunodeficiency virus (HIV)- and hepatitis C (HCV)-seropositive males: predictors of the success of viral removal after sperm washing. *Hum Reprod*. 2005;20(4):1028–34.

117. Savasi V, Ferrazzi E, Lanzani C, Oneta M, Parrilla B, Persico T. Safety of sperm washing and ART outcome in 741 HIV-1-serodiscordant couples. *Hum Reprod*. 2007;22(3):772–7.

118. Semprini AE, Fiore S. HIV and reproduction. *Curr Opin Obstet Gynecol*. 2004;16(3):257–62.

119. Nicopoullos JD, Almeida PA, Ramsay JW, Gilling-Smith C. The effect of human immunodeficiency virus on sperm parameters and the outcome of intrauterine insemination following sperm washing. *Hum Reprod*. 2004;19(10):2289–97. Epub 2004 Jul 8.

120. Ohl J, Partisani M, Wittemer C, Schmitt MP, Cranz C, Stoll-Keller F, Rongieres C, Bettahar-Lebugle K, Lang JM, Nisand I. Assisted reproduction techniques for HIV serodiscordant couples: 18 months of experience. *Hum Reprod*. 2003;18(6):1244–9.

47

The Prediction and Management of Poor Responders in ART

Hassan N. Sallam, Botros R. M. B. Rizk, Juan A. Garcia-Velasco

INTRODUCTION

Although the first successful in vitro fertilization (IVF) reported in 1978 resulted from a natural (unstimulated) cycle, it became subsequently clear that ovarian stimulation resulted in a higher number of oocytes retrieved and higher pregnancy rates (1). In the following years, various stimulation protocols were suggested and used in patients treated with IVF and intracytoplasmic sperm injection (ICSI). Today, controlled ovarian stimulation prior to IVF or ICS is the universally accepted practice. However, in some instances, the female partner's response to ovarian stimulation is less than optimal, resulting in the retrieval of a small number of oocytes. These patients have been termed poor responders.

Poor responders have a higher incidence of cycle cancellation, lower fertilization, and lower pregnancy and implantation rates. In a study by Saldeen et al, poor responders, defined as those from whom less than five oocytes were retrieved, and who were above thirty-seven years of age, had a significantly lower pregnancy rate per ovum pick-up (OPU) compared to normal responders in the same age-group (3.0 versus 22.1 percent, $p < 0.05$). In addition, 43.6 percent of these women did not receive an embryo transfer (ET), compared to 13.2 percent of normal responders in the same age-group ($p < 0.05$). Poor responders who were thirty-seven years of age or younger had a significantly lower pregnancy rate per OPU compared to normal responders of the same age-group (14.0 versus 34.5 percent, $p < 0.05$) together with a higher cancellation rate (40.1 versus 10.5 percent) (2).

DEFINITION

There is no universally accepted definition of "poor responders." In a review by Surrey and Schoolcraft, the authors reported that at least twenty-seven definitions have been used to define poor responders and that no more than four sets of investigators have used any single definition (3). These definitions were based on the number of mature (i.e., 18 mm) follicles observed on ultrasonography (4–12), the measurement of early–follicular phase FSH level (13–17), the calculation of the FSH/LH ratio (18), the measurement of basal plasma E2 level (6, 9, 16, 19–21), the calculation of the mean daily HMG dose necessary to achieve a preset response (5, 13, 22, 23), the total dose of HMG used (14, 24), the number of days of HMG administration (5, 14, 15), or the number of

oocytes retrieved (9, 25, 26). Moreover, for each of these criteria used to define poor responders, different cutoff levels have been used. For example, Surrey et al, Chong et al, and Rombauts et al defined poor responders as those patients from whom lesser than or equal to three, lesser than or equal to four, or lesser than six oocytes were retrieved, respectively (9, 25, 26).

The absence of a standard definition for poor responders makes the interpretation and comparison of various tests used for the prediction and management of the condition very difficult. In an attempt to establish an objective definition for poor responders, we have reasoned that if the aim of performing IVF or ICSI is to achieve a clinical pregnancy, the definition of poor responders should be based on the least number of oocytes retrieved below which the clinical pregnancy rate is significantly diminished compared to those patients from whom a higher number of oocytes is retrieved. In a study published in 2005, we analyzed the data from all 782 consecutive patients attending our unit. They included 584 patients treated with ICSI, 112 patients treated with IVF, and 78 patients treated with freshly obtained testicular sperm extraction followed by ICSI (TESE/ICSI). Cycles with ICSI using frozen ejaculated or testicular sperm and cycles with frozen ET were excluded from the analysis. As expected, there was an excellent correlation between the number of oocytes retrieved and the clinical pregnancy rate ($r = 0.90$) (Figure 47.1). In order to determine the optimal number of oocytes below which the clinical pregnancy rate would be significantly diminished, receiver-operator characteristic (ROC) curves were constructed. When the patients were taken collectively, the cutoff point was eight oocytes (Figure 47.2). However, subgroup analysis showed that the cutoff point was five for patients treated with ICSI, six for those treated with IVF, and eight for those treated with TESE/ICSI. These findings reflect the higher fertilization rate usually achieved in ICSI compared to IVF when failure of fertilization may surprisingly occur in some patients with apparently "normal semen parameters." The sensitivities and specificities at these cutoff points were 78.5 percent and 43.4, 86.7, and 41.5 percent, and 77.8 and 66.7 percent, respectively (Figures 47.3–47.5). In our unit, we therefore define poor responders as those patients undergoing treatment with ICSI, IVF, or TESE/ICSI from whom less than five, six, or eight oocytes are retrieved, respectively (27).

The definition of poor responders depends therefore on the success rate of the specific unit and on the technique used. Why should we aim at obtaining eight oocytes from a patient

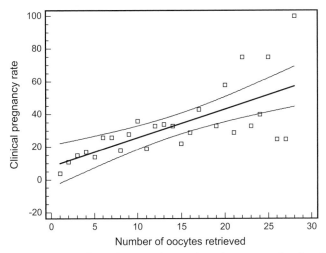

Figure 47.1. Correlation between the number of oocytes retrieved and the clinical pregnancy rate in all patients studied ($n = 782$, $r = 0.90$) (from Sallam et al, 2005).

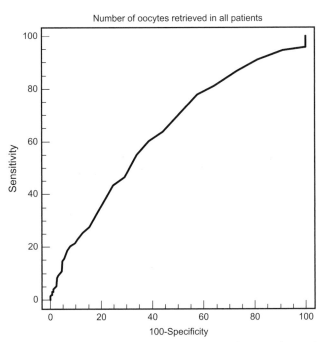

Figure 47.2. ROC curve showing the relationship between the sensitivity and specificity in all the patients undergoing treatment with assisted reproduction ($n = 782$, cutoff point = 8 oocytes, sensitivity = 60.2 percent, specificity = 61.3 percent) (from Sallam et al, 2005).

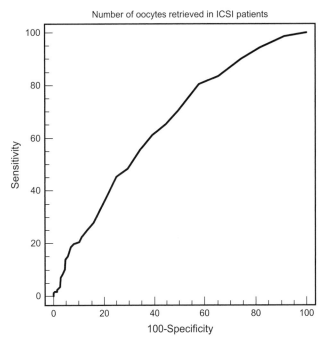

Figure 47.3. ROC curve showing the relationship between the sensitivity and specificity in the group of patients undergoing treatment with ICSI ($n = 584$, cutoff point = 5 oocytes, sensitivity = 78.5 percent, specificity = 43.4 percent) (from Sallam et al, 2005).

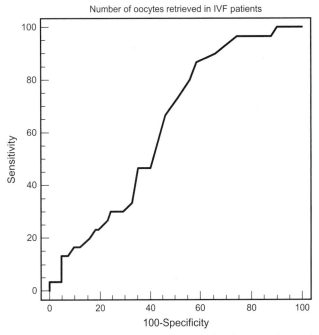

Figure 47.4. ROC curve showing the relationship between the sensitivity and specificity in the group of patients undergoing treatment with IVF ($n = 112$, cutoff point = 6 oocytes, sensitivity = 86.7 percent, specificity = 41.5 percent) (from Sallam et al, 2005).

undergoing ICSI when the success rate will be the same if we obtain five oocytes? Nevertheless, there is a need for a standard universal definition in order to allow proper comparison of various methods of prediction and management protocols for these unfortunate patients by performing a similar analysis using the average international success rates.

INCIDENCE

The exact incidence of poor responders is not exactly known but is thought to represent 10 percent of the ART population

(28). This is partly due to the lack of a universal definition. Data from the ASRM/SART register show that 14.1 percent of initiated cycles are canceled, and it is assumed that at least 50 percent of those were poor responders (29).

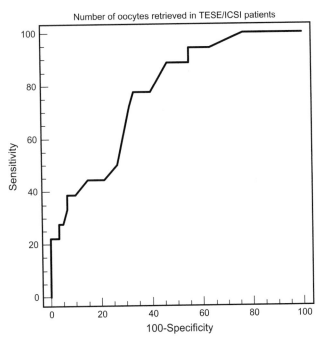

Figure 47.5. ROC curve showing the relationship between the sensitivity and specificity in the group of patients undergoing treatment with TESE/ICSI (*n* = 78, cutoff point = 8 oocytes, sensitivity = 77.8 percent, specificity = 66.7 percent) (from Sallam et al 2005).

ETIOLOGY

The etiology of poor response to ovarian stimulation is not exactly known, but ovarian response is a function of age. Many studies have confirmed that the pregnancy rates in IVF diminish with increasing age (30–34). In a study by Galey-Fontaine et al, the cutoff age above which the pregnancy rate started to diminish significantly was found to be thirty-six years (35). In younger patients, the cause of poor response remains a mystery but may represent a step toward early menopause and ovarian aging with fewer antral follicles remaining in the ovarian pool (36–38).

In order to understand the mechanism underlying this condition, various substances were analyzed in the follicular fluid of poor and normal responders. Owen et al measured IGF-I and IGF-II concentrations in the follicular fluid and suggested that poor responders may have an abnormality of growth factor response (39). Similar results were reported by Bahceci et al (40). On the contrary, Hamori et al, found no significant differences in IGF or IGFBP in the follicular fluid between normal and poor responders (41). Nishimura et al found that gonadotropins lead to an increase in ovarian macrophage colony-stimulating factor (MCSF) production and that this production in response to HMG administration was lost in poor ovarian responders (42), while Battaglia et al found elevated follicular fluid levels of vascular endothelial growth factor (VEGF) concentrations in those patients (43). Similarly, Luisi et al found lower follicular fluid levels of inhibin B (*p* < 0.001) but not of activin A in poor compared to normal responders (44). In Contrast, there was no significant difference in follicular fluid concentrations of soluble Fas and soluble Fas ligand between poor and normal responders (45). Lower expression of FSH receptors was also associated with poor ovarian response to gonadotropin stimulation (46), while Luborsky et al suggested that ovar-

ian antibodies may play a role in this process (47). Whether these changes are the cause or the result of poor response remains to be seen, and these findings represent small attempts at solving the big puzzle.

PREDICTION OF POOR RESPONDERS

Although age is a strong predictor of ovarian response (48, 49), numerous tests have been suggested for the prediction of poor response in patients undergoing assisted reproductive therapy (IVF or ICSI). These include static as well as dynamic tests. Static tests depend on the measurement of the concentrations of specific markers in blood or serum during the early follicular phase of the menstrual cycle (usually day 3) or the use of ultrasound imaging, while dynamic tests assess the response of the ovary to a defined dose of an ovarian stimulation agent.

Static Tests

Static tests for the prediction of poor responders include day 3 measurement of the concentration of serum FSH (31, 50), serum inhibin B (51, 52), serum estradiol (E2) (53, 54), and serum anti-Müllerian hormone (AMH) (55) as well as the determination of the antral follicle count (AFC) (56), the ovarian volume (OVVOL) (5, 57, 58), and the ovarian blood flow (59).

As serum FSH concentration starts rising with approaching menopause, the measurement of basal FSH concentration in the early follicular phase was used as a test to predict ovarian response in assisted reproduction, with higher levels of FSH indicating a poorer response (31, 60). The test is performed on day 3 during a cycle preceding the actual treatment cycle. An arbitrary cutoff level has been variously taken as greater than 10, greater than 12, or greater than 15 mIU/mL by various authors. Many studies have shown that basal FSH levels are significantly higher in poor responders compared to normal responders (50, 61–65), and Toner et al found it a better predictor of ovarian response compared to age (31). However, the test has been shown to be of limited value as some women exhibit a good ovarian response despite elevated basal FSH levels and vice versa. Indeed, in patients with elevated FSH levels and older than forty years, Bassil et al reported a pregnancy rate of 16 percent per egg retrieval when three or more developing follicles were observed by ultrasound (61). Similarly, in patients older than forty years with high basal FSH levels (>15 IU/L), van Rooij et al reported higher ongoing pregnancy rates despite more cycle cancellations compared to those with normal basal FSH levels (66). Repeated testing of basal FSH levels was also performed in order to improve the predictive value of the test, but this proved to be of no value (67). In an attempt to further evaluate the test, a meta-analysis was performed by Bancsi et al ROC curves were constructed and showed that the test had a moderate predictive performance. The authors concluded that basal FSH cannot be regarded as a useful routine test for the prediction of ovarian response or IVF outcome (68). A high FSH:LH ratio has also been described as a predictor of poor response despite the presence of normal basal FSH levels (62, 69), and Mukherjee et al suggested that the rise in FSH:LH ratio predates the elevation of FSH levels (69). However, these findings have not been further evaluated.

The measurement of basal (day 3) serum concentration of inhibin B was also used as a method for the prediction of ovarian response. Inhibin B is a glycoprotein member of the transforming growth factor beta (TGF-β) superfamily. It is secreted by the granulosa cells surrounding the oocyte and inhibits the production of FSH by the anterior pituitary gland. Various studies found that low levels of inhibin B were associated with poor response (44, 48, 49, 51, 52, 63, 64, 70–72). Luisi et al found that serum inhibin B levels correlated very well with developing follicles measuring 10 mm or more (p = 0.000) (44), and Muttukrishna et al found that the mean inhibin B levels were significantly lower (p < 0.001) in poor responders (70 ± 12.79 pg/mL) compared to normal responders (126.9 ± 8.8 pg/mL) (63). However, the test was also shown to be of limited value as some women exhibit a good ovarian response despite low basal levels of inhibin B and vice versa (48, 73).

Basal (day 3) levels of E2 were also used as predictors of ovarian response. Liccardi et al found that in patients undergoing IVF without GnRH analog, oocyte numbers and pregnancy rates decrease with increasing levels of day 3 E2. No pregnancies occurred when the E2 level was more than 75 pg/mL. Combining day 3 FSH and E2 improved the prognostic ability of either of these hormones used alone (53). Similar results were reported by Smotrich et al, Evers et al, and Costello et al (54, 74, 75), but other studies could not confirm these results. Vázquez et al found that elevated basal estradiol levels have no negative prognosis in young women undergoing ART cycles, and Phophong et al found that basal 17beta-estradiol levels do not correlate with the ovarian response or the treatment outcome (76, 77).

Basal levels of AMH have also been used to predict poor response in IVF and ICSI. AMH is a glycoprotein hormone that belongs to the TGF-β superfamily. It is synthesized by the Sertoli cell of the testis but also by the granulosa cells surrounding the oocyte. The basal levels of AMH were also found to be statistically lower in poor responders compared to normal responders (55, 63, 78–80). In the study by Muttukrishna et al, the mean AMH levels were significantly lower (p < 0.01) in the poor responders (0.175 ± 0.04 ng/mL) compared to the controls (1.13 ± 0.2 ng/mL) (63). More recently, Elgindy et al reported a good discriminatory potential for basal AMH levels with an area under the ROC curve of 90 percent (80). However, in a systematic review, Broekmans et al found the test to be of limited predictive value (81). More studies are necessary to further evaluate this test.

AFC during the early follicular phase of the cycle is also used for the prediction of ovarian response to stimulation. The technique was first described by Tomas et al (82), who calculated the number of antral follicles measuring 2–5 mm in both ovaries, using transvaginal ultrasound after ovarian suppression with GnRH agonist and before starting FSH stimulation. They found that the number of small follicles (2–5 mm) predicted the number of oocytes collected (82). Patients with less than five follicles in both ovaries were found to have a poor response to ovarian stimulation, and this was a better predictor to ovarian response compared to age and ovarian volume. This paper was followed by numerous publications, confirming the predictive value of the AFC (48, 55, 56, 58, 64, 80, 83–87). Although most of these studies have found the predictive value of AFC to be better than other parameters, a recent systematic review concluded that the test has only a moderate predictive value (81). In order to improve the predictive value of the test, Bancsi et al suggested repeating it and Durmusoglu et al

suggested combining it with day 7 follicle count (88, 89). More studies are needed to confirm the enthusiasm currently expressed with this test.

Ultrasound measurement of OVVOL is also used for the prediction of poor responders (48, 57, 58, 64, 73, 81, 82, 84). The measurements are made in the early follicular phase (day 3 or 4), preferably with transvaginal sonography (57). The ovarian volume is calculated from the formula $OVVOL = (4/3 \pi D_1 \times D_2 \times D_3)/8$ (D_1, D_2, and D_3 being the three diameters of the ovary measured in two perpendicular planes). Alternatively, 3D or 4D ultrasound can be used where the OVVOL is computed by the ultrasound machine (56). Tomas et al reported a good correlation between OVVOL and the AFC, and some studies have found it to have a good predictive value (64, 82). In contrast, other studies found it less predictable. For example, Bancsi et al and Kwee et al found it less predictable than the AFC (48, 84, 90), while Eldar-Giva et al and Elgindy et al found it less predictable than basal AMH (80, 84). A recent meta-analysis concluded that the predictive performance of ovarian volume toward poor response was inferior compared with that of AFC (91).

Dynamic Tests

In order to improve the predictive value of the static tests, dynamic tests have been suggested and used. These tests assess the response of the ovary to a defined dose of an ovarian stimulation agent. They include the clomiphene citrate (CC) challenge test (92), the FSH stimulation test (93, 94), as well as the gonadotrophin agonist stimulation test (95, 96).

The clomiphene citrate challenge test (CCCT) was first described by Navot et al (92). A daily dose of 100 mg of CC is administered on days 5–9 of the menstrual cycle. Serum FSH is measured before (days 2–3 of the menstrual cycle) and after (days 9–11) administration of CC. The increment in FSH is then calculated. Various studies have reported that the test has a good predictive value, and Erdem et al found it the only independent significant factor in predicting ovarian response compared to four other parameters (AFC, OVVOL, basal FSH, and basal and induced inhibin-B) (64, 97, 98). Kwee et al found the test to have a good predictive value and that 18 IU/L was the best cutoff point (99). On the contrary, Vladimirof et al found it less predictable than AFC (85), and Hendricks et al suggested repeating the test to improve its predictive value (100). In a variant of the test, Scott et al measured serum E2 levels before and after administration of CC but found that this could not predict ovarian responsiveness (98). Similarly, Hofmann et al measured inhibin B before and after the test and found that women with diminished ovarian reserve had reduced granulosa cell inhibin B production in response to the CCCT. They suggested that the lower inhibin B concentrations in these patients may be responsible for the elevated FSH concentrations and may be indicative of the aging follicular apparatus (71). A recent meta-analysis failed to reach a definite conclusion because of heterogeneity of the studies analyzed (101).

The FSH stimulation test is also used to predict the ovarian response in assisted reproduction. In this test, a dose of 150 IU of urinary or recombinant FSH is administered daily from day 3 to day 6 of the menstrual cycle preceeding the IVF cycle. Serum E2 is measured before and after FSH administration, and the increment in E2 calculated. Fanchin et al described a variant of the test and termed it EFORT (exogenous FSH ovarian reserve test) (102). In EFORT, 300 IU of FSH is administered IM on day 3 of the cycle. Plasma E2 is measured in two blood samples withdrawn just before and twenty-four hours after FSH administration. The plasma E2 increment is then calculated. The cutoff point was set at 30 pg/mL, with lower levels indicating poor response (102). In their study, Fanchin et al found the test to be predictive of ovarian response and that its combination with basal FSH measurement increased the predictive value significantly (102). Various studies have also confirmed that the E2 increments were significantly lower in poor responders (84, 94, 103), and Fábregues et al found that the test had a better predictive power compared to age and basal hormone values of FSH or inhibin (94). In addition, Kwee et al found the test to have minimal intercycle variability compared to basal FSH and the CCCT (104). In a variant of the test, Dzik et al measured the inhibin B increment in response to FSH stimulation and found the increment in inhibin B to be predictive of ovarian response (105). However, Fábregues et al questioned the clinical value of the test considering the discomfort and cost it entails (94).

The GnRH stimulation test was also used to predict ovarian response in patients treated with IVF or ICSI (95, 106). A flare-up dose of GnRH agonist is administered on day 2 or 3 of an unstimulated menstrual cycle. Basal and poststimulation E2 levels are measured and the increment in E2 calculated. Following an early enthusiasm with the test, it was later abandoned due to its low sensitivity. In an attempt to improve this sensitivity, Hendricks et al suggested repeating the test but found no advantage in this practice (107).

Comparison of Indices

Various studies have been conducted to compare the predictive value of these tests, with little agreement between the studies. For example, Bancsi et al compared the predictive value of various static indices by performing ROC curves and found the AFC to be the best predictor compared to the total OVVOL and the basal levels of FSH, E2, and inhibin B. The area under the ROC curve was 0.87. Addition of the basal FSH and inhibin B to a logistic model improved the predictive value significantly, with an area under the ROC curve of 0.92. The addition of basal E2 and total OVVOL did not improve the predictive value of the test (48).

However, Erdem et al found the CCCT and OVVOL to be better predictors of ovarian response compared to basal (day 3) FSH, estradiol (E2), inhibin B, and the AFC (64). In a different study, Vladimirov et al conducted a logistic regression analysis and found that the CCCT (cutoff point >12.5 mIU/mL) was a better single predictor of poor ovarian response than AFC and inhibin B. The areas under the ROC curves were 0.90, 0.85, and 0.79, respectively. However, they concluded that the addition of the CCCT to the much simpler AFC does not improve the predictive value of AFC alone (85). On the contrary, Hendricks et al found that the predictive value of the CCCT was not better than that of basal FSH in combination with an AFC (108). In a different study, the same authors compared the predictive value of the GAST test to the day 3 AFC and inhibin B tests and found it to be less predictive than each of them (107). In a third study, the same group compared the predictive value of AFC to day 3 basal FSH levels and found it significantly better. They suggested that AFC should be considered the test

of first choice in the assessment of ovarian reserve prior to IVF (108).

Muttukrishna et al compared the predictive value of AFC, AMH, and inhibin B and found that basal AMH was the single best predictor of poor response (109). More recently, McIlveen et al, using multivariate logistic regression, found that day 3 inhibin B levels were the best predictor of cycle cancellation with an area under the ROC (ROC AUC) of 0.78. When only baseline variables were considered, the mean ovarian volume was the best predictor of cycle cancellation (ROC AUC = 0.78), while AMH concentrations were the best predictor of a poor response (110).

In another study, Kwee et al compared the AFC, the basal ovarian volume, the EFORT, and the CCCT, with respect to their ability to predict poor and hyper-responders. They found that AFC performs well as a test for ovarian response, being superior or at least similar to complex, expensive, and time-consuming endocrine tests (90). In a different study, the same group compared the CCCT to the EFORT test and found that the CCCT was better in predicting poor, while the EFORT test was better in predicting hyperstimulation (99). On the contrary, Fanchin et al found that day 3 serum AMH was more strongly related to ovarian follicular status than serum inhibin B, E2, FSH, and LH (78).

In a recent systematic review, Broekmans et al provided an integrated ROC analysis and curve of each test in all individual evaluated published papers and concluded that the ORTs known to date have only modest-to-poor predictive properties and are therefore far from suitable for relevant clinical use (81). They suggested that entering the first cycle of IVF without any prior testing seems to be the preferable strategy (81).

Combination of Indices

Combining various indices has been suggested as a method to improve their predictive values. For example, in their study, Bancsi et al found that the addition of the basal FSH and inhibin B to a logistic model improved the predictive value significantly, with an area under the ROC curve of 0.92. However, the addition of basal E2 and total ovarian volume did not improve the predictive value of the test (48). Similarly, Vladimirov et al found that the addition of the CCCT to the much simpler AFC does not improve the predictive value of AFC alone (85). Muttukrishna has also found that the combination of basal FSH, AMH, and inhibin B test improved the predictive value over AMH alone (Muttukrishna et al, 2004). In a different study, Muttikrishna et al devised a cumulative score using basal FSH, basal AMH, delta E2 (levels of estradiol on day 4 minus day 3), delta inhibin B, AFC, and age and found it to give the best predictive statistics to identify poor responders with 87 percent sensitivity and 80 percent specificity and a positive likelihood ratio of 4.36 (109).

To summarize, there is currently no full proof test or combination of tests to predict poor response in ART patients. In an elegant review, Bukulmez and Arici concluded that there is currently no clinically useful predictive test sufficiently accurate and distinct in time from controlled ovarian stimulation to assess ovarian reserve accurately (111). Similarly, in their systematic review, Broekmans et al reached the same conclusion. In fact, they advised that entering the first cycle of IVF without any prior testing seems to be the preferable strategy (81). This policy is supported by the findings of Klinkert et al that a poor response in the first IVF cycle is not necessarily related to a poor prognosis in subsequent cycles (112).

MANAGEMENT

Regardless of the definition used, various modifications of the stimulation protocols have been suggested for the treatment of poor responders. These include increasing the dose of HMG or FSH, using purified or recombinant FSH as opposed to HMG, diminishing the dose or shortening the duration of the GnRH agonist, using GnRH antagonists, performing IVF in natural (unstimulated) cycles, adding CC, human growth hormone (hGH), or other adjuvant therapies to the stimulating agents, or pretreating the patient with oral contraceptives or androgenic hormones (testosterone or DHEA). In all cases, proper counseling of the couple at each step of the IVF procedure is a cornerstone of good medical practice as cancellation of the cycle can still occur at any step.

Tailoring the FSH Administration

Increasing the dose of HMG or FSH has been reported by many authors (113–117). The daily dose is increased to six or eight ampoules per day (450 or 600 IU). Using this approach, Land et al reported a significant increase in the mean number of retrieved oocytes and Hofman et al reported a significant diminution in the cancellation rate (113, 117). However, none of these studies found an improvement in the clinical pregnancy rate. Another randomized study confirmed that doubling the dose of HMG in low responders did not enhance the ovarian response in those patients (118). Similarly, Khalaf et al found that increasing the gonadotrophin dose in the course of an IVF cycle does not rectify an initial poor response, confirming an initial observation by Hershlag et al (119, 120). A recent randomized trial confirmed that expected poor responders, defined as patients with an AFC less than 5, do not benefit from a higher starting dose of gonadotrophins in IVF (121).

Using purified or recombinant FSH (rFSH) was also suggested for the management of poor responders (4, 122–125). In a randomized study, Raga et al found that rFSH was more effective than uFSH in inducing multifollicular development and achieving pregnancy in young low responders (4). These results were confirmed by the studies of De Placido et al and Lisi et al (122, 123). However, the clinical importance of these findings are not of great value as recombinant preparations are now becoming the main preparations used for ovarian stimulation in all patients, normal and poor responders alike.

Tailoring GnRH Agonist Protocols

Although standard GnRH protocols have been first suggested as a treatment for poor responders, it soon became clear that a different regimen may need to be used in those patients (126). The tailoring of this regimen may take the form of diminishing the dose of the agonist, shortening the duration (in days) of its administration or simply to stop the agonist altogether once realized that the ovaries are not responding properly.

Lowering the dose of the GnRH agonist in poor responders was reported by various authors. Feldberg et al found that a minidose of GnRH-a (0.1 mg daily until menstruation, fol-lowed by 0.05 mg daily) resulted in higher E2 levels and lower P levels on the day of hCG and lower cancelation rates. Furthermore, a higher number of oocytes were recovered and fertilized and more embryos were transferred. The trend indicated improved pregnancy and implantation rates with a lower miscarriage rate (127). Similar results were reported by Scott and Navot, Olivennes et al, and Surrey et al (128–130). In addition, in a randomized trial, Weissman et al found that a modified long "minidose" protocol was superior to a modified megadose protocol in terms of oocyte yield and cycle outcome, while the improvement in pregnancy rate did not reach statistical significance (131).

Shortening the duration of GnRH agonist administration was also proposed as a better regimen for poor responders. This "flare-up" protocol was first reported by Howles et al GnRH agonist was administered to seven poor responders in a dose of 500 μg/day on days 1–3 of the menstrual cycle followed by gonadotrophin stimulation. All seven patients had oocytes recovered and embryos replaced, and three became pregnant (132). This study was followed by numerous publications that showed that the flare-up protocol, usually combined with higher doses of FSH, was associated with higher peak E2 levels, more oocytes, and more embryos but without a significant improvement in the pregnancy rate (133–138).

Cessation of the GnRH agonist once it is realized that the ovaries are not responding or with the onset of menses, followed by high doses of FSH or HMG stimulation, is another alternative (139). This policy was described by Faber et al who reported a nonsignificant increase in pregnancy rates (140). Similar results were reported by Dirnfeld et al, Schachter et al, and Wang et al (141–143).

GnRH Antagonists for Poor Responders

The use of GnRH antagonists was also proposed in cases of poor responders, and the initial studies were promising (143–145). GnRH antagonists are associated with simpler stimulation regimens, lower gonadotrophin requirements, reduced patients costs, and shorter downtimes between consecutive cycles (146). Daily administration of 0.25 mg of Cetrorelix or Ganirelix is usually started when the leading follicle reaches 14 mm. The treatment is continued until the day of HCG administration. Nikolettos et al suggested that the multiple-dose protocol was the protocol of choice for poor responders (144). However, randomized trials failed to confirm these initial findings (145, 147–150). In addition, a recent meta-analysis has shown no differences in clinical outcomes except a significantly higher number of oocytes with the GnRH antagonist protocol compared to the GnRH agonist protocol (151), while another meta-analysis showed that the GnRH antagonist protocol was superior to the long protocol but inferior to the flare-up protocol in term of oocytes retrieved (152).

Variants on the classical GnRH antagonist protocol have been described. Frankfurter et al used two single 3-mg doses of cetrorelix acetate together with medroxyprogesterone acetate to achieve complete ovarian suppression before the start of FSH stimulation (153) and D'Amato et al used GnRH antagonist in combination with high doses of recombinant FSH together with CC (154). The use of estrogen priming with oral estradiol valerate (155) or estradiol patches (156) prior to gonadotrophin stimulation has also been described. All these nonrandomized studies reported promising initial results in terms of oocyte yield, but further work is needed to show whether these protocols will result in higher pregnancy rates.

Natural Cycle IVF for Poor Responders

Natural (unstimulated) cycle IVF (NC-IVF) was also proposed as a good alternative for poor responders. In a study by Bassil et al, the authors reported that an encouraging number of pregnancies could be achieved by IVF during natural cycles in those patients (157). Similar results were reported by Feldman et al (158), and in a randomized study, Morgia et al found that NC-IVF was at least as effective as with standard stimulation protocols, especially in younger patients (159). In an attempt to eliminate any LH surge that may occur during NC-IVF, Elizur et al proposed the addition of GnRH antagonists and found that this "modified natural IVF cycle" was a feasible alternative to ovarian stimulation protocols in those patients (160). Frydman recommended that the GnRH antagonist should be started at day 8, at a daily dose of 0.5 mg (161). However, in a recent study, Kolibianakis et al could not confirm these results (162).

Adjuvant Therapy

Various adjuvant therapies have been suggested for improving the results of IVF and ICSI in poor responders. They include pretreatment with oral contraceptives or testosterone or the addition of CC, letrozole, growth hormone, or aspirin to the stimulation protocol.

Pretreatment with oral contraceptives (OC) was first suggested by Gonen et al who found that this regimen prevented LH surges and diminished the FSH dose required (163). Two studies published in 1996 supported these findings (164, 165). However, this early enthusiasm could not be confirmed by subsequent studies (166–169). In a randomized trial published in 2005, Bramat et al found that although the OC pretreatment with recombinant FSH/GnRH-antagonist protocols provided a patient-friendly regimen, no difference was seen in the number of 2PN embryos, cryopreserved embryos, embryos transferred, implantation, and pregnancy rates compared to the classical stimulation protocol (170).

Pretreatment with testosterone was also proposed. In a non-controlled trial, Balasch et al administered transdermal testosterone (20 µg/kg per day) during the five days preceding gonadotrophin treatment to twenty-five poor responders. Twenty patients (80 percent) showed a fivefold increase in the number of recruited follicles, with a clinical pregnancy rate of 30 percent per oocyte retrieval (171). However, in a randomized trial, Massin et al administered testosterone gel for fifteen days prior to ovarian stimulation to a group of poor responders but could not confirm these results. They suggested that more clinical trials are needed to determine whether an optimal dose and/or a longer duration of testosterone administration may be helpful (172). Dehydroepiandrosterone (DHEA) administration prior to ovarian stimulation has also been suggested. In two case series, pretreatment with DHEA was found to improve the response to ovarian stimulation (173, 174). However, this work has not been confirmed by larger controlled studies.

CC was also proposed as a better stimulation protocol for poor responders either alone (175) or as an adjuvant to HMG stimulation (176). In a different, but nonrandomized trial,

D'Amato et al administered a combination of CC, high-dose recombinant human FSH, and a delayed, multidose GnRH antagonist to eighty-five poor responders. They found that this regimen was associated with lower cancellation rates, higher E2 levels, more oocyte retrieved, and higher pregnancy (22.2 vs. 15.3 percent) and implantation rates (13.5 vs. 7.6 percent) compared with those receiving the long protocol (177). However, these promising results could not be confirmed by Ashrafi et al and randomized studies are clearly needed to further evaluate these regimens (178).

hGH (0.1 IU/kg body weight per day) was also proposed as an adjuvant therapy in poor responders as it was found to facilitate ovarian response to gonadotrophin stimulation, probably mediated through IGF-I (179–181). Initial studies were encouraging (172, 182, 183). However, subsequent work including two randomized trials failed to confirm these results (184–189). In a Cochrane review published in 2003, Harper et al concluded that although the meta-analysis showed a significant improvement in live birth rate, the results were only just significant and were obtained from three small trials and suggested that more randomized trials were necessary before recommending this expensive therapy (190). A recent study has reported that the coadministration of GH and aspirin to poor ovarian responders was effective in increasing the rates of oocyte retrieval, promoting oocyte maturation, and improving the fertilization rate (191). Adjuvant therapy with the growth hormone–releasing factor was also tried. In a small randomized study, Busacca et al reported an increase in the number of developing follicles with no improvement in the pregnancy rate (5).

It has also been suggested that the administration of aspirin may improve the results of assisted reproduction in poor responder ART patients. However, two recent studies have failed to support this claim (192, 193). In the randomized study by Lok et al, supplementation with low-dose aspirin failed to improve neither ovarian nor uterine blood flow or ovarian responsiveness in poor responders undergoing IVF (192). A more recent study, however, suggested that the coadministration of GH and aspirin to poor ovarian responders was effective in increasing the rates of oocyte retrieval, promoting oocyte maturation, and improving the fertilization rate but not the pregnancy rate in patients undergoing IVF-ET therapy (191).

Letrozole was also suggested for the management of poor responders (194). However, no definite advantage has been shown so far. In a randomized trial, Goswami et al compared the use of letrozole and rFSH versus the long stimulation protocol. They found that the adjunctive use of letrozole was a lower cost IVF protocol, but offered no improvement in pregnancy rates (195). Similarly, Schoolcraft et al compared the use of a microdose GnRH agonist flare-up protocol with a GnRH antagonist/letrozole protocol in poor responders and found a trend toward higher ongoing pregnancy rates and superior implantation rates with the flare-up protocol (196).

Other adjuvant therapies were also suggested. In a randomized study, low-dose dexamethasone together with aspirin was shown to reduce the incidence of poor response in an initial stimulation cycle. Preliminary studies using pyridostigmine and L-arginine in established poor responders reported encouraging results, but these require confirmation in adequately powered studies (197).

In summary, no single regimen or combination of regimens has so far proven its superiority in the management of poor responders. This situation was highlighted in a systematic review by Tarlatzis et al in 2003 (198). More recently, a Cochrane review reiterated this state of affairs and reported that, so far, there is insufficient evidence to support the routine use of any particular intervention for pituitary downregulation, ovarian stimulation, or adjuvant therapy in the management of poor responders in IVF (199).

Oocyte Donation

Oocyte donation remains the final cornerstone for the management of poor responders. The pregnancy rate in these women is as good as in normal responders (200). Unfortunately, this treatment option is not available for women in many parts of the world due to cultural or religious reasons (201).

CONCLUSIONS

The evaluation and treatment of low responders in ART remains a challenge. No single test or combination of tests has been shown to accurately predict the condition. Similarly, there is no universally accepted policy for the management of these patients.

Understanding the underlying etiology and pathophysiology of this disorder is necessary in order to help the clinician to manage this problem successfully. Currently, little is being done in this domain and there is a great need for basic research in this area. There is also a need for a standard definition for poor responders, and this is currently being sought (Nargund and Frydman, personal communications). This will form the basis of multicenter trials for comparing the various management options in order to offer better chances of pregnancy for these unfortunate women. Currently, poor responders younger than thirty-seven years can expect a pregnancy rate of about 14 percent, while about 3 percent of older patients become pregnant after IVF/ICSI (2).

KEY POINTS FOR CLINICIANS

■ About 10 percent of patients attempting IVF or ICSI respond poorly to ovarian stimulation. The incidence increases with advancing age.

■ There is no standard definition for poor responders. This is needed in order to properly compare predictive tests and management policies.

■ A working definition is that poor responders are patients from whom less than five, six, or eight oocytes are retrieved when undergoing ICSI, IVF, or TESE/ICSI, respectively.

■ The exact etiology is not known, but insensitivity of FSH receptors or the development of antibodies are possible causes.

■ There is no universally accepted test or combination of tests for the prediction of the condition. Of the static tests, the best are probably the AFC and the measurement of day 3 serum AMH levels.

■ Of the dynamic tests for prediction, the CCCT is probably the best to predict poor response, while the EFORT test is better in predicting hyperresponses.

■ Randomized trials have not confirmed the superiority of any management protocol. Promising regimens are the use of recombinant FSH (as opposed to urinary FSH and HMG), the low-dose flare-up protocol, and the modified NC-IVF (i.e., natural cycle + GnRH antagonist). Supplementing the treatment with hGH is not beneficial.

■ Using these therapies, 14 percent of young poor responders (younger than thirty-seven years) and 3 percent of older patients (thirty-seven years or older) can expect to become pregnant.

REFERENCES

1. Jones HW Jr. IVF: past and future. *Reprod Biomed Online.* 2003;6(3):375–81.
2. Saldeen P, Källen K, Sundström P. The probability of successful IVF outcome after poor ovarian response. *Acta Obstet Gynecol Scand.* 2007;86(4):457–61.
3. Surrey ES, Schoolcraft WB. Evaluating strategies for improving ovarian response of the poor responder undergoing assisted reproductive techniques. *Fertil Steril.* 2000;73(4):667–76.
4. Raga F, Bonilla-Musoles F, Casan EM, et al. Recombinant follicle stimulating hormone stimulation in poor responders with normal basal concentrations of follicle stimulating hormone and oestradiol: improved reproductive outcome. *Hum Reprod.* 1999;14(6):1431–4.
5. Busacca M, Fusi FM, Brigante C, et al. Use of growth hormone-releasing factor in ovulation induction in poor responders. *J Reprod Med.* 1996;41(9):699–703.
6. Feldberg D, Farhi J, Ashkenazi J, et al. Minidose gonadotropin-releasing hormone agonist is the treatment of choice in poor responders with high follicle-stimulating hormone levels. *Fertil Steril.* 1994;62(2):343–6.
7. Fridstrom M, Akerlof E, Sjoblom P, et al. Serum levels of luteinizing and follicle-stimulating hormones in normal and poor-responding patients undergoing ovarian stimulation with uro-follitropin after pituitary down regulation. *Gynecol Endocrinol.* 1997;11(1):25–8.
8. Serafini P, Stone B, Kerin J, et al. An alternate approach to controlled ovarian hyperstimulation in "poor responders": pretreatment with a gonadotropin-releasing hormone analog. *Fertil Steril.* 1988;49(1):90–5.
9. Surrey ES, Bower J, Hill DM, et al. Clinical and endocrine effects of a microdose GnRH agonist flare regimen administered to poor responders who are undergoing in vitro fertilization. *Fertil Steril.* 1998;69(3):419–24.
10. Lindheim SR, Sauer MV, Francis MM, et al. The significance of elevated early follicular-phase follicle stimulating hormone (FSH) levels: observations in unstimulated in vitro fertilization cycles. *J Assist Reprod Genet.* 1996;13(1):49–52.
11. Land JA, Yarmolinskaya MI, Dumoulin JC, et al. High-dose human menopausal gonadotropin stimulation in poor responders does not improve in vitro fertilization outcome. *Fertil Steril.* 1996;65(5):961–5.
12. Lashen H, Ledger W, Lopez-Bernal A, et al. Poor responders to ovulation induction: is proceeding to in-vitro fertilization worthwhile? *Hum Reprod.* 1999;14(4):964–9.
13. Faber BM, Mayer J, Cox B, et al. Cessation of gonadotropin-releasing hormone agonist therapy combined with high-dose gonadotropin stimulation yields favorable pregnancy results in low responders. *Fertil Steril.* 1998;69(5):826–30.
14. Karande V, Morris R, Rinehart J, et al. Limited success using the "flare" protocol in poor responders in cycles with low basal follicle-stimulating hormone levels during in vitro fertilization. *Fertil Steril.* 1997;67(5):900–3.

15. Toth TL, Awwad JT, Veeck LL, et al. Suppression and flare regimens of gonadotropin-releasing hormone agonist. Use in women with different basal gonadotropin values in an in vitro fertilization program. *J Reprod Med.* 1996;41(5):321–6.

16. Brzyski RG, Muasher SJ, Droesch K, et al. Follicular atresia associated with concurrent initiation of gonadotropin-releasing hormone agonist and follicle-stimulating hormone for oocyte recruitment. *Fertil Steril.* 1998;50(6):917–21.

17. Karande VC, Jones GS, Veeck LL, et al. High-dose follicle-stimulating hormone stimulation at the onset of the menstrual cycle does not improve the in vitro fertilization outcome in low-responder patients. *Fertil Steril.* 1990;53(3):486–9.

18. Yang JH, Wu MY, Chao KH, Chen SU, Ho HN, Yang YS. Long GnRH-agonist protocol in an IVF program. Is it appropriate for women with normal FSH levels and high FSH/LH ratios? *J Reprod Med.* 1997;42(10):663–8.

19. Salat-Baroux J, Rotten D, Alvarez S, et al. Comparison of growth hormone responses to growth hormone-releasing factor and clonidine in women with normal or poor ovarian response to gonadotropin stimulation. *Fertil Steril.* 1993;60(5):791–9.

20. Ibrahim ZH, Matson PL, Buck P, et al. The use of biosynthetic human growth hormone to augment ovulation induction with buserelin acetate/human menopausal gonadotropin in women with a poor ovarian response. *Fertil Steril.* 1991;55(1):202–4.

21. Manzi DL, Thornton KL, Scott LB, et al. The value of increasing the dose of human menopausal gonadotropins in women who initially demonstrate a poor response. *Fertil Steril.* 1994;62(2):251–6.

22. Hofmann GE, Toner JP, Muasher SJ, et al. High-dose follicle-stimulating hormone (FSH) ovarian stimulation in low-responder patients for in vitro fertilization. *J In Vitro Fert Embryo Transf.* 1989;6(5):285–9.

23. Hughes SM, Huang ZH, Morris ID, et al. A double-blind cross-over controlled study to evaluate the effect of human biosynthetic growth hormone on ovarian stimulation in previous poor responders to in-vitro fertilization. *Hum Reprod.* 1994;9(1):13–18.

24. Shaker AG, Fleming R, Jamieson ME, et al. Absence of effect of adjuvant growth hormone therapy on follicular responses to exogenous gonadotropins in women: normal and poor responders. *Fertil Steril.* 1992;58(5):919–23.

25. Chong AP, Rafael RW, Forte CC. Influence of weight in the induction of ovulation with human menopausal gonadotropin and human chorionic gonadotropin. *Fertil Steril.* 1986;46(4):599–603.

26. Rombauts L, Suikkari AM, MacLachlan V, et al. Recruitment of follicles by recombinant human follicle-stimulating hormone commencing in the luteal phase of the ovarian cycle. *Fertil Steril.* 1998;69(4):665–9.

27. Sallam HN, Ezzeldin F, Agameya AF, Rahman AF, El-Garem Y. Defining poor responders in assisted reproduction. *Int J Fertil Womens Med.* 2005;50(3):115–20.

28. Fasouliotis SJ, Simon A, Laufer N. Evaluation and treatment of low responders in assisted reproductive technology: a challenge to meet. *J Assist Reprod Genet.* 2000;17(7):357–73.

29. Society for Assisted Reproductive Technology; American Society for Reproductive Medicine. Assisted reproductive technology in the United States: 2001 results generated from the American Society for Reproductive Medicine/Society for Assisted Reproductive Technology registry. *Fertil Steril.* 2007;87(6):1253–66. Epub 2007 Feb 2.

30. Tan SL, Royston P, Campbell S, Jacobs HS, Betts J, Mason B, Edwards RG. Cumulative conception and livebirth rates after in-vitro fertilisation. *Lancet.* 1992;339(8806):1390–4.

31. Toner JP, Philput CB, Jones GS, et al. Basal follicle-stimulating hormone level is a better predictor of in vitro fertilization performance than age. *Fertil Steril.* 1991;55(4):784–91.

32. Check JH, Lurie D, Callan C, Baker A, Benfer K. Comparison of the cumulative probability of pregnancy after in vitro fertilization-embryo transfer by infertility factor and age. *Fertil Steril.* 1994;61(2):257–61.

33. Engmann L, Maconochie N, Bekir JS, Jacobs HS, Tan SL. Cumulative probability of clinical pregnancy and live birth after a multiple cycle IVF package: a more realistic assessment of overall and age-specific success rates? *Br J Obstet Gynaecol.* 1999;106(2):165–70.

34. Ulug U, Ben-Shlomo I, Turan E, Erden HF, Akman MA, Bahceci M. Conception rates following assisted reproduction in poor responder patients: a retrospective study in 300 consecutive cycles. *Reprod Biomed Online.* 2003;6(4):439–43.

35. Galey-Fontaine J, Cédrin-Durnerin I, Chaïbi R, Massin N, Hugues JN. Age and ovarian reserve are distinct predictive factors of cycle outcome in low responders. *Reprod Biomed Online.* 2005;10(1):94–9.

36. Beckers NG, Macklon NS, Eijkemans MJ, Fauser BC. Women with regular menstrual cycles and a poor response to ovarian hyperstimulation for in vitro fertilization exhibit follicular phase characteristics suggestive of ovarian aging. *Fertil Steril.* 2002;78(2):291–7.

37. Nikolaou D, Lavery S, Turner C, Margara R, Trew G. Is there a link between an extremely poor response to ovarian hyperstimulation and early ovarian failure? *Hum Reprod.* 2002;17(4):1106–11.

38. Lawson R, El-Toukhy T, Kassab A, Taylor A, Braude P, Parsons J, Seed P. Poor response to ovulation induction is a stronger predictor of early menopause than elevated basal FSH: a life table analysis. *Hum Reprod.* 2003;18(3):527–33.

39. Owen EJ, Torresani T, West C, Mason BA, Jacobs HS. Serum and follicular fluid insulin like growth factors I and II during growth hormone co-treatment for in-vitro fertilization and embryo transfer. *Clin Endocrinol (Oxf).* 1991;35(4):327–34.

40. Bahceci M, Ulug U, Turan E, Akman MA. Comparisons of follicular levels of sex steroids, gonadotropins and insulin like growth factor-1 (IGF-1) and epidermal growth factor (EGF) in poor responder and normoresponder patients undergoing ovarian stimulation with GnRH antagonist. *Eur J Obstet Gynecol Reprod Biol.* 2007;130(1):93–8. Epub 2006 May 23.

41. Hamori M, Blum WF, Török A, Stehle R, Waibel E, Cledon P, Ranke MB. Insulin-like growth factors and their binding proteins in human follicular fluid. *Hum Reprod.* 1991;6(3):313–8.

42. Nishimura K, Tanaka N, Kawano T, Matsuura K, Okamura H. Changes in macrophage colony-stimulating factor concentration in serum and follicular fluid in in-vitro fertilization and embryo transfer cycles. *Fertil Steril.* 1998;69(1):53–7.

43. Battaglia C, Genazzani AD, Regnani G, Primavera MR, Petraglia F, Volpe A. Perifollicular Doppler flow and follicular fluid vascular endothelial growth factor concentrations in poor responders. *Fertil Steril.* 2000;74(4):809–12.

44. Luisi S, Palumbo M, Calonaci G, De Leo V, Razzi S, Inaudi P, Cobellis G, Petraglia F. Serum inhibin B correlates with successful ovulation in infertile women. *J Assist Reprod Genet.* 2003;20(6):241–7.

45. Onalan G, Selam B, Onalan R, Ceyhan T, Cincik M, Pabuccu R. Serum and follicular fluid levels of soluble Fas and soluble Fas ligand in IVF cycles. *Eur J Obstet Gynecol Reprod Biol.* 2006;125(1):85–91.

46. Cai J, Lou HY, Dong MY, Lu XE, Zhu YM, Gao HJ, Huang HF. Poor ovarian response to gonadotropin stimulation is associated

with low expression of follicle-stimulating hormone receptor in granulosa cells. *Fertil Steril.* 2007;87(6):1350–6.

47. Luborsky JL, Thiruppathi P, Rivnay B, Roussev R, Coulam C, Radwanska E. Evidence for different aetiologies of low estradiol response to FSH: age-related accelerated luteinization of follicles or presence of ovarian autoantibodies. *Hum Reprod.* 2002;17(10): 2641–9.

48. Bancsi LF, Broekmans FJ, Eijkemans MJ, de Jong FH, Habbema JD, te Velde ER. Predictors of poor ovarian response in in vitro fertilization: a prospective study comparing basal markers of ovarian reserve. *Fertil Steril.* 2002;77(2):328–36.

49. Kligman I, Rosenwaks Z. Differentiating clinical profiles: predicting good responders, poor responders, and hyperresponders. *Fertil Steril.* 2001;76(6):1185–90.

50. Klein NA, Illingworth PJ, Groome NP, McNeilly AS, Battaglia DE, Soules MR. Decreased inhibin B secretion is associated with the monotropic FSH rise in older, ovulatory women: a study of serum and follicular fluid levels of dimeric inhibin A and B in spontaneous menstrual cycles. *J Clin Endocrinol Metab.* 1996;81(7):2742–5.

51. Burger HG, Groome NP, Robertson DM. Both inhibin A and B respond to exogenous follicle-stimulating hormone in the follicular phase of the human menstrual cycle. *J Clin Endocrinol Metab.* 1998;83(11):4167–9.

52. Welt CK, Adams JM, Sluss PM, Hall JE. Inhibin A and inhibin B responses to gonadotropin withdrawal depends on stage of follicle development. *J Clin Endocrinol Metab.* 1999;84(6): 2163–9.

53. Licciardi FL, Liu HC, Rosenwaks Z. Day 3 estradiol serum concentrations as prognosticators of ovarian stimulation response and pregnancy outcome in patients undergoing in vitro fertilization. *Fertil Steril.* 1995;64(5):991–4.

54. Smotrich DB, Widra EA, Gindoff PR, et al. Prognostic value of day 3 estradiol on in vitro fertilization outcome. *Fertil Steril.* 1995;64(6):1136–40.

55. de Vet A, Laven JS, de Jong FH, Themmen AP, Fauser BC. Antimüllerian hormone serum levels: a putative marker for ovarian aging. *Fertil Steril.* 2002;77(2):357–62.

56. Pellicer A, Ardiles G, Neuspiller F, Remohí J, Simón C, Bonilla-Musoles F. Evaluation of the ovarian reserve in young low responders with normal basal levels of follicle-stimulating hormone using three-dimensional ultrasonography. *Fertil Steril.* 1998; 70(4):671–5.

57. Lass A, Skull J, McVeigh E, et al. Measurement of ovarian volume by transvaginal sonography before ovulation induction with human menopausal gonadotrophin for in-vitro fertilization can predict poor response. *Hum Reprod.* 1997;12(2):294–7.

58. Kwee J, Elting ME, Schats R, McDonnell J, Lambalk CB. Ovarian volume and antral follicle count for the prediction of low and hyper responders with in vitro fertilization. *Reprod Biol Endocrinol.* 2007;5:9.

59. Kan A, Ng EH, Yeung WS, Ho PC. Perifollicular vascularity in poor ovarian responders during IVF. *Hum Reprod.* 2006;21(6): 1539–44.

60. Scott RT, Toner JP, Muasher SJ, Oehninger S, Robinson S, Rosenwaks Z. Follicle-stimulating hormone levels on cycle day 3 are predictive of in vitro fertilization outcome. *Fertil Steril.* 1989; 51(4):651–4.

61. Bassil S, Godin PA, Gillerot S, Verougstraete JC, Donnez J. In vitro fertilization outcome according to age and follicle-stimulating hormone levels on cycle day 3. *J Assist Reprod Genet.* 1999;16(5):236–41.

62. Barroso G, Oehninger S, Monzo A, Kolm P, Gibbons WE, Muasher SJ. High FSH:LH ratio and low LH levels in basal cycle

day 3: impact on follicular development and IVF outcome. *J Assist Reprod Genet.* 2001;18(9):499–505.

63. Muttukrishna S, Suharjono H, McGarrigle H, Sathanandan M. Inhibin B and anti-Mullerian hormone: markers of ovarian response in IVF/ICSI patients? *BJOG* 2004;111(11):1248–53.

64. Erdem M, Erdem A, Gursoy R, Biberoglu K. Comparison of basal and clomiphene citrate induced FSH and inhibin B, ovarian volume and antral follicle counts as ovarian reserve tests and predictors of poor ovarian response in IVF. *J Assist Reprod Genet.* 2004;21(2):37–45.

65. Onagawa T, Shibahara H, Ayustawati Machida S, Hirano Y, Hirashima C, Takamizawa S, Suzuki M. Prediction of ovarian reserve based on day-3 serum follicle stimulating hormone concentrations during the pituitary suppression cycle using a gonadotropin releasing hormone agonist in patients undergoing in vitro fertilization-embryo transfer. *Gynecol Endocrinol.* 2004; 18(6):335–40.

66. van Rooij IA, Bancsi LF, Broekmans FJ, Looman CW, Habbema JD, te Velde ER. Women older than 40 years of age and those with elevated follicle-stimulating hormone levels differ in poor response rate and embryo quality in in vitro fertilization. *Fertil Steril.* 2003;79(3):482–8.

67. Abdalla H, Thum MY. Repeated testing of basal FSH levels has no predictive value for IVF outcome in women with elevated basal FSH. *Hum Reprod.* 2006;21(1):171–4.

68. Bancsi LF, Broekmans FJ, Mol BW, Habbema JD, te Velde ER. Performance of basal follicle-stimulating hormone in the prediction of poor ovarian response and failure to become pregnant after in vitro fertilization: a meta-analysis. *Fertil Steril.* 2003; 79(5):1091–100.

69. Mukherjee T, Copperman AB, Lapinski R, Sandler B, Bustillo M, Grunfeld L. An elevated day three follicle-stimulating hormone:luteinizing hormone ratio (FSH:LH) in the presence of a normal day 3 FSH predicts a poor response to controlled ovarian hyperstimulation. *Fertil Steril.* 1996;65(3):588–93.

70. Seifer DB, Lambert-Messerlian G, Hogan JW, et al. Day 3 serum inhibin-B is predictive of assisted reproductive technologies outcome. *Fertil Steril.* 1997;67(1):110–1104.

71. Hofmann GE, Danforth DR, Seifer DB. Inhibin-B: the physiologic basis of the clomiphene citrate challenge test for ovarian reserve screening. *Fertil Steril.* 1998;69(3):474–7.

72. Urbancsek J, Hauzman EE, Murber A, Lagarde AR, Rabe T, Papp Z, Strowitzki T. Serum CA-125 and inhibin B levels in the prediction of ovarian response to gonadotropin stimulation in in vitro fertilization cycles. *Gynecol Endocrinol.* 2005;21(1):38–44.

73. Corson SL, Gutmann J, Batzer FR, Wallace H, Klein N, Soules MR. Inhibin-B as a test of ovarian reserve for infertile women. *Hum Reprod.* 1999;14(11):2818–21.

74. Evers JL, Slaats P, Land JA, Dumoulin JC, Dunselman GA. Elevated levels of basal estradiol-17-beta predict poor response in patients with normal basal levels of follicle-stimulating hormone undergoing in vitro fertilization. *Fertil Steril.* 1998;69:1010–4.

75. Costello MF, Hughes GJ, Garrett DK, Steigrad SJ, Ekangaki A. Prognostic value of baseline serum oestradiol in controlled ovarian hyperstimulation of women with unexplained infertility. *Aust N Z J Obstet Gynaecol.* 2001;41(1):69–74.

76. Vázquez ME, Verez JR, Stern JJ, Gutierrez Najar A, Asch RH. Elevated basal estradiol levels have no negative prognosis in young women undergoing ART cycles. *Gynecol Endocrinol.* 1998;12(3):155–9.

77. Phophong P, Ranieri DM, Khadum I, Meo F, Serhal P. Basal 17beta-estradiol did not correlate with ovarian response and in vitro fertilization treatment outcome. *Fertil Steril.* 2000;74(6): 1133–6.

78. Fanchin R, Schonauer LM, Righini C, Guibourdenche J, Frydman R, Taieb J. Serum anti-Mullerian hormone is more strongly related to ovarian follicular status than serum inhibin B, estradiol, FSH and LH on day 3. *Hum Reprod.* 2003;18(2):323–7.

79. Hazout A, Bouchard P, Seifer DB, Aussage P, Junca AM, Cohen-Bacrie P. Serum antimullerian hormone/mullerian-inhibiting substance appears to be a more discriminatory marker of assisted reproductive technology outcome than follicle-stimulating hormone, inhibin B, or estradiol. *Fertil Steril.* 2004;82(5):1323–9.

80. Elgindy EA, El-Haieg DO, El-Sebaey A. Anti-Müllerian hormone: correlation of early follicular, ovulatory and midluteal levels with ovarian response and cycle outcome in intracytoplasmic sperm injection patients. *Fertil Steril.* 2007. Epub ahead of print.

81. Broekmans FJ, Kwee J, Hendriks DJ, Mol BW, Lambalk CB. A systematic review of tests predicting ovarian reserve and IVF outcome. *Hum Reprod Update.* 2006;12(6):685–718.

82. Tomas C, Nuojua-Huttunen S, Martikainen H. Pretreatment transvaginal ultrasound examination predicts ovarian responsiveness to gonadotrophins in in-vitro fertilization. *Hum Reprod.* 1997;12(2):220–3.

83. Chang MY, Chiang CH, Hsieh TT, Soong YK, Hsu KH. Use of the antral follicle count to predict the outcome of assisted reproductive technologies. *Fertil Steril.* 1998;69(3):505–10.

84. Eldar-Geva T, Ben-Chetrit A, Spitz IM, Rabinowitz R, Markowitz E, Mimoni T, Gal M, Zylber-Haran E, Margalioth EJ. Dynamic assays of inhibin B, anti-Mullerian hormone and estradiol following FSH stimulation and ovarian ultrasonography as predictors of IVF outcome. *Hum Reprod.* 2005;20(11):3178–83.

85. Vladimirov IK, Tacheva DM, Kalinov KB, Ivanova AV, Blagoeva VD. Prognostic value of some ovarian reserve tests in poor responders. *Arch Gynecol Obstet.* 2005;272(1):74–9. Epub 2005 Jan 20.

86. Hendriks DJ, Broekmans FJ, Bancsi LF, Looman CW, de Jong FH, te Velde ER. Single and repeated GnRH agonist stimulation tests compared with basal markers of ovarian reserve in the prediction of outcome in IVF. *J Assist Reprod Genet.* 2005;22(2):65–73.

87. Haadsma ML, Bukman A, Groen H, Roeloffzen EM, Groenewoud ER, Heineman MJ, Hoek A. The number of small antral follicles (2-6 mm) determines the outcome of endocrine ovarian reserve tests in a subfertile population. *Hum Reprod.* 2007;22(7):1925–31. Epub 2007 Apr 16.

88. Bancsi LF, Broekmans FJ, Looman CW, Habbema JD, te Velde ER. Impact of repeated antral follicle counts on the prediction of poor ovarian response in women undergoing in vitro fertilization. *Fertil Steril.* 2004;81(1):35–41.

89. Durmusoglu F, Elter K, Yoruk P, Erenus M. Combining cycle day 7 follicle count with the basal antral follicle count improves the prediction of ovarian response. *Fertil Steril.* 2004;81(4):1073–8.

90. Kwee J, Elting ME, Schats R, McDonnell J, Lambalk CB. Ovarian volume and antral follicle count for the prediction of low and hyper responders with in vitro fertilization. *Reprod Biol Endocrinol.* 2007;5:9.

91. Hendriks DJ, Kwee J, Mol BW, te Velde ER, Broekmans FJ. Ultrasonography as a tool for the prediction of outcome in IVF patients: a comparative meta-analysis of ovarian volume and antral follicle count. *Fertil Steril.* 2007;87(4):764–75. Epub 2007 Jan 18.

92. Navot D, Rosenwaks Z, Margalioth EJ. Prognostic assessment of female fecundity. *Lancet.* 1987;2(8560):645–7.

93. Fanchin R, De Ziegler D, Olivennes F, Taieb J, Dzik A, Frydman R. Exogenous follicle stimulating hormone ovarian reserve test (EFORT) (a simple and reliable screening test for detecting "poor responders" in in-vitro fertilization). *Hum Reprod.* 1994;9:1607–1611.

94. Fábregues F, Balasch J, Creus M, Carmona F, Puerto B, Quintó L, Casamitjana R, Vanrell JA. Ovarian reserve test with human menopausal gonadotropin as a predictor of in vitro fertilization outcome. *J Assist Reprod Genet.* 2000;17(1):13–19.

95. Padilla SL, Smith RD, Garcia JE. The Lupron screening test (tailoring the use of leuprolide acetate in ovarian stimulation for in vitro fertilization). *Fertil Steril.* 1991;56:79–83.

96. Karande V, Gleicher N. A rational approach to the management of low responders in in-vitro fertilization. *Hum Reprod.* 1999;14(7):1744–8.

97. Loumaye E, Billion JM, Mine JM, et al. Prediction of individual response to controlled ovarian hyperstimulation by means of a clomiphene citrate challenge test. *Fertil Steril.* 1990;53(2):295–301.

98. Scott RTJr, Illions EH, Kost ER, et al. Evaluation of the significance of the estradiol response during the clomiphene citrate challenge test. *Fertil Steril.* 1993;60(2):242–6.

99. Kwee J, Schats R, McDonnell J, Schoemaker J, Lambalk CB. The clomiphene citrate challenge test versus the exogenous follicle-stimulating hormone ovarian reserve test as a single test for identification of low responders and hyperresponders to in vitro fertilization. *Fertil Steril.* 2006;85(6):1714–22.

100. Hendriks DJ, Broekmans FJ, Bancsi LF, de Jong FH, Looman CW, Te Velde ER. Repeated clomiphene citrate challenge testing in the prediction of outcome in IVF: a comparison with basal markers for ovarian reserve. *Hum Reprod.* 2005;20(1):163–9.

101. Hendriks DJ, Mol BW, Bancsi LF, te Velde ER, Broekmans FJ. The clomiphene citrate challenge test for the prediction of poor ovarian response and nonpregnancy in patients undergoing in vitro fertilization: a systematic review. *Fertil Steril.* 2006;86(4):807–18. Epub 2006 Sep 7. Review.

102. Fanchin R, de Ziegler D, Olivennes F, et al. Exogenous follicle stimulating hormone ovarian reserve test (EFORT): a simple and reliable screening test for detecting poor responders in in-vitro fertilization. *Hum Reprod.* 1994;9(9):1607–11.

103. Iwase A, Ando H, Kuno K, Mizutani S. Use of follicle-stimulating hormone test to predict poor response in in vitro fertilization. *Obstet Gynecol.* 2005;105(3):645–52.

104. Kwee J, Schats R, McDonnell J, Lambalk CB, Schoemaker J. Intercycle variability of ovarian reserve tests: results of a prospective randomized study. *Hum Reprod.* 2004;19(3):590–5.

105. Dzik A, Lambert-Messerlian G, Izzo VM, Soares JB, Pinotti JA, Seifer DB. Inhibin B response to EFORT is associated with the outcome of oocyte retrieval in the subsequent in vitro fertilization cycle. *Fertil Steril.* 2000;74(6):1114–7.

106. Winslow KL, Toner JP, Brzyski RG, Oehninger SC, Acosta AA, Muasher SJ. The gonadotropin-releasing hormone agonist stimulation test—a sensitive predictor of performance in the flare-up in vitro fertilization cycle. *Fertil Steril.* 1991;56(4):711–7.

107. Hendriks DJ, Broekmans FJ, Bancsi LF, Looman CW, de Jong FH, te Velde ER. Single and repeated GnRH agonist stimulation tests compared with basal markers of ovarian reserve in the prediction of outcome in IVF. *J Assist Reprod Genet.* 2005;22(2): 65–73.

108. Hendriks DJ, Mol BW, Bancsi LF, Te Velde ER, Broekmans FJ. Antral follicle count in the prediction of poor ovarian response and pregnancy after in vitro fertilization: a meta-analysis and

comparison with basal follicle-stimulating hormone level. *Fertil Steril.* 2005;83(2):291–301.

109. Muttukrishna S, McGarrigle H, Wakim R, Khadum I, Ranieri DM, Serhal P. Antral follicle count, anti-mullerian hormone and inhibin B: predictors of ovarian response in assisted reproductive technology? *BJOG* 2005;112(10):1384–90.

110. McIlveen M, Skull JD, Ledger WL. Evaluation of the utility of multiple endocrine and ultrasound measures of ovarian reserve in the prediction of cycle cancellation in a high-risk IVF population. *Hum Reprod.* 2007;22(3):778–85.

111. Bukulmez O, Arici A. Assessment of ovarian reserve. *Curr Opin Obstet Gynecol.* 2004;16(3):231–7.

112. Klinkert ER, Broekmans FJ, Looman CW, Te Velde ER. A poor response in the first in vitro fertilization cycle is not necessarily related to a poor prognosis in subsequent cycles. *Fertil Steril.* 2004;81(5):1247–53.

113. Hofmann GE, Toner JP, Muasher SJ, Jones GS. High-dose follicle-stimulating hormone (FSH) ovarian stimulation in low-responder patients for in vitro fertilization. *J In Vitro Fert Embryo Transf.* 1989;6(5):285–9.

114. Pantos C, Thornton SJ, Speirs AL, Johnston I. Increasing the human menopausal gonadotropin dose—does the response really improve? *Fertil Steril.* 1990;53(3):436–9.

115. Karande VC, Jones GS, Veeck LL, Muasher SJ. High-dose follicle-stimulating hormone stimulation at the onset of the menstrual cycle does not improve the in vitro fertilization outcome in low-responder patients. *Fertil Steril.* 1990;53(3):486–9.

116. Manzi DL, Thornton KL, Scott LB, Nulsen JC. The value of increasing the dose of human menopausal gonadotropins in women who initially demonstrate a poor response. *Fertil Steril.* 1994;62(2):251–6.

117. Land JA, Yarmolinskaya MI, Dumoulin JC, Evers JL. High-dose human menopausal gonadotropin stimulation in poor responders does not improve in vitro fertilization outcome. *Fertil Steril.* 1996;65(5):961–5.

118. van Hooff MH, Alberda AT, Huisman GJ, Zeilmaker GH, Leerentveld RA. Doubling the human menopausal gonadotrophin dose in the course of an in-vitro fertilization treatment cycle in low responders: a randomized study. *Hum Reprod.* 1993;8(3):369–73.

119. Hershlag A, Asis MC, Diamond MP, DeCherney AH, Lavy G. The predictive value and the management of cycles with low initial estradiol levels. *Fertil Steril.* 1990;53(6):1064–7.

120. Khalaf Y, El-Toukhy T, Taylor A, Braude P. Increasing the gonadotrophin dose in the course of an in vitro fertilization cycle does not rectify an initial poor response. *Eur J Obstet Gynecol Reprod Biol.* 2002;103(2):146–9.

121. Klinkert ER, Broekmans FJ, Looman CW, Habbema JD, te Velde ER. Expected poor responders on the basis of an antral follicle count do not benefit from a higher starting dose of gonadotrophins in IVF treatment: a randomized controlled trial. *Hum Reprod.* 2005;20(3):611–5. Epub 2004 Dec 9.

122. De Placido G, Alviggi C, Mollo A, Strina I, Varricchio MT, Molis M. Recombinant follicle stimulating hormone is effective in poor responders to highly purified follicle stimulating hormone. *Hum Reprod.* 2000;15(1):17–20.

123. Lisi F, Rinaldi L, Fishel S, Lisi R, Pepe G, Picconeri MG, Campbell A, Rowe P. Use of recombinant FSH and recombinant LH in multiple follicular stimulation for IVF: a preliminary study. *Reprod Biomed Online.* 2001;3(3):190–4.

124. Eskandar M, Jaroudi K, Jambi A, Archibong EI, Coskun S, Sobande AA. Is recombinant follicle-stimulating hormone more effective in IVF poor responders than human menopausal gonadotrophins? *Med Sci Monit.* 2004;10(1):PI6–9.

125. Berkkanoglu M, Isikoglu M, Aydin D, Ozgur K. Clinical effects of ovulation induction with recombinant follicle-stimulating hormone supplemented with recombinant luteinizing hormone or low-dose recombinant human chorionic gonadotropin in the midfollicular phase in microdose cycles in poor responders. *Fertil Steril.* 2007;88(3):665–9. Epub 2007 Feb 12.

126. Belaisch-Allart J, Testart J, Frydman R. Utilization of GnRH agonists for poor responders in an IVF programme. *Hum Reprod.* 1989;4(1):33–4.

127. Feldberg D, Farhi J, Ashkenazi J, Dicker D, Shalev J, Ben-Rafael Z. Minidose gonadotropin-releasing hormone agonist is the treatment of choice in poor responders with high follicle-stimulating hormone levels. *Fertil Steril.* 1994;62(2):343–6.

128. Scott RT, Navot D. Enhancement of ovarian responsiveness with microdoses of gonadotropin-releasing hormone agonist during ovulation induction for in vitro fertilization. *Fertil Steril.* 1994;61(5):880–5.

129. Olivennes F, Righini C, Fanchin R, et al. A protocol using a low dose of gonadotrophin-releasing hormone agonist might be the best protocol for patients with high follicle-stimulating hormone concentrations on day 3. *Hum Reprod.* 1996;11(6):1169–72.

130. Surrey ES, Bower J, Hill DM, Ramsey J, Surrey MW. Clinical and endocrine effects of a microdose GnRH agonist flare regimen administered to poor responders who are undergoing in vitro fertilization. *Fertil Steril.* 1998;69(3):419–24.

131. Weissman A, Farhi J, Royburt M, Nahum H, Glezerman M, Levran D. Prospective evaluation of two stimulation protocols for low responders who were undergoing in vitro fertilization-embryo transfer. *Fertil Steril.* 2003;79(4):886–92.

132. Howles CM, Macnamee MC, Edwards RG. Short term use of an LHRH agonist to treat poor responders entering an in-vitro fertilization programme. *Hum Reprod.* 1987;2(8):655–6.

133. Padilla SL, Dugan K, Maruschak V, Shalika S, Smith RD. Use of the flare-up protocol with high dose human follicle stimulating hormone and human menopausal gonadotropins for in vitro fertilization in poor responders. *Fertil Steril.* 1996;65(4):796–9.

134. Karande V, Morris R, Rinehart J, Miller C, Rao R, Gleicher N. Limited success using the "flare" protocol in poor responders in cycles with low basal follicle-stimulating hormone levels during in vitro fertilization. *Fertil Steril.* 1997;67(5):900–3.

135. Surrey ES, Bower J, Hill DM, Ramsey J, Surrey MW. Clinical and endocrine effects of a microdose GnRH agonist flare regimen administered to poor responders who are undergoing in vitro fertilization. *Fertil Steril.* 1998;69(3):419–24.

136. Karacan M, Erkan H, Karabulut O, Sarikamiş B, Camlibel T, Benhabib M. Clinical pregnancy rates in an IVF program. Use of the flare-up protocol after failure with long regimens of GnRH-a. *J Reprod Med.* 2001 May;46(5):485–9.

137. Confino E, Zhang X, Kazer RR. GnRHa flare and IVF pregnancy rates. *Int J Gynaecol Obstet.* 2004;85(1):36–9.

138. Orvieto R, Kruchkovich J, Rabinson J, Zohav E, Anteby EY, Meltcer S. Ultrashort gonadotropin-releasing hormone agonist combined with flexible multidose gonadotropin-releasing hormone antagonist for poor responders in in vitro fertilization/embryo transfer programs. *Fertil Steril.* 2007. Epub ahead of print.

139. Rizk B (Ed.). Ultrasonography in reproductive medicine and infertility. Cambridge: United Kingdom, Cambridge University Press (in press).

140. Faber BM, Mayer J, Cox B, Jones D, Toner JP, Oehninger S, Muasher SJ. Cessation of gonadotropin-releasing hormone agonist therapy combined with high-dose gonadotropin stimulation yields favorable pregnancy results in low responders. *Fertil Steril*. 1998;69(5):826–30.

141. Dirnfeld M, Fruchter O, Yshai D, Lissak A, Ahdut A, Abramovici H. Cessation of gonadotropin-releasing hormone analogue (GnRH-a) upon down-regulation versus conventional long GnRH-a protocol in poor responders undergoing in vitro fertilization. *Fertil Steril*. 1999;72(3):406–11.

142. Schachter M, Friedler S, Raziel A, Strassburger D, Bern O, Ron-el R. Improvement of IVF outcome in poor responders by discontinuation of GnRH analogue during the gonadotropin stimulation phase—a function of improved embryo quality. *J Assist Reprod Genet*. 2001;18(4):197–204.

143. Wang PT, Lee RK, Su JT, Hou JW, Lin MH, Hu YM. Cessation of low-dose gonadotropin releasing hormone agonist therapy followed by high-dose gonadotropin stimulation yields a favorable ovarian response in poor responders. *J Assist Reprod Genet*. 2002;19(1):1–6.

144. Craft I, Gorgy A, Hill J, Menon D, Podsiadly B. Will GnRH antagonists provide new hope for patients considered 'difficult responders' to GnRH agonist protocols? *Hum Reprod*. 1999; 14(12):2959–62.

145. Nikolettos N, Al-Hasani S, Felberbaum R, Demirel LC, Kupker W, Montzka P, Xia YX, Schopper B, Sturm R, Diedrich K. Gonadotropin-releasing hormone antagonist protocol: a novel method of ovarian stimulation in poor responders. *Eur J Obstet Gynecol Reprod Biol*. 2001;97(2):202–7.

146. Fasouliotis SJ, Laufer N, Sabbagh-Ehrlich S, Lewin A, Hurwitz A, Simon A. Gonadotropin-releasing hormone (GnRH)-antagonist versus GnRH-agonist in ovarian stimulation of poor responders undergoing IVF. *J Assist Reprod Genet*. 2003; 20(11):455–60.

147. Mahutte NG, Arici A. Role of gonadotropin-releasing hormone antagonists in poor responders. *Fertil Steril*. 2007; 87(2):241–9. Epub 2006 Nov 16.

148. Akman MA, Erden HF, Tosun SB, Bayazit N, Aksoy E, Bahceci M. Addition of GnRH antagonist in cycles of poor responders undergoing IVF. *Hum Reprod*. 2000;15(10):2145–7.

149. Cheung LP, Lam PM, Lok IH, Chiu TT, Yeung SY, Tjer CC, Haines CJ. GnRH antagonist versus long GnRH agonist protocol in poor responders undergoing IVF: a randomized controlled trial. *Hum Reprod*. 2005;20(3):616–21. Epub 2004 Dec 17.

150. Malmusi S, La Marca A, Giulini S, Xella S, Tagliasacchi D, Marsella T, Volpe A. Comparison of a gonadotropin-releasing hormone (GnRH) antagonist and GnRH agonist flare-up regimen in poor responders undergoing ovarian stimulation. *Fertil Steril*. 2005;84(2):402–6.

151. De Placido G, Mollo A, Clarizia R, Strina I, Conforti S, Alviggi C. Gonadotropin-releasing hormone (GnRH) antagonist plus recombinant luteinizing hormone vs. a standard GnRH agonist short protocol in patients at risk for poor ovarian response. *Fertil Steril*. 2006;85(1):247–50.

152. Griesinger G, Diedrich K, Tarlatzis BC, Kolibianakis EM. GnRH-antagonists in ovarian stimulation for IVF in patients with poor response to gonadotrophins, polycystic ovary syndrome, and risk of ovarian hyperstimulation: a meta-analysis. *Reprod Biomed Online*. 2006;13(5):628–38.

153. Franco JG Jr, Baruffi RL, Mauri AL, Petersen CG, Felipe V, Cornicelli J, Cavagna M, Oliveira JB. GnRH agonist versus GnRH antagonist in poor ovarian responders: a meta-analysis. *Reprod Biomed Online*. 2006;13(5):618–27.

154. Frankfurter D, Dayal M, Dubey A, Peak D, Gindoff P. Novel follicular-phase gonadotropin-releasing hormone antagonist stimulation protocol for in vitro fertilization in the poor responder. *Fertil Steril*. 2007. Epub ahead of print.

155. D'Amato G, Caroppo E, Pasquadibisceglie A, Carone D, Vitti A, Vizziello GM. A novel protocol of ovulation induction with delayed gonadotropin-releasing hormone antagonist administration combined with high-dose recombinant follicle-stimulating hormone and clomiphene citrate for poor responders and women over 35 years. *Fertil Steril*. 2004;81(6): 1572–7.

156. Fisch JD, Keskintepe L, Sher G. Gonadotropin-releasing hormone agonist/antagonist conversion with estrogen priming in low responders with prior in vitro fertilization failure. *Fertil Steril*. 2007. Epub ahead of print.

157. Dragisic KG, Davis OK, Fasouliotis SJ, Rosenwaks Z. Use of a luteal estradiol patch and a gonadotropin-releasing hormone antagonist suppression protocol before gonadotropin stimulation for in vitro fertilization in poor responders. *Fertil Steril*. 2005;84(4):1023–6.

158. Bassil S, Godin PA, Donnez J. Outcome of in-vitro fertilization through natural cycles in poor responders. *Hum Reprod*. 1999;14(5):1262–5. CCT – Our findings demonstrate that an encouraging number of pregnancies can be achieved by IVF during natural cycles in poor responders to ovarian stimulation.

159. Feldman B, Seidman DS, Levron J, Bider D, Shulman A, Shine S, Dor J. In vitro fertilization following natural cycles in poor responders. *Gynecol Endocrinol*. 2001;15(5):328–34. CCT—We conclude that poor responders are a unique group of patients who may benefit from natural-cycle IVF treatment.

160. Morgia F, Sbracia M, Schimberni M, Giallonardo A, Piscitelli C, Giannini P, Aragona C. A controlled trial of natural cycle versus microdose gonadotropin-releasing hormone analog flare cycles in poor responders undergoing in vitro fertilization. *Fertil Steril*. 2004;81(6):1542–7. (RCT) In poor responders.

161. Elizur SE, Aslan D, Shulman A, Weisz B, Bider D, Dor J. Modified natural cycle using GnRH antagonist can be an optional treatment in poor responders undergoing IVF. *J Assist Reprod Genet*. 2005;22(2):75–9. Retrospective study.

162. Frydman R. [GnRH antagonists in natural cycles]. [Article in French]. *J Gynecol Obstet Biol Reprod (Paris)*. 2004;33(6 Pt. 2): 3S46–9.

163. Kolibianakis E, Zikopoulos K, Camus M, Tournaye H, Van Steirteghem A, Devroey P. Modified natural cycle for IVF does not offer a realistic chance of parenthood in poor responders with high day 3 FSH levels, as a last resort prior to oocyte donation. *Hum Reprod*. 2004;19(11):2545–9. Epub 2004 Oct 7.

164. Gonen Y, Jacobson W, Casper RF. Gonadotropin suppression with oral contraceptives before in vitro fertilization. *Fertil Steril*. 1990;53(2):282–7.

165. Lindheim SR, Barad DH, Witt B, Ditkoff E, Sauer MV. Short-term gonadotropin suppression with oral contraceptives benefits poor responders prior to controlled ovarian hyperstimulation. *J Assist Reprod Genet*. 1996;13(9):745–7.

166. Fisch B, Royburt M, Pinkas H, Avrech OM, Goldman GA, Bar J, Tadir Y, Ovadia J. Augmentation of low ovarian response to superovulation before in vitro fertilization following priming with contraceptive pills. *Isr J Med Sci*. 1996;32(12): 1172–6.

167. al-Mizyen E, Sabatini L, Lower AM, Wilson CM, al-Shawaf T, Grudzinskas JG. Does pretreatment with progestogen or oral contraceptive pills in low responders followed by the GnRHa

flare protocol improve the outcome of IVF-ET? *J Assist Reprod Genet.* 2000;17(3):140–6.

168. Kovacs P, Barg PE, Witt BR. Hypothalamic-pituitary suppression with oral contraceptive pills does not improve outcome in poor responder patients undergoing in vitro fertilization-embryo transfer cycles. *J Assist Reprod Genet.* 2001;18(7):391–4.

169. Bendikson K, Milki AA, Speck-Zulak A, Westphal LM. Comparison of GnRH antagonist cycles with and without oral contraceptive pretreatment in potential poor prognosis patients. *Clin Exp Obstet Gynecol.* 2006;33(3):145–7.

170. Keltz MD, Gera PS, Skorupski J, Stein DE. Comparison of FSH flare with and without pretreatment with oral contraceptive pills in poor responders undergoing in vitro fertilization. *Fertil Steril.* 2007;88(2):350–3.

171. Barmat LI, Chantilis SJ, Hurst BS, Dickey RP. A randomized prospective trial comparing gonadotropin-releasing hormone (GnRH) antagonist/recombinant follicle-stimulating hormone (rFSH) versus GnRH-agonist/rFSH in women pretreated with oral contraceptives before in vitro fertilization.

172. Balasch J, Fábregues F, Peñarrubia J, Carmona F, Casamitjana R, Creus M, Manau D, Casals G, Vanrell JA. Pretreatment with transdermal testosterone may improve ovarian response to gonadotrophins in poor-responder IVF patients with normal basal concentrations of FSH. *Hum Reprod.* 2006;21(7):1884–93. Epub 2006 Mar 3.

173. Massin N, Cedrin-Durnerin I, Coussieu C, Galey-Fontaine J, Wolf JP, Hugues JN. Effects of transdermal testosterone application on the ovarian response to FSH in poor responders undergoing assisted reproduction technique—a prospective, randomized, double-blind study. *Hum Reprod.* 2006;21(5):1204–11. Epub 2006 Feb 13.

174. Casson PR, Lindsay MS, Pisarska MD, Carson SA, Buster JE. Dehydroepiandrosterone supplementation augments ovarian stimulation in poor responders: a case series. *Hum Reprod.* 2000;15(10):2129–32.

175. Barad D, Gleicher N. Effect of dehydroepiandrosterone on oocyte and embryo yields, embryo grade and cell number in IVF. *Hum Reprod.* 2006;21(11):2845–9.

176. Awonuga AO, Nabi A. In vitro fertilization with low-dose clomiphene citrate stimulation in women who respond poorly to superovulation. *J Assist Reprod Genet.* 1997;14(9):503–7.

177. Benadiva CA, Davis O, Kligman I, Liu HC, Rosenwaks Z. Clomiphene citrate and hMG: an alternative stimulation protocol for selected failed in vitro fertilization patients. *J Assist Reprod Genet.* 1995;12(1):8–12.

178. D'Amato G, Caroppo E, Pasquadibisceglie A, Carone D, Vitti A, Vizziello GM. A novel protocol of ovulation induction with delayed gonadotropin-releasing hormone antagonist administration combined with high-dose recombinant follicle-stimulating hormone and clomiphene citrate for poor responders and women over 35 years. *Fertil Steril.* 2004;81(6):1572–7.

179. Ashrafi M, Ashtiani SK, Zafarani F, Samani RO, Eshrati B. Evaluation of ovulation induction protocols for poor responders undergoing assisted reproduction techniques. *Saudi Med J.* 2005;26(4):593–6.

180. Homburg R, West C, Torresani T, Jacobs HS. Co-treatment with human growth hormone and gonadotropins for induction of ovulation: a controlled clinical trial. *Fertil Steril.* 1990;53(2):254–60.

181. Bergh C, Carlstrom K, Selleskog U, Hillensjo T. Effect of growth hormone on follicular fluid androgen levels in patients treated with gonadotropins before in vitro fertilization. *Eur J Endocrinol.* 1996;134(2):190–6.

182. Orvieto R, Homburg R, Farhi J, Bar-Hava I, Ben-Rafael Z. A new concept of cotreatment with human growth hormone and menotropins in ovulation induction protocols. *Med Hypotheses.* 1997;49(5):413–15.

183. Ibrahim ZH, Matson PL, Buck P, Lieberman BA. The use of biosynthetic human growth hormone to augment ovulation induction with buserelin acetate/human menopausal gonadotropin in women with a poor ovarian response. *Fertil Steril.* 1991;55(1):202–4.

184. Wu MY, Chen HF, Ho HN, Chen SU, Chao KH, Huang SC, Lee TY, Yang YS. The value of human growth hormone as an adjuvant for ovarian stimulation in a human in vitro fertilization program. *J Obstet Gynaecol Res.* 1996;22(5):443–50.

185. Shaker AG, Fleming R, Jamieson ME, Yates RW, Coutts JR. Absence of effect of adjuvant growth hormone therapy on follicular responses to exogenous gonadotropins in women: normal and poor responders. *Fertil Steril.* 1992;58(5):919–23.

186. Levy T, Limor R, Villa Y, Eshel A, Eckstein N, Vagman I, Lidor A, Ayalon D. Another look at co-treatment with growth hormone and human menopausal gonadotrophins in poor ovarian responders. *Hum Reprod.* 1993;8(6):834–9.

187. Bergh C, Hillensjö T, Wikland M, Nilsson L, Borg G, Hamberger L. Adjuvant growth hormone treatment during in vitro fertilization: a randomized, placebo-controlled study. *Fertil Steril.* 1994;62(1):113–20.

188. Hughes SM, Huang ZH, Morris ID, Matson PL, Buck P, Lieberman BA. A double-blind cross-over controlled study to evaluate the effect of human biosynthetic growth hormone on ovarian stimulation in previous poor responders to in-vitro fertilization. *Hum Reprod.* 1994;9(1):13–8.

189. Dor J, Seidman DS, Amudai E, Bider D, Levran D, Mashiach S. Adjuvant growth hormone therapy in poor responders to in-vitro fertilization: a prospective randomized placebo-controlled double-blind study. *Hum Reprod.* 1995;10(1):40–3.

190. Suikkari A, MacLachlan V, Koistinen R, Seppala M, Healy D. Double-blind placebo controlled study: human biosynthetic growth hormone for assisted reproductive technology. *Fertil Steril.* 1996;65(4):800–5.

191. Harper K, Proctor M, Hughes E. Growth hormone for in vitro fertilization. *Coch Database Syst Rev.* 2003;(3):CD000099.

192. Guan Q, Ma HG, Wang YY, Zhang F. [Effects of co-administration of growth hormone(GH) and aspirin to women during in vitro fertilization and embryo transfer (IVF-ET) cycles]. [Article in Chinese]. *Zhonghua Nan Ke Xue.* 2007;13(9):798–800.

193. Lok IH, Yip SK, Cheung LP, Yin Leung PH, Haines CJ. Adjuvant low-dose aspirin therapy in poor responders undergoing in vitro fertilization: a prospective, randomized, double-blind, placebo-controlled trial. *Fertil Steril.* 2004;81(3):556–61.

194. Frattarelli JL, McWilliams GD, Hill MJ, Miller KA, Scott RT Jr. Low-dose aspirin use does not improve in vitro fertilization outcomes in poor responders. *Fertil Steril.* 2007. Epub ahead of print.

195. Mitwally MF, Casper RF. Aromatase inhibition improves ovarian response to follicle-stimulating hormone in poor responders. *Fertil Steril.* 2002;77(4):776–80.

196. Goswami SK, Das T, Chattopadhyay R, Sawhney V, Kumar J, Chaudhury K, Chakravarty BN, Kabir SN. A randomized single-blind controlled trial of letrozole as a low-cost IVF protocol in women with poor ovarian response: a preliminary report. *Hum Reprod.* 2004;19(9):2031–5. Epub 2004 Jun 24.

197. Schoolcraft WB, Surrey ES, Minjarez DA, Stevens JM, Gardner DK. Management of poor responders: can outcomes be improved with a novel gonadotropin-releasing hormone antagonist/letrozole protocol? *Fertil Steril.* 2007; Epub ahead of print.

198. Keay SD. Poor ovarian response to gonadotrophin stimulation the role of adjuvant treatments. *Hum Fertil (Camb).* 2002;5(1 Suppl.):S46–52.

199. Tarlatzis BC, Zepiridis L, Grimbizis G, Bontis J. Clinical management of low ovarian response to stimulation for IVF: a systematic review. *Hum Reprod Update.* 2003;9(1):61–76.

200. Shanbhag S, Aucott L, Bhattacharya S, Hamilton MA, McTavish AR. Interventions for 'poor responders' to controlled ovarian hyperstimulation (COH) in in-vitro fertilisation IVF). *Coch Database Syst Rev.* 2007;(1):CD004379. Review.

201. Devroey P, Wisanto A, Camus M, Van Waesberghe L, Bourgain C, Liebaers I, Van Steirteghem AC. Oocyte donation in patients without ovarian function. *Hum Reprod.* 1988;3(6): 699–704.

202. Kolibianakis E, Zikopoulos K, Camus M, Tournaye H, Van Steirteghem A, Devroey P. Modified natural cycle for IVF does not offer a realistic chance of parenthood in poor responders with high day 3 FSH levels, as a last resort prior to oocyte donation. *Hum Reprod.* 2004;19(11):2545–9. Epub 2004 Oct 7.

48

OOCYTE DONATION

E. Bosch, S. Reis, J. Domingo, J. Remohí

INTRODUCTION

Oocyte donation (OD) is defined as the assisted reproduction technique (ART) in which the female gamete is provided by a different woman than the one who will receive it or the resulting embryo. Its diffusion has grown progressively due to both its excellent results and the increase of its indications, ranging from the initial indication of premature ovarian failure (POF) (1, 2) to a number of possibilities that are detailed in Table 48.1.

In the Instituto Valenciano de Inferrtilidad (IVI), age of patients (35 percent), background of low response to gonadotropin stimulation (21 percent), and POF (18 percent) are the three most frequent indications of OD (Figure 48.1).

OOCYTE DONORS

According to Spanish legislation, donated oocytes can have different origins:

1. Women willing to donate their oocytes in an altruistic way.
2. Patients with high response to gonadotropin stimulation for in vitro fertilization (IVF) who donate part of the recovered oocytes.
   - Donation must be anonymous and lacking of any lucrative or commercial character.
   - Age of oocyte donors is limited to be between eighteen and thirty-five years old.
   - Oocyte donors must be on healthy physical and psychological condition. They must not have any of personal or familiar background of genetically transmittable disease.
   - All women willing to donate their oocytes must have negative blood evaluation of syphilis, toxoplasm, rubella, chlamydia, CMV, hepatitis B and C, and HIV (3).
   - Negative vaginal culture.
   - In our clinic, we also include blood test for discharging cystic fibrosis mutation and fragile X syndrome and karyotyping.
   - It is the responsibility of the institution to match donors and recipients as much as possible, according to blood groups, phenotype, and physical characteristics in general (4).

RESULTS OF OOCYTE DONATION

During the decade of the 1990s, OD has become a successful ART for treating couples that had very low prognosis through other techniques. Pregnancy rates obtained with OD are the highest when compared to any other ART (5). In the IVI groups clinics, 3,851 OD cycles were performed during 2006, with a total of 3,462 embryo transfers (Table 48.2).

Our policy is to perform OD with a sufficient number of oocytes to ensure the transfer of good quality embryos. When compared to results previously reported, there has been a significant reduction in the mean number of embryos transferred (from 4.3 to 2.1), without affecting pregnancy rates, but diminishing dramatically multiple pregnancy rates. This is the trend in the majority of first-line reproduction centers, and it has been possible through the increase of implantation rates due to the improvement in culture conditions.

An added risk of OD is unnoticed cosanguinity. To minimize it, the number of newborns coming from a particular donor is limited. The development of international regulations could further reduce this risk in the future.

LESSONS LEARNED FROM OOCYTE DONATION

The relative inaccessibility of female gametes and the difficulty on the synchronization of the ovulatory cycle of the donor with the endometrial cycle of the recipient have delayed OD almost one century with respect to sperm donation. Nevertheless, once these problems have been solved, OD has grown exponentially in a very short lap of time. OD is not only the solution for many infertile couples but also a reference model for obtaining useful knowledge of the physiology of reproduction and consequently to be applied in other ART. The possibility of evaluating separately ovarian and uterine function allows to elucidate the relationship of different variables with both components of the reproductive system.

Oocyte Recovery in Donors

One of the controversies regarding ovarian stimulation for IVF regards the impact that successive cycles could have on oocyte recovery in terms of quality and quantity of the obtained oocytes. In this sense, our group evaluated the effect of successive ovarian stimulation cycles in oocyte donors on the number of obtained oocytes, fertilization rate, embryo development,

Table 48.1: Indications for Oocyte Donation

Women without ovarian function

   Primary ovarian failure: Swyer syndrome, Turner syndrome

   Premature ovarian failure: autoimmune, iatrogenic, metabolic, infectious

   Menopause

Women with ovarian function

   Genetic or chromosomal alterations

   Repeated IVF-ICSI failure:
   low response, poor
   oocyte quality, implantation failure

   Women younger
   than forty years

   Recurrent pregnancy loss

   Unaccessible ovaries
   for ovum pickup:
   severe adhesion pelvis disease

Table 48.2: General Results of Oocyte Donation Program of IVI Team in 2006

Cycles with embryo transfer	3,462
Mean age of recipient	40
Mean number of embryos transferred	1.99
Pregnancies (%)	59.4
Implantation (%)	35.7

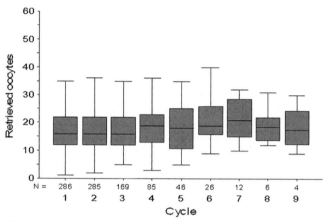

Figure 48.2. Oocyte recovery after successive ovarian stimulation cycles in oocyte donors.

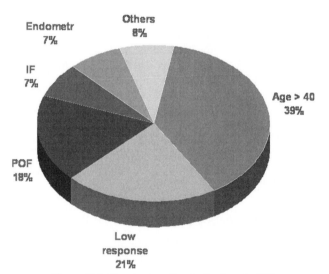

Figure 48.1. Oocyte donation indications in IVI.

and implantation and pregnancy rates (6). No significant differences were observed in any of these variables, depending on the ordinal cycle evaluated (Figure 48.2; Table 48.3). In a similar study performed on the different type of patients, a progressive decrease in ovarian response was observed in patients with endometriosis, while patients with tubal infertility showed similar ovarian response across the cycle, as we observed in oocyte donors (7).

   These data reflect that ovarian stimulation with high doses of FSH allows the rescue of follicles that were destined to atresia, and there is no accelerated decline of ovarian reserve. Therefore, there is no detrimental effect on follicular population, neither is there a progressive ovarian resistance to gonadotrophin stimulation. Oocyte quality, according to fertilization rate, embryo morphology, and implantation and pregnancy

rates, does not change because of repeating cycles of ovarian stimulation (6) (Table 48.3).

Factors Influencing Embryo Implantation

Age of Recipient

   The effect of the age of the recipient on uterine receptivity has been evaluated using the OD model, with controversial results (8–12). There is no agreement in the literature due to the performance of studies with too small sample sizes to detect differences among age-groups. In 2002, a retrospective study of data of OD donation cycles performed in the United States showed that implantation and pregnancy rates were maintained until the age of forty-five and that they declined significantly after that age (sharper after the age of fifty). It was also observed that there was a trend of an increase in miscarriage incidences in these age ranges (13). This study was strongly powered due to the enormous sample size (more than 17,000 cases), but it was lacking control of the protocols and information used as it often happens in multicentre studies.

   In 2005, our group published data from the longest series reported from a single center regarding age of recipient and OD results (more than 3,000 cycles) (14). The potential sources of bias were controlled through the strict definition of a uniform group of patients, excluding cases with severe male factor, including a unique protocol of endometrial preparation, and controlling for the quality and the number of embryos

Table 48.3: Recipients Outcome after Five Consecutive Stimulation Cycles in Oocyte Donors

Variables	Cycle 1	Cycle 2	Cycle 3	Cycle 4	Cycle 5	p value
Fertilization (%)	77.9 ± 18.3	77.2 ± 17	81.8 ± 17.2	78.7 ± 15.0	72.6 ± 21	NS
Mean of blastomeres on day 2	2.9 ± 0.5	2.9 ± 0.5	3.0 ± 0.5	3.1 ± 0.7	3.0 ± 0.6	NS
Embryo fragmentation degree	1.5 ± 0.4	1.6 ± 0.5	1.6 ± 0.4	1.8 ± 0.5	1.8 ± 0.4	NS
Mean of embryos transferred	3.0 ± 1.1	3.4 ± 0.9	3.0 ± 1.1	3.2 ± 1.0	2.9 ± 1.2	NS
Implantation rate (%)	23.9 ± 28.1	26.5 ± 21.6	32.3 ± 34.1	25.1 ± 25.4	30.7 ± 38.3	NS
Pregnancy rate (%)	35.5 ± 40.3	47.0 ± 38.4	35.1 ± 38.3	43.1 ± 41.7	42.7 ± 39.4	NS

Table 48.4: Oocyte Donation Outcome according to Recipients' Age

	Age-group (years)	
	Less than forty-five	Greater than or equal to forty-five
Number of cycles	2,683	406
Donors' age[a]	2.0 ± 4.3	25.5 ± 4.2
Pregnancy rate (%)[b]	49.8 (1.333/2.683)	44.4 (180/406)
Implantation rate (%)[c]	20.7 (1.555/7.512)	16.8 (191/1.137)
Miscarriage rate (%)[d]	16.8 (224/1.333)	23.3 (42/180)
Mean number of embryos transferred[a]	2.8 ± 0.7	2.8 ± 0.7
Mean number of good-quality embryos transferred[a]	1.6 ± 0.6	1.7 ± 0.5
Duration of endometrial preparation (weeks)[a]	5.1 ± 2.5	5.0 ± 2.5

[a]NS.
[b]$p = 0.045$.
[c]$p = 0.02$.
[d]$p = 0.03$.

transferred. Our results were similar to those observed in the above-mentioned multicentre study, showing undoubtedly that implantation, pregnancy, and miscarriage rates were significantly worse after the age of forty-five (Table 48.4).

Body Mass Index (BMI)

Most of the studies that have analyzed IVF results in patients with high BMI agree that obese patients show lower success rates with this kind of treatments (15–18).

Some authors have evaluated the impact of a uterine factor in these lower results, analyzing the relationship between BMI and OD outcome. Two studies did not observe any significant association between these two variables. In the first of them, only ninety-six OD cycles were included, and patients were divided into four BMI groups, and the only analyzed variable was implantation rate (19). The second one of these studies included a considerably higher number of cycles ($n = 536$) (20). Authors reported general pregnancy, implantation, and miscarriage rates higher than those that usually appear in literature (73, 54, and 23 percent, respectively). Miscarriage rate in obese patients was 29.8 and increased to 45.0 percent when day 3 embryo transfers were analyzed.

We have analyzed this issue in a large series of 2,597 OD cycles, in which other miscarriage risk factors were excluded. We observed a trend to lower implantation and pregnancy rates, and higher miscarriage rates in obese patients, leading to a significant diminished ongoing pregnancy rate in patients with BMI 30 kg/m or greater (2, 21). These data suggest that BMI determines a clinically relevant decreased uterine receptivity.

Smoking

Although the negative impact of smoking on female fertility is well known, in both natural and IVF cycles (22–26), the association between cigarette consuming and uterine receptivity has not been analyzed.

We have recently published the impact of smoking in the probability of recipients' pregnancy. Data from 785 OD embryo transfers were analyzed (27). All potential confounding variables were controlled, such as male and oocyte-donor smoking, recipient's BMI, duration of endometrial preparation, and number and quality of the transferred embryos. Recipients that smoked more than ten cigarettes per day obtained significantly lower pregnancy rate (34.1 vs 52.2 percent), although twin pregnancy rate was significantly higher in this subgroup of patients (60.0 vs 31.0 percent). This surprising paradox has led to analyze the hypothesis that smoking could display different endometrial gene profile among patients. Further studies are currently being conducted to elucidate this issue.

Endometriosis

IVF outcome in patients with endometriosis is clearly poorer compared to those obtained in patients without this pathology (28, 29). All parameters are negatively affected and show the impact of endometriosis on ovarian reserve and oocyte quality. Nevertheless, the lower implantation rate could be also related to an endometrial factor.

Endometriosis could affect uterine receptivity through alteration of the local environment by means of endocrine and paracrine mechanisms or due to changes in immune response.

Several studies have demonstrated that serum and peritoneal fluid of women with endometriosis have altered levels of cytokines and growth factors (30–32). In contrast, luteal phase deficiency has also been described in this type of patients (33, 34) and a higher incidence of alterations in cell and humoral immunity compared to other infertile patients has also been observed (32).

Despite the above-mentioned data, OD cycles have consistently shown that outcome in patients with endometriosis is similar to those obtained in general population: pregnancy, implantation, miscarriage, and delivery rates are not different from the rest of infertile patients. This could be explained because of the following:

1. None of the previously described alterations affects uterine receptivity.
2. Protocols of endometrial preparation for OF restore uterine cavity environment.

In this sense, it is interesting to notice that there is some "in vivo" and "in vitro" evidence (35, 36) that GnRH analogs could have a positive effect on the physiology of endometrial cells of patients with endometriosis (33, 34, 37–39). Moreover, the substitutive hormonal therapy with estrogens and progesterone could compensate the luteal deficiency described in these patients.

REFERENCES

1. Trouson A, Leeton J, Besako M et al. Pregnancy established in an infertile patient after transfer of a donated embryo fertilized in vitro. *Br Med J* 1983;286:835–8.
2. Lutjen P, Trouson A, Leeton J et al. The establishment and maintenance of pregnancy using in vitro fertilization and embryo donation in a patient with primary ovarian failure. *Nature* 1984;307:104–5.
3. World Health Organization. Guidelines for gamete donation. *Fertil Steril* 1993;59:5–9s.
4. Ley 35/1988, de 33 de noviembre, sobre Técnicas de Reproducción Asistida. BOE núm. 282. Jueves, 24 de noviembre de 1988. 33373–8.
5. Remohí J, Gartner B, Gallardo E et al. Pregnancy and birth rates after oocyte donation. *Fertil Steril* 1997;67:717–23.
6. Caligara C, Navarro J, Vargas G et al. The effect of repeated controlled ovarian stimulation in donors. *Hum Reprod* 2001;16:2320–3.
7. Al-Azemi M, Bernal AL, Steele J. Ovarian response to repeated controlled stimulations in in-vitro fertilization cycles in patients with ovarian endometriosis. *Hum Reprod* 2000;15:72–5.
8. Yaron Y, Ochshorn Y, Amit A et al. Oocyte donation in Israel: a study of 1001 initiated treatment cycles. *Hum Reprod* 1998; 13:1819–24.
9. Moomjy M, Cholst I, Mangieri R et al. Oocyte donation: insights into implantation. *Fertil Steril* 1999;71:15–21.
10. Legro RS, Wong IL, Paulson RJ et al. Recipient's age does not adversely affect pregnancy outcome after oocyte donation. *Am J Obstet Gynecol* 1995;172:96–100.
11. Paulson RJ, Hatch IE, Lobo RA et al. Cumulative conception and live birth rates after oocyte donation: implications regarding endometrial receptivity. *Hum Reprod* 1997;12:835–9.
12. Noyes N, Hampton BS, Berkeley A et al. Factors useful in predicting the success of oocyte donation: a 3-year retrospective analysis. *Fertil Steril* 2001;76:92–7.
13. Toner JP, Grainger DA, Frazier LM. Clinical outcomes among recipients of donated eggs: an analysis of the U.S. national experience, 1996–1998. *Fertil Steril* 2002;78:1038–45.
14. Soares SR, Troncoso C, Bosch E et al. Age and uterine receptiveness: predicting the outcome of oocyte donation cycles. *J Clin Endocrinol Metab* 2005;90:4399–404.
15. Fedorcsak P, Dale PO, Storeng R et al. The impact of obesity and insulin resistance on the outcome of IVF or ICSI in women with polycystic ovarian syndrome. *Hum Reprod* 2001;16:1086–91.
16. Nichols JE, Crane MM, Higdon HL et al. Extremes of body mass index reduce in vitro fertilization pregnancy rates. *Fertil Steril* 2003;79:645–7.
17. Fedorcsak P, Dale PO, Storeng R et al. Impact of overweight and underweight on assisted reproduction treatment. *Hum Reprod* 2004;19:2523–8.
18. Van Swieten EC, van der Leeuw-Harmsen L, Badings EA et al. Obesity and clomiphene challenge test as predictors of outcome of in vitro fertilization and intracytoplasmic sperm injection. *Gynecol Obstet Invest* 2005;59:220–4.
19. Wattanakumtornkul S, Damario MA, Stevens Hall SA et al. Body mass index and uterine receptivity in the oocyte donation model. *Fertil Steril* 2003;80:336–40.
20. Styne-Gross A, Elkind-Hirsch K, Scott RT Jr. Obesity does not impact implantation rates or pregnancy outcome in women attempting conception through oocyte donation. *Fertil Steril* 2005;83:1629–34.
21. Bellver J, Melo M, Bosch E et al. Obesity and poor reproductive outcome: the subtle role of the endometrium. *Fertil Steril* 2007. In press.
22. Augood C, Duckitt K, Templeton AA. Smoking and female infertility: a systematic review and meta-analysis. *Hum Reprod* 1998;13:1532–9.
23. Jick H, Porter J, Morrison AS. Relation between smoking and age of natural menopause. Report from the Boston Collaborative Drug Surveillance Program, Boston University Medical Center. *Lancet* 1977;309:1354–5.
24. Crha I, Hruba D, Fiala J et al. The outcome of infertility treatment by in-vitro fertilisation in smoking and non-smoking women. *Cent Eur J Public Health* 2001;9:64–8.
25. Klonoff-Cohen H, Natarajan L, Marrs R et al. Effects of female and male smoking on success rates of IVF and gamete intrafallopian transfer. *Hum Reprod* 2001;16:1382–90.
26. El-Nemr A, Al-Shawaf T, Sabatini L et al. Effect of smoking on ovarian reserve and ovarian stimulation in in-vitro fertilization and embryo transfer. *Hum Reprod* 1998;13:2192–8.
27. Soares SR, Simon C, Remohi J et al. Cigarette smoking affects uterine receptiveness. *Hum Reprod*. E-pub 2006 Nov 9.
28. Barnhart K, Dunsmoor-Su R, Coutifaris C. Effect of endometriosis on in vitro fertilization. *Fertil Steril* 2002;77:1148–55.
29. Kuivasaari P, Hippeläinen M, Anttila M et al. Effect of endometriosis on IVF/ICSI outcome: stage III/IV endometriosis worsens cumulative pregnancy and live-born rates. *Hum Reprod* 2005;20:3130–5.
30. Sharpe-Timms K, Keisler LW, McIntush EW et al. Tissue inhibitor of metalloproteinase-1 concentrations are attenuated in peritoneal fluid and sera of women with endometriosis and restored in sera by gonadotropin-releasing hormone agonist therapy. *Fertil Steril* 1998;69:1128–34.

31. Taketani Y, Kuo TM, Mizuno M. Comparison of cytokine levels and embryo toxicity in peritoneal fluid in infertile women with untreated or treated endometriosis. *Am J Obstet Gynecol* 1992; 167:265–70.

32. Ulukus M, Arici A. Immunology of endometriosis. *Minerva Ginecol* 2005;57:237–48.

33. Cunha-Filho JS, Gross JL, Bastos de Souza CA et al. Physiopathological aspects of corpus luteum defect in infertile patients with mild/minimal endometriosis. *J Assist Reprod Genet* 2003;20:117–21.

34. Ayers JW, Birenbaum DL, Menon KM. Luteal phase dysfunction in endometriosis: elevated progesterone levels in peripheral and ovarian veins during the follicular phase. *Fertil Steril* 1987;47: 925–9.

35. Surrey ES, Silverberg KM, Surrey M *et al.* Effect of prolonged gonadotropin-releasing hormone agonist therapy on the outcome of in vitro fertilization-embryo transfer in patients with endometriosis. *Fertil Steril* 2002;78:699–704.

36. Sallam H, Garcia-Velasco J, Dias S et al. Long-term pituitary down-regulation before in vitro fertilization (IVF) for women with endometriosis. *Cochrane Database Syst Rev* 2006;25(1):CD004635.

37. Simón C, Gutiérrez A, Vidal A et al. Outcome of patients with endometriosis in assisted reproduction: results from in-vitro fertilization and oocyte donation. *Hum Reprod* 1994;9: 725–9.

38. Sung L, Mukherjee T, Takeshige T et al. Endometriosis is not detrimental to embryo implantation in oocyte recipients. *J Assist Reprod Genet* 1997;14:152–6.

39. Díaz I, Navarro J, Blasco L et al. Impact of stage III-IV endometriosis on recipients of sibling oocytes: matched case-control study. *Fertil Steril* 2000;74:31–4.

40. Imai A, Takagi A, Tamaya T. Gonadotropin-releasing hormone analog repairs reduced endometrial cell apoptosis in endometriosis in vitro. *Am J Obstet Gynecol* 2000;182:1142–6.

49

In Vitro Maturation of Human Oocytes

Ezgi Demirtas, Hananel Holzer, Shai Elizur, Yariv Gidoni, Ri-Cheng Chian, Seang Lin Tan

DEVELOPMENT OF IN VITRO MATURATION

The history of in vitro maturation (IVM) of oocytes goes back to as far as the 1930s (1) to Pincus, Enzman, and Saunders who studied the maturation of mammalian oocytes including human oocytes in vivo and in vitro (1, 2). Pincus and his colleagues observed that when oocytes were removed from the follicles and cultured in the laboratory without hormones, they spontaneously resumed meiosis and progressed to the mature stage, metaphase II (MII), as they do in vivo. In 1965, Edwards (3, 4) described the kinetics of in vitro oocyte maturation both in animals – mice, sheep, cows, pigs, and rhesus monkeys – and in humans. He introduced tissue culture medium 199 (TCM-199) for IVM and showed that meiosis is resumed in 80 percent of immature oocytes independent of cycle day and gonadotropin support. He subsequently concluded that "human oocytes can be fertilized after maturation in-vitro."

In 1983, Veeck et al. reported two pregnancies resulting from in vitro matured oocytes (5). These morphologically immature oocytes were recovered from human menopausal gonadotropin and/or follicle-stimulating hormone (FSH) and human chorionic gonadotropin (hCG) primed cycles in an in vitro fertilization (IVF) program.

Cha et al. published the first birth resulting from the fertilization of in vitro matured oocytes, which were harvested from an unstimulated ovary on cycle day 13 in an oocyte donation program (6). They also mentioned in the same report that immature oocytes were recovered from unstimulated ovaries both in proliferative and secretory phases. In the following year, the same group published maturation and fertilization outcomes of immature oocytes recovered from women undergoing gynecologic surgery or cesarean section and reported that immature oocytes can be matured and fertilized in vitro and that secretory-phase immature oocytes had an even higher maturation rate (7). This group also reported live births resulting from the transfer of embryos generated from in vitro matured oocytes, which were recovered from oocyte donors during cesarean section.

In 1994, the first pregnancy in a woman with anovulatory infertility using her own immature oocytes was reported by Trounson et al. from Australia (8), and in 1995, the same group reported a further pregnancy in a woman with polycystic ovary syndrome (PCOS) through the use of IVM combined with intracytoplasmic sperm injection (ICSI), assisted hatching, and blastocyst culture (9). Trounson et al. placed IVM firmly in the clinical realm when they developed an outpatient technique for immature oocyte retrieval using a specially designed aspiration needle manipulated under transvaginal USG guidance (8).

Clinical Need for IVM and Advantages

Since the birth of the first IVF baby in 1978 (10), assisted reproductive technologies (ART) have helped thousands of couples to have children through the use of ovarian stimulation (11). However, certain risks are associated with IVF, the most important one being ovarian hyperstimulation syndrome (OHSS), which is a potentially life-threatening condition associated with ovarian stimulation. Women with polycystic ovaries (PCO) and/or PCOS undergoing IVF have an increased risk of OHSS from ovarian stimulation with gonadotropins compared to women with normal ovaries (12). Severe OHSS affects 1–2 percent of all women undergoing ART and up to 6 percent of women with PCO or PCOS (13). The only way to eliminate the risk of OHSS is to avoid ovarian stimulation altogether (14). Furthermore, ovarian stimulation is an expensive treatment, especially due to the high cost of gonadotropin preparations. Patients must also be meticulously monitored by repeated ultrasonography with serum estradiol measurement, which also adds to the cost of treatment. Other disadvantages of ovarian stimulation include the inconvenience of daily injections and symptoms such as bloating, breast tenderness, and nausea. All these factors can be major deterrents to potential oocyte donors, who may decline due to the inherent risks involved (15). IVM of oocytes seems to provide a good alternative as it eliminates the risk of OHSS syndrome, simplifies patient monitoring, reduces the cost of treatment, and results in fair pregnancy outcomes.

OOCYTE MATURATION: IN VIVO AND IN VITRO

In Vivo Maturation

Ovarian follicles begin their development as primordial structures, which consist of an oocyte arrested at the diplotene stage of the first meiotic division, surrounded by a few flattened granulosa cells (16). At birth, the oocytes remain in the prolonged resting phase and each ovary has around 500,000 healthy nongrowing or primordial follicles. At puberty, these follicles start growing gradually and continuously. During early development, the oocyte grows, granulosa cells proliferate, and primordial follicles transform into preantral follicles. Once the follicles reach a specific size, they form a fluid-filled space called the antrum and antral follicles are formed. For further development of the follicles, gonadotropins are required.

Oocyte maturation is defined as the reinitiation and completion of the first meiotic division from the germinal vesicle (GV) stage to metaphase II, with accompanying cytoplasmic maturation necessary for fertilization and early embryonic development (17).

Oocyte maturation in vivo is classically divided into two parts: nuclear and cytoplasmic maturation. Nuclear maturation of the oocytes can be divided into six specific mechanistic events (18):

1. *Meiotic resumption (GVBD).* Gonadotropins are required for oocyte maturation in vivo. Under the influence of FSH, the follicles develop from the early antral stage to the preovulatory stage. A surge of gonadotropins preceding ovulation releases the oocyte from its quiescent state and signals the reinitiation of meiosis, characterized by dissolution of the GV known as germinal vesicle breakdown (GVBD), and this swollen nucleus can easily be recognized under microscope.
2. *Chromatin condensation.* During completion of prophase of the first meiotic division, homologous chromosomes undergo a process of pairing and recombination, and then homologs condense for a reductional division.
3. *Formation of the meiotic spindle.* The bipolar meiotic spindle attaches to homolog chromosomes at their centromeres.
4. *Separation and segregation of homologs.* Physical contact between the homologs' ends and the alignment of the chromosomes along the metaphase plate occurs. Here, metaphase I is completed and homolog chromosomes are pulled toward opposite poles at the beginning of anaphase.
5. *Disproportionate cytokinesis/polar body extrusion.* The process continues with telophase and the first polar body is extruded by a disproportionate cytokinesis.
6. *Meiotic rearrest.* The oocyte remains in meiotic rearrest stage until fertilization occurs, and it is surrounded by closely associated granulosa cells, known as cumulus cells, forming the cumulus-oocyte complex (COC).

Cytoplasmic maturation refers to preparation of oocyte cytoplasm for fertilization and embryonic development. Cytoplasmic maturation includes relocation of organelles, synthesis and modification of proteins and mRNAs, proper storage and timely reactivation of molecules and biochemical processes essential for supplying building materials required for successful fertilization, and pronuclear formation (18).

Cumulus cells are important for oocyte maturation. They respond to gonadotropins and secrete various substances. Not only do these substances control nuclear maturation but they also perform an important role in cytoplasmic maturation (19). The protein synthesis pattern is different between oocytes with and without cumulus cells, and FSH modulates the protein synthesis patterns of cumulus cell–intact oocytes (20).

In Vitro Maturation

Once immature oocytes are recovered from the follicles, they are cultured with the surrounding cumulus cells in the maturation medium. Oocyte maturation in vitro is profoundly affected by culture conditions. Different media have been used for in vitro oocyte maturation. TCM-199 was introduced by Edwards (3, 4) and has most often been used as the in vitro oocyte maturation medium (8, 9, 21–24). Other media such as Ham's-F10 and Chang's medium buffered with bicarbonate or HEPES supplemented with serum, gonadotropins, and estradiol have also been used for IVM, but no one medium among these has clearly been shown to be superior to the others (25, 26). Based on animal studies, a new IVM medium was developed and shown to be beneficial for nuclear and cytoplasmic maturation of immature human oocytes derived from stimulated IVF and ICSI cycles (27).

IVM medium includes major beneficial components: different energy substrates (glucose, pyruvate, lactate, and amino acids), serum, gonadotropins, steroids, and growth factors. Gonadotropins are required for oocyte maturation in vivo; however, any requirement in vitro is unclear. Currently, most IVM media do supplement gonadotropins. The idea to use FSH and luteinizing hormone (LH) for IVM is based on the physiological role of FSH and LH in oocyte maturation in vivo. Although it is clear that the LH surge triggers the resumption of meiosis in vivo, COCs can be spontaneously induced to resume meiosis when they are released from follicles into the in vitro culture. The actions of the endocrine, paracrine, and autocrine factors that control oocyte maturation in vitro are mediated by the cumulus cells. Although FSH and LH play an important role in the development and maturation of preantral, antral, and preovulatory follicles in vivo, they may not serve the same function in promoting oocyte maturation in vitro. Most IVM applications are performed using oocytes from small follicles; however, these follicles are in many aspects different from preovulatory oocytes.

The presence of estradiol in the culture medium of immature oocytes has no effect on the progression of meiosis, but improves fertilization and cleavage rates (28). The ratio of progesterone to estradiol in follicular fluid may be an indicator of oocyte maturity (29); however, the role of progesterone in oocyte maturation is not fully understood. Culture medium supplemented with FSH and LH stimulates estrogen and progesterone secretions from the cultured granulosa and cumulus cells (30). Therefore, it is likely that one of the actions of gonadotropins is mediated by estrogen or progesterone, which may control oocyte maturation in vitro.

It is well known that many growth factors are contained in follicular fluid. These factors must be secreted from the cumulus cells that respond to gonadotropins and subsequently act on the oocyte via paracrine and autocrine pathways. Since oocytes are cultured with the surrounding cumulus cells for maturation in vitro, it seems that only denuded oocytes require the supplementation of growth factors in the culture medium (27). The culture medium is supplemented with human serum or serum albumin as a protein source, both of which are a rich source of growth factors. Therefore, it seems that there is no need for additional growth factors in the IVM culture medium.

DEVELOPMENTAL COMPETENCE OF ASPIRATED IMMATURE OOCYTES

Immature Oocytes from Unstimulated Cycles

In IVF treatment cycles, mature oocytes are recovered in the follicular phase. LH surge is avoided by the use of GnRH agonists or antagonists. Oocyte retrieval in IVM cycles is also largely performed in the follicular phase in routine practice. It was advocated that the selection of a dominant follicle may induce endocrine changes in the remaining cohort that may be detrimental to their subsequent fertilization and embryonic development (31); therefore, in the past ten years, oocyte retrievals were largely performed before the dominant follicle reached 10 mm. However, the size of follicles may be important for subsequent embryonic development, but it appears that the developmental competence of the oocytes derived from the small antral follicles is not adversely affected by the presence of a dominant follicle (32). It seems that atresia does not occur in the nondominant follicles even after the dominant follicle is selected during folliculogenesis. Immature oocytes retrieved from nondominant follicles have been successfully matured in vitro and fertilized and have resulted in several pregnancies and healthy live births (33, 34). Animal studies also support these results; oocyte quality and early embryonic developmental competence of immature oocytes following maturation were not detrimentally affected by the presence of the dominant follicle in cattle and bovine models (35, 36). As a possible explanation for these findings, recently two new studies have suggested that there are two or three waves of ovarian follicular development in women during each menstrual cycle, based on daily transvaginal ultrasonography. This suggestion is indeed challenging the traditional theory of a single cohort of antral follicles that grow only during the follicular phase. At the McGill Reproductive Centre, we currently use the threshold of 14 mm for the dominant follicle diameter for hCG administration. An additional theoretical advantage of this approach is for endometrium to have the adequate thickness until the day of hCG.

Immature human oocytes can be recovered from the ovaries during both the follicular and luteal phase (6, 7). The first IVM baby was conceived from immature oocytes retrieved from a donor during gynecologic surgery. In this oocyte donation program, oocytes were recovered during gynecologic operations, regardless of the cycle day, or during cesarean sections. Interestingly, immature oocytes from the luteal phase had an even significantly higher maturation rate than those obtained during the follicular phase in this oocyte donation program (7). The possibility of immature oocyte retrieval, regardless of the ovulatory phase, provides very flexible and useful treatment opportunities for oocyte donors and for cancer patients who do not have time to wait for the next follicular phase. However, we prefer follicular-phase oocyte retrieval for patients who are undergoing classical IVM with embryo transfer in the fresh cycle so as to have the endometrium prepared for the transfer in that cycle.

Immature Oocytes from Stimulated Cycles

Although large numbers of MII oocytes are retrieved in stimulated cycles, approximately 15 percent of recovered oocytes are still immature, whether at GV or MI stage (17) because ovarian stimulation results in follicular asynchrony (37). It would be very useful if these immature oocytes from stimulated cycles could be matured in vitro as they are capable of undergoing spontaneous nuclear maturation in vitro and then normal fertilization; however, there is a question about their developmental competence when they are denuded from the surrounding granulosa cells at GV stage (19). The IVM rates of these oocytes were reported as disappointingly low, yet a few

pregnancies have been obtained (5, 38–41). However, the idea can also be used in high responders to ovarian stimulation. More recently, Lim et al. reported seventeen patients with a high risk of developing OHSS during the course of their IVF cycles (42). Instead of canceling the cycles, they administered hCG before the usual scheduled time, before estradiol increased, and oocyte retrieval was performed when the leading follicle reached 12–14 mm in diameter. In all, 11.6 percent of the oocytes recovered were already mature at the time of retrieval. In this group, eight of seventeen (47.1 percent) patients became pregnant after IVM, ICSI and embryo transfer (ET), and no patient had OHSS.

FSH Pretreatment

It was postulated that pretreatment with FSH in the early days of folliculogenesis may increase the number of the oocytes and/ or their maturational potential. Theoretically, the provision of additional FSH could promote follicular granulosa cell proliferation and steroid production; therefore, it can be hypothesized that this approach may help to improve and prepare the endometrium for implantation. However, because the data have not been analyzed with regard to the endometrium, this suggestion is only a possibility at present. It has been suggested that one other advantage of FSH priming is that it facilitates oocyte retrieval and leads to a higher number of recovered oocytes because of the increased size of the follicles, which may, in turn, result in better pregnancy rates.

Although Suikkari et al. did not have any pregnancies in twelve patients with PCOS to whom they administered low-dose rFSH (37.5 IU) from the previous luteal phase until the leading follicle reached 10 mm in diameter (43), Mikkelsen et al. achieved improved implantation and pregnancy rates in the FSH-primed group (21.6–29 percent) compared to the non-primed group (0–0 percent) in their randomized controlled study of patients with PCOS.

In women with regular cycles and normal ovaries, FSH priming did not increase the number of oocytes recovered, and no benefit of FSH priming compared to the natural cycle on the maturation rate could be demonstrated (44). However, further research is required to confirm the possible beneficial effect of FSH priming on IVM cycles.

hCG Pretreatment

In women with PCO or PCOS, the time course and maturation rates are different when GV-stage oocytes were divided into different groups based on the morphology of cumulus cells after hCG priming (45). It seems that hCG priming promotes some GV-stage oocytes to reach the MI stage when derived from relatively larger follicles and enhances other GV-stage oocytes from smaller follicles to acquire maturational and developmental competence. Pretreatment with hCG 10,000 IU thirty-six hours prior to IVM oocyte retrieval increases the maturation rate of oocytes in vitro (46), hastens the maturation process, and shortens the maturation duration (22). A prospective, randomized, controlled trial demonstrated no improvement in oocyte maturation rates with 20,000 IU of hCG compared with 10,000 IU of hCG and therefore no benefit of the higher dose (47). With use of pretreatment, implantation and pregnancy rates have increased to 10–15 and 30–35 percent, respectively (19, 48).

IVM INDICATIONS

PCO/PCOS Patients

The majority of IVM pregnancies in the literature have been in women with PCOS, and pregnancy rates in women with normal ovaries appear to be lower (49). The reason for this difference is that the pregnancy rate in IVM has a direct relation to the number of immature oocytes retrieved (50, 51). The number of immature oocytes retrieved can be predicted by the number of 2- to 8-mm antral follicles, ovarian volume, and peak ovarian stromal velocity measured by doppler ultrasound during the early follicular phase. Additionally, the antral follicular count is the most important independent ultrasonographic predictor of the number of immature oocytes recovered (51). The advantage of IVM for PCO and/or PCOS patients is that they have higher number of antral follicles than women with normal ovaries and they are at a high risk of developing OHSS. According to our study, the clinical pregnancy rate per cycle in relation to the antral follicle count is as follows: less than twenty follicles, 6 percent; twenty–twenty nine follicles, 15 percent; more than twenty nine follicles, 44 percent ($p < 0.001$) (50).

PCO and/or PCOS patients having the highest risk of OHSS, and the best chance for pregnancy due to a higher antral follicle count (AFC) have been the most appropriate candidates for routine IVM treatment. At the McGill Reproductive Centre, ART candidates having an AFC of more than twenty are routinely offered IVM.

Poor Responders

Oocyte donation offers the best chance for pregnancy to poor responders because ovarian stimulation for IVF has high cancellation rates, and no single protocol seems to benefit poor responders. Immature oocyte retrieval and IVM of the retrieved oocytes followed by ICSI and ET can be an option for selected patients who want to use their own oocytes but do not respond to gonadotropins. In a study by Child et al. (52), eight women with a history of poor response to IVF underwent oocyte retrieval thirty-six hours after hCG administration without ovarian stimulation. ET was performed in six and pregnancy was achieved in one woman. The numbers of embryos produced and available were similar to those in previous IVF cycles. In another study, Liu et al. reported three pregnancies out of eight poor responders (37.5 percent) who underwent immature oocyte retrieval before cancellation of the cycle owing to poor response to gonadotropins (53). In this study, hCG was not used before oocyte retrieval. In such poor responders, hCG administration may optimize the successful pregnancy rate; some already matured oocytes can be recovered and the transfer of embryos obtained from these mature oocytes pooled together with in vitro matured ones maximizes the treatment outcome.

Natural-cycle IVF is another option for women with poor ovarian reserve. In this treatment, women who still have their regular cycles despite poor ovarian reserve undergo oocyte retrieval for the in vivo matured oocyte of the dominant follicle. Cumulative pregnancy rate after four cycles was reported to be 46 percent with a live birth rate of 32 percent in natural-cycle IVF (54). One possibility to increase the success rate of natural-cycle IVF treatment is to combine it with immature oocyte retrieval and IVM of the immature oocytes. The mature oocyte from the dominant follicle with other in vitro matured oocytes may produce more than one embryo and may increase the chance of pregnancy. Three successful pregnancies were reported before with this method, one of the women being a poor responder (55). A preliminary report of a series of 129 patients who underwent natural-cycle IVF combined with IVM has recently been published (56). One hundred twenty three of the 129 patients completed the treatment, and 10.4 percent of implantation and 29.3 percent of clinical pregnancy rates were achieved. However, in the latter report, patients were not poor responders; all were younger than forty and have serum FSH level of less than 10 IU/L. It seems that mature and immature oocyte retrieval followed by IVF and IVM is an efficient treatment; however, its benefit for poor responders has not been established yet.

IVM Oocyte Donation

Cumulative pregnancy rates after four transfers by ovarian stimulation followed by oocyte donation may increase up to 94.8 percent. However, the risk of OHSS, complications associated with the procedure, concerns about the side effects of the gonadotropins, and the long-term risks of ovarian stimulation may deter some potential oocyte donors. Up to three quarters of potential donors may change their mind after receiving information about the procedures involved (15). Avoiding ovarian stimulation would eliminate most of the concerns and reduce the cost as well.

The first IVM baby was delivered by a woman who received oocytes from a donor who underwent gynecologic surgery on day 13 of her cycle (6). In this oocyte donation program, donors were chosen from the patients who were undergoing gynecologic surgery regardless of the cycle day or cesarean section. Oocyte retrieval was performed during surgery by direct aspiration of the follicles at the time of laparotomy, and several pregnancies were reported (6, 7). In our center, twelve oocyte donors with high antral follicle counts (mean: 29.6) underwent immature oocyte retrieval in the follicular phase of folliculogenesis without ovarian stimulation (57). A mean number of 12.8 GV oocytes were retrieved, forty-eight embryos were transferred to twelve recipients and six conceived (50 percent). Although two miscarried, four women gave birth to five healthy babies.

Fertility Preservation

While female cancer incidence increases, antineoplastic regimens have become more successful (58). As a result, an increasing number of women with cancer survive to endure the long-term consequences of chemotherapy. One of the most important long-term effects of cancer treatments in young females is premature ovarian failure and infertility. Because of the increasing survival rate, many of these young women are seeking methods to preserve their fertility. For patients who have sufficient time and no contraindication for ovarian stimulation, embryo or oocyte cryopreservation following controlled ovarian stimulation appears to be the most suitable approach (59). In cases where estrogen-sensitive tumors and/or time constraints are involved, IVM has been suggested as ovarian stimulation is not required and much less time is required than for IVF treatment (60). Oocyte retrieval may be performed at any time for anovulatory patients and prior to ovulation for ovulatory patients (60, 61). Although it is not routinely used, immature oocyte retrieval after ovulation or in the secretory phase has also yielded promising IVM results (7, 62).

The retrieved immature oocytes can be fertilized and vitrified for future use, or for patients without partners, in vitro matured oocytes can be vitrified to be thawed and fertilized when the woman is ready for pregnancy. Although pregnancy rates appear to be lower compared to in vivo matured and vitrified oocytes, we have obtained a pregnancy rate approximately of 20 percent per embryo transfer from in vitro matured oocytes followed by vitrification, thawing, and ICSI (unpublished data). Vitrification of oocytes retrieved from unstimulated ovaries seems to be a promising procedure for the preservation of fertility as this technique avoids hormonal stimulation and is not associated with considerable delay in cancer treatment.

Another novel approach involves the retrieval of immature oocytes from excised ovarian tissue, maturation in vitro, and cryopreservation by vitrification. This new fertility preservation method could be combined with ovarian tissue banking. Twenty-two patients with various cancers underwent ovarian tissue cryobanking at the McGill Reproductive Centre. Recently, four of these patients underwent retrieval of immature oocytes from ovarian tissue. Eight of the eleven oocytes recovered using this method have been matured in vitro and vitrified besides cryopreservation of the ovarian tissue (63). Indications for fertility preservation are not limited to cancer. Any reason for a decrease in ovarian reserve can be an indication. Apart from the above-mentioned cryobank users, more recently, a 16-year-old girl underwent ovarian wedge resection for fertility preservation because of Turner's syndrome, and before the ovarian tissue was cryopreserved, eleven immature oocytes were aspirated from the surface follicles and eight matured following IVM, resulting in eight vitrified oocytes for future use (unpublished data).

OVERVIEW OF AN IVM CYCLE

Monitoring of the Cycle and hCG Timing

The treatment cycle is initiated by progesterone administration in women with oligo- or amenorrhea. On days 2–4 of the withdrawal bleeding, a baseline ultrasound is performed to ensure that there is no ovarian cyst. Transvaginal ultrasound is repeated on days 7–9 of the cycle to plan immature oocyte retrieval. At the McGill Reproductive Centre, we wait until endometrial thickness reaches 8 mm before hCG administration. In women with oligomenorrhea, retrieval can be delayed to the third week of the cycle. However, ovulatory women with regular menstrual cycles will grow a dominant follicle; for these women, our cutoff for the diameter of the dominant follicle is 14 mm on the day of hCG. Women are primed with 10,000 IU hCG thirty-six to thirty-eight hours prior to oocyte retrieval depending on the size of the leading follicle.

Immature Oocyte Retrieval

Transvaginal ultrasound-guided follicular aspiration has now become the preferred procedure for oocyte retrieval in IVM cycles; it requires certain modifications compared to conventional IVF oocyte retrieval.

Anesthesia/Analgesia

The mode of anesthesia is decided according to the accessibility of the ovaries. Although the initial cases were performed under general or spinal anesthesia, they are not needed for most of the cases. At the McGill Reproductive Centre, intravenous sedation with 2 mg midazolam and 50–200 mg fentanyl for pain control, and paracervical block with 10–20 mL of 0.5 percent bupivacaine, are used for immature oocyte retrieval. For patients who have previously experienced poor pain relief during oocyte retrieval or for those where ovarian access is difficult, a general or spinal anesthesia may be more appropriate and in our experience is needed more frequently than for conventional IVF retrievals.

Cleaning and Antisepsis

The vagina is cleaned with saline.

Preparation

Compared to oocyte retrieval in stimulated cycles, a smaller gauge needle (19G or 20G) is preferable. The aspiration vacuum pressure is reduced to 75–80 mmHg, which is approximately half of conventional IVF aspiration pressure. The aspiration tubes are prepared with 2 mL heparinized saline before the collection in the warm blocks. Heparinized saline is also used as aspiration medium for flushing the needle.

Aspiration Technique

The needle is introduced into the follicle at 90° to the follicle wall; otherwise, it easily slips into the surrounding stroma. Also, the needle is frequently removed to realign it with the small follicles. The follicle should be completely emptied; rotating the needle could be of help. Multiple ovarian punctures are generally needed for IVM retrievals; it is almost always impossible to reach all the follicles from the same puncture site. In addition, the volume of the fluid aspirated from the follicles is very small and the single lumen aspiration needle tends to be blocked easily. The needle is generally withdrawn after aspirating several follicles and flushed with the heparinized saline. Collection takes, on average, longer than IVF oocyte retrieval because of the repeated flushing and the tubing of the needle in order to prevent blockage (64, 65).

Good ultrasonographic visualization is the key point for successful immature oocyte retrieval. Follicular sizes vary, and certain follicles may be difficult to aspirate, or even if they are aspirated, the oocyte may not be recovered especially from the very small size follicles (< 4 mm).

In Vitro Oocyte Maturation

Follicles are isolated from follicular aspirates and collected in tubes containing heparinized saline in the laboratory by using a stereomicroscope. Oocytes are evaluated for the presence or absence of a GV in the cytoplasm; if no GV is seen in an immature oocyte, it is defined as GVBD. The mature (MII) oocytes are determined by the presence of the first polar body. The follicular aspirate is then filtered and rechecked for oocytes. Immature oocytes are transferred into IVM medium (27) supplemented with 75 mIU FSH and LH for culture at 37 °C in an atmosphere of 5 percent CO_2 and 95 percent air with high humidity. Maturity is determined twenty-four hours after retrieval, and at this time, the mature oocytes are denuded from the surrounding granulosa cells and ICSI is performed. Those that have not reached to MII stage are cultured in the medium for another twenty-four hours and rechecked.

Endometrial Preparation and Luteal Support

Estradiol valerate is given to the women for endometrial preparation at a dosage depending on the endometrial thickness on the day of oocyte retrieval. If endometrial thickness is less than 6 mm, 12 mg of estradiol valerate is given at 2 mg tid p.o. and 2 mg tid vaginal, starting from the day of retrieval. If endometrial thickness is 6–8 mm, total 8–10 mg daily, and in cases where thickness is more than 8 mm, 2 mg of estradiol valerate tid p.o. is recommended.

Luteal support is started on the day that maturation is achieved and ICSI is performed. We use 50 mg daily intramuscular progesterone injections for luteal support. ET is performed according to the maturation and fertilization of the oocytes. Retrieved oocytes may not have matured synchronously; therefore, the developmental stages of the embryos may be different at the time of ET.

OUTCOME OF IVM TREATMENT CYCLES

IVM Success Rates

All centers performing conventional IVF and IVM report higher clinical pregnancy rates with IVF. One case-matched controlled study, which compared IVF and IVM pregnancy outcomes in women with PCOS or PCO, reported a 38 percent clinical pregnancy rate with conventional IVF and 26 percent with IVM. Still, IVM pregnancy rates are higher than those of natural-cycle IVF (54).

The AFC is the best indicator of the number of immature oocytes that may be retrieved and of clinical pregnancy (51). Therefore, clinical pregnancy rates in PCOS/PCO patients are expected to be higher than in women who have regular menses and normal ovaries. Recent data indicate that IVM using hCG priming before immature oocyte retrieval leads to clinical pregnancy and implantation rates of 30–35 and 10–15 percent, respectively (19). Furthermore, current data show that in women with higher numbers of antral follicles, pregnancy rates are also higher and reach 30–40 percent (51). As mentioned before, the clinical pregnancy rate per cycle in relation to the AFC was reported as less than twenty follicles, 6 percent; twenty–twenty nine follicles, 15 percent; and more than twenty nine follicles, 44 percent (50). As with IVF, clinical pregnancy and implantation rates decrease with increasing age. In women younger than thirty-five years, we have achieved a clinical pregnancy rate of 38 percent per oocyte retrieval and an implantation rate of 13 percent at McGill Reproductive Center. In women between thirty-six and forty years, the clinical pregnancy rate is 21 percent per retrieval and the implantation rate 5 percent.

Clinical pregnancy rate per oocyte retrieval in United States was announced to be 38.2 percent in fresh IVF cycles in the Society for Assisted Reproductive Technology registry report, according to the data collected from 385 clinics on procedures performed in the year 2001 (66). Results from the Canadian ART Register were also similar; per cycle started, the clinical pregnancy rate was 31.2 percent and it was reported to be 37.3 percent per ET procedure (67). Implantation, clinical preg-

nancy, and delivery rates will differ between individual centers; however, when outcome total is considered, the above-mentioned IVM results seem to compete with the fresh-cycle IVF results for the selected patient groups.

IVM Babies

Any new method of assisted reproduction must be accompanied by data concerning congenital abnormality and perinatal outcome. Early data concerning IVM pregnancies have generally been reassuring (68–70). Recent studies also support those reports. From a total of 150 babies born following IVM, six major congenital anomalies have been reported (71); omphalocele, one case; cleft palate, two cases; ventriculo-septal defect, two cases; and 45XO/46XY mosaic, one case. This rate is similar to that reported following other ARTs (72) and slightly higher than those in spontaneously conceived controls. A comparative study shows a similar odds ratio when IVM is compared with IVF and with ICSI (71). The odds ratio of any congenital abnormality following conception with IVF was reported to be 1.01; with IVM, 1.19; and with ICSI, 1.41. There are no significant differences in the multiple pregnancy rates between IVM and other ART pregnancies, either. The obstetric and perinatal outcomes of pregnancies following IVM are comparable to established ART data and may even be associated with fewer low-birth-weight babies according to a study comparing the neonatal outcomes of 55 IVM, 217 IVF, and 160 ICSI babies (73). However, continued data collection and matched studies are needed in order to obtain more detailed information.

KEY POINTS

- IVM of oocytes has become an alternative treatment to conventional IVF in women with PCO/PCOS. The AFC is the most important independent ultrasonographic predictor of the number of immature oocytes recovered. In general, implantation and the clinical pregnancy rates have reached 10–15 and 30–35 percent, respectively, in infertile women with PCO/PCOS.
- Besides women with PCO/PCOS, IVM seems to become a promising treatment alternative particularly for women who are seeking fertility preservation and for women who are candidates for oocyte donation. Poor responders may also benefit from IVM treatment if they refuse oocyte donation as they do not need to receive large doses of gonadotropins.
- The most important advantage of IVM is that it avoids or minimizes gonadotropin use and therefore avoids OHSS, reduces cost, and simplifies the treatment.
- Although oocyte retrieval for IVM has widely been performed in the follicular phase and before the dominant follicle reaches 10 mm in diameter, it has been shown that the size of follicles may be important for the subsequent embryonic development, but the developmental competence of the oocytes derived from the small antral follicles is not adversely affected by the presence of a dominant follicle.
- Although IVM is relatively a new treatment, early evidence from pregnancy outcome studies suggest that there is unlikely to be a significant risk to children conceived with this treatment.

REFERENCES

1. Pincus G, Enzmann EV. The comparative behavior of mammalian eggs in vivo and in vitro. I. The activation of ovarian eggs. *J Exp Med* 1935;62:665–75.

2. Pincus G, Saunders B. The comparative behavior of mammalian eggs in vivo and in vitro. VI. The maturation of human ovarian ova. *Anat Rec* 1939;75:537–45.

3. Edwards RG. Maturation in vitro of mouse, sheep, cow, pig, rhesus monkey and human ovarian oocytes. *Nature* 1965;208:349–51.

4. Edwards RG. Maturation in vitro of human ovarian oocytes. *Lancet* 1965;286:926–9.

5. Veeck LL, Wortham JW Jr., Witmyer J, et al. Maturation and fertilization of morphologically immature human oocytes in a program of in vitro fertilization. *Fertil Steril* 1983;39(5):594–602.

6. Cha KY, Koo JJ, Ko JJ, Choi DH, Han SY, Yoon TK. Pregnancy after in vitro fertilization of human follicular oocytes collected from nonstimulated cycles, their culture in vitro and their transfer in a donor oocyte program. *Fertil Steril* 1991;55(1):109–13.

7. Cha KY, Do BR, Chi HJ, et al. Viability of human follicular oocytes collected from unstimulated ovaries and matured and fertilized in vitro. *Reprod Fertil Dev* 1992;4(6):697–701.

8. Trounson A, Wood C, Kausche A. In vitro maturation and the fertilization and developmental competence of oocytes recovered from untreated polycystic ovarian patients. *Fertil Steril* 1994;62(2):353–62.

9. Barnes FL, Crombie A, Gardner DK, et al. Blastocyst development and birth after in-vitro maturation of human primary oocytes, intracytoplasmic sperm injection and assisted hatching. *Hum Reprod* 1995;10(12):3243–7.

10. Steptoe PC, Edwards RG. Birth after the reimplantation of a human embryo. *Lancet* 1978;2(8085):366.

11. Tan SL, Royston P, Campbell S, et al. Cumulative conception and livebirth rates after in-vitro fertilisation. *Lancet* 1992; 339(8806):1390–4.

12. MacDougall MJ, Tan SL, Jacobs HS. In-vitro fertilization and the ovarian hyperstimulation syndrome. *Hum Reprod* 1992;7(5): 597–600.

13. MacDougall MJ, Tan SL, Balen A, Jacobs HS. A controlled study comparing patients with and without polycystic ovaries undergoing in-vitro fertilization. *Hum Reprod* 1993;8(2):233–7.

14. Buckett W, Chian RC, Tan SL. Can we eliminate severe ovarian hyperstimulation syndrome? Not completely. *Hum Reprod* 2005;20(8):2367; author reply 8.

15. Murray C, Golombok S. Oocyte and semen donation: a survey of UK licensed centres. *Hum Reprod* 2000;15(10):2133–9.

16. Thomas FH, Vanderhyden BC. Oocyte growth and developmental competence. In: Tan SL, Chian RC, Buckett WM, eds. *In-vitro Maturation of Human Oocytes, Basic Science to Clinical Application*. London: Informa Healthcare; 2007:1–14.

17. Cha KY, Chian RC. Maturation in vitro of immature human oocytes for clinical use. *Hum Reprod Update* 1998;4(2):103–20.

18. Swain JE, Smith GD. Mechanism of oocyte maturation. In: Tan SL, Chian RC, Buckett WM, eds. *In-vitro Maturation of Human Oocytes, Basic Science to Clinical Application*. London: Informa Healthcare; 2007:83–12.

19. Chian RC, Buckett WM, Tan SL. In-vitro maturation of human oocytes. *Reprod Biomed Online* 2004;8(2):148–66.

20. Chian RC, Sirard MA. Effects of cumulus cells and follicle-stimulating hormone during in vitro maturation on parthenogenetic activation of bovine oocytes. *Mol Reprod Dev* 1995;42(4): 425–31.

21. Chian RC, Buckett WM, Too LL, Tan SL. Pregnancies resulting from in vitro matured oocytes retrieved from patients with polycystic ovary syndrome after priming with human chorionic gonadotropin. *Fertil Steril* 1999;72(4):639–42.

22. Chian RC, Buckett WM, Tulandi T, Tan SL. Prospective randomized study of human chorionic gonadotrophin priming before immature oocyte retrieval from unstimulated women with polycystic ovarian syndrome. *Hum Reprod* 2000;15(1):165–70.

23. Mikkelsen AL, Lindenberg S. Influence of the dominant follicle on in-vitro maturation of human oocytes: a prospective non-randomized study. *Reprod Biomed Online* 2001;3(3):199–204.

24. Mikkelsen AL, Host E, Blaabjerg J, Lindenberg S. Maternal serum supplementation in culture medium benefits maturation of immature human oocytes. *Reprod Biomed Online* 2001;3(2):112–16.

25. Trounson A, Anderiesz C, Jones G. Maturation of human oocytes in vitro and their developmental competence. *Reproduction* 2001;121(1):51–75.

26. Trounson A, Anderiesz C, Jones GM, Kausche A, Lolatgis N, Wood C. Oocyte maturation. *Hum Reprod* 1998;13(Suppl. 3):52–62.

27. Chian RC, Tan SL. Maturational and developmental competence of cumulus-free immature human oocytes derived from stimulated and intracytoplasmic sperm injection cycles. *Reprod Biomed Online* 2002;5(2):125–32.

28. Tesarik J, Mendoza C. Nongenomic effects of 17 beta-estradiol on maturing human oocytes: relationship to oocyte developmental potential. *J Clin Endocrinol Metab* 1995;80(4):1438–43.

29. Kreiner D, Liu HC, Itskovitz J, Veeck L, Rosenwaks Z. Follicular fluid estradiol and progesterone are markers of preovulatory oocyte quality. *Fertil Steril* 1987;48(6):991–4.

30. Chian RC, Ao A, Clarke HJ, Tulandi T, Tan SL. Production of steroids from human cumulus cells treated with different concentrations of gonadotropins during culture in vitro. *Fertil Steril* 1999;71(1):61–6.

31. Cobo AC, Requena A, Neuspiller F, et al. Maturation in vitro of human oocytes from unstimulated cycles: selection of the optimal day for ovum retrieval based on follicular size. *Hum Reprod* 1999;14(7):1864–8.

32. Chian RC, Lim JH, Tan SL. State of the art in in-vitro oocyte maturation. *Curr Opin Obstet Gynecol* 2004;16(3):211–19.

33. Paulson RJ, Sauer MV, Francis MM, Macaso T, Lobo RA. Factors affecting pregnancy success of human in-vitro fertilization in unstimulated cycles. *Hum Reprod* 1994;9(8):1571–5.

34. Thornton MH, Francis MM, Paulson RJ. Immature oocyte retrieval: lessons from unstimulated IVF cycles. *Fertil Steril* 1998; 70(4):647–50.

35. Smith LC, Olivera-Angel M, Groome NP, Bhatia B, Price CA. Oocyte quality in small antral follicles in the presence or absence of a large dominant follicle in cattle. *J Reprod Fertil* 1996; 106(2):193–9.

36. Chian RC, Chung JT, Downey BR, Tan SL. Maturational and developmental competence of immature oocytes retrieved from bovine ovaries at different phases of folliculogenesis. *Reprod Biomed Online* 2002;4(2):127–32.

37. Bomsel-Helmreich O, Huyen LV, Durand-Gasselin I, Salat-Baroux J, Antoine JM. Mature and immature oocytes in large and medium follicles after clomiphene citrate and human menopausal gonadotropin stimulation without human chorionic gonadotropin. *Fertil Steril* 1987;48(4):596–604.

38. Nagy ZP, Cecile J, Liu J, Loccufier A, Devroey P, Van Steirteghem A. Pregnancy and birth after intracytoplasmic sperm injection of in vitro matured germinal-vesicle stage oocytes: case report. *Fertil Steril* 1996;65(5):1047–50.

39. Edirisinghe WR, Junk SM, Matson PL, Yovich JL. Birth from cryopreserved embryos following in-vitro maturation of oocytes and intracytoplasmic sperm injection. *Hum Reprod* 1997;12(5): 1056–8.

40. Liu J, Katz E, Garcia JE, Compton G, Baramki TA. Successful in vitro maturation of human oocytes not exposed to human chorionic gonadotropin during ovulation induction, resulting in pregnancy. *Fertil Steril* 1997;67(3):566–8.

41. Jaroudi KA, Hollanders JM, Elnour AM, Roca GL, Atared AM, Coskun S. Embryo development and pregnancies from in-vitro matured and fertilized human oocytes. *Hum Reprod* 1999;14(7):1749–51.

42. Lim KS, Son WY, Yoon SH, Lim JH. IVM/F-ET in stimulated cycles for the prevention of OHSS. *Fertil Steril* 2002;78(Suppl. 1):S10.

43. Suikkari AM, Tulppala M, Tuuri T, Hovatta O, Barnes F. Luteal phase start of low-dose FSH priming of follicles results in an efficient recovery, maturation and fertilization of immature human oocytes. *Hum Reprod* 2000;15(4):747–51.

44. Mikkelsen AL. FSH priming in IVM cycles. In: Tan SL, Chian RC, Buckett W, eds. *In-vitro Maturation of Human Oocytes, Basic Science to Clinical Application*. London: Informa Healthcare; 2007.

45. Yang SH, Son WY, Yoon SH, Ko Y, Lim JH. Correlation between in vitro maturation and expression of LH receptor in cumulus cells of the oocytes collected from PCOS patients in HCG-primed IVM cycles. *Hum Reprod* 2005;20(8):2097–103.

46. Chian RC, Gulekli B, Buckett WM, Tan SL. Priming with human chorionic gonadotropin before retrieval of immature oocytes in women with infertility due to the polycystic ovary syndrome. *N Engl J Med* 1999;341(21):1624, 6.

47. Gulekli B, Buckett WM, Chian RC, Child TJ, Abdul-Jalil AK, Tan SL. Randomized, controlled trial of priming with 10,000 IU versus 20,000 IU of human chorionic gonadotropin in women with polycystic ovary syndrome who are undergoing in vitro maturation. *Fertil Steril* 2004;82(5):1458–9.

48. Lin YH, Hwang JL, Huang LW, et al. Combination of FSH priming and hCG priming for in-vitro maturation of human oocytes. *Hum Reprod* 2003;18(8):1632–6.

49. Mikkelsen AL, Smith S, Lindenberg S. Impact of oestradiol and inhibin A concentrations on pregnancy rate in in-vitro oocyte maturation. *Hum Reprod* 2000;15(8):1685–90.

50. Child TJ, Gulekli B, Tan SL. Success during in-vitro maturation (IVM) of oocyte treatment is dependent on the numbers of oocytes retrieved which are predicted by early follicular phase transvaginal ultrasound measurement of the antral follicular count and peak ovarian stromal blood flow velocity. *Hum Reprod* 2001;16(Abstract book 1):41.

51. Tan SL, Child TJ, Gulekli B. In vitro maturation and fertilization of oocytes from unstimulated ovaries: predicting the number of immature oocytes retrieved by early follicular phase ultrasonography. *Am J Obstet Gynecol* 2002;186(4):684–9.

52. Child TJ, Gulekli B, Chian RC, Abdul Jalil AK, Tan SL. In-vitro maturation of oocytes from unstimulated normal ovaries of women with a previous poor response to IVF. *Fertil Steril* 2000;74(3 Suppl. 1):S45.

53. Liu J, Lu G, Qian Y, Mao Y, Ding W. Pregnancies and births achieved from in vitro matured oocytes retrieved from poor responders undergoing stimulation in in vitro fertilization cycles. *Fertil Steril* 2003;80(2):447–9.

54. Nargund G, Waterstone J, Bland J, Philips Z, Parsons J, Campbell S. Cumulative conception and live birth rates in natural (unstimulated) IVF cycles. *Hum Reprod* 2001;16(2):259–62.

55. Chian RC, Buckett WM, Abdul Jalil AK, et al. Natural-cycle in vitro fertilization combined with in vitro maturation of immature oocytes is a potential approach in infertility treatment. *Fertil Steril* 2004;82(6):1675–8.

56. Lim JH, Park SY, Yoon SH, Yang SH, Chian RC. Combination of natural cycle IVF with IVM as infertility treatment. In: Tan SL, Chian RC, Buckett W, eds. *In-Vitro Maturation of Oocytes, Basic Science to Clinical Application*. London: Informa Healthcare; 2007.

57. Holzer H, Scharf E, Chian RC, Demirtas E, Buckett W, Tan SL. In vitro maturation of oocytes collected from unstimulated ovaries for oocyte donation. *Fertil Steril* 2007. In press.

58. Hayat MJ, Howlader N, Reichman ME, Edwards BK. Cancer statistics, trends, and multiple primary cancer analyses from the Surveillance, Epidemiology, and End Results (SEER) Program. *Oncologist* 2007;12(1):20–37.

59. Lee SJ, Schover LR, Partridge AH, et al. American Society of Clinical Oncology recommendations on fertility preservation in cancer patients. *J Clin Oncol* 2006;24(18):2917–31.

60. Rao GD, Chian RC, Son WS, Gilbert L, Tan SL. Fertility preservation in women undergoing cancer treatment. *Lancet* 2004;363(9423):1829–30.

61. Holzer HE, Tan SL. Fertility preservation in oncology. *Minerva Ginecol* 2005;57(1):99–109.

62. Oktay K, Demirtas E, Son W, Lostritto K, Chian RC, Tan SL. In vitro maturation of germinal vesicle oocytes recovered post-premature LH surge: description of a novel approach to fertility preservation. *Fertil Steril* 2007. In press.

63. Huang JYJ, Holzer H, Tulandi T, Tan SL, Chian RC. Combining ovarian tissue cryobanking with retrieval of immature oocytes by in vitro maturation and vitrification: a noble method of fertility preservation. *Fertil Steril* 2007. In press.

64. Child TJ, Abdul-Jalil AK, Gulekli B, Tan SL. In vitro maturation and fertilization of oocytes from unstimulated normal ovaries, polycystic ovaries, and women with polycystic ovary syndrome. *Fertil Steril* 2001;76(5):936–42.

65. Child TJ, Phillips SJ, Abdul-Jalil AK, Gulekli B, Tan SL. A comparison of in vitro maturation and in vitro fertilization for women with polycystic ovaries. *Obstet Gynecol* 2002;100(4):665–70.

66. Assisted reproductive technology in the United States: 2001 results generated from the American Society for Reproductive Medicine/Society for Assisted Reproductive Technology registry. *Fertil Steril* 2007.

67. Gunby J, Daya S. Assisted reproductive technologies (ART) in Canada: 2003 results from the Canadian ART Register. *Fertil Steril* 2007.

68. Mikkelsen AL, Ravn SH, Lindenberg S. Evaluation of newborns delivered after in vitro maturation. *Hum Reprod* 2003;18(Suppl. 1):xviii5.

69. Buckett WM, Chian RC, Barrington K, Dean N, Abdul Jalil AK, Tan SL. Obstetric, neonatal and infant outcome in babies conceived by in vitro maturation (IVM): initial five-year results 1998–2003. *Fertil Steril* 2004;82(Suppl. 2):S133.

70. Cha KY, Chung HM, Lee DR, et al. Obstetric outcome of patients with polycystic ovary syndrome treated by in vitro maturation and in vitro fertilization-embryo transfer. *Fertil Steril* 2005;83(5):1461–5.

71. Buckett WM. Pregnancy and neonatal outcome following IVM. In: Tan SL, Chian RC, Buckett WM, eds. *In-vitro Maturation of Human Oocytes, Basic Science to Clinical Application*. London: Informa Healthcare; 2007:313–18.

72. Hansen M, Kurinczuk JJ, Bower C, Webb S. The risk of major birth defects after intracytoplasmic sperm injection and in vitro fertilization. *N Engl J Med* 2002;346(10):725–30.

73. Buckett W, Chian RC, Holzer H, Dean N, Tan SL. Congenital abnormalities and perinatal outcome in pregnancies following IVM, IVF, and ICSI delivered in a single center. *Fertil Steril* 2006;85(Suppl. 2):S11–12.

50

Oocyte and Embryo Freezing

Eleonora Porcu, Patrizia Maria Ciotti, Giuseppe Damiano, Maria Dirodi, Stefano Venturoli

Reproductive cryopreservation has recently gained an increasing importance in in vitro fertilization (IVF) programs throughout the world and is probably going to play a significant role over the next few years.

The main vantages of this technique include storage for future use without repeating ovarian stimulation, chance of fertility for neoplastic patients who are going to receive chemotherapy, low risk of multiple pregnancies by reducing the number of fresh embryos transferred, and low risk, without canceling the cycle, of developing ovarian hyperstimulation syndrome (1), which still represents the most serious complication of the superovulation regimes.

Since the first pregnancy and the first birth achieved from human embryo cryopreservation were reported (2, 3), several methods have been developed to make cryopreservation, thawing, and transfer of human embryos more safe, embryo freezing being now routinely used in many IVF programs all over the world.

However, the debate on the safety of cryopreservation is still open, and many authors have expressed their concerns about it, especially after the alarming report in 1995 of morphological and development alteration in mice born from frozen-thawed embryos (4). Moreover, many mutations may be difficult to evaluate since they can have minimal phenotypic effects, with respect viability and macromorphological appearance of offsprings, thus altering behavior and cognitive functions through biochemical and microstructular changes.

Actually, the major concern is expressed about potential long-time risk to children born from embryo freezing and oocyte freezing.

EMBRYO CRYOPRESERVATION

Embryo cryopreservation was applied for the first time in mammalians in 1972 (5) and in humans in the early 1980s (6).

The first pregnancy from human embryo cryopreservation was reported in 1983 (2), whereas the first birth in 1984 (3).

Till date, both freezing and thawing techniques result greatly improved and not only transfer of freezed-thawed embryos is widely and successfully practiced all over the world but there also has been a consistent enhancement of IVF efficiency, thanks to cryopreservation.

In 1993, an increase of 5.2 percent in the birth rate, of 13.2 percent in the ongoing pregnancy rate, and of 11.6 percent in the number of viable fetuses was reported by a study performed on 485 women treated with IVF programs of which 124 were frozen embryo transfer (FRET) cycles (7).

The ongoing pregnancy rate in 2,707 couples entering an IVF program was increased by 4 percent (8). In the same year, an analysis on 610 patients who performed 1,000 fresh cycles and 373 FRET cycles demonstrated an enhancement of 6.6 percent on the ongoing pregnancy rate (9).

In 1998, an 8 percent of additional births were observed in 5,032 FRET cycles, with a 12 percent of live births per transfer, and a 6 percent per transferred embryo (10). The latest world report estimated more than 80,000 embryos frozen and more than 4,000 pregnancies conceived with embryo cryopreservation during 1995 (11).

Cryopreservation of human embryos is then a rapidly expanding field needing maximal attention by scientists in order to assess the safety of this procedure.

A comparison between transfers of fresh and frozen embryos with similar quality is necessary in order to test the reliability of embryo freezing-thawing procedures.

The capacity of human frozen-thawed embryos to implant appeared significantly reduced compared with fresh embryos in a study performed in 1990 (12) in which donor eggs were fertilized and embryos obtained distributed to recipients randomly chosen to transfer either fresh or frozen-thawed embryos. Twenty-four percent of the fresh embryos and only 7.7 percent of the frozen-thawed embryos were successfully implanted.

A similar study (13) reported an implantation rate of 12.6 percent for fresh embryo transfer cycles versus 8.1 percent for FRET cycles.

In a recent retrospective study (14), a significantly higher implantation and pregnancy rate was reported in fresh embryo tranfers compared with frozen-thawed embryo transfers. Keeping in mind that the ability of embryos to implant is directly reflected by their ability to survive the freezing-thawing process, an important factor for the implantation capacity of human embryos is the morphological aspect at the time of freezing (15, 16).

A retrospective analysis of the implantation and in vivo development of frozen-thawed embryos (17) demonstrated a higher implantation rate after transfer of fully intact embryos (11,4 percent) compared with the transfer of partially damaged embryos (3.5 percent).

Another retrospective study reported a significantly higher pregnancy rate after transfer of frozen-thawed embryos with intact blastomeres compared with embryos in which not all blastomeres were intact (18).

A matter of concern results in the observation that even if on the whole the pregnancy rate is lower in FRET cycles compared with fresh cycles, the multiple pregnancy rate is significantly higher: 13 percent (10) or 17 percent (19). An explanation for this can be found in a slightly improved endometrial receptivity in FRET cycles, compensating for the decreased quality of frozen-thawed embryos (20, 21).

Many studies suggest that the insemination method can interfere with the outcome of cryopreservation. Intracytoplasmatic sperm injection (ICSI) is supposed either to allow to obtain higher post-thawing survival rates, implantation rates, and delivery rates (22) or to cause a lower implantation rate and a higher incidence of preclinical abortions due to the damage inflicted to the zona pellucida during the ICSI, which could sensitize the embryo to the chemical and physical changes associated with freezing and thawing (23, 24). According to other authors, there would be no difference between ICSI FRET and normal IVF FRET in post-thawing survival, implantation rates, preclinical abortion rates, and clinical pregnancy rates (24–29).

The length of cryostorage (30–32) does not influence the outcome of cryopreservation. Indeed, a successful pregnancy in a forty-four-year-old woman has been described after the transfer of embryos cryopreserved for 7.5 years (33). In addition, a twin birth of two healthy children from cryopreserved embryos stored for twelve years has been reported in a thirty-nine-year-old woman (34). Further, the transfer of embryos kept in liquid nitrogen for thirteen years gave rise to the birth of a normal child in a patient at the age of forty (35).

The potential risks of damage for cryopreserved-thawed embryos include exposure to medium biochemical contaminants, ice crystal formation within the embryo, toxic effect of cryoprotectants, damage during thawing process, physical damage during embryo manipulation, and DNA damage during embryo storage (36); but freezing itself cannot be considered a mutagenic procedure. Many studies showed in the past that embryo cryopreservation was related with reduced fetal weight (37) and increased frequency of early postimplantation fetal loss (37–39); actually, these alterations may be related to the high incidence of multiple pregnancies in IVF cycles, even if a more adverse perinatal outcome has been observed also in singleton IVF pregnancies compared with spontaneous pregnancies (40, 41).

In 1989, the first descriptive study was performed over a two-year period on fifty pregnancies obtained after transfer of frozen-thawed embryos (42). One pregnancy was terminated at twenty-two weeks gestation for a severe fetal malformation, one delivery was premature, and a high incidence of breech presentation (12 percent) in singleton pregnancies occurred.

Major chromosomal anomalies, such as trisomy of chromosome 13, 18, and 21, were found in fetuses and babies conceived from frozen-thawed embryos, with a higher incidence compared with spontaneously conceived babies, as reported by two studies (43, 44). A retrospective study performed in 1994 (45) considered 232 babies conceived from cryopreserved embryos between 1985 and 1991 and an equivalent number of babies born after standard IVF programs used as controls. In the two groups, mean gestational age, birth weight, and perinatal mortality rates were similar and major malformations were found to be even lower in the cryopreserved group than in the control group. Actually, it is possible that a "filtering" effect occurred by not counting "chemical" pregnancy and early spontaneous abortions as a sign of congenital abnormality.

An observational study was performed in 1995 on thirty pregnancies following transfer of frozen-thawed embryos (46). All babies presented an over-average birth weight (45 percent of singletons weighting more than the 75th percentile); no major congenital anomalies, only two minor malformations (lubfeet and undescended testicle), a low prematurity rate (4 percent), and a high breech presentation rate (14 percent) were found in singleton pregnancies as well.

In the same year, genetic effects have been reported also in bacteria and somatic cells undergoing freezing and thawing procedure (4).

A group of ninety-one children (sixty-eight singletons, twenty twins, and three triplets) conceived after cryopreservation was compared with a control group of eighty-three normally conceived children between 1989 and 1994 (47). In the study group, a higher incidence of perinatal problems such as longer periods spent in special care baby units and the presence of three children with major congenital abnormalities was noted. However, the frequency of minor and major congenital anomalies was similar between the two groups (31.9 vs. 21.7 percent and 3.3 vs. 2.4 percent, respectively) and the relative risk in the cryopreserved embryo group compared with the control group was 1.7 for minor congenital anomalies and 1.4 for major congenital anomalies. The minor congenital malformations included naevi and hemangiomas in both groups; the major congenital anomalies were Down's syndrome, Beckwith-Widenmann syndrome, and hypophosphatemic rickets in the cryopreserved embryos and hydronephrosis and gastroschisis in the controls.

The same results were confirmed in 1996 by a study of eighty-nine children born after transfer on cryopreserved-thawed embryos without controls (48). This study showed a high incidence of multiple births and premature births (14.7 percent for singleton pregnancies and 85.7 percent for twin pregnancies), whereas the malformation rate (1.1 percent with only one child with a short ureter) was comparable to that observed in general population, even considering the two therapeutic abortions that occurred for Down's syndrome and polymalformation (3.4 percent).

A complete cohort study in 1997 observed 270 pregnancies (163 singleton, 98 twins, and 9 triplets), both from the obstetric and the neonatal point of view (49). The pregnancy rate per embryo transfer was 21 percent, the frequency of spontaneous abortions 23 percent, the frequency of ectopic pregnancy 4 percent, and the frequency of multiple births 24.2 percent, (22.8 percent twins and 1.4 triplets); the incidence of preterm births was 5.6 percent for singletons, 44.9 percent for twins, and 100 percent for triplets; the incidence of major malformations was 2.7 percent and the perinatal mortality occurred in 8 percent of these children. The comparison with two control groups (standard IVF and normally conceived) showed no significant differences in pregnancy rate, delivery, and perinatal outcome; the only emergent differences were a significantly lower mean birth weight and a higher incidence of cesarean sections in the IVF group, compared with the normally conceived group.

The same results were confirmed by a study performed in the same year by Wood (50).

A study was performed in 1998 on 255 children from cryopreserved embryos, matched with 255 children from fresh IVF and 252 children normally conceived for maternal age, parity, single or twin pregnancy, and date of delivery (51). The main outcome of this study was prenatal growth, which showed similar growth features for both singleton and twin pregnancies in the three groups. The frequency of major malformations was 2.4 percent for the first group, 3.5 percent for the second one, and 3.2 percent for the third one.

In 1999, the Swedish IVF National Registry performed a cohort study that reported a lower birth weight and incidence of preterm birth in FRET cycles, compared with fresh cycles, and a twenty fold increased risk of multiple pregnancy, at high risk for preterm birth and low birth weight, in IVF babies, compared with general population (52).

Actually, it is difficult to distinguish genotoxic and teratogenic effects, which are caused by embryo freezing-thawing techniques from those caused by exposure to toxic substances: for example, preimplantation exposure to ammonium ions has been related to retarded fetal development and neural tube defects in mice (53), whereas lamb birth weight can be affected by the medium in which embryos were cultivated (54); it is clear then that the findings of a cytotoxic and mutagenic chemical such as formaldehyde in cryoprotectant solutions (55, 56) can be considered a very serious matter of concern. Also the ICSI method has been considered as a potential cause of functional disorders, even if paternal inherited factors may be involved (57, 58). It is thus important not to confuse these alteration with those caused by cryopreservation.

Concluding, as far as now, there is no sufficient scientific evidence to support the hypothesis of a negative impact of embryo cryopreservation on obstetric outcome and on congenital malformations, but it must be considered that the power of most of the studies to detect any difference in malformation rate is very low.

Although there is no evidence that embryo cryopreservation increases the frequency of birth defects as the incidence of chromosomal anomalies such as Down's syndrome, and of minor congenital malformations, is similar to that in standard IVF, it is possible that even more severe chromosomal alterations, such as cellular aneuploidy, derive from cryopreservation methods and that they are not clinically evident because of implantation failure or early abortion.

The incidence of tetraploidy in human abortive tissues and in born babies naturally conceived is between 4 and 8 percent (59, 60), and it is probably due to genome duplication and suppression of the early cleavage divisions (59); on the contrary, in frozen-thawed embryos, the principal mechanism leading to aneuploidy seems to be spontaneous blastomere fusion.

The early embryos frailty and their sensitivity to many exogenous factors, such as viruses, polyethylene glycol, or electric fields, is well known (61, 62); indeed, it is easy to suppose that also the freezing-thawing process may determine cellular damage, particularly to early-stage embryos. Cracks in the zona pellucida and injuries to the cell membranes or to intracellular components have been observed as a consequence of cryopreservation in many studies (63, 64).

The first study on cellular blastomere fusion, conducting to cellular aneuploidy, was performed in 1984 (65) and showed no difference between different cryoprotectants used in determining cellular damage (except glycerol soon abandoned because of its high harmfullness); instead, it attributed more importance to a previous poor quality of embryos.

However, the use of propanediol as cryoprotectant has been related to the formation of polyploid cells by the mechanism of spontaneous blastomere fusion, as demonstrated by a study performed in 1991 (66), whereas rapid freezing methods (vitrification) may cause increased mitotic crossing overs (67, 68) and chromosomal damage (69).

Cryoprotectants probably contribute to determine spontaneous blastomere fusion by causing cell dehydration and osmotic swelling; cytoplasmatic bridges may be the other important factor to initiate the fusion process, but they were never detected on electron microscope examination of early human embryos (70, 71).

A study of aneuploidy and mosaicism of chromosomes X and Y and one in frozen human embryos in days 2 and 3 of development were performed in 1998 using fluorescence in situ hybridization and showed that 57 percent of thawed embryos that presented cleavage arrest during the first twenty-four hours had chromosomal abnormalities (72).

In 2000, a report pointed out the presence of spontaneous blastomere fusion, leading to polyploidy and chromosomal mosaicism, in a group of 1,141 embryos frozen on day 2 and 873 embryos frozen on day 3 using the standard propanediol technique (73). The process of fusion was observed with a frequency of 4.6 percent in day 2 and 1.5 percent in day 3; this leading to the conclusion that early human embryos are more susceptile to cryodamage than older embryos because fluidity and other properties of cell membranes are changing during embryo development. The fusion of two or more blastomeres conduced to the formation of multinucleated hybrid cells, a clear signal of ploidy alteration, and to either entirely polyploid embryos (with tetraploid, hexaploid, or more complex aberrations) or mosaics embryos with both polyploid and normal cells. The numerical chromosomal changes in human frozenthawed embryos were demonstrated within mosaics using fluorescence in situ hybridization analysis with DNA probes targeting unique sequences on chromosomes 9, 15, 17, and 22, which indicated the presence of tetraploid and diploid fluorescence signals in the interphase nuclei. The creation of entirely polyploid embryos was less frequent (16 percent) than the creation of mosaics (84 percent) among the altered embryos. Moreover, 70 percent of altered embryos were morphologically good, in contrast to that reported by previous studies.

The development potential of embryos affected by fusion is unclear. In this study, 7 percent of these embryos left in suboptimal culture conditions reached the blastocyst stage, 56 percent cleaved, and 37 percent were totally arrested. Fifteen mosaic normal-looking embryos were transferred, leading to two spontaneous abortions and one chemical pregnancy. So, it is highly probable that embryos affected by fusion are eliminated either before implantation or by early abortion; however, it is possible that protective mechanisms correct embryonic errors or that abnormal cells are sequestered to the trophoblast and later to the placenta since polyploid cells are often found in these extraembryonic tissues (74).

Only one case was reported of a twin pregnancy of two empty tetraploid sacks after the transfer of frozen-thawed zygotes (75), but tetraploid mouse embryos resulted, capable of advanced postimplantation development and could possibly be viable (76).

In conclusion, it is possible to admit that cryopreservation may cause cellular damage, leading to aneuploidy; but, at present, the clinical outcome of these events seems not relevant; further studies must be performed on this issue.

Very few studies have focused by now on long-term effects of human embryo cryopreservation as the appropriate clinical parameters are difficult to find and evaluate and can easily be influenced by environment or other confounding factors; moreover, a close follow-up might become an element of disturbance in the life of these children and might be accepted with difficulty by their parents, who often want to keep secret the origin of the conception.

An increased incidence of psychomotorial and language delay, development and mental disability, cerebral palsy, mental retardation, sensory impairments, learning difficulties, and attention and behavioral problems were found in children born from twin and triple pregnancies compared with singletons (77).

In 1995, a study followed up ninety-two children born after embryo freezing beyond the postnatal period and compared them with eighty-three naturally conceived children, concluding that the overall QI, assessed with the Griffith scale, was higher in the studied children compared with controls, but this was probably due to their parents' slightly higher social class; a lower but significant difference in hearing and speech was found in the cryopreserved group after the analysis of the Griffith scale subquotients (36).

A cohort study of eighty-nine children, one to nine years old, was performed in 1996 but did not use controls (48). All the children studied, except three of them, aged one and two years, were normal for height and weight, even those who were prematurely delivered.

The frequency of chronic diseases was of no interest. Only 7.9 percent of children received temporary psychological support; five of these had learning difficulties and two sleeping problems. No pathological features in the major psychomotor acquisitions were found in children younger than five years old, and only one (prematurely born) presented psychomotor delay. A normal intelligence was found, based on retrospective assessments of scholastic achievement in those children older than five years: only one presented learning difficulties, whereas 24.4 percent were one year in advance or ahead in their class.

In 1998, an important study was conducted on 255 children from cryopreserved embryos, matched with 255 children from fresh IVF and with 252 children normally conceived for maternal age, parity, single or twin pregnancy, and date of delivery (51). The main end point of this study was growth; the secondary end points were major malformations, chronic illness, cumulative incidence of common diseases, and development during the first eighteen months. The frequency of chronic diseases at eighteen months of age in the cryopreserved group was 17 percent; a slightly higher frequency in the cryopreserved group, compared with the standard IVF and the naturally conceived groups, was found for neurological disorders (1.2 vs. 0 vs. 0 percent), food allergy (4.3 vs. 2.4 vs. 2.8 percent), and lactose intolerance (1.6 vs. 0.4 vs. 0.8 percent).

No significant difference was found between the three groups for common disease. The conclusions were that cryopreservation did not affect growth negatively and did not seem to cause minor handicaps, behavioral disturbances, learning difficulties, and dysfunction of attention and perception; however, if the power of this study was strong enough for the main end point, minimal cognitive disturbances could probably not be ruled out in such young children.

In conclusion, children born after transfer of frozen-thawed embryos seem healthy; but studies performed until now are few and size limited, and so no definitive conclusions can be drawn at this point.

Conventional embryo freezing concerns multicell embryos. However, recent studies focused on cryopreserving early-stage embryos such as zygotes, before or after the pronuclei fusion (pronuclear embryos and syngamic zygotes, respectively).

Cryopreservation of pronuclear embryos (or two PN oocytes) has resulted to be an effective method for the utilization of supernumerary embryos, being a very simple technique and implicating less ethical problems than freezing conventional multicell embryos or syngamic zygotes, within which genetic identity has already been shaped by pronuclei fusion. Moreover, two studies showed that the age of zygotes at the time of freezing was crucial to determine the success of implantation after thawing and that the optimal implantation rate was achieved with zygotes frozen at the time of completion of pronuclear migration (twenty to twenty-two hours after insemination) before pronuclei fusion since, approaching syngamy, frozen IVF zygotes gradually lost their implantation capability (78, 79).

However, the optimal time for freezing ICSI-conceived zygotes is still unclear.

A study performed in 1997 (26) compared thirty-nine embryos from ICSI with sixty embryos from standard IVF, which were cryopreserved at the pronuclear stage. This study showed no significant differences between the two groups for survival rate (93.2 vs. 94.8 percent) and pregnancy rate (14 vs. 17.4 percent).

Similar results were obtained by a previous study performed in 1996, which compared ICSI-conceived embryos with standard IVF-conceived embryos frozen at pronuclear stage (80).

Actually, in ICSI oocytes, pronuclei appear much earlier than in standard IVF oocytes (as oocytes are quickly activated after direct insertion of spermatozoon into cytoplasm); so the onset of syngamy (signaled by the disappearance of pronuclei) takes place earlier too. This suggests the necessity to shorten the interval between insemination and freezing in ICSI cycles. This has been confirmed by a cohort study performed in 1998 (27), which compared the survival, implantation, and embryonic loss rates of frozen human zygotes obtained from ICSI with frozen human zygotes obtained from standard IVF. Survival rates were similar in the two groups (87.7 vs. 89.1 percent), whereas a lower implantation rate (10.9 vs. 25 percent) and a higher abortion rate (57.1 vs. 11.8 percent) were found after transfer of ICSI frozen-thawed zygotes. The timing of zygote freezing (after pronuclei fusion in the ICSI group) was considered the principal reason for the lower implantation capability of the frozen-thawed ICSI zygotes in this study.

As for conventional embryo freezing, the length of cryopreservation does not seem to influence negatively the development and implantation potential of frozen zygotes. Indeed, live births have been reported after transfer of a zygote cryopreserved for eight years (81).

Therefore, cryopreservation of early-stage embryos can be considered a valid alternative to conventional embryo cryopreservation.

OOCYTE CRYOPRESERVATION

Cryopreservation of unfertilized oocytes presents more technical problems than early-stage embryo cryopreservation, but also less ethical and legal implications; moreover, it gives women the possibility of preserving fertility after pelvic diseases, surgery, and radiochemotherapy, which determines ovarian damage (82).

Normal living offsprings after oocyte cryopreservation were obtained in the mouse and in the rabbit (83).

It is well known that the oocytes are particularly vulnerable to the low temperature.

The main alterations inflicted to the oocytes by the freezing process include possible alterations to the zona pellucida, which may become harder, reducing the fertilization rate (64, 84, 85); possible alterations to the cortical granules, which may be released prematurely, increasing the risk of polyspermy (86); possible alterations to the meiotic spindle, which might increase the risk of aneuploidy (32, 87, 88); alterations to the ooplasm organelles due to the formation of intracellular ice crystal (89); and alterations of oocyte volume due to the different osmotic pressures between intracellular and extracellular solutions (90).

The most alarming risk related with oocyte cryopreservation is aneuploidy in embryos conceived with this method.

The fact is that oocyte meiotic spindle depolymerizes with low temperature and, even if repolymerization takes place after warming, genetic anomalies leading to embryo aneuploidy can occur when the oocyte, arrested at the metaphase of the second meiotic division (MII stage), completes its division at the moment of fertilization (91). The entity of spindle disassembly depends on the extent of temperature decrease and on its duration, and cryoprotectants themselves can increase the alteration of spindle structure (92).

Kola et al. (93) found a higher incidence of aneuploidy after mouse oocytes freezing compared with controls (32 vs. 12 percent), even if no malformed implanted fetuses were observed.

An important factor in the assessment of the risk of aneuploidy is represented by maternal age as the meiotic spindle is frequently abnormal in forty-year-old women (94) and more nondysjunction and predivision of chromatids are found in these women (95).

The effects of cryoprotectants on the oocyte meiotic spindle have been studied by many authors. In 1987, the exposure of unfertilized oocytes to dimethyl sulphoxide (DMSO) was related to spindle disassembly (96). 1,2-Propanediol was found to have an additional effect on DMSO as its presence after rewarming prevented the spindles to become normal, even if it showed no effect on fertilization (97). Another study performed in 1988 (98) showed that cooling to 0°C in the presence of DMSO did not provide a stabilization of the spindle.

Contrasting results were found by other studies. In 1993, the use of propanediol as a cryoprotectant allowed 64 percent of MII oocytes to survive the slow-freeze-rapid-thaw procedure, with normal spindles and no evidence of freezing-associated aneuploidy (99). In 1994, similar results were found comparing 182 cryopreserved MII oocytes with 268 control oocytes: the survival rate using a slow freezing protocol with propanediol sucrose as cryoprotectants was 65 percent and there were no increased abnormal karyotypes in cryopreserved oocytes (86).

In 2001, a study of fifty-five in vitro matured oocytes (100) showed that spindle damage in metaphase II stage is time dependent: minimal after one minute and complete disappearance after ten minutes.

Vitrification was first introduced in order to avoid crystallization damage by the total elimination of ice crystal formation, both intra- and extracellulary. Another advantage of this method is that it is very simple: it is based on direct contact between the vitrification solution containing cryoprotectants and liquid nitrogen (101).

Cryopreservation of immature oocytes at prophase I (GV stage) has also been proposed as an alternative to standard oocyte cryopreservation as it was thought that these oocytes were less sensitive to cryoinjury, due to the missing spindle and different membrane permeability (10, 102, 103). Actually, no advantage seems to derive from immature oocyte cryopreservation in terms of survival rate, fertilization rate, and developmental ability; moreover, this method requires oocyte in vitro maturation after thawing and has also been related to an increased incidence of chromosomal abnormalities. A study performed in 1997 (104) comparing 128 frozen immature oocytes with 91 control oocytes showed an increased frequency of chromosomal anomalies (77.8 vs. 31.8 percent) and spindle anomalies (70 vs. 22.2 percent); these percentages were similar (70 vs. 22 percent of spindle anomalies) in another more recent study (105). On the contrary, other authors did not find differences in spindle anomalies between cryopreserved MII or GV-stage oocytes (106, 107). However, as far as now, only one child has been born from early-stage cryopreserved oocytes matured in vitro and fertilized by ICSI (108).

The first human pregnancies and live births were announced in 1986–1988 (109–111). Apparently, those children were normal and healthy. Chen (109) reported this result obtained with a technique involving the reduction in size of the oocyte/cumulus-oophorus complex, the addition of DMSO as a one-step procedure, slow cooling between −7°C and −36°C after seeding, and rapid freezing to −196°C before storage in liquid nitrogen. Thawing was rapidly achieved by warming in a 37°C water bath, followed by dilution of the cryoprotectant as a single step. The oocytes were examined for morphological evidence of survival. Further development of the gametes required the transfer to the regular culture medium, and at appropriate time insemination was carried out.

Van Uem (111) obtained the second birth reported in the literature after oocyte cryopreservation, with a freezing technique different from the one described by Chen. In attempt to overcome cell damage due to super cooling, he developed a computer-controlled "open-vessel" freezing device (CTE 8100). This device permits seeding to take place automatically in the ideal temperature range around the freezing point of the medium (self-seeding). Further, van Uem adopted the technique of slow freezing and slow thawing. As Chen did, Van Uem also reduced the cumulus by needle dissection, but he used a freezing medium of phosphate-buffered saline containing 10 percent heat-inactivated fetal cord serum and 1.5-mol/L DMSO not chilled before the addition to the oocyte.

Subsequently, it was only after several years that another birth of a healthy female conceived with cryopreserved human oocytes was reported (112). This was the first child born after ICSI of oocytes cryopreserved with the propandiol slow-freezing technique. ICSI appeared to be a winning choice for the insemination of cryopreserved eggs as several additional pregnancies were obtained shortly after by the same team (113–118) and by other groups adopting the same technique (119–123). In the same period and with the same technique, Tucker et al. (108) obtained the first birth of a healthy child from a cryopreserved germinal vesicle oocyte. The following year,

Kuleshova (124) announced the birth of the first child from oocytes stored by vitrification. Also in this case, the newborn was normal and healthy. Subsequently, vitrification was successfully adopted by other authors with the publication of ten additional pregnancies (125, 126). Other technical variations such as the use of low-sodium-content medium resulted in normal children (127, 128).

Pregnancies from frozen eggs inseminated with epididymal and testicular (113) spermatozoa were published as well as the birth of a child conceived with frozen eggs and frozen sperms (115). Recently, the combination of both frozen eggs and frozen sperms ejaculated, epididymal, or testicular was successfully adopted by some authors (129–131) published the birth of a child conceived with a frozen embryo derived from frozen eggs and frozen testicular spermatozoa. These cases document that reproductive storage increases the flexibility of assisted reproduction routine and, even in the most complex combination, is apparently safe.

The recent literature often reports high pregnancy rates, ranging from 33 to 57 percent with the slow-freezing protocol (123, 127, 128, 132). However, these authors report studies done in a limited number of cycles with a low number of oocytes and probably in selected populations. Very recently, larger studies documented a pregnancy rate of 17 percent in 501 thawing cycles (133), 8.9 percent in 201 thawing cycles (134), 11.3 percent in 159 cycles (135), and 3.8 percent in 502 cycles (136).

In contrast, the performances of egg storage by means of vitrification do not seem to be more efficient so far. Yoon et al., (125) in thirty-four thawing cycles of 474 vitrified oocytes, reported a pregnancy rate of 21.4 percent per transfer and of 17.6 percent per cycle. The higher pregnancy rate reported by Katayama (126) (33 percent per transfer) and by Kuwayama (137) (41.4 percent per transfer) were, however, related to the thawing of a very small number of oocytes: forty-six and sixty-four, respectively. The same is true for the paper of Lucena (138) reporting a pregnancy rate of 56.5 percent in twenty-three transfers of embryos derived from vitrified oocytes. The patients of this report are very young, and the mean number of transferred embryos (4.63) is very high.

Finally, the application of oocyte cryopreservation to store the reproductive potential in cancer patients (139) appears promising.

It is crucial to perform the follow-up of the children from frozen eggs. The international register of frozen-egg babies has recently started to collect data.

KEY POINTS FOR CLINICAL PRACTICE

Embryo Cryopreservation

■ Embryo cryopreservation is crucial for both the efficiency and the safety of assisted reproduction treatments.

■ Storage of supernumerary embryos allows a significant increase in the cumulative pregnancy rate per patient.

■ Elective cryopreservation of all embryos and postponement of the embryo transfer is mandatory to avoid severe ovarian hyperstimulation syndrome in high-risk cases.

■ Cryopreserved embryos can be viable, and their transfer can be clinically successful even after more than ten years of storage.

■ Children born from cryopreserved embryos should be accurately monitored to ascertain the correct growth and development and to exclude possible genetic anomalies and malformations.

■ Legal and moral problems may arise from the long-term storage of cryopreserved embryos, and therefore, a detailed informed consent should be signed by the two partners.

Oocyte Cryopreservation

■ Oocyte freezing is an additional tool in the armamentarium of reproductive cryopreservation devoted from ethical and legal problems.

■ Egg freezing increases the flexibility of everyday IVF routine and can be used to rescue a treatment cycle in cases of failure to produce or retrieve the semen.

■ Storage of supernumerary oocytes allows an increase in the cumulative pregnancy rate per patient.

■ Elective cryopreservation of all the retrieved oocytes and postponement of the egg fertilization and embryo transfer avoid the development of severe ovarian hyperstimulation syndrome in high-risk cases and has no legal or ethical implications.

■ Oocyte cryopreservation should be taken into consideration in cancer patients (particularly, in partnerless women) undergoing antineoplastic treatments.

■ Egg freezing allows to perform quarantine in cases of egg donation.

■ Children born from cryopreserved oocytes should be accurately monitored to ascertain the correct growth and development and to exclude possible genetic anomalies and malformations.

REFERENCES

1. Wada I., Matson P.L., Troup S.A. et al. Does elective cryopreservation of all embryos from women at risk of ovarian hyperstimulation reduce the incidence of the condition? *Br. J. Obstet. Gynaecol.* 1993; 100: 265–9.

2. Trounson, Mohr L. Human pregnancy following cryopreservation, thawing and transfer of an eight-cell embryo. *Nature* 1983; 305: 707–9.

3. Zeilmaker G.H., Alberta A.T., Gent Van, I. et al. Two pregnancies following transfer of intact frozen–thawed embryos. *Fertil. Steril.* 1984; 42: 293–6.

4. Dulioust E., Toyama K., Busnel M.C., et al. Long term effects of embryo freezing in mice. *Proc. Natl. Acad. Sci. USA* 1995; 92: 589–93.

5. Whittingham D.G., Leibo S.P., Mazur P. Survival of mouse embryos frozen to −196° and −269°C. *Science* 1972; 178: 411–14.

6. Edwards R.G., Steptoe P.C. *Matter of Life*. Hutchinson, London, UK; 1980.

7. Kahn J.A., von During V., Sunde A., Sordal T., Molne K. The efficacy and efficiency of an in-vitro fertilization programme including embryo cryopreservation: a cohort study. *Hum. Reprod.* 1993; 8: 247–52.

8. Wang X.J., Ledger W., Payne D., Jeffrey R. Matthews C.D. The contribution of embryo cryopreservation to in-vitro fertilization/gamete intra-fallopian transfer: 8 years experience. *Hum. Reprod.* 1994; 9: 103–9.

9. Van Voorhis B.J., Syrop C.H., Allen B.D., Sparks A.E., Stovall D.W. The efficacy and cost effectiveness of embryo cryopreservation

compared with other assisted reproductive techniques. *Fertil. Steril.* 1995; 64: 647–50.

10. Mandelbaum, Belaisch-Allart J., Junca A.M., Antoine J.M., Plachot M., Alvarez S., et al. Cryopreservation in human assisted reproduction is now routine for embryos but remains a research procedure for oocytes. *Hum. Reprod.* 1998; 13 (Suppl. 3): 161–74.

11. Mouzon De, Lancaster P. International working group for registers on assisted reproduction. *J. Assist. Reprod. Gen.* 1997; 14: 251S–65.

12. Levran D., Dor J., Rudak E., Nebel L., Ben-Shlomo I., Ben-Rafael Z., Mashiach S. Pregnancy potential of human oocytes—the effect of cryopreservation. *N. Engl. J. Med.* 1990; 323: 1153–6.

13. Selick C.E., Hofmann G.E., Albano C., Horowitz G.M., Copperman A.B., Garrisi G.J., Navot D. Embryo quality and pregnancy potential of fresh compared with frozen embryos—is freezing detrimental to high quality embryos? *Hum. Reprod.* 1995; 10: 392–5.

14. Check J.H., Choe J.K., Nazari A., Fox F., Swenson K. Fresh embryo transfer is more effective than frozen for donor oocyte recipients but not for donors. *Hum. Reprod.* 2001; 16: 1403–8.

15. Mandelbaum J., Junca A.M., Plachot M., Alnot M.O., Alvarez S., Debache C., Salat-Baroux J., Cohen J. Human embryo cryopreservation, extrinsic and intrinsic parameters of success. *Hum. Reprod.* 1987; 2: 709–15.

16. Karlstrom P.O., Bergh T., Forsberg A.S., Sandkvist U., Wikland M. Prognostic factors for the success rate of embryo freezing. *Hum. Reprod.* 1997; 12: 1263–6.

17. Van den Abbeel E., Camus M., Van Waesberghe L., Devroey P., Van Steirteghem A.C. Viability of partially damaged human embryos after cryopreservation. *Hum. Reprod.* 1997; 12: 2006–10.

18. Burns W.N., Gaudet T.W., Martin M.B., Leal Y.R., Schoen H., Eddy C.A., Schenken R.S. Survival of cryopreservation and thawing with all blastomeres intact identifies multicell embryos with superior frozen embryo transfer outcome. *Fertil. Steril.* 1999; 72: 527–32.

19. Wang J.X., Yap Y.Y., Matthews C.D. Frozen–thawed embryo transfer: influence of clinical factors on implantation rate and risk of multiple conception. *Hum. Reprod.* 2001; 16: 2316–19.

20. Check J.H., O'Shaughnessy A., Lurie D., Fisher C., Adelson H.G. Evaluation of the mechanism for higher pregnancy rates in donor oocyte recipients by comparison of fresh with frozen embryo transfer pregnancy rates in a shared oocyte programme. *Hum. Reprod.* 1995; 10: 3022–7.

21. Check J.H., Choe J.K., Katsoff D., Summers-Chase D., Wilson C. Controlled ovarian hyperstimulation adversely affects implantation following in vitro fertilization-embryo transfer. *J. Assist. Reprod. Genet.* 1999; 16: 416–20.

22. Hu Y., Maxson W.S., Hoffman D.I., Ory S.J., Eager S. A comparison of post-thaw results between cryopreserved embryos derived from intracytoplasmic sperm injection and those from conventional IVF. *Fertil. Steril.* 1999; 72: 1045–8.

23. Van Steirteghem A.C., Van der Elst J., Van den Abbeel E., Joris H., Camus M., Devroey P. Cryopreservation of supernumerary multicellular human embryos obtained after intracytoplasmic sperm injection. *Fertil. Steril.* 1994; 62: 775–80.

24. Kowalik A., Palermo G.D., Barmat L., Veeck L., Rimarachin J., Rosenwaks Z. Comparison of clinical outcome after cryopreservation of embryos obtained from intracytoplasmic sperm injection and in-vitro fertilization. *Hum. Reprod.* 1998; 13: 2848.

25. Palermo, Cohen J., Alikani M., Adler A., Rosenwaks Z. Intracytoplasmic sperm injection: a novel treatment for all forms of male factor infertility. *Fertil. Steril.* 1995; 63: 1231–40.

26. Hoover L., Baker A., Check J.H., Lurie D., Summers D. Clinical outcome of cryopreserved human pronuclear stage embryos

resulting from intracytoplasmic sperm injection. *Fertil. Steril.* 1997; 67: 621–4.

27. Macas E., Imthurn B., Borsos M., Rosselli M., Maurer-Major E., Keller P.J. Impairment of the developmental potential of frozen–thawed human zygotes obtained after intracytoplasmic sperm injection. *Fertil. Steril.* 1998; 69: 630–5.

28. Damario M.A., Hammitt D.G., Galanits T.M., Session D.R., Dumesic D.A. Pronuclear stage cryopreservation after intracytoplasmic sperm injection and conventional IVF: implications for timing of the freeze. *Fertil. Steril.* 1999; 72: 1049–54.

29. Wennerholm W.B. Cryopreservation of embryos and oocytes: obstetric outcome and health in children. *Hum. Reprod.* 2000; 15 (Suppl. 5): 18–25.

30. Schalkoff M.E., Oskowitz S.P., Powers R.D. A multifactorial analysis of the pregnancy outcome in a successful embryo cryopreservation program. *Fertil. Steril.* 1993; 59: 1070–4.

31. Lin Y., Cassidenti D., Chacon R., et al. Successful implantation of frozen sibling embryos is influenced by the outcome of the cycle from which they were derived. *Fertil. Steril.* 1995; 63: 262–7.

32. Wang W.H., Meng L., Hackett R.J., Odenbourg R., Keefe D.L. Limited recovery of meiotic spindle in living human oocytes after cooling–rewarming observed using polarized light microscopy. *Hum. Reprod.* 2001a; 16: 2374–8.

33. Ben-Ozer S., Vermesh M. Full term delivery following cryopreservation of human embryos for 7. 5 years. *Hum. Reprod.* 1999; 14(6): 1650–2.

34. Revel A., Safran A., Laufer N., Lewin A., Reubinov B.E., Simon A. Twin delivery following 12 years of human embryo cryopreservation: case report. *Hum. Reprod.* 2004; 19(2): 328–9.

35. Lopez Teijon M., Serra O., Olivares R., Moragas M., Castello C., Alvarez J.G. Delivery of a healthy baby following the transfer of embryos cryopreserved for 13 years. *Reprod. Biomed. Online* 2006; 13(6): 821–2.

36. Sutcliffe A., D'Souza S., Cadman J., et al. Minor congenital anomalies, major congenital malformations and development in children conceived from cryopreserved embryos. *Hum. Reprod.* 1995a; 10: 3332–7.

37. Shaw J.M., Trounson A. Effect of dimethylsulfoxide and protein concentration on the viability of two-cell mouse embryos frozen with a rapid freezing technique. *Cryobiology* 1989; 26: 413–21.

38. Rall W.F., Wood M.J., Kirby C., et al. Development of mouse embryos cryopreserved by vitrification. *J. Reprod. Fertil.* 1987; 80: 499–504.

39. Liu J., Van Den Abbeel E., Van Steirteghem A. Assessment of ultrarapid and slow freezing procedures for 1-cell and 4-cell mouse embryos. *Hum. Reprod.* 1993; 7: 1115–19.

40. Olivennes F., Rufat P., Andre B., Pourade A., Quiros M.C., Frydman R. The increased risk of complication observed in singleton pregnancies resulting from in-vitro fertilization (IVF) does not seem to be related to the IVF method itself. *Hum. Reprod.* 1993; 8(8): 1297–300.

41. Tanbo Dale, P.O., Lunde O., Moe N., übyholm T. Obstetric outcome in singleton pregnancies after assisted reproduction. *Obstet. Gynecol.* 1995; 86: 188–92.

42. Frydman R., Forman R.G., Belaisch-Allart J., et al. An obstetric analysis of fifty consecutive pregnancies after transfer of cryopreserved human embryos. *Am. J. Obstet. Gynecol.* 1989; 160: 209–13.

43. Rizk B., Edwards R.G., Nicolini U., et al. Edward's syndrome after the replacement of cryopreserved-thawed embryos. *Fertil. Steril.* 1991; 55: 208–10.

44. Deffontaines D., Logerot-Lebrun H., Sele B., et al. Comparaison des grossesses issues de transferts d'embryons congeles aux

grossesses issues de transferts d'embryons frais en fecondation in vitro. *Contracept. Fertil. Sex.* 1994; 22: 287–91.

45. Wada I., Macnamee M.C., Wick K., Bradfield J.M., Brinsden P.R. Birth characteristics and perinatal outcome of babies conceived from cryopreserved embryos. *Hum. Reprod.* 1994; 9: 543–6.

46. Heijnsbroek I., Helmerhorst F.M., van den Berg-Helder A.F., van der Zwan K.J., Naaktgeboren N., Keirse, M.J. Follow-up of 30 pregnancies after embryo cryopreservation. Eur. *J. Obstet. Gynecol. Reprod. Biol.* 1995; 59(2): 201–4.

47. Sutcliffe A.G., D'Souza S.W., Cadman J., et al. Outcome in children from cryopreserved embryos. *Arch. Dis. Child.* 1995b; 72: 290–3.

48. Olivennes F., Schneider Z., Remy V., et al. Perinatal outcome and follow-up of 82 children aged 1–9 years old conceived from cryopreserved embryos. *Hum. Reprod.* 1996; 11: 1565–8.

49. Wennerholm Hamberger, L., Nilsson L., Wennergren M., Wikland M. Bergh C. Obstetric and perinatal outcome of children conceived from cryopreserved embryos. *Hum. Reprod.* 1997; 12: 1819–25.

50. Wood M.J. Embryo freezing: is it safe? *Hum. Reprod.* 1997; 12 (Natl Suppl. 1): 32–7.

51. Wennerholm U.B., Albertsson-Wikland K., Bergh C., et al. Postnatal growth and health in children born after cryopreservation as embryos. *Lancet* 1998; 351: 1085–90.

52. Bergh T., Ericson A., Hillensjo T., Nygren K.G., Wennerholm U.B. Deliveries and children born after in-vitro fertilisation in Sweden 1982-95: a retrospective cohort study. *Lancet* 1999; 354(9190): 1579–85.

53. Lane M., Gardner D.K. Increase in postimplantation development of cultured mouse embryos by amino acids and induction of fetal retardation and exencephaly by ammonium ions. *J. Reprod. Fertil.* 1994; 102: 305–12.

54. Thompson J.G., Gardner D.K., Pugh P.A., et al. Lamb birth weight is affected by culture system utilized during in vitro pre-elongation development of ovine embryos. *Biol. Reprod.* 1995; 53: 1385–91.

55. Karran G., Legge M. Non-enzymatic formation of formaldehyde in mouse oocyte freezing mixtures. *Hum. Reprod.* 1996; 11: 2691–86.

56. Mahadevan M.M., McIntosh A., Miller M.M., et al. Formaldehyde in cryoprotectant propanediol and effect on mouse zygotes. *Hum. Reprod.* 1998; 13: 979–82.

57. Bonduelle M., Joris H., Hofmans K., et al. Mental development of 201 ICSI children at 2 years of age. *Lancet* 1998; 351: 1553.

58. Bowen J., Gibson F.L., Leslie G.I., Saunders D.M. Medical and developmental outcome at 1 year for children conceived by intracytoplasmic sperm injection. *Lancet* 1998; 351: 1529–34.

59. Sheppard D.M., Fisher R.A., Lawler S.D., Povey S. Tetraploid conceptus with three paternal contributions. *Hum. Genet.* 1982; 62: 371–4.

60. Warburton D., Byrne J., Canki N. (eds) Chromosome Anomalies and Prenatal Development: An Atlas. *Oxford Monographs on Medical Genetics.* No. 21, Oxford University Press; 1991.

61. Hui S.W., Stewart T.P., Boni L.T., Yeagle P.L. Membrane fusion through point defects in bilayers. *Science* 1981; 212: 921–3.

62. Zimmermann U., Vienken J. Electric field-induced cell-to-cell fusion. *J. Memb. Biol.* 1982; 67: 165–82.

63. Ng S.C., Sathananthan A.H., Wong P.C., et al. Fine structure of early human embryos frozen with 1,2 propanediol. *Gamete Res.* 1988; 19: 253–63.

64. Dumoulin J.C., Bergers-Janssen J.M., Pieters M.H., Enginsu M.E., Geraedts J.P., Evers J.L. The protective effects of polymers in the cryopreservation of human and mouse zonae pellucidae and embryos. *Fertil. Steril.* 1994; 62: 793–8.

65. Trounson A. In vitro fertilization and embryo preservation. In: Trounson A., Wood C. (eds). *In Vitro Fertilization and Embryo Transfer.* Churchill Livingstone, Edinburgh; 1984; pp. 111–30.

66. Balakier H., Zenzes M., Wang P., et al. The effect of cryopreservation on development of S- and G2-phase mouse embryos. *J. In Vitro Fertil. Embryo Transfer* 1991; 8: 89–95.

67. Bongso A., Chye N.S., Sathananthan H., et al. Chromosome analysis of two-cell mouse embryos frozen by slow and ultra-rapid methods using two different cryoprotectants. *Fertil. Steril.* 1988; 49: 908–12.

68. Ishida G.M., Saito H., Ohta N., et al. The optimal equilibration time for mouse embryos frozen by vitrification with trehalose. *Hum. Reprod.* 1997; 12: 1259–62.

69. Shaw J.M., Kola I., MacFarlane D.R., Trounson A.O. An association between chromosomal abnormalities in rapidly frozen 2-cell mouse embryos and the ice-forming properties of the cryoprotective solution. *J. Reprod. Fertil.* 1991; 91: 9–18.

70. Dale B., Gualtieri R., Talevi R., et al. Intercellular communication in the early human embryo. *Mol. Reprod. Dev.* 1991; 29: 22–8.

71. Mottla G.L., Adelman M.R., Hall J.L., et al. Lineage tracing demonstrates that blastomeres of early cleavage-stage human pre-embryos contribute to both trophectoderm and inner cell mass. *Hum. Reprod.* 1995; 10: 384–91.

72. Laverge H., Van der Elst J., De Sutter P., et al. Fluorescent in situ hybridization on human embryos showing cleavage arrest after freezing and thawing. *Hum. Reprod.* 1998; 13: 425–9.

73. Balakier H., Cabaca O., Bouman D., Shewchuk A.B., Laskin C., Squire J.A. Spontaneous blastomere fusion after freezing and thawing of early human embryos leads to polyploidy and chromosomal mosaicism. *Hum. Reprod.* 2000; 15(11): 2404–10.

74. James R.M., West J.D. A chimaeric animal model for confined placental mosaicism. *Hum. Genet.* 1994; 93: 603–4.

75. Ginsburg K.A., Johnson M.P., Sacco A.G., et al. Tetraploidy after frozen embryo transfer: cryopreservation may interfere with first mitotic division. 39th Annual Meeting of the Pacific Coast Fertility Society. 1991P-196, Abstracts of oral and poster presentations. Program Supplement, S169.

76. Henery C., Bard J.B.L., Kaufman M.H. Tetraploidy in mice, embryonic cell number, and the grain of the developmental map. *Dev. Biol.* 1992; 152: 233–41.

77. Tanbo T., Abyholm T. Obstetric and perinatal outcome in pregnancies after assisted reproduction. *Curr. Opin. Obstet. Gynecol.* 1996; 8(3): 193–8.

78. Wright G., Wiker S., Elsner C., Kort H., Massey J., Mitchell D., Toledo A., Cohen J. Observations on the morphology of pronuclei and nucleoli in human zygotes and implications for cryopreservation. *Hum. Reprod.* 1990; 5(1): 109–15.

79. Van der Auwera I., Meuleman C., Koninckx P.R. Human menopausal gonadotrophin increases pregnancy rate in comparison with clomiphene citrate during replacement cycles of frozen/thawed pronucleate ova. *Hum. Reprod.* 1994; 9(8): 1556–60.

80. Al-Hasani S., Ludwig M., Gagsteiger F., Kupker W., Sturm R., Yilmaz A., Bauer O., Diedrich K. Comparison of cryopreservation of supernumerary pronuclear human oocytes obtained after intracytoplasmic sperm injection (ICSI) and after conventional in-vitro fertilization. *Hum. Reprod.* 1996; 11: 604–7.

81. Go K., Corson S., Batzer F., et al. Live birth from a zygote cryopreserved for 8 years. *Hum. Reprod.* 1998; 13: 2970–1.

82. Porcu E., Fabbri R., Damiano G., Fratto R., Giunchi S., Venturoli S. Oocyte cryopreservation in oncological patients. *Eur. J. Obstet. Gynecol. Reprod. Biol.* 2004;113 (Suppl. 1): S14–16.

83. Whittingham D.G. Fertilization in vitro and development to term of unfertilized mouse oocytes previously stored at—196 degrees C. *J. Reprod. Fertil.* 1977; 49(1): 89–94.

84. Vincent C., Johnson M.H.Cooling, cryoprotectants, and the cytoskeleton of the mammalian oocyte. *Oxf. Rev. Reprod. Biol.* 1992; 14: 73–100.

85. Kazem R., Thompson L.A., Srikantharajah A., Laing M.A., Hamilton M.P.R., Templeton A. A Cryopreservation of human oocytes and fertilization by two techniques in-vitro fertilization and intracytoplasmic sperm injection. *Hum. Reprod.* 1995; 10: 2650–4.

86. Van Blerkom, Davis P. Cytogenetic, cellular and developmental consequences of cryopreservation of immature and mature mouse and human oocytes. *Microsc. Res. Tech.* 1994; 27: 165–93.

87. Pickering S.J., Brande P.R., Johnson M.H. Transient cooling to room temperature can cause irreversible disruption to the meiotic spindle in human oocytes. *Fertil. Steril.* 1990; 54: 102–8.

88. Wang W.H., Cao B., Meng L., Hackett R.J., Keefe D.L. Imaging living, human MII oocytes with the polscope reveals a high proportion of abnormal meiotic spindles. *Fertil. Steril.* 2001b; 76 (Suppl. 1): S2.

89. Mazur P., Rall W.F., Leibo S.P. Kinetics of water loss and the likelihood of intracellular freezing in mouse ova: influence of the method of calculating the temperature dependence of water permeability. *Cell Biophys.* 1984; 6: 197–213.

90. Bernard A., McGrath J.J., Fuller B.J., Imoedemhe D., Shaw R.W. Osmotic response of oocytes using a microscope diffusion chamber: a preliminary study comparing murine and human ova. *Cryobiology* 1988; 25: 495–501.

91. Magistrini M., Szollosi D. Effects of cold and of isopropyl-N-phenylcarbamate on the second meiotic spindle of mouse oocytes. *Eur. J. Cell Biol.* 1980; 22(2): 699–707.

92. Mandelbaum J., Anastasiou O., Levy R., Guerin J.F., de Larouziere V., Antoine J.M. Effects of cryopreservation on the meiotic spindle of human oocytes. *Eur. J. Obstet. Gynecol. Reprod. Biol.* 2004; 113 (Suppl. 1): S17–23.

93. Kola I., Cirby C., Shaw J., Davey A., Trouson A. Vitrification of mouse oocytes results in aneuploid zygotes and malformed fetuses. *Teratology* 1988; 38: 467–74.

94. Battaglia D.E., Goodwin P., Klein N.A., Soules M.R. Influence of maternal age on meiotic spindle assembly in oocytes from naturally cycling women. *Hum. Reprod.* 1996; 11: 2217–22.

95. Sandalinas Marquez, C., Munne S. Spectral karyotyping of fresh, non-inseminated oocytes. *Mol. Hum. Reprod.* 2002; 8: 580–5.

96. Johnson MH, Pickering SJ. The effect of dimethylsulphoxide on the microtubular system of the mouse oocyte. *Development* 1987; 100(2): 313–24.

97. Van der Elst J, Van den Abbeel E, Jacobs R, Wisse E, Van Steirteghem A. Effect of 1,2-propanediol and dimethylsulphoxide on the meiotic spindle of the mouse oocyte. *Hum. Reprod.* 1988; 3(8): 960–7.

98. Sathananthan, Trounson A., Freeman L., Brady T. The effects of cooling human oocytes. *Hum. Reprod.* 1988; 3: 968–77.

99. Gook, Osborn S.M., Johnston W.I. Cryopreservation of mouse and human oocytes using 1,2-propanediol and the configuration of the meiotic spindle. *Hum. Reprod.* 1993; 8: 1101–9.

100. Zenzes, Bielecki R., Casper R.F., Leibo S.P. Effects of chilling to 0 °C on the morphology of meiotic spindles in human metaphase II oocytes. *Fertil. Steril.* 2001; 75: 769–77.

101. Fahy, McFarlane D.R., Angell C.A., Meryman H.A.T. Vitrification as an approach to cryopreservation. *Cryobiology* 1984; 21: 407–26.

102. Toth, Lanzendorf S.E., Sandow B.A., Veeck L.L., Hassen W.A., Hansen K., et al. Cryopreservation of human prophase I oocytes collected from unstimulated follicles. *Fertil. Steril.* 1994; 61: 1077–82.

103. Son, Park S.E., Lee K.A., Lee W.S., Ko J.J., Yoon T.K., et al. Effects of 1,2-propanediol and freezing-thawing on the in vitro developmental capacity of human immature oocytes. *Fertil. Steril.* 1996; 66: 995–9.

104. Park, Son W.Y., Lee S.H., Lee K.A., Ko J.J., Cha K.Y. Chromosome and spindle configurations of human oocytes matured in vitro after cryopreservation at the germinal vesicle stage. *Fertil. Steril.* 1997; 68: 920–6.

105. Boiso I., Marti M., Santalo J., Ponsa M., Barri P.N., Veiga A. A confocal microscopy analysis of the spindle and chromosome configurations of human oocytes cryopreserved at the germinal vesicle and metaphase II stage. *Hum. Reprod.* 2002; 17(7): 1885–91.

106. Baka, Toth T.L., Veeck L.L., Jones H.W. Jr., Muasher S.J. Lanzendorf S.E. Evaluation of the spindle apparatus of in-vitro matured human oocytes following cryopreservation. *Hum. Reprod.* 1995; 10: 1816–20.

107. Cobo A., Rubio C., Gerli S., Ruiz A., Pellicer A., Remohi J. Use of fluorescence in situ hybridization to assess the chromosomal status of embryos obtained from cryopreserved oocytes. *Fertil. Steril.* 2001; 75: 354–60.

108. Tucker, Wright G., Morton P.C., Massey J.B. Birth after cryopreservation of immature oocytes with subsequent in vitro maturation. *Fertil. Steril.* 1998; 70: 578–9.

109. Chen C. Pregnancy after human oocyte cryopreservation. *Lancet* 1986; i: 884–6.

110. Chen C. Pregnancies after human oocyte cryopreservation. *Ann. N.Y. Acad. Sci.* 1988; 54: 541–9.

111. Van Uem J.F., Siebzehnrubl E.R., Schuh B., Koch R., Trotnow S., Lang N. Birth after cryopreservation of unfertilized oocytes. *Lancet* 1987; i: 752–3.

112. Porcu E., Fabbri R., Seracchioli R., Ciotti P.M., Magrini O., Flamigni C. Birth of a healthy female after intracytoplasmic sperm injection of cryopreserved human oocytes. *Fertil. Steril.* 1997; 68: 724–6.

113. Porcu E., Fabbri R., Petracchi S., Ciotti P.M., Flamigni C. Ongoing pregnancy after intracytoplasmic sperm injection of testicular spermatozoa into cryopreserved human oocytes. *Am. J. Obstet. Gynecol.* 1999a; 180: 1044–5.

114. Porcu E., Fabbri R., Ciotti P.M., Petracchi S., Seracchioli R., Flamigni C. Ongoing pregnancy after intracytoplasmic sperm injection of epididymal spermatozoa into cryopreserved human oocytes. *J. Assist. Reprod. Genet.* 1999b; 16: 283–5.

115. Porcu E., Fabbri R., Damiano G., Giunchi S., Fratto R., Ciotti P.M., Venturoli S., Flamigni C. Clinical experience and applications of oocyte cryopreservation. *Mol. Cell. Endocrinol.* 2000; 169: 33–7.

116. Porcu E., Fabbri R., Seracchioli R., De Cesare R., Giunchi S., Caracciolo D. Obsterics, perinatal outcome and follow up of children conceived from cryopreserved oocytes. *Fertil. Steril.* 2000a; 74 (n.3S, Suppl. 1): S48.

117. Porcu E. Oocyte freezing. *Semin. Reprod. Med.* 2001a; 19: 221–30.

118. Porcu E., Fabbri R., Ciotti P.M., Frau F., De Cesare R., Venturoli S. Oocytes or embryo storage? *Fertil. Steril.* 2002; 169 (Suppl. 1): S15.

119. Polak de Fried E., Notrica J., Rubinstein M., Marazzi A., Gomez Gonzalez M. Pregnancy after human donor oocyte cryopreservation and thawing in association with intracytoplasmic sperm injection in a patient with ovarian failure. *Fertil. Steril.* 1998; 69(3): 555–7.

120. Young E., Kenny A., Puigdomenech E., Van Thillo G., Tiveron M., Piazza A. Triplet pregnancy after intracytoplasmic sperm injection of cryopreserved oocytes: case report. *Fertil. Steril.* 1998; 70(2): 360–1.

121. Nawroth F., Kissing K. Pregnancy after intracytoplasmatic sperm injection (ICSI) of cryopreserved human oocytes. *Acta Obstet. Gynecol. Scand.* 1998; 77(4): 462–3.

122. Chen S.U., Lien I.R., Tsai Y.Y., Hanh L.I. Successful pregnancy occurred from slowly freezing human oocytes using the regime of 1.5 mol/l 1,2-propanediol with 0.3 mol/l sucrose. *Hum. Reprod.* 2002; 17(5): 1412.

123. Fosas N., Marina F., Torres P.J., Jove I., Martin P., Perez N., Arnedo N., Marina S. The births of five Spanish babies from cryopreserved donated oocytes. *Hum. Reprod.* 2003; 18(7): 1417–21.

124. Kuleshova L., Gianaroli L., Magli C., Ferraretti A., Trounson A. Birth following vitrification of a small number of human oocytes: case report. *Hum. Reprod.* 1999; 14(12): 3077–9.

125. Yoon T.K., Kim T.J., Park S.E., Hong S.W., Ko J.J., Chung H.M., Cha K.Y. Live births after vitrification of oocytes in a stimulated in vitro fertilization-embryo transfer program. *Fertil. Steril.* 2003; 79(6): 1323–6.

126. Katayama K.P., Stehlik J., Kuwayama M., Kato O., Stehlik E. High survival rate of vitrified human oocytes results in clinical pregnancy. *Fertil. Steril.* 2003; 80(1): 223–4.

127. Quintans C.J., Donaldson M.J., Bertolino M.V., Pasqualini R.S. Birth of two babies using oocytes that were cryopreserved in a choline-based freezing medium. *Hum. Reprod.* 2002; 17(12): 3149–52.

128. Boldt J., Cline D., McLaughlin D. Human oocyte cryopreservation as an adjunct to IVF-embryo transfer cycles. *Hum. Reprod.* 2003; 18(6): 1250–5.

129. Azambuja R., Badalotti M., Teloken C., Michelon J., Petracco A. Case report: successful birth after injection of frozen human oocytes with frozen epididymal spermatozoa. *Reprod. BioMed. Online* 2005; 11: 449–51.

130. Ching-Ching Tjer G., Tak-Yu Chiu T., Cheung L., Lok I.H., Haines C.J. Birth of a healthy baby after transfer of blastocysts derived from cryopreserved human oocytes fertilized with frozen spermatozoa. *Fertil. Steril.* 2005; 83: 1547.e1–e3.

131. Levi Setti P.E., Albani E., Novara P.V., Cesana A., Bianchi S., Negri L. Normal birth after transfer of cryopreserved human embryos generated by microinjection of cryopreserved testicular spermatozoa into cryopreserved human oocytes. *Fertil. Steril.* 2006; 83: 1041.e9–10.

132. Chen S.U., Lien Y.R., Chen H.F., Chang L.J., Tsai Y.Y., Yang Y.S. Observational clinical follow-up of oocyte cryopreservation using a slow-freezing method with 1,2-propanediol plus sucrose followed by ICSI. *Hum. Reprod.* 2005; 20(7): 1975–80.

133. Porcu E. Cryopreservation of oocytes: indications, risks and outcome. *Hum. Reprod.* 2005; 20: 50.

134. Borini A., Sciajno R., Bianchi V., Sereni E., Flamigni C., Coticchio G. Clinical outcome of oocyte cryopreservation after slow cooling with a protocol utilizing a high sucrose concentration. *Hum. Reprod.* 2006; 21(2): 512–17.

135. Levi Setti P.E., Albani E., Novara P.V., Cesana A., Morreale G. Cryopreservation of supernumerary oocytes in IVF/ICSI cycles. *Hum. Reprod.* 2006; 21(2): 370–5.

136. La Sala G.B., Nicoli A., Villani M.T., Pescarini M., Gallinelli A., Blickstein I. Outcome of 518 salvage oocyte-cryopreservation cycles performed as a routine procedure in an in vitro fertilization program. *Fertil. Steril.* 2006; 86(5): 1423–7.

137. Kuwayama M., Vajta G., Kato O., Leibo S. Highly efficient vitrification method for cryopreservation of human oocytes. *Reprod. BioMed. Online* 2005; 11(3): 300–8.

138. Lucena E., Bernal D.P., Lucena C., Rojas A., Moran A., Lucena A. Successful ongoing pregnancies after vitrification of oocytes. *Fertil. Steril.* 2006; 85(1): 108–11.

139. Porcu E., Fabbri R., Damiano G., Fratto R., Giunchi S., Venturoli S. Oocyte cryopreservation in oncological patients. *Eur. J. Obstet. Gynecol. Reprod. Biol.* 2004; 113 (Suppl. 1): S14–16.

51

CRYOPRESERVATION OF MALE GAMETES

Amjad Hossain, Manubai Nagamani

INTRODUCTION

Cryopreservation of male gametes is an important aspect of human fertility preservation. With the advancement in assisted reproductive technology, indication for sperm cryopreservation is expanding. The exciting developments that have occurred over the years in this field have resulted in frozen sperm being as good as fresh sperm in fertilizing oocytes. Our objective is to provide the readers with the latest available information on cryopreservation of human spermatozoa including the sperm retrieved by epididymal aspiration and testicular biopsies. Conceptual, methodological, as well as regulatory information are provided so that the readers can obtain comprehensive knowledge about human sperm cryopreservation. Since American Society for Reproductive Medicine (ASRM) is the leading organization worldwide that is professionally involved with the assisted reproduction, ASRM's stance on ethical, professional, and patient safety issues related to cryopreservation of human sperm and their utilization are discussed. The techniques, methodology, and procedures described in this chapter are highly relevant to the current practice of assisted human reproduction and sperm banking.

HISTORICAL BACKGROUND

It has been known for more than a decade that the fertilization capacity of mammalian spermatozoa can be preserved by cryopreservation technology (1, 2). It was an Italian physician who first proposed in 1866 the concept of human sperm bank to store semen specimens (1, 3, 4). The first successful human pregnancy by cryopreserved spermatozoa was reported by Bunge et al. in 1954 (1). This cryopreservation-related early discoveries and subsequent successful pregnancies (4–11) led to the gradual clinical application of frozen human sperm and the establishment of sperm bank (1). Sherman, in 1978 (12), and David and Lansac, in 1980 (13), were the pioneers who advocated using cryopreserved sperm for treating infertility. There have been numerous reviews of sperm cryopreservation and banking over time, but the reviews of human sperm cryopreservation by Trounson et al. (5), Crister (9), Leibo et al. (2), and Fuller and Paynter (2) are noteworthy since they cover the major historical events that occurred in the field of human sperm cryopreservation.

DIFFERENCES BETWEEN CLIENT AND DONOR SPERM CRYOPRESERVATION

Donor sperm banking involves semen donated to women who are not intimate partners. Some of the relevant internationally accepted terminologies used in sperm banking are listed in Table 51.1. Sperm donor can be either anonymous or known (directed donor) to the recipient. A client depositor is one whose sperm is cryopreserved for use by his intimate partner. Regulations are similar yet different in many ways between the sperm donor and the client depositor. There is no mandatory requirement for testing and quarantine in case of the client depositor's sperm. It is argued that since the client has intimate relationship with the partner, the risk of sexually transmitted infection is already there. Food and Drug Administration FDA recommends, but does not require, disease testing and quarantine when stored reproductive tissues are used between sexually intimate partners (11).

CURRENT CONSIDERATION OF DONOR SPERM BANKING

Based on the current scientific understanding, fresh semen is no longer appropriate for therapeutic use in utilization of donor sperm for artificial insemination (AI). It is not only the recommendation, it is also the regulatory requirement that only cryopreserved sperm from the donor can be used and the specimen has to be tested for disease, quarantined for six months, and retested before specimens can be released for use. Reproductive tissue banks are required to register with FDA for oversight of their practices. FDA and other federal and state regulatory agencies are enforcing mandatory good tissue practices in reproductive tissue processing, handling, and utilization (14–18). The level of donor screening and quarantine requirements is not uniform. In the United States, it, to some extent, varies between the states. New York State probably implements the most stringent rules for donor sperm banks. In the private sector, ASRM, AATB (American Association of Tissue Bank), CAP (College of American Pathologist), AAB (American Association of Bioanalyst), and JCAHO (Joint Commission of Accreditation of Healthcare Organizations) have established standards and oversight for reproductive tissue industries.

The semen donor is selected based on established selection criteria and screening processes. The minimum semen parameters recommended for donor sperm cryopreservation are shown in Table 51.2. The initial screening should include

Table 51.1: Terminologies Used in Semen Banking

Donor	One who provides his own semen for cryobanking for artificial insemination of a recipient other than his wife or intimate partner
Anonymous donor	A donor whose identity is unknown to the recipient
Directed donor	A donor who is known to the recipient and who directs his semen for use by a particular recipient
Client depositor	One who cryopreserved his semen for deferred insemination of a sexually intimate partner
Cryobank	An entity that collects, processes, stores, and/or distributes human sperm for use in assisted reproductive procedures
Quarantine	Temporary storage/isolation of cryopreserved semen in a physically separate area identified for such use to prevent improper release in order to prevent the spread of communicable disease agent
Cryopreservation	The branch of cryobiology that deals with the brining of reversible suspension of life activities in the frozen state at ultra low temperatures with the help of cryoprotectant

Table 51.2: Minimal Semen Parameters Recommended for Sperm Donor Whose Semen Is Intended for Cryopreservation

Volume	>2.0 mL
Sperm motility	>50 percent
Sperm concentration	>50 × 10^6 motile sperm/mL
Sperm morphology	Normal range
Cryosurvival	>50 percent

Source: Supplement to Fertility and Sterility, September 2004, Vol. 82 (Suppl. 1).

individual's personal history, sexual and social history, and family's medical and genetic history. The next screening step includes physical examination with specific examination of the individual's urogenital tract. Finally, specific blood tests and semen cultures are performed (4, 9, 19–21). Examples of general screening tests for semen donors are shown in Table 51.3, and recommended genetic screenings for gamete donor (egg donor as well as sperm donor) are listed in Table 51.4.

INDICATIONS FOR SPERM CRYOPRESERVATION

With the advancement of knowledge in assisted reproduction, the indications for sperm cryopreservation are expanding.

Table 51.3: Major Tests Used for Screening Semen Donors

1. Physical examination
2. Genetical screening
3. Syphillis serology
4. Hepatitis B and C
5. HIV
6. Chlamydia
7. Cytomegalovirus
8. Gonorrhea
9. Special test/screening; specific genetic disorder based on family history and ethnicity.

With advances in gene chip technology, it may be possible to eliminate donors if they carry certain genetic risk factors.

Table 51.4: Genetic Screening for Gamete Donors in Various Ethnic Groups

Ethnic group	Disorder	Test
Ashkenazi Jews	Tay-Sachs disease	Serum hexosaminidase-A
	Canavan disease	Analysis of alleles
African American	Sickle cell anemia	Sickle cell hemoglobin
Mediterranean and Southeast Asians	Beta-thalassemia	Hemoglobin electrophoresis
All ethnic groups	Cystic fibrosis	Analysis of a panel of 25 CFTR mutations

Source: Supplement to Fertility and Sterility, September 2004, Vol. 82 (Suppl. 1).

Since intracytoplasmic sperm injection (ICSI) has proved to be a successful method of fertilization, virtually any ejaculate, aspirate, no matter how poor the quality, is worthy of freezing. Cryopreservation of sperm cut down the necessity of obtaining fresh sperm for subsequent ART cycles. Abundant evidence exists in literature indicating that frozen sperm are as good as fresh sperm in fertilizing oocytes and subsequent developments (8, 22–24). Currently, known traditional as well as nontraditional indications of sperm cryopreservation can be summarized as below (24–29).

1. Cancer patients: Cancer therapy is well documented to have profound effects on testicular function. The duration of this effect can be variable or be permanent. It is important to offer sperm cryopreservation to male cancer patient who will be undergoing gonadotoxic therapy for the treatment of cancer.
2. Vasectomy: Prevasectomy sperm freeze can act as reproductive insurance in case of remarriage or accidentally becoming childless by natural catastrophe affecting children after vasectomy. Vasectomy reversal that is used as an

alternative for prevasectomy sperm freezing is very expensive, exposes the man to anesthetic and surgical risk, and is not always successful.

3. Spinal cord injured patient: Electroejaculation specimen can be cryopreserved and successfully used in assisted reproduction for spinal cord injured patient.
4. Oligozoospermic/asthenozoospermic sample: Anticipation of enriching the number of motile sperm by pooling several cryopreserved samples.
5. MESA, TESE, and TESA (see explanation of terminologies in appropriate section): to avoid multiple biopsies/surgeries.

Other less common indications for sperm cryopreservation and storage include:

6. Vassal and vasoepididymal reconstruction procedures.
7. Transurethral resection of the ejaculatory ducts.
8. Postmortem sperm retrieval and storage.

All men have the natural desire to have their own biological children. Both men and women may face unexpected circumstances in real life, which make them to plan for fertility preservation with the help of cryopreservation technology. Figure 51.1 outlines the current cryopreservation options available for male fertility preservation of infertility patients and cancer patients who need radiation or chemotherapy.

CRYOBIOLOGY OF HUMAN SPERMATOZOA

The laws of thermodynamics that dictate the principles of cryopreservation of human sperm cells are similar to the cryopreservation of other cells (30–35). The sperm cryopreservation process involves four major steps, namely temperature reduction, cellular dehydration, freezing, and thawing. The function of a cryoprotectant is to remove or reduce the water content from a sperm cell, which in turn helps to minimize intracellular ice formation during freezing. Exposure of spermatozoa to cryoprotectant solution initially causes them to shrink because of losing intracellular water due to increased extracellular osmolarity. The sperm cells return to its original volume by allowing the penetration of cryoprotectant into their intracellular space. In actual freezing, the addition of a cryoprotectant is usually accompanied by the reduction of temperature. In the cooling process, when the temperature reaches -5 to $-15°C$, extracellular ice formation occurs and it induces the development of an extracellular solid phase (35). The sperm cell remains unfrozen but supercooled. The supercooled intracellular water diffuses out of the cell osmotically, and freezing continues extracellularly, resulting in hypertonicity and a further reduction of water from sperm cell, leading to dehydration in fulfilling the goal of freezing. At the time of thawing, the sperm cells undergo the same hydration/dehydration process but in reverse. Spermatozoa that have undergone a slow freezing rate should also be warmed slowly during thawing, while sperms that have been frozen rapidly should be thawed rapidly (33, 35).

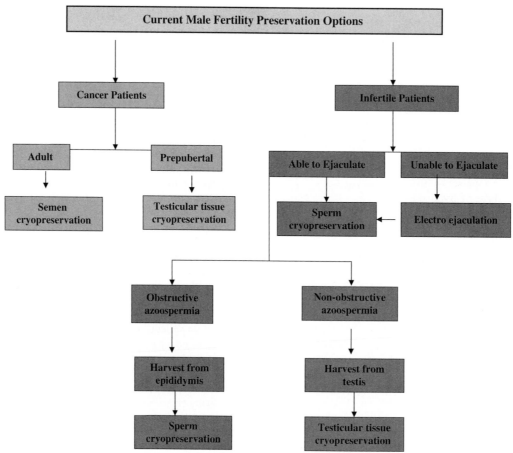

Figure 51.1. Current approaches to male fertility preservation.

Human sperm like other mammalian sperm apparently are not adapted to endure low temperatures. All mammalian sperms are sensitive to cooling. It has been shown that cold shock (cooling above 0°C) has an impact on motility, membrane permeability, and other metabolic functions. A reduction in temperature can cause forced transition of the membrane phospholipids from liquid crystalline to gel. These detrimental effects of cold shock can be prevented with the help of a cryoprotectant and by controlling the rate of cooling. Freezing related injury is different from that of cold shock. At subzero temperature (-5 to -10°C) and further below, disruption of cellular structures from mechanical stress of ice crystal formation can occur. Controlled rate of cooling and cryoprotectants are utilized to prevent the impact of ice crystals on the integrity of the cell as much as possible.

The success of cryopreservation is affected by many factors including membrane permeability, amount of intracellular water, type of cryoprotectant, and the method of freezing and thawing (7, 31, 33, 35, 36). Two important parameters that influence cryopreservation the most are cell membrane permeability and amount of intracellular water. Thus, the outcome of cryopreservation can be considered as cell specific. Theoretically, spermatozoa are ideal cells to cryopreserve since they have relatively small volume, a large surface area, very little cytoplasm, and contain less intracellular water than other cells (35). However, cryosurvival rate of human spermatozoa of around 50 percent does not fully support this theoretical notion. Such low cryosurvival rate indicates the necessity of more understanding of sperm cryobiology in order to improve cryosurvival. The effectiveness of a cryoprotectant that is used in cryopreservation plays a vital role in controlling cryosurvival. The characteristics of an ideal cryoprotectant should be 1) low molecular weight, 2) high solubility, 3) cell permeability, and 4) being nontoxic at high intracellular concentration. Glycerol was accidentally discovered to possess cryoprotecting property, and glycerol still remains as the most widely used cryoprotectant for freezing spermatozoa. Human spermatozoa have been cryopreserved since 1953, using glycerol as the cryoprotectant (1).

CRYOPROTECTANT RECIPE SUITABLE FOR HUMAN SPERM CRYOPRESERVATION

The survival of cryopreserved cells became a reality only after the discovery and use of cryoprotective agents. Cryoprotectants can be classified as permeating or nonpermeating, depending on whether or not they enter the cell. The majority of cryoprotectants that have been discovered so far are permeating agents. Four cryoprotectants that are most often used for cryopreservation of human spermatozoa are shown in Table 51.5. However, glycerol is the cryoprotectant of choice for human spermatozoa (1, 35–38). Glycerol, at a concentration of 5–10 percent, has been used to cryopreserve human sperm. The cryosurvival rates reported to fluctuate depending on the glycerol cocktail (glycerol with more complex buffer media extenders) used in the freezing method. Many different glycerol cocktails are in use for cryopreserving human spermatozoa (Table 51.6). Zwitterions, TES and TRIS, sodium citrate, and egg yolk have been reported to be superior to others as buffering and stabilizing agents for maintaining sperm viability. The use of zwitterion buffers has been attributed to their ability to bind free hydrogen and hydroxyl ions in the surrounding medium, aiding in the dehydration process, while the addition of egg yolk

Table 51.5: Cryoprotectants and Different Ingredients in Cryoprotective Media

Glycerol	Most widely used and successful cryoprotectant for human spermatozoa. About 7 percent (vol/vol) appears to be optimum concentration
Dimethylsulfoxide (DMSO)	Temperature sensitive
Ethylene glycol	Possesses fast rate of penetration
Propanediol (PROH)	Most successful for early-cleavage human embryos but seen little application with human spermatozoa
Egg yolk	Usually included in the cryoprotectant medium but is not itself a cryoprotectant. It helps to maintain membrane fluidity
Buffering agents (TES, Tris, glycine, citrate)	For maintaining pH of cryoprotectant media to avoid acidity/alkalinity related damage to spermatozoa

helps sperm viability by improving membrane fluidity. Egg yolk is routinely included in cryopreservation protocols for human semen, domestic animals, and exotic species. Yolk is regarded as a protection against cold shock. However, in the current need of disease control, there is a pressing requirement to find an egg yolk substitute. TEST yolk buffer freezing medium (Irvine Scientific), human sperm preservation medium HSPM (39), and IUI-ready cryoprotectant (40) are some of the many commercially available cryopreservation medium for human sperm cryopreservation.

CRYOPRESERVATION PROTOCOLS

General Protocol

There are many variations in protocols for cryopreservation (8, 41–45). However, any protocol is found to be equally efficient for cryopreservation of ejaculated (human semen, semen-recovered spermatozoa), epididymal, or testicular sperm (35).

In all the protocols, the cryoprotectant medium (glycerol cocktail) is added drop wise to the semen/sperm solution at ambient temperature until a 1:1 sample to medium ratio is obtained. Microshaking the vial is helpful to mix the cryoprotectant with the sample. The mixture is refrigerated (2–4°C) for a short time (ten to sixty minutes) to allow for slow cooling. Several cooling devices are in use to perform sperm freezing (Table 51.7). In manual method, the sample vial is then placed in liquid nitrogen vapor for freezing and then plunged into liquid nitrogen for storing. The rate of freezing is controlled by the distance above the surface of the liquid nitrogen.

The vials containing the samples can be handled in the liquid nitrogen vapor in different ways. One way is placing the cryovials on a metal cane and then inserting the cane into fully liquid nitrogen charged dry shipper for about thirty minutes, followed by plunging the cane into liquid nitrogen. Another simple method is to suspend the sample approximately 4 cm above the liquid nitrogen surface (approximately

Table 51.6: Glycerol Cocktails Currently Used as Cryoprotectants

Glycerol alone	Final concentration of 7.5 percent
Citrate-egg yolk-glycerol	325 mOsm sodium citrate, 20 percent (vol/vol) fresh egg yolk, 2 percent (vol/vol) 325 mOsm fructose, and glycerol (7.5 percent final concentration), pH adjusted at 7.0
TEST-C-I	A zwitterionic buffer system composed of 325 mOsm TES, 325 mOsm TRIS, 48 percent (vol/vol) TEST, 30 percent sodium citrate, 20 percent egg yolk, 2 percent fructose, and glycerol (6 percent final concentration)
TEST-C-II	70 percent (vol/vol) TEST, 12.5 percent sodium citrate, 17.5 percent egg yolk, and glycerol (10 percent final concentration)
TEST milk	30 percent (vol/vol) TEST, 30 percent 325 mOsm powdered milk, 18 percent sodium citrate, 20 percent egg yolk, 2 percent fructose, osmolality and pH 325 mOsm and 7.0, respectively, and glycerol (6 percent final concentration)
HSPM	Modified Tyrode's medium with glycerol (15 percent final concentration)
HEPES-KOH-G	325 mOsm HEPES, 325 mOsm KOH to adjust pH to 7.0, 40 percent 325 mOsm glucose, 20 percent egg yolk, and glycerol (6 percent final concentration)

Table 51.7: Different Cooling Methods and Devices for Sperm Freezing

Natural vapor-phase cooling

The vapor phase that naturally exists in the liquid nitrogen tank found sufficiently ideal to provide desired cooling. In this device, the cryovials/straws are placed at predetermined heights above liquid phase for predetermined periods so the desired cooling curve is attached

Mechanically assisted vapor-phase cooling

In this device, the machine causes liquid nitrogen vapor to flow around the samples at a controlled rate, thus an expected cooling rate can be achieved

Programmable freezing machine

Not widely used for human sperm cryopreservation probably because such automated device is not needed for sperm freezing. It does not produce any better result than manual method

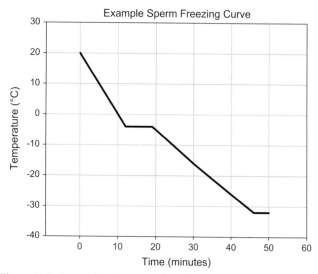

Figure 51.2. Sperm freezing curve (Cryologic, Biogenic, California).

less than −150°C) around twenty to thirty minutes before plunging into liquid nitrogen. A third option is placing the sample at 20 cm above liquid nitrogen (approximately −2°C) for twenty to thirty minutes, lowered to 14 cm (approximately −40°C) for about ten minutes, and finally lowering to 10–12 cm (approximately −90°C) for another ten minutes before plunging into liquid nitrogen.

Programmable freezers that are used routinely for freezing human embryos can also be used for freezing sperm. A freezing program defines how temperature changes with time in the freezing operation. Such changes are controlled by a temperature controller. In other words, a freezing program contains a series of steps that are executed in sequence by the temperature controller. Kaminski's group (35) describes a programmable freezer, which uses a cooling rate of 0.5°C/minute from room temperature to −5°C and a freezing rate of −10°C/minute from −5°C to −80°C, followed by plunging into liquid nitrogen for storage. Many commercial companies are marketing computer chip–controlled programmable freezers, which use controlled cooling program for sperm freezing. Figure 51.2 demonstrates an example of a freezing curve that these computer chip–controlled freezers execute in freezing human sperm (Biogenic, California).

Processing of Cryopreserved Sperm for Utilization

Utilization of cryopreserved sperm is possible only after the cryoprotectant is removed from the sperm and their motility is restored. This is accomplished by properly thawing the cryosample and post-thaw washing. Cryopreserved sperm are removed from liquid nitrogen for thawing, warming, and removing cryoprotectant to restore their motility. Frozen samples can be thawed in numerous ways. They can be either slowly thawed at ambient temperature for thirty to sixty minutes or rapidly thawed at 37°C for five to ten minutes before they are ready to remove cryoprotectants. Discontinuous gradient column or direct media (e.g., modified human tubal fluid) wash is usually used to remove cryoprotectant from thawed sample. Protocols for gradient column or other wash techniques for cryopreserved sperm are well described in the literature (7, 23, 46–48).

Cryopreservation of Epididymal and Testicular Sperm

The outcome (fertilization, embryo development, blastocyst formation rate, and pregnancy) following the ICSI of oocytes with ejaculated, epididymal, and testicular sperm is similar (6, 24, 46, 49, 50). When the ejaculated sperm is not available for any reason, use of epididymal or testicular sperm is the alternate choice. If freshly harvested epididymal and testicular sperm is used, sperm-harvesting procedure has to be performed to coincide with oocyte harvesting (47, 48). This can create logistical problem for the urologist, who has to be on call to perform sperm retrieval as needed. The cryopreservation and storage of epididymal and testicular sperm would alleviate the logistical concerns for both urologist and ART laboratory personnel. More importantly, sperm can be stored for multiple ART cycles and therefore avoiding the need for multiple surgical procedures to retrieve sperm (47, 48). When the use of ejaculated sperm is not an option, sperm retrieval can be achieved from two distinct anatomical locations, epididymis and testis, by using the following four microsurgical techniques. These procedures are performed as open biopsy or percutaneously (23, 51–53).

- MESA: Microsurgical epididymal sperm aspiration
- PESA: Percutaneous epididymal sperm aspiration
- TESE: Testicular sperm extraction
- TESA: Testicular sperm aspiration

The type of microsurgical procedure to be used obtaining sperm will depend on the availability of sperm in the two primary reservoirs: epididymis and testis. The epididymis is the first choice for the urologist since it provides more motile sperm. MESA is preferred over PESA probably because the former yield cleaner specimen and more sperm (51, 54, 55). Similarly, TESA is more preferable over TESE for the same reason. However, in case of nonobstructive azoospermia and maturation arrest or sertoli cell only syndrome, TESE is considered to be the most reliable option (8, 23, 51, 55).

The epididymal sperm is obtained by isolating a small amount of fluid (MESA or PESA) from epididymis using a twenty-seven-gauge butterfly set. Aspirated fluid is then diluted with any base media, for example, modified human tubal fluid (mHTF), supplemented with human serum albumin or serum substitute and examined for sperm under dissecting microscope. After confirmation of sperm, the sample is cryopreserved.

For harvesting sperm from testis (TESA or TESE), the testicular biopsy tissue can be processed manually or enzymatically. In manual method, the biopsy tissue is minced into fine pieces in Petri dish under dissecting microscope using a needle attached to the syringe or a scalpel. Tissues can also be meshed with appropriate tissue homogenizer (manual). Minced/smashed tissues are vigorously pipetted in appropriate volume of base media (e.g., mHTF) to release sperm. Volume of tissue homogenate and concentration of sperm in it can be adjusted by centrifuging (300 g) and removing extra supernatant.

Biopsy tissue can also be processed enzymatically. In enzymatic method, the testicular tissue is cut into small pieces and incubated in collagenase (1 mg/mL) for a short time (ten to twenty minutes) at 37°C. The seminiferous tubules are separated from interstitial tissue by repeated aspiration with pasture pipette. Collagenase is removed by repeated wash and centrifugation. The collagenase-treated tissue is then treated with trypsin (5 μg/mL) for ten to fifteen minutes at 37°C. Pipetting is done to further disaggregate. The enzymatic activity can be halted by adding trypsin inhibitor. The centrifuged pellet (testicular tissue disaggregates) can be resuspended in the required volume for cryopreservation.

The protocol for cryopreservation of testicular sperm is very similar to that of ejaculated sperm (56). Adding of cryoprotectant to the testicular sperm at 37°C instead of at ambient temperature produces superior recovery results. The following specific recommendations have also been made in the protocols for testicular sperm cryopreservation to obtain better cryosurvival: 1) adding equal volume of prewarmed (37°C) cryoprotectant drop by drop with gentle mixing, 2) holding at 37°C for another thirty minutes, 3) incubation at 4°C for ninety minutes, 4) incubation in the liquid nitrogen vapor for fifteen minutes, and 5) then plunging into liquid nitrogen for storage (56, 57). If cryomachine is used to freeze the testicular disaggregates, the freezing program similar to the one shown below is recommended (43, 56).

Start temp	Ambient
Ramp 1	Cool at 2°C/minute to 6–7°C
Soaking	Ten minutes
Seeding	At 6–7°C
Hold	Ten minutes
Ramp 2	0.3°C/minute to below –35°C
End of program	
Plunging into liquid nitrogen	

Thawing of testicular tissue aggregates is done following standard rapid-thaw procedure, which usually includes holding at ambient air for about one minute and higher temperature (30–37°C) for few minutes. Cryoprotectant is removed by repeated wash (two times) and centrifugation. Incubation of the cell/tissue isolates for few hours helps to recuperate the sperm motility. If motile sperm are not visible, the sample can be treated with pentoxifyline (2.5 mM). If pentoxifyline is used, it is recommended that the sperm be washed further before it is used in ICSI. Some studies find improvement in post-thaw motility if short-term culture of testicular sperm is done before cryopreservation.

Male fertility preservation may be considered for individuals who will require chemotherapy or radiation therapy particularly at early ages. Testicular germ cells are highly susceptible to both types of treatment. If germ cells are destroyed, fertility will be irreversibly lost. Isolation of spermatogonial germ cells/ stem cell spermatogonia from testicular biopsies and their cryopreservation for future autotransplantation has been proposed (28, 58, 59). The cryopreserved germ cells are expected to be infused to resume spermatogenesis when the patient is free from the disease. Experiments dealing with the restoration of fertility by infusion of germ cells in mouse have been encouraging. Cryopreservation of spermatogonial germ cells in humans could be considered a viable option for germ cell banking with the hope that reliable methods for autotransplantation will emerge in near future. The possible future use of the reproductive tissue will depend on future advances in reproductive technology. Ethical and legal considerations will require more evaluation.

Special Cryopreservation Procedures

Cryopreservation techniques for single or small number of sperms were introduced in the field of ART by Cohen et al. and coworkers (60, 61). The method involves injection of spermatozoa into empty zona pellucidae of human oocyte before they are brought under treatment of cryoprotectant. The sperm-containing zona is then stored in cryostraw or vial. This special procedure is indicated for individuals who have extremely few sperms in their semen. Conventional method of cryopreservation is not suitable because of harvesting such few sperm from the frozen sample. It is crucial to remove all cellular material from the zona and wash well before the spermatozoa are inserted into it. The theoretical possibility of transgenesis must be considered with this method.

Another approach for cryopreservation of a small number of sperms is use of alginic acid capsules, which has been found to be very effective. Herrler et al. (62) developed a method of freezing small amounts of spermatozoa in polymerized alginic acid drops, which can be liquefied after thawing for recovery of the spermatozoa. This device eliminates the chance of contamination of sperm with foreign biological materials.

Another new method emerging in the field that deals with cryopreservation of spermatozoa without a cryoprotectant is by a method called vitrification. Vitrification cannot be considered as a new method; rather the application of vitrification was dormant until recently (63–67). In one of such vitrification protocols, Isachenko et al. (67) successfully vitrified human sperm in copper cryoloop loaded with sperm suspension. Experiments show that the vitrification approach can preserve the sperm motility and their ability to fertilize the oocytes. Presently, vitrification is more extensively used in oocyte, embryo, and blastocyst freezing than sperm freezing.

INDIVIDUAL VARIABILITY AND VARIABLES AFFECTING CRYOPRESERVATION

Human pregnancy using cryopreserved semen occurred around fifty years ago. Since then, hundreds of thousands of children have been born as a result of this simple procedure of assisted reproduction. Despite this success, the cryopreservation procedure can hardly be considered standardized (11, 19, 36, 67, 68). The mechanisms responsible for damage to sperm resulting from exposure to CPAs, from cooling, from thawing, or from removing CPAs are not well understood. It is also not known why sperms of different individual respond differently to the same cryopreservation procedure. It is also not clear why around 50 percent sperm of most men are damaged or destroyed by freeze-thaw cycle.

Even though hundreds of thousands of children were born as a result of insemination with cryopreserved sperm indicate success of cryopreservation technology in human reproduction, current cryopreservation technology is not very efficient. The cryosurvival data reported in the literature suggest that 50 percent of sperm cells damaged or destroyed by freezing and thawing, limiting the overall efficiency and efficacy of sperm cryopreservation (2, 4, 9, 41, 68). The obvious question that comes to mind is why sperm freezing is so less efficient.

The answer to this question is not very clear at this time. Spermatozoa of different males exhibit widely different responses to the same cryopreservation protocol. Such differences in sensitivity to cryopreservation among males have profound practical implications on the successes of cryopreservation method. McLaughlin et al. (21) conducted experiments that produced strong evidence of such individual variation of sensitivity to cryopreservation. Their (21) results show that the response of spermatozoa to cryopreservation is consistent among different ejaculates from the same individual, but the spermatozoa from different men responded quite differently to cryopreservation. Coefficient of variation in sperm parameters between individual males is much higher than that of the ejaculates of the same individual. Several studies have addressed if the male-to-male difference in sperm freezing sensitivity reflects properties of membranes and if these properties are genetically determined (1). The available data indicate that characteristics of sperm membranes may be genetically determined. Since the membranes of sperm of different individuals differ, their permeability characteristics also differ. Such compounding differences in membrane will cause significant differences in chilling as well as freezing sensitivity of spermatozoa.

Hormonal differences have also been implicated with the individual differences in cryosensitivity. Males of different ages have differences in concentrations of hormones. Since hormones affect the structure of the cellular cytoskeleton, the endocrinological differences among individuals may influence susceptibility of their sperm to cryoinjuries at different ages (69, 70).

Cryopreservation protocols may influence the survival of sperm during cryopreservation. The rate of dilution of sperm sample with freezing solution (cryoprotectant), cooling from ambient temperature to 5°C, and cooling rate that brings sample to subzero temperature are important for sustaining satisfactory viability and motility. Other notable factors are concentration of CPA, thawing rate, and post-thaw dilution method. It should be reemphasized that the motility of sperm in cryopreservation varies significantly as a function of cooling rate and also of warming rate.

STABILITY OF FROZEN SPECIMEN AND CROSS-CONTAMINATION

Available information related to stability of the frozen specimens is less contradictory. Most literatures indicated that cryopreserved sperm as well as embryos can be stored for decades with no loss of function (71, 72). Previous reports show that bull sperm stored frozen for thirty-seven years is capable of fertilizing oocytes that subsequently developed into blastocysts (1). In humans, sperm cryopreserved for more than fifteen years has been reported to produce viable pregnancy. Some early studies reported decays in the stored cryopreserved specimens (73, 74). Suboptimal cryopreservation techniques may be responsible for these results. Recent cryoliteratures indicate that there is probably no limit to the length of time that spermatozoa remain alive in liquid nitrogen.

Cryopreserved sperm is stored in liquid nitrogen in a specially designed cryotank. Samples from a large number of individuals are usually stored together in a tank. Questions have been raised about possible cross-contamination during long-term storage of cryopreserved sperm (75–78). Some studies demonstrated that plastic straws commonly used for cryopreserving semen may leak their contents, thus increasing the possibility of cross-contamination (75, 76, 79, 80). Broken, cracked, and exploded cryovials are also occasionally found in storage tank (7, 11, 19). Concern has been expressed about the possible transmission of infectious agents during cryostorage, particularly viruses like HIV and hepatitis B. Special straws manufactured by ionomeric resin has been recommended to combat the risk of cross-contamination because this type of straw does not crack or become brittle at subzero temperatures. Another alternative to prevent cross-contamination between samples has been implemented by some programs by storing cryopreserved specimens in the vapor phase above boiling liquid nitrogen at about −180°C.

Liquid nitrogen, like water, can act as a vehicle for transmission of viruses, bacteria, and fungi (11). Previous studies show that viruses in semen can survive in liquid nitrogen without loss of activity during routine cryobanking. If an individual is identified to be positive for viruses, it has been suggested that the specimens from such groups of individuals be stored in a separate tank. Separate tank for specimens of each type of disease would be ideal but are logistically impractical. Many facilities have adopted some practical methods to minimize the potential for transmission within a cryotank. These practical considerations include 1) liquid nitrogen vapor storing, 2) use of special secure straws, and 3) use of extra wraps for cryovials. Pathogens are less likely to move in and out of storage vials in vapor phase. Some have suggested that if specimens are to be maintained in liquid nitrogen, vials can be covered with impervious plastic wrapping. The Conception Technologies (San Diego, California) came up with high-security straw for cryopreservation of sperm, which claimed to eliminate the risk of cross-contamination in liquid nitrogen. These straws have been evaluated and shown to be nonabsorbent, nonporous, and nontoxic to embryos and sperm and are guaranteed to be shatterproof at any subzero temperature. The objective is that appropriate measures should be taken to eliminate risks of contamination within a storage tank.

STORAGE OF CRYOPRESERVED SPERM IN VAPOROUS NITROGEN

Guidelines have emerged advocating that liquid nitrogen should never come into direct contact with the specimen, vials should be sealed and free of external contamination, and unscreened semen should not be stored in the same container with screened and infection-free semen. These recommendations can easily be achieved by storing samples in the vaporous phase of liquid nitrogen (10, 81). In vapor-phase method, there is no direct contact between the specimen and liquid nitrogen in the storage Dewar tanks since the sample is never immersed in liquid nitrogen. Literature shows no difference in the viability parameters between semen specimens stored in either liquid nitrogen or vaporous nitrogen (45, 81, 82). Therefore, it has been proposed that storage in vaporous phase is a viable alternative to storage in liquid nitrogen. Support is growing for storing cryopreserved sperm in vaporous phase nitrogen as a method of preventing cross-contamination of semen samples.

The disadvantage of vapor storing of cryopreserved sperm should also be taken into consideration. The need for constant surveillance is crucial in vapor-phase storage. The liquid nitrogen must be maintained at a certain level in order to provide stable vapor phase and less fluctuating temperature gradients, which requires dedicated commitment.

CRYOPACKAGING AND STORAGE MATERIALS

Usually, three types of packaging materials are used in packaging human semen/sperm for cryopreservation, namely glass ampoules, plastic cryovials, and plastic straws. Glass ampoules were originally used for semen cryopreservation but discontinued or became less popular on safety grounds. Cryovials (screw caps, 1- to 2-mL size) and straws (0.25- to 0.5-mL size) are equally popular and widely used. The following materials/devices are used for storing and safe handling of cryopreserved specimens.

1. Metal (aluminum) cane: for stacking plastic cryovials.
2. Goblet (plastic): for stacking cryostraws.
3. Canister: barrel-shaped steel container to hold several canes/goblet.
4. Cryotank: usually holds several canisters.
5. Cryosensors: device to monitor the level of liquid nitrogen in the cryotank.

CRYOINVENTORY TRACKING

All cryopreserved sperm samples in a clinic must be positively identifiable. The inventory control system used depends on the type of storage containers being used and other resources available. Labeling of cryopackages (vials and straws) must be permanent type and particularly cryoresistant. Vials are usually attached to metal canes, which stand free inside the canisters of the storage tank. Cryostraws are grouped in plastic tubes (visotubes)/goblets that can be attached with the cane, which then can be in the canister of the storage tank. Mortimer (7) proposed several basic principles in organizing cryosamples in the tank as summarized below:

1. Each cryospecimen (straw or vial) must be individually identifiable, so there will not be any chance of mix up if more than one sample is handled simultaneously.
2. Cryoinformation must be available in several documents kept in different locations.
3. Cryospecimens should be organized in the tank following a system/pattern.
4. Use of color-coded vials, cane, and canister advisable.

TRANSPORTATION OF CRYOSPECIMENS

Human spermatozoa can be transported anywhere in the world by the advantage of cryopreservation. Cryostraws as well as cryovials can be sent to distant locations using a dry shipper, a special Dewar minitank that holds low temperature for four to five days and are easy to carry. The commercial donor sperm banks are taking advantage of this so-called "dry shipper" technology and speedy transportation services of UPS, Fed-X, in distribution of donor sperm to their clients worldwide. The ART clinics are also utilizing dry shipping to relocate patients' sperm from one clinic to another.

SAFETY RELATED TO LIQUID NITROGEN USE

Liquid nitrogen is an essential component of cryopreservation. It is a cryogenic liquid (−196°C), its contact with body parts like finger, eye, and so on may cause freezing injuries similar to frostbite. Laboratory personnel handling liquid nitrogen should be familiar with safe practices in its use; some such safety measures are listed below:

1. Protective devices: wear apron to cover body and legs, use gloves to protect hand, and wear goggles to protect eye.
2. Liquid nitrogen should be handled in containers specifically designed for that purpose.
3. Use cover for the liquid nitrogen container during filling with liquid nitrogen to minimize splashing and also during carrying the container from one location to another.
4. The room used for liquid nitrogen and cryotank storage should be adequately ventilated.
5. Appropriate carrier like roller board should be used for heavy cryovessels like cryotank.
6. Commercially available sensors can be used for detecting the level of oxygen in the liquid nitrogen–handling area.

GENETIC CONSEQUENCES OF CRYOPRESERVATION

Most literature indicates that cryopreservation has no genetic consequences. Some literatures actually argue that defective sperm are eliminated by cryopreservation, indicating the evidence of fewer spontaneous abortions and birth defects from the inseminations with frozen sperm. Most investigators report no significant differences in chromosomal anomalies before and after cryopreservation and no evidence of altered sex ratio caused by cryopreservation. Cytogenetic investigation of the effects of cryopreservation on human spermatozoa, using hamster oocyte to reveal sperm chromosome, has reported no alteration in the frequency of chromosomal abnormalities. In contrast, some literature reported increased frequency of trisomic births by AI with frozen sperm. No strong evidence is available in the cryoliterature to indicate any detrimental genetic consequences directly linked to cryopreservation (1, 27, 36, 83–88).

ASRM RECOMMENDATIONS RELATED TO SPERM CRYOPRESERVATION

The ASRM is the forefront organization of the human infertility specialists in America. This organization like similar organizations in other countries deals with the emerging issues related to human reproduction in the era of ART. The ASRM has established practice committee and ethics committee to review the issues and set guidelines, recommendations, and minimum standards for different aspects of reproductive medicine (2004 compendium of ASRM practice committee and ethics committee) (89). Since the assisted reproduction is not fully regulated, the reproductive specialist, public and even government agencies, put emphasis on ASRM's view on all aspects of assisted reproduction including rational use of cryopreservation technology. In this section, the ASRM recommendations related to reproductive donation, rational utilization of cryopreservation technology particularly male gamete cryopreservation, are summarized.

Donor sperm has been used in the treatment of male infertility for more than hundred years. The ASRM practice committee recommends evaluations of potential sperm donors incorporating recent information about optimal screening and testing for sexually transmitted infections, genetic diseases, and psychological assessments. The committee recommends the utilization of information from the Centers for Disease Control and Prevention, FDA, and AATB. The ASRM practice committee indicated that leukocyte-rich semen donation poses unique risks.

In United States, DI is ethically and legally permissible for females without male partners or when the male partner for any reason is unable to provide genetically competent sperm. The use of only cryopreserved sperm for donor insemination is permissible. Frozen sperm are required to be quarantined for 180 days and the donor should be retested for seronegitivity before the specimen is used. Commercial sperm banks in United States are required to comply with federal, state, and local regulations, which are designed to prevent sexually transmitted diseases and other issues. Appropriate informed consent form is essential for any DI. It is essential to maintain permanent records of the specimen and its utilization to the extent possible. A mechanism should exist to maintain the records as a future medical and legal resource. At the same time, the individuals participating in donor program should be assured of protection of confidentiality. Donors as well as the recipients are obliged to execute documents that define or limit their rights and duties.

The ASRM practice committee recommends psychological assessment by a qualified mental health professional for sperm donors and recipients. The psychological assessment should address the potential psychological risks and evaluate the evidence of coercion (financial and emotional). Recipients of donor sperm should get counseling of all potential psychological implications.

The ASRM practice committee has also set recommendations for minimal genetic screening for gamete donors. The major highlights of the recommendations are that the donor should not have any major Mendelian disorder, should not carry any known karyotypic abnormality, and should not carry any significant familial disease. The committee considers some ethnic groups as potential high risk and recommends screening to determine heterozygosity for certain conditions (Table 51.4). The list of tests may change as new test(s) for other disorders are developed.

ASRM identified and summarized the elements to be considered in the informed consent form to be used for donor sperm cryopreservation and other ART procedures. ASRM suggests that all consents must be in writing, signed by all parties involved, and witnessed. Parties should be sufficiently informed of all required aspects. Besides ASRM, the fertility drug manufacturers like Organon and Serono and a nonprofit organization like Embryo Donation Society developed more comprehensive consent forms targeting ART procedures, which require sometime more than one regulatory compliance.

The ethics committee of ASRM expresses opinion on infertility treatment of patients who have human immunodeficiency virus (HIV), which cover cryopreservation of sperm of HIV-infected males. About 86 percent of HIV-infected persons are of reproductive age, and ironically majority of this population is male. There is evidence of occupational transmission of HIV. According to ASRM, the risk associated to HIV is not a sufficient reason to deny reproductive services to HIV-infected individuals and couples. The ethics committee states that the clinicians have the same obligation to care for those infected with HIV as to care for patients with other chronic diseases.

The andrology laboratory personnel should have sufficient training to safely cryopreserve and utilize semen of HIV-infected males.

KEY POINTS

- The developments in the field of human sperm cryopreservation have been analyzed by reviewing published literatures.
- Readers are provided with the latest available information on cryopreservation of human spermatozoa including epididymal and testicular sperm.
- All possible indications for sperm cryopreservation have been listed.
- Current approaches to male fertility preservation have been illustrated.
- Conceptual, methodological, as well as regulatory information are provided so that the readers can obtain comprehensive knowledge about human sperm cryopreservation.
- Techniques and methodology described are highly relevant to the current practice of assisted human reproduction and sperm banking.
- Transportation and safety of cryopreserved specimens were discussed.

ACKNOWLEDGMENT

The authors are very thankful to Collin Osuamkpe, M.Sc., for the technical help with the manuscript.

REFERENCES

1. Leibo SP, Picton HM, Gosden RG. (2001). Cryopreservation of human spermatozoa. In: *Current Practices and Controversies in Assisted Reproduction: A WHO Sponsored Symposium, Switzerland, September 17–21, 2001*, World Health Organization, WHO headquarters, Geneva, Switzerland.
2. Fuller B, Paynter S. (2004). Fundamentals of cryobiology in reproductive medicine. *RBM Online*, 9(6): 680–91.
3. Bunge RG, Keettel WC, Sherman JK. (1954). Clinical use of frozen semen. *Ferti Steril*, 5: 520–9.
4. Royere D, Barthelemy C, Hamamah S, et al. (1996). Cryopreservation of spermatozoa: a 1996 review. *Hum Reprod*, 2: 553–9.
5. Trounson AO, et al. (1981). Artificial insemination by frozen donor semen: results of multicentre Australian experience. *Intern J Androl*, 4: 227–32.
6. Wolf D, Patton P. (1989). Sperm cryopreservation: state of the ART. *J In Vitro Fertil Emb Trans*, 6: 325–7.
7. Mortimer D. (1994). *Practical Laboratory Andrology*. New York: Oxford University Press.
8. Watson PF. (1995). Recent developments and concepts in the cryopreservation of spermatozoa and the assessment of their post-thawing function. *Reprod Fertil Dev*, 7: 871–91.
9. Crister JK. (1998). Current status of semen banking in the USA. *Hum Reprod*, 13(Suppl. 2): 55–67.
10. Tomlinson M, Sakkas D. (2000). Is a review of standard procedures for cryopreservation needed? Safe and effective cryopreservation – should sperm banks and fertility centres move toward storage in nitrogen vapour? *Hum Reprod*, 15: 2460–3.
11. Centola GM. (2002). The art of donor gamete cryobanking: current considerations. *J Androl*, 174–9.
12. Sherman JK. (1978). Banks for frozen human semen: current status and prospects. In: Graham E, ed. *The Integrity of Frozen Spermatozoa*. Washington: National Academy of Sciences; pp. 78–91.
13. David G, Lansac J. (1980). The organization of the centers for the study and preservation of semen in France. In: David G, Price WS, eds. *Human Artificial Insemination and Semen Preservation*. New York: Plenum Press; pp. 15–26.
14. Centola GM. (1997). Update on the use of donor gametes, sperm and oocytes involvement in the FDA regulation of gamete banking: the FDA proposed rule to include reproductive tissue. *ASRM News. Fall.*
15. Federal Registry (2002). Eligibility determination for donors of human cells, tissues, and cellular and tissue-based products. 21 CFR parts 210, 211, 820, and 1271.
16. Food and Drug Administration (2004). Eligibility determination for donors of human cells, tissues, and cellular and tissue-based products. Posting in FDA Web site www.FDA.GOV.
17. ASRM (2005). Postgraduate course 21: FDA and ART—how to comply with the new regulations. ASRM annual meeting, Montreal, Canada.
18. Reglera (2005). Human cells, tissues, and cellular and tissue based products: registration, donor eligibility, and current good tissue practices final rules of FDA: Registration Final Rule and Donor Eligibility Final Rule, 21 CFR Part 1271, www.reglera.com.
19. AATB (1995). *Standards for Semen Banking*. Revision draft. MCLean, VI: American Association of Tissue Bank.
20. Bick D, et al. (1998). Screening semen donors for hereditary diseases. The Fairfax cryobank experience. *J Reprod Med*, 43: 423–8.
21. McLaughlin EA. (1999). British Andrology Society guidelines for the screening of semen donor for donor insemination. *Hum Reprod*, 14: 1823–6.
22. Carson SA, Gentry WL, Smith AL, Buster JE. (1991). Feasibility of semen collection and cryopreservation during chemotherapy. *Hum Reprod*, 6: 992–4.
23. Verheyen G, De Croco I, Tournaye H, et al. (1995). Comparison of four mechanical methods to retrieve spermatozoa from testicular tissue. *Hum Reprod*, 10: 2956–9.
24. Davis NS. (1997). The hows, whys and when of sperm cryopreservation. In: *ASRM 30th Postgraduate Program Course on Andrologic Practices*; pp. 83–9, American Society for Reproductive Medicine, Burmingham, Alabama, USA.
25. Averette HE, Boike GM, Jarrell MA. (1990). Effects of cancer chemotherapy on gonadal function and reproductive capacity. *Cancer J Clin*, 40: 199–209.
26. Costabile RA. (1993). The effects of cancer and cancer therapy on male reproductive function. *J Urol*, 149: 1327–30.
27. Arnon J, Meirow D, Lewis-Roness H, Ornoy A. (2001). Genetic and teratogenic effects of cancer treatments on gametes and embryos. *Hum Reprod Update*, 7: 394–403.
28. Lee SJ, Schover LR, Partridge AH, et al. (2006). American Society of Clinical Oncology recommendations on fertility preservation in cancer patients. *J Clin Oncol*, 24: 2917–31.
29. Oktay K, Meirow D. (2007). Planning for fertility preservation before cancer treatment. *Sexuality, Reproduction and Menopause (srm) – A Clinical Publication of American Society of Reproductive Medicine*, 5(1): 17–22.
30. Mazur P. (1963). Kinetics of water loss from cells at subzero temperatures and the likelihood of intracellular freezing. *J Gen Physiol*, 47: 347–69.
31. Mazur P. (1984). Freezing of living cells: mechanisms and implications. *Am J Physiol*, 247: C125–42.
32. Wolfinbarger L, Sutherlan V, Braendle L, Sutherlan G. (1996). Engineering aspects of cryobiology. *Adv Cryogenic Eng*, 41: 1–12.

33. Gao DY, Mazur P, Crister JK. (1997). Fundamental cryobiology of mammalian spermatozoa. In: Karow A, Crister JK, eds. *Reproductive Tissue Banking*. San Diego, CA: Academic Press; pp. 263–328.

34. Leibo SP, Bradley L. (1999). Comparative cryobiology of mammalian spermatozoa. In: Gagnon C, ed. *The Male Gamete*. Vienna II: Cache River Press; pp. 501–16.

35. Kaminski J, Centola G, Lamb DJ. (2003). Sperm cryopreservation. *Androl Embryol Rev Course*, 13.1–13.8.

36. Sophonsritsuk A, Rojanasakul A. (2003). Cryopreservation of human spermatozoa. *Ramathibodi Med J*, 126: 156–62.

37. Weidel L, Prins GS. (1987). Cryosurvival of human spermatozoa frozen in eight different buffer systems. *J Androl*, 8: 41.

38. Crister JK, et al. (1998). Cryopreservation of human spermatozoa. III. The effect of cryoprotectants on motility. *Fertil Steril*, 50: 314–20.

39. Mahadevan M, Trounson AO. (1983). Effects of cryopreservative media and dilution methods on the preservation of human spermatozoa. *Andrologia*, 15: 355–66.

40. Larson JM, et al. (1998). An intrauterine insemination-ready cryopreservation method compared with sperm recovery after conventional freezing and post-thaw processing. *Fertil Steril*, 68: 143–8.

41. Taylor PJ, et al. (1982). A comparison of freezing and thawing methods for the cryopreservation of human semen. *Fertil Steril*, 37: 100–3.

42. Fiser PS, Fairfull RW, Marcus GJ. (1986). The effect of thawing velocity on survival and acrosomal integrity of spermatozoa frozen at optimal and suboptimal rates in straws. *Cryobiology*, 23: 141–9.

43. Henry M, et al. (1993). Cryopreseravation of human spermatozoa. IV. The effects of cooling rate and warming rate on the maintenance of motility, plasma membrane integrity, and mitochondrial function. *Fertil Steril*, 60: 911–18.

44. Gao DY, et al. (1995). Prevention of osmotic injury to human spermatozoa during addition and removal of glycerol. *Hum Reprod*, 10: 1109–22.

45. Medeiros CM, Forell F, Oliveira AT, et al. (2002). Current status of sperm cryopreservation: Why isn't it better? *Theriogenology*, 57: 327–44.

46. Cohen J, Felten P, Zeilmaker GH. (1981). Fertilizing capacity of fresh and frozen human sperm: a comparative study. *Fertil Steril*, 36: 356–62.

47. Hossain A, Osuamkpe C, Nagamani M. (2007a). Extended culture of human sperm in the laboratory may have practical value in the assisted reproductive procedures. *Fertil Steril, 2008* Jan; 89(1): 237–9. Epub 2007 May 4.

48. Hossain A, Osuamkpe C, Nagamani M. (2007b). Sole use of sucrose in human sperm cryopreservation. *Arch Androl*, 53: 1–5.

49. Bunge RG, Sherman JK. (1953). Fertilizing capacity of frozen human spermatozoa. *Nature*, 172: 767.

50. Gil-Salmon M, Romero J, Minguez Y. (1996). Pregnancies after ICSI with cryopreserved testicular spermatozoa. *Hum Reprod*, 11: 1309–13.

51. Craft I, Tsirigotis M. (1995). Simplified recovery, preparation and cryopreservation of testicular spermatozoa. *Hum Reprod*, 10: 1623–7.

52. Salzbrunn A, Benson D, Holstein A, et al. (1996). A new concept for the extraction of testicular spermatozoa as a tool for assisted fertilization (ICSI). *Hum Reprod*, 11: 752–5.

53. Van Perperstraten A, Proctor M, Phillipson G. (2002). Techniques for surgical retrieval of sperm prior to ICSI for azoospermia (Cochrane review). In: *Cochrane Library, Oxford, The Cochrane Collaborations*, John Wiley and Sons Ltd., Baltimore, Maryland.

54. Buch J, Philips K, Kolon T. (1994). Cryopreservation of microsurgically extracted ductal sperm: pentoxyfylline enhancement of motility. *Fertil Steril*, 62: 418–20.

55. Oates R, Lobel S, Harris D, et al. (1996). Efficacy of intracytoplasmic sperm injection using cryopreserved epididymal sperm. *Hum Reprod*, 11: 133–8.

56. Freeman MR. (2002). Cryopreservation of epididymal and testicular sperm. In: *ASRM 35th postgraduate program course on recent advances in cryopreservation*; 37–44, American Society for Reproductive Medicine, Burmingham, Alabama, USA.

57. Sharma R, et al. (1997). Factors associated with the quality before freezing and after thawing of sperm obtained by microsurgical epididymal aspiration. *Fertil Steril*, 68: 626–31.

58. Schover L, Brey K, Litchin A, et al. (2002). Knowledge and experience regarding cancer and sperm banking in younger male survivors. *J Clin Oncol*, 20: 1880–9.

59. Orwig KE, Schlatt S. (2005). Cryopreservation and transplantation of spermatogonia and testicular tissue for preservation of male fertility. *J Natl Cancer Inst Monogr*. 34: 51–6.

60. Cohen J, et al. (1997). Cryopreservation of single human spermatozoa. *Hum Reprod*, 12: 994–1001.

61. Liu J, et al. (2000). Cryopreservation of a small number of fresh human testicular spermatozoa and testicular spermatozoa cultured in vitro for 3 days in an empty zona pellucida. *J Androl*, 21: 409–13.

62. Herrler A, et al. (2006). Cryopreservation of spermatozoa in alginic acid capsules. *Fertil Steril*, 85: 208–13.

63. Luyet BJ, Hodapp A. (1938). Revival of frog spermatozoa vitrified in liquid air. *Proc Soc Exp Biol*, 39: 433–4.

64. Polge C, Smith AU, Parkes AS. (1949). Revival of spermatozoa after vitrification and dehydration at low temperatures. *Nature*, 169: 626–7.

65. Nawroth F, Isachenko V, Dessole S, et al. (2002). Vitrification of human spermatozoa without cryoprotectant. *Cryoletters*, 23: 93–102.

66. Schuster G, Keller L, Dunn R, et al. (2003). Ultra-rapid freezing of very low number of sperm using cryoloops. *Hum Reprod*, 18: 788–95.

67. Isachenko V, Isachenko E, KatkovII, et al. (2004). Cryoprotectant-free cryopreservation of human sperm by vitrification and freezing in vapour: effect on motility, DNA integrity and fertilization ability. *Biol Reprod*, 71: 1167–73.

68. Centola GM, Raubertas RF, Mattox JH. (1992). Cryopreservation of human semen. Comparison of cryopreservatives, sources of variability, and prediction of post-thaw survival. *J Androl*, 13: 283–8.

69. Robinson J. (1975). Effects of age and season on sexual behavior and plasma testosterone concentrations of laboratory rhesus monkeys. *Biol Reprod*, 13: 203–10.

70. Wickings E, Nieschlag R. (1980). Seasonality in endocrine and exocrine testicular function in adult rhesus monkey. *Int J Androl*, 3: 87–104.

71. Leibo SP, Semple M, Kroetsch T. (1994). In vitro fertilization of oocytes by 37 year old cryopreserved bovine spermatozoa. *Theriogenology*, 42: 1257–62.

72. Fogarty NM, et al. (2000). The viability of transferred sheep embryos after long term cryopreservation. *Reprod Fertil Dev*, 12: 31–7.

73. Freund M, Wiederman J. (1996). Factors affecting dilution, freezing and storage of human semen. *J Reprod Fertil*, 11: 1–7.

74. Smith KD, Steinberger E. (1973). Survival of spermatozoa in a human sperm bank. Effects of long-term storage in liquid nitrogen. *J Am Med Assoc*, 223: 774–7.

75. Tedder R, Zuckerman M, Goldstone A. (1995). Hepatitis B transmission from a contaminated cryopreservation tank. *Lancet*, 346: 137–40.

76. Russell P, et al. (1997). The potential transmission of infectious agents by semen packaging during storage for artificial insemination. *Anim Reprod Sci*, 47: 337–42.

77. British Andrology Society (1999). Guidelines for the screening of semen donors for donor insemination. *Hum Reprod*, 14: 1823–6.

78. Clarke GN. (1999). Sperm cryopreservation: is there a significant risk of cross-contamination? *Hum Reprod*, 14: 2941–3.

79. Sherman J, Menna J. (1986). Cryosurvival of herpes simplex virus during cryopreservation of human sperm. *Cryobiology*, 23: 383–5.

80. Fountain D, Ralston M, Higgins N, et al. (1997). Liquid nitrogen freezers: a potential source of microbial contamination of hematopoetic stem cell components. *Transfusion*, 37: 585–91.

81. Amesse LS, et al. (2003). Comparison of cryopreserved sperm in vaporous and liquid nitrogen. *J Reprod Med*, 48: 319–24.

82. Saritha K, Bongso A. (2001). Comparative evaluation of fresh and washed sperm cryopreserved in vapor and liquid phases of liquid nitrogen. *J Androl*, 22: 857–62.

83. Mattei JF, Lemarec B. (1983). Genetic aspects of artificial insemination by donor (AID): indications, surveillance, and results. *Clin Genet*, 23: 132–8.

84. Chernos J, Martin H. (1989). A cytogenetic investigation of the effects of cryopreservation on human sperm. *Am J Hum Genet*, 45: 766–77.

85. Martin RH, et al. (1991). Effect of cryopreservation on the frequency of chromosomal abnormalities and sex ratio in human sperm. *Mol Reprod Dev*, 30: 159–63.

86. Donnelly E, Steele K, McClure N, et al. (2001). Assessment of DNA integrity and morphology of ejaculated sperm before and after cryopreservation. *Hum Reprod*, 16: 1191–9.

87. Rizk B, Edwards RG, Nicolini U, et al. (1991). Edwards syndrome after the replacement of cryopreserved thawed embryos. *Fertil Steril*, 55(1): 208–10.

88. Rizk B. (2007). Outcome of assisted reproductive technology. In: Rizk B, Abdalla H, eds. *Infertility and Assisted Reproductive Technology*. Oxford, UK: Health Press. pp. 214–16.

89. Rizk B (Ed.) (2008). Ultrasonography in reproductive medicine and infertility. Cambridge: United Kingdom, Cambridge University Press (in press).

■ 52 ■

THE MANAGEMENT OF AZOOSPERMIA

S. Friedler, A. Raziel, D. Strassburger, M. Schachter, O. Bern, E. Kasterstein,
D. Komarovsky, R. Ron-El

The ability to treat azoospermic men to become genetic fathers of children represents one of the most dramatic revolutions that have occurred in the field of infertility treatment during the past two decades. Use of donor sperm is no longer the first and only treatment option in these cases. The discovery that one may use a single sperm cell and achieve normal embryos, pregnancy, and delivery after assisted fertilization by intracytoplasmic sperm injection (ICSI) changed many of the previous axiomas in the field of andrology (Palermo et al., 1992; Van Steirteghem et al., 1993). For men with no sperm in the ejaculate, surgical retrieval of sperm cells from the epididymis or testicular seminiferous tubules in combination with ICSI opened new avenues for fulfilling their fatherhood.

DEVELOPMENT OF METHODS FOR SURGICAL SPERM RETRIEVAL (SSR)

The first to be treated were patients with obstructive azoospermia (OA), where viable spermatozoa were retrieved from the testis with testicular sperm extraction (TESE) or testicular biopsy and used for ICSI (Craft et al., 1993; Schoysman et al., 1993a, b; Devroey et al., 1994; Nagy et al., 1995; Abuzeid et al., 1995; Silber et al., 1995a, b, c; Tucker et al., 1995) or epididymal sperm retrieval by an open surgery aimed at the epididymis named microepididymal sperm aspiration (MESA) (Temple-Smith et al., 1985; Silber et al., 1994; Tournaye et al., 1994).

Following the remarkable results in patients with obstructive azoospermia, a less invasive method of sperm retrieval was introduced, the percutaneous aspiration by fine needle, aiming at the epididymis (percutaneous epididymal sperm aspiration, PESA) (Craft and Shrivastav, 1994; Shrivastav et al., 1994; Craft et al., 1995a, b) or testis (testicular sperm aspiration, TESA) (Craft and Tsirigotis, 1995; Tsirigotis and Craft, 1995). Alternatively, in OA, efficient retrieval of testicular spermatozoa by closed percutaneous testicular biopsy was reported, using a modified twenty-gauge Menghini testicular biopsy needle (Bourne et al., 1995) or a biopsy gun (Hovatta et al., 1995) or testicular biopsy gun needle (Tuuri et al., 1999).

While in obstructive cases, spermatozoa are abundant in the epididymal or testicular tubuli, permitting a high rate of retrieval success, in patients with nonobstructive azoospermia (NOA), the epididymis is devoid of spermatozoa and only a few foci with spermatogenesis may be found in the testicles. Publication of successful sperm retrieval by testicular open biopsy in a case of partial tubular atrophy and severely reduced spermatogenesis, but normal gonadotrophins (Yemini et al., 1995), and another case with Sertoli cell–only (SCO) syndrome and hypergonadotrophic hypogonadism (Gil-Salom et al., 1995), was complemented almost simultaneously by a report on a series of successful attempts in extraction of spermatozoa from testicular tissue by multiple open biopsies with testicular sperm extraction in nonobstructive azoospermic patients (Devroey et al., 1995a). Since then, the use of TESE and ICSI has become the first-line treatment in NOA (Tournaye et al., 1995, 1996; Devroey et al., 1996; Kahraman et al., 1996a; Silber et al., 1996; Schlegel et al., 1997; Friedler et al., 1997a). Testicular fine-needle aspiration (TEFNA) was also offered as a less invasive but efficient methodology of sperm retrieval for NOA (Lewin et al., 1996, 1999). The last novel microsurgical technique was introduced by Schlegel et al. (1998). First, the microsurgical multiple testicular biopsies (Micro TESE) using an operating microscope to identify regions containing spermatozoa in the testes of men with NOA. Subsequently, Schlegel (1999) achieved better retrieval rates using a microdissection technique (Microdissection TESE) while the amount of testicular tissue excised was reduced. This technique is based on the observation that seminiferous tubules in cases with SCO are thinner than tubules containing sperm cells, and difference between the larger and smaller tubules is visible with optical magnification.

THE IMPORTANCE OF A PROPER DIAGNOSIS OF THE AZOOSPERMIC PATIENT

As per the definition, an azoospermic patient fails to produce sperm cells in sufficient quantity to be detected when examining the ejaculate in the camera under the microscope. In some patients, surgical sperm retrieval may be avoided as sperm cells may be found in the ejaculate after high-velocity centrifugation and thorough examination of the pellets in multiple droplets and used for ICSI (Ron-El et al., 1997). These patients should be classified as suffering from cryptozoospermia.

It is imperative to pursue in every azoospermic patient a proper diagnostic process, during which one should classify the patients according to the etiology of their azoospermia due to pretesticular, testicular, or post-testicular causes. This will help to group the patients to obstructive or nonobstructive azoospermia, allowing to counsel them and estimate their prognosis and optimal treatment plan.

Pretesticular Azoospermia

Patients with pretesticular causes have insufficient hormonal drive to produce spermatozoa usually combined with hypoandrogenism. Their treatment is medical, using hormonal replacement therapy with gonadotropins (Bouloux et al., 2002). The details concerning the various medical treatment protocols used are not within the scope of this chapter.

Testicular Azoospermia

Patients with testicular failure do not produce sperm cells at all or at least not in sufficient numbers to appear in the ejaculate. Nonobstructive azoospermia is characterized by hypergonadotropic hypogonadism, in which bilateral normal or small testes and elevated levels of follicle-stimulating hormone (FSH) are found. As NOA may exist also in the presence of normal gonadotrophin levels, the gold standard for the definitive diagnosis of testicular failure is a testicular biopsy evaluation in which normal spermatogenesis is ruled out and hypospermatogenesis, maturation arrest, germ cells aplasia, or tubular hyalinization with Leydig cells hypertrophy is confirmed.

Genetic evaluation with Y-chromosome microdeletion analysis and karyotype testing provides prognostic information in these men. Among infertile men, the prevalence of Y microdeletions is approximately 6.5–8.2 percent (Foresta et al., 2002; Teng et al., 2007), with a range of 1–55 percent depending on the patients selected for study and study techniques. More than 80 percent of deletions were associated with azoospermia.

In a recent publication by Teng et al. (2007) comprising 629 patients, the overall deletion frequency was 6.5 percent (41/627). The deletion rate was 11.6 percent (34/293) in patients with sperm concentration less than 1×10^6/mL or azoospermia, 4.5 percent (5/110) in patients with sperm concentration between 1×10^6/mL and 5×10^6/mL, and 0.9 percent (2/224) in patients with sperm concentration more than 5×10^6/mL. Most Y chromosome microdeletions occur on the long arm (q) and are subdivided into three azoospermic factor (AZF) regions: a, b, and c (Figure 52.1).

Genes encoded in the AZF regions might be important in spermatogenesis. However, a small portion (up to 2 percent) (Foresta et al., 2001) of the fertile male population might also harbor very small microdeletions of the Y chromosome, likely involving noncoding regions.

In a study comprising seventeen patients with Y microdeletions who attempted IVF/ICSI cycles, following TESE, sperm was only obtained from patients with AZFc microdeletions (and from one patient with a partial AZFb microdeletion). A trend toward lower fertilization rates in patients with Y microdeletions was noted, which did not reach statistical significance. Clinical pregnancy rates per cycle and per transfer were similar to those for controls. Patients with AZFc microdeletions seem to have IVF/ICSI outcomes comparable to those of controls with normal Y chromosomes. Presence of AZFa or b microdeletion is a bad prognostic factor (Choi et al., 2002). A comprehensive review concerning the current knowledge and the possible risks involved in the transmission of male infertility linked to the Y chromosome was published by Silber and Repping (2002).

No doubt that the most dramatic advancement in the field of azoospermia treatment was the finding that unlike previous believes, 40–50 percent of these patients do pro-

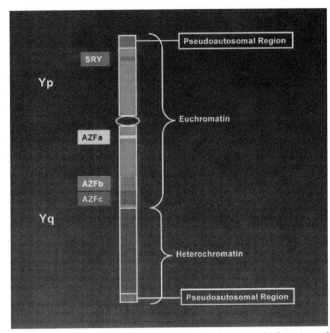

Figure 52.1. Diagram of the Y chromosome depicting the location of AZF regions a, b, and c. SRY, sex-determining region of the Y chromosome. From Choi et al. (2002).

duce some sperm cells, which may be surgically retrieved, used for ICSI, and result in pregnancy and delivery (Jow et al., 1993; Devroey et al., 1995a; Silber et al., 1995a, b, c; Tournaye et al., 1997a, b). Several studies of patients with NOA found a sperm extraction rate of 30–90 percent (Friedler et al., 1997a; Tournaye et al., 1997a, b; Ezeh et al., 1998a; Amer et al., 1999; Schlegel, 1999; Turek et al., 1999; Tsujimura et al., 2002) (Table 52.1).

These testicular sperm cells may be present in minute foci (focal spermatogenesis) and not dispersed in a homogenous fashion throughout the testicular tissue (Hauser et al., 1998; Silber, 2000; Ezeh and Moore, 2001).

Post-testicular Azoospermia

These patients have normal testicular spermatogenesis. However, there are no sperm cells in their ejaculate due to a blockage in the trajectory of sperm expulsion. This defect could be congenital, that is, absence of bilateral vas deferens (CABVD) or idiopathic epididymal obstruction, or acquired such as after orchiepididymitis, after vasectomy or vasectomy reversal failure or other injury to the vas deferens or epididymis. Couples in whom the man has congenital reproductive tract obstruction should have cystic fibrosis (CF) gene mutation analysis also for the female partner because of the high risk of the male being a CF carrier.

This group of patients characterized by normal serum gonadotrophin levels combined with normal sized testicles is classified as suffering from OA. Evidently, complete retrograde ejaculation has to be ruled out.

Prevalence of Azoospermia

The prevalence of azoospermia is estimated to be 10 percent of male infertility cases and is caused by a testicular insufficiency

Table 52.1: Frequency of Successful Testicular Sperm Retrieval in Patients with NOA Literature Survey

Reference	Sperm available on TESE, n/N (percent)
Devroey et al. (1995)	13/15 (87)
Kahraman et al. (1996)	14/29 (48)
Schlegel et al. (1997)	10/16 (62)
Silber et al. (1997)	39/63 (62)
Ostad et al. (1998)	47/81 (58)
Rosenlund et al. (1998)	6/12 (50)
Schlegel et al. (1999)	10/22 (45)
Ben Yosef et al. (1999)	33/55 (60)
Westlander et al. (1999)	27/86 (31)
Ezeh et al. (1998)	22/35 (63)
Turek et al. (1999)	20/21 (95)
Kahraman et al. (1999)	22/86 (31)
Von Eckardstein et al. (1999)	34/52 (65)
Hauser et al. (2006)	54/87 (62)
Seo and Ko. (2001)	94/178 (53)
Friedler et al. (2002)	50/123 (41)
Everaert et al. (2006)	17/48 (35)
Total	512/1009 (51)

in the majority of patients. In 20 percent, a bilateral obstruction of the male genital tract is responsible for the azoospermia.

METHODS OF SSR

Methods of SSR include epididymal and testicular sperm retrieval, which can be open, close, or with microdissection.

MESA Procedure

MESA involves the opening of the scrotal sac, exposing the testicle and the epididymis, visualization of the engorged epididymal ducts, and aspirating their content by a glass tube or syringe preferably from the caudal part of the epididymis. The methodology of MESA was published by several investigators (Schlegel et al., 1994; Silber et al., 1994; Tournaye et al., 1994).

PESA Procedure

The technique of PESA has been described by Craft and Shrivastav (1995) and performed by several authors, with some minor variations. According to Friedler et al. (1998), PESA is performed using twenty three-gauge butterfly needles attached to a 20-mL plastic syringe serving as an aspiration device. While holding the testicle between the index finger and the thumb, the epididymis is palpated and the butterfly needle

is directly passed through the scrotal skin into the epididymis. As much epididymal fluid as possible is aspirated, and before retrieving the needle from the epididymis, a small artery forceps is used to clamp the butterfly's microtubing. If aspiration is not successful on one side, the contralateral epididymis is aspirated.

TEFNA/TESA Procedure

Alternatively, one may try closed testicular biopsies with needles of various diameters (Bourne et al., 1995) or a biopsy gun (Hovatta et al., 1995) or percutaneous fine-needle testicular sperm aspiration (Lewin et al., 1996).

The variation on the technique of TEFNA described by Friedler et al. (1998) includes using twenty one-gauge butterfly needles attached to a 20-mL plastic syringe serving as an aspiration device. The butterfly needle is passed directly through the scrotal skin, into the testis, moved up and down at various sites, directing the needle into the rete testis. While holding the testicle between the index finger and the thumb, six or more different entries may be done in each testicle, allowing to sample various locations. Before retrieving the needle from the testis, a small artery forceps is used to clamp the butterfly's microtubing. Following each aspiration, the needle is flushed with Earle's balanced salt solution into one of a four-well plate. For each puncture, a new butterfly needle is used. The aspirates are examined under an inverted microscope at ×200 and ×400 magnification to detect the presence of spermatozoa. This preliminary search under the microscope helps the surgeon to make his decision when to stop aspiration. Later on, the aspirate is then examined after appropriate laboratory processing.

The TESA procedure has several advantages: it is technically easier to perform and requires fewer surgical skills and training. The procedure is shorter and can be performed under local anesthesia (Belker et al., 1998; Gorgy et al., 1998). The healing process may be easier and more rapid because there are no skin scars and sutures. Nevertheless, insofar as the procedure is painful, local anesthesia or some form of sedation or even general anesthesia is always required (Gorgy et al., 1998). In our program, the routine is general anesthesia for all surgical sperm retrieval procedures.

Testicular Sperm Extraction

The first technique for surgical sperm retrieval that was introduced included open testicular biopsy with TESE. At the moment, this procedure is still the first line of treatment for NOA in most of the centers. TESE requires a fully equipped operating theater, general anesthesia, and a skillful surgeon. In the open biopsy technique, large amounts of testicular tissue are extracted in an effort to find spermatozoa. Some authors have suggested a single large biopsy, others perform multiple smaller biopsies taken from different regions of the testicle, three to four biopsies from each testicle representing an optimal number (Hauser et al., 1998; Amer et al., 1999), and still others have reported excising a majority of the volume of the testis (Silber et al., 1996, 1997a; Tournaye et al., 1996). Moreover, the duration of the procedure is relatively short (about twenty to forty-five minutes) and is performed on a day-clinic basis.

Conventional TESE

The technique for standard biopsies has been previously described in detail by several authors (Silber et al., 1996; Schlegel et al., 1997; Tournaye et al. 1997a; Ostad et al., 1998).

In brief, usually under general anesthesia, after stabilization of the testicle that is larger (usually the right testicle) or showed better histological evidence of spermatogenesis in diagnostic biopsy, an incision of approximately 1 cm is made through the skin and underlying layers, cutting through the scrotal skin, tunica vaginalis, and the tunica albuginea. Then, a gentle pressure is applied to the testicular mass, and a small specimen of 150–500 mg (depending on the testicular volume) of the protruding testicular mass is removed using a pair of small curved scissors, washed by medium to remove blood traces, and placed in a Petri dish, containing approximately 1–3 mL HEPES-buffered Earle's medium with 0.5 percent human serum albumin and heparin 0.4 percent. In the laboratory, a wet preparation is conducted for examination. Testicular tissue is vigorously fragmented and minced by using two glass microscope slides in the Petri dish and immediately examined under an inverted microscope (×200 or ×400) to look for the presence of spermatozoa.

Once spermatozoa were found, the surgical procedure can be terminated. If spermatozoa are not observed, up to three biopsies may be taken, in different areas in the same testicle and subsequently from the contralateral one. During surgery, a single randomly taken biopsy of each testis should be sent for histological examination.

After vigorous tissue shredding and homogenization by repeated aspiration and spilling out maneuver into a tuberculin syringe, human tubal fluid medium supplemented with 7.5 percent synthetic serum is added to the suspension obtained and incubated for two hours. Then, the overlaying pellet is collected and separated from the underlying tissue and centrifuged. The remaining pellet is isolated, resuspended, and finally examined in multiple droplets under oil. Also, the remains of the underlying pellet is processed and examined in multiple droplets. After performance of ICSI for all the available mature oocytes, the remaining testicular cell suspension may be frozen for later use.

Microdissection TESE

As an ultimate goal to reduce the amount of testicular tissue removed and also to improve the sperm recovery, a direct microdissection technique was developed (Schlegel, 1999).

This technique uses an operating microscope that allows identification of subtunical vessels and helps to detect rare foci of spermatogenesis.

In brief, optical magnification (six to eight power) is used to visualize blood vessels under the surface of the tunica vaginalis, allowing placement of biopsy incisions in avascular regions of the testis. However, instead of planning for multiple incisions in the tunica albuginea, a single wide incision in the tunica albuginea near its midportion is made to allow visualization of the testicular parenchyma, without affecting the testicular blood supply. Direct examination of the testicular parenchyma is then performed at ×20 magnification under the operating microscope to identify individual seminiferous tubules that are larger than other tubules in the testicular parenchyma. Small (2- to 10-mg) samples are removed containing tubules that were larger and typically more opaque (whiter). Each excised testicular tissue specimen is further cut into smaller pieces to allow spermatozoa to be released from the inside of the seminiferous tubules. The resulting suspension is examined for spermatozoa. The procedure is terminated when spermatozoa are retrieved or all areas of testicular tissue had been examined and representative samples taken.

THE CHANCES OF SPERM RETRIEVAL WITH DIFFERENT METHODS

In patients with OA, MESA or PESA yielded approximately 100 percent success rate (Silber et al., 1994; Mansour et al., 1997; Tournaye et al., 1997a; Palermo et al., 1999; Friedler et al., 2002a; Nicopoullos et al., 2004a). If sperm cells are not found in the epidydimal aspirate, fine-needle TESA will result in retrieval of testicular sperm in virtually all cases of OA.

In patients with NOA, epidydimal aspiration is useless and the patients should be offered surgical retrieval of testicular sperm, preferably performing an open biopsy (Friedler et al., 1997a).

With TESE, the failure to extract spermatozoa may occur in up to 57 percent of the attempts (Devroey et al., 1995a; Kahraman et al., 1996a, 1996b; Friedler et al., 1997a, 2002b; Schlegel et al., 1997; Hauser et al., 1998; Rosenlund et al., 1998; Seo and Ko, 2001).

WHICH IS THE MOST EFFICIENT SSR METHOD FOR PATIENTS WITH OA AND NOA?

The optimal surgical procedure to obtain epididymal spermatozoa in patients with obstructive azoospermia is in debate (Craft and Shrivastav, 1995; Schlegel et al., 1995; Tsirigotis and Craft, 1995, 1996; Tsirigotis et al., 1995; Khalifa and Grudzinskas, 1996; Silber, 1996).

Advocating open surgery (MESA), Schlegel et al. (1994, 1995) argued that blood cells may contaminate percutaneous fine-needle aspiration specimens and affect fertilization rates and that a cleaner specimen may be retrieved by microsurgical retrieval. Silber (1996) stressed the possibility to cryopreserve enough spermatozoa for twenty future ICSI cycles following MESA. One might argue that the freezability of epididymal sperm specimens retrieved by MESA could be different from those retrieved by PESA. Although PESA in patients with OA was shown to be efficient (Craft and Shrivastav, 1995; Craft et al., 1995a, b; Tsirigotis and Craft, 1995; Meniru et al., 1997a, b), reports concerning cryopreservation of spermatozoa retrieved by PESA are scarce. Our results (Friedler et al., 1998) showed that not only is the fertilization rate of ICSI with fresh or cryopreserved-thawed epididymal spermatozoa retrieved by PESA comparable to that retrieved by MESA but also the clinical outcome does not differ significantly between the groups. Therefore, as PESA has definitive clinical advantages compared with the open surgery required in MESA, it may be offered as the treatment of choice for patients with obstructive azoospermia. Epididymal micropuncture with perivascular nerve stimulation was suggested by Yamamoto et al. and compared to the routine MESA (Yamamoto et al., 1996, 1997), but a recent updated Cochrane analysis could not recommend any specific technique as superior to be used for OA, and in the absence of evidence to support more invasive or more technically difficult methods, the reviewers recommend the least invasive and simplest technique available (Van Perperstraten et al., 2006).

Presently, only a few studies performed well-conducted comparisons of the efficiency of TESA with TESE, using the same subjects as their own controls. Whereas some studies

Table 52.2: Studies Published in the Literature Comparing Sperm Recovery Using Both TESE and TESA Procedures in the Same Men with NOA

Study	No. of men with NOA	Sperm recovery rate by TESE, % (n)	Sperm recovery rate by TESA (21-gauge*needle), % (n)	P value
Friedler et al. (1997a)	37	43 (16)	11 (4)	0.02
Rosenlund et al. (1998)	12	50 (6)	16.7 (2)	—
Ezeh et al. (1998a)	35	63 (22)	14 (5)	0.0001
Tournaye (1999)	14	64.3 (9)	7.1 (1)	—
Hauser et al. (2006)	87	62.1 (54)	24.1 (21)	0.001
Qublan et al. (2002)	27	33 (9)	30 (8)	NS
Aridogan et al. (2003)	38	40.8 (31)	39.5 (30)	NS

Modified from Hauser et al. (2006).

found comparable results (Rosenlund et al., 1998; Qublan et al., 2002; Aridogan et al., 2003), most of the studies reported better results performing TESE (Friedler et al., 1997a; Ezeh et al., 1998a; Tournaye, 1999) (Table 52.2).

Recently, Hauser et al. (2006) reported a study including eighty-seven patients with NOA, showing again that multifocal TESE is significantly more efficient than multifocal TESA for sperm detection and recovery.

The TESE procedure enables a better histopathological evaluation of intact testicular tissue, including the peritubular space.

Some investigators reported success using TESE after previous failure of sperm retrieval with TESA (Mercan et al., 2000; Khadra et al., 2003).

Numerous studies have compared conventional versus microdissection TESE (Schlegel, 1999; Amer et al., 2000; Okada et al., 2002; Tsujimura et al., 2002), showing that the sperm retrieval rate with microdissection TESE is higher than with an open biopsy, in which even multiple samples are obtained (conventional TESE).

In Schlegel's hands, the microdissection TESE resulted in an improvement of sperm retrieval rates from 45 to 63 percent. In men where no spermatozoa were found in a nonmicrosurgical single testicular biopsy procedure, the retrieval rate was 35 percent (Schlegel, 1999). Ramasamy et al. (2005) from the same group have compared the retrieval rates between the two retrieval approaches, conventional and microdissection TESE, in 435 men with NOA with different histological diagnoses, who had undergone 543 TESE attempts. The initial 83 attempts were done using the conventional open technique and the remaining 460 attempts were performed by microdissection. The retrieval rate by the conventional technique was 32 percent and by microdissection was 57 percent ($P = 0.0002$). A significant difference was found in sperm retrieval between the two procedures in patients with hypospermatogenesis ($P = 0.03$). The other histopathological types showed no statistically significant difference, although a trend toward higher retrieval rates was seen in this study.

Other studies have reported significant benefits for patients with SCO syndrome (Silber 2000; Okada et al., 2002). Sperm retrieval rate using microdissection technique in the hands of other investigators was reported as less efficient compared to

results of Schlegel et al., being only 47 percent (Amer et al., 2000), 42.9 percent (Tsujimiura et al., 2002), and 44.6 percent (Okada et al., 2002).

In some centers, microdissection TESE has become a standard treatment for patients with NOA.

Among patients with NOA, in whom no spermatozoa were found following a microepididymal sperm aspiration and a simple testicular biopsy, we were able to retrieve spermatozoa in 35 percent by means of multiple microsurgical testis biopsies or testicular microdissection. The per couple take-home baby rate was 24 percent (Everaert et al., 2006).

Some alternative strategies to TESE have been offered, such as needle aspiration mapping (Turek et al., 1999; Hussein et al., 2005) and Doppler-guided TESE (Tunc et al., 2005; Herwig et al., 2006). These methods are under constant development, and their clinical value requires still further validation.

WHAT FACTORS INFLUENCE THE OUTCOME OF ICSI USING NONEJACULATED SPERM?

Male Factors

According to Friedler et al. (2002a), the parameters linked to the male partner, which influence the ICSI outcome include age, serum FSH, and testicular histology that may reflect upon the quality of the surgically retrieved sperm cells. The injected sperm cell quality and viability may also be related to the etiology of azoospermia, that is, obstructive or nonobstructive, the site of sperm origin, that is, epididymis or testis, expressing the developmental stage of the sperm cell (Bachtell et al., 1999), as well as the status of the sperm being fresh or cryopreserved-thawed. Efficient nonejaculated sperm preservation may allow the independence of the surgical sperm retrieval from the controlled ovarian stimulation and oocyte retrieval (Oates et al., 1996; Nudell et al., 1998; Ben-Yosef et al., 1999).

Female Factors

Parameters determined by the female partner such as age and ovarian reserve may also have a significant contribution to the success of ICSI in these patients (Oehninger et al. 1995; Silber et al., 1997b). Female factors such as age (less than thirty seven years) and ovarian reserve (less than five oocytes retrieved) have significant negative impact upon clinical success rates (Silber et al., 1997b; Friedler et al., 2002a).

Friedler et al. (2002a) analyzed the outcome of ICSI after surgical sperm retrieval by percutaneous epididymal sperm aspiration (55 cycles) or testicular sperm extraction (142 cycles) in 52 and 123 patients with OA and NOA, respectively.

Occurrence of pregnancy was significantly correlated with female age (90th quantile: thirty eight years), number of oocytes retrieved (10th quantile: five oocytes), and number of oocytes injected (10th quantile: four oocytes). Sperm origin (epididymal versus testicular), status (fresh or thawed), male partner's age, and serum FSH had no significant effect upon implantation rate, pregnancy rate per embryo transfer, or spontaneous miscarriage rate.

Successful outcome of ICSI measured by live birth rates has been shown to be independent of the type of the procedure (Nicopoullos et al., 2004b).

ETIOLOGY OF AZOOSPERMIA INFLUENCING ICSI OUTCOME

Although there is a general agreement that ICSI using nonejaculated sperm cells yields lower fertilization rates compared with ejaculated spermatozoa (De Vos and Van Steirteghem, 1999; Van Steirteghem et al., 2000), there is still controversy about which type of azoospermia yields better outcome.

The underlying etiology of azoospermia could influence the viability of the retrieved sperm cells as well as determine their maturational status being from epididymal or testicular source, in OA or NOA, respectively. Viability of sperm, at least as judged by motility, may be influenced by their source (Bachtell et al., 1999). Several reports did not find a significant difference in the 2PN fertilization rate between patients with OA and NOA, as well as the clinical pregnancy rate, early miscarriage rate, and the ongoing pregnancy/delivery rates. Although the last was higher in patients with OA, they did not reach a statistically significant difference.

The ESHRE ICSI Task Force reported their experience for the year 1995 (Tarlatzis and Bili, 1998, 2000) and found a tendency for lower fertilization rates following ICSI in NOA compared with OA patients. A total of 339 ICSI cycles performed in 298 patients with OA and 287 ICSI cycles in 247 patients with NOA resulted in a 2PN fertilization rate of 54.7 and 46.7 percent, respectively; similar results reported by Friedler et al. (1997a, b), were 56 and 51 percent, respectively. Clinical pregnancy, early miscarriage, and ongoing pregnancy/delivery rates, although higher in patients with OA, did not reach a statistically significant difference (Friedler et al., 1997a, b; Tarlatzis and Bili, 1998, 2000).

Silber et al. (1997b) reported data concerning outcome of ICSI in 186 patients with OA and 163 patients with NOA. Neither the pathology nor the sperm source and neither the quality nor the quantity had any effect on fertilization or pregnancy rates. Comparing the outcome of thirty and thirty-nine ICSI cycles in OA and NOA patients, respectively, Vicari et al. (2001) reported similar fertilization and pregnancy rates in OA, significantly higher abortion rates for NOA, resulting in a significantly higher ongoing/delivery rates for OA.

Despite the above-mentioned results, many other authors reported superior results following ICSI using sperm from OA compared to NOA patients. Mansour et al. (1997) compared the outcome of ICSI using epididymal sperm from patients with OA (44 cycles) and the use of testicular sperm in NOA (106 cycles) and found a significantly lower fertilization rate in the latter group (59.5 vs. 39 percent), significantly lower clinical pregnancy rate per cycle (27.3 vs. 11.3 percent), and lower pregnancy rate per embryo transfer (27.3 vs. 15.2 percent). Palermo et al. (1999) reported a significantly higher fertilization rate of 73 percent in 241 cycles of OA – acquired and congenital – using epididymal sperm compared with 57 percent in 53 cycles of NOA as well as a significantly higher clinical pregnancy rate of 56 percent (135/241) compared with 49.1 percent (26/53) for OA and NOA cases, respectively. Ubaldi et al. (1999) compared the outcome of ICSI using testicular sperm from OA (thirty three cycles), NOA (twenty nine cycles), and patients with ejaculated sperm. They found a significantly lower implantation rate (13.4 vs. 24.5 percent, for NOA and OA, respectively, $P = 0.05$).

In a retrospective analysis involving 139 patients with OA and 54 with NOA who underwent ICSI using testicular sperm, fertilization rates were significantly lower in patients with NOA. However, pregnancy and embryo implantation rates were similar (De Croo et al., 2000). In patients with NOA, pregnancy rates were lowest for maturation arrest (20 percent), but not significantly different from SCO or hypoplasia. Implantation rate was lowest in germ-cell hypoplasia (15.8 percent).

Other authors reported also higher fertilization rates and higher pregnancy rates after ICSI in OA compared with NOA (Kahraman et al., 1996b; Aboulghar et al., 1997; Fahmy et al., 1997; Ghazzawi et al., 1998; Schwarzer et al., 2003; Vernaeve et al., 2003). A recent meta-analysis of five studies including 833 patients and comparing OA and NOA showed significantly better fertilization rates among OA patients (Ghanem et al., 2005). However, pregnancy rates did not differ significantly.

Considering the possible increased incidence of genetic abnormalities among the testicular sperm in patients with NOA (Palermo et al., 2002; Silber et al., 2003), these findings are not surprising. Oates et al. (2002) concluded that this is not related to the presence of AZFc microdeletion.

PROGNOSTIC FACTORS

In order to make the best decision concerning the treatment in patients with azoospermia, clarification of their actual prognosis is important for the clinical decision to perform surgical sperm retrieval.

In OA patients, sperm retrieval is possible in most cases.

In a patient with NOA, it is not possible to predict with certainty successful sperm retrieval or failure to find mature testicular sperm following TESE, as no good noninvasive predictors are available including patients' age, testicular size, or serum FSH level (Ezeh et al., 1998a; Jezek et al., 1998; Friedler et al., 2002a).

Testicular histopathology on a previous biopsy or fine-needle aspiration cytology (Bettella et al., 2005) was suggested as the strongest indicator for the chance of finding sperm for ICSI, which was significantly higher in cases with severe hypospermatogenesis, according to some of the reports in the literature (Tournaye et al., 1996, 1997b; Friedler et al., 1997a, 2002a; Mulhall et al., 1997; Gil-Salom et al., 1998; Jezek et al., 1998; Amer et al., 1999; Schulze et al., 1999; Mercan et al., 2000; Silber, 2000; Seo and Ko, 2001; Vicari et al., 2001; Tsujimura et al., 2002). According to a recent minireview by McLachlan et al.

(2007), the lack of clarity may well arise from inaccurate identification of germ cells and confusing and not uniform categorization of biopsies.

Of course, testicular biopsy is an invasive procedure; so the search for a noninvasive marker still continues. Serum inhibin B levels, as a measure of Sertoli cell function, may correlate with the chance of finding sperm in NOA patients, being significantly higher in patients with successful TESE (Ballesca et al., 2000; Bohring et al., 2002). However, controversy concerning its clinical value still exists as some reports (Von Eckardstein et al., 1999; Vernaeve et al., 2002; Tunc et al., 2006) failed to corroborate the previous findings and showed that inhibin B failed to predict the presence of testicular sperm in patients with NOA. Also, Doppler ultrasonography has recently been used to correlate testicular blood flow with successful sperm recovery in azoospermic men (Souza et al., 2005). However, at the present time, none of the markers or the combinations between them proved to be of sufficient clinical value to accurately predict presence or lack of presence of some foci of testicular spermatogenesis, warranting the performance of TESE in patients with NOA (Tunc et al., 2006).

COMPLICATIONS OF TESA/TESE/ MICROSURGICAL TESE

Surgical sperm retrieval is generally tolerated well, and the complication rate is low from both PESA and TESE (Wood et al., 2003). Following TESA, complications of both procedures are relatively rare. Gorgy et al. (1998) used local anesthesia for needle aspiration procedures and reported vasovagal reflex in two men (6 percent) and anxiety in thirteen others (39 percent).

TESE appears to affect testicular damage both structurally and functionally.

In humans, the testicular artery enters the testis posteriorly beneath the epididymis at the midpole, continues inferiorly to the lower pole, and then courses superiorly along the anterior surface, where it gives rise to branches that supply the parenchyma (Jarow, 1991). Therefore, multiple testicular biopsies can result in the loss of significant amounts of testicular tissue and can interrupt the testicular blood supply underneath the tunica albuginea with risks of testicular devascularization and subsequent atrophy of the testis (Schlegel and Su, 1997, 1998; Schlegel et al., 1997). Indeed, Schlegel and Su (1997) reported complete testicular atrophy in two out of sixty-four patients following nonmicrosurgical TESE. Although intratesticular bleeding can be better controlled in TESE due to the full exposure of the tissue, TESE is sometimes complicated by infection or hematoma (Friedler et al., 1997a; Hauser et al., 1998). Many studies reported ultrasonographic evidence of residual testicular damage after TESE (reviewed in Schill et al., 2003). Schlegel and Su (1997) reported that 82 percent of the patients who underwent a TESE procedure had intratesticular abnormalities on ultrasound as long as three months afterward. Most of the lesions seemed to disappear six months after TESE, leaving only linear scars visible on ultrasound. In a study by Ron El et al. (1998) involving patients with OA and NOA, testicular volumes remained unchanged during the follow-up period in both the nonobstructive and obstructive groups. Of the nonobstructive group, focal testicular lesions were seen in twenty of the twenty-six testes (77 percent) five days after the procedure and in 54 percent by six

months. Ten were hypoechoic, of which six converted to echogenic foci, three remained hypoechoic, and one disappeared at six months. The other ten were echogenic lesions, three of which were no longer visible at six months and the remainder was unchanged. In the obstructive azoospermic group, focal lesions were not found. Extratesticular abnormality consistent with hematoma was demonstrated in four nonobstructive cases, which disappeared at the six-month examination, and in none of the obstructive azoospermic patients. Whether residual focal lesions in the testes have long-term effects remains to be evaluated. In the obstructive azoospermic group, the aspirations performed did not leave any sonographic abnormalities.

Damage may be caused also due to pressure atrophy from intratesticular swelling and hematoma (Silber, 2000). Both procedures may have a deleterious effect on testicular histology. A post-TESE decrease in seminiferous tubular volume within the testicular parenchyma adjacent to the biopsy site has been reported (Tash and Schlegel, 2001).

In the largest study regarding micro-TESE by Ramasamy et al. (2005), following 543 TESE attempts including 83 using the conventional open TESE technique and 460 by microdissection TESE, despite involving a large transverse incision in the tunica albuginea, ultrasound findings demonstrated fewer acute and chronic changes in the microdissection group than in the conventional group ($P = 0.05$).

Furthermore, multiple testicular biopsies involving vascular damage can lead to a decrease of Leydig cell function causing a decrease of serum testosterone (T) level. This may result in T deficiency, requiring lifelong androgen supplementation as androgen deficiency may have serious long-term health consequences (Comhaire, 2000).

Manning et al. (1998) found that T levels decreased initially after conventional TESE in most patients with NOA, with partial recovery one year after the procedure. Schill et al. (2003) reported no decrease in serum T levels in patients with azoospermia after an average of eighteen months following conventional TESE. However, the same study indicated that patients with NOA had lower serum T levels and that T response to human chorionic gonadotrophin stimulation was more frequently impaired compared to men with OA (Bouloux et al., 2002). Therefore, they concluded that patients with NOA show an increased risk of androgen deficiency following nonmicrosurgical TESE and recommended long-term follow-up in this group of patients (16). According to Komori et al. (2004), alterations in serum total T and free T are similar between patients undergoing conventional TESE and those undergoing microdissection TESE. A decrease in the serum T concentrations after eighty-three conventional TESE procedures was noted also in the study by Ramasamy et al. (2005). The initial decrease was followed by a return to 95 percent of the pre-TESE T levels at the end of eighteen months of follow-up. Considering the number of patients undergoing TESE presently, there are relatively few data on the long-term effects of TESE performed by microsurgery.

Needle aspiration of testicular spermatozoa had no adverse effect on serum T after up to nine months of follow-up (Westlander et al., 2001).

To assess the functional changes to the testis, Tash et al. (2000) analyzed the T levels preoperatively and at three to six, twelve, and eighteen months after micro-TESE. Although previous reports found no decrease in serum T one month after microdissection TESE in four patients (Hibi et al., 2002), at three to six months after surgery, the T levels had dropped to 80 percent of their pre-TESE levels in both groups ($P = 0.01$). The levels rose back to 85 percent after twelve months and to 95 percent after eighteen months. The mean FSH levels increased from 22 ± 2 to 30 ± 3 IU/L after TESE ($P = 0.02$), but no difference was found in FSH levels between those patients in whom sperms were retrieved and those in whom no sperm was found. The change in FSH levels may have been a result of the scar tissue left behind in the testis, with local germ-cell loss near the scar after the procedure (Tash et al., 2000). No significant difference in the LH levels was noted between the preoperative and postoperative groups. According to Ramasamy et al. (2005), TESE has effects on testicular function, but the microdissection procedure is relatively safer than the conventional technique and improves the sperm retrieval rate significantly in patients with NOA.

These findings corroborate those of studies reported earlier (Amer et al., 2000; Okada et al., 2002). In a recent report by Everaert et al. (2006), microsurgical TESE was associated with a significant long-term decrease of serum T levels. A relatively high incidence of T deficiency was recorded preoperatively (8 percent), and after an average of 2.4 years of follow-up, a de novo androgen deficiency occurred in 16 percent of the male patients undergoing micro-TESE, indicating that in men with NOA, long-term hormonal follow-up is recommended after TESE (Everaert et al., 2006). It is unlikely that age per se was a major contributing factor to T deficiency in their patients since they were relatively young, with a mean age of thirty-four years.

Men with NOA are more prone to develop premature "andropause" due to the presence of testicular pathology, the effects of which on serum T may be additive to those of the TESE procedure (Everaert et al., 2006). When the testosterone level declines, one should consider also factors, other than the micro-TESE surgery, which can gradually compromise the Leydig cell function (e.g., cryptorchidism, testicular torsion, and chemotherapy).

Evidently, patients need to be informed on the long-term consequences of TESE, including possible androgen deficiency and its therapy. Before starting substitution therapy, it seems advisable to wait for about one year after the surgery since some degree of spontaneous recovery may occur (Manning et al., 1998).

SHOULD FRESH OR CRYOPRESERVED SPERM BE USED?

Proving the efficiency of ICSI using nonejaculated sperm after cryopreservation is of paramount importance. Cryopreservation of nonejaculated sperm following surgical sperm retrieval allows us to perform further ICSI cycles, thus avoiding the repetition of SSR. Furthermore, efficient nonejaculated sperm preservation allows the independence of the SSR from the controlled ovarian stimulation and oocyte retrieval (Oates et al., 1996; Nudell et al., 1998; Ben-Yosef et al., 1999; Janzen et al., 2000). Thus, unnecessary ovarian stimulation is prevented in cases where no sperm can be retrieved, and oocyte retrieval planning is possible in the others.

Whereas in OA a greater number of motile sperm may usually be aspirated and cryopreserved than in cases of NOA, usually in NOA, only a small number of sperm cells are identified in the testicular biopsies and remain available for cryopreservation.

Comparing fresh with cryopreserved-thawed sperm, in either the OA or NOA groups, successful cryopreservation of epididymal sperm in OA patients was reported by many investigators, showing comparable implantation rate or clinical or ongoing pregnancy rates achieved following embryo transfer (Devroey et al., 1995b; Nagy et al., 1995; Oates et al., 1996; Holden et al., 1997; Silber et al., 1997b; Madgar et al., 1998; Palermo et al., 1999; Tournaye et al., 1999; Janzen et al., 2000; Cayan et al., 2001). Also, successful testicular sperm cryopreservation has been reported (Fischer et al., 1996; Gil-Salom et al., 1996; Hovatta et al., 1996; Romero et al., 1996; Liu et al., 1997; Oates et al., 1997; Perraguin-Jayot et al., 1997; DeCroo et al., 1998; Marmar, 1998; Ben Yosef et al., 1999; Tuuri et al., 1999; Gil-Salom et al., 2000).

For example, examining outcome of ICSI in patients suffering from OA, using fresh epididymal sperm (seventy-five cycles) and frozen epidydimal sperm (twenty-seven cycles), Silber et al. (1997) found no significant differences in 2PN fertilization (58 vs. 48 percent), implantation (20 vs. 14 percent), clinical pregnancy rate/embryo transfer (49 vs. 41 percent), and delivery rate/embryo transfer (36 vs. 37 percent). Comparing the use of fresh or cryopreserved-thawed epididymal sperm in patients undergoing their first ICSI cycle (108 fresh and 33 cryopreserved), Janzen et al. (2000) reported similar fertilization rates (78.2 and 76.9 percent), clinical pregnancy rates (67 and 61 percent), and delivery rates (57 and 51 percent, respectively). Van Steirteghem et al. (1998) summarized the five-year experience of the Brussels group performing ICSI and reported no significant differences in the fertilization and, embryo cleavage rates when using fresh epididymal, cryopreserved epididymal or testicular sperm. The delivery rate per embryo transfer was 31.3 and 27.2 percent, respectively.

Several studies aiming to control for oocyte factor by comparing outcome of ICSI in the same couples found no significant differences in fertilization or clinical pregnancy rates when using fresh or frozen-thawed epididymal sperm (Friedler et al., 1998; Tournaye et al., 1999). Palermo et al. reported no difference in fertilization rate after cryopreservation using epididymal sperm (72 vs. 74 percent, fresh vs. thawed, respectively), but a significant decrease in the clinical pregnancy rate (64.3 vs. 46.4 percent accordingly) (Palermo et al., 1999). Using testicular sperm, no difference was noted in fertilization or clinical pregnancy rates following cryopreservation. Also, Ben-Yosef et al. (1999) found no significant difference in 2PN fertilization, pregnancy, or implantation rates (59 vs. 61 percent, 26.7 vs. 21.7 percent, and 12.5 vs. 8.5 percent, using fresh or cryopreserved-thawed testicular sperm, respectively) in patients with NOA. Also, Habermann et al. (2000) reported no differences in the outcome of all parameters using fresh or frozen-thawed epididymal or testicular sperm, in OA or NOA patients.

One has to note, however, that lack of motility after thawing resulted in significantly lower fertilization rates (Friedler et al., 1997b; Liu et al., 1997).

To investigate the outcome of ICSI with fresh and cryopreserved-thawed testicular spermatozoa in the first cycle in patients with OA and NOA, a total of ninety cases, forty-eight OA and forty-two NOA, were studied (Ghanem et al., 2005). All patients underwent TESE. Sperm status (fresh or thawed), male partner's age, female age, and male serum FSH had no significant effect upon fertilization, implantation, or pregnancy rate. The results of meta-analysis indicate that although fertilization rate was significantly superior in patients with OA compared to NOA, there was no statistically significant difference in clinical pregnancy rates between the two groups.

In thirteen couples who underwent both, a treatment with fresh testicular sperm that were retrieved shortly beforehand were injected and a consecutive cycle, with frozen-thawed sperm that were retrieved in the original TESE procedure, fertilization and pregnancy rates were not significantly compromised. These results took place, although cryopreservation did impair motility (Hauser et al., 2005).

It seems that epididymal as well as testicular sperm may be successfully cryopreserved, irrespective of the specific histological diagnosis of the biopsy.

In patients with NOA, as sperm retrieval rate is lower, but the performance of ICSI using thawed sperm is similar to that using fresh ones, elective surgical sperm retrieval may be offered to patients prior to ovarian stimulation of their partners, especially when donor backup is not an alternative for the couple. The main benefit of this policy would be the avoidance of ovarian hyperstimulation in cases where no sperm are found for ICSI following sperm retrieval. However, in some men, only very few sperm may be found in their testicular biopsy for cryopreservation, or in others, the risk of repeated surgery – in case the sperm cells do not survive cryopreservation – is unacceptable. In these cases, elective sperm cryopreservation may not serve the patient's best interest (Friedler et al., 2002a).

METHODS OF TESTICULAR SPERM CRYOPRESERVATION

Cryopreservation of the remaining testicular tissue after sperm extraction or of individual sperm cells isolated after TESE represents a technical challenge. The small amount of testicular supernatant/tissue may be cryopreserved under a layer of paraffin oil with glycerol (Craft and Tsirigotis, 1995), in a mixture called "testicular pill" (Romero et al., 1996), or isolated sperm cells may be injected into an empty zona pellucida of a hamster oocyte and placed between two air bubbles inside a straw, to help in post-thaw localization (Cohen et al, 1997; Hsieh et al., 2000). For ethical reasons, the last mentioned method was abandoned.

However, the cryopreservation methodology used in our center is quite simple (Friedler et al., 1997a, b, 1998). In brief, in cases following ICSI using fresh epididymal or testicular spermatozoa, the remaining spermatozoa are cryopreserved using a freezing protocol with test yolk buffer freezing medium (Irvine Scientific). The spermatozoa-containing extract is diluted dropwise, 1:1, with the freezing medium and sealed in freezing straws (0.5 mL, Instruments de Médicine Veterinaire, IMV, l'Aigle, France). A simple two-step cryopreservation protocol is used. The straws are dropped in a nitrogen vapor chamber stabilized at –80°C for twenty minutes (cooling rate of –10°C/minute) prior to immersion into liquid nitrogen for sperm storage at –196°C.

Regarding thawing, following removal of the straws from the liquid nitrogen, rapid thawing occurs at room temperature. Then the frozen-thawed sperm mixture containing cryoprotectant is diluted with insemination medium and centrifuged at 300 g for seven minutes, and the pellet is processed for examination in multiple droplets.

WHAT ARE THE RESULTS IN REPETITIVE SSR?

Pregnancy rates were limited following ICSI using testicular sperm found in patients with NOA (Vernaeve et al., 2003; Nicopoullos et al., 2004b); so cryopreservation of the remaining testicular tissue is a valid option to avoid repeated surgery. However, cryopreservation is not always feasible in NOA, and sperms will not be found after thawing in about 20 percent of patients. In these cases, a repeated TESE procedure, therefore, should be considered on the day of oocyte retrieval (Verheyen et al., 2004).

Some couples may also need a repeated procedure to achieve a second pregnancy.

Because the quantity of testicular tissue is limited and some authors have cautioned for possible testicular damage after TESE (Schlegel and Su, 1997; Ron-El et al., 1998), the true prognosis of repetitive TESE is of paramount importance to adequately counsel patients.

Only three studies, based on a limited number of cases, examined the possibility of finding sperm in repeated testicular biopsies in patients with azoospermia (Westlander et al., 2001b; Friedler et al., 2002b; Kamal et al., 2004). In cases of OA, it is widely accepted that sperm can be recovered in all patients. Regarding the feasibility of repeating testicular sperm aspiration in twenty-two men suffering from OA, Westlander et al. (2001b) found a sufficient number of spermatozoa to be able to inject all the oocytes of each patient up to the third procedure. In a large recent report by Vernaeve et al. (2006), overall, sperm could be retrieved in all procedures in the 598 cycles performed in OA men (100 percent). A total of 117, 57, 24, 11, 7, and 1 men underwent, respectively, two, three, four, five, six, and seven sperm retrievals; all were successful.

Regarding the outcome of repeated TESE procedures in patients with NOA, the study by Westlander et al. (2001b) included thirty-four patients. They found that, in one patient, repeating the procedure up to the sixth attempt was feasible. However, their definition of NOA was not based on histology. The study by Friedler et al. (2002b) examined repeated TESE in twenty-two patients with NOA, defined according to histology. They found that repeating the procedure up to the fourth trial was justified. In few cases where the fifth TESE procedure was performed, no sperm were found and histology revealed no seminiferous tubuli. These findings were corroborated by Kamal et al. (2004), with a study on forty-one patients with NOA. Repeated TESE trials were successful in 91.5 percent of patients, if sperm was recovered during the first procedure. These findings were recently corroborated by Vernaeve et al. (2006), reporting the Brussel Free University IVF team's results on their success rate following SSR. A total of 1,066 azoospermic men had their first sperm recovery between January 1, 1995, and December 31, 2003. A total of 381 men had OA, 628 had NOA, and 57 showed hypospermatogenesis. Of the 784 procedures performed on the 628 men with NOA, sperm could be retrieved in 384 procedures (49 percent). During the first TESE procedure, sperms could be extracted in 261 men with NOA (41.6 percent). In repeated procedures, sperm could be extracted in 123 of the 156 TESE procedures in NOA men (78.8 percent). A total of 103 men had a second attempt, 34 had a third attempt, 11 had a fourth attempt, 6 had a fifth attempt, and 2 had a sixth attempt. In these cycles, sperms could be extracted in, respectively, 77 (74.7 percent), 28 (82.3 percent), 11 (100 percent), 5 (83.3 percent), and 2 (100 percent) men.

Although it is our policy not to repeat a TESE in case of previous failed surgery, two patients who had had a first successful and a second unsuccessful TESE chose to undergo a third one. In both the cases, the third biopsy was also unsuccessful.

Overall, these results indicate that repeated TESE ensures a high sperm recovery rate even in patients with NOA. However, in NOA patients, studies reporting on TESE may therefore overestimate the retrieval rate by reallocating successful patients.

Moreover, the retrieval rate fell by 30 percent in repeated needle aspiration procedures in cases in which there had been successful sperm retrieval in the first attempt (Lewin et al., 1999). This may indicate damage to the testis related to the methodology of the procedure.

SHOULD VARICOCELECTOMY BE RECOMMENDED IN AZOOSPERMIC PATIENTS?

Over the years, some rare and conflicting reports appeared in the literature regarding the beneficial effect of varicocelectomy in patients with NOA (Mehan, 1976; Czaplicki et al., 1979; D'Ottavio et al., 1987; Matthews et al., 1998; Kim et al., 1999). As some of these studies were performed before the era of special techniques to find sperm cells after extensive sperm preparation (Ron-El et al., 1997; Jaffe et al., 1998), it is difficult to evaluate their clinical value today. Clearly, most of these men will require performance of TESE and ICSI. In a recent study comprising thirty-one patients with NOA and clinical varicocele, Schlegel and Kaufmann (2004) reported that men with clinical varicocele who were associated with NOA will rarely have adequate sperm in the ejaculate after varicocele repair to avoid TESE. A history of prior varicocele repair does not appear to affect the chance of sperm retrieval by TESE. They have reached the conclusion that the benefits of varicocelectomy in men with NOA may be less than previously reported.

In conclusion, we reviewed the current literature regarding the management of patients with azoospermia. After a correct presumptive diagnosis including genetic counseling and informed consent regarding the possible short- and long-term complications of SSR, one may offer a very efficient method of sperm retrieval in OA, whereas in NOA, success of sperm retrieval is still uncertain. Once sperm cells are available, the technique of ICSI offers satisfactory pregnancy rates, limited mainly by female factors. Surgically retrieved sperm cryopreservation is efficient and offers a mean to reduce the number of surgical procedures needed. Repetition of SSR provides satisfactory results, up to about four trials, but long-term complications should be considered in each case. There is no satisfactory evidence that varicocelectomy has a place in the treatment of azoospermia.

REFERENCES

Aboulghar M.A., Mansour R.T., Serour G.I., Fahmy I., Kamal A., Tawab N.A., Amin Y. (1997). Fertilization and pregnancy rates after intracytoplasmic sperm injection using ejaculate semen and surgically retrieved sperm. *Fertil Steril* 68: 108–11.

Abuzeid M., Chan Y., Sasy M.A. et al. (1995). Fertilization and pregnancy achieved by intracytoplasmic injection of sperm retrieved from testicular biopsies. *Fertil Steril* 64: 644–6.

Amer M., Ateyah A., Hany R., Zohdy W. (2000). Prospective comparative study between microsurgical and conventional testicular sperm extraction in non-obstructive azoospermia: follow-up by serial ultrasound examinations. *Hum Reprod* 15: 653–6.

Amer M., Haggar S.E., Moustafa T., Abd El-Naser T., Zohdy W. (1999). Testicular sperm extraction: impact of testicular histology on outcome, number of biopsies to be performed and optimal time for repetition. *Hum Reprod* 14: 3030–4.

Aridogan I.A., Bayazit Y., Yaman M., Ersoz C., Doran S. (2003). Comparison of fine-needle aspiration and open biopsy of testis in sperm retrieval and histopathologic diagnosis. *Andrologia* 35: 121–5.

Bachtell N.E., Conaghan J., Turek P.J. (1999). The relative viability of human spermatozoa from the vas deferens, epididymis and testis before and after cryopreservation. *Hum Reprod* 14: 3048–51.

Ballesca J., Balasch J., Calfell J.M., Alvarez R., Fabregues F., Osaba M.J. et al. (2000). Serum inhibin B determination is predictive of successful testicular sperm extraction in men with non-obstructive azoospermia. *Human Reprod* 15(8): 1734–8.

Belker A.M., Sherins R.J., Dennison-Lagos L., Thorsell L.P., Schulman J.D. (1998). Percutaneous testicular sperm aspiration: a convenient and effective office procedure to retrieve sperm for in vitro fertilization with intracytoplasmic sperm injection. *J Urol* 160: 2058–62.

Ben Yosef D., Yogev L., Hauser R., Yavetz H., Azem F., Yovel I., Lessing J.B., Amit A. (1999). Testicular sperm retrieval and cryopreservation prior to initiating ovarian stimulation as the first line approach in patients with non-obstructive azoospermia. *Hum Reprod* 14: 1794–801.

Bettella A., Ferlin A., Menegazzo M., Ferigo M., Tavolini I.M., Bassi P.F. et al. (2005). Testicular fine needle aspiration as a diagnostic tool in non-obstructive azoospermia. *Asian J Androl* 7(3): 289–94.

Bohring C., Printzen I.S., Weidner W., Krause W. (2002). Serum levels of inhibin B and follicle-stimulating hormone may predict successful sperm retrieval in men with azoospermia who are undergoing testicular sperm extraction. *Fertil Steril* 78(6): 1195–8.

Bouloux, P., Warne, D., Loumaye, E; FSH Study Group in Men's Infertility. (2002). Efficacy and safety of recombinant human follicle stimulating hormone in men with isolated hypogonadotropic hypogonadism. *Fertil Steril* 77: 270–3.

Bourne H., Watkins W., Speirs A., Baker H.W.G. (1995). Pregnancies after intracytoplasmic injection of sperm collected by fine needle biopsy of the testis. *Fertil Steril* 64: 433–6.

Cayan S., Lee D., Conaghan J., Givens C.A., Ryan I.P., Schriock E.D., Turek P.J. (2001). A comparison of ICSI outcomes with fresh and cryopreserved epididymal spermatozoa from the same couples. *Hum Reprod* 16(3): 495–9.

Choi M.J., Chung P., Veeck L., Mielnik A., Palermo G.D., Schlegel P.N. (2002). AZF microdeletions of the Y chromosome and in vitro fertilization outcome. *Hum Reprod* 17(3): 570–5.

Cohen J., Garrisi G.J., Congedo-Ferrara T.A., Kieck K.A., Schimmel T.W., Scott R.T. (1997). Cryopreservation of single human spermatozoa. *Hum Reprod* 12: 994–1001.

Comhaire F.H. (2000). Andropause: hormone replacement therapy in the ageing male. *Euro Urol* 38: 655–62.

Craft I., Bennett V., Nicholson N. (1993). Fertilising ability of testicular spermatozoa (Letter). *Lancet* 342: 864.

Craft I., Shrivastav P. (1994). Treatment of male infertility. *Lancet* 344: 191–2.

Craft I., Shrivastav P. (1995). Value of percutaneous epididymal sperm aspiration? *Fertil Steril* 63: 208–9.

Craft I., Tzirigotis M. (1995). Simplified recovery, preparation and cryopreservation of testicular spermatozoa. *Hum Reprod* 10: 1623–7.

Craft I.L., Tzirigotis M., Bennet V. et al. (1995a). Percutaneous epididymal sperm aspiration and intracytoplasmic sperm injection in the management of infertility due to obstructive azoospermia. *Fertil Steril* 63: 1038–42.

Craft I.L., Khalifa Y., Boulos A. et al. (1995b). Factors influencing the outcome of in-vitro fertilization with percutaneous aspirated epididymal spermatozoa and intracytoplasmic sperm injection in azoospermic men. *Hum Reprod* 10: 1791–4.

Czaplicki M., Bablok L., Janczewski Z. (1979). Varicocelectomy in patients with azoospermia. *Arch Androl* 3: 51–5.

De Croo I., Van der Elst J., Everaert K., De Sutter P., Dhont M. (1998). Fertilization, pregnancy and embryo implantation rates after ICSI with fresh or frozen-thawed testicular spermatozoa. *Hum Reprod* 13: 1893–7.

De Croo I., Van der Elst J., Everaert K., De Sutter P., Dhont M. (2000). Fertilization, pregnancy and embryo implantation rates after ICSI in cases of obstructive and non-obstructive azoospermia. *Hum Reprod* 15, 1383–8.

De Vos A., Van Steirteghem A. (1999). Assisted reproduction techniques for male factor infertility: current status of intracytoplasmic sperm injection. In: *In Vitro Fertilization and Assisted Reproduction*, 2nd edn (Brinsdern P., ed.) The Parthenon Publishing Group, London, pp. 219–36.

Devroey P., Liu J., Nagy A., Goossens A., Tournaye H., Camus M. et al. (1995a). Pregnancies after testicular sperm extraction and intracytoplasmic sperm injection in non-obstructive azoospermia. *Hum Reprod* 10: 1457–60.

Devroey P., Liu J., Nagy Z. et al. (1994). Normal fertilization of human oocytes after testicular sperm extraction and intracytoplasmatic sperm injection (TESE and ICSI). *Fertil Steril* 62: 639–41.

Devroey P., Nagy Z., Tournaye H. et al. (1996). Outcome of intracytoplasmatic sperm injection with testicular spermatozoa in obstructive and non-obstructive azoospermia. *Hum Reprod* 11: 1015–8.

Devroey P., Silber S., Nagy Z., et al. (1995b). Ongoing pregnancies and birth after intracytoplasmic sperm injection with frozen–thawed epididymal spermatozoa. *Hum Reprod* 10: 903–6.

D'Ottavio G., Lagana A., Pozza D., Mezzetti M., Toscana C. (1987). Results of the surgical treatment of varicocelectomy in patients with azoospermia. *Minerva Chir* 426: 489–91.

Everaert K., Croo De, Kerckhaert W., Dekuyper P., Dhont M., Van der Elst J., De Sutter P., Comhaire F., Mahmoud A., Lumen N. (2006). Long term effects of micro-surgical testicular sperm extraction on androgen status in patients with non obstructive azoospermia. *BMC Urol* 6: 9.

Ezeh U.I.O., Moore H.D.M., Cooke I.D. (1998a). Correlation of testicular sperm extraction with morphological, biophysical and endocrine profiles in men with azoospermia due to primary gonadal failure. *Hum Reprod* 14: 2020–4.

Ezeh U.I., Moore H.D., Cooke I.D. (1998b). A prospective study of multiple needle biopsies versus a single open biopsy for testicular sperm extraction in men with nonobstructive azoospermia. *Hum Reprod* 13: 3075–80.

Ezeh U.I.O., Moore H.M.D. (2001). Redefining azoospermia and its implications. *Fertil Steril* 75: 213–14.

Fahmy I., Mansour R., Aboulghar M., Serour G., Kamal A., Tawab N.A., Ramzy A.M., Amin Y. (1997). Intracytoplasmic sperm injection using surgically retrieved epididymal and testicular spermatozoa in cases of obstructive and non-obstructive azoospermia. *Int J of Androl* 20: 37–44.

Fischer R., Baukloh V., Naether O.G.J., Schulze W., Salzbrunn A., Benson D.M. (1996). Pregnancy after intracytoplasmic sperm injection of spermatozoa from frozen-thawed testicular biopsy. *Hum Reprod* 11: 2197–9.

Foresta C., Moro E., Ferlin A. (2001). Y chromosome microdeletions and alterations of spermatogenesis. *Endocr Rev* 22: 226–39.

Friedler S., Raziel A., Schachter M., Strassburger D., Bern O., Ron-el R. (2002b). Outcome of first and repeated testicular sperm extraction and ICSI in patients with non-obstructive azoospermia. *Hum Reprod* 17: 2356–61.

Friedler S., Raziel A., Soffer Y., Strassburger D., Komaroversusky D., Ron-El R. (1997b). Intracytoplasmic injection of fresh and cryopreserved testicular spermatozoa in patients with non-obstructive azoospermia—a comparative study. *Fertil Steril* 68: 892–7.

Friedler S., Raziel A., Soffer Y., Strassburger D., Komaroversusky D., Ron-El R. (1998). The outcome of intracytoplasmic injection of fresh and cryopreserved epididymal spermatozoa in patients with obstructive azoospermia—a comparative study. *Hum Reprod* 13: 1872–7.

Friedler S., Raziel A., Strassburger D., Schachter M., Soffer Y., Ron-El R. (2002a). Factors influencing the outcome of ICSI in patients with obstructive and non-obstructive azoospermia: a comparative study. *Hum Reprod* 17: 3114–21.

Friedler S., Raziel A., Strassburger D., Soffer Y., Komaroversusky D., Ron-El R. (1997a). Testicular sperm retrieval by percutaneous fine needle sperm aspiration compared with testicular sperm extraction by open biopsy in men with non-obstructive azoospermia. *Hum Reprod* 12: 1488–93.

Ghanem M., Bakr N.I., Elgayaar M.A., El-Mongy S., Fathy H., Ibrahim A.H.A. (2005). Comparison of the outcome of intracytoplasmic sperm injection in obstructive and non-obstructive azoospermia in the first cycle: a report of case series and meta-analysis. *Int J of Androl* 28: 16–21.

Ghazzawi I.M., Sarraf M.G., Taher M.R., Khalifa F.A. (1998). Comparison of fertilizing capability of spermatozoa from ejaculates, epididymal aspirates and testicular biopsies using intracytoplasmic sperm injection. *Hum Reprod* 13: 348–52.

Gil-Salom M., Remohi J., Minguez Y. et al. (1995). Pregnancy in an azoospermic patient with markedly elevated serum follicle stimulating hormone levels. *Fertil Steril* 64: 1218–20.

Gil-Salom M., Romero J., Minguez Y., Rubio C., De los Santos M.J., Remohi J., Pellicer A. (1996). Pregnancies after intracytoplasmic sperm injection with cryopreserved testicular spermatozoa. *Hum Reprod* 11(6): 1309–13.

Gil-Salom M., Romero J., Rubio C., Ruiz A., Remohi J., Pellicer A. (2000). Intracytoplasmic sperm injection with cryopreserved testicular spermatozoa. *Mol Cell Endocrinol* 169: 15–19.

Gorgy A., Meniru G.I., Naumann N., Beski S., Bates S., Craft I.L. (1998). The efficacy of local anaesthesia for percutaneous epididymal sperm aspiration and testicular sperm aspiration. *Hum Reprod* 13: 646–50.

Habermann H., Seo R., Cieslak J., Niederberger C., Prins G.S., Ross L. (2000). In vitro fertilization outcomes after intracytoplasmic sperm injection with fresh or frozen-thawed testicular spermatozoa. *Fertil Steril* 73(5): 955–60.

Hauser R., Botchan A., Amit A., Ben-Yosef D., Gamzu R., Paz G., Lessing J.B., Yogev L., Yavetz H. (1998). Multiple testicular sampling in non-obstructive azoospermia—is it necessary? *Hum Reprod* 13: 3081–5.

Hauser R., Yogev L., Amit A., Yavetz H., Botchan A., Azem F., Lessing J.B., Ben-Yosef D. (2005). Severe hypospermatogenesis in cases of nonobstructive azoospermia: should we use fresh or frozen testicular spermatozoa? *J Androl* 26: 772–8.

Hauser R., Yogev L., Paz G., Yavetz H., Azem F., Lessing J.B., Botchan A. (2006). Comparison of efficacy of two techniques for testicular sperm retrieval in nonobstructive azoospermia: multifocal testicular sperm extraction versus multifocal testicular sperm aspiration. *J Androl* 27: 28–33.

Herwig R., Tosun K., Schuster A., Rehder P., Glodny B., Wildt L., Illmensee K., Pinggera G.M. (2006). Tissue perfusion-controlled guided biopsies are essential for the outcome of testicular sperm extraction. *Fertil Steril* Dec 13; [Epub ahead of print].

Hibi H., Taki T., Yamada Y., Honda N., Fukatsu H., Yamamoto M., Asada Y. (2002). Testicular sperm extraction using microdissection for non-obstructive azoospermia. *Reprod Med Biol* 1: 31–4.

Holden C.A., Fuscaldo G.F., Jackson, P. et al. (1997). Frozen–thawed epididymal spermatozoa for intracytoplasmic sperm injection. *Fertil. Steril.* 67: 81–7.

Hovatta O., Foudila T., Siegberg R., Johansson K., von Smitten K., Reima I. (1996). Pregnancy resulting from intracytoplasmic injection of spermatozoa from a frozen-thawed testicular biopsy specimen. *Hum Reprod* 11(11): 2472–3.

Hovatta O., Moilanen J., Von Smitten K., Reima I. (1995). Testicular needle biopsy, open biopsy, epididymal aspiration and intracytoplasmic sperm injection in obstructive azoospermia. *Hum Reprod* 10: 2595–9.

Hsieh Y.Y., Tsai H.D., Chang C.C., Lo H.Y. (2000). Cryopreservation of human spermatozoa within human or mouse empty zona pellucidae. *Fertil Steril* 73: 694–7.

Hussein M.R., Bedaiwy M.M., Ezat A., Ibraheem A.F., Nayel M. (2005). Role of fine needle aspirate mapping and touch imprint preparations in the evaluation of azoospermia. *Anal Quant Cytol Histol* 27(2): 67–70.

Jaffe T., Kim E.D., Hoekstra T., Lipshultz L.I. (1998). Semen pellet analysis: a technique to detect the presence of sperm in men considered azoospermic by routine semen analysis. *J Urol* 159: 1548–50.

Janzen N., Goldstein M., Schlegel P.N., Palermo G.D., Rosenwaks Z., Hariprashad J. (2000). Use of electively cryopreserved microsurgically aspirated epididymal sperm with IVF and intracytoplasmic sperm injection for obstructive azoospermia. *Fertil Steril* 74(4): 696–701. Erratum in: Fertil Steril 2001; 75(1): 230.

Jarow J.P. (1991). Clinical significance of intratesticular arterial anatomy. *J Urol* 145: 777–9.

Jezek D., Knuth U.A., Schulze W. (1998). Successful testicular sperm extraction (TESE) in spite of high serum follicle stimulating hormone and azoospermia: correlation between testicular morphology, TESE results, semen analysis and serum hormone values in 103 infertile men. *Hum Reprod* 13: 1230–4.

Jow W.W., Steckel J., Schlegel P.N., Magid M.S., Goldstein M. (1993). Motile sperm in human testis biopsy specimens. *J Androl* 14: 194–8.

Kahraman S., Ozgur S., Alatas C., Aksoy S., Tasdemir M., Nuhoglu A. et al. (1996a). Fertility with testicular sperm extraction and intracytoplasmic sperm injection in non-obstructive azoospermic men. *Hum Reprod* 11: 756–60.

Kahraman S., Ozgur S., Alatas C. et al. (1996b). High implantation and pregnancy rates with testicular sperm extraction and intracytoplasmic sperm injection in obstructive and non-obstructive azoospermia. *Hum Reprod* 11: 673–6.

Kamal A., Fahmy I., Mansour R., Abou-Setta A., Serour G., Aboulghar M. (2004). Outcome of repeated testicular sperm extraction and ICSI in patients with non-obstructive azoospermia. *MEFSJ* 9: 42–6.

Khadra A.A., Abdulhadi I., Ghunain S., Kilani Z. (2003). Efficiency of percutaneous testicular sperm aspiration as a mode of sperm collection for intracytoplasmic sperm injection in nonobstructive azoospermia. *J Urol* 169: 603–5.

Khalifa Y., Grudzinkas J.G. (1996). Microepididymal sperm aspiration or percutaneous epididymal sperm aspiration? The dilemma. *Hum Reprod* 11: 680.

Kim E.D., Leibman B.B., Grinblat D.M., Lipshultz L.I. (1999). Varicocele repair improves semen parameters in azoospermic men with spermatogenic failure. *J Urol* 162: 737–40.

Komori K., Tsujimura A., Miura H. et al. (2004). Serial follow-up study of serum testosterone and antisperm antibodies in patients with non-obstructive azoospermia after conventional or microdissection testicular sperm extraction. *Int J Androl* 27: 32–6.

Lewin A., Reubinoff B., Porat-Katz A., Weiss D., Eisenberg V., Arbel R., Bar-el H., Safran A. (1999). Testicular fine needle aspiration: the alternative method for sperm retrieval in non-obstructive azoospermia. *Hum Reprod* 14: 1785–90.

Lewin A., Weiss D.B., Friedler S., Ben-Shachar I., Porat-Katz A., Meirow D., Schenker J.G., Safran A. (1996). Delivery following intracytoplasmic injection of mature sperm cells recovered by testicular fine needle aspiration in a case of hypergonadotropic azoospermia due to maturation arrest. *Hum Reprod* 11: 769–71.

Liu J., Tsai Y., Kats E., Compton G., Garcia J.E., Baramki T.A. (1997). Outcome of in-vitro culture of fresh and frozen-thawed human testicular spermatozoa. *Hum Reprod* 12: 1667–72.

Madgar I., Hourvitz A., Levron J., Seidman D.S., Shulman A., Raviv G.G., Levran D., Bider D., Mashiach S., Dor J. (1998). Outcome of in vitro fertilization and intracytoplasmic injection of epididymal and testicular sperm extracted from patients with obstructive and nonobstructive azoospermia. *Fertil Steril* 69(6): 1080–4.

Manning M., Junemann K., Alken P. (1998). Decrease in testosterone blood concentrations after testicular sperm extraction for intracytoplasmic sperm injection in azoospermic men. *Lancet* 352: 37.

Mansour R.T., Kamal A., Fahmy I., Tawab N., Serour G.I., Aboulghar M.A. (1997). Intracytoplasmic sperm injection in obstructive and non-obstructive azoospermia. *Hum Reprod* 12: 1974–9.

Marmar J.L. (1998). The emergence of specialized procedures for the acquisition, processing, and cryopreservation of epididymal and testicular sperm in connection with intracytoplasmic sperm injection. *J Androl* 19(5): 517–26. Review.

Matthews G.J., Matthews E.D., Goldstein M. (1998). Induction of spermatogenesis and achievement of pregnancy after microsurgical varicocelectomy in men with azoospermia and severe oligoasthenospermia. *Fertil Steril* 70: 71–5.

McLachlan R.I., Rajpert-De Meyt E., Hoei-Hansen C.E., de Kretser D.M., Skakkebaek N.E. (2007). Histological evaluation of the human testis—approaches to optimizing the clinical value of the assessment: Mini Review. *Hum Reprod* 22(1): 2–16.

Mehan D.J. (1976). Results of ligation of internal spermatic vein in the treatment of infertility in azoospermic patients. *Fertil Steril* 271: 110–14.

Meniru G.I., Forman R.G., Craft I. (1997a). Utility of percutaneous epididymal sperm aspiration in situations of unexpected obstructive azoospermia. *Hum Reprod* 12: 1013–14.

Meniru G.I., Tsirigotis M., Zhu J., Craft I. (1997b). Successful percutaneous epididymal sperm aspiration (PESA) after more than 20 years of acquired obstructive azoospermia. *J. Ass. Reprod. Genet.* 13: 449–50.

Mercan R., Urman B., Alatas C., Aksoy S., Nuhoglu A., Isiklar A., Balaban B. (2000). Outcome of testicular sperm retrieval procedures in non-obstructive azoospermia: percutaneous aspiration versus open biopsy. *Hum Reprod* 15: 1548–51.

Mulhall J.P., Burgess C.M., Cunningham D., Carson R., Harris D., Oates R.D. (1997). Presence of mature sperm in testicular parenchyma of men with nonobstructive azoospermia: prevalence and predictive factors. *Urology* 49: 91–5.

Nagy Z., Liu J., Janssenswillen C. et al. (1995). Using ejaculated, fresh and frozen–thawed epididymal and testicular spermatozoa gives rise to comparable results after intracytoplasmic sperm injection. *Fertil Steril* 63: 808–15.

Nicopoullos J.D., Gilling-Smith C., Almeida P.A., Norman-Taylor J., Grace I., Ramsay J.W. (2004b). Use of surgical sperm retrieval in azoospermic men: a meta-analysis. *Fertil Steril* s82: 691–701.

Nicopoullos J.D., Gilling-Smith C., Ramsay J.W. (2004a). Does the cause of obstructive azoospermia affect the outcome of intracytoplasmic sperm injection: a meta-analysis. *BJU* Int 93: 1282–6.

Nudell D.M., Conaghan J., Pedersen R.A., Givens C.R., Schriock E.D., Turek P.J. (1998). The mini-micro-epididymal sperm aspiration for sperm retrieval: a study of urological outcomes. *Hum Reprod* 13(5): 1260–5.

Oates R.D., Lobel S.M., Harris D.H. et al. (1996). Efficacy of intracytoplasmic sperm injection using intentionally cryopreserved epididymal sperm. *Hum Reprod* 11: 133–8.

Oates R.D., Mulhall J., Burgess C., Cunningham D., Carson R. (1997). Fertilization and pregnancy using intentionally cryopreserved testicular tissue as the sperm source for intracytoplasmic sperm injection in 10 men with non-obstructive azoospermia. *Hum Reprod* 12: 734–9.

Oates R.D., Silber S., Brown L.G., Page D.C. (2002). Clinical characterization of 42 oligospermic or azoospermic men with microdeletion of the AZFc region of the Y chromosome, and of 18 children conceived via ICSI. *Hum Reprod* 17: 2813–24.

Oehninger S., Veeck L., Lanzendorf S., Maloney M., Toner J., Muasher S. (1995). Intracytoplasmic sperm injection: achievement of high pregnancy rates in couples with severe male factor infertility is dependent primarily upon female and not male factors. *Fertil Steril* 64: 977–81.

Okada H., Dobashi M., Yamazaki T. et al. (2002). Conventional versus microdissection testicular sperm extraction for nonobstructive azoospermia. *J Urol* 168: 1063–7.

Ostad M., Liotta D., Ye Z. et al. (1998). Testicular sperm extraction for nonobstructive azoospermia: results of a multibiopsy approach with optimized tissue dispersion. *Urology* 52: 692–6.

Palermo G., Joris H., Devroey P., Van Steirteghem A.C. (1992). Pregnancies after intracytoplasmic injection of single spermatozoon into an oocyte. *Lancet* 340: 17–18.

Palermo G.D., Colombero L.T., Hariprashad J.J., Schlegel P.N., Rosenwaks Z. (2002). Chromosome analysis of epididymal and testicular sperm in azoospermic patients undergoing ICSI. *Hum Reprod* 17(3): 570–5.

Palermo G.D., Schlegel P.N., Hariprashad J.J., Ergun B., Mielnik A., Zaninovic N., Veeck L.L., Rosenwaks Z. (1999). Fertilization and pregnancy outcome with intracytoplasmic sperm injection for azoospermic men. *Hum Reprod* 14: 741–8.

Perraguin-Jayot S., Audebert A., Emperaire J.C., Parneix I. (1997). Ongoing pregnancies after intracytoplasmic injection using cryopreserved testicular spermatozoa. *Hum Reprod* 12(12): 2706–9.

Qublan H.S., Al-Jader K.M., Al-Kaisi N.S., Alghoweri A.S., Abu-Khait S.A., Abu-Qamar A.A., Haddadin E. (2002). Fine needle aspiration cytology compared with open biopsy histology for the diagnosis of azoospermia. *J Obstet Gynaecol* 22: 527–31.

Ramasamy R., Yagan N., Schlegel P.N. (2005). Structural and functional changes to the testis after conventional versus microdissection testicular sperm extraction. *Urology* 65: 1190–4.

Romero J., Remohi J., Minguez Y., Rubio C., Pellicer A., Gil-Salom M. (1996). Fertilization after intracytoplasmic sperm injection with cryopreserved testicular spermatozoa. *Fertil Steril* 65: 877–9.

Ron-EL, R., Stassburger D., Friedler S., Komarovsky D., Bern O., Soffer Y., Bukovsky I., Raziel A. (1997). Extended sperm preparation (ESP) may save testicular sperm extraction (TESE) from the testis in non-obstructive azoospermia. *Hum Reprod* 12(6): 1222–6.

Ron-El R., Strauss S., Friedler S., Strassburger D., Komarovsky D., Raziel A. (1998). Serial sonography and colour flow Doppler imaging following testicular and epididymal sperm extraction. *Hum Reprod* 13: 3390–3.

Rosenlund B., Kvist U., Ploen L., Rozell B.L., Sjoblom P., Hillensjo T. (1998). A comparison between open and percutaneous needle biopsies in men with azoospermia. *Hum Reprod* 13: 1266–71.

Schill T., Bals-Pratsch M., Kupker W., Sandmann J., Johannison R., Diederich K. (2003). Clinical and endocrine follow-up of patients after testicular sperm extraction. *Fertil Steril* 79: 281–6.

Schlegel P. (1999). Testicular sperm extraction: microdissection improves sperm yield with minimal tissue excision. *Hum Reprod* 14: 131–135.

Schlegel P., Berkeley A.S., Goldstein M. et al. (1994). Epididymal micropuncture with *in vitro* fertilization and oocyte micromanipulation for the treatment of unreconstructable obstructive azoospermia. *Fertil Steril* 61: 895–901.

Schlegel P., Berkeley A.S., Goldstein M. et al. (1995). Value of percutaneous epididymal sperm aspiration. *Fertil Steril* 63: 209–10.

Schlegel P.N., Kaufmann J. (2004). Role of varicocelectomy in men with nonobstructive azoospermia. *Fertil Steril* 81: 1585–8.

Schlegel P.N., Li P.S. (1998). Microdissection TESE: sperm retrieval in non-obstructive azoospermia. *Hum Reprod Update* 4: 439.

Schlegel P.N., Palermo G.D., Goldstein M., Menendez S., Zaninovic N., Veeck L.L., et al. (1997). Testicular sperm extraction with intracytoplasmic sperm injection for nonobstructive azoospermia. *Urology* 49: 435–40.

Schlegel P.N., Su L. (1997). Physiologic consequences of testicular sperm extraction. *Hum Reprod* 12: 1688–92.

Schlegel P.N., Su L.M. (1998). Physiological consequences of testicular sperm extraction. *Hum Reprod* 13: 505–6.

Schoysman R., Vanderzwalmen P., Nijs M. et al. (1993a). Pregnancy after fertilization of human testicular sperm. *Lancet* 342: 1237.

Schoysman R., Vanderzwalmen P., Nijs M., Segal-Bertin C., Geerts L., Van de Casseye M. (1993b). Successful fertilization by testicular spermatozoa in an in-vitro fertilization programme. *Hum Reprod* 8: 1339–40.

Schulze W., Thoms F., Knuth U.A. (1999). Testicular sperm extraction: comprehensive analysis with simultaneously performed histology in 1418 biopsies from 766 subfertile men. *Hum Reprod* 14(Suppl. 1.): 82–96.

Schwarzer J.U., Fiedler K., Hertwig I., Krusmann G., Wurfel W., Muhlen B., et al. (2003). Male factors determining the outcome of intracytoplasmic sperm injection with epididymal and testicular spermatozoa. *Andrologia* 35: 220–6.

Seo J.T., Ko W.J. (2001). Predictive factors of successful testicular sperm recovery in non-obstructive azoospermia patients. *Int J Androl* 24: 306–10.

Shrivastav P., Nadkarni P., Wensvoort S., Craft I. (1994). Percutaneous epididymal sperm aspiration for obstructive azoospermia. *Hum Reprod* 9: 2058–61.

Silber J.S., Repping S. (2002). Transmisson of male infertility to future generations: lessons from the Y chromosome. *Hum Reprod Update* 8(3): 217–29.

Silber S.J. (1996). Microepididymal sperm aspiration or percutaneous epididymal sperm aspiration? The dilemma. *Hum Reprod* 11: 681.

Silber S.J. (2000). Microsurgical TESE and the distribution of spermatogenesis in non-obstructive azoospermia. *Hum Reprod* 15: 2278–84.

Silber S.J., Devroey P., Van Steirteghem A.C. (1994). Conventional in-vitro fertilization versus intracytoplasmic sperm injection for patients requiring microsurgical sperm aspiration. *Hum Reprod* 9: 1905–9.

Silber S.J., Escudero T., Lenahan K., Abdelhadi I., Kilani Z., Munne S. (2003). Chromosomal abnormalities in embryos derived from testicular sperm extraction. *Fertil Steril* 79: 30–8.

Silber S.J., Nagy Z., Devroey P., Camus M., Van Steirteghem A.C. (1997b). The effect of female age and ovarian reserve on pregnancy rate in male infertility: treatment of azoospermia with sperm retrieval and intracytoplasmic sperm injection. *Hum Reprod* 12: 2693–700.

Silber S.J., Nagy Z., Devroey P., Tournaye H., Van Steirteghem A.C. (1997a). Distribution of spermatogenesis in the testicles of azoospermic men: the presence or absence of spermatids in the testes of men with germinal failure. *Hum Reprod* 12: 2422–8.

Silber S.J., Nagy Z., Liu J. et al. (1995a). The use of epididymal and testicular sperm for ICSI: the genetic implications for male infertility. *Hum Reprod* 10: 2031–43.

Silber S.J., Van Steirteghem A.C., Devroey P. et al. (1995c). Sertoli cell only revisited. *Hum Reprod* 10: 1031–2.

Silber S.J., Van Steirteghem A.C., Liu J. et al. (1995b). High fertilization and pregnancy rates after ICSI with spermatozoa obtained from testicle biopsy. *Hum Reprod* 10: 148–52.

Silber S.J., Van Steirteghem A.C., Nagy Z., Liu J., Tournaye H., Devroey P. (1996). Normal pregnancies resulting from testicular sperm extraction and intracytoplasmatic sperm injection for azoospermia for maturation arrest. *Fertil Steril* 66: 110–17.

Souza C.A., Cunha-Filho J.S., Fagundes P., Freitas F.M., Passos E.P. (2005). Sperm recovery prediction in azoospermic patients using Doppler ultrasonography. *Int Urol Nephrol* 37: 535–40.

Tarlatzis B., Bili H. (1998). Survey on intracytoplasmic sperm injection: report from the ESHRE ICSI Task Force. *Hum Reprod* 13(Suppl. 1): 165–77.

Tarlatzis B.C., Bili H. (2000). Intracytoplasmic sperm injection. Survey of world results. *Ann N Y Acad Sci* 900: 336–44.

Tash J.A., McGovern J.H., Schlegel P.N. (2000). Acquired hypogonadotropic hypogonadism presenting as decreased seminal volume. *Urology* 56: 669.

Tash J.A., Schlegel P.N. (2001). Histologic effects of testicular sperm extraction on the testicle in men with nonobstructive azoospermia. *Urology* 57: 334–7.

Temple Smith P.D., Southwick G.J., Yates C.A. et al. (1985). Human pregnancy by *in vitro* fertilisation (IVF) using sperm aspirated from the epididymis. *J In Vitro Fert Embryo Transfer* 2: 112–22.

Teng Y.N., Lin Y.U., Tsai Y.C., Hsu C.C., Kuo P.L., Lin Y.M. (2007). A simplified gene-specific screen for Y chromosome deletions in infertile men. *Fertil Steril*. Epub ahead of print.

Tournaye H. (1999). Surgical sperm recovery for intracytoplasmic sperm injection: which method is to be preferred? *Hum Reprod* 14(Suppl. 1): 71–81.

Tournaye H., Camus C., Vandervorst M., Nagy Z., Joris H., Van Steirteghem A., Devroey P. (1997a). Surgical sperm retrieval for intracytoplasmic sperm injection. *Int J Androl* 20(Suppl. 3): 69–73.

Tournaye H., Camus M., Goossens, A. et al. (1995). Recent concepts in the management of infertility because of non-obstructive azoospermia. *Hum Reprod* 10(Suppl. 1): 115–19.

Tournaye H., Devroey P., Liu J. et al. (1994). Microsurgical epididymal sperm aspiration and intracytoplasmatic sperm injection: a new effective approach to infertility as a result of congenital bilateral absence of the vas deferens. *Fertil Steril* 61: 1045–51.

Tournaye H., Liu J., Nagy P.Z. et al. (1996). Correlation between testicular histology and outcome after intracytoplasmatic sperm injection using testicular spermatozoa. *Hum Reprod* 11: 127–32.

Tournaye H., Verheyen G., Nagy P., Goossens A., Ubaldi F., Silber S., Van Steirteghem A., Devroey P. (1997b). Are there any predictive factors for successful testicular sperm recovery in azoospermic patients? *Hum Reprod* 12: 80–6.

Tsirigotis M., Craft I. (1995). Sperm retrieval methods and ICSI for obstructive azoospermia. *Hum Reprod* 10: 758–60.

Tsirigotis M., Craft I. (1996). Microepididymal sperm aspiration or percutaneous epididymal sperm aspiration? The dilemma. *Hum Reprod* 11: 1680–1.

Tsirigotis M., Pelekanos M., Yazdani N. et al. (1995). Simplified sperm retrieval and intracytoplasmic sperm injection in patients with azoospermia. *Br J Urol* 76: 765–8.

Tsujimura A., Matsumiya K., Miyagawa Y., Tohda A., Miura H., Nishimura K., Koga M., Takeyama M., Fujioka H., Okuyama A. (2002). Conventional multiple or microdissection testicular sperm extraction: a comparative study. *Hum Reprod* 17: 2924–9.

Tucker M.J., Morton P.C., Witt M.A., Wright G. (1995). Intracytoplasmic injection of testicular and epididymal spermatozoa for treatment of obstructive azoospermia. *Hum Reprod* 10: 486–9.

Tunc L., Alkibay T., Kupeli B., Tokgoz H., Bozkirli I., Yucel C. (2005). Power Doppler ultrasound mapping in nonobstructive azoospermic patients prior to testicular sperm extraction. *Arch Androl* 51(4): 277–83.

Tunc L., Kirac M., Gurocak S., Yucel A., Kupeli B., Alkibay T., Bozkirli I. (2006). Can serum inhibin B and FSH levels, testicular histology and volume predict the outcome of testicular sperm extraction in patients with non-obstructive azoospermia? *Int Urol Nephrol*. Epub ahead of print.

Turek P.J., Givens C.R., Schriock E.D., Meng M.V., Pedersen R.A., Conaghan J. (1999). Testis sperm extraction and intracytoplasmic sperm injection guided by prior fine-needle aspiration mapping in patients with nonobstructive azoospermia. *Fertil Steril* 71(3): 552–7.

Tuuri T., Moilanen J., Kaukoranta S., Makinen S., Kotola S., Hovatta O. (1999). Testicular biopsy gun needle biopsy in collecting spermatozoa for intracytoplasmic injection, cryopreservation and histology. *Hum Reprod* 14: 1274–8.

Tzirigotis M., Craft I. (1995). Sperm retrieval methods and ICSI for obstructive azoospermia. *Hum Reprod* 10: 758–60.

Ubaldi F., Nagy Z.P., Rienzi L., Tesarik J., Anniballo R., Franco G., Menchini-Fabris F., Greco E. (1999). Reproductive capacity of spermatozoa from men with testicular failure. *Hum Reprod* 14: 2796–80.

Van Perperstraten A.M., Proctor M.L., Phillipson G., Johnson N.P. (2001). Techniques for surgical retrieval of sperm prior to ICSI for azoospermia. *Cochrane Database Syst Rev* 4: CD002807.

Van Perperstraten A.M., Proctor M.L., Phillipson G., Johnson N.P. (2006). Techniques for surgical retrieval of sperm prior to ICSI for azoospermia. Update. *Cochrane Database Syst Rev* 3: CD002807.

Van Steirteghem A., Devroey P., Liebaers I. (2000). Microinjection. In: *Manual in Assisted Reproduction*, 2nd update (Rabe, Diedrich V.T.K., Runnebaum B., eds). Springer-Verlag, Berlin; 377–87.

Van Steirteghem A., Nagy P., Joris H., Janssenswillen C., Staessen C., Verheyen G., Camus M., Tournaye H., Devroey P. (1998). Results of intracytoplasmic sperm injection with ejaculated, fresh and frozen-thawed epididymal and testicular spermatozoa. *Hum Reprod* 13 (Suppl. 1): 134–42. Review.

Van Steirteghem A.C., Nagy Z., Joris H. et al. (1993). High fertilization and implantation rates after intracytoplasmic sperm insemination. *Hum Reprod* 8: 1061–6.

Verheyen G., Vernaeve V., Van Landuyt L., Tournaye H., Devroey P., Van Steirteghem A. (2004). Should diagnostic testicular sperm retrieval followed by cryopreservation for later ICSI be the procedure of choice for all patients with non-obstructive azoospermia? *Hum Reprod* 19(12): 2822–30.

Vernaeve V., Tournaye H., Osmanagaoglu K., Verheyen G., Van Steirteghem A., Devroey P. (2003). Intracytoplasmic sperm injection with testicular spermatozoa is less successful in men with nonobstructive azoospermia than in men with obstructive azoospermia. *Fertil Steril* 79: 529–533.

Vernaeve V., Tournaye H., Schiettecatte J., Verheyen G., Steirteghem A.C., Devroey P. (2002). Serum inhibin B cannot predict testicular sperm retrieval in patients with non-obstructive azoospermia. *Hum Reprod* 17(4): 971–6.

Vernaeve V., Verheyen G., Goossens A., Van Steirteghem A., Devroey P., Tournaye H. (2006). How successful is repeat testicular sperm extraction in patients with azoospermia? *Hum Reprod* 21(6): 1551–4.

Vicari E., Grazioso C., Burrello N., Cannizzaro M., D'Agata R., Calogero A.E. (2001). Epididymal and testicular sperm retrieval in azoospermic patients and the outcome of intracytoplasmic sperm injection in relation to the etiology of azoospermia. *Fertil Steril* 75: 215–16.

Von Eckardstein S., Simoni M., Bergmann M., Weinbauer G.F., Gassner P., Schepers A.G. et al. (1999). Serum inhibin B in combination with serum follicle stimulating hormone (FSH) is a more sensitive marker than serum FSH alone for impaired spermatogenesis in men, but cannot predict the presence of sperm in testicular tissue samples. *J Clin Endocrinol Metab* 84: 2496–501.

Westlander G., Ekerhovd E., Granberg S., Lycke N., Nilsson L., Werner C., Bergh C. (2001a). Serial ultrasonography, hormonal profile and antisperm antibody response after testicular sperm aspiration. *Hum Reprod* 16: 2621–7.

Westlander G., Rosenlund B., Soderlund B., Wood M., Bergh C. (2001b). Sperm retrieval, fertilization, and pregnancy outcome in repeated testicular sperm aspiration. *J Assist Reprod Genet* 18: 171–7.

Wood S., Thomas K., Sephton V., Troup S., Kingsland C., Lewis-Jones I. (2003). Postoperative pain, complications, and satisfaction rates in patients who undergo surgical sperm retrieval. *Fertil Steril* 79: 56–62.

Yamamoto M., Hibi H., Asada Y., Suganuma N., Tomoda Y. (1997). Epididymal sperm retrieval by epididymal micropuncture combined with intracytoplasmic sperm injection: difference between acquired and congenital irreparable obstructive azoospermia. *Urol Int* 58(3): 177–8.

Yamamoto M., Hibi H., Miyake K., Asada Y., Suganuma N., Tomoda Y. (1996). Microsurgical epididymal sperm aspiration versus epididymal micropuncture with perivascular nerve stimulation for intracytoplasmic sperm injection to treat unreconstructable obstructive azoospermia. *Arch Androl* 36(3): 217–24.

Yavetz H., Hauser R., Botchan A., Azem F., Yovel I., Lessing J.B., Amit A., Yogev L. (1998). Pregnancy resulting from frozen-thawed embryos achieved by intracytoplasmic injection of cryopreserved sperm cells extracted from an orchidectomized, seminoma bearing testis, causing obstructive azoospermia. *Hum Reprod* 12: 2836–8.

Yemini M., Vanderzwalmen P., Mukaida T. et al. (1995). Intracytoplasmatic sperm injection, fertilization and embryo transfer after retrieval of spermatozoa by testicular biopsy from an azoospermic male with testicular tubular atrophy. *Fertil Steril* 63: 1118–20.

53

Spermatid Injection: Current Status

Rosália Sá, Nieves Cremades, Joaquina Silva, Alberto Barros, Mário Sousa

DEFINITION OF SECRETORY AZOOSPERMIA AND MAIN HISTOPATHOLOGICAL SYNDROMES

Secretory azoospermia (nonobstructive azoospermia) is diagnosed by the absence of sperm in semen after centrifugation, a normal seminal pH, and absence of extratesticular genital duct obstruction, as detected by physical, biochemical, ultrasonography, and surgical inspection. Secretory azoospermia may be primary or secondary, and the absence of sperm in semen is caused by inefficient, deficient, or absent germ cell proliferation, meiosis, and differentiation.

Based on the diagnostic testicular biopsy, three major histopathological syndromes are recognized in secretory azoospermia, Sertoli cell–only syndrome, maturation arrest, and hypospermatogenesis. Sertoli cell–only syndrome is characterized by the exclusive presence of Sertoli cells and complete absence of germ cells; maturation arrest is characterized by the presence of Sertoli cells and diploid germ cells (spermatogonia or/and primary spermatocytes); and hypospermatogenesis is characterized by a global reduction in the number of germ cells, causing a decreased production of spermatids and spermatozoa (Figure 53.1).

Microscopical observation of at least 100 seminiferous tubule sections per patient with secretory azoospermia shows that Sertoli cell–only syndrome, maturation arrest, and hypospermatogenesis may be complete or incomplete syndromes (Figure 53.2). In complete syndromes, all seminiferous tubules present the same cell types, whereas in incomplete syndromes a minority of the seminiferous tubules (at least one of a hundred) present a different cytologic picture. This indicates that the diagnostic testicular biopsy is just representative of the clinical situation, once a single isolated testicular biopsy might eventually not reflect the entire testicular situation (Figure 53.3). The presence of spermatids and sperm in the diagnostic testicular biopsy from cases with incomplete maturation arrest and incomplete Sertoli cell–only syndrome thus suggests that a multiple and bilateral treatment testicular open biopsy might eventually enable the recovery of spermatids and spermatozoa for treatments in secretory azoospermia. In this reasoning, the treatment testicular biopsy was also thought to be applicable to cases of complete Sertoli cell–only syndrome and complete maturation arrest.

In a clinical series of 148 patients with secretory azoospermia (Table 53.1), testicular histopathology showed that complete syndromes were found in 44 (100 percent) cases with

hypospermatogenesis, in 15/47 (32 percent) of cases with maturation arrest, and in 35/57 (61 percent) of cases with Sertoli cell–only syndrome. Incomplete syndromes were found in cases with maturation arrest (32/47, 68 percent), 17/47 (36 percent) with one focus of germ cells up to the round spermatid stage, and 15/47 (32 percent) with one focus of germ cells up to the elongated spermatid/spermatozoon stages; and in cases with Sertoli cell–only syndrome (22/57, 39 percent), 3/57 (5 percent) with one focus of diploid germ cells, 17/57 (30 percent) with one focus of germ cells up to the round spermatid stage, and 2/57 (4 percent) with one focus of germ cells up to the elongated spermatid/spermatozoon stages (1).

DEVELOPMENT OF SPERMATID MICROINJECTION

After the introduction of the intracytoplasmic sperm injection technique (2) and its subsequent developments (3), extraction of testicular sperm became successfully applied to the clinical treatment of azoospermic patients (4). However, several patients with secretory azoospermia did not show spermatozoa in testicular samples after the treatment biopsy. For these cases, the alternative use of round, elongating, and elongated spermatid microinjection was envisaged, as all are haploid germ cells (Figures 53.4 and 53.5). Elongating spermatid microinjection is rarely applied as most cases also have elongated spermatids; elongated spermatid microinjection showed to be a very successful approach; and round spermatid microinjection, unfortunately, was proved to be seldom useful (1, 5–15).

SPERMATID WORLD SERIES REVIEW OF CLINICAL TREATMENTS

Most of the clinical series in secretory azoospermia describe the clinical outcomes associated with treatment testicular biopsy and intracytoplasmic sperm injection, either with fresh or frozen-thawed sperm. Overall, and in comparison with ejaculated sperm, testicular sperm showed a relatively lower fertilization rate (38–67 percent; zygotes with two pronuclei and two polar bodies) and a normal total pregnancy rate (40–60 percent). In detail, the fertilization rate varied between 39 and 69 percent, the embryo cleavage rate varied between 66 and 97 percent, the rate of embryos with high morphological grade varied between

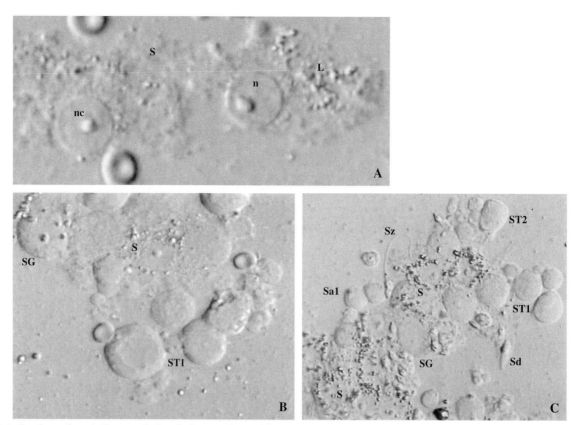

Figure 53.1. Cytology of seminiferous tubule cells from patients with secretory azoospermia. Live cells observed at the inverted microscope with Normarsky optics after being released from the seminiferous tubules by mechanical teasing. Cells appear flattened due to the compression by the glass cover slide. (A) Sertoli cell–only syndrome. Note the characteristics of Sertoli cells (S), with a large nucleus with an elevated border (n), a large round nucleolus (nc) and a very large cytoplasm rich in lipid droplets and lysosomes (L). (B) Maturation arrest. (C) Hypospermatogenesis. Spermatogonia (SG), primary spermatocytes (ST1), secondary spermatocytes (ST2), round spermatids (Sa1), late spermatids (Sd), spermatozoa (Sz). ×40, ×20, and ×10 objective, respectively.

56 and 77 percent, and the mean total pregnancy rate per embryo transfer cycle was about 33 percent.

Per type of testicular histopathology, hypospermatogenesis showed 67 percent of fertilization rate, 83 percent of embryo cleavage rate, 71 percent of embryos with high morphological grade, and 54–60 percent of mean total pregnancy rate per embryo transfer cycle; in maturation arrest, the fertilization rate (42–46 percent) and the embryo cleavage rate (61 percent) were lower, the rate of embryos with high morphological grade was higher (80–86 percent), and the mean total pregnancy rate per embryo transfer cycle was similar (57 percent); in Sertoli cell–only syndrome, the fertilization rate was lower (38–44 percent), and the embryo cleavage rate (79 percent), the rate of embryos with high morphological grade (57–61 percent), and the mean total pregnancy rate per embryo transfer cycle (40 percent) were slightly lower (16–23).

Our results with treatment testicular biopsy and intracytoplasmic sperm injection (eighty-seven cycles) appeared quite similar, with 71 percent of fertilization rate, 79 percent of embryos with high morphological grade, and 32 percent of term pregnancy rate per embryo transfer cycle (Table 53.2). Per testicular histopathology, our data revealed higher fertilization rates (75 percent in hypospermatogenesis, 66 percent in maturation arrest, and 63 percent in Sertoli cell–only syndrome), higher rates of embryos with high morphological grade (82 percent in hypospermatogenesis, 72 percent in maturation

arrest, and 75 percent in Sertoli cell–only syndrome), and higher term pregnancy rates per embryo transfer cycle (33 percent in hypospermatogenesis, 35 percent in maturation arrest, and 20 percent in Sertoli cell–only syndrome). Although data with frozen-thawed testicular sperm showed lower fertilization rates (65 percent), lower rates of embryos with high morphological grade (71 percent), and lower term pregnancy rates per embryo transfer cycle (27 percent), the differences to fresh testicular sperm were not significant. Similarly, no significant differences were found between hypospermatogenesis, maturation arrest, and Sertoli cell–only syndrome cases (1, 8, 9, 15).

Elongating and Elongated Spermatids

In comparison to testicular sperm intracytoplasmic microinjection, the largest clinical series of testicular elongated spermatid intracytoplasmic microinjection (sixty-two cycles) demonstrates (Table 53.2) that although elongated spermatids appeared associated with significant lower fertilization rates (53 percent), they were able to elicit normal and similar rates of embryos with high morphological grade (78 percent) and of term pregnancy per embryo transfer cycle (31 percent). This observation was confirmed by analysis per type of testicular histopathology, which revealed lower fertilization rates (48 percent in hypospermatogenesis, 56 percent in maturation arrest, and 46 percent in Sertoli cell–only syndrome) but similar rates

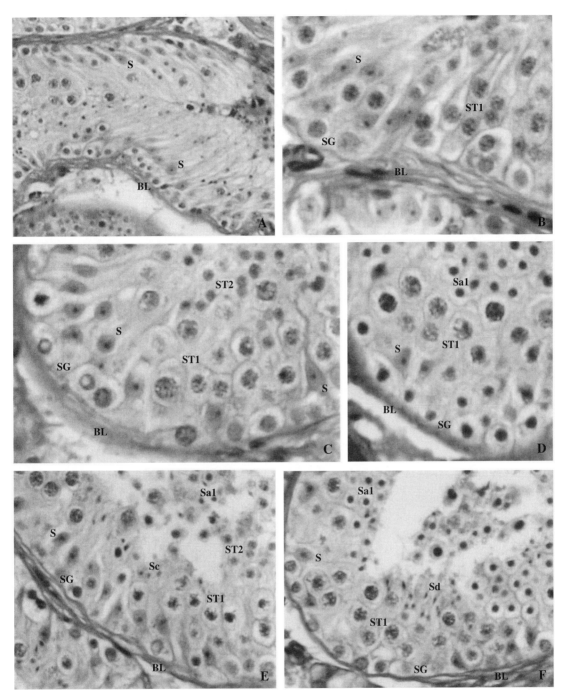

Figure 53.2. Diagnostic testicular biopsy from patients with secretory azoospermia. Histology may reveal different cell stages in different seminiferous tubule sections. (A) Tubule with predominance of Sertoli cells (S). (B) Tubule with spermatogenesis up to the primary spermatocyte stage (ST1). (C) Tubule with spermatogenesis up to the secondary spermatocyte stage (ST2). (D) Tubule with spermatogenesis up to the round spermatid stage (Sa1). (E) Tubule with spermatogenesis up to the elongating spermatid stage (Sc). (F) Tubule with spermatogenesis up to the elongated spermatid stage (Sd). Spermatogonia (SG), basal lamina (BL). ×4, ×20, ×20, ×20, ×10, ×10 objective, respectively.

of embryos with high morphological grade (72 percent in hypospermatogenesis, 77 percent in maturation arrest, and 96 percent in Sertoli cell–only syndrome) and of term pregnancy per embryo transfer cycle (42 percent in hypospermatogenesis, 25 percent in maturation arrest, and 44 percent in Sertoli cell–only syndrome). The use of fresh elongated spermatids was also associated with lower fertilization rates (54 percent) and a normal term pregnancy rate per embryo transfer cycle (35 per-

cent), with no significant differences being found between hypospermatogenesis, maturation arrest, and Sertoli cell–only syndrome. On the contrary, frozen-thawed testicular elongated spermatids evidenced significant lower rates of fertilization (45 percent) and of embryos with high morphological grade (48 percent), with no term pregnancy being achieved. This may be explained by the low number of cases studied (six cycles) but probably is related to the fact that frozen-thawed late

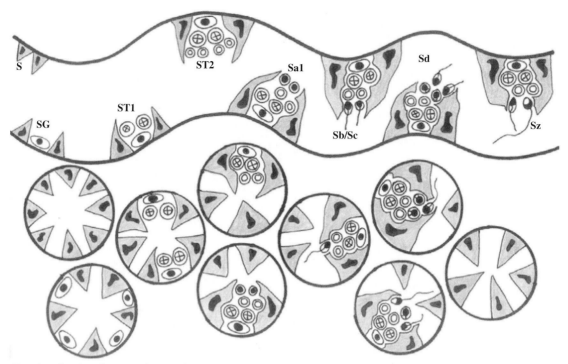

Figure 53.3. Drawing showing the assynchrony of the human male germinal epithelium along the seminiferous tubule. Sertoli cells (S), spermatogonia (SG), primary spermatocytes (ST1), secondary spermatocytes (ST2), round spermatids (Sa1), early (Sb) and late (Sc) elongating spermatids, elongated spermatids (Sd), and spermatozoa (Sz).

spermatids very easily loose their in situ or slowly progressive motility (1, 8, 9, 15).

Confirming population-based studies with children conceived by in vitro fertilization and intracytoplasmic sperm microinjection (24–26), all our newborn conceived by intracytoplasmic elongated spermatid microinjection are healthy, with absence of congenital malformations, chromosome aberrations, cancer, or retarded development (1, 8, 9, 11, 12, 15). We strongly believe that this achievement is associated with the fact that we follow strict morphological selection criteria, using only morphologically normal spermatids (in head and tail). On the contrary (27, 28), we always use donor sperm whenever only morphologically abnormal spermatids are found (Figure 53.6).

Analysis of all world-reported cases (189 cycles) with intracytoplasmic elongating spermatid microinjection and intracytoplasmic elongated spermatid microinjection (Table 53.3) confirmed that these spermatids exhibit lower fertilization rates (52 percent), although with normal embryo cleavage rates (72 percent) and term pregnancy rates per embryo transfer cycle (28 percent) (1, 8, 9, 15, 29–46). In those studies are included the first pregnancy achieved with early elongating spermatids (8) and the first pregnancy achieved after in vitro maturation of early elongating spermatids (15). The first pregnancies obtained after in vitro maturation of pachytene primary spermatocytes and round spermatids are also included, although controversy exists as maturation was achieved in a too short (two days) period of time (42–44, 46).

Round Spermatids

In comparison to intracytoplasmic testicular sperm microinjection and intracytoplasmic testicular elongated spermatid mi-

croinjection, the largest clinical series of intracytoplasmic testicular round spermatid microinjection (ninety-one cycles) showed very low fertilization rates (14 percent), normal rates of embryos with high morphological grade (89 percent), and an absence of pregnancy achievement (Table 53.2). This observation was confirmed by analysis per specific type of testicular histopathology, which revealed lower fertilization rates (17 percent in maturation arrest and 12 percent in Sertoli cell–only syndrome) and normal rates of embryos with high morphological grade (82 percent in maturation arrest and 95 percent in Sertoli cell–only syndrome). No significant differences were also found between fresh (14 percent of fertilization rate and 88 percent of embryos with high morphological grade) and frozen-thaw cycles (19 percent of fertilization rate and 100 percent of embryos with high morphological grade). There were also no significant differences between cycles using round spermatids retrieved from the semen and from the testicular tissue (1, 8, 9). We also did not observe any significant differences regarding the fertilization rate, the rate of embryos with high morphological grade, and the term pregnancy rate between original intracytoplasmic testicular round spermatid microinjection cases and intracytoplasmic testicular round spermatid microinjection cycles performed in patients previously treated by intracytoplasmic testicular elongated spermatid/sperm microinjection and in whom intracytoplasmic testicular round spermatid microinjection was needed in the second trial due to the absence of further mature spermatids (1).

Analysis of all world-reported cases (354 cycles) using intracytoplasmic round spermatid microinjection (Table 53.4) confirmed the significant lower rates of fertilization (22 percent) and term pregnancy (3 percent) in comparison with intracytoplasmic testicular sperm microinjection and

Table 53.1: Histopathological Syndromes in Secretory Azoospermia

	DTB	DTB-subtypes			
Syndromes	N (percent)	SC	DGC	Sa	SdSz
HP	44 (30)	—	—	—	44 (100)
MA	47 (32)	—	15 (32)	17 (36)	15 (32)
SO	57 (39)	35 (61)	3 (5)	17 (30)	2 (4)

DTB, diagnostic testicular biopsy. Testicular histopathological syndromes: HP, hypospermatogenesis; MA, maturation arrest; SO, Sertoli cell–only syndrome. More mature cells found after analysis of 100 seminiferous tubule sections: SC, Sertoli cells, DGC, diploid germ cells; Sa, round spermatids; SdSz, elongated spermatids/spermatozoa.

intracytoplasmic testicular elongated spermatid microinjection (1, 8, 9, 29, 34, 35, 37–39, 41, 42, 45, 47–56). Although pregnancies with round spermatids were described using unipronucleated zygotes reported to form from precociously formed two pronuclei/two polar bodies zygotes, in our experience unipronucleated zygotes exhibit a haploid set of chromosomes (12).

Other studies also confirmed that intracytoplasmic round spermatid microinjection is significantly associated with higher rates of embryo cleavage arrest (41 percent) and of embryo poor morphology (79 percent), as well as with significant lower rates of blastocyst formation (8 percent) and of high-quality blastocyst morphology (3 percent), although the rate of formation of blastocysts with high-quality morphology (37 percent) from embryos cleaved with high-quality morphology was normal (52, 53, 55–58). However, even with transfer of blastocysts with high-quality morphology (55) or of embryos with a normal chromosomal set, as ascertained by preimplantation genetic diagnosis with aneuploidy screening (56), no patient conceived. These results thus suggest a developmental failure of embryos derived from round spermatid microinjection.

Round spermatid nucleus injection in humans has been suggested to be a better alternative to intracytoplasmic intact round spermatid microinjection (40, 49, 59). Round spermatid nucleus injection was introduced by Japanese groups as they

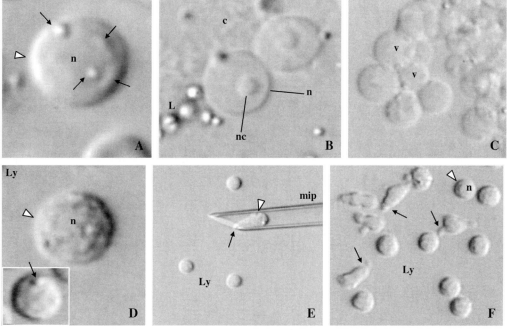

Figure 53.4. Strict morphological criteria for round spermatid recognition. (A) Round spermatid at the Golgi phase (6–8 μm in diameter). The cell is flattened and pale and has smooth periphery and contents. Nucleus (n), proacrosomal vesicles (arrows), and short rim of cytoplasm (arrowhead). (B–F) Round organelles and cells that can be confounded as round spermatids. (B) Released nuclei (n), cytoplasmic debris (c), and lipid droplets (L) from ruptured Sertoli cells. The round nucleus has an elevated border (n) and contains a large nucleolus (nc). Sertoli cell nuclei lack a cytoskeleton and shrink in PVP. (C) Round cytoplasmic fragments released from degenerating Sertoli cells through blebbing. These round structures have no internal organelles and shrink in PVP. (D–F) Small lymphocytes from the testicular tissue. (D) The small lymphocyte (Ly) is dense and irregular, either in the periphery and contents. Nucleus (n), with irregular contents (chromatin clumps); lipid droplet or lysosome resembling an acrosomal vesicle (arrow); short rim of cytoplasm (arrowhead). (E) Aspiration of isolated lymphocytes (Ly) with a 8-μm microinjection pipette (mip). The lymphocyte sticks at the micropipette tip (arrow) and stretches (arrowhead). Note the irregular surface and contents of the stretched cell inside the micropipette. (F) Isolated lymphocytes (Ly) after one-day culture. Lymphocytes become irregular, the nucleus appears more eccentric (n), and the cytoplasm sticks to the bottom of the plastic culture dish and stretches (arrows). Inverted microscopy with Hoffman optics. ×40 objective.

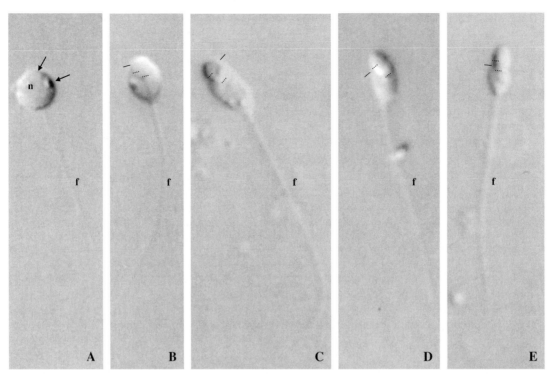

Figure 53.5. Strict morphological criteria for the distinction of spermatids with tail. (A) Late round spermatid (Sa2). The dense acrosomal vesicle is still extending (arrows) over the round central nucleus (n). (B) Early elongating spermatid (Sb). The nucleus is round but condensed (smaller), eccentric, and slightly protruding on the cell periphery. The cytoplasm is elongating and displaced to the basal pole of the cell. The upper limit of the cytoplasm (dense line) is well above the base of the acrosomal vesicle (dashed line inside the nucleus). The dashed line at the base of the nucleus marks the site of the future posterior ring (point of the occluding junction between the cytoplasmic membrane of the head and the nuclear envelope). (C) Late elongating spermatid (Sc). The nucleus is oval and densificated and further protrudes on the cell periphery. The basal cytoplasm is fully elongated. The upper limit of the cytoplasm is slightly above the base of the acrosomal vesicle (upper limit of the equatorial region). (D) Early elongated spermatid (Sd1). The nucleus is elongated and dense and further protrudes on the cell periphery. The basal elongated cytoplasm is reduced. The upper limit of the cytoplasm is below the base of the acrosomal vesicle. (E) Late elongated spermatid (Sd2). The nucleus is fully elongated, condensed, and now totally protruded on the cell periphery. The basal elongated cytoplasm is further reduced. The upper limit of the cytoplasm is slightly above the base of the nucleus. Flagellum (f). Inverted microscopy with Hoffman optics. ×40 objective.

considered that the use of a larger microinjection pipette, such as that used for intact round spermatids, would cause oocyte injury and also because they supposed that an intact cytoplasmic membrane and the large cytoplasm of round spermatids could cause serious difficulties in male pronucleus formation. However, experience with round spermatid nucleus injection as applied to humans remains scarce and all achieved pregnancies have ended into early abortions.

The intracytoplasmic intact round spermatid microinjection technique was envisaged for the relief of male infertility in those cases where no elongating spermatids, elongated spermatids, or spermatozoa could be found in semen and at the treatment testicular biopsy of patients with secretory azoospermia (1, 5–15). However, intracytoplasmic intact round spermatid microinjection was first applied to patients who had spermatozoa in semen and then recently became azoospermic (29, 38, 47). Analysis restricted to these special cases (seven cycles) showed a normal term pregnancy rate (29 percent), but this type of clinical situation is rare (Table 53.4).

When intracytoplasmic intact round spermatid microinjection was applied to the more frequent situation of men with absence of elongating spermatids, elongated spermatids, or spermatozoa in semen and at the treatment testicular biopsy of patients with secretory azoospermia, all trials (347 cycles)

failed to demonstrate the generalized usefulness of intracytoplasmic intact round spermatid microinjection treatments as the rates of term pregnancy were extremely low (2 percent). For this reason, intracytoplasmic intact round spermatid microinjection is now restricted to special cases, those patients with severe oligozoospermia and who recently became azoospermic and patients with secretory azoospermia who do not accept donor sperm (1, 15).

PREDICTIVE FACTORS FOR SUCCESSFUL SPERMATID RETRIEVAL

As many patients with secretory azoospermia have no successful sperm/spermatid retrieval at the treatment testicular biopsy, several studies were conducted to disclose if there was any factor that could establish a successful prognosis before treatment. Present data suggest that only the presence of elongated spermatids/spermatozoa in the histopathological analysis of the diagnostic testicular biopsy appears highly correlated with successful sperm/spermatid retrieval at the treatment testicular biopsy (1, 9, 15–19, 23, 60).

In a small clinical series, the prognosis of finding elongated spermatids/sperm at the treatment testicular biopsy was shown to vary according to major histopathological syndromes, being

Table 53.2: Outcomes in Secretory Azoospermia Using Spermatid Microinjection

		ICSI			ELSI			ROSI		
		F	FT	Total	F	FT	Total	F	FT	Total
HP										
	C	33	20	53	11	1	12	0	0	—
	iMII	194	104	298	76	6	82			
	2PN	157	66	223	37	2	39			
	AB	134	48	182	27	1	28			
	TP	13/32	4/20	17/52	5/11	0/1	5/12			
MA										
	C	11	11	22	35	5	40	37	3	40
	iMII	52	52	104	273	41	314	192	26	218
	2PN	34	35	69	156	19	175	33	5	38
	AB	27	23	50	126	9	135	26	5	31
	TP	4/11	3/9	7/20	10/35	0/5	10/40	0/22	0/3	0/25
SO										
	C	6	6	12	10	0	10	51	0	51
	iMII	33	30	63	56		56	348		348
	2PN	21	19	40	26		26	43		43
	AB	16	14	30	25		25	41		41
	TP	0/6	2/4	2/10	4/9		4/9	0/42		0/42
Total										
	C	50	37	87	56	6	62	88	3	91
	iMII	279	186	465	405	47	452	540	26	566
	2PN	212	120	332	219	21	240	76	5	81
	AB	177	85	262	178	10	188	67	5	72
	TP	17/49	9/33	26/82	19/55	0/6	19/61	0/64	0/3	0/67

ELSI, elongated spermatids; F, fresh gametes; FT, frozen-thawed gametes; ICSI, intracytoplasmic microinjection of sperm; ROSI, round spermatids. Testicular histopathological syndromes: HP, hypospermatogenesis; MA, maturation arrest; SO, Sertoli cell–only syndrome. C, treatment cycles; iMII, injected and intact mature MII oocytes. Normally fertilized oocytes: zygotes with two pronuclei and two polar bodies (2PN); embryos cleaved from 2PN zygotes, with high-quality morphology (AB); term pregnancies per embryo transfer cycle (TP).

about 74 percent for hypospermatogenesis, 48 percent for maturation arrest, and 25 percent for Sertoli cell–only syndrome (16, 17), or, according to further histopathological subdivisions, 100 percent in incomplete maturation arrest and in incomplete Sertoli cell–only syndrome, and 0 percent in complete maturation arrest and in complete Sertoli cell–only syndrome (17). In larger clinical series, the probability of finding elongated spermatids/sperm at the treatment testicular biopsy showed mean values of 95 percent for hypospermatogenesis, 69 percent for incomplete maturation arrest, 52 percent for complete maturation arrest, 90 percent for incomplete Sertoli cell–only syndrome, and 22 percent for complete Sertoli cell–only syndrome (19, 23).

Our results from 148 consecutive patients with secretory azoospermia (Table 53.5) revealed very similar figures in the case of hypospermatogenesis (98 percent) and maturation arrest (60 percent; 63 percent in incomplete maturation arrest and 53 percent in complete maturation arrest) but showed divergent results regarding Sertoli cell–only syndrome cases (30 percent; 73 percent in incomplete Sertoli cell–only syndrome and 3 percent in complete Sertoli cell–only syndrome). These results confirm the importance of a very strict histopathological analysis of at least 100 seminiferous tubules in the diagnostic testicular biopsy. In fact, incomplete maturation arrest cases showing one focus of early spermiogenesis (presence of round spermatids) had a similar rate of elongated spermatid/sperm retrieval (41 percent) as cases with complete maturation arrest, whereas incomplete maturation arrest cases with one focus of late spermiogenesis (presence of elongated spermatids/sperm)

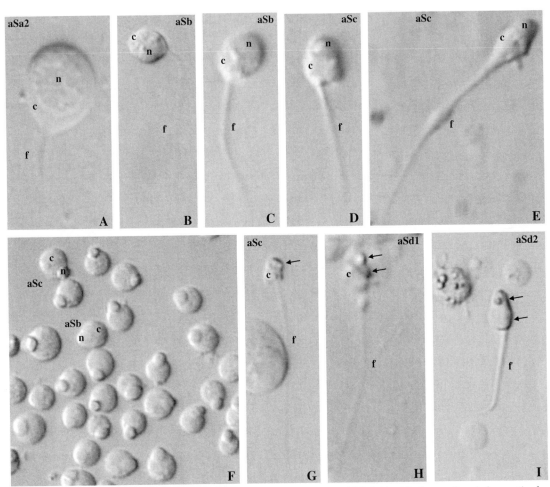

Figure 53.6. Morphologically abnormal spermatids. (A) Abnormal late round spermatid (aSa2) with short tail and chromatin decondensation. (B) Abnormal early elongating spermatid (aSb) with basal displacement of the nucleus (n) and apical displacement of the cytoplasm (c). (C Abnormal early elongating spermatid (aSb) with short and thickened tail (f). (D) Abnormal late elongating spermatid (aSc) with short and thickened tail and abnormal condensed nucleus. (E) Abnormal late elongating spermatid (aSc) with thickened tail. (F) Abnormal early (aSb) and late (aSc) elongating spermatids without tails. (G) Abnormal late elongating spermatid (aSc) with abnormal nucleus (arrow). (H) Abnormal early elongated spermatid (aSd1) with fragmented nucleus (arrows) and thickened tail. (I) Abnormal late elongated spermatid (aSd2) with short and thickened tail, and giant amorphous nucleus (arrows). Inverted microscopy with Hoffman optics. ×40 objective.

had a much higher chance of success (87 percent); similarly, incomplete Sertoli cell–only syndrome cases with a focus of diploid germ cells (100 percent), with a focus containing round spermatids (71 percent), or with a focus of elongated spermatids/sperm (50 percent) had a very high chance of success for elongated spermatids/sperm retrieval at the treatment testicular biopsy (1, 8, 9, 12, 14, 15, 60).

Based on the results presented in Tables 53.1 and 53.5, we here suggest that the histopathological diagnosis made from the diagnostic testicular biopsy should reclassify the three main syndromes, hypospermatogenesis, maturation arrest, and Sertoli cell–only syndrome, according to the more mature cell found in at least 1 out of 100 seminiferous tubule sections studied and not on the cell that predominates in most of the seminiferous tubules. With this new classification (Table 53.6), hypospermatogenesis should incorporate all incomplete maturation arrest cases (those with presence of round spermatids and elongated spermatids/sperm) and the incomplete Sertoli cell–only syndrome cases, with a focus of round spermatids and with a focus of elongated spermatids/sperma-

tozoa; maturation arrest should incorporate all complete maturation arrest cases and the incomplete Sertoli cell–only syndrome cases with a focus of diploid germ cells; Sertoli cell–only syndrome should incorporate only the cases presenting as complete Sertoli cell–only syndrome cases. The application of this new diagnostic testicular biopsy classification to our clinical series gave extraordinary results. First, most of the male population with normal karyotypes and secretory azoospermia are diagnosed as having hypospermatogenesis (64 percent vs 30 percent); second, much fewer patients subsequently present with the more severe syndromes of complete maturation arrest (12 vs. 32 percent) and complete Sertoli cell–only syndrome (24 vs. 39 percent). According to this new diagnostic testicular biopsy classification, the general prognosis for a successful treatment testicular biopsy was thus lowered in hypospermatogenesis (80 vs. 98 percent), kept in maturation arrest (61 vs. 60 percent), and lowered in Sertoli cell–only syndrome (3 vs. 30 percent). This new diagnostic testicular biopsy classification enables the clinician to give the patient a prognosis that is more adapted to each

Table 53.3: World Series Outcomes in Secretory Azoospermia Using Elongating and Elongated Spermatid Microinjection

References	Cycles	MII	2PN	EC	TP
29	4 (a)	23	14	14	0
30, 31	1	10	1	1	1
32	1 (b)	13	4	2	0
33	15 (c)	105	40	—	2
34	3	34	19	18	2
35	17	123	71	55	3
36	9	130	55	55	3
	14	—	—	—	5
37	8	36	23	23	3
38	13	137	49	—	0
8	1 (d)	7	3	3	1
39	3	31	24	17	2
40	13	79	52	41	2
41	2	18	10	—	2
9	20 (e)	148	78	63	7
42	1 (f)	6	6	6	1
	1 (fg)	—	—	—	0
	2 (h)	—	—	—	1
43	1	5	1	1	0
	1 (i)	6	5	5	1
1	39	289	155	119	10
44	4 (j)	25	16	14	1
	9 (k)	76	51	48	2
	1 (l)	7	4	4	1
45	3	—	—	—	1
46	1 (j)	—	—	—	1
15	2 (m)	8	4	3	1
Total (percent)	189	1,316	685/1,316 (52)	492/685 (72)	53/189 (28)

ELSI, intracytoplasmic elongated spermatid microinjection; ROSI, intracytoplasmic round spermatid microinjection. Injected mature MII oocytes (MII); normally fertilized oocytes: zygotes with two polar bodies and two pronuclei (2PN); embryos cleaved from 2PN zygotes (EC); term pregnancies (TP).

(a) Late elongated spermatids retrieved from centrifuged semen in men who had severe oligozoospermia and recently became azoospermic.

(b) Case of obstructive azoospermia without sperm at microsurgical epididymal aspiration.

(c) Four ELSI cycles (two live born) and eleven mixed ELSI/ROSI cycles.

(d) Cycle with early elongating spermatids.

(e) There were a total of nine clinical pregnancies, of which two ended in first trimester abortions.

(f) Cycle with late elongating spermatids in vitro matured after two days culture of pachytene primary spermatocytes.

(g) Ectopic pregnancy.

(h) Cycles with late elongating and late elongated (pregnancy) spermatids in vitro matured after two days' culture of round spermatids.

(i) Cycle with late elongated spermatids in vitro matured after one day culture of early elongated spermatids (born November 2000).

(j) Cycles with late elongated spermatids in vitro matured after two days culture of pachytene primary spermatocytes.

(k) Cycles with late elongated spermatids in vitro matured after two days culture of early elongating spermatids.

(l) Cycle with late elongating spermatids in vitro matured after two days culture of round spermatids.

(m) One cycle (pregnancy with birth at May 2000) with late elongated spermatids in vitro matured after five days culture of early elongating spermatids.

Table 53.4: World Series Outcomes in Secretory Azoospermia Using Round Spermatid Microinjection

References	Cycles	MII	2PN	EC	TP
29, 47	7 (a)	39	14	14	2
34	56 (b)	610	110	79	0
35, 48	21	150	82	62	3
37	32	260	57	49	1
49	9	53	34	30	0
38	8 (c)	37	10	—	1
39	20	199	51	31	0
8	8 (d)	59	7	7	0
50	1	—	—	—	1
51	1	—	—	—	1
41	4	49	9	—	0
42	1 (e)	2	2	2	0
9	50	325	43	42	0
52	17	—	—	—	0
53	6	—	—	—	0
54	1	—	—	—	1
45	7	—	—	—	0
55	58	1,021	202	144	0
1	33 (f)	182	31	23	0
56	14	143	52	11	0
					10/354 (3)
					2/7 (29) (a)
Total (percent)	354	3,129	704/3, 129 (22)	494/704 (70)	8/347 (2) (g)

ELSI, intracytoplasmic elongated spermatid microinjection; ICSI, intracytoplasmic sperm microinjection; ROSI, intracytoplasmic round spermatid microinjection; TESE, treatment testicular biopsy. Injected mature MII oocytes (MII); normally fertilized oocytes: zygotes with two polar bodies and two pronuclei (2PN); embryos cleaved from 2PN zygotes (EC); term pregnancies (TP).
(a) Round spermatids retrieved from semen in men who had severe oligozoospermia and recently became azoospermic and in whom TESE was not performed.
(b) Twenty-five cycles with round spermatids retrieved from semen; thirty-one cycles with TESE-ROSI.
(c) Six cycles with round spermatids retrieved from semen after hormonal stimulation; two cycles with TESE-ROSI.
(d) Six cycles with round spermatids retrieved from semen and in vitro cultured for one day; two cycles with TESE-ROSI.
(e) Testicular round spermatids matured in vitro after two days culture of pachytene primary spermatocytes.
(f) Fourteen cycles with testicular round spermatids from patients with previous TESE-ELSI/ICSI treatments and in whom no further mature spermatids were found for the second treatment cycle.
(g) Cycles with confirmed past and present absence of elongating spermatids/elongated spermatids/sperm in semen.

individual. Furthermore, it respects the cell biology of the testis as the former diagnostic testicular biopsy classification could not explain the disparity of the results obtained at the treatment testicular biopsy in the different histopathological syndromes that presented similar types of spermatogenic foci (Tables 53.1 and 53.5). As examples, the successful rate of elongated spermatid/sperm recovery was 41 percent in incomplete maturation arrest cases with a focus of round spermatids and 71 percent in incomplete Sertoli cell–only syndrome cases with a focus of round spermatids, or 53 percent in complete maturation arrest cases and 100 percent in incomplete Sertoli cell–only syndrome cases with a focus of diploid germ cells. Similarly, inside the same histopathological syndrome diagnosis, the successful rate of elongated spermatid/sperm recovery was not

Table 53.5: Prognosis for Successful Elongated Spermatid/Spermatozoa Retrieval at the Testicular Treatment Biopsy Based on the Diagnostic Testicular Biopsy

TESE	N (percent)	DTB			
		SC	DGC	Sa	SdSz
HP	44	—	—	—	44 (100)
SC	1				1 (2)
DGC	—				—
Sa	—				—
SdSz	43				43 (98)
MA	47	—	15 (32)	17 (36)	15 (32)
SC	—		—	—	—
DGC	7 (15)		3 (20)	3 (18)	1 (7)
Sa	12 (26)		4 (27)	7 (41)	1 (7)
SdSz	28 (60)		8 (53)	7 (41)	13 (87)
SO	57	35 (61)	3 (5)	17 (30)	2 (4)
SC	32 (56)	31 (89)	—	—	1 (50)
DGC	—	—	—	—	—
Sa	8 (14)	3 (9)	—	5 (29)	—
SdSz	17 (30)	1 (3)	3 (100)	12 (71)	1 (50)

DTB, diagnostic testicular biopsy for histopathology analysis; TESE, treatment testicular biopsy.
Histopathological syndromes: HP, hypospermatogenesis; MA, maturation arrest; SO, Sertoli cell–only syndrome.
More mature cells found after analysis of 100 seminiferous tubule sections (DTB) or at TESE: Sertoli cells (SC), diploid germ cells (DGC), round spermatids (Sa), and elongated spermatids/spermatozoa (SdSz).

Table 53.6: Proposed New Histopathological Classification of the Diagnostic Testicular Biopsy in Secretory Azoospermia

New DTB classification		Probability of SdSz at TESE
Syndromes/subtypes	N (percent)	
HP	95 (64)	76 (80)
HP	44	43
iMA (Sa)	17	7
iMA (SdSz)	15	13
iSO (Sa)	17	12
iSO (SdSz)	2	1
MA	18 (12)	11 (61)
cMA	15	8
iSO(DGC)	3	3
SO cSo	35 (24)	1 (3)

DTB, diagnostic testicular biopsy; TESE, treatment testicular biopsy.
Testicular histopathological syndromes: HP, hypospermatogenesis; MA, maturation arrest; SO, Sertoli cell–only syndrome. Syndromes may be complete (cMA and cSO) or incomplete (iMA and iSO).
HP includes all cases where after analysis of 100 seminiferous tubule sections, the more mature cells found were any type of haploid germ cell, round spermatids (Sa), elongated spermatids (Sd), and spermatozoa (Sz).
MA includes all cases where after analysis of 100 seminiferous tubule sections, the more mature cells found were diploid germ cells (DGC).
SO includes all cases where after analysis of 100 seminiferous tubule sections, all had only Sertoli cells (SC).

related to the specific kind of germ cell found, being frequently associated with a worse prognosis. As examples, the successful rate of elongated spermatid/sperm recovery at the treatment testicular biopsy was 53 percent in complete maturation arrest cases and 41 percent in incomplete maturation arrest cases with a focus of round spermatids, or 100 percent in incomplete Sertoli cell–only syndrome cases with a focus of diploid germ cells, 71 percent in incomplete Sertoli cell–only syndrome cases with a focus of round spermatids, and 50 percent in incomplete Sertoli cell–only syndrome cases with a focus of elongated spermatids/sperm.

KEY POINTS FOR CLINICAL PRACTICE

In secretory (nonobstructive) azoospermia, the patient should undergo a full andrological evaluation. This will enable to establish a correct diagnosis and offer a proper prognosis. This includes a clinical familial and personal history, a physical examination, an ultrasound evaluation of the scrotum (testis, epididymis, and spermatic cord structures), biochemical assays in peripheral venous blood (including hormone levels and serologies), genetic screenings (karyotype, Yq11.2-AZF/DAZ microdeletions), and a histopathology analysis of the testicular tissue. In histopathology, the most mature germ cell found in at least one seminiferous tubule section should make the final diagnosis: Sertoli cell–only syndrome (SO), if only Sertoli cells are present, maturation arrest (MA), if spermatogonia or spermatocytes are the only germ cells present, and hypospermatogenesis (HP), if spermatids or spermatozoa are observed. In patients with primary nonobstructive azoospermia and normal karyotypes, the probability of finding late spermatids or spermatozoa for clinical treatments after multiple bilateral testicular biopsy (TESE) is about 3 percent in SO, 61 percent in MA, and 80 percent in HP. Deletion of the entire AZFa region is associated with SO, and deletion of the entire AZFb region is associated with MA. On the contrary, deletion of the entire AZFc region or of the *DAZ1* and *DAZ2* gene copies are associated with a strong probability of finding spermatids or spermatozoa at TESE. Analysis of world clinical series using elongating and elongated spermatids retrieved by TESE shows 28 percent of mean term pregnancy rate. On the contrary, only 3 percent of term pregnancy rate is achieved with round spermatids. In this latter case, we thus suggest to culture round spermatids before microinjection to test, if they are able to mature in vitro. If they do not mature, donor sperm is a better option. In order to avoid any fetal abnormalities, strict criteria should be used to select morphologically normal spermatids for microinjection. SO cases will need donor sperm for treatment. In MA cases not associated with AZF microdeletions, we strongly suggest to perform in vitro maturation of diploid germ cells.

ACKNOWLEDGMENTS

Rosália Sá (Ph.D. student) was responsible for literature search on Medline, PubMed, and ISI databases; performed the statistical analyses; and reviewed the manuscript. Nieves Cremades (Ph.D., Chief Embryologist) and Joaquina Silva (M.D., Chief Embryologist) were responsible for the IVF work. Alberto Barros (M.D., Ph.D.) was responsible for recruitment, treatment, and follow-up of the patients and manuscript review. Mário Sousa (MD, PhD) planned and designed the study; was responsible for spermatid recognition, isolation, culture, and injection; and wrote the final manuscript.

We acknowledge the contribution of C. Oliveira and J. Teixeira-Silva (Gynecology and Obstetrics); L. Ferrás (Urology); P. Viana, A. Gonçalves, M. Cunha, C. Osório, and S. Sousa (IVF and Andrology Laboratories); and the staff of the Department of Genetics, Faculty of Medicine, University of Porto, for karyotypes (S. Dória, C. Alves, M.J. Pinto, and C. Almeida), Y chromosome screening (J. Marques, C. Ferraz, and S. Fernandes), and *CFTR* screening (A. Grangeia and F. Carvalho).

This work was partially supported by the Foundation for Science and Technology of the Ministry for Science, Technology and Superior Education (SFRH/BD/23616/2005; POCI/SAU-MMO/60709/04, 60555/04, 59997/04; UMIB). The sponsors of the study had no role in study design, data collection, data analysis, data interpretation, or writing of the report.

REFERENCES

1. Sousa M, Cremades N, Silva J et al. Predictive value of testicular histology in secretory azoospermic subgroups and clinical outcome after microinjection of fresh and frozen-thawed sperm and spermatids. *Hum Reprod* 2002;17:1800–10.
2. Palermo G, Joris H, Devroey P, Van Steirteghem AC. Pregnancies after intracytoplasmic injection of a single spermatozoon into an oocyte. *Lancet* 1992;340:17–8.
3. Tesarik J, Sousa M. Key elements of a highly efficient intracytoplasmic sperm injection technique: Ca²⁺ fluxes and oocyte cytoplasmic dislocation. *Fertil Steril* 1995;64:770–6.
4. Schoysman R, Vanderzwalmen P, Nijs P et al. Pregnancy after fertilization with human testicular spermatozoa. *Lancet* 1993; 342:1237.
5. Sousa M, Barros A, Tesarik K. Human oocyte activation after intracytoplasmic injection of leucocytes, spermatocytes and round spermatids: comparison of calcium responses. *Mol Hum Reprod* 1996;2:853–7.
6. Sousa M, Barros A, Tesarik J. Current problems with spermatid conception. *Hum Reprod* 1998;13:255–8.
7. Tesarik J, Sousa M, Greco E, Mendoza C. Spermatids as gametes: indications and limitations. *Hum Reprod* 1998;13 (Suppl. 3): 89–111.
8. Bernabeu R, Cremades N, Takahashi K, Sousa M. Successful pregnancy after spermatid injection. *Hum Reprod* 1998;13: 1898–900.
9. Sousa M, Barros A, Takahashi K, Oliveira C, Silva J, Tesarik J. Clinical efficacy of spermatid conception. Analysis using a new spermatid classification scheme. *Hum Reprod* 1999;14:1279–86.
10. Cremades N, Bernabeu R, Barros A, Sousa M. In-vitro maturation of round spermatids using coculture on Vero cells. *Hum Reprod* 1999;14:1287–93.
11. Cremades N, Sousa M, Bernabeu R, Barros A. Developmental potential of elongating and elongated spermatids obtained after in-vitro maturation of isolated round spermatids. *Hum Reprod* 2001;16:1938–44.
12. Sousa M, Cremades C, Alves C, Silva J, Barros A. Developmental potential of human spermatogenic cells cocultured with Sertoli cells. *Hum Reprod* 2002;17:161–72.
13. Sá R, Sousa M, Cremades N et al. In-vitro maturation of sperm. In: Gurgan T, Demirol A, eds. *In Vitro Fertilization, Assisted Reproduction and Genetics*. Bologna, Italy: Medimond, 2005:79–82.
14. Sousa M, Cremades N, Silva J et al. Spermatid injection and beyond. In: Gurgan T, Demirol A, eds. *In Vitro Fertilization, Assisted Reproduction and Genetics*. Bologna, Italy: Medimond, 2005:83–6.
15. Sá R, Sousa M, Cremades N, Alves C, Silva J, Barros A. In vitro maturation of spermatozoa. In: Oehninger SC, Kruger TF, eds. *Male Factor Infertility. Diagnosis and Treatment*. Oxon, UK: Informa, 2007:425–52.
16. Devroey P, Liu J, Nagy Z et al. Pregnancies after testicular sperm extraction and intracytoplasmic sperm injection in non-obstructive azoospermia. *Hum Reprod* 1995;10:1457–60.
17. Gil-Salom M, Minguez Y, Rubio C, De los Santos MJ, Remohi J, Pellicer A. Efficacy of intracytoplasmic sperm injection using testicular spermatozoa. *Hum Reprod* 1995;10:3166–70.
18. Silber SJ, Van Steirteghem A, Nagy Z, Liu J, Tournaye H, Devroey P. Normal pregnancies resulting from testicular sperm extraction and intracytoplasmic sperm injection for azoospermia due to maturation arrest. *Fertil Steril* 1996;66:110–17.
19. Tournaye H, Liu J, Nagy PZ et al. Correlation between testicular histology and outcome after intracytoplasmic sperm injection using testicular spermatozoa. *Hum Reprod* 1996;11:127–32.
20. Romero J, Remohi J, Minguez Y, Rubio C, Pellicer A, Gil-Salom M. Fertilization after intracytoplasmic sperm injection with cryopreserved testicular spermatozoa. *Fertil Steril* 1996;65:877–9.
21. Devroey P, Nagy P, Tournaye H, Liu J, Silber S, Van Steirteghem A. Outcome of intracytoplasmic sperm injection with testicular spermatozoa in obstructive and non-obstructive azoospermia. *Hum Reprod* 1996;11:1015–18.
22. Gil-Salom M, Romero J, Minguez Y, Rubio C, De los Santos MJ, Remohi J, Pellicer A. Pregnancies after intracytoplasmic sperm injection with cryopreserved testicular spermatozoa. *Hum Reprod* 1996;11:1309–13.
23. Tournaye H, Verheyen G, Nagy P et al. Are there any predictive factors for successful testicular sperm recovery in azoospermic patients? *Hum Reprod* 1997;12:80–6.
24. Van Steirteghem AC, Bonduelle M, Devroey P, Liebaers I. Follow-up of children born after ICSI. *Hum Reprod Update* 2002; 8:111–16.
25. Lidegaard O, Pinborg A, Andersen AN. Imprinting diseases and IVF: Danish National IVF cohort study. *Hum Reprod* 2005;20: 950–4.
26. Marques CJ, Carvalho F, Sousa M, Barros A. Altered genomic imprinting in disruptive spermatogenesis. *Lancet* 2004;363: 1700–2.
27. Hansen M, Kurinczuk JJ, Bower C, Webb S. The risk of major birth defects after intracytoplasmic sperm injection and in vitro fertilization. *N Engl J Med* 2002;346:725–30.

28. Zech H, Vanderzwalmen P, Prapas Y, Lejeune B, Duba E, Schoysman R. Congenital malformations after intracytoplasmic injection of spermatids. *Hum Reprod* 2000;15:969–71.

29. Tesarik J, Rolet F, Brami C, Sedbon E, Thorel J, Tibi C, Thebault A. Spermatid injection into human oocytes. II. Clinical application in the treatment of infertility due to non-obstructive azoospermia. *Hum Reprod* 1996;11:780–3.

30. Fishel S, Green S, Bishop M, Thornton S, Hunter A, Fleming S, Al-Hassan S. Pregnancy after intracytoplasmic injection of spermatid. *Lancet* 1995;345:1641–2.

31. Fishel S, Aslam I, Tesarik J. Spermatid conception: a stage too early, or a time too soon? *Hum Reprod* 1996;11:1371–5.

32. Chen S-U, Ho H-N, Chen H-F, Tsai T-C, Lee T-Y, Yang Y-S. Fertilization and embryo cleavage after intracytoplasmic spermatid injection in an obstructive azoospermic patient with defective spermiogenesis. *Fertil Steril* 1996;66:157–60.

33. Mansour RT, Aboulghar MA, Serour GI et al. Pregnancy and delivery after intracytoplasmic injection of spermatids into human oocytes. *Middle East Fertil Soc J* 1996;1:223–5.

34. Amer M, Soliman E, El-Sadek M, Mendoza C, Tesarik J. Is complete spermiogenesis failure a good indication for spermatid conception? *Lancet* 1997;350:116.

35. Antinori S, Versaci C, Dani G, Antinori M, Pozza D, Selman HA. Fertilization with human testicular spermatids: four successful pregnancies. *Hum Reprod* 1997;12:286–91.

36. Araki Y, Motoyama M, Yoshida A, Kim S-Y, Sung H, Araki S. Intracytoplasmic injection with late spermatids: a successful procedure in achieving childbirth for couples in which the male partner suffers from azoospermia due to deficient spermatogenesis. *Fertil Steril* 1997;67:559–61.

37. Vanderzwalmen P, Zech H, Birkenfeld A et al. Intracytoplasmic injection of spermatids retrieved from testicular tissue: influence of testicular pathology, type of selected spermatids and oocyte activation. *Hum Reprod* 1997;12:1203–13.

38. Barak Y, Kogosowski A, Goldman S, Soffer Y, Gonen Y, Tesarik J. Pregnancy and birth after transfer of embryos that developed from single-nucleated zygotes obtained by injection of round spermatids into oocytes. *Fertil Steril* 1998;70:67–70.

39. Kahraman S, Polat G, Samli M, Sozen E, Ozgun OD, Dirican K, Ozbicer T. Multiple pregnancies obtained by testicular spermatid injection in combination with intracytoplasmic sperm injection. *Hum Reprod* 1998;13:104–10.

40. Sofikitis NV, Yamamoto Y, Miyagawa I et al. Ooplasmic injection of elongating spermatids for the treatment of non-obstructive azoospermia. *Hum Reprod* 1998;13:709–14.

41. Al-Hasani S, Ludwig M, Palermo I et al. Intracytoplasmic injection of round and elongated spermatids from azoospermic patients: results and review. *Hum Reprod* 1999;14(Suppl. 1):97–107.

42. Tesarik J, Bahceci M, Ozcan C, Greco E, Mendoza C. Restoration of fertility by in vitro spermatogenesis. *Lancet* 1999;353:555–6.

43. Tesarik J, Cruz-Navarro N, Moreno E, Canete MT, Mendoza C. Birth of healthy twins after fertilization with in vitro cultured spermatids from a patient with massive in vivo apoptosis of postmeiotic germ cells. *Fertil Steril* 2000;74:1044–6.

44. Tesarik J, Nagy P, Abdelmassih R, Greco E, Mendoza C. Pharmacological concentrations of follicle-stimulating hormone and testosterone improve the efficacy of in vitro germ cell differentiation in men with maturation arrest. *Fertil Steril* 2002;77:245–51.

45. Khalili MA, Aflatoonian A, Zavos PM. Intracytoplasmic injection using spermatids and subsequent pregnancies: round versus elongated spermatids. *J Assist Reprod Genet* 2002;19:84–6.

46. Tesarik J., Overcoming maturation arrest by in vitro spermatogenesis: search for the optimal culture system. *Fertil Steril* 2004;81:1417–19.

47. Tesarik J, Mendoza C, Testart J. Viable embryos from injection of round spermatids into oocytes. *N Engl J Med* 1995;333:525.

48. Antinori S, Versaci C, Dani G, Antinori M, Selman HA. Successful fertilization and pregnancy after injection of frozen-thawed round spermatids into human oocytes. *Hum Reprod* 1997;12:554–6.

49. Yamanaka K, Sofikitis NV, Miyagawa I et al. Ooplasmic round spermatid nuclear injection procedures as a experimental treatment for non-obstructive azoospermia. *J Assist Reprod Genet* 1997;14:55–62.

50. Gianaroli L, Selman HA, Magli MC, Colpi G, Fortini D, Ferraretti AP. Birth of a healthy infant after conception with round spermatids isolated from cryopreserved testicular tissue. *Fertil Steril* 1999;72:539–41.

51. Choavaratana R, Suppinyopong S, Chaimahaphruksa P. ROSI from TESE the first case in Thailand: a case report. *J Med Assoc Thai* 1999;82:938–41.

52. Levran D, Nahum H, Farhi J, Weissman A. Poor outcome with round spermatid injection in azoospermic patients with maturation arrest. *Fertil Steril* 2000;74:443–9.

53. Vicdan K, Isik AZ, Delilbasi L. Development of blastocyst-stage embryos after round spermatid injection in patients with complete spermiogenesis failure. *J Assist Reprod Genet* 2001;18:78–86.

54. Saremi A, Esfandiari N, Salehi N, Saremi MR. The first successful pregnancy following injection of testicular round spermatid in Iran. *Arch Androl* 2002;48:315–19.

55. Urman B, Alatas C, Aksoy S et al. Transfer at the blastocyst stage of embryos derived from testicular round spermatid injection. *Hum Reprod* 2002;17:741–3.

56. Benkhalifa M, Kahraman S, Biricik A, Serteyl S, Domez E, Kumtepe Y, Qumsiyeh MB. Cytogenetic abnormalities and the failure of development after round spermatid injections. *Fertil Steril* 2004;81:1283–8.

57. Aslam I, Fishel S. Evaluation of the fertilization potential of freshly isolated, in vitro cultured and cryopreserved human spermatids by injection into hamster oocytes. *Hum Reprod* 1999;14:1528–33.

58. Balaban B, Urman B, Isiklar A, Alatas C, Aksoy S, Mercan R, Nuhoglu A. Progression to the blastocyst stage of embryos derived from testicular round spermatids. *Hum Reprod* 2000;15:1377–82.

59. Hannay T. New Japanese IVF method finally made available in Japan. *Nat Med* 1995;1:289–90.

60. Sousa M, Fernandes S, Barros A. Prognostic factors for successful testicle spermatid retrieval. *Mol Cell Endocrinol* 2000;166:37–43.

54

OPTIMIZING EMBRYO TRANSFER

Hassan N. Sallam

Despite numerous developments in assisted reproduction, the implantation rate of the replaced embryos in IVF and ICSI remains low. In 1995, Edwards observed that despite the replacement of good quality embryos, 85 percent of these embryos do not implant (1). These low success rates have been variously blamed on compromised endometrial receptivity, compromised implantation capacity of the embryo, or a suboptimal embryo transfer (ET) technique. The aim of this review is to describe the technique of ET, to evaluate the various modifications proposed in order to maximize the chances of pregnancy, and to discuss the different approaches available for managing difficult ETs.

THE TECHNIQUE OF ET

ET is usually performed two to five days after oocyte retrieval. Although the knee-chest position was originally recommended by some authors, most of the transfers are now performed in the lithotomy position (2, 3). The procedure is performed under sterile conditions; the patient is draped, a speculum is inserted in the vagina, and the cervix exposed. The cervical mucus is aspirated using a mucus aspirator and the cervix is then cleansed with a swab soaked with saline or culture medium.

Different types of plastic catheters are used for ET varying in length, diameter, stiffness, and memory and are checked for embryo toxicity. Catheters are either preloaded or afterloaded, depending on whether embryos are loaded directly into the catheter or whether the outer sheath is first placed in the uterine cavity using a guide wire or obturator.

At the time of transfer, the catheter is fitted with a 1-mL tuberculin-type syringe and flushed with culture medium. The embryos are then loaded in the distal end of the catheter in a volume of 15–25 µL of culture medium. If a preloading-type catheter is used, the catheter is passed through the cervix to approximately 1–2 cm below the uterine fundus. This is determined by markings 1 cm apart on the catheter. The length of the uterine cavity should have been measured previously using a uterine sound or by ultrasound. The embryos are then delivered into the uterine cavity by gently pressing the syringe plunger. The catheter is then left in situ for about thirty seconds and then withdrawn gently. The catheter is then checked under the dissecting microscope for retained embryos. If these are found, they can be reloaded and transferred again.

If an afterloading catheter is used, the outer sheath is passed first through the cervix until to approximately 1 cm above the internal cervical os (4). The inner catheter containing the embryos is then advanced inside the outer catheter to 1–2 cm below the uterine fundus. The embryos are then gently deposited into the uterine cavity.

In the early days of IVF, the patients were asked to remain in bed for up to twelve hours (2, 3). Later, they were asked to rest for thirty minutes following the procedure. However, many recent studies have shown that this is not necessary (5–7).

FACTORS AFFECTING ET

Despite its apparent simplicity, the technique of ET is of utmost importance in maximizing the chances of pregnancy, if meticulously performed. More information is now available on the various factors involved in optimizing its success, and these will now be discussed in the light of recent evidence.

Before ET

Before embarking on an ET, the following factors should be considered.

Embryo Selection

The introduction of IVF and ICSI in infertility treatment has been accompanied by an increase in multiple pregnancies with various medical, social, and economical consequences (8). In response, most IVF/ICSI programs have now introduced policies to restrict the number of embryos transferred, usually to two or three. More recently, a policy of single embryo transfer has been called for and many studies reported that this practice did not diminish the success rate (9).

The implementation of these policies necessitates proper embryo selection, and various criteria have been used for this purpose. Selection is mainly based on morphological criteria (10, 11). A graduated embryo score was also described by Fisch et al., (12) and we have recently experimented with a computer-assisted system for embryo selection (13). Other criteria used for embryo selection are early cleavage, (14, 15) prolonging embryo culture to the blastocyst stage, (16, 17) as well as performing preimplantation diagnosis for embryo selection (18). More recently, de Boer et al. combined two selection criteria by performing PGD on day 5 and 6 blastocysts before the transfer of a single embryo (19). Other methods of embryo selection include the embryo's respiratory rate (20), glucose consumption (21), and amino acid turnover rate (22), but these are still in the experimental phase.

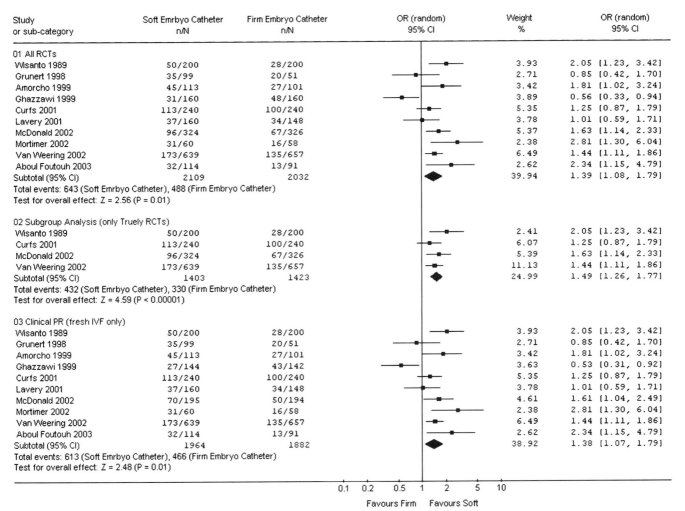

Study or sub-category	Soft Emrbyo Catheter n/N	Firm Embryo Catheter n/N	OR (random) 95% CI	Weight %	OR (random) 95% CI
01 All RCTs					
Wisanto 1989	50/200	28/200		3.93	2.05 [1.23, 3.42]
Grunert 1998	35/99	20/51		2.71	0.85 [0.42, 1.70]
Amorcho 1999	45/113	27/101		3.42	1.81 [1.02, 3.24]
Ghazzawi 1999	31/160	48/160		3.89	0.56 [0.33, 0.94]
Curfs 2001	113/240	100/240		5.35	1.25 [0.87, 1.79]
Lavery 2001	37/160	34/148		3.78	1.01 [0.59, 1.71]
McDonald 2002	96/324	67/326		5.37	1.63 [1.14, 2.33]
Mortimer 2002	31/60	16/58		2.38	2.81 [1.30, 6.04]
Van Weering 2002	173/639	135/657		6.49	1.44 [1.11, 1.86]
Aboul Foutouh 2003	32/114	13/91		2.62	2.34 [1.15, 4.79]
Subtotal (95% CI)	2109	2032		39.94	1.39 [1.08, 1.79]
Total events: 643 (Soft Emrbyo Catheter), 488 (Firm Embryo Catheter) Test for overall effect: Z = 2.56 (P = 0.01)					
02 Subgroup Analysis (only Truely RCTs)					
Wisanto 1989	50/200	28/200		2.41	2.05 [1.23, 3.42]
Curfs 2001	113/240	100/240		6.07	1.25 [0.87, 1.79]
McDonald 2002	96/324	67/326		5.39	1.63 [1.14, 2.33]
Van Weering 2002	173/639	135/657		11.13	1.44 [1.11, 1.86]
Subtotal (95% CI)	1403	1423		24.99	1.49 [1.26, 1.77]
Total events: 432 (Soft Emrbyo Catheter), 330 (Firm Embryo Catheter) Test for overall effect: Z = 4.59 (P < 0.00001)					
03 Clinical PR (fresh IVF only)					
Wisanto 1989	50/200	28/200		3.93	2.05 [1.23, 3.42]
Grunert 1998	35/99	20/51		2.71	0.85 [0.42, 1.70]
Amorcho 1999	45/113	27/101		3.42	1.81 [1.02, 3.24]
Ghazzawi 1999	27/144	43/142		3.63	0.53 [0.31, 0.92]
Curfs 2001	113/240	100/240		5.35	1.25 [0.87, 1.79]
Lavery 2001	37/160	34/148		3.78	1.01 [0.59, 1.71]
McDonald 2002	70/195	50/194		4.61	1.61 [1.04, 2.49]
Mortimer 2002	31/60	16/58		2.38	2.81 [1.30, 6.04]
Van Weering 2002	173/639	135/657		6.49	1.44 [1.11, 1.86]
Aboul Foutouh 2003	32/114	13/91		2.62	2.34 [1.15, 4.79]
Subtotal (95% CI)	1964	1882		38.92	1.38 [1.07, 1.79]
Total events: 613 (Soft Emrbyo Catheter), 466 (Firm Embryo Catheter) Test for overall effect: Z = 2.48 (P = 0.01)					

0.1 0.2   0.5   1   2   5   10

Favours Firm   Favours Soft

Figure 54.1. Meta-analysis of clinical pregnancy rates for all RCTs (random effects model), truly RCTs (fixed-effect model), and fresh IVF cycles only (random-effect model) (from Abou-Setta et al., with kind permission of the editor of *Human Reproduction*) (23).

Choice of the Catheter

The choice of catheter used for ET has been a matter of debate, with some studies showing that soft catheters are superior to firm catheters; other studies showing the opposite while a third group of studies found no difference in outcome between different catheters used for ET. However, recently two meta-analyses of randomized controlled trials (RCTs) have shown that soft catheters are associated with a higher clinical pregnancy rate compared to firm catheters (23, 24). In the meta-analysis of Abou-Setta et al., the OR (95 percent CI) for clinical pregnancy using the soft catheters was 1.49 (1.26–1.77), while in the Bucket's meta-analysis this was 1.34 (1.17–1.53) (Figure 54.1) (23, 24). The ongoing pregnancy/take-home baby rate was also significantly increased [OR = 1.25 (95 percent CI = 1.02–1.53)] (23).

Mock ET

It has been suggested that performing a trial (mock or dummy) ET before the actual transfer diminishes the incidence of difficult transfers and increases the pregnancy and implantation rates (25). This can be performed during the luteal phase of the preceding cycle (26), at the time of oocyte retrieval (27) or immediately before the real transfer (28). The technique is thought to work by allowing the physician to choose the best

catheter suitable for the particular uterus and helps mapping the direction of the uterine axis (29).

A recent publication challenged the value of performing a mock ET and showed that a retroverted uterus at mock ET will often change position during the actual procedure (30). The authors suggested that ultrasound guidance during the real ET is a better method of judging the direction of the uterine axis, as shown in an earlier publication by our group (31). In contrast, Shamonki et al. suggested that performing the mock ET under ultrasound guidance may be beneficial in preparation for the actual ET (32, 33).

ET Medium

The ET medium is usually supplemented with a high concentration of the patient's decomplemented serum (34), synthetic serum substitute (SSS) (35), human serum albumin (36), and even fetal cord serum (37). In a recent publication, Simon et al. compared two types of ET media: one supplemented with 10 percent SSS and the other supplemented with 0.5 mg/mL hyaluronic acid and reported comparable pregnancy and implantation rates (38). In a different study, Loutradi et al. evaluated the use of an ET medium with a high concentration of hyaluronan and found that it had no statistically significant effect on pregnancy rates (39). These two studies form an important step toward the development of ET media free of blood-derived additives.

A fibrin sealant has also been added to the ET medium in an attempt to improve the outcome of IVF, and two RCTs have been conducted. One study showed a nonsignificant improvement in pregnancy rate (40), while the second study showed benefit in elderly patients (41). Recently, a third RCT found that treating the embryo with a fibrin glue (EmbryoGlue) prior to ET resulted in a significant improvement in clinical, implantation, and ongoing pregnancy rates (42).

Ultrasound Before ET

Ultrasound is used before ET to study the configuration and contents of the endometrial cavity. Two recent reports showed that ultrasonography before ET was useful in detecting newly developed hydrometra in patients with hydrosalpinges. Aspiration of the uterine fluid did not help because of its rapid reaccumulation, and the authors recommended cryopreservation of the embryos for future transfer after removal of the hydrosalpinges (43, 44).

Ultrasound is also used to measure the endometrial thickness before ET. A thickness of 8 mm has been suggested as a cutoff point below which implantation cannot take place and an excessively thick endometrial has always been thought to hinder implantation. However, a recent publication reported the occurrence of successful pregnancies in two women who had a thick endometrium measuring 16 and 20 mm, respectively (45). Ultrasound is also used to measure the endometrial pattern before ET. Jarvela et al. found that the presence of a homogeneous endometrial pattern seems to predict an adverse outcome in IVF, while a triple-line pattern and a decrease in endometrial volume appear to be associated with conception (46). Similarly, the endometrial volume can be measured with 3D ultrasound and an endometrial volume of less than 2.5 mL on the day of ET was associated with a poor likelihood of implantation (47).

Ultrasound has also been used to study endometrial receptivity before ET by measuring the endometrial-subendometrial blood flow by transvaginal color Doppler (48) as well as 3D power Doppler (49). Recently, Chien et al. performed ultrasound Doppler examinations before ET and found that the mean uterine arterial resistance index and pulsatility index values were significantly lower in the pregnant compared to the nonpregnant group (50). Similarly, Ng et al. found that in women treated with IVF or ICSI, endometrial and subendometrial vascularity was significantly higher in those who achieved a live birth than in those who suffered a miscarriage (51). In a different study, the same group had reported that endometrial and subendometrial blood flows measured by 3D power Doppler ultrasound were not good predictors of pregnancy per se during IVF treatment (52), contradicting the findings of earlier studies (53, 54). Obviously, more work is needed in this area to evaluate the role of ultrasound before ET and whether the embryos should be frozen and transferred in a subsequent cycle if poor implantation is predicted.

The Necessity of a Full Bladder

It has been suggested by Lewin et al. that performing ET with a full bladder results in "straightening" the uterus during the procedure and increases the clinical pregnancy rate (55). However, in a recent study by Lorusso et al., these results could not be confirmed (56). There is now a need for larger RCTs to evaluate the necessity of a full bladder during ET.

Flushing the Cervical Mucus Before ET

It has been suggested in a nonrandomized trial that vigorous flushing of the cervical canal with culture medium prior to ET increases the clinical pregnancy rate after IVF (57). However, in an RCT, we could not confirm these results (58). On the contrary, concern had been expressed that, following this practice, some of the culture medium may enter the uterine cavity and adversely affect the implantation of the embryos. In a recent RCT, Berkkanoglu et al. found that the presence of culture medium inside the uterine cavity at the time of ET does not affect the pregnancy or implantations rates (59).

Experience of the Provider

The physician factor may be an important variable in ET technique. In a retrospective study of 854 fresh ETs by Hearns-Stokes et al., a significant difference in the pregnancy rate was found between the ten clinicians involved (60). Similar results were reported by Angelini et al. (61). On the contrary, two studies found that properly trained nurses were as good as clinicians in performing ET, with no significant differences in pregnancy and implantation rates (62, 63). This was recently confirmed in an RCT (64). In an attempt to establish the minimal number of ETs necessary to acquire proper experience, Papageogriou et al. found that the clinical pregnancy rates achieved by fellows in training who had performed fifty ETs were similar to those achieved by more experienced senior clinicians (65).

During ET

Once the previous factors have been considered, the following steps may be taken in order to maximize the outcome of ET:

Position of the Patient

In 1986, Englert et al. conducted an RCT comparing the knee-chest position to the dorsal position during ET. They found no significant difference in the clinical pregnancy rate in both groups of patients studied (66). This early work has not been repeated. In an attempt to investigate the relation between the position of the patient during ET and the incidence of ectopic pregnancy, Rubic-Pujcelj et al. found that the incidence was 3.5 percent when the ET was performed in the knee-chest position compared to 5.4 percent when performed in the lithotomy position, but this difference was not statistically significant (67).

Gentle and Atraumatic Technique

Some but not all publications reported that a gentle and atraumatic ET technique is necessary for maximizing the chances of pregnancy. Difficulties during ET include difficulty in negotiating the cervical canal, the necessity of using a volsellum (tenaculum), and the presence of blood after ET. In a recent publication, Alvero et al. found that out of these factors, only the presence of blood on or in the catheter decreased the clinical pregnancy and implantation rates significantly (68), confirming the findings of previous studies (69, 70). Similarly, Tomas et al. found that the degree of difficulty was an independent factor for predicting pregnancy (71). On the contrary, Silberstien et al. found that cannulation of a resistant internal os by the malleable outer sheath and blood on the transfer

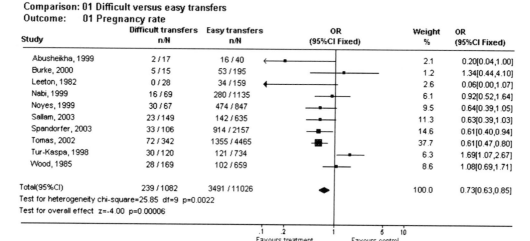

Figure 54.2. Meta-analysis of controlled trials showing that difficult ETs are associated with a significant reduction in pregnancy rate (from Sallam, with kind permission of the editor of *Current Opinion in Obstetrics and Gynecology*) (146).

catheter after ET do not have an adverse effect on implantation rate or clinical pregnancy rate (72).

In order to help resolve the issue, we have conducted a meta-analysis of ten controlled trials and found that difficult ETs were associated with diminished pregnancy rates [OR = 0.73 (95 percent CI = 0.63–0.85)] (Figure 54.2). The effect of difficult transfers on the pregnancy and implantation rates is thought to be due to trauma to the endocervix and endometrium. Cevrioglu et al. performed office hysteroscopy immediately after a mock embryo transfer and found a statistically significant concordance between the perceived difficulty of transfer and degree of endometrial damage. Difficult transfers were associated with more endocervical and endometrial damage and more blood on the catheter (73). In another study, Marconi et al. had used microhysteroscopy to visualize any possible lesions made by various ET catheters and found that the Wallace catheter was less traumatic to the endometrium compared to the Tomcat catheter and the Frydman's set (74). Contrary to these findings, Murray et al. used hysteroscopy and found that there was no clear association between perceived difficulty of transfer and amount of endometrial damage (75). The cause of diminished pregnancy and implantation rates associated with difficult transfers remains therefore a matter of speculation. In fact a non-published study found that a higher pregnancy rate was achieved when the endometrium was scratched with the ET catheter before performing the actual transfer (Ben-Rafael Z, personal communication).

Reducing Uterine Contractility

In an attempt to improve the implantation rate, various medications have been suggested in order to diminish uterine contractility during ET. In 2001, Fanchin et al. showed in an RCT that vaginal progesterone administration starting on the day of oocyte retrieval decreased the frequency of uterine contraction on the day of ET and increased the implantation rate (76). On the contrary, in another RCT, Baruffi et al. compared the administration of 400 mg of vaginal progesterone from the evening of the day of oocyte retrieval to starting it on the evening of ET and found no significant difference in pregnancy and implantation rates between the two regimens

(77). Other drugs used to diminish uterine contractility include glyceryl trinitrate (GTN), piroxicam, and atosiban. In an RCT, Shaker et al. found that the sublingual administration of GTN before ET resulted in a smoother technique, a shorter time of cervical manipulation, and a higher pregnancy rate (78). More recently, in a RCT, Moon et al. found that the oral administration of 10 mg of piroxicam one to two hours before ET increased the clinical pregnancy and implantation rates significantly (79).

Analgesia and Anesthesia

It has been suggested that various methods of analgesia or even anesthesia during ET may be associated with higher pregnancy rates. In 1988, van der Ven et al. found no significant difference in pregnancy rates between patients who had general anesthesia during ET and those who did not (80).

Acupuncture and hypnosis have also been used during ET. In an RCT published in 2002, Paulus et al. found that patients who received acupuncture during ET had a significantly higher pregnancy rate than those who did not (81). Two further RCTs were recently conducted (82, 83). The first study confirmed these results (82), while the second reported a trend for increased pregnancy rates with acupuncture, which fell short of statistical significance (83). Similarly, but in a nonrandomized trial, Levitas et al. reported that hypnosis during ET resulted in significantly higher implantation and clinical pregnancy rates (84).

Ultrasound-Guided ET

Abdominal ultrasound-guided ET was first suggested by Strickler et al. in 1985 (85). The technique allows the clinician to visualize the tip of the ET catheter and the exact site of embryo deposition and also to confirm that the embryo-associated air bubble is not displaced after ET (86). Catheters with echodense tips have been used to help their immediate ultrasound visualization and minimize intrauterine manipulations (87). Ultrasound can also be used to measure the uterocervical angle immediately prior to ET (Figure 54.3) and bend the catheter accordingly in order to minimize trauma to the cervical canal and/or the endometrium (31). Numerous studies evaluating the technique have been published, and two recent meta-analyses

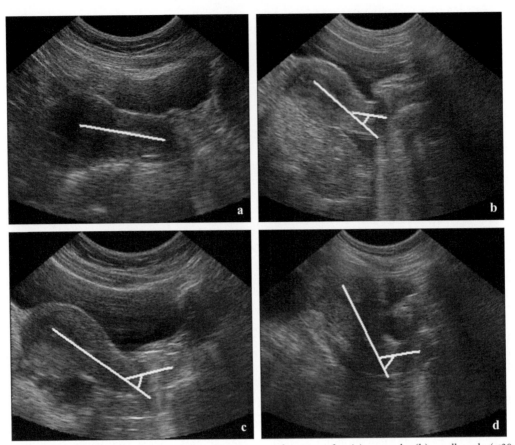

Figure 54.3. Measuring the uterocervical angle prior to embryo transfer: (a) no angle, (b) small angle (<30 degrees), (c) moderate angle (30–60 degrees), (d) large angle (>60 degrees) (from Sallam et al. With the kind permission of the editor of *Human Reproduction*) (31).

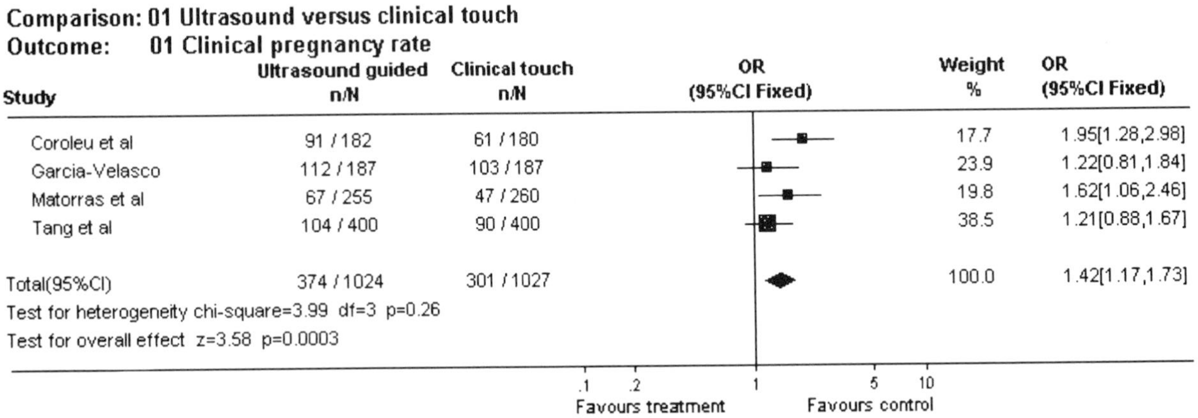

Comparison: 01 Ultrasound versus clinical touch
Outcome: 01 Clinical pregnancy rate

Study	Ultrasound guided n/N	Clinical touch n/N	OR (95%CI Fixed)	Weight %	OR (95%CI Fixed)
Coroleu et al	91 / 182	61 / 180		17.7	1.95[1.28,2.98]
Garcia-Velasco	112 / 187	103 / 187		23.9	1.22[0.81,1.84]
Matorras et al	67 / 255	47 / 260		19.8	1.62[1.06,2.46]
Tang et al	104 / 400	90 / 400		38.5	1.21[0.88,1.67]
Total(95%CI)	374 / 1024	301 / 1027		100.0	1.42[1.17,1.73]

Test for heterogeneity chi-square=3.99 df=3 p=0.26
Test for overall effect z=3.58 p=0.0003

.1   .2   1   5   10
Favours treatment   Favours control

Figure 54.4. Meta-analysis of RCTs showing that transabdominal ultrasound-guided ETs are associated with an increased clinical pregnancy rate in IVF and ICSI (from Sallam and Sadek, with the kind permission of the editor of *Fertility and Sterility*) (88).

confirmed that abdominal ultrasound-guided ET increased the clinical [OR = 1.42 (95 percent CI = 1.17–1.73)] (Figure 54.4) and ongoing pregnancy rates [OR=1.49 (95 percent CI = 1.22–1.82)] (Figure 54.5) significantly compared to the "clinical touch" method (88, 89).

Transvaginal ultrasound-guided ET has also been described. Woolcott and Stanger used the technique to observe

the movements of the embryo-associated air bubble and follow the subendometrial myometrial contractions during ET (90), while Anderson et al. found that it improves outcome in patients with previous failed in vitro fertilization cycles (91). More recently, 3D and 4D have also been described by Letterie and by Gergely et al. (92, 93). Both studies suggest that these advanced techniques give a better accuracy in locating the best

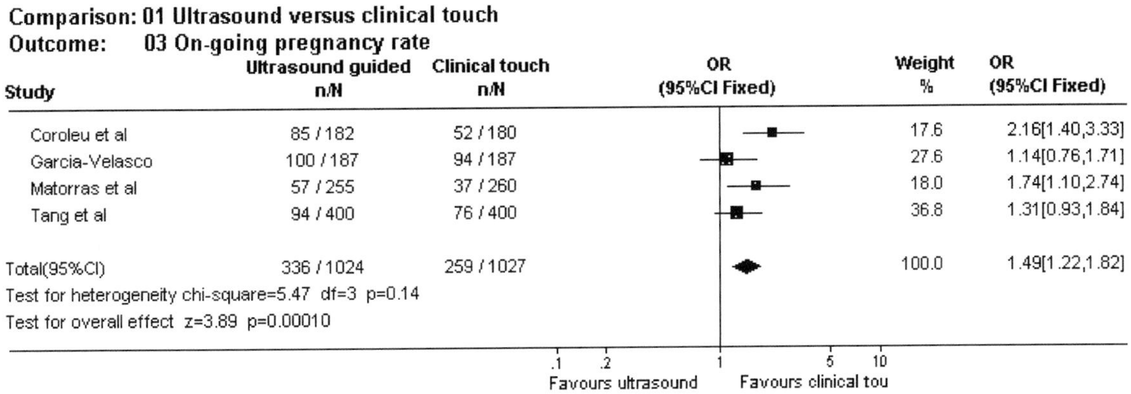

Comparison: 01 Ultrasound versus clinical touch
Outcome: 03 On-going pregnancy rate

Study	Ultrasound guided n/N	Clinical touch n/N	OR (95%CI Fixed)	Weight %	OR (95%CI Fixed)
Coroleu et al	85 / 182	52 / 180		17.6	2.16[1.40,3.33]
Garcia-Velasco	100 / 187	94 / 187		27.6	1.14[0.76,1.71]
Matorras et al	57 / 255	37 / 260		18.0	1.74[1.10,2.74]
Tang et al	94 / 400	76 / 400		36.8	1.31[0.93,1.84]
Total(95%CI)	336 / 1024	259 / 1027		100.0	1.49[1.22,1.82]

Test for heterogeneity chi-square=5.47 df=3 p=0.14
Test for overall effect z=3.89 p=0.00010

.1   .2   1   5   10
Favours ultrasound   Favours clinical tou

Figure 54.5. Meta-analysis of RCTs showing that transabdominal ultrasound-guided ETs are associated with an increased ongoing pregnancy rate in IVF and ICSI (from Sallam HN and Sadek, with the kind permission of the editor of *Fertility and Sterility*) (88).

site for embryo deposition (92, 93). In an interesting study, Baba et al. used transabdominal and transvaginal 3D ultrasound to study the site of embryo implantation in relation to the site of embryo deposition. They found that 80 percent of the embryos implant in the areas to which they were initially transferred (94).

Air in the ET Catheter

In 1995, Krampl et al. suggested that bracketing the embryo-containing medium by air bubbles offers several advantages, especially the possibility of tracking the air on the ultrasound monitor to localize the embryos after the ET, and found that this technique did not affect the pregnancy rate (95). These findings were confirmed in a recent RCT conducted by Moreno et al. (96). On the contrary, using a transparent laboratory model of the uterine cavity, Eytan et al. found that the presence of air blocked the transport of the transferred liquid toward the fundus and suggested that the ET catheter should contain minimal volumes of air in order to enhance the embryo's chances of reaching the site of implantation (97). Whether this model mimics the live conditions of ET remains to be seen, and larger RCTs are needed to clarify the issue.

Time Interval between Embryo Loading and Discharging

The effect of the time interval from loading the ET catheter to depositing the embryos in the uterine cavity on the success rates has recently been studied by Matorras et al. (98). These authors found that the longer this time interval, the lower the pregnancy and implantation rates and that an interval of more than 120 seconds carries a poor prognosis. They recommended speeding up the ET process, whenever possible.

Site of Embryo Deposition

The best site for embryo deposition has been a matter of debate, but most of the studies seem to agree that depositing the embryos in the miduterine cavity away from the fundus is associated with better implantation. In an RCT, Coroleu et al. found that the implantation rate was significantly higher when the embryos were deposited 2 cm below the uterine fundus compared to when deposited 1 cm below the fundus (99). Recently, Pope et al. confirmed these results by performing a multivariate logistic regression analysis on 699 ETs and found

that for every additional millimeter embryos are deposited away from the fundus, the odds of clinical pregnancy increased by 11 percent (100). Similar findings were reported by Frankfurter et al. who studied videotaped ETs (101) and conducted a prospective cohort study (102).

Other studies suggested that the best site for embryo deposition is the middle part of the uterine cavity. In an RCT, Franco et al. found no statistically significant differences in clinical pregnancy or implantation rates when the embryos were deposited in the upper half compared to the lower half of the uterus (103). Subsequently, the same group conducted a prospective study and found that implantation and pregnancy rates were higher when the catheter tip was positioned close to the middle area of the endometrial cavity. They concluded that the relative position of the catheter tip within the uterine cavity was more important than its exact distance from the fundus (104). More recently, they reported that when embryos were transferred to the central area of the uterine cavity, there was an increase in implantation rate in the middle region compared with the rate expected in naturally conceived pregnancies (105).

Using 3D ultrasound guidance, Gergely et al. attempted to deposit the embryos at the maximum implantation potential point (MIP), defined as the point of intersection of the two imaginary lines formed by extending the Fallopian tube course inside the uterine cavity. They found that embryos deposited at the MIP were associated with good implantation and pregnancy rates (93). Similarly, Silberstein et al. found that by depositing the embryos in the miduterine cavity, the incidence of embryo retention in the transfer catheter was diminished (106).

The site of embryo deposition was also found to influence the incidence of ectopic pregnancies in two nonrandomized studies. In 1993, Nazari et al. reported a lower incidence of ectopic pregnancies when the embryos were deposited away from the fundus (107). The same findings were recently confirmed by Pope et al. (100).

The Use of a Volsellum (Tenaculum)

Holding the cervix with a tenaculum (volsellum) during ET may sometimes be necessary in order to negotiate of the cervical canal with the catheter's tip. This practice was found to increase oxytocin release and junctional zone contractions (108, 109). At the same time, a nonrandomized study had suggested that a high frequency of uterine contractions on the day of ET hinders the outcome of IVF, possibly by expelling embryos out of the uterine cavity, but this work has not been confirmed (110). More studies are therefore needed to evaluate the true effect of holding the cervix with a volsellum on the outcome of IVF and ICSI.

Immediate Removal of the ET Catheter

Since the early days of IVF, it has been customary to leave the catheter inside the uterine cavity for thirty seconds after ET in an attempt to improve the pregnancy and implantation rates. However, an RCT found no statistically significant differences in pregnancy rates between immediately removing of the catheter after ET and leaving it for thirty seconds. The authors concluded that either the waiting interval is insufficient to detect any difference or the retention time before withdrawing the catheter is not a factor that influences pregnancy rate (111).

Gentle Pressure on the Cervix to Minimize Embryo Expulsion

It has been suggested that gentle pressure on the cervix during ET may minimize expulsion of the replaced embryos. In a recent RCT, Mansour found that applying gentle mechanical pressure on the portiovaginalis of the cervix using the vaginal speculum during and for seven minutes after ET significantly improved clinical pregnancy and implantation rates (112). However, this interesting work has not been repeated.

Retained Embryos and Double ETs

Retention of one or more embryos in the catheter following IVF presents the physician with a difficult choice as retransferring them immediately may dislodge the embryos already inside the uterine cavity (113). However, Lee et al. conducted a retrospective study and found that immediate retransfer of the retained embryos did not have an adverse effect on the pregnancy outcome (114).

In line with these findings, recently published studies have suggested that embryos can be transferred on two separate occasions in order to maximize the pregnancy rate, confirming an early work by Abramovici et al. (115). Phillips et al. and Loutradis et al. found that the consecutive ET of cleavage-stage embryos and of blastocysts in the same cycle protects against failure to reach ET and maximizes the chances of pregnancy (116, 117). Similar results were reported by Goto et al. and Machtinger et al. (118, 119).

After ET

Once the ET has been performed, the following factors should be considered:

Bed Rest after ET

In the early days of IVF, prolonged bed rest was advised in an attempt to improve pregnancy rates. However, subsequent studies have shown that this is not necessary (5–7, 120). This has recently been confirmed by an RCT by Amarin and Obeidat (2004), who found no statistically significant difference in clinical pregnancy rate between patients who had one hour of bed rest (21.5 percent) and those who had twenty-four hours of bed rest (18.2 percent) following ET. Interestingly, the implantation rate was significantly higher in those who rested for one hour only (14.4 versus 9 percent) (121).

Sexual Intercourse after ET

The effect of sexual intercourse after ET has also been a matter of debate for fear that this may lead to uterine contractions and/or the introduction of infection. However, in an RCT, Tremellen et al. found that in women who had intercourse during the peritransfer period, the pregnancy rate was not significantly different compared to women who abstained from intercourse during that period. Interestingly, the implantation rate was significantly higher in the intercourse group compared to the abstinence group (122).

Medication after ET

Various medications have been proposed and used after ET in an attempt to improve the outcome of IVF and ICSI. In an RCT, Waldenstrom et al. studied the effect of routine administration of low-dose aspirin (75 mg/day) following ET and found that the birth rate was significantly increased in women receiving the medication (123). However, two recent RCTs could not confirm these results (124, 125).

Sildenafil administration has also been suggested for improving endometrial receptivity at the time of ET. However, Check et al. found that in women whose endometrium did not reach 8 mm in thickness, neither vaginal E2 nor sildenafil significantly improved endometrial thickness or blood flow in a subsequent cycle (126).

Several studies have shown that infection in the cervix or at the tip of the ET catheter was associated with a diminished pregnancy rate (127–129). Consequently, the routine administration of antibiotics following ET has been suggested; but so far, this suggestion has not been confirmed by any RCT (130).

DIFFICULT ETS

Despite all these precautions, in some patients, ET cannot be accomplished due to the presence of a tight or closed cervix or due to anatomical distortion caused by fibromyomata or previous surgical interference. In these cases, one can consider one or more of the following procedures:

1. *Transabdominal transmyometrial ET.* Transabdominal ET has been tried by some clinicians after failing to introduce the catheter in the uterine cavity. In 1987, Lenz et al. performed ultrasound-guided transabdominal ET in ten patients, but none of them became pregnant (131). In contrast, Groutz et al. used ultrasound-guided transmyometrial and transcervical ET in forty patients with cervical stenosis or repeated implantation failures after IVF. Four patients became pregnant: one after transmyometrial ET and three after transcervical ET (132). These poor results have been blamed on the increased junctional zone contractions, which occur after this procedure (133).

2. *Transvaginal transmyometrial ET.* Ultrasound-guided transvaginal transmyometrial ET was also used. Kato et al. performed the procedure in 104 patients and reported a clinical pregnancy rate of 36.5 percent per attempt (134). In 1996, Sharif et al. performed the same procedure in thirteen patients who had difficult or impossible mock transcervical ET immediately before the real transfer. Four patients became pregnant, including three with clinical pregnancies (135). More recently, Lai et al. reported a successful pregnancy in a patient with congenital cervical

atresia who had simultaneous transmyometrial and trans-tubal ET after IVF (136).

3. *Cervical dilatation.* Cervical dilatation is another solution for patients with cervical stenosis or with previously failed ETs and should better be performed in a cycle preceding the treatment cycle. Abusheikha et al. performed cervical dilatation in fifty-seven patients who failed to conceive after a previous difficult ET due to cervical stenosis. Eighteen women (31.6 percent) achieved pregnancy, and in forty patients (70.2 percent), the subsequent ET was classified as "easy," whereas in the other seventeen (29.8 percent), it remained difficult (137). More recently, in an RCT, Prapas et al. performed cervical dilatation one to three months prior to IVF in patients with prior difficult ET and reported significantly higher pregnancy, implantation, and live birth rates (138). Cervical dilatation has also been performed on the day of oocyte retrieval in patients with suspected cervical stenosis, but the results are unsatisfactory. Groutz et al. performed the procedure in forty-one treatment cycles in twenty-two patients with a history of extremely difficult ET. Only one clinical and one extrauterine pregnancy resulted (139).

4. *Hysteroscopic correction of cervical stenosis.* Hysteroscopic canalization for patients with a history of difficult transfers has also been suggested. Noyes et al. performed surgical correction of cervical stenosis in eight patients with a history of extremely difficult ETs. Twelve postoperative IVF-ET in these women resulted in eight clinical pregnancies. The embryo implantation rate of these cycles was 42.2 percent (140). Similar results were recently reported by Pabucco et al. (141).

5. *The use of hygroscopic rods for slow cervical dilatation.* Slow dilatation of the cervical canal using hygroscopic rods for patients with a history of difficult transfers has also been reported. Glatstein et al. used laminaria tents in two patients with cervical stenosis and a history of multiple failed cycles of IVF. Both patients became pregnant (142). More recently, Serhal et al. used hygroscopic cervical rods in fifty-four patients. Of those, 79.5 percent has a subsequent easy ET and 55 percent of them became pregnant (143).

6. *Using special ET catheters.* Various attempts have been made to design special catheters for difficult ETs (144, 145). However, so far, no ideal catheter has acquired wide-use acceptance in these cases.

7. *Freezing the embryos and retransferring in a subsequent cycle.* Obviously, if one is to embark on one of the above-mentioned procedure, freezing the embryos and transferring them in a subsequent cycle is always a logical choice (146).

CONCLUSIONS

ET is arguably the most critical step in assisted reproduction and must be performed gently and meticulously. A minimum of fifty transfers is usually necessary for clinicians to acquire experience. The best site for embryo deposition is the midcavity of the uterus, 2 cm below the fundus, and a trial (mock) ET results in easier transfers. Difficult transfers and cervical infection are associated with low pregnancy rates, but immediate retransfer of any retained embryos is not detrimental. Randomized trials have shown that ultrasound guidance and the use of soft catheters as opposed to firm catheters are associated with higher pregnancy rates. They have also shown that the presence of air in the catheter, its immediate removal, bed rest after ET, sexual intercourse, and the administration of aspirin after ET do not affect the results. Further studies are needed to evaluate the necessity of a full bladder, flushing the cervical canal before ET, the best transfer medium, and the best position of the patient. Studies are also needed to find out whether analgesia or anesthesia is beneficial and whether any particular medication to reduce uterine contractility or increase endometrial blood flow can improve the success rates in these unfortunate ladies.

KEY POINTS FOR CLINICAL PRACTICE

- ET is a critical step in assisted reproduction.
- ET should be performed under ultrasound guidance and soft catheters perform better than firm ones.
- The best site for embryo deposition is the midcavity of the uterus, 2 cm below the fundus.
- Difficult transfers and cervical infection affect the results negatively.
- Air in the catheter, its immediate removal, and retransferring the retained embryos do not affect the results.
- There is no need for bed rest after ET and sexual intercourse is permitted.
- Aspirin after ET has no effect on the results but the routine use of antibiotics, uterine relaxants, and medication to increase uterine blood flow await further evaluation.
- Young clinicians should perform at least fifty ETs before claiming experience.

More RCTs are needed to evaluate the necessity of a full bladder, flushing the cervical canal before ET, the best transfer medium, the best position of the patient, and the necessity of analgesia or anesthesia.

REFERENCES

1. Edwards RG. Clinical approaches to increasing uterine receptivity during human implantation. *Hum Reprod* 1995;10 (Suppl. 2): 60–6.
2. Edwards RG, Steptoe PC, Purdy JM. Establishing full-term human pregnancies using cleaving embryos grown in vitro. *Br J Obstet Gynaecol* 1980;87:737–56.
3. Jones HW Jr., Acosta AA, Garcia JE, Sandow BA, Veeck L. On the transfer of conceptuses from oocytes fertilized in vitro. *Fertil Steril* 1983;39:241–3.
4. Neithardt AB, Segars JH, Hennessy S, James AN, McKeeby JL. Embryo afterloading: a refinement in embryo transfer technique that may increase clinical pregnancy. *Fertil Steril* 2005;83: 710–14.
5. Sharif K, Afnan M, Lenton W, et al. Do patients need to remain in bed following embryo transfer? The Birmingham experience of 103 in-vitro fertilization cycles with no bed rest following embryo transfer. *Hum Reprod* 1995;10:1427–9.
6. Botta G, Grudzinskas G. Is a prolonged bed rest following embryo transfer useful? *Hum Reprod* 1997;12:2489–92.
7. Sharif K, Afnan M, Lashen H, Elgendy M, Morgan C, Sinclair L. Is bed rest following embryo transfer necessary? *Fertil Steril* 1998;69:478–81.
8. El-Toukhy T, Khalaf Y, Braude P. IVF results: optimize not maximize. *Am J Obstet Gynecol* 2006;194:322–31.
9. Gerris JM. Single embryo transfer and IVF/ICSI outcome: a balanced appraisal. *Hum Reprod Update* 2005;11:105–21.

10. Kovacs G, MacLachlan V, Rombauts L, Healy D, Howlett D. Replacement of one selected embryo is just as successful as two embryo transfer, without the risk of twin pregnancy. *Aust N Z J Obstet Gynaecol* 2003;43:369–71.

11. De Neubourg D, Gerris J. Single embryo transfer—state of the art. *Reprod Biomed Online* 2003;7:615–22.

12. Fisch JD, Sher G, Adamowicz M, Keskintepe L. The graduated embryo score predicts the outcome of assisted reproductive technologies better than a single day 3 evaluation and achieves results associated with blastocyst transfer from day 3 embryo transfer. *Fertil Steril* 2003;80:1352–8.

13. Manna C, Patrizi G, Rahman A, Sallam H. Experimental results on the recognition of embryos in human assisted reproduction. *Reprod Biomed Online* 2004;8:460–9.

14. Van Montfoort AP, Dumoulin JC, Kester AD, Evers JL. Early cleavage is a valuable addition to existing embryo selection parameters: a study using single embryo transfers. *Hum Reprod* 2004;19:2103–8.

15. Ciray HN, Ulug U, Bahceci M. Transfer of early-cleaved embryos increases implantation rate in patients undergoing ovarian stimulation and ICSI-embryo transfer. *Reprod Biomed Online* 2004;8:219–23.

16. Gardner DK, Surrey E, Minjarez D, et al. Single blastocyst transfer: a prospective randomized trial. *Fertil Steril* 2004;81:551–5.

17. Milki AA, Hinckley MD, Westphal LM, Behr B. Elective single blastocyst transfer. *Fertil Steril* 2004;81:1697–8.

18. Gianaroli L, Magli MC, Ferraretti AP, et al. Preimplantation genetic diagnosis increases the implantation rate in human in vitro fertilization by avoiding the transfer of chromosomally abnormal embryos. *Fertil Steril* 1997;68:1128–31.

19. De Boer KA, Catt JW, Jansen RP, et al. Moving to blastocyst biopsy for preimplantation genetic diagnosis and single embryo transfer at Sydney IVF. *Fertil Steril* 2004;82:295–8.

20. Lopes AS, Greve T, Callesen H. Quantification of embryo quality by respirometry. *Theriogenology* 2007;67:21–31.

21. Sallam HN, El-Kassar Y, Hany Abdel-Rahman A, Agameya A, Farrag A, Shams A. Glucose consumption and total protein production by preimplantation embryos in pregnant and non-pregnant women—possible methods for embryo selection. *Fertil Steril* 2006;86 (3) (Suppl.): S114.

22. Houghton FD, Hawkhead JA, Humpherson PG, Hogg JE, Balen AH, Rutherford AJ, Leese HJ. Non-invasive amino acid turnover predicts human embryo developmental capacity. *Hum Reprod* 2002;17:999–1005.

23. Abou-Setta AM, Al-Inany HG, Mansour RT, Serour GI, Aboulghar MA. Soft versus firm embryo transfer catheters for assisted reproduction: a systematic review and meta-analysis. *Hum Reprod* 2005;20:3114–21.

24. Buckett WM. A review and meta-analysis of prospective trials comparing different catheters used for embryo transfer. *Fertil Steril* 2006;85:728–34.

25. Mansour R, Aboulghar M, Serour G. Dummy embryo transfer: a technique that minimizes the problems of embryo transfer and improves the pregnancy rate in human in vitro fertilization. *Fertil Steril* 1990;54:678–81.

26. Knutzen V, Stratton CJ, Sher G, et al. Mock embryo transfer in early luteal phase, the cycle before in vitro fertilization and embryo transfer: a descriptive study. *Fertil Steril* 1992;57:156–62.

27. Sallam HN. Embryo transfer—the elusive step. In: *Progress in Obstetrics and Gynaecology*. Studd John, Ed. Edinburgh and London: Churchill Livingstone; 2003:363–80.

28. Sharif K, Afnan M, Lenton W. Mock embryo transfer with a full bladder immediately before the real transfer for in-vitro fertilization treatment: the Birmingham experience of 113 cases. *Hum Reprod* 1995;10:1715–18.

29. Urman B, Aksoy S, Alatas C, et al. Comparing two embryo transfer catheters. Use of a trial transfer to determine the catheter applied. *J Reprod Med* 2000;45:135–8.

30. Henne MB, Milki AA. Uterine position at real embryo transfer compared with mock embryo transfer. *Hum Reprod* 2004;19:570–2.

31. Sallam HN, Agameya AF, Rahman AF, et al. Ultrasound measurement of the uterocervical angle before embryo transfer: a prospective controlled study. *Hum Reprod* 2002;17:1767–72.

32. Shamonki MI, Spandorfer SD, Rosenwaks Z. Ultrasound-guided embryo transfer and the accuracy of trial embryo transfer. *Hum Reprod* 2005;20:709–16.

33. Shamonki MI, Schattman GL, Spandorfer SD, Chung PH, Rosenwaks Z. Ultrasound-guided trial transfer may be beneficial in preparation for an IVF cycle. *Hum Reprod* 2005;20:2844–9.

34. Feichtinger W, Kemeter P, Menezo Y. The use of synthetic culture medium and patient serum for human in vitro fertilization and embryo replacement. *J In Vitro Fert Embryo Transf* 1986;3:87–92.

35. Psalti I, Loumaye E, Pensis M, Depreester S, Thomas K. Evaluation of a synthetic serum substitute to replace fetal cord serum for human oocyte fertilization and embryo growth in vitro. *Fertil Steril* 1989;52:807–11.

36. Khan I, Staessen C, Devroey P, Van Steirteghem AC. Human serum albumin versus serum: a comparative study on embryo transfer medium. *Fertil Steril* 1991;56:98–101.

37. Laverge H, De Sutter P, Desmet R, Van der Elst J, Dhont M. Prospective randomized study comparing human serum albumin with fetal cord serum as protein supplement in culture medium for in-vitro fertilization. *Hum Reprod* 1997;12:2263–6.

38. Simon A, Safran A, Revel A, et al. Hyaluronic acid can successfully replace albumin as the sole macromolecule in a human embryo transfer medium. *Fertil Steril* 2003;79:1434–8.

39. Loutradi KE, Prassas I, Bili E, Sanopoulou T, Bontis I, Tarlatzis BC. Evaluation of a transfer medium containing high concentration of hyaluronan in human in vitro fertilization. *Fertil Steril* 2006.

40. Feichtinger W, Strohmer H, Radner KM, Goldin M. The use of fibrin sealant for embryo transfer: development and clinical studies. *Hum Reprod* 1992;7:890–3.

41. Ben-Rafael Z, Ashkenazi J, Shelef M, et al. The use of fibrin sealant in in vitro fertilization and embryo transfer. *Int J Fertil Menopausal Stud* 1995;40:303–6.

42. Valojerdi MR, Karimian L, Yazdi PE, Gilani MA, Madani T, Baghestani AR. Efficacy of a human embryo transfer medium: a prospective, randomized clinical trial study. *J Assist Reprod Genet* 2006;23:207–12.

43. Hinckley MD, Milki AA. Rapid reaccumulation of hydrometra after drainage at embryo transfer in patients with hydrosalpinx. *Fertil Steril* 2003;80:1268–71.

44. Hofmann GE, Warikoo P, Jacobs W. Ultrasound detection of pyometra at the time of embryo transfer after ovum retrieval for in vitro fertilization. *Fertil Steril* 2003;80:637–8.

45. Quintero RB, Sharara FI, Milki AA. Successful pregnancies in the setting of exaggerated endometrial thickness. *Fertil Steril* 2004;82:215–17.

46. Jarvela IY, Sladkevicius P, Kelly S, Ojha K, Campbell S, Nargund G. Evaluation of endometrial receptivity during in-vitro fertilization using three-dimensional power Doppler ultrasound. *Ultrasound Obstet Gynecol* 2005;26:765–9.

47. Zollner U, Zollner KP, Specketer MT, et al. Endometrial volume as assessed by three-dimensional ultrasound is a predictor of pregnancy outcome after in vitro fertilization and embryo transfer. *Fertil Steril* 2003;80:1515–17.

48. Zaidi J, Campbell S, Pittrof R, Tan SL. Endometrial thickness, morphology, vascular penetration and velocimetry in predicting implantation in an in vitro fertilization program. *Ultrasound Obstet Gynecol* 1995;6:191–8.

49. Kupesic S, Bekavac I, Bjelos D, Kurjak A. Assessment of endometrial receptivity by transvaginal color Doppler and three-dimensional power Doppler ultrasonography in patients undergoing in vitro fertilization procedures. *J Ultrasound Med* 2001; 20:125–34.

50. Chien LW, Lee WS, Au HK, Tzeng CR. Assessment of changes in utero-ovarian arterial impedance during the peri-implantation period by Doppler sonography in women undergoing assisted reproduction. *Ultrasound Obstet Gynecol* 2004;23:496–500.

51. Ng EH, Chan CC, Tang OS, Yeung WS, Ho PC. Endometrial and subendometrial vascularity is higher in pregnant patients with livebirth following ART than in those who suffer a miscarriage. *Hum Reprod* 2006.

52. Ng EH, Chan CC, Tang OS, Yeung WS, Ho PC. The role of endometrial and subendometrial blood flows measured by three-dimensional power Doppler ultrasound in the prediction of pregnancy during IVF treatment. *Hum Reprod* 2006;21: 164–70.

53. Chien LW, Au HK, Chen PL, Xiao J, Tzeng CR. Assessment of uterine receptivity by the endometrial-subendometrial blood flow distribution pattern in women undergoing in vitro fertilization-embryo transfer. *Fertil Steril* 2002;78:245–51.

54. Maugey-Laulom B, Commenges-Ducos M, Jullien V, Papaxanthos-Roche A, Scotet V, Commenges D. Endometrial vascularity and ongoing pregnancy after IVF. *Eur J Obstet Gynecol Reprod Biol* 2002;104:137–43.

55. Lewin A, Schenker JG, Avrech O, et al. The role of uterine straightening by passive bladder distension before embryo transfer in IVF cycles. *J Assist Reprod Genet* 1997;14:32–4.

56. Lorusso F, Depalo R, Bettocchi S, Vacca M, Vimercati A, Selvaggi L. Outcome of in vitro fertilization after transabdominal ultrasound-assisted embryo transfer with a full or empty bladder. *Fertil Steril* 2005;84:1046–8.

57. MacNamee P. Vigorous flushing the cervical canal with culture medium prior to embryo transfer. Paper presented at the World Congress of IVF, Sydney 1999.

58. Sallam HN, Farrag F, Ezzeldin A, Agameya A, Sallam AN. The importance of flushing the cervical canal with culture medium prior to embryo transfer. *Fertil Steril* 2000;3 (Suppl. 1):64–5.

59. Berkkanoglu M, Isikoglu M, Seleker M, Ozgur K. Flushing the endometrium prior to the embryo transfer does not affect the pregnancy rate. *Reprod Biomed Online* 2006;13:268–71.

60. Hearns-Stokes RM, Miller BT, Scott L, et al. Pregnancy rates after embryo transfer depend on the provider at embryo transfer. *Fertil Steril* 2000;74:80–6.

61. Angelini A, Brusco GF, Barnocchi N, El-Danasouri I, Pacchiarotti A, Selman HA. Impact of physician performing embryo transfer on pregnancy rates in an assisted reproductive program. *J Assist Reprod Genet* 2006;23:329–32.

62. Barber D, Egan D, Ross C, et al. Nurses performing embryo transfer: successful outcome of in-vitro fertilization. *Hum Reprod* 1996;11:105–8.

63. Sinclair L, Morgan C, Lashen H, et al. Nurses performing embryo transfer: the development and results of the Birmingham experience. *Hum Reprod* 1998;13:699–702.

64. Bjuresten K, Hreinsson JG, Fridstrom M, et al. Embryo transfer by midwife or gynecologist: a prospective randomized study. *Acta Obstet Gynecol Scand* 2003;82:462–6.

65. Papageorgiou TC, Hearns-Stokes RM, Leondires MP, Miller BT, Chakraborty P, Cruess D, Segars J. Training of providers in

66. embryo transfer: what is the minimum number of transfers required for proficiency? *Hum Reprod* 2001;16:1415–19.

66. Englert Y, Puissant F, Camus M, Van Hoeck J, Leroy F. Clinical study on embryo transfer after human in vitro fertilization. *J In Vitro Fert Embryo Transf* 1986;3:243–6.

67. Ribic-Pucelj M, Tomazevic T, Vogler A, Meden-Vrtovec H. Risk factors for ectopic pregnancy after in vitro fertilization and embryo transfer. *J Assist Reprod Genet* 1995;12:594–8.

68. Alvero R, Hearns-Stokes RM, Catherino WH, Leondires MP, Segars JH. The presence of blood in the transfer catheter negatively influences outcome at embryo transfer. *Hum Reprod* 2003; 18:1848–52.

69. Sallam HN, Agameya AF, Rahman AF, et al. Impact of technical difficulties, choice of catheter, and the presence of blood on the success of embryo transfer—experience from a single provider. *J Assist Reprod Genet* 2003;20:135–42.

70. Goudas VT, Hammitt DG, Damario MA, et al. Blood on the embryo transfer catheter is associated with decreased rates of embryo implantation and clinical pregnancy with the use of in vitro fertilization-embryo transfer. *Fertil Steril* 1998;70:878–82.

71. Tomas C, Tikkinen K, Tuomivaara L, Tapanainen JS, Martikainen H. The degree of difficulty of embryo transfer is an independent factor for predicting pregnancy. *Hum Reprod* 2002;17: 2632–5.

72. Silberstein T, Weitzen S, Frankfurter D, et al. Cannulation of a resistant internal os with the malleable outer sheath of a coaxial soft embryo transfer catheter does not affect in vitro fertilization-embryo transfer outcome. *Fertil Steril* 2004;82:1402–6.

73. Cevrioglu AS, Esinler I, Bozdag G, Yarali H. Assessment of endocervical and endometrial damage inflicted by embryo transfer trial: a hysteroscopic evaluation. *Reprod Biomed Online* 2006;13:523–7.

74. Marconi G, Vilela M, Bello J, et al. Endometrial lesions caused by catheters used for embryo transfers: a preliminary report. *Fertil Steril* 2003;80:363–7.

75. Murray AS, Healy DL, Rombauts L. Embryo transfer: hysteroscopic assessment of transfer catheter effects on the endometrium. *Reprod Biomed Online* 2003;7:583–6.

76. Fanchin R, Righini C, de Ziegler D, et al. Effects of vaginal progesterone administration on uterine contractility at the time of embryo transfer. *Fertil Steril* 2001;75:1136–40.

77. Baruffi R, Mauri AL, Petersen CG, et al. Effects of vaginal progesterone administration starting on the day of oocyte retrieval on pregnancy rates. *J Assist Reprod Genet* 2003;20:517–20.

78. Shaker AG, Fleming R, Jamieson ME, Yates RW, Coutts JR. Assessments of embryo transfer after in-vitro fertilization: effects of glyceryl trinitrate. *Hum Reprod* 1993;8:1426–8.

79. Moon HS, Park SH, Lee JO, Kim KS, Joo BS. Treatment with piroxicam before embryo transfer increases the pregnancy rate after in vitro fertilization and embryo transfer. *Fertil Steril* 2004;82:816–20.

80. van der Ven H, Diedrich K, Al-Hasani S, Pless V, Krebs D. The effect of general anaesthesia on the success of embryo transfer following human in-vitro fertilization. *Hum Reprod* 1988;3 (Suppl. 2):81–3.

81. Paulus WE, Zhang M, Strehler E, El-Danasouri I, Sterzik K. Influence of acupuncture on the pregnancy rate in patients who undergo assisted reproduction therapy. *Fertil Steril* 2002; 77:721–4.

82. Westergaard LG, Mao Q, Krogslund M, Sandrini S, Lenz S, Grinsted J. Acupuncture on the day of embryo transfer significantly improves the reproductive outcome in infertile women: a prospective, randomized trial. *Fertil Steril* 2006;85:1341–6.

83. Smith C, Coyle M, Norman RJ. Influence of acupuncture stimulation on pregnancy rates for women undergoing embryo transfer. *Fertil Steril* 2006;85:1352–8.

84. Levitas E, Parmet A, Lunenfeld E, Bentov Y, Burstein E, Friger M, Potashnik G. Impact of hypnosis during embryo transfer on the outcome of in vitro fertilization-embryo transfer: a case-control study. *Fertil Steril* 2006;85:1404–8.

85. Strickler RC, Christianson C, Crane JP, et al. Ultrasound guidance for human embryo transfer. *Fertil Steril* 1985;43: 54–61.

86. Coroleu B, Barri PN, Carreras O, Belil I, Buxaderas R, Veiga A, Balasch J. Effect of using an echogenic catheter for ultrasound-guided embryo transfer in an IVF programme: a prospective, randomized, controlled study. *Hum Reprod* 2006;21:1809–15.

87. Letterie GS, Marshall L, Angle M. A new coaxial catheter system with an echodense tip for ultrasonographically guided embryo transfer. *Fertil Steril* 1999;72:266–8.

88. Sallam HN, Sadek SS. Ultrasound-guided embryo transfer: a meta-analysis of randomized controlled trials. *Fertil Steril* 2003;80:1042–6.

89. Buckett WM. A meta-analysis of ultrasound-guided versus clinical touch embryo transfer. *Fertil Steril* 2003;80:1037–41.

90. Woolcott R, Stanger J. Potentially important variables identified by transvaginal ultrasound-guided embryo transfer. *Hum Reprod* 1997;12:963–6.

91. Anderson RE, Nugent NL, Gregg AT, Nunn SL, Behr BR. Transvaginal ultrasound-guided embryo transfer improves outcome in patients with previous failed in vitro fertilization cycles. *Fertil Steril* 2002;77:769–75.

92. Letterie GS. Three-dimensional ultrasound-guided embryo transfer: a preliminary study. *Am J Obstet Gynecol* 2005;192: 1983–7; discussion 1987–8.

93. Gergely RZ, DeUgarte CM, Danzer H, Surrey M, Hill D, DeCherney AH. Three dimensional/four dimensional ultrasound-guided embryo transfer using the maximal implantation potential point. *Fertil Steril* 2005;84:500–3.

94. Baba K, Ishihara O, Hayashi N, Saitoh M, Taya J, Kinoshita K. Where does the embryo implant after embryo transfer in humans? *Fertil Steril* 2000;73:123–5.

95. Krampl E, Zegermacher G, Eichler C, Obruca A, Strohmer H, Feichtinger W. Air in the uterine cavity after embryo transfer. *Fertil Steril* 1995;63:366–70.

96. Moreno V, Balasch J, Vidal E, et al. Air in the transfer catheter does not affect the success of embryo transfer. *Fertil Steril* 2004; 81:1366–70.

97. Eytan O, Elad D, Zaretsky U, Jaffa AJ. A glance into the uterus during in vitro simulation of embryo transfer. *Hum Reprod* 2004;19:562–9.

98. Matorras R, Mendoza R, Exposito A, Rodriguez-Escudero FJ. Influence of the time interval between embryo catheter loading and discharging on the success of IVF. *Hum Reprod* 2004;19: 2027–30.

99. Coroleu B, Barri PN, Carreras O, et al. The influence of the depth of embryo replacement into the uterine cavity on implantation rates after IVF: a controlled, ultrasound-guided study. *Hum Reprod* 2002;17:341–6.

100. Pope CS, Cook EK, Arny M, et al. Influence of embryo transfer depth on in vitro fertilization and embryo transfer outcomes. *Fertil Steril* 2004;81:51–8.

101. Frankfurter D, Silva CP, Mota F, et al. The transfer point is a novel measure of embryo placement. *Fertil Steril* 2003;79: 1416–21.

102. Frankfurter D, Trimarchi JB, Silva CP, Keefe DL. Middle to lower uterine segment embryo transfer improves implantation and pregnancy rates compared with fundal embryo transfer. *Fertil Steril* 2004;81:1273–7.

103. Franco JG Jr, Martins AM, Baruffi RL, et al. Best site for embryo transfer: the upper or lower half of endometrial cavity? *Hum Reprod* 2004;19:1785–90.

104. Oliveira JB, Martins AM, Baruffi RL, et al. Increased implantation and pregnancy rates obtained by placing the tip of the transfer catheter in the central area of the endometrial cavity. *Reprod Biomed Online* 2004;9:435–41.

105. Cavagna M, Contart P, Petersen CG, Mauri AL, Martins AM, Baruffi RL, Oliveira JB, Franco JG Jr. Implantation sites after embryo transfer into the central area of the uterine cavity. *Reprod Biomed Online* 2006;13:541–6.

106. Silberstein T, Trimarchi JR, Shackelton R, Weitzen S, Frankfurter D, Plosker S. Ultrasound-guided miduterine cavity embryo transfer is associated with a decreased incidence of retained embryos in the transfer catheter. *Fertil Steril* 2005;84: 1510–12.

107. Nazari A, Askari HA, Check JH, O'Shaughnessy A. Embryo transfer technique as a cause of ectopic pregnancy in in vitro fertilization. *Fertil Steril* 1993;60:919–21.

108. Dorn C, Reinsberg J, Schlebusch H, et al. Serum oxytocin concentration during embryo transfer procedure. *Eur J Obstet Gynecol Reprod Biol* 1999;87:77–80.

109. Lesny P, Killick SR, Robinson J, et al. Junctional zone contractions and embryo transfer: is it safe to use a tenaculum? *Hum Reprod* 1999;14:2367–70.

110. Fanchin R, Righini C, Ayoubi JM, et al. [Uterine contractions at the time of embryo transfer: a hindrance to implantation?] [Article in French]. *Contracept Fertil Sex* 1998;26:498–505.

111. Martinez F, Coroleu B, Parriego M, et al. Ultrasound-guided embryo transfer: immediate withdrawal of the catheter versus a 30 second wait. *Hum Reprod* 2001;16:871–4.

112. Mansour R. Minimizing embryo expulsion after embryo transfer: a randomized controlled study. *Hum Reprod* 2005;20:170–4.

113. Visser DS, Fourie FL, Kruger HF. Multiple attempts at embryo transfer: effect on pregnancy outcome in an in vitro fertilization and embryo transfer program. *J Assist Reprod Genet* 1993;10: 37–43.

114. Lee HC, Seifer DB, Shelden RM. Impact of retained embryos on the outcome of assisted reproductive technologies. *Fertil Steril* 2004;82:334–7.

115. Abramovici H, Dirnfeld M, Weisman Z, et al. Pregnancies following the interval double-transfer technique in an in vitro fertilization-embryo transfer program. *J In Vitro Fert Embryo Transf* 1988;5:175–6.

116. Phillips SJ, Dean NL, Buckett WM, Tan SL. Consecutive transfer of day 3 embryos and of day 5-6 blastocysts increases overall pregnancy rates associated with blastocyst culture. *J Assist Reprod Genet* 2003;20:461–4.

117. Loutradis D, Drakakis P, Dallianidis K, et al. A double embryo transfer on days 2 and 4 or 5 improves pregnancy outcome in patients with good embryos but repeated failures in IVF or ICSI. *Clin Exp Obstet Gynecol* 2004;31:63–6.

118. Goto S, Shiotani M, Kitagawa M, Kadowaki T, Noda Y. Effectiveness of two-step (consecutive) embryo transfer in patients who have two embryos on day 2: comparison with cleavage-stage embryo transfer. *Fertil Steril* 2005;83:721–3.

119. Machtinger R, Dor J, Margolin M, et al. Sequential transfer of day 3 embryos and blastocysts after previous IVF failures despite adequate ovarian response. *Reprod Biomed Online* 2006;13:376–9.

120. Bar-Hava I, Kerner R, Yoeli R, Ashkenazi J, Shalev Y, Orvieto R. Immediate ambulation after embryo transfer: a prospective study. *Fertil Steril* 2005;83:594–7.

121. Amarin ZO, Obeidat BR. Bed rest versus free mobilisation following embryo transfer: a prospective randomised study. *BJOG* 2004;111:1273–6.

122. Tremellen KP, Valbuena D, Landeras J, et al. The effect of intercourse on pregnancy rates during assisted human reproduction. *Hum Reprod* 2000;15:2653–8.

123. Waldenstrom U, Hellberg D, Nilsson S. Low-dose aspirin in a short regimen as standard treatment in in vitro fertilization: a randomized, prospective study. *Fertil Steril* 2004;81:1560–4.

124. Pakkila M, Rasanen J, Heinonen S, et al. Low-dose aspirin does not improve ovarian responsiveness or pregnancy rate in IVF and ICSI patients: a randomized, placebo-controlled double-blind study. *Hum Reprod* 2005;20:2211–14.

125. Duvan CI, Ozmen B, Satiroglu H, Atabekoglu CS, Berker B. Does addition of low-dose aspirin and/or steroid as a standard treatment in nonselected intracytoplasmic sperm injection cycles improve in vitro fertilization success? A randomized, prospective, placebo-controlled study. *J Assist Reprod Genet* 2006;23:15–21.

126. Check JH, Graziano V, Lee G, et al. Neither sildenafil nor vaginal estradiol improves endometrial thickness in women with thin endometria after taking oral estradiol in graduating dosages. *Clin Exp Obstet Gynecol* 2004;31:99–102.

127. Egbase PE, al-Sharhan M, al-Othman S, et al. Incidence of microbial growth from the tip of the embryo transfer catheter after embryo transfer in relation to clinical pregnancy rate following in-vitro fertilization and embryo transfer. *Hum Reprod* 1996;11:1687–9.

128. Moore DE, Soules MR, Klein NA, Fujimoto, et al. Bacteria in the transfer catheter tip influence the live-birth rate after in vitro fertilization. *Fertil Steril* 2000;74:1118–24.

129. Wittemer C, Bettahar-Lebugle K, Ohl J, et al. [Abnormal bacterial colonisation of the vagina and implantation during assisted reproduction]. [Article in French]. *Gynecol Obstet Fertil* 2004;32:135–9.

130. Egbase PE, Udo EE, Al-Sharhan M, Grudzinskas JG. Prophylactic antibiotics and endocervical microbial inoculation of the endometrium at embryo transfer. *Lancet* 1999;354:651–2.

131. Lenz S, Leeton J, Rogers P, Trounson A. Transfundal transfer of embryos using ultrasound. *J In Vitro Fert Embryo Transf* 1987;4:13–17.

132. Groutz A, Lessing JB, Wolf Y, Azem F, Yovel I, Amit A. Comparison of transmyometrial and transcervical embryo transfer in patients with previously failed in vitro fertilization-embryo transfer cycles and/or cervical stenosis. *Fertil Steril* 1997;67:1073–6.

133. Biervliet FP, Lesny P, Maguiness SD, Robinson J, Killick SR. Transmyometrial embryo transfer and junctional zone contractions. *Hum Reprod* 2002;17:347–50.

134. Kato O, Takatsuka R, Asch RH. Transvaginal-transmyometrial embryo transfer: the Towako method; experiences of 104 cases. *Fertil Steril* 1993;59:51–3.

135. Sharif K, Afnan M, Lenton W, Bilalis D, Hunjan M, Khalaf Y. Transmyometrial embryo transfer after difficult immediate mock transcervical transfer. *Fertil Steril* 1996;65:1071–4.

136. Lai TH, Wu MH, Hung KH, Cheng YC, Chang FM. Successful pregnancy by transmyometrial and transtubal embryo transfer after IVF in a patient with congenital cervical atresia who underwent uterovaginal canalization during Caesarean section: case report. *Hum Reprod* 2001;16:268–71.

137. Abusheikha N, Lass A, Akagbosu F, Brinsden P. How useful is cervical dilatation in patients with cervical stenosis who are participating in an in vitro fertilization-embryo transfer program? *The Bourn Hall experience. Fertil Steril* 1999;72:610–12.

138. Prapas N, Prapas Y, Panagiotidis Y, Prapa S, Vanderzwalmen P, Makedos G. Cervical dilatation has a positive impact on the outcome of IVF in randomly assigned cases having two previous difficult embryo transfers. *Hum Reprod* 2004;19:1791–5.

139. Groutz A, Lessing JB, Wolf Y, Yovel I, Azem F, Amit A. Cervical dilatation during ovum pick-up in patients with cervical stenosis: effect on pregnancy outcome in an in vitro fertilization-embryo transfer program. *Fertil Steril* 1997;67:909–11.

140. Noyes N, Licciardi F, Grifo J, Krey L, Berkeley A. In vitro fertilization outcome relative to embryo transfer difficulty: a novel approach to the forbidding cervix. *Fertil Steril* 1999;72:261–5.

141. Pabuccu R, Ceyhan ST, Onalan G, Goktolga U, Ercan CM, Selam B. Successful treatment of cervical stenosis with hysteroscopic canalization before embryo transfer in patients undergoing IVF: a case series. *J Minim Invasive Gynecol* 2005;12:436–8.

142. Glatstein IZ, Pang SC, McShane PM. Successful pregnancies with the use of laminaria tents before embryo transfer for refractory cervical stenosis. *Fertil Steril* 1997;67:1172–4.

143. Serhal P, Ranieri DM, Khadum I, Wakim RA. Cervical dilatation with hygroscopic rods prior to ovarian stimulation facilitates embryo transfer. *Hum Reprod* 2003;18:2618–20.

144. El Danasouri I, Milki A. A new cervical introducer for embryo transfer with soft open-end catheters. *Fertil Steril* 1992;57:939–41.

145. Patton PE, Stoelk EM. Difficult embryo transfer managed with a coaxial catheter system. *Fertil Steril* 1993;60:182–3.

146. Sallam HN. Embryo transfer: factors involved in optimizing the success. *Curr Opin Obstet Gynecol* 2005;17:289–98.

55

SINGLE EMBRYO TRANSFER

Jan Gerris, Petra De Sutter

INTRODUCTION

It has always been silently accepted that a high proportion of iatrogenic twins and high-order multiple pregnancies (HOMPs) was the price to be paid for a reasonable success rate of a treatment that is physically and emotionally demanding and, in many cases, expensive (Rizk et al. 1989). Even though many twins are delivered healthy and advances in neonatal medicine have decreased mortality and morbidity of premature babies from multiple pregnancies, there remains an important increase in the absolute numbers of (severe) pathologies. Tan et al. also pointed to the possible increase in *average* costs for multiple pregnancies, deliveries, and neonatal care (Rizk et al. 1991; Tan et al. 1992; Hidlebaugh et al. 1997; Wølner-Hanssen and Rydhstroem 1998; De Sutter et al. 2002; Ericson et al. 2002; Garceau et al. 2002; Ellison and Hall 2003); severe stress experienced by parents of multiples (Ostfeld et al. 2000; Glazebrook et al. 2004); and the lifelong support needed for mildly or severely disabled children.

MP causes several well-documented pathologies, extensively reviewed elsewhere (Dhont et al. 1997, 1999; Pons et al. 1998a,b; Senat et al. 1998; Bergh et al. 1999; Koudstaal et al. 2000a,b; Wennerholm and Bergh 2000, 2004a,b; Rydhstroem and Heraib 2001; Klemetti et al. 2002; Lynch et al. 2002; Strömberg et al. 2002; Wang et al. 2002; Helmerhorst et al. 2004), comprising both maternal and fetal/neonatal risks and complications. Apart from medical considerations, there has been a strong philosophical argumentation putting the responsibility for our children's good health at their start of life with all those involved in IVF/ICSI (Pennings 2000; ESHRE Task Force on Ethics and Law 2003). Recently, authors from different parts of the world have voiced their opinions and convictions regarding single-embryo transfer (SET), indicating a worldwide understanding of the problem of iatrogenic twinning and HOMPs.

CLINICAL DATA ON SET

Published Randomized Trials Comparing Outcome of Infertility Treatment

Five truly prospective randomized trials have been published, four European studies, of which two utilized day 3 SET (Gerris et al. 1999; Martikainen et al. 2001) and two mostly day 2 SET (Thurin et al. 2004; van Montfoort et al. 2006), and one American study using single blastocyst transfers (Gardner et al. 2004) (Table 55.1). It is, however, not fully appropriate to make a reliable meta-analysis of these trials. All five have a randomized design, but they compare different things. In our own study, patients were randomized between receiving one versus two top-quality embryos, strictly defined as an embryo with more than 20 percent fragmentation, four or five blastomeres on day 2 and greater than or equal to seven blastomeres on day 3 after fertilization, and no multinucleation in any of the blastomeres. Such embryos were shown to have an ongoing implantation potential of about 40 percent (Van Royen et al. 1999). The aim of this study was to find out what would be the difference in pregnancy rate when one or two embryos of documented *similar* high implantation potential are transferred in a homogenous group of ideal patients (younger than thirty-four years, first IVF/ICSI cycle). In the four-center Martikainen study, including patients in different treatment ranks and using traditional criteria of embryo selection, the aim was to show that single- and two-embryo transfers yield similar results. The conclusion of the study that a 32.4 percent pregnancy rate after SET is not significantly different from a 47.1 percent pregnancy rate after double-embryo transfer (DET) was statistically valid, but does not convince because the difference between the pregnancy rate after SET and DET was very substantial (34 vs. 47 percent). The Thurin study is an eleven-center Scandinavian study in women younger than thirty-six years in their first or second treatment cycles who were randomized to receive one excellent fresh embryo *and* one frozen/thawed embryo $(1 + 1)$ in case no pregnancy occurred versus two fresh embryos (2). Embryos were selected on the basis of fragmentation, number of blastomeres, and multinucleation. It showed that a strategy of $1 + 1$ transfer (39.7 percent) did not result in a substantial reduction in ongoing pregnancy rate when compared with two-embryo transfer (43/5 percent). However, the fresh PR was $91/330 = 27.6$ percent after SET versus $142/330 = 43$ percent after DET (OR $= 1.56$; 95 percent CI $= 1.26–1.93$). The Gardner study compared the transfer of one with two day 5 embryos in a selected good-prognosis group. In the most recent study by van Montfoort, eSET was compared in unselected patients with DET; all twins were prevented in the SET group but the pregnancy rate after DET was twice as high (40.3 percent) as after SET (20.4 percent) (van Montfoort et al. 2006).

Taken together, the mean *fresh* pregnancy rate after SET in the four studies was 31.3 percent with 1.58 percent twins and 47.6 percent after DET with 29.8 percent twins. A formal Cochrane meta-analysis came to a similar conclusion (Pandian et al. 2005).

Table 55.1: Randomized Studies and Cohort Studies Comparing SET with DET. (Data for the Martikainen 2001 Study and the Thurin 2004 Study Show Both the Fresh and the Cryoaugmented Pregnancy Rates)

Randomised trials

Author, year	N cycles	PR SET (%)	Twins (%)	PR DET (%)	Twins (%)
Gerris et al., 1999	53	10/26 (38.5)	1/10	20/27 (74)	6/20 (30.0)
Martikainen et al., 2001	144	24/74 (32.4)	1/24	33/70 (47.1)	6/33 (18.2)
Gardner et al., 2004	48	14/23 (60.9)	0/14	19/25 (76)	9/19 (47.4)
Thurin et al., 2004	661+ cryo	91/330 (27.6) 131/330 (39.7)	1/91 1/131	144/331 (43.5)	52/144 (36.1)
van Montfoort et al., 2006	308	51/154 (33.)	0/51	73/154 (47.4)	13/73 (17.8)
Total	906	190/607 (31.3)	3/190 (1.58)	289/607 (47.6)	86/289 (29.8)

Cohort studies

Author, year	N cycles	PR SET (%)	Twins (%)	PR DET (%)	Twins + HOMPs (%)
Gerris et al., 2002	1,152	105/299 (35.1)	1/124	309/853 (36.2)	105 + 5/309 (35.6)
De Sutter et al., 2003	2,898	163/579 (28.2)	1/163	734/2319 (31.7)	219 + 4/734 (30.4)
Tiitinen et al., 2003	1,494	162/470 (34.5)	2/162	376/1,024 (36.7)	113/376 (30.1)
Catt et al., 2003	385	49/111 (44.1)	1/49	161/274 (58.8)	71/161 (44.1)
Gerris et al., 2004	367	83/206 (40.3)	0	65/161 (40.4)	20/65 (30.8)
Martikainen et al., 2004	1,111	107/308 (34.7) 187/308 (60.7)	1/107	255/803 (31.8)	n.a.
Total	7,407	669/1,973 (33.9)	6/591 (1.0)	1,900/5,434 (35.0)	537/1,645 (32.6)

Published Cohort Studies Describing Fertility Treatment Outcome after SET and DET

A summary of results from a total of 7,407 cycles published in six cohort studies comparing single with two-embryo transfer is also shown in Table 55.1. The mean pregnancy rate after SET was 33.9 percent with 1.0 percent twins versus 35.0 percent after DET with 32.6 percent multiple pregnancies. In most of these studies, SET was elective, that is, SET was performed on the condition that an excellent-quality embryo was available from a cohort of several embryos. Taken together, these data suggest that *elective* SET (transfer of a high-competence embryo) yields the same pregnancy rate as indiscriminate two-embryo transfer. This is because the high success rate after the transfer of two high-competence embryos is balanced down by the low success rate after the transfer of two poor-quality embryos. This is where the importance of optimal embryo selection and of a validated definition of a high competence embryo becomes most obvious.

Recently, excellent results have been published from prospective nonrandomized studies in selected patients (Criniti et al. 2005; Henman et al. 2005) where use has been made of single blastocyst transfer in selected good-prognosis patients.

Opinion Papers

Recently, some authors have spoken in defense, whereas others have been criticizing the application of SET. In a paper entitled "One at a time" the authors stated that a review of abstracts presented at the 2004 Annual Meeting of the American Society

for Reproductive Medicine clearly demonstrate that good-prognosis patients should be given the option of an SET (Flisser and Licciardi 2006). Others have stressed the importance of counseling and educating patients as well as staff members (Wang et al. 2006). In contrast, some have argued that according to U.S. guidelines, eSET appears to represent an appropriate transfer option for only a small minority of IVF patients. They consider argument in favor of indiscriminate SET appears unrealistic and should be reconsidered (Gleicher and Barad 2006).

Arguments against SET are mostly of a nonmedical nature but can be very understandable. Several reviews have given balanced arguments to optimize, not maximize, IVF results (Bergh 2005; Gerris 2005; El-Toukhy et al. 2006).

A Balanced Appraisal of Published Results

These data illustrate two points of paramount importance with respect to SET. First, cryopreservation is a very important tool in reducing twins after IVF/ICSI. Second, transferring the "two best" embryos always yields more pregnancies than transferring "the" best embryo. There is no point in saying that SET equals DET. This is clearly shown when comparing the results after SET versus DET between the randomized and the cohort studies. In the former, there is a clear difference between both (DET: 216/453 versus SET: 139/453; OR = 1.55; 99 percent CI = 1.24–1.94).

This is also illustrated in the recent Dutch study by van Montfoort et al. (2006). This study in our reading did not serve to defend SET in all cycles but precisely to warn against an overzealous application of SET, which would damage the interest of the patients. We have always defended a *judicious* application of SET and have taken a *balanced* view of the possibilities and limits of SET. Essential in a good understanding of these is the link between optimal embryo (and patient) selection and SET.

The fine point in *elective* SET is that it is closely tied up with optimal embryo selection and that it should only be applied if an embryo with putative high competence is available. We have defined it in our way (Van Royen et al. 1999), others in another way. It can be applied to a smaller or to a larger proportion of the patient population. The essential point should not be missed: optimized embryo selection, however and for whomever it is performed, is a tool that can be used in two opposite directions. It can be used to perform SET in a substantial proportion of patients, maintaining an overall PR in the vicinity of the natural conception rate for a normally fertile couple (approximately 30 percent) but lowering the twinning rate substantially. Or it can be used to perform optimized two-embryo transfer in that same patient population, increasing the overall PR to well over 30 percent but "accepting" an elevated twinning rate of the program. It is understandable that to some centers, primarily looking at the PR, SET appears to be a step back, whereas for others, looking primarily at safety, it is a step forward. For many, it could be a step forward from both points of view. The decision is a matter of judgment and trade-off.

Generally, randomization is a valuable method for clinical research aims, resulting in a similar distribution of confounding variables over the study arms. It is an excellent tool to demonstrate *efficacy* of a particular treatment in a patient population fulfiling specified inclusion criteria. However, in a clinical IVF/ICSI program, which cannot be a never-ending randomized trial, one needs clear criteria to transfer one or two embryos in real-life situations, utilizing a validated selection method.

The difference between SET and DET in randomized trials could be anticipated; only the extent of the difference is correctly made clearer (~50 percent more pregnancies after DET). In the real-life cohort studies, no difference between SET and DET exists because SET means the *elective* transfer of a highly selected embryo of predictable implantation potential, whereas DET means a mix of transfers of two embryos with excellent, intermediate, or poor implantation potential. These trials are useful to establish what is the trade-off point at which a mean physiological PR can be reached with an acceptably low (<10 percent) twinning rate. In addition, the significant difference found in the randomized studies disappears when one cryopreservation cycle is added to the fresh SET cycle (Thurin et al. 2004).

In summary, the only reasonable interpretation of the combined data of these and other studies can be no other than favoring the use of SET of the appropriate embryo in the appropriate patient.

The European Experience with eSET

In Belgium, from July 1, 2003 onward, a reimbursement system for six IVF/ICSI cycles in a lifetime has been set up, based on the clinical experience of Belgian groups. Beneficiaries are patients who fall under the Belgian health insurance provisions up to less than forty-three years of age. For each oocyte recovery, the hospital receives approximately 1,200 on a central account, which is booked by the center for reproductive

Table 55.2: Results from the BELRAP Showing Results after the First Full Year of Implementation of the Reimbursement Regulation in Belgium (July 2003–June 2004)

	<36 years				36–40 years			
Rank	1	2	3–6	7	1	2	3–6	7
No. of cycles	5,728	2,033	732	183	1,497	594	278	92
No. of transfers	5,384	1,921	691	170	1,371	546	259	87
		(94%)				(93%)		
No. of embryos transferred								
1	4,918	807	98	71	344	135	55	13
2	426	1,103	581	82	968	382	114	58
3	28	7	12	14	50	28	86	13
No. of cycles with +hCG								
	1,880	697	213	74	419	135	66	34
% per cycle	33	34	29	40	28	23	24	37
% per ET	35	36	31	43	31	25	26	39

medicine. This amount covers the collection of both oocytes and spermatozoa, including MESA/TESE, laboratory costs of fresh and frozen/thawed transfers resulting from each oocyte harvest, and related costs for registration and follow-up. The medical costs (consultations, sonographies, oocyte recovery, and embryo transfer) and drugs are covered by the standard system of third-party reimbursement through the health insurance companies. The crux is that (mainly neonatal) savings from the reduction in twins and the disappearance of triplets make up for the money needed to cover six cycles, thus providing access to treatment to all who need it and at the same time ensure quality outcome (Ombelet et al. 2005). There is also compulsory online registration of all cycles.

Pivotal in the whole exercise is the judicious application of SET. Depending on the woman's age and the rank of the trial, the maximum number of embryos to transfer is regulated. All women younger than thirty-six years in their first cycle receive one embryo, independent of its morphological assessment. In older women or in subsequent cycles, the number of embryos to transfer never exceeds two except in women older than thirty-nine years, where there is no imposed maximum.

Table 55.2 shows data from the Belgian Registry of Artificial Reproduction (BELRAP) on the first year after the reimbursement regulation. There has been a tremendous rise in the number of SET cycles and a drastic reduction of twins. The evolution of the number of embryos transferred, of multiple pregnancies, and of children born in one particular center are shown in Figures 55.1 and 55.2, whereas the evolution over a longer period of time for the whole of Belgium is illustrated in Figures 55.3 and 55.4.

In Finland, SET has been applied widely since several years. On a national level, the incidence of IVF/ICSI twins has significantly decreased and even the total national birth registry shows a decrease in the proportion of twins (Vilska and Tiitinen 2004). SET has been combined very successfully

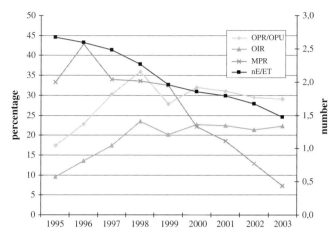

Figure. 55.1. Evolution of the overall pregnancy rate per oocyte pick-up (OPR/OPU), the ongoing implantation rate (OIR), the multiple pregnancy rate (MPR), and the mean number of embryos transferred (nE/ET) in one IVF centre, Antwerp, Belgium, 1995–2003.

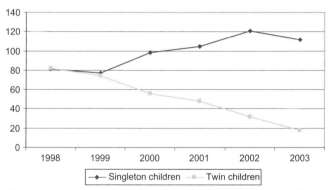

Figure. 55.2. Evolution in the number of children born as a singleton or as part of a twin in the Centre for Reproductive Medicine, Middelheim Hospital, Antwerp, Belgium, 1998–2003.

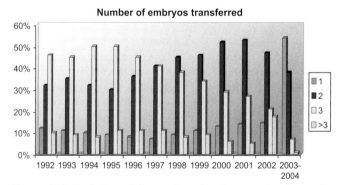

Figure. 55.3. Evolution of the number of embryos replaced over the years 1992–2004 in Belgium.

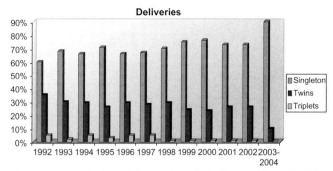

Figure. 55.4. Evolution of the number of singleton, twin, and triplet deliveries over the years 1992–2004 in Belgium.

practice seems to be in concordance with the regulation of the National Board on Health and Welfare stating that in principle only one embryo should be replaced apart from exceptional circumstances, which seem to be loosely defined.

In Germany, the Embryo Protection Act rules that no more than three oocytes can be cultured further than the two pronuclear (2PN) stage and no embryos can be frozen. This compels the German embryologists to select the embryos for transfer at the 2PN stage, which is not only likely to be suboptimal, but also hinders the application of SET because the average implantation rate of embryos selected at the 2PN stage seems to be lower than for early-cleavage embryos or blastocysts. Switzerland and Austria have a similar ruling.

In Italy, the situation at present is even more restrictive since no more than three oocytes can be fertilized and all the embryos that result have *to* be replaced. Ethical concerns about respect of human life and protection of the family and offspring have the deplorable effect of burdening women with a legislation that is not reflecting biomedical reality (Robertson et al. 2004).

Dutch IVF centers seem convinced of the value of SET as testified by an increasing number of Dutch publications addressing clinical or health-economic aspects of SET (Lukassen et al. 2004; van Montfoort et al., 2004; 2006).

In the United Kingdom, there is at present legal restriction of the number of embryos to transfer to two, unless there are exceptional circumstances. The British Human Fertilization and Embryology Authority has stated that it would like to move to SET and has installed a SET working group, which is studying how and when to implement SET. Several recent papers from British authors sustain the introduction of SET (El-Toukhy et al. 2006; Ledger et al. 2006).

Southern European countries (France, Spain, Portugal, Greece) have until now not produced clear evidence of a substantial proportion of SET cycles or do have a legislation that puts no maximum to the number of embryos transferred.

INDICATIONS AND EXCEPTIONS: SET FOR WHOM?

The essential prerequisites to introduce elective SET are simple. There must be a high base line ongoing PR of the program in the group of good-prognosis patients (e.g., first and second cycles in women younger than thirty-eight years) in combination with a compellingly high MPR, and there must be an efficient cryopreservation program.

We should make a distinction between compulsory, medical, and elective SET. Obviously, if only one embryo is

with cryopreservation (Tiitinen et al. 2001) and was shown to be very successful in oocyte donation (Söderström-Anttila et al. 2003).

The Scandinavian prospective randomized trial, mentioned earlier (Thurin et al. 2004), which was performed in five Swedish, two Norwegian, and four Danish centers, has made SET to be now largely accepted in these countries. In Sweden, the

Table 55.3: Published Results of Compulsory SETs.

Author, year	N of compulsory SETs	N of implantations	IR (%)	N Live Births	LBR (%)
Giorgetti et al., 1995	858	88	10.3	62	7.2
Vilska et al., 1999	94	19	20.2	15	16.0
Gerris et al., 2002	86	26	30.2	19	22.1
Tiitinen et al., 2003	205	39	19.0	31	15.1
De Sutter et al., 2003	211	21	10.0	19	9.0
Total	1454	193	13.3	146	10.1

IR: implantation rate; LBR: live birth rate

available for transfer, SET is compulsory (cSET). Because in the majority of these cases, the only available embryo is of poor quality, mean implantation rates in published series of cSET are low (Table 55.3) (Giorgetti et al. 1995; Vilska et al. 1999; Gerris et al. 2001, 2002; De Sutter et al. 2003a; Tiitinen et al. 2003). These poor results are due to the fact that the majority of these cycles occur in poor prognosis patients (poor responders, older women, and intrinsic fertilization defects).

There are women in whom a multiple pregnancy represents an a priori increased risk compared to the overall population. Congenital anomalies of the uterus, bad obstetrical history, previous loss of a twin, previous severe prematurity in a singleton, insufficiency of the cervical isthmus, severe systemic disease (e.g., insulin-dependent diabetes), and the explicit wish of recipients to avoid a twin pregnancy constitute absolute contraindications against two-embryo transfer.

By definition, elective SET means that there is choice from among two or more embryos suitable for transfer, with the purpose of transferring only one embryo.

Therefore, embryo criteria for eligibility must be defined and validated, so that selection is optimized. This should be done using one or a set of criteria in a prospective setting where the outcome of each individual embryo is documented, ideally using only SET, which creates the possibility of one-to-one observations.

The theoretical possibility to transfer only one embryo in all cycles can for the present be discarded. Hence, the challenge is to define the subgroup of patients who should receive one embryo. A number of older retrospective studies examined which *clinical* factors correlate with the chance for pregnancy or MP (Staessen et al. 1992; Roseboom et al. 1995; Svendsen et al. 1996; Templeton and Morris 1996; Commenges-Ducos et al. 1998; Minaretzis et al. 1998; Hsu et al. 1999; Shapiro et al. 2000, 2001). These were based on the transfer of two or more embryos. Most of the factors that were found to correlate (age being the most important one) are in fact themselves correlated with intrinsic embryo implantation potential (e.g., number of oocytes, number of normally fertilized 2PN zygotes, number of "good-looking" embryos, low dose of FSH needed, and good ovarian response), emphasizing the dominant impact of the embryo factor as compared to the patient factor.

Others have approached the problem using theoretical mathematical prediction models (Martin and Welch 1998; Trimarchi 2001; Hunault et al. 2002) or made recommendations

toward two-embryo transfer (Staessen et al. 1993; Vauthier-Brouzes et al. 1994; Tasdemir et al. 1995; Roest et al. 1997; Templeton and Morris 1998; Milki et al. 1999; Dean et al. 2000; Ozturk et al. 2001).

One study tried to identify patients most suitable for SET on the basis of a multivariate analysis of more than 2000 IVF/ICSI cycles with two-embryo transfers. These were found to be women younger than thirty-five to thirty-seven years in their first or second treatment cycles, with at least two embryos and without tubal pathology as an indication for IVF (Strandell et al. 2000).

A specific group that in our opinion should be actively counseled toward SET is women who obtained a non-ongoing pregnancy in a first IVF/ICSI cycle. For psychological reasons, these patients often ask for two embryos in a second cycle, and it may be difficult to convince them to accept SET, although there is evidence that these are very good-prognosis patients (Croucher et al. 1998; Bates and Ginsburg 2002).

Even with SET as standard policy for IVF/ICSI, there will always remain a subgroup of patients in whom the transfer of more than one embryo is acceptable as an exception, based on sound medical considerations.

Cost for the patient is not a *medical* exception, but in many countries the high cost of IVF/ICSI for the patient causes an understandable objection to SET, although of course the health economic considerations remain the same.

A real exception is female age. In some countries, SET is performed up to thirty-eight or even forty years of age. Above that age, the transfer of more than one embryo is performed more liberally. Further clinical research has to elucidate which are the optimal transfer algorithms in this age-group. The potential advantage of aneuploidy screening may also be situated here.

In patients with nonobstructive azoospermia, the recovery by TESE of spermatozoa for ICSI at times is so extremely low that only one or two treatment trials can be performed. Should against all odds more than one embryo be obtained in such unfavorable circumstances, the transfer of more than one embryo may be warranted. Other circumstances where only very small amounts of sperm are available, for example, freezing before chemotherapy or "end of stock" of a particular sperm donor, may be considered exceptions as well.

Patients undergoing preimplantation diagnosis because of genetic disease frequently just have one or two unaffected embryos available to them after a long and technically complicated and expensive treatment, perhaps creating a relative contraindication to limit the number of embryos to one, although this should be weighed against the odds of an MP during the counseling.

Another example is oocyte donation. Depending on the availability of oocytes, which in some countries is much lower than the demand, or due to practical arrangements, where oocytes from one donor are shared by more than one acceptor, a dilemma may arise between the transfer of more than one embryo versus cryopreservation. However, a Finnish group has reported excellent results with SET in an oocyte donation program (Söderström-Anttila et al. 2003).

SET AND EMBRYO SELECTION

Opinions do vary whether SET should or should not be accompanied by some strategy of optimized selection of the embryo

Table 55.4: Implanted Fraction of Embryos without Observed Multinucleation, Assessed by the Number of Blastomeres on Day 2 (44–46 hours) and Day 3 (66–69 hours) and the Percentage of Fragmentation (1: <10%; 2: <20%) (≥10 Embryos in Each Group; Only Embryos with an Observed Implantation Rate of ≥20% Shown) (Adapted from Van Royen et al., 2001)

Fragmentation	Cells on day 2	Cells on day 3	100% Implantation	0% + 100% implantion	Implanted fraction (%)
1	4	8	187	429	43.6
1	4	9	12	30	40.0
2	4	9	8	20	40.0
2	4	8	50	129	38.8
1	5	9	13	38	34.2
1	5	8	10	31	32.3
1	2	7	4	13	30.8
1	2	8	6	20	30.0
2	5	10	3	11	27.3
1	6	10	3	11	27.3
2	5	9	10	38	26.3
1	5	10	5	19	26.3
2	5	8	5	20	25.0
1	2	6	3	13	23.1
1	4	7	19	83	22.9
2	4	7	10	45	22.2
2	5	7	4	20	20.0
1	3	5	2	10	20.0

to transfer. If embryo selection is pushed too hard and embryos considered as having a high implantation potential are too strictly defined or if the proposed technique is too complicated or expensive, the number of SET cycles will remain low and the impact on the twinning rate limited. If, on the other hand, only one embryo is transferred without using strict selection criteria, the PR might drop below what is acceptable.

Documented ongoing implantation is the gold standard for a particular embryo's competence. Published data show it to be a gradual biological variable, varying between 0 percent for the "worst" and about 60 percent for the "best" embryos. Labeling an embryo as a "top-quality embryo" or a "high–implantation potential embryo" or a "putative high-competence embryo" remains a clinically useful (when communicating with patients) but intrinsically oversimplifying representation of this gradual implantation potential. This is illustrated in Table 55.4 (adapted from Van Royen et al. 2001) showing the observed implantation rates of embryos with certainly known outcome (one-to-one observations). Is has been previously shown that embryos with multinucleated blastomeres have very low implantation rates of approximately 5 percent (Pickering et al. 1995; Kligman et al. 1996; Jackson et al. 1998; Palmstierna et al. 1998; Pelinck et al. 1998; Van Royen et al. 2003).

Morphological and functional characteristics that have been studied comprise the following: morphology of the oocyte; ATP content and mitochondrial distribution in oocytes; pronuclear body breakdown; number and symmetry of distribution of nucleolar bodies in zygote pronuclei; early (twenty-five to twenty-seven hours after fertilization) or late first cleavage for day 2 embryos; number and symmetry of blastomeres, fragmentation, and presence or absence of multinucleation in early-cleaving embryos; number of blastomeres undergoing compaction; and the morphology of the compaction process in day 4 morulas and blastocyst morphology in day 5 or day 6 embryos. Dynamic characteristics such as pyruvate and glucose metabolism or amino acid turnover have also been studied but not in an immediate clinical context.

Morphology alone cannot disclose whether *a particular* embryo will implant or not because we are looking at a statistical correlation, not at an individual measurement and because morphology alone cannot disclose all the information contained in the embryo.

In many studies that have tried to correlate particular morphological characteristics with implantation potential, selection for transfer was not based on the criterion studied but on traditional day 2 and/or day 3 observations. Some studies are clinical, either randomized comparisons or cohort studies, which clearly stated the embryo selection technique. Others are retrospective analyses correlating PR and IR with particular recorded embryo characteristics either used or not used as a selection method. Some studies concern the overall IVF/ICSI population, others only very good-prognosis patients. Therefore, comparison is flawed and conclusions hard to draw. There appears to be more than one valid selection method. It cannot be concluded at this time which is the optimal selection method when it comes to SET.

Studies focusing on early first cleavage are in agreement that this is a good indicator discerning embryos with high from embryos with low implantation potential, but, excluding the one study that clearly states actual selection took place on the basis of day 2 morphology (Salumets et al. 2003), the average reported IR varies between 14 and 28 percent. This is lower than the IR reported in studies where routine selection was based on day 2 or 3 characteristics, varying between 27 and 48 percent, averaging about 35 percent. Another realm of IR (60 percent) is reported in studies utilizing day 5 embryo transfers, which is usually in highly selected patients (Gardner et al. 2004; Criniti et al. 2005; Stillman et al. 2005). When used as a routine selection stage, IR for day 5 embryos seem to average about 35 percent as well. Culturing several high-quality day 3 embryos, if available, to blastocysts may add selective power, increasing the chance to transfer the best embryo available, but this subgroup of patients is limited to those with at least four good-quality embryos on day 3 (Papanikolaou et al. 2005).

No single static observation gives all the information contained in an embryo's morphology. It is more logical to consider that a combination of different observations, preferably reflecting different aspects of implantation potential, should be used; for example, it is likely that blastomere asymmetry and multinucleation are both associated with aneuploidy (Hardarson et al. 2001). From the point of view of the prevention of MP, including twins, the discussion regarding the optimal stage to transfer in our opinion remains largely academic. It seems more important to get started implementing SET rather than wait for any final proof of which selection technique is "better" because the question will always be: better for whom? Better for the average patient or for particular subgroups of patients?

Although some centers proclaim excellent results after single blastocyst transfer (Gardner et al. 2004; Criniti et al. 2005; Stillman et al. 2005), others found the merits of blastocyst versus cleavage-stage embryo transfer not to exist for the overall population (Coskun et al. 2000; Kolibianakis and Devroey 2002; Rienzi et al. 2002; Bungum et al. 2003; Blake et al. 2004; Kolibianakis et al. 2004; Utsunomiya et al. 2004).

In summary, the introduction of SET compels embryologists to optimize their embryo selection procedure. It appears that much can be improved with respect to cleavage-stage selection and that in certain circumstances blastocyst culture may facilitate the acceptance by patients of just a single embryo.

Whether routine preimplantation aneuploidy screening is superior to (a combination of) morphology characteristics remains equally unproven. Limited available evidence suggests that preimplantation genetic diagnosis serves mainly as prevention of miscarriage, and after PGD, the about 35 percent "limit" seems to appear again (Obasaju et al. 2001).

It should be underlined that to obtain a high ongoing pregnancy, other factors than embryo competence play a role in the IVF/ICSI treatment chain, for example, ovarian stimulation, optimized laboratory conditions at oocyte retrieval and embryo transfer, transfer technique, and endometrial receptivity.

THE ROLE OF CRYOPRESERVATION

One benefit of SET is an increase in the number of embryos available for cryopreservation (De Neubourg et al. 2003). Optimized cryopreservation of embryos after SET is part of the strategy to decrease multiple pregnancies (Jones et al. 1995, 1997a,b; Gerris et al. 2003). It increases the cumulative PR per oocyte harvest and ideally allows patients who "desire" a twin pregnancy to have their "delayed" twin.

In a group of 127 Finnish patients who had a fresh SET, forty-nine became pregnant (38.6 percent) and thirty-four delivered (26.8 percent); those without ongoing pregnancy had a total of 129 frozen-embryo transfers, resulting in another thirty-two pregnancies and thirty-two deliveries. This increased the PR per patient to 62.4 percent and the delivery rate to 52.8 percent (Tiitinen et al. 2001, 2003).

In a Swedish study, the transfer of one frozen/thawed embryo after a failed fresh cycle was able to increase the cumulative PR (39.5 percent) to the same as after the transfer of two embryos (43.5 percent) (Thurin et al. 2004).

In a Dutch study (van Montfoort et al. 2004), the cumulative ongoing PR rose from 24 to 34 percent in SET patients and from 34 to 38 percent after DET, loosing significance between SET and DET.

An Australian group performed a fresh transfer of either a single blastocyst or two blastocysts (PRs of 44 and 59 percent, respectively) followed by a frozen/thaw cycle of maximum two embryos, rising the PR per patient to 74 percent in the SET group and 70 percent in the DET group, respectively (Catt et al. 2003). The twinning rates were 2 versus 44 percent for the fresh SET versus the fresh DET, respectively, and 5 versus 28 percent after cryoaugmentation. A small, recent Japanese study of sixty-six patients (Uchiyama et al. 2004) obtained a fresh PR of 44.9 percent in sixty-six fresh SET cycles and a cryoaugmented PR of 72.4 percent after twenty-nine patients underwent a subsequent transfer of one frozen/thawed blastocyst. In this study, embryos had been cryopreserved by vitrification.

Further development of cryotechnology and increasing application of frozen/thawed cycles is becoming an integral part of every IVF/ICSI program applying SET.

eSET: NOT ONLY LESS TWINS BUT ALSO BETTER SINGLETONS

It has been shown (Helmerhorst et al. 2004; Jackson et al. 2004) that the outcome of singletons but not of twins after IVF/ICSI in a standard two-embryo program is worse than that of naturally conceived singleton or twins.

However, these studies analyzed pregnancies before the introduction of SET. Therefore, the groups were very heterogeneous and comprised both young good-prognosis patients, who, for example, conceived twins in a first treatment cycle and, on the other hand, older women with poor prognosis who conceived a singleton after multiple-embryo transfer in high rank trials.

Recently, we have shown that singletons after eSET do not compare unfavorably with spontaneously conceived singletons (De Neubourg et al. 2006).

In another study, we also found that ongoing IVF/ICSI pregnancies showing first-trimester blood loss had an inferior obstetrical and neonatal outcome than if no first-trimester blood loss occurred (De Sutter et al. 2006a) and that there was an almost linear relationship between the number of embryos transferred and the incidence of first-trimester blood loss. First-trimester bleeding is frequent in assisted reproductive technique (ART) pregnancies. It was not previously known whether first-trimester bleeding, if not ending in a spontaneous abortion, negatively influences further pregnancy outcome in ART in singletons. We obtained data from our ART database (1993–2002), with 1,432 singleton ongoing pregnancies being included in this study. The outcome measures – second-trimester and third-trimester bleeding, preterm contraction rates, pregnancy duration, birth weight, cesarean section rates, intrauterine growth retardation (IUGR), preterm prelabor rupture of membranes (P-PROM), neonatal intensive care unit (NICU) admission, and perinatal mortality – were compared in the groups with and without first-trimester bleeding. We found that significantly more singleton pregnancies resulted from a vanishing twin in the group with first-trimester bleeding (8.7 percent) than in the controls (4.0 percent). A correlation was found between the incidence of first-trimester bleeding and the number of embryos transferred. First-trimester bleeding led to increased second-trimester (OR = 4.56; 95 percent CI = 2.76–7.56) and third-trimester bleeding rates (OR = 2.85; 95 percent CI = 1.42–5.73), P-PROM (OR = 2.44; 95 percent CI = 1.38–4.31), preterm contractions (OR = 2.27; 95 percent CI = 1.48–3.47), and NICU admissions (OR = 1.75; 95 percent CI = 1.21–2.54). First-trimester bleeding increased the risk for preterm birth (OR = 1.64; 95 percent CI = 1.05–2.55) and extreme preterm birth (OR = 3.05; 95 percent CI = 1.12–8.31). Therefore, we hold the opinion that first-trimester bleeding in an ongoing singleton pregnancy following ART increases the risk for pregnancy complications. The association between first-trimester bleeding, the number of embryos transferred, and adverse pregnancy outcome provides a further argument in favor of SET.

In yet another study, we found that the birth weight of singletons born after eSET (3,324.6 ± 509.7g) was significantly higher than after two-embryo transfer (3,204.3 ± 617.5) (p < 0.01) (De Sutter et al. 2006b), that the incidence of prematurity less than thirty-seven weeks was 6.2 percent for singletons after SET versus 10.4 percent after DET (adjusted odds 1.77; 95 percent CI = 1.06–2.94), and that the incidence of low birth weight (<2,500 g) was lower for singletons after SET (4.2 percent) versus DET (11.6 percent) (adjusted odds = 3.38; 95 percent CI = 1.86–6.12).

These observations are in line with the fact that there appears to be more vanishing twins after IVF than previously suspected (Pinborg et al. 2005) and that in utero competition for implantation may play a role in the final outcome of these pregnancies. Hence, eSET does not only prevent the well-known and documented complications of twin pregnancies but actually improves the outcome of singleton pregnancies.

HEALTH-ECONOMIC CONSIDERATIONS

Although the main reason to apply SET is the health of the children at their start of life, financial considerations are paramount. The increased utilization of hospital care in ART children is the consequence of MP (Ericson et al. 2002). The estimated cost for an IVF singleton after IVF was calculated to be three times that of a twin (Wølner-Hanssen et al. 1998); an American group found a twin twice and a triplet fifteen times as expensive as a singleton (Hidlebaugh et al. 1997). Others have used a health-economic model to establish that SET and DET are financially equivalent per live born child. SET needs more cycles and yields less children per cycle, but DET yields higher obstetrical and mainly neonatal costs per child (De Sutter et al. 2002, 2003b) and these effects balance out each other. They conclude SET is hence to be preferred because most of the extra cost and care start only after birth.

A Dutch retrospective cost analysis showed that an IVF twin pregnancy costs on average 10,000€ more than an IVF singleton pregnancy (Lukassen et al. 2004). In a real-life prospective comparison between elective SET versus DET in women younger than thirty-eight years in their first IVF/ICSI cycle, elective SET of one high competence embryo was as efficient as two-embryo transfer (40 percent PR on both groups), but the cost per child was only approximately half after elective SET (Gerris et al. 2004). In all studies, as in the models, the major cost driver was the higher neonatal cost for premature born children.

Cost-effectiveness is also strongly dependent on the age of the female partner (Mol et al. 2000). An international survey of IVF costs revealed huge differences, both in accessibility and cost per cycle between countries (Collins 2002). In the United States, the existence of (partial) insurance coverage had a decreasing effect on the number of embryos transferred (Jain et al. 2002; Reynolds et al. 2003), although the mean number of embryos transferred in centers in states with complete coverage was still high. Reimbursement is not the whole story, although it incites a sense of responsibility in patients, serves as a leverage to overrule short-sighted considerations for quick success, and puts the quality of the child in the center of the debate.

In Belgium, it has been calculated that the money saved by avoiding half of the MP would suffice to finance all IVF/ICSI cycles in a year (Ombelet et al. 2005). This is the basis for the Belgian reimbursement system. Although the figures both for pregnancy rates, multiple pregnancy rates, and number of embryos transferred have evolved positively, the health-economic calculations still are to follow. The Achilles tendon of the system is the number of cycles, which has initially shown a sharp rise; but this has now topped off.

A British study also found that multiple pregnancies after IVF are associated with high direct costs to the National Health System (NHS). Redirection of money saved by implementation of a mandatory "two-embryo transfer" policy into increased provision of IVF treatment could double the number of NHS-funded IVF treatment cycles at no extra cost. Further savings could be made if a selective "SET" policy were to be adopted (Ledger et al. 2006).

Different countries are using or considering different systems of (partial) reimbursement of IVF. This is very much influenced by historical considerations, by fundamental choices made in society, and by political agendas. All of these seem to have a significant impact on the introduction of SET.

THE PATIENT'S PERSPECTIVE: INFORMATION AND COUNSELING

One of the most important challenges for a future toward a safe IVF/ICSI treatment resides in the proper counseling of patients. Patients need proper and complete information (Buckett and Tan 2004; D'Alton 2004) about the fact that prevention is possible without serious decline in the chances for pregnancy, especially if combined with cryopreservation and if results are expressed (and patients or health insurers charged) per oocyte harvest and not per cycle or per transfer.

There are differences among patients, embryologists, and clinicians in their perceptions of the desirability of MP (Hartshorne and Lilford 2002). These have different origins and are determined by a mix of objective elements (statistics of chances for success versus risks for complications) and subjective factors (hope versus bad obstetrical experience and the "happy twin" illusion in the patient; wanting to perform versus a sense of responsibility in the professionals). Decisions imply a trade-off between the informed patients' autonomy and the physicians' clinical judgment, increasingly including medicolegal considerations.

This takes time, patience, commitment, and personal conviction from those who treat and counsel. It also gives an insight into how patients think, or feel, about their chances and about risks they do not always understand (Ryan and Van Voorhis 2004).

A British study investigated whether patients' willingness to accept a hypothetical policy of SET changed with the method of providing information. The information that their chance for a pregnancy would not decrease due to SET and that fresh and frozen transfers would imply a fixed charge led to acceptance in a similar proportion of respondents who received a standard information pack (82 percent), an additional information leaflet (83 percent), or a personal discussion session (87 percent) (Murray et al. 2004). It thus did not seem that counseling could easily change the patients' views.

A Danish group analyzed attitudes of IVF/ICSI-twin mothers toward twins and embryo transfers and found that only a quarter of these mothers agreed to SET (Pinborg et al. 2003). They also found that the delivery of a child with very low birth weight and hence morbidity was predictive of high acceptance of SET. It is noteworthy that not much was known about

20 percent of women who did not respond to the questionnaire and who may have been the ones with a bad obstetrical outcome. They conclude that SET requires extensive counseling. It also illustrates that mothers of twins even with some degree of disability always *love* their children and would go through the same efforts and risks again to have them. As long as they are under the erroneous conviction that their twin was the result of a choice between either twins versus no children, they will not easily agree with SET.

The importance of full counseling of patients was recently stressed by an Australian group (Wang et al. 2006).

CONCLUSIONS AND FUTURE PERSPECTIVES

Elective SET, combined with subsequent transfer of frozen/thawed embryos, can maintain a high PR with a dramatic decrease in MP rate. This leads to a similar proportion of infertile patients who will become pregnant. The medical complications, human suffering, and expense that can thus be avoided should be sufficiently strong arguments to demand a reimbursement of IVF/ICSI costs, linked to a strict embryo transfer policy to avoid MP as well as a strict policy of acceptance to treatment to avoid overconsumption.

It has been argued that in the near future, SET should be the default policy for good-prognosis IVF/ICSI patients. If at least one high competence embryo is available, only one should be transferred. Its definition should preferably be based on a large and ever increasing number of one-to-one observations (Table 55.3), so that selection is refined by experience. Since criteria cannot be extrapolated from one lab to another, the best option seems to let centers build their own expertise. The pioneering groups in SET have a proportion of SET cycles well exceeding 60 percent; hence, the exception is non-SET. This is probably the way to go on a global scale and we should welcome that evolution. In contrast, there will always remain a substantial subgroup of patients in whom the transfer of more than one embryo remains unavoidable or even acceptable.

An alternative to elective SET is the use of natural-cycle IVF/ICSI (Pelinck et al. 2002). Although this approach has its attractive sides (easy, cheap, repeatable, and no ovarian hyperstimulation syndrome), its efficacy per cycle is low. The strength of elective SET resides in the fact that ovarian stimulation allows selection of the putative most competent embryo. Nevertheless, not much is known about implantation potential of embryos from natural cycles as compared with stimulated cycles (Ziebe et al. 2004) and the possibility of natural cycle IVF/ICSI should perhaps be included as a possibility in some patients. Ovarian stimulation schemes might be adapted toward a lower dose approach, without compromising the possibility of choice. The search for "the" best embryo to transfer should remain within reasonable limits, dictated by the intrinsic genetic limitations of human embryos.

The impact of SET will depend on the size of the group in whom it is applied. If criteria are very strict, the impact will be small, but the overall pregnancy rate is likely not to decrease. If the inclusion criteria are very liberal, the twinning rate will drop dramatically, but the overall pregnancy rate might somewhat decrease, although the decrease appears to be much less than what was feared and it can be compensated by improved cryoaugmentation. To find the optimal trade-off between ongoing PR and twinning rate is the foremost clinical challenge for each IVF center.

Clinical judgments regarding SET differ between centers and countries. It should be underlined that it has been no one's intention to implement SET in all or even in the large majority of IVF/ICSI cycles, as insinuated by some authors (Gleicher and Barad 2006). It is also clear that in large parts of the world, none of the players are "ripe" for SET. This is the best reason to continue the search for optimized embryo selection and to exchange clinical experience with SET between different types of medical practice.

KEY POINTS FOR CLINICAL PRACTICE

■ More and more data are published indicating the feasibility to perform SET. This is definitely the case in good-prognosis patients (younger than thirty-six years, first or second IVF/ICSI trial) and if there is a choice from several embryos. Embryo selection, still on the basis of an optimized morphology assessment using strict criteria and time intervals, is essential. Apart from the preventive effect on the (complications associated with many but not all) twin pregnancies, both health-economic considerations and neonatal outcome consideration also underpin the value of SET. Cryopreservation is a useful tool in an optimal strategy and management of all oocyte harvests.

REFERENCES

Bates GW, Ginsburg ES (2002) Early pregnancy loss in in vitro fertilization (IVF) is a positive predictor of subsequent IVF success. *Fertil Steril* 77, 337–341.

Bergh C (2005) Single embryo transfer: a mini-review. *Hum Reprod* 20, 323–327.

Bergh T, Ericson A, Hillensjö T, Nygren KG, Wennerholm UB (1999) Deliveries and children born after in-vitro fertilization in Sweden 1982–95: a retrospective cohort study. *Lancet* 453, 1579–1585.

Blake D, Proctor M, Johnson N, Olive D (2004) The merits of blastocyst versus cleavage stage embryo transfer: a Cochrane Review. *Hum Reprod* 19, 795–807.

Buckett W, Tan SL (2004) What is the most relevant standard of success in assisted reproduction? The importance of informed choice. *Hum Reprod* 19, 1043–1045.

Bungum M, Bungum L, Humaidan P, Yding Andersen C (2003) Day 3 versus day 5 embryo transfer: a prospective randomized study. *Reprod BioMed Online* 7, 98–104.

Catt J, Wood T, Henman M, Jansen R (2003) Single embryo transfer in IVF to prevent multiple pregnancies. *Twin Res* 6, 536–539.

Collins JA (2002) An international survey of the health economics of IVF and ICSI. *Hum Reprod Update* 8, 265–277.

Commenges-Ducos M, Tricaud S, Papaxanthos-Roche A, Dallay D, Horovitz J, Commenges D (1998) Modelling of the probability of success of the stages of in-vitro fertilization and embryo transfer: stimulation, fertilization and implantation. *Hum Reprod* 13, 78–83.

Coskun S, Hollanders J, Al-Hassan S, Al-Sufyan H, Al-Mayman H, Jaroudi K (2000) Day 5 versus day 3 embryo transfer: a controlled randomized trial. *Hum Reprod* 15, 1947–1952.

Criniti A, Thyer A, Chow G, Lin P, Klein N, Soules M (2005) Elective single blastocyst transfer reduces twin rates without compromising pregnancy rates. *Fertil Steril* 84, 1613–1619.

Croucher CA, Lass A, Margara R, Winston RM (1998) Predictive value of the results of a first in-vitro fertilization cycle on the outcome of subsequent cycles. *Hum Reprod* 13, 403–408.

D'Alton M (2004) Infertility and the desire for multiple births. *Fertil Steril* 81, 523–525.

Dean NL, Philips SJ, Buckett WM, Biljan MM, Lin Tan S (2000) Impact of reducing the number of embryos transferred from three to two in women under the age of 35 who produced three or more high-quality embryos. *Fertil Steril* 74, 820–823.

De Neubourg D, Mangelschots K, Van Royen E, Vercruyssen M, Ryckaert G, Valkenburg M, Barudy-Vasquez J, Gerris J (2003) Impact of patients' choice for single embryo transfer of a top quality embryo versus double transfer in the first IVF/ICSI cycle. *Hum Reprod* 17, 2621–2625.

De Neubourg D, Mangelschots K, Van Royen E, Vercruyssen M, Gerris J (2004) Singleton pregnancies are equally affected by ovarian hyperstimulation syndrome as twin pregnancies. *Fertil Steril* 82, 1691–1693.

De Neubourg D, Gerris J, Mangelschots K, Van Royen E, Vercruyssen M, Steylemans A, Elseviers M (2006) The obstetrical and neonatal outcome of babies born after single-embryo transfer in IVF/ICSI compares favourably to spontaneously conceived babies. *Hum Reprod* 21, 1041–1046.

De Sutter P, Gerris J, Dhont M (2002) A health-economic decision-analytic model comparing double with single embryo transfer in IVF/ICSI. *Hum Reprod* 17, 2891–2896.

De Sutter P, Van der Elst J, Coetsier T, Dhont M (2003a) Single embryo transfer and multiple pregnancy rate reduction after IVF/ICSI: a 5-year appraisal. *Reprod Biomed Online* 18, 464–469.

De Sutter P, Gerris J, Dhont M (2003b) A health-economic decision-analytic model comparing double with single embryo transfer in IVF/ICSI: a sensitivity analysis. *Hum Reprod* 18, 1361.

De Sutter P, Bontinck J, Schutysers V, Van der Elst J, Gerris J, Dhont M (2006a) First-trimester bleeding and pregnancy outcome in singletons after assisted reproduction. *Hum Reprod (advance access publication)*.

De Sutter P, Delbaere I, Gerris J, Goetgeluk S, Van der Elst J, Temmerman M, Dhont M (2006b) Birth weight of singletons in ART is higher after single than after double embryo transfer. *Hum Reprod (advance access publication)*.

Dhont M, De Neubourg F, Van Der Elst J, De Sutter P (1997) Perinatal outcome of pregnancies after assisted reproduction: a case-control study. *J Assist Reprod Genet* 14, 575–580.

Dhont M, De Sutter P, Ruyssinck G, Martens G, Bekaert A (1999) Perinatal outcome of pregnancies after assisted reproduction: a case-control study. *Am J Obstet Gynecol* 181, 688–695.

Ellison MA, Hall JE (2003) Social stigma and compound losses: quality-of-life issues for multiple-birth families. *Fertil Steril* 80, 405–414.

El-Toukhy T, Khalaf Y, Peter Braude (2006) IVF results: optimize not maximize. *Am J Obstet Gynecol* 194, 322–331.

Ericson A, Nygren KG, Otterblad Olausson P, Källén B (2002) Hospital care utilization of infants born after IVF. *Hum Reprod* 17, 929–932.

ESHRE Task Force on Ethics and Law (2003) Ethical issues related to multiple pregnancies in medically assisted procreation. *Hum Reprod* 18, 1976–1979.

Flisser E, Licciardi F (2006) One at a time. *Fertil Steril* 85, 555–558.

Garceau L, Henderson J, Davis LJ, Petrou S, Henderson LR, Mc Veigh DH, Barlow DH, Davidson LL (2002) Economic implications of assisted reproductive techniques: a systematic review. *Hum Reprod* 17, 3090–3109.

Gardner DK, Surrey E, Minjarez D, Leitz A, Stevens J, Schoolcraft W (2004) Single blastocyst transfer: a prospective randomized trial. *Fertil Steril* 81, 551–555.

Gerris J. (2005) Single embryo transfer and IVF/ICSI outcome: a balanced appraisal *Hum Reprod Update* 11, 105–121.

Gerris J, De Neubourg D, Mangelschots K, Van Royen E, Van de Meersche M, Valkenburg M (1999) Prevention of twin pregnancy after in-vitro fertilization or intracytoplasmic sperm injection based on strict embryo criteria: a prospective randomized clinical trial. *Hum Reprod* 14, 2581–2587.

Gerris J, Van Royen E, De Neubourg D, Mangelschots K, Valkenburg M, Ryckaert G (2001) Impact of single embryo transfer on the overall and twin-pregnancy rates of an IVF/ICSI programme. *RBM Online* 2, 172–177.

Gerris J, De Neubourg D, Mangelschots K, Van Royen E, Vercruyssen M, Barudy-Vasquez J, Valkenburg M, Ryckaert G (2002) Elective single day-3 embryo transfer halves the twinning rate without decrease in the ongoing pregnancy rate of an IVF/ICSI programme. *Hum Reprod* 17, 2621–2626.

Gerris J, De Neubourg D, De Sutter P, Van Royen E, Mangelschots K, Vercruyssen M (2003) Cryopreservation as a tool to reduce multiple birth. *Reprod BioMed Online* 7, 286–294.

Gerris J, De Sutter P, De Neubourg D, Van Royen E, Van der Elst J, Mangelschots K, Vercruyssen M, Kok P, Elseviers M, Annemans L, et al. (2004) A real-life prospective health economic study of elective single embryo transfer versus two-embryo transfer in first IVF/ICSI cycles. *Hum Reprod* 19, 917–923.

Giorgetti C, Terriou P, Auquier P, Hans E, Spach J-L, Salzmann J, Roulier R (1995) Embryo score to predict implantation after in-vitro fertilization: based on 957 single embryo transfers. *Hum Reprod* 10, 2427–2431.

Glazebrook C, Sheard C, Cox S, Oates M, Ndukwe G (2004) Parenting stress in first-time mothers of twins and triplets conceived after in vitro fertilization. *Fertil Steril* 81, 505–511.

Gleicher N, Barad D. The relative myth of elective single embryo transfer. *Hum Reprod (advance access publication)*.

Hardarson T, Hanson C, Sjögren A, Lundin K (2001) Human embryos with unevenly sized blastomeres have lower pregnancy and implantation rates: indications for aneuploidy and multinucleation. *Hum Reprod* 16, 313–18.

Hartshorne GM, Lilford RJ (2002) Different perspectives of patients and health care professionals on the potential benefits and risks of blastocyst culture and multiple embryo transfer. *Hum Reprod* 17, 1023–1030.

Helmerhorst FM, Perquin DAM, Donker D, Keirse MJNC (2004) Perinatal outcome of singletons and twins after assisted conception: a systematic review of controlled studies. *BMJ* 328, 261–264.

Henman M, Catt JW, Wood T, Bowman MC, de Boer KA, Jansen RPS (2005) Elective transfer of single fresh blastocysts and later transfer of cryostored blastocysts reduces the twin pregnancy rate and can improve the in vitro fertilization live birth rate in younger women. *Fertil Steril* 84, 1620–1627.

Hidlebaugh DA, Thompson IE, Berger MJ (1997) Cost of assisted reproductive technologies for a health maintenance organization. *J Reprod Med* 42, 570–574.

Hsu M-I, Mayer J, Aronshon M, Lanzendorf S, Muasher S, Kolm P, Oehninger S (1999) Embryo implantation in in vitro fertilization and intracytoplasmic sperm injection: impact of cleavage status, morphology grade, and number of embryos transferred. *Fertil Steril* 72, 679–685.

Jackson KV, Ginsburg ES, Hornstein MD, Rein MS, Clarke RN (1998) Multinucleation in normally fertilized embryos is associated with an accelerated ovulation induction response and lower implantation and pregnancy rates in in vitro fertilization-embryo transfer cycles. *Fertil Steril* 70, 60–66.

Jackson RA, Gibson KA, Wu YW, Croughan MS (2004) Perinatal outcome in singletons following in vitro fertilization: a meta-analysis. *Obstet Gynecol* 103, 551–563.

Jain T, Harlow BL, Horstein MD (2002) Insurance coverage and outcomes of in vitro fertilization. *N Engl J Med* 347, 661–666.

Jones HW, Schnorr JA (2001) Multiple pregnancies: a call for action. *Fertil Steril* 75, 11–17.

Jones HW Jr., Veeck LL, Muasher SJ (1995) Cryopreservation: the problem of evaluation. *Hum Reprod* 10, 2136–2138.

Jones HW Jr., Jones D, Kolm P (1997a) Cryopreservation: a simplified method of evaluation. *Hum Reprod* 12, 584–553.

Jones HW Jr., Out HJ, Hoomans EHM, Driessen GAJ, Coelingh Bennink HJT (1997b) Cryopreservation: the practicalities of evaluation. *Hum Reprod* 12, 1522–1524.

Klemetti R, Gissler M, Hemminski E (2002) Comparison of perinatal health of children born from IVF in Finland in the early and late 1990s. *Hum Reprod* 17, 2192–2198.

Kligman I, Benadiva C, Alikani M, Munné S (1996) The presence of multinucleated blastomeres in human embryos is correlated with chromosomal abnormalities. *Hum Reprod* 11, 1492–1498.

Kolibianakis EM, Devroey P (2002) Blastocyst culture: facts and fiction. *Reprod Biomed Online* 5, 285–293.

Kolibianakis EM, Zikopoulos K, Verpoest W, Joris H, Van Steirteghem AC, Devroey P (2004) Should we advise patients undergoing IVF to start a cycle leading to a day 3 or a day 5 transfer? *Hum Reprod.* In press.

Koudstaal J, Bruinse HW, Helmerhorst FM, Vermeiden JPW, Willemsen WNP, Visser GHA (2000a) Obstetric outcome of twin pregnancies after in-vitro fertilization: a matched control study in four Dutch University hospitals. *Hum Reprod* 15, 935–940.

Koudstaal J, Braat DDM, Bruinse HW, Naaktgeboren N, Vermeiden JPW, Visser GHA (2000b) Obstetric outcome of singleton pregnancies after in-vitro fertilization: a matched control study in four Dutch University hospitals. *Hum Reprod* 15, 1819–1825.

Ledger WL, Anumba D, Marlow N, Thomas CM, Wilson ECF; the Cost of Multiple Births Study Group (COMBS Group) (2006) The costs to the NHS of multiple births after IVF treatment in the UK. *BJOG* 113, 21–25.

Lukassen HGM, Schönbeck Y, Adang EMM, Braat DDM, Zielhuis GA, Kremer JAM (2004) Cost analysis of singleton versus twin pregnancies after in vitro fertilization. *Fertil Steril* 81, 1240–1246.

Lynch A, McDuffie R Jr, Murphy J, Faber K, Orleans M (2002) Preeclampsia in multiple gestation: the role of assisted reproductive technologies. *Obstet Gynecol* 99, 445–451.

Martikainen H, Tiitinen A, Tomàs C, Tapanainen J, Orava M, Tuomivaara L, Vilska S, Hydèn-Granskog C, Hovatta O, Finnish (2001) One versus two embryo transfers after IVF and ICSI: randomized study. *Hum Reprod* 16, 1900–1903.

Martin PM, Welch HG (1998) Probabilities for singleton and multiple pregnancies after in vitro fertilization. *Fertil Steril* 70, 478–481.

Milki AA, Fisch JD, Behr B (1999) Two-blastocyst transfer has similar pregnancy rates and a decreased multiple gestation rate compared with three-blastocyst transfer. *Fertil Steril* 72, 225–228.

Minaretzis D, Harris D, Alper MM, Mortola JF, Berger MJ, Power D (1998) Multivariate analysis of factors predictive of successful live births in in vitro fertilization (IVF) suggests strategies to improve IVF outcome. *J Assist Reprod Genet* 15, 365–371.

Murray S, Shetty A, Rattray A, Taylor V, Bhattacharya S (2004) A randomized comparison of alternative methods of information provision on the acceptability of elective single embryo transfer. *Hum Reprod* 19, 911–916.

Obasaju M, Kadam A, Biancardi T, Sultan K, Munné S (2001) Pregnancies from single normal embryo transfer in women older than 40 years. *Reprod BioMed Online* 2, 98–101.

Ombelet W, De Sutter P, Van der Elst J, Martens G (2005) Multiple gestation and infertility treatment: registration, reflection and reaction—the Belgian project. *Hum Reprod Update* 11, 3–14.

Ostfeld BM, Smith RH, Hiatt M, Hegyi T (2000) Maternal behavior toward premature twins: implications for development. *Twin Res* 3, 234–241.

Ozturk O, Bhattacharya S, Templeton A (2001) Avoiding multiple pregnancies in ART. Evaluation and implementation of new strategies. *Hum Reprod* 16, 1319–1321.

Palmstierna M, Murkes D, Cseminczky Andersson O, Wramby H (1998) Zona pellucida thickness variation and occurrence of visible mononucleated blastomeres in preembryos are associated with a high pregnancy rate in IVF treatment. *J Assist Reprod Genet* 15, 70–74.

Pandian Z, Templeton A, Serour G, Bhattacharya S. (2005) Number of embryos for transfer after IVF and ICSI: a Cochrane review. *Hum Reprod* 20, 2681–2687.

Papanikolaou EG, D'haeseleer E, Verheyen G, Van de Velde H, Camus M, Van Steirteghem A, Devroey P, Tournaye H (2005) Live birth rate is significantly higher after blastocyst transfer than after cleavage-stage embryo transfer when at least four embryos are available on day 3 of embryo culture. A randomized prospective study. *Hum Reprod* 20, 3198–3203.

Pelinck MJ, De Vos M, Dekens M, Van der Elst J, De Sutter P, Dhont M (1998) Embryos cultured *in vitro* with multinucleated blastomeres have poor implantation potential in human in-vitro fertilization and intracytoplasmic sperm injection. *Hum Reprod* 13, 960–963.

Pelinck MJ, Hoek A, Simmons AHM, Heineman MJ (2002) Efficacy of natural cycle IVF: a review of the literature. *Hum Reprod* 8, 129–139.

Pennings G (2000) Multiple pregnancies: a test case for the moral quality of medically assisted reproduction. *Hum Reprod* 15, 2466–2469.

Pickering BJ, Taylor A, Johnson MH, Braude PR (1995) An analysis of multinucleated blastomere formation in human embryos. *Mol Hum Reprod* 10, 1912–1922.

Pinborg A, Loft A, Schmidt L, Andersen NA (2003) Attitudes of IVF/ICSI-twin mothers towards twins and single embryo transfer. *Hum Reprod* 18, 621–627.

Pinborg A, Lidegaard Ø, la Cour Freiesleben N, Andersen AN (2005) Consequences of vanishing twins in IVF/ICSI pregnancies. *Hum Reprod* 20, 2821–2829.

Pons JC, Charlemaine C, Dubreuil E, Papiernik E, Frydman R (1998a) Management and outcome of triplet pregnancy. *Eur J Obstet Gynecol Reprod Biol* 76, 131–139.

Pons JC, Suares F, Duyme M, Pourade A, Vial M, Papiernik E, Frydman R (1998b) Prévention de la prématurité au cours du suivi de 842 grossesses gémellaires consécutives. *J Gynecol Obstet Biol Reprod* 27, 319–328.

Reynolds MA, Schieve L, Jeng G, Peterson HB (2003) Does insurance coverage decrease the risk for multiple births associated with assisted reproductive technology? *Fertil Steril* 80, 16–22.

Rienzi L, Ubaldi F, Iacobelli M, Ferrero S, Minasi MG, Martinez F, Tesarik J, Greco E (2002) Day 3 embryo transfer with combined evaluation at the pronuclear and cleavage stages compares favourably with day 5 blastocyst transfer. *Hum Reprod* 17, 1852–1855.

Rizk B, Aboulghar MA, Mansour RT, et al. (1991) Severe ovarian hyperstimulation syndrome: analytical study of twenty-one cases. *Hum Reprod* 6, S368–9.

Rizk B, Davies M, Kingsland C, et al. (1989) *How many embryos should be replaced in an in vitro fertilization programme?*. *6th World Congress for In Vitro Fertilization and Alternate Conception Techniques.* Jerusalem, Israel. Abstract Book, p. 97.

Roberston JA (2004) Protecting embryos and burdening women: assisted reproduction in Italy. *Hum Reprod* 19, 1693–1696.

Roest J, van Heusden AM, Verhoeff A, Mous HVH, Zeilmaker GH (1997) A triplet pregnancy after in vitro fertilization is a procedure-related complication that should be prevented by replacement of two embryos only. *Fertil Steril* 67, 290–295.

Roseboom TJ, Vermeiden JPW, Schoute E, Lens JW, Schats R (1995) The probability of pregnancy after embryo transfer is affected by the age of the patient, cause of infertility, number of embryos transferred and the average morphology score, as revealed by multiple logistic regression analysis. *Hum Reprod* 10, 3035–3041.

Ryan GL, Van Voorhis BJ (2004) The desire of infertile patients for multiple gestations—do they know the risks. *Fertil Steril* 81, 526.

Rydhstroem H, Heraib F (2001) Gestational duration, and fetal and infant mortality for twins vs. singletons. *Twin Res* 4, 227–231.

Salumets A, Hydén-Granskog C, Mäkinen S, Suikkari A-M, Tiitinen A, Tuuri T (2003) Early cleavage predicts the viability of human embryos in elective single embryo transfer procedure. *Hum Reprod* 18, 821–825.

Senat M-V, Ancel P-Y, Bouvier-Colle M-H, Bréart G (1998) How does multiple pregnancy affect maternal mortality and morbidity? *Clin Obstet Gynaecol* 41, 79–83.

Shapiro BS, Harris DC, Richter KS (2000) Predictive value of 72-hour blastomere cell number on blastocyst development and success of subsequent transfer based on the degree of blastocyst development. *Fertil Steril* 73, 582–586.

Shapiro BS, Richter KS, Harris DC, Daneshmand ST (2001) Dramatic declines in implantation and pregnancy rates in patients who undergo repeated cycles of in vitro fertilization with blastocyst transfer after one or more failed attempts. *Fertil Steril* 76, 538–542.

Söderström-Anttila V, Vilska S, Mäkinen S, Foudila T, Suikkari AM (2003) Elective single embryo transfer yields good delivery rates in oocyte donation. *Hum Reprod* 18, 1858–1863.

Staessen C, Camus M, Bollen N, Devroey P, Van Steirteghem A (1992) The relationship between embryo quality and the occurrence of multiple pregnancies. *Fertil Steril* 57, 626–630.

Staessen C, Janssenswillen C, Van Den Abbeel E, Devroey P, Van Steirteghem A (1993) Avoidance of triplet pregnancies by elective transfer of two good quality embryos. *Hum Reprod* 8, 1650–1653.

Stillman RJ, Richter KS, Tucker MJ, Kearns WG, Widra EA (2005) Preliminary experience with elective single embryo transfer (eSET). *Fertil Steril* 84(Suppl. 1), S81.

Strandell A, Bergh C, Lundin K (2000) Selection of patients suitable for one-embryo transfer may reduce the rate of multiple births by half without impairment of overall birth rates. *Hum Reprod* 15, 2520–2525.

Strömberg B, Dahlquist G, Ericson A, Finnström O, Köster M, Stjernqvist K (2002) Neurological sequelae in children born after in-vitro fertilization: a population-based study. *Lancet* 359; 461–465.

Svendsen TO, Jones D, Butler L, Muasher SJ (1996) The incidence of multiple gestations after in vitro fertilization is dependent on the number of embryos transferred and maternal age. *Fertil Steril* 65, 561–563.

Tan SL, Doyle P, Campbell S, et al. (1992) Obstetric outcome of in vitro fertilization pregnancies compared with normally conceived pregnancies. *Am J Obstet Gynecol* 167(3), 778–784.

Tasdemir M, Tasdemir I, Kodama H, Fukuda J, Tanaka T (1995) Two instead of three embryo transfer in in-vitro fertilization. *Hum Reprod* 10, 2155–2158.

Templeton A, Morris JK (1996) Factors that affect outcome of in-vitro fertilization treatment. *Lancet* 348, 1402–1406.

Templeton A, Morris JK (1998) Reducing the risk of multiple birth by transfer of two embryos after *in vitro* fertilization. *N Engl J Med* 339, 573–577.

Thurin A, Hausken J, Hillensjö T, Jablonowska B, Pinborg A, Strandell A, Bergh C (2004) Elective single embryo transfer in IVF, a randomized study. *N Engl J Med* 351, 2392–2402.

Tiitinen A, Halttunen M, Härkki P, Vuoristo P, Hydén-Granskog C (2001) Elective embryo transfer: the value of cryopreservation. *Hum Reprod* 16, 1140–1144.

Tiitinen A, Unkila-Kallio L, Halttunen M, Hydén-Granskog C (2003) Impact of elective single embryo transfer on the twin pregnancy rate. *Hum Reprod* 18, 1449–1453.

Trimarchi JR (2001) A mathematical model for predicting which embryos to transfer – an illusion of control or a powerful tool? *Fertil Steril* 76, 1286–1288.

Uchiyama K, Aono F, Kuwayama M, Osada H, Kato O (2004) The efficacy of single embryo transfer with vitrification. *Hum Reprod* 19(Suppl. 1), i135.

Utsunomiya T, Ito H, Nagaki M, Sato J (2004) A prospective, randomized study: day 3 versus hatching blastocyst stage. *Hum Reprod* 19, 1598–1603.

van Montfoort APA, Janssen JM, Fiddelers AAA, Derhaag JG, Dirksen CD, Evers JLH, Dumoulin JCM (2004) Single versus double embryo transfer: a randomized study. *Hum Reprod* 19(Suppl. 1), i134.

van Montfoort APA, Fiddelers AAA, Janssen JM, Derhaag JG, Dirksen CD, Dunselman GAJ, Land JA, Geraedts JPM, Evers JLH, Dumoulin JCM (2006) In unselected patients, elective single embryo transfer prevents all multiples, but results in significantly lower pregnancy rates compared with double embryo transfer: a randomized controlled trial. *Hum Reprod* 21, 338–343.

Van Royen E, Mangelschots K, De Neubourg D, Valkenburg M, Van de Meerssche M, Ryckaert G, Eestermans W, Gerris J (1999) Characterization of a top quality embryo, a step towards single-embryo transfer. *Hum Reprod* 14, 2345–2349.

Van Royen E, Mangelschots K, De Neubourg D, Laureys I, Ryckaert G, Gerris J (2001) Calculating the implantation potential of day 3 embryos in women younger than 38 years of age: a new model. *Hum Reprod* 16, 326–332.

Van Royen E, Mangelschots K, Vercruyssen M, De Neubourg D, Valkenburg M, Ryckaert G, Gerris J (2003) Multinucleation in cleavage stage embryos. *Hum Reprod* 18, 1062–1069.

Vauthier-Brouzes D, Lefebvre G, Lessourd S, Gonzales J, Darbois Y (1994) How many embryos should be transferred in in vitro fertilization? A prospective randomized study. *Fertil Steril* 62, 339–342.

Vilska S, Tiitinen A (2004) National experience with elective single-embryo transfer: Finland. In Gerris J, Olivennes F, De Sutter P (eds.) *Assisted Reproduction Technologies. Quality and Safety.* The Parthenon Publishing Group, New York, pp. 106–112.

Vilska S, Tiitinen A, Hydèn-Granskog C, Hovatta O (1999) Elective transfer of one embryo results in an acceptable pregnancy rate and eliminates the risk of multiple birth. *Hum Reprod* 14, 2392–2395.

Wang J, Lane M, Norman RJ (2006) Reducing multiple pregnancy from assisted reproduction treatment: educating patients and medical staff. *Med J Aust* 184, 180–181.

Wang JX, Norman RJ, Kristiansson P (2002) The effect of various infertility treatments on the risk of preterm birth. *Hum Reprod* 17, 945–949.

Wennerholm UB (2004) Obstetric risks and neonatal complications of twin pregnancy and higher-order multiple pregnancy. In Gerris J, Olivennes F, De Sutter P (eds.) *Assisted Reproduction Technologies. Quality and Safety*. The Parthenon Publishing Group, New York, pp. 23–38.

Wennerholm UB, Bergh C (2000) Obstetric outcome and follow-up of children born after in vitro fertilisation (IVF). *Hum Reprod* 3, 52–64.

Wennerholm UB, Bergh C (2004a,b) Outcome of IVF pregnancies. *Fetal Maternal Med Rev* 15, 27–57.

Wølner-Hanssen P, Rydhstroem H (1998) Cost-effectiveness analysis of in-vitro fertilization: estimated costs per successful pregnancy after transfer of one or two embryos. *Hum Reprod* 13, 88–94.

Ziebe S, Bangsbøll S, Schmidt KLT, Loft A, Lindhard A, Nyboe Andersen A (2004) Embryo quality in natural versus stimulated cycles. *Hum Reprod* 19, 1457–1460.

56

Blastocyst Transfer

David K. Gardner

INTRODUCTION

Over the past three decades basic research has culminated in many significant advances in human assisted conception (Edwards 2004). An example of this is the relatively recent development of more physiological culture conditions. By employing such conditions, it has become possible to culture the human embryo to the blastocyst stage as a matter of routine (Gardner and Lane 1997). Clinics now have more options regarding the day of embryo transfer, giving increased flexibility in scheduling. Subsequently, the question raised is, is there an optimal day for embryo transfer following IVF in the human? In this chapter, the probable advantages of blastocyst transfer are discussed and the clinical data reviewed.

There are numerous potential benefits of blastocyst transfer in human IVF, which are summarized in Table 56.1. Not all sperm or oocytes are destined to give rise to a viable embryo (Tesarik 1994). By culturing the human embryo past the cleavage stages, that is, past embryonic genome activation (Braude et al. 1988), it is feasible to study the embryo properly. A key factor in determining transfer outcome in animal models is the synchronization of the embryo with the female reproductive tract. In all mammalian species studied to date, including nonhuman primates (Marston et al. 1977), the transfer of embryos to the uterus prior to compaction (and, therefore, before the generation of the first transporting epithelium) results in greatly reduced pregnancy rates compared to the transfer of morulae or blastocysts. The significance of transferring embryos post-compaction is that the embryo has greater control of its homeostasis due to the presence of an epithelium (Gardner and Lane, 2005) and synchronizes the metabolism of the embryo with the nutrients available (Gardner et al. 1996). Although the human cleavage-stage embryo can develop in the uterus, in vivo the cleavage-stage embryo resides in the Fallopian tube until day 4 (Croxatto et al. 1978), that is, asynchronous transfers are being performed in the majority of IVF cases. Embryo and uterine asynchrony in all animal models is not consistent with optimal transfer outcome (Barnes 2000). Furthermore, it has been demonstrated in animal models that the environment within the female tract following gonadotropin treatment of the female is not as supportive to embryonic development as that within a female during a natural cycle (Van der Auwera et al. 1999; Ertzeid and Storeng 2001; Kelley et al. 2006). Such observations raise concerns regarding the suitability of the uterine environment following a patient's exposure to exogenous gonadotropins. Clinical data also support the hypothesis that the uterine milieu is compromised following hyperstimulation (Pellicer et al. 1996; Simon et al. 1998). Therefore, it may be preferable to expose embryos to such an altered uterine environment for as short a period as possible, which can be achieved through blastocyst transfer. Finally, it has been demonstrated that there exist significant uterine contractions post-hCG, which greatly diminish over time (Lesny et al. 1998; Fanchin et al. 2001). By day 5 of embryo development, these contractions have ceased, thereby minimizing the chance of mechanical expulsion from the uterus. Subsequently, it would appear that the transfer of human embryos at the blastocyst stage has a sound physiological basis.

HOW CAN VIABLE HUMAN BLASTOCYSTS BE OBTAINED IN THE IVF LABORATORY?

In order to optimize embryo culture and blastocyst transfer, one needs to consider all aspects of a treatment cycle, as exemplified in Figure 56.1 (Gardner and Lane 2003). Improvements in the environment and the quality in the embryology laboratory (Cohen et al. 2007), in culture media (Gardner and Lane 1997, 2005, 2007; Summers and Biggers 2003; Lane and Gardner 2005, 2007), and in the equipment used to produce embryos and embryo selection methods (Ebner et al. 2003; Sakkas and Gardner 2005) have all had positive impacts on the results of embryo transfers. Subsequently, in order to obtain results established by other programs, changes other than culture media alone will almost certainly be required.

CLINICAL DATA ON BLASTOCYST TRANSFER

Huisman et al., (1994) compared day 2, day 3, and day 4 transfers in a retrospective analysis. It was determined that the overall implantation and pregnancy rates were not significantly different. Of interest, when cavitating morula were present on day 4, an implantation rate of 41 percent was attained. In contrast, if there were no cavitating morula, implantation rates on day 2, day 3, or day 4 ranged between 12.7 and 14.4 percent. Scholtes and Zeilmaker (1996) performed a randomized trial comparing day 3 versus day 5 embryo transfer. The implantation and pregnancy rates were 23 and 40 percent for day 5 transfers compared to 15 and 28 percent for day 3 transfers. These studies indicate that if an embryo has developed to the appropriate stage on day 4 or 5, then viability is increased compared to when embryos are transferred on either day 2 or

Table 56.1: Potential Benefits of Blastocyst Transfer in Human IVF

- Ability to identify those embryos with limited as well as those with the highest, developmental potential through morphological assessment and grading

- Assessment of the embryo post genome activation

- Synchronization of embryonic stage with the female tract to reduce cellular stress on the embryo

- Minimizing exposure of the embryo to a hyperstimulated uterine environment

- Reduction in uterine contractions by day 5, thereby reducing the chance of the embryo being expelled

- Higher implantation rates leading to a reduction in the number of embryos transferred

- Ability to undertake cleavage-stage embryo biopsy without the need for cryopreservation when the biopsied blastomere has to be sent to a different locale for analysis

- Ability to undertake trophectoderm biopsy rather than cleavage-stage biopsy, thereby increasing the number of cells analyzed (typically six to ten) and overcoming ethical/religious concerns of sampling embryonic tissue

- Increased ability to survive cryopreservation

- Increase in overall efficiency of IVF

---

day 3. Interestingly, the studies above used a mixture of Earle's and Ham's F10 media for culture, neither of which have physiological concentrations of a number of components, and these could not be described as sequential even though technically two media were employed. Therefore, care must be taken when comparing data from different studies as different culture conditions can support similar rates of blastocyst development, but result in dramatically different implantation rates (Gardner and Lane 1997; Gardner 1998).

With the introduction of sequential media, designed to account for physiological changes in the human embryo and maternal milieu, there have been numerous studies on human blastocyst transfer in IVF. The use of more physiological culture systems to support human blastocyst development was initially offered to patients with either a good response to gonadotropins (Gardner et al. 1998) or with more than 4 eight-cell embryos on day 3 (Milki et al. 2000). This approach for good-prognosis patients was associated with a significant increase in implantation rates and facilitated the establishment of high pregnancy rates (70 percent), while the number of embryos transferred was reduced. Subsequently, blastocyst transfer has been used effectively to reduce the incidence of high-order multiple gestations and could greatly facilitate the move to single embryo transfer (SET) in human assisted conception (Gardner et al. 2004a; Kissin et al. 2005).

Blastocyst transfer has now been used successfully to treat patients with poor-quality embryos (Balaban et al. 2001a; Langley et al. 2001), patients with multiple IVF failures (Cruz et al. 1999; Levitas et al. 2004; Guerif et al. 2005), patients with low numbers of oocytes and embryos (Wilson et al. 2002; Trokoudes et al. 2005), and oocyte donors (Schoolcraft and

Gardner 2000). Blastocyst transfer has even been proposed as an alternative, or at least a complement, to preimplantation genetic diagnosis (Menezo et al. 2001). Although the examples listed above show that extended embryo culture has been associated with an increase in IVF success rates, there are a number of reports that question the merits of extended culture (Alikani et al. 2000; Coskun et al. 2000; Kolibianakis and Devroey 2002; Rienzi et al. 2002).

Parental factors also affect blastocyst development and subsequent implantation rates. As maternal age increases, both the number and quality of the oocytes retrieved is reduced, thus affecting the outcome of blastocyst transfer (Scholtes and Zeilmaker 1998; Pantos et al. 1999). The success of blastocyst culture has also been shown to be under paternal influence (Janny and Menezo 1994). Blastocyst formation is affected by the source of spermatozoa utilized for intracytoplasmic sperm injection. In close relation to this, implantation and clinical pregnancy rates with blastocyst transfers decrease with the increase in severity of the spermatogenic disorder (Balaban et al. 2001b).

Seventeen prospective randomized trials using sequential media have examined the effect of day of transfer on IVF cycle outcome (Table 56.2) (Gardner et al. 1998; Coskun et al. 2000; Karaki et al. 2002; Levron et al. 2002; Rienzi et al. 2002; Utsunomiya et al. 2002; Van der Auwera et al. 2002; Bungum et al. 2003; Emiliani et al. 2003; Frattarelli et al. 2003; Margreiter et al. 2003; Hreinsson et al. 2004; Kolibianakis et al.2004; Levitas et al. 2004; Pantos et al. 2004; Papanikolaou et al. 2005, 2006a). Of these seventeen trials, eight reported a significant benefit in outcome as defined by either increased implantation rate or pregnancy rates (one study only reported pregnancy rates) when embryos were transferred at the blastocyst stage on day 5 rather than at the cleavage stage. In contrast, only one study found a significant advantage in transferring embryos at the cleavage stage (Levron et al. 2002). The remaining eight trials reported no difference in implantation rate with respect to day of transfer. Interestingly, in a Cochrane review on cleavage-stage versus blastocyst-stage embryo transfer (Blake et al. 2003), it was concluded that in clinical trials in which sequential media were used there was "a substantial improvement in implantation rates" following blastocyst transfer.

So how can such discrepancies in outcome be resolved? Seven of the trials that showed a benefit of day 5 transfer (Table 56.2) were based on relatively good-prognosis patients. So from this, it would appear that in younger patients, or those with good ovarian reserve, that blastocyst transfer is a viable effective treatment. Certainly, there are growing data to support this hypothesis (Papanikolaou et al. 2005, 2006b).

Regrettably, of the seventeen trials listed in Table 56.2, there is limited information on the culture system (as described in Figure 56.1) used. Although the media types are listed in most cases, there is limited information available on other components of the culture system used. Also, important laboratory information is missing, such as the number and type of incubators, the types of air-handling systems, and so on. It would be extremely valuable to start documenting such parameters in order to determine the impact of such variables on IVF outcome.

With the exception of just one study out of the seventeen listed in Table 56.2, there is no negative impact on blastocyst transfer with regard to implantation and pregnancy rates. Therefore, certain programs have taken the philosophy that blastocyst transfer is beneficial for all patients. In such clinics,

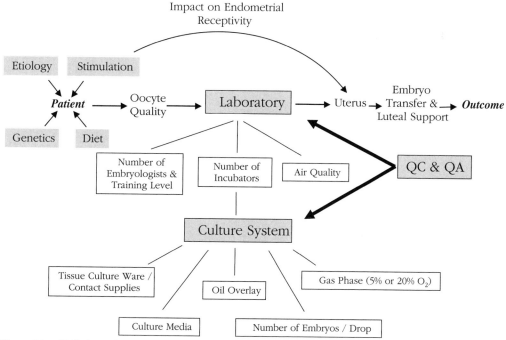

Figure 56.1. Holistic analysis of human IVF. This figure serves to illustrate the complex and interdependent nature of human IVF treatment. For example, the stimulation regimen not only impacts oocyte quality (hence embryo physiology and viability) (Hardy et al. 1995) but also can affect subsequent endometrial receptivity (Simon et al. 1998; Van der Auwera et al. 1999; Ertzeid and Storeng 2001; Kelley et al. 2006). It is also apparent that a patient's etiology and genetics will impact their cycle outcome. Furthermore, the health and dietary status of the patient can have a profound effect on the subsequent developmental capacity of the oocyte and embryo. The dietary status of patients attending IVF is typically not considered as a compounding variable, but growing data would indicate that nutrition can have a profound effect on oocyte and embryo quality (Kwong et al. 2000; Armstrong et al. 2001; Gardner et al. 2004b, 2004c). In this schematic, the laboratory can be broken down into its core components, only one of which is the culture system. The culture system can be broken down into its components, only one of which is the culture media. Therefore, it would appear rather simplistic to assume that the results of a given laboratory or clinic can be mimicked by changing only one part of the culture system (i.e., culture media). A major determinant of the success of a laboratory and culture system is the level of quality control and quality assurance in place (Mortimer et al. 2005). For example, one should never assume that anything coming into the laboratory that has not been pretested with a relevant bioassay (e.g., mouse embryo assay) is safe merely because a previous lot has performed satisfactorily. Only a small percentage of the contact supplies and tissue culture ware used in IVF comes suitably tested. Therefore, it is essential to assume that everything entering the IVF laboratory without a suitable pretest is embryo toxic until proven otherwise. In our program, the one-cell mouse embryo assay (MEA) is employed to prescreen every lot of tissue culture ware that enters the program, that is, plastics that are approved for tissue culture. Around 25 percent of all such material fails the one-cell MEA (in a simple medium lacking protein after the first twenty-four hours) (Gardner et al. 2005). Therefore, if one does not perform QC to this level, one in four of all contact supplies used clinically could compromise embryo development. In reality, many programs cannot allocate the resources required for this level of QC; and when embryo quality is compromised in the laboratory, it is the media that are held responsible, when in fact the tissue culture ware is more often the culprit. Adapted from Gardner and Lane (2003), with permission from Reproductive Healthcare Ltd.

the move to extended culture and day 5 transfer resulted in increases in IVF outcome, although such analyses have been retrospective (Marek et al. 1999; Wilson et al. 2002).

SELECTION OF EMBRYOS

By culturing the human embryo to the blastocyst stage, one is not only looking at the embryo postgenome activation, but one can evaluate the two cell types that have differentiated, specifically the inner cell mass (ICM) and trophectoderm. Grading systems have been developed to accommodate the degree of blastocoel expansion, differentiation of the ICM, together with the shape of the ICM (Dokras et al. 1993; Gardner and Schoolcraft 1999; Richter et al. 2001; Kovacic et al. 2004; Gardner et al. 2007). In a randomized trial, it was established that a grading system that took into account ICM differentiation rather than simply blastocyst expansion alone was more effective in selecting embryos of higher implantation potential (Balaban et al. 2006). The use of image analysis systems to further capture and characterize the key morphological characteristics associated with subsequent pregnancy should also lead to improvements in blastocyst selection. Figure 56.2 presents a human blastocyst

Table 56.2: Prospective Randomized Trials on the Transfer of Either Cleavage-Stage Embryos or Blastocysts following Culture in Similar Media Types

Author	Patient population	Cleavage stage			Blastocyst		
		Embryos transferred	Implantation rate (%)	Pregnancy (%)	Embryos transferred	Implantation rate (%)	Pregnancy (%)
Gardner et al. (1998)	More than ten follicles of >12 mm on day of hCG	3.7	37.0	66	2.2	55.4**	71
Coskun et al. (2000)	Greater than or equal to four 2PN	2.3	21	39	2.2	24	39
Karaki et al. (2002)	Greater than or equal to five 2PN	3.5	13	26	2.0	26**	29
Levron et al. (2002)	Younger than thirty-eight years and more than five 2PN	3.1	38.7**	45.5	2.3	20.2	18.6
Utsonomiya et al. (2002)	All	2.9	11.7	26.3	3.0	9.2	24.9
Rienzi et al. (2002)	Younger than thirty-eight years and greater than or equal to eight 2PN by ICSI	2	35	58	2	38	62
Van der Auwera et al. (2002)	All (day 2 transfers)	1.86	29	32	1.87	46*	44
Fratarelli et al. (2003)	Younger than thirty-five years, no previous IVF, and greater than or equal to ten follicles of ≥14 mm on day of hCG	2.96	26.1	43.5	2.04	43.4*	69.2
Emiliani et al. (2003)	Younger than thirty-nine years (day 2 transfers)	2.1	29	49	1.9	30	44

Study	Patient selection						
Magreiter et al. (2003)	Mean age of 32.1 years with a mean of seven pronucleate oocytes (days 1–5 transfers)			20 on day 1 and 30.4 on days 2 and 3			50 * on days 4 and 5
Bungum et al. (2003)	Younger than forty years, FSH <12 IU/L, more than two 8-cell embryo with <20 percent fragmentation	2.0	43.9	61	1.96	36.7	51
Pantos et al. (2004)	Younger than forty years, less than four previous failures, days 2 and 3	4.0	15.7 and 16	46.9 and 48.1	3.39	15.6	37
Levitas et al. (2004)	Younger than thirty-seven years and three failed IVF attempts	3.4	6.0	12.9	1.9	21.2 **	21.7
Hreinsson et al. (2004)	More than five follicles, days 2 and 3	1.8	20.9	36.7	1.9	21.1	32.5
Kolibianakis et al. (2004)	Younger than forty-three years	1.9	24.5	33.1	1.8	24.5	33.2
Papanikolaou et al. (2005)	Younger than thirty-seven years, more than three embryos with >5-cell and <20 percent fragmentation	2.0	20.6	27.4	1.97	37.3 **	51.3 **
Papanikolaou et al. (2006a)	Younger than thirty-six, first or second cycle, FSH <12	1.0	24.0	22.2	1.0	34.3 *	34.3 **

Significantly different to cleavage-stage transfer; *P < 0.05; **P < 0.01.

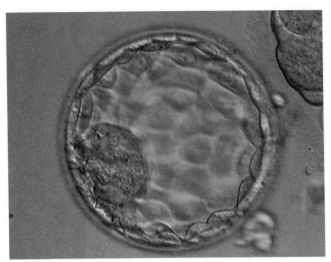

Figure 56.2. Photomicrograph of a day 5 human blastocyst. The embryo in the figure was cultured for four days from the pronucleate oocyte stage: forty-eight hours in medium G1, followed by forty-eight hours in medium G2. The gas phase was 6 percent carbon dioxide and 5 percent oxygen, the remaining 89 percent of the gas being nitrogen. The blastocyst was graded as 4AA.

with a grade of 4AA, which reflects an implantation potential of more than 60 percent. It is evident that such embryos should be transferred individually.

However, assessment of morphology alone provides little insight into the physiology of the embryo. Further increases in implantation rates will come from the application of noninvasive methods to assess the metabolism of the blastocyst (Lane and Gardner 1996; Gardner and Leese 1999) together with the identification of specific factors produced by the embryo at stage-specific times (Sakkas et al. 2003; Noci et al. 2005; Katz-Jaffe et al. 2006). It is envisaged that the analysis of blastocyst physiology will greatly assist in the move to SET.

CUMULATIVE PREGNANCY RATES AND THE IMPACT OF CRYOPRESERVATION

The initial introduction of blastocyst culture was not well received by many clinics due to their poor success with blastocyst cryopreservation (Alper et al. 2001). However, with the development of more suitable freezing procedures, it is now possible to obtain implantation and ongoing pregnancy rates (OPR) of greater than 30 and 60 percent, respectively, using frozen-thawed blastocysts (Gardner et al. 2003; Veeck et al. 2004; Kosasa et al. 2005). Such data reveal that blastocyst cryopreservation is actually highly effective. Indeed, two studies have indicated that blastocyst cryopreservation is more effective than that of cleavage-stage embryo (Veeck 2003; Anderson et al. 2004). These data, therefore, indicate that appropriate blastocyst cryopreservation will assist in increasing the overall efficiency of a given IVF cycle.

Further advances in the cryopreservation of human blastocysts will come in the form of vitrification (Vajta and Nagy 2006). Vitrification is now already the preferred method of cryopreserving embryos of the mouse and cow, and it is only a matter of time before this elegant procedure supercedes slow freezing in the clinical laboratory. Excellent data have now been published on the vitrification of human blastocysts (Takahashi

et al. 2005). Concerns regarding the direct contact of the embryo with liquid nitrogen during the vitrification process have been alleviated (Larman et al. 2006), and new closed systems are being made available.

THE MOVE TO SET

The move to blastocyst transfer has already had a significant impact on reducing the number of embryos required for transfer, thereby greatly reducing the incidence of high-order multiple gestations (Gardner et al. 1998; Kissin et al. 2005). However, although triplets can now be confined to the archives of IVF, the overall multiple rate of many programs has not decreased dramatically as the incidence of twins remains high when two blastocysts are transferred. The only means to avoid this problem is to implement single blastocyst transfer.

In the first prospective randomized trial of single versus two blastocyst transfers, in a population of patients with a day 3 FSH 10 mIU/mL or less and at least ten follicles larger than 12 mm in diameter on day of hCG administration (age range twenty-six to forty-three years), it was possible to establish an ongoing pregnancy rate of 60.9 percent without any incidence of twins (Gardner et al. 2004a). Significantly, when two blastocysts were transferred, the pregnancy rate rose to 76 percent, but with a 47.4 percent incidence of twins.

One group of patients where blastocyst transfer should already become the preferred treatment option is oocyte donors. Schoolcraft and Gardner (2000) determined that it was feasible to attain a 65 percent implantation rate (fetal heart beat) in donor oocyte cycles having a blastocyst transfer, compared to 42 percent implantation rates for recipients having a day 3 transfer. The resultant pregnancy rates were 80 versus 68 percent for transfers on days 5 and 3, respectively. To date, at the Colorado Center for Reproductive Medicine, day 5 transfer has been used on close to 1,000 donor cases, with a resultant implantation and pregnancy rate of 68 and 85 percent. However, of those donors that conceived, only 40 percent had a singleton pregnancy, clearly highlighting the need for SET in such cases.

In a previously reported prospective randomized trial of SET versus double embryo transfer (DET) on day 3 performed on good-prognosis patients (younger than thirty-four years, no previous IVF, and who had at least two top-quality embryos at the time of embryo transfer), an OPR of 38.5 percent was attained in the SET group (Gerris et al. 1999). The implantation rate reported for the SET group was 42.3 percent. Clearly, such implantation and pregnancy rates are excellent, but do fall somewhat short of those obtained with the transfer of a single blastocyst.

Therefore, the move to single blastocyst transfer appears a more viable alternative to SET on day 3 in good-prognosis patients. Papanikolaou and colleagues showed in a prospective randomized trial on SET that not only were higher ongoing pregnancy rates established with SBT but also pregnancy loss was lower and birth rate higher than that obtained with SET (Papanikolaou et al. 2006a, 2006b).

CONCERNS ABOUT MONOZYGOTIC TWINNING AND BLASTOCYST TRANSFER

When blastocyst transfer was introduced on a wider scale toward the end of the twentieth century, there were isolated reports of greatly increased monozygotic twinning rates.

Behr et al. (2000) reported a 5 percent monozygotic twining rate in 199 pregnancies conceived through blastocyst transfer. However, in 2007, the same senior author reported that the monozygotic rate had decreased to 2.3 percent in a subsequent 932 blastocyst transfer cases (Moayeri et al. 2007). This rate was not statistically different to that observed with day 3 transfers in the same program (1.8 percent). It remains unclear why one group would start with a high rate of monozygotic twinning and then have it reduced to the levels typically observed with other modes of assisted conception. However, such observations do support the holistic analysis of IVF concept (Gardner and Lane 2003), in that many variables can impact the outcome of a given IVF cycle.

CONCLUSIONS

The cost-effectiveness of IVF has been analyzed (Collins 2001), and the negative impacts of IVF on the community include heavy medical and financial costs associated with twin, triplet, and quadruplet deliveries (Adashi et al. 2003). Looking at the cost-effectiveness of an SET compared to a DET on day 3 has revealed that even though more ART cycles are required when employing SET, the overall cost per child born is the same as, or cheaper than, DET due to the increased costs associated with multiple births in the latter group (Wolner-Hanssen and Rydhstroem 1998; De Sutter et al. 2002). Therefore, except in countries where the patient has to carry the costs of an IVF treatment but where insurance carriers cover delivery and neonatal care, there are no financial reasons not to elect to move to SET.

Single blastocyst transfer appears to be the most effective treatment for oocyte donors (Schoolcraft and Gardner 2000), for good-prognosis patients (Gardner et al. 1998), and those younger than thirty-six years (Papanikolaou et al. 2006a). It remains to be determined whether blastocyst transfer is effective for all patients, although there are some programs electing to perform day 5 transfers on all patients, with improved overall outcome (Marek et al. 1999; Wilson et al. 2004).

At this time of rapid developments in human assisted conception, it is appropriate to ponder the future of patient treatment. Given the documented evidence for the detrimental effect of exogenous gonadotropins on endometrial function, combined with more effective methods of embryo cryopreservation, that is, ultrarapid vitrification, the day may fast be approaching where we no longer transfer in the retrieval cycle. Rather, embryos are cultured to the blastocyst stage, their morphology graded, their physiology assessed, and their complete karyotype determined through either comparative genome hybridization or gene array technology, following trophectoderm biopsy. Once the blastocyst is biopsied, and therefore collapsed, it is vitrified. Subsequently, a single euploid blastocyst with the highest developmental potential, as determined through morphological grading and noninvasive assays of physiology, is transferred to a natural uterus. What an elegant and effective way to establish a normal singleton pregnancy!

REFERENCES

Adashi E.Y., Barri P.N., Berkowitz R. et al. (2003). Infertility therapy-associated multiple pregnancies (births): an ongoing epidemic. *Reprod Biomed Online* 7, 515–542.

Alikani M., Calderon G., Tomkin G. et al. (2000). Cleavage anomalies in early human embryos and survival after prolonged culture in-vitro. *Hum Reprod* 15, 2634–2643.

Alper M.M., Brinsden P., Fischer R. et al. (2001). To blastocyst or not to blastocyst? That is the question. *Hum Reprod* 16, 617–619.

Anderson A.R., Weikert M.L., and Crain J.L. (2004). Determining the most optimal stage for embryo cryopreservation. *Reprod Biomed Online*, 8, 207–211.

Armstrong D.G., McEvoy T.G., Baxter G. et al. (2001). Effect of dietary energy and protein on bovine follicular dynamics and embryo production in vitro: associations with the ovarian insulin-like growth factor system. *Biol Reprod*, 64, 1624–1632.

Balaban B., Urman B., Alatas C. et al. (2001a) Blastocyst-stage transfer of poor-quality cleavage-stage embryos results in higher implantation rates. *Fertil Steril* 75, 514–518.

Balaban B., Urman B., Isiklar A. et al. (2001b). Blastocyst transfer following intracytoplasmic injection of ejaculated, epididymal or testicular spermatozoa. *Hum Reprod* 16, 125–129.

Balaban B., Yakin K., and Urman B. (2006). Randomized comparison of two different blastocyst grading systems. *Fertil Steril* 85, 559–563.

Barnes F.L. (2000). The effects of the early uterine environment on the subsequent development of embryo and fetus. *Theriogenology*, 53, 649–658.

Behr B., Fisch J.D., Racowsky C. et al. (2000). Blastocyst-ET and monozygotic twinning. *J Assist Reprod Genet* 17, 349–351.

Blake D., Proctor M., Johnson N. et al (2003). Cleavage stage versus blastocyst stage embryo transfer in assisted conception. *Cochrane Database Syst Rev* 1, 1–92.

Braude P., Bolton V., and Moore S. (1988). Human gene expression first occurs between the four- and eight-cell stages of preimplantation development. *Nature* 332, 459–461.

Bungum M., Bungum L., Humaidan P. et al (2003). Day 3 versus day 5 embryo transfer: a prospective randomized study. *Reprod Biomed Online* 7, 98–104.

Cohen J., Gilligan A., and Garris J. (2007). Setting up an ART laboratory. In Gardner D.K., Weissman A., Howles C.M. et al. (eds), *Textbook of Assisted Reproductive Techniques; Laboratory and Clinical Perspectives*. Taylor and Francis, London, pp. 17–24.

Collins J. (2001). Cost-effectiveness of in vitro fertilization. *Semin Reprod Med* 19, 279–289.

Coskun S., Hollanders J., Al Hassan S. et al. (2000). Day 5 versus day 3 embryo transfer: a controlled randomized trial. *Hum Reprod* 15, 1947–1952.

Croxatto H.B., Ortiz M.E., Diaz S. et al. (1978). Studies on the duration of egg transport by the human oviduct. II. Ovum location at various intervals following luteinizing hormone peak. *Am J Obstet Gynecol* 132, 629–634.

Cruz J.R., Dubey A.K., Patel J. et al. (1999). Is blastocyst transfer useful as an alternative treatment for patients with multiple in vitro fertilization failures? *Fertil Steril* 72, 218–220.

De Sutter P., Gerris J., and Dhont M. (2002). A health-economic decision-analytic model comparing double with single embryo transfer in IVF/ICSI. *Hum Reprod* 17, 2891–2896.

Dokras A., Sargent I.L., and Barlow D.H. (1993). Human blastocyst grading: an indicator of developmental potential? *Hum Reprod* 8, 2119–2127.

Ebner T., Moser M., Sommergruber M. et al. (2003). Selection based on morphological assessment of oocytes and embryos at different stages of preimplantation development: a review. *Hum Reprod Update* 9, 251–262.

Edwards R.G. (2004). The beginnings of human in vitro fertilization. In Gardner D.K., Weissman A., Howles C.M. et al. (eds), *Textbook of Assisted Reproductive Techniques: Laboratory and Clinical Perspectives*. Taylor and Francis, London, pp. 1–15.

Emiliani S., Delbaere A., Vannin A.S. et al. (2003). Similar delivery rates in a selected group of patients, for day 2 and day 5 embryos both cultured in sequential medium: a randomized study. *Hum Reprod* 18, 2145–2150.

Ertzeid G. and Storeng R. (2001). The impact of ovarian stimulation on implantation and fetal development in mice. *Hum Reprod* 16, 221–225.

Fanchin R., Ayoubi J.M., Righini C., et al. (2001). Uterine contractility decreases at the time of blastocyst transfers. *Hum Reprod* 16, 1115–1119.

Frattarelli J.L., Leondires M.P., McKeeby J.L. et al. (2003). Blastocyst transfer decreases multiple pregnancy rates in in vitro fertilization cycles: a randomized controlled trial. *Fertil Steril* 79, 228–230.

Gardner D.K. (1998). Changes in requirements and utilization of nutrients during mammalian preimplantation embryo development and their significance in embryo culture. *Theriogenology* 49, 83–102.

Gardner D.K. and Lane M. (1997). Culture and selection of viable blastocysts: a feasible proposition for human IVF? *Hum Reprod Update* 3, 367–382.

Gardner D.K. and Lane M. (2003). Towards a single embryo transfer. *Reprod Biomed Online* 6, 470–481.

Gardner D.K. and Lane M. (2005). Ex-vivo early embryo development and effects on gene expression and imprinting. *Reprod Fertil Dev* 17, 361–370.

Gardner D.K. and Lane M. (2007). Embryo culture systems. In Gardner D.K. (ed), *In Vitro Fertilization: A Practical Approach.* Informa Healthcare, New York, pp. 221–282.

Gardner D.K. and Leese H.J. (1999). Assessment of embryo metabolism and viability. In Trounson A. and Gardner D.K. (eds), *Handbook of In Vitro Fertilization*, Second Ed. CRC Press, Inc., Boca Raton, pp. 347–372.

Gardner D.K. and Schoolcraft W.B. (1999). In-vitro culture of human blastocysts. In Jansen R. and Mortimer D. (eds), *Towards Reproductive Certainty: Fertility and Genetics Beyond* 1999. Parthenon Press, Carnforth, pp. 378–388.

Gardner D.K., Lane M., Calderon I. et al. (1996). Environment of the preimplantation human embryo in vivo: metabolite analysis of oviduct and uterine fluids and metabolism of cumulus cells. *Fertil Steril* 65, 349–353.

Gardner D.K., Schoolcraft W.B., Wagley L. et al. (1998). A prospective randomized trial of blastocyst culture and transfer in in-vitro fertilization. *Hum Reprod* 13, 3434–3440.

Gardner D.K., Lane M., Stevens J. et al. (2003). Changing the start temperature and cooling rate in a slow-freezing protocol increases human blastocyst viability. *Fertil Steril* 79, 407–410.

Gardner D.K., Surrey E., Minjarez D. et al. (2004a). Single blastocyst transfer: a prospective randomized trial. *Fertil Steril* 81, 551–555.

Gardner D.K., Stilley K., and Lane M. (2004b). High protein diet inhibits inner cell mass formation and increases apoptosis in mouse blastocysts developed in vivo by increasing the levels of ammonium in the reproductive tract. *Reprod Fertil Dev* 16, 190.

Gardner D.K., Hewitt E.A., and Linck D. (2004c). Diet affects embryo imprinting and fetal development. *Hum Reprod* 19, i27.

Gardner D.K., Reed L., Linck D. et al. (2005). Quality control in human IVF. *Semin Reprod Med* 23, 319–324.

Gardner D.K., Stevens J., Sheehan C.B. et al. (2007). Analysis of blastocyst morphology. In Elder K., Coehn J. (eds) *Human Preimplantation Embryo Selection.* Informa Healthcare, London, pp. 79–87.

Gerris J., De Neubourg D., Mangelschots K. et al. (1999). Prevention of twin pregnancy after in-vitro fertilization or intracytoplasmic sperm injection based on strict embryo criteria: a prospective randomized clinical trial. *Hum Reprod* 14, 2581–2587.

Guerif F., Bidault R., Gasnier O. et al. (2005). Efficacy of blastocyst transfer after implantation failure. *RBM Online* 9, 630–636.

Hardy K., Robinson F.M., Paraschos T. et al. (1995). Normal development and metabolic activity of preimplantation embryos in vitro from patients with polycystic ovaries. *Hum Reprod* 10, 2125–2135.

Hreinsson J., Rosenlund B., Fridstrom M. et al. (2004). Embryo transfer is equally effective at cleavage stage and blastocyst stage: a randomized prospective study. *Eur J Obstet Gynecol Reprod Biol* 117, 194–200.

Huisman G.J., Alberda A.T., Leerentveld R.A. et al. (1994). A comparison of in vitro fertilization results after embryo transfer after 2, 3, and 4 days of embryo culture. *Fertil Steril* 61, 970–971.

Janny L. and Menezo Y.J. (1994). Evidence for a strong paternal effect on human preimplantation embryo development and blastocyst formation. *Mol Reprod Dev* 38, 36–42.

Karaki R.Z., Samarraie S.S., Younis N.A. et al. (2002). Blastocyst culture and transfer: a step toward improved in vitro fertilization outcome. *Fertil Steril* 77, 114–118.

Katz-Jaffe M.G., Schoolcraft W.B., Gardner D.K. (2006). Analysis of protein expression (secretome) by human and mouse preimplantation embryos. *Fertil Steril* 86, 678–685.

Kelley R.L., Kind K.L., Lane M. et al. (2006). Recombinant human follicle stimulating hormone (rhFSH) alters maternal ovarian hormone concentrations and the uterus, and perturbs fetal development in mice. *Am J Physiol Endocrinol Metab* 291, E761–E770.

Kissin D.M., Schieve L.A., and Reynolds M.A. (2005). Multiple-birth risk associated with IVF and extended embryo culture: USA, 2001. *Hum Reprod* 20, 2215–2223.

Kolibianakis E.M. and Devroey P. (2002). Blastocyst culture: facts and fiction. *Reprod Biomed Online* 5, 285–293.

Kolibianakis E.M., Zikopoulos K., Verpoest W. et al. (2004). Should we advise patients undergoing IVF to start a cycle leading to a day 3 or a day 5 transfer? *Hum Reprod* 19, 2550–2554.

Kosasa T.S., McNamee P.I., Morton C. et al. (2005). Pregnancy rates after transfer of cryopreserved blastocysts cultured in a sequential media. *Am J Obstet Gynecol* 192, 2035–2039.

Kovacic B., Vlaisavljevic V., Reljic M. et al. (2004). Developmental capacity of different morphological types of day 5 human morulae and blastocysts. *Reprod Biomed Online*, 8, 687–694.

Kwong W.Y., Wild A.E., Roberts P. et al. (2000). Maternal undernutrition during the preimplantation period of rat development causes blastocyst abnormalities and programming of postnatal hypertension. *Development* 127, 4195–4202.

Lane M. and Gardner D.K. (1996). Selection of viable mouse blastocysts prior to transfer using a metabolic criterion. *Hum Reprod* 11, 1975–1978.

Lane M. and Gardner D.K. (2005). Understanding the cellular disruptions during early embryo development that cause perturbed viability and fetal development. *Reprod Fertil Dev* 17, 371–378.

Lane M. and Gardner D.K. (2007). Embryo culture medium: which is the best? *Best Pract Res Clin Obstet Gynaecol* 21, 83–100.

Langley M.T., Marek D.M., Gardner D.K. et al. (2001). Extended embryo culture in human assisted reproduction treatments. *Hum Reprod* 16, 902–908.

Larman M.G., Sheehan C.B., and Gardner D.K. (2006). Vitrification of mouse pronuclear oocytes with no direct liquid nitrogen contact. *Reprod Biomed Online*, 12, 66–69.

Lesny P., Killick S.R., Tetlow R.L. et al. (1998). Uterine junctional zone contractions during assisted reproduction cycles. *Hum Reprod Update* 4, 440–445.

Levitas E., Lunenfeld E., Har-Vardi I. et al. (2004). Blastocyst-stage embryo transfer in patients who failed to conceive in three or more day 2-3 embryo transfer cycles: a prospective, randomized study. *Fertil Steril* 81, 567–571.

Levron J., Shulman A., Bider D. et al. (2002). A prospective randomized study comparing day 3 with blastocyst-stage embryo transfer. *Fertil Steril* 77, 1300–1301.

Marek D., Langley M., Gardner D.K. et al. (1999). Introduction of blastocyst culture and transfer for all patients in an in vitro fertilization program. *Fertil Steril* 72, 1035–1040.

Margreiter M., Weghofer A., Kogosowski A. et al. (2003). A prospective randomised multicenter study to evaluate the best day for embryo transfer: Does the outcome justify prolonged embryo culture? *J Assis Reprod Genet*, 20, 91–93.

Marston J.H., Penn R., and Sivelle P.C. (1977). Successful autotransfer of tubal eggs in the rhesus monkey (Macaca mulatta). *J Reprod Fertil*, 49, 175–176.

Menezo Y., Chouteau J., and Veiga A. (2001). In vitro fertilization and blastocyst transfer for carriers of chromosomal translocation. *Eur J Obstet Gynecol Reprod Biol* 96, 193–195.

Milki A.A., Hinckley M.D., Fisch J.D. et al. (2000). Comparison of blastocyst transfer with day 3 embryo transfer in similar patient populations. *Fertil Steril* 73, 126–129.

Moayeri S.E., Behr B., Lathi R.B. et al. (2007). Risk of monozygotic twinning with blastocyst transfer decreases over time: an 8-year experience. *Fertil Steril* 87, 1028–1032.

Mortimer D. and Mortimer S.T. (2005). *Quality and Risk Management in the IVF Laboratory*. Cambridge University Press, Cambridge.

Noci I., Fuzzi B., Rizzo R. et al. (2005). Embryonic soluble HLA-G as a marker of developmental potential in embryos. *Hum Reprod* 20, 138–146.

Pantos K., Athanasiou V., Stefanidis K. et al. (1999). Influence of advanced age on the blastocyst development rate and pregnancy rate in assisted reproductive technology. *Fertil Steril* 71, 1144–1146.

Pantos K., Makrakis E., Stavrou D. et al. (2004). Comparison of embryo transfer on day 2, day 3, and day 6: a prospective randomized study. *Fertil Steril* 81, 454–455.

Papanikolaou E.G., Camus M., Kolibianakis E.M. et al. (2006a). In vitro fertilization with single blastocyst-stage versus single cleavage-stage embryos. *N Engl J Med* 354, 1139–1146.

Papanikolaou E.G., Camus M., Fatemi H.M. et al. (2006b). Early pregnancy loss is significantly higher after day 3 single embryo transfer than after day 5 single blastocyst transfer in GnRH antagonist stimulated IVF cycles. *Reprod Biomed Online* 12, 60–65.

Papanikolaou E.G., D'haeseleer E., Verheyen G. et al. (2005). Live birth rate is significantly higher after blastocyst transfer than after cleavage-stage embryo transfer when at least four embryos are available on day 3 of embryo culture. A randomized prospective study. *Hum Reprod* 20, 3198–3203.

Pellicer A., Valbuena D., Cano F. et al. (1996). Lower implantation rates in high responders: evidence for an altered endocrine milieu during the preimplantation period. *Fertil Steril* 65, 1190–1195.

Richter K.S., Harris D.C., Daneshmand S.T. et al. (2001). Quantitative grading of a human blastocyst: optimal inner cell mass size and shape. *Fertil Steril* 76, 1157–1167.

Rienzi L., Ubaldi F., Iacobelli M. et al. (2002). Day 3 embryo transfer with combined evaluation at the pronuclear and cleavage stages compares favourably with day 5 blastocyst transfer. *Hum Reprod* 17, 1852–1855.

Sakkas D. and Gardner D.K. (2005). Noninvasive methods to assess embryo quality. *Curr Opin Obstet Gynecol* 17, 283–288.

Sakkas D., Lu C., Zulfikaroglu E. et al. (2003). A soluble molecule secreted by human blastocysts modulates regulation of HOXA10 expression in an epithelial endometrial cell line. *Fertil Steril* 80, 1169–1174.

Scholtes M.C. and Zeilmaker G.H. (1996). A prospective, randomized study of embryo transfer results after 3 or 5 days of embryo culture in in vitro fertilization. *Fertil Steril* 65, 1245–1248.

Scholtes M.C. and Zeilmaker G.H. (1998). Blastocyst transfer in day-5 embryo transfer depends primarily on the number of oocytes retrieved and not on age. *Fertil Steril* 69, 78–83.

Schoolcraft W.B. and Gardner D.K. (2000). Blastocyst culture and transfer increases the efficiency of oocyte donation. *Fertil Steril* 74, 482–486.

Simon C., Garcia Velasco J.J., Valbuena D. et al. (1998). Increasing uterine receptivity by decreasing estradiol levels during the preimplantation period in high responders with the use of a follicle-stimulating hormone step-down regimen. *Fertil Steril* 70, 234–239.

Summers M.C. and Biggers J.D. (2003). Chemically defined media and the culture of mammalian preimplantation embryos: historical perspective and current issues. *Hum Reprod Update* 9, 557–582.

Takahashi K., Mukaida T., Goto T. et al. (2005). Perinatal outcome of blastocyst transfer with vitrification using cryoloop: a 4-year follow-up study. *Fertil Steril* 84, 88–92.

Tesarik J. (1994). Developmental failure during the preimplantation period of human embryogenesis. In Van Blerkom J. (ed), *In the Biological Basis of Early Human Reproductive Failure*. OUP, New York, pp. 327–344.

Trokoudes K.M., Minbattiwalla M.B., Kalogirou L. et al. (2005). Controlled natural cycle IVF with antagonist use and blastocyst transfer. *Reprod Biomed Online*, 11, 685–689.

Utsunomiya T., Naitou T., and Nagaki M. (2002). A prospective trial of blastocyst culture and transfer. *Hum Reprod*, 17, 1846–1851.

Vajta G. and Nagy Z.P. (2006). Are programmable freezers still needed in the embryo laboratory? Review on vitrification. *Reprod Biomed Online* 12, 779–796.

Van der Auwera I., Pijnenborg R., and Koninckx P.R. (1999). The influence of in-vitro culture versus stimulated and untreated oviductal environment on mouse embryo development and implantation. *Hum Reprod* 14, 2570–2574.

Van der Auwera I., Debrock S., Spiessens C. et al. (2002). A prospective randomized study: day 2 versus day 5 embryo transfer. *Hum Reprod* 17, 1507–1512.

Veeck L. (2003). Does the developmental stage at freeze impact on clinical results post-thaw? *RBM Online* 6, 367–374.

Veeck L.L., Bodine R., Clarke R.N. et al. (2004). High pregnancy rates can be achieved after freezing and thawing human blastocysts. *Fertil Steril* 82, 1418–1427.

Wilson M., Hartke K., Kiehl M. et al. (2002). Integration of blastocyst transfer for all patients. *Fertil Steril*, 77, 693–696.

Wilson M., Hartke K., Kiehl M. et al. (2004). Transfer of blastocysts and morulae on day 5. *Fertil Steril* 82, 327–333.

Wolner-Hanssen P. and Rydhstroem H. (1998). Cost-effectiveness analysis of in-vitro fertilization: estimated costs per successful pregnancy after transfer of one or two embryos. *Hum Reprod* 13, 88–94.

57

CLINICAL SIGNIFICANCE OF EMBRYO MULTINUCLEATION

Carlos E. Sueldo, Florencia Nodar, Mariano Lavolpe, Vanesa Y. Rawe

INTRODUCTION

Among the changes in assisted reproductive technology (ART) that have taken place over the past decade, there has been a steady effort to decrease the incidence of multiple pregnancies, widely recognized as one of the most serious complications in ART. Several European countries, and more recently the United States, pushed for lowering the number of embryos transferred in order to cut down the rates of high-degree multiple gestations. In order to accomplish this objective, in some European countries, physicians are electively transferring only one embryo (1), while in other countries including the Unites States, transferring two embryos, in good-prognosis IVF patients has been the norm (2).

Rizk and Abdalla pointed to the importance of keeping the right balance between decreasing the multiple pregnancies in ART and maintaining a reasonable overall implantation and clinical pregnancy rate (3). This means learning to identify the best-quality embryo(s) with a high implantation potential.

The process of embryo selection has been a long-time goal among reproductive endocrinologists and embryologists; in the initial days of IVF, embryos selected for transfer were those with the appropriate cleavage after a set time in culture, as well as those embryos without significant fragmentation (4). More recently, the identification of a nucleolar pattern alignment in day 1 preembryos, at the pronuclear stage (5), became another morphological parameter of embryo quality that was found to be clinically useful.

At about the same time, it was reported that those embryos that showed early cleavage, identified as the presence of two-cell embryos at twenty-four to twenty-seven hours after ICSI or IVF (6), provided an excellent marker of good embryo quality. This soon became a well-established morphological parameter, when it was reproduced by several other investigators (7, 8).

Among these various morphological assessment tools, embryo multinucleation (MNC) as a sign of embryo quality has been recognized in many publications (9, 10). Sathananthan et al. (11) was the first to report this feature back in 1982; soon thereafter, other investigators reported on the same findings (12, 13). Recently, Morikawi et al. (14) reported that MNC was a better predictor of embryo quality, compared to the degree of fragmentation or symmetry of the blastomeres.

Hardy et al. (15) published an interesting paper on the possible mechanisms and pathophysiology of embryo MNC and explored other aspects that provided knowledge on the true clinical significance of this embryo abnormality. After all these years, many questions still remain and are the main focus of our chapter: are the mechanisms that generate binucleated or micronucleated embryos different? How common are the chromosomal anomalies present in binucleated or micronucleated embryos? Do we have an acceptable classification of multinucleated embryos that will allow for a good communication and interaction between embryologists and clinicians? Are the nonmultinucleated embryos in the same cohort affected? Are transferred multinucleated embryos able to establish a normal pregnancy? These and many other important issues about embryo MNC constitute the essence of our chapter, with the purpose of clarifying the true clinical significance of this embryological finding in ART today.

PATHOPHYSIOLOGY OF EMBRYO MNC

Embryo MNC can be defined as the presence of two or more nuclei, within a blastomere, in a given embryo under in vitro culture. In contrast, the norm is to have a single nucleus per blastomere, as in normal mononucleated embryos (Figure 57.1A). When two nuclei are present, we use the term binucleated blastomere or embryo (Figure 57.1B). In contrast, when more than two nuclei are present, we name this finding micronucleated blastomere or embryo (Figure 57.1C and D). The significance of separating these two types of MNC relates to the fact that they seem to be different in their potential to reach blastocysts in culture, in their chromosomal anomaly rates, as well as in their potential to establish a pregnancy if transferred in ART procedures (16–18).

Despite efforts by a number of investigators to disclose how these abnormal blastomeres are developed, the mechanism that leads to their formation is still unknown (15, 19). Since cleavage divisions successively subdivide the cytoplasm of the embryo without cellular growth, blastomeres become proportionately smaller at later stages (15). These findings were recently confirmed by computer-controlled morphometric analysis of blastomere size (20); studying mononuclear embryos, the authors determined that the average volume of a blastomere in a two-cell embryo was $0.28 \times 10^6 \ \mu m^3$, while it was $0.15 \times 10^6 \ \mu m^3$ at the four-cell stage ($p < 0.01$). In contrast, multinucleated blastomeres were significantly larger, both at the two- and four-cell stages, compared to their sibling non-multinucleated blastomeres (51.5–73.1 percent smaller, respectively), $p < 0.001$ (19).

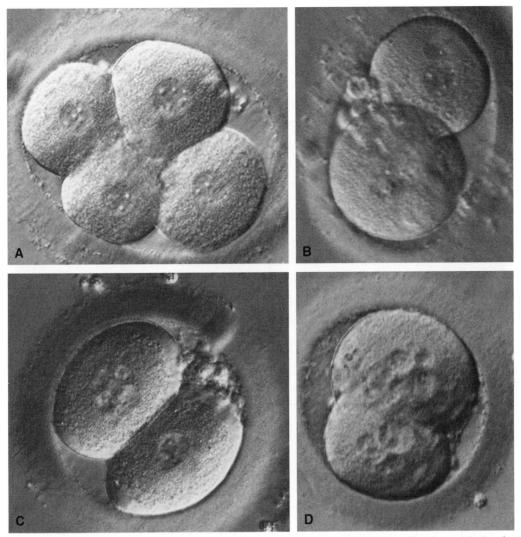

Figure 57.1. Contrast-phase microscopy of human embryos. (A) Mononucleated four-cell embryo. (B) Binucleated two-cell embryo. (C) Micronucleated two-cell embryo with mixed patterns of MNC (micronucleated upper blastomere and binucleated lower blastomere). (D) Severely affected micronucleated two-cell embryo.

By reference to the volume of blastomeres from normal embryos that had uniformly and evenly completed particular cleavage divisions, it has been possible to determine how many divisions a blastomere has undergone. After comparing blastomere sizes in binucleated and mononucleated cells within the same embryo, Hardy et al. (15) concluded that binucleated cells are formed by a failure of cytokinesis at the second, third, or fourth cleavage and that the persistence of some binucleated blastomeres for one or two days after their initial formation suggests that they may have undergone cleavage arrest. After considering other mechanisms, these authors postulated that binucleation may develop after a failure during cytokinesis, giving rise to cleavage arrest (15).

Different mechanisms may exist to explain micronucleation; this nuclear abnormality could be formed by continued karyokinesis, and these fragmenting nuclei may represent a form of cell death similar to apoptosis, where further degradation of these fragments would produce at times an anucleate blastomere, another variant of embryonic cell abnormality. What triggers these abnormal cell behaviors is a matter of debate, but less than adequate culture conditions, chromosomal abnormalities, defective cell surface properties, or lack of molecular components that trigger cell division are possible candidates, either working alone or in combination.

Intracellular restructuring, remodeling, and imprinting are of paramount importance to the developing oocyte and eventual embryo; any interruption in these delicate processes may cause errors during division, resulting in abnormal embryos with the potential to express multinucleate phenotypes (19).

Meriano et al. (19) performed time-lapse photography studies of binucleated and micronucleated embryos and concluded that separate nuclei on both types of multinucleated embryos dissolve independently with intervals of several minutes. These authors also noticed that larger nuclei tended to dissolve before the smaller ones and that there was a trend toward fasting disappearance of micronucleated nuclei compared to binucleated ones. Since few embryos were monitored in this study, it is difficult to draw any meaningful clinical conclusions at this time.

In order to further help elucidate a possible cellular pathway that operates during embryo binucleation and micronucleation in humans, we studied different cytoskeletal structures under confocal microscopy (Figure 57.2). In more than fifty multinucleated embryos studied (unpublished observations), we analyzed the distribution of key components, like F-actin, microtubules (α and β tubulins) and actin-related proteins (Arps), like Profilin, that promotes incorporation of actin monomers into filaments and whose nucleation is catalyzed by the Arps 2/3 complex (21). Microtubules serve as an intracellular scaffold, and their unique polymerization dynamics are critical for many cellular functions, such as embryo cleavage. If defects in cytokinesis are present during embryo MNC, one would expect to observe abnormalities in cytoskeletal components.

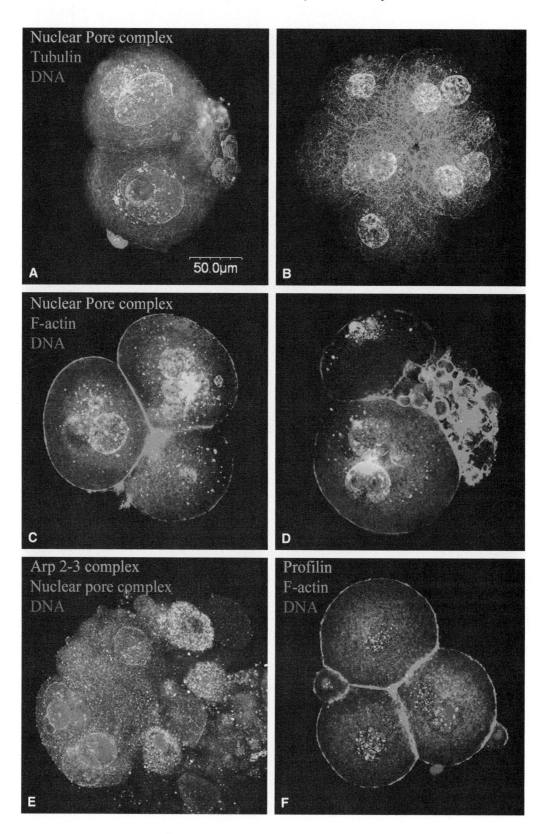

Our preliminary work showed an incidence of F-actin disorganization (accumulation in distinct areas or lack of homogeneous distribution) in 46 percent of the studied embryos (Figure 57.2D), only when more than two nuclei were present (micronucleated embryo). Contrarily to what we observed in the majority of binucleated blastomeres (nuclear envelopes normally organized, Figure 57.2B), micronucleated blastomeres showed a high incidence of apoptotic characteristics, like nuclear envelope disassembling and lack or spread of DNA (Figure 57.2A, C, and D).

Trying to elucidate the possible mechanisms involved in the formation of multinucleated blastomeres, we asked ourselves if this phenomenon was already present at the time of pronuclear formation. For this purpose, we randomly selected supernumerary pronucleated zygotes with normal aspect under light microcopy and performed a visualization of its DNA content. To our surprise, we detected that approximately 30 percent showed the presence of small clusters of DNA outside the pronuclear area (arrows, Figure 57.3A).

Figure 57.3B and D shows a schematic representation of one of the proposed mechanisms of micronuclei formation; small fragments of DNA seen dispersed outside the pronuclear area (Figure 57.3B) remain there without being monitorized by deficient checkpoints, and after nuclear envelope breakdown (Figure 57.3C), first cleavage takes place (Figure 57.3D) and displaced DNA is surrounded by a new nuclear envelope, forming visible micronuclei (by light microscopy) in the newly formed embryo.

In summary, there may be more than one mechanism to explain embryo MNC; some investigators believe that the pathophysiology involved in binucleation and micronucleation may be different (19). It is possible that karyokinesis without cytokinesis may be the likely source of binucleation, while continued karyokinesis or fragmenting of the nuclei may be involved in micronucleation. The triggering factors involved in causing these nuclear abnormalities appear to be very diverse, from suboptimal culture conditions to inherent oocyte chromosomal anomalies related or not to the type of ovarian response, observed after the controlled ovarian hyperstimulation protocols.

CHROMOSOMAL ANOMALIES IN MULTINUCLEATED EMBRYOS

Chromosomal defects occurring during early cleavage stages of human embryo development are common and result in embryos with limited developmental capacity and potential to implant when transferred during ART procedures (22).

In general, there is a correlation between chromosomal anomalies and poor morphological embryo features. Thus, embryos presenting slow growth in vitro, signs of fragmentation, asymmetric blastomeres, and so on are more likely to be chromosomally abnormal (23). The incidence of chromosomal anomalies present in multinucleated embryos has shown differences in embryos with binucleation when compared to those presenting micronucleation. Kligman et al. (17) studied the incidence of chromosomal anomalies in multinucleated embryos and found that 76.6 percent of the embryos were abnormal, while only 32.3 percent were abnormal in the control group of mononucleated embryos ($p < 0.05$) after aneuploidy was excluded; other types of abnormalities among multinucleated embryos were polyploidy, mosaicism, monosomy, or mixed pattern.

Aneuploidy may arise through two mechanisms: chromosome loss and nondisjunction. Chromosome loss takes place by lagging of chromosomes at metaphase by, for example, failure of the spindle fibers to attach to a chromosome. If the chromosome remains behind in the metaphase plate, it can give origin to micronuclei. Nondisjunction is the failure of two sister chromatids to segregate normally, resulting in one daughter cell that gains a chromosome, while the other loses a chromosome (24). Hence, nondisjunction will not lead to micronuclei formation.

Of significance is the fact that the action of genotoxic agents, like aneugens (agents that affect cell division and mitotic spindle, thereby generating aneuploidies), could be inducers of embryo micronuclei.

Meriano et al. (19) studied a total of sixty-nine multinucleated blastomeres from twenty-three embryos with multinucleation on day two and reported results in a total of fifty-five cells analyzed by FISH; micronucleated embryos showed a 96.3 percent abnormality rate, while binucleated embryos showed only 68 percent of chromosomal anomalies ($p < 0.01$). These authors speculated that these results explain the reason why embryos with binucleated cells are more likely to advance in vitro to blastocyst stage (25), as well as being able to produce a pregnancy if transferred (26).

In summary, the rate of chromosomal anomalies in multinucleated embryos needs to be better studied; the data available so far seem to show a high incidence of chromosomal anomalies in micronucleated embryos, while binucleated embryos

---

Figure 57.2. Confocal microscopy of different cytoskeletal components of multinucleated human embryos. All the studied embryos developed from normally fertilized eggs and showed at least one blastomere with more than two nuclei on day 2. (A) Microtubules (red) are uniformly distributed throughout the cytoplasm and concentrated in different fragments. Note that this embryo has asymmetric binucleated blastomeres (two uneven-sized interphase nuclei) with disorganized nuclear envelopes (green). (B) This binucleated embryo has microtubules (red) uniformly distributed throughout the cytoplasm. No abnormal patterns can be seen. In this case, smooth and organized nuclear envelopes are visualized in each even-sized nuclei. (C) F-actin is distributed in the cytoplasm and enriched at the cortex of a three-cell multinucleated embryo. As seen in A, nuclear envelopes are disorganized resembling the features of an apoptotic cell. (D) Two-cell embryo with abnormal distribution and absence of homogenous actin filaments (red). The upper blastomere has just a very small amount of spread DNA surrounded by disorganized nuclear envelopes. The presence of four nuclei can be seen in the lower blastomere. Anucleate fragments enriched with actin are also visualized. (E) Arp 2/3 complex (green) is present in the cytoplasm and inside each nuclei taking part of "the nucleoskeleton." Variable intense fluorescence signal can be observed in each blastomere. (F) Profilin (green) is dispersed in the cytoplasm and is present inside each nuclei in a punctuated pattern. This pattern resembles what has been observed in normal bovine embryos (20). Actin filaments seem to be normally distributed. Embryos were examined under a spectral confocal microscope (Olympus), using laser lines at 488, 568, and 633 nm wavelengths (University of Buenos Aires, Faculty of Exact and Natural Sciences). Images were edited using Adobe Photoshop 7.0.

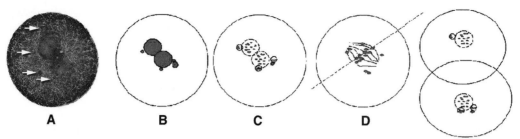

Figure 57.3. Confocal image and schematic representation of a proposed mechanism of micronuclei formation. (A) Presence of small clusters of DNA outside the pronuclear area. (B–D) Fragments of DNA are dispersed outside the pronuclear area, and after nuclear envelope breakdown, cleavage takes place and displaced DNA is surrounded by new nuclear envelopes forming a micronucleated embryo.

are showing an incidence within the range reported for normal mononucleated embryos (26). These findings are compatible with the capacity of these types of embryos to reach blastocyst stage, under in vitro culture conditions. Meriano et al. (19) recently reported that 38 percent of binucleated embryos reached blastocyst stage (38/102), while only 8.6 percent of micronucleated embryos (7/81; $p < 0.05$) achieved that stage of development. Also, Yakin et al. (24) reported on the blastocyst formation capability of 5,982 embryos; multinucleated embryos reached blastocyst at a rate of 11.4 percent, which was significantly lower than nonmultinucleated embryos, forming blastocysts in 51 percent of the extended cultures ($p < 0.05$).

CLASSIFICATION OF EMBRYO MNC

We are lacking a satisfactory classification of embryo MNC that will enable embryologists and clinicians to interact properly, using a language that not only will easily determine the significance of the embryological findings in the ART laboratory but also will offer the clinician a clear picture that will be helpful in his/her communication with patients.

We feel that a useful classification should take into account two major parameters: first, the type of multinucleation present, either binucleation or micronucleation, since they have been shown to be clinically different, and second, the number of blastomeres involved with multinucleation in a given embryo since it appears that a greater surface involvement of the embryo with MNC carries a worse prognosis than lighter involvement (19).

We propose using the number 1 to define binucleation, and 2 to be applied to micronucleation, subsequently using a number that will proportionately define the embryo percentage involved with the nuclear defect. Since the identification of MNC will be best established on day 2 of embryo culture, most embryos will be either at the two-, three-, or four-cell stage (17).

For example, a two-cell embryo with only one blastomere involved with binucleation will be classified as multinucleated two-cell embryo 1/50, the 1 identifying the binucleation and 50 the percentage of blastomeres involved with the MNC. A three-cell embryo presenting micronucleation in two of its cells will be defined as multinucleated three-cell embryo 2/66, 2 representing the micronucleation and 66 the percentage involved with the nuclear defect.

This is indeed a very simplistic classification and is not covering all the possible variants found in clinical embryology;

for example, it does not consider the presence of mixed patterns (binucleation and MNC in the same embryo), although it makes sense to label the embryo by the pattern with a worse prognosis.

Also, it does not consider the presence of variants within a given pattern; for example, the binucleated embryos may have two nuclei of equal size or one larger than the other. We feel that asymmetric binucleation has a worse prognosis than symmetric ones (unpublished observation) and as such worth differentiating, yet the data are not as yet conclusive and therefore for now, and until more clinical data document this suspicion, we should include both patterns under the same group. That is why, in our center, we were using a classification based on numbering each blastomere, 0 for symmetric binucleation, 1 for asymmetric binucleation, and 3 or more depending on the number of micronuclei present. For example, a two-cell embryo with one symmetric binucleated blastomere and one normal will be 0/−, if the binucleated blastomere was asymmetric would be 1/−, and so forth.

In summary, we need a comprehensive classification of embryo MNC to help communicate embryologists and clinicians, clinicians and patients, and also as a tool for future scientific reporting on these frequent embryological findings. This proposed classification is simply an initial step in that direction.

EMBRYO MNC IN THE ART LABORATORY

Embryo MNC is a frequent finding in the embryology laboratory. Although Hardy et al. (15) reported a 17.5 percent incidence of binucleation, she did not include other nuclear abnormalities. Later, Jackson et al. (26) showed an incidence of 31 percent MNC in all embryos studied and at least one multinucleated embryo in 74 percent of all cycles. Van Royen et al. (27) also showed the presence of multinucleation in 33.6 percent of all embryos and at least the presence of one multinucleated embryo in 79.6 percent of all cycles.

During 2005, we studied a total of 1,785 embryos in patients using their own oocytes and found multinucleated embryos in 33.5 percent and the presence of at least one multinucleated embryo in 61.3 percent of all cycles (28). Somewhat surprisingly, in 2006 (in patients using their own oocytes), the incidence so far has been significantly lower, with MNC present in only 19.5 percent of all embryos studied, and one multinucleated embryo was present in 50 percent of the cycles.

Regarding the type of MNC present, Meriano et al. (19) showed that in all 183 multinucleated embryos reported, 55.7 percent (102/183) were binucleated, while 44.3 percent (81/183) showed micronucleation. Based on this fact, we looked at our own data for 2006 (total = 1,569 embryos studied) and found 35.6 percent binucleation, 49.6 percent micronucleation, and 14.7 percent mixed pattern, again in patients using their own oocytes.

We also studied the incidence of MNC among oocyte donors in 2006 (a total of 722 embryos) and found a slightly lower incidence (16.9 percent, 122/722) of multinucleated embryos, also the individual types of MNC were reversed (46.8 percent binucleation, 34.4 percent micronucleation, and 18.8 percent mixed) in relation to the incidence found among patients using their own oocytes. Of interest, during 2005 in all our egg donation cycles, we observed that the presence of MNC in the embryo cohort did not have an impact on the overall pregnancy rates (cycles with MNC or not-MNC had the same CPR and IR), yet if the percentage of multinucleation was more than 50 percent of all embryos, the CPR = 10 percent, and IR = 9.6 percent were significantly lower than in cases where the multinucleation rate was below 50 percent, CPR = 52.1 percent, and IR = 34.2 percent, respectively. Further analysis of the type of MNC present in oocyte donation and its potential impact on pregnancy rate is mandatory since in the data shown above, all types of MNC were included.

It is important to emphasize that our egg donation program is based on what we called split cycles or egg sharing (29), where the oocytes retrieved from a single donor are shared among several recipients. During 2005, an average of 2.5 recipients shared oocytes from a single donor (average number of mature oocytes received per recipient was 5.0).

Based on the high incidence of chromosomal anomalies, as well as the coexistence of other embryo-morphology abnormalities, like asymmetric blastomeres (30), high degree of fragmentation (27), or slow rate of embryo development in vitro (27), multinucleated embryos are typically excluded from the embryo transfer (17). Yet, at times, multinucleated embryos is all the patient may have for transfer, and a joint decision (patients and doctors) has to be made about transferring those embryos.

We reviewed our own data on pregnancies generated after transferring only multinucleated embryos during 2005. From almost 500 cycles, where patients used their own oocytes, we studied twenty-two cycles where only multinucleated embryos were transferred; the average age of the patient was 37.5 years and the average number of embryos transferred was 1.47 per patient. A total of five pregnancies took place (22.7 percent), although one aborted during the first trimester.

Of the four ongoing pregnancies, all resulted in healthy newborns at term: two cases from transferring binucleated embryos (50 percent MNC); in one case, we failed to document the type of MNC; and finally, the last case was what we believed to be the first reported case of a healthy newborn at term after transferring only micronucleated embryos (two micronucleated embryos resulting in a singleton healthy newborn) (31).

During the first half of 2006, we transferred only multinucleated embryos in eight cases (out of 236 total) and obtained three pregnancies, one aborted in the first trimester, and the other two are ongoing, one case after transferring a two-cell embryo having binucleation and, in the other case, after trans-

ferring two micronucleated embryos, resulting in an ongoing gestation (single sac).

Other reported pregnancies after transferring only multinucleated embryos were those of Jackson et al. (26), with a clinical pregnancy rate of 8 percent and a live birth rate of 4 percent in twenty-five cases; Balakier et al. (32), one twin pregnancy in nineteen cases, and Pelinck et al. (33), only one pregnancy in eight cases; although Jackson et al. (26) did not report the type of MNC present, the other investigators (32, 33) transferred only binucleated embryos.

DISCUSSION

Embryo MNC is a common event in human clinical embryology. It has been reported to take place in vivo (34), but clearly the in vitro culture conditions of human embryos have given us an opportunity to fully identify and study different aspects of this fascinating cell nuclear-cytoplasmic abnormality.

We have accumulated enough clinical data to report that both types of MNC, binucleation, and micronucleation probably arise through different mechanisms (although the triggering factors may or may not be the same); that both have different capability to continue to cleave and reach the stage of blastocyst in vitro; and that both have different prognoses in terms of establishing a pregnancy if transferred as part of the ART procedure.

Our own personal experience with MNC in human embryos has shown that the presence of MNC may not be related to exaggerated ovarian response, as reported by others to controlled ovarian hyperstimulation (26) since young healthy egg donors, presenting high-serum estradiols on the day of HCG administration in our program, do not show a higher incidence of embryo MNC when compared to age-matched ART patients using their own oocytes (32).

It remains to be shown, if young ART patients with ovarian dysfunction and exaggerated ovarian response to COH (like PCOS patients) have a higher incidence of multinucleated embryos in comparison to young egg donors having a normal ovarian reserve and function.

As already mentioned, we suspect that the mechanisms leading to binucleation or MNC are probably different, and these differences are probably reflected in the chromosomal abnormality rates seen with each type of MNC. Meriano et al. (19), using time-lapse photography, observed that nuclei break down independently, confirming that each set of chromosomal material will be distinct and attached to separate mitotic spindles, resulting in the continuous development of abnormal daughter cells if there are preexisting chromosomal abnormalities. This brings into account another important clinical aspect, which is that binucleated embryos may not affect the rest of the embryo cohort not showing MNC, while it appears that micronucleated embryos do affect the rest of the cohort (19). This would explain why the pregnancy expectancy is different when transferring nonmultinucleated embryos, under those two different set of circumstances.

As suggested earlier, the presence of embryo MNC can be the cellular manifestation of suboptimal culture conditions. An interesting observation is that an increase in the frequency of micronuclei, in a population of somatic cells (micronuclei are particularly apparent in red blood cells, which lack DNA in the nucleus), is indicative of genotoxicity. The "micronucleation test" was developed over two decades ago (24) as a mean to establish in vivo the presence of chromosomal damage. The test is based on the observation that displaced chromatin induced by different mutagens (chemical or radiation) can result in chromosomal loss or breakage, resulting in a secondary nucleus (micronucleus) outside the main nucleus of a dividing cell, following telophase.

We strongly believe that a classification of embryo MNC is badly needed, mainly to uniformly report on these nuclear abnormalities, as well as to compare different events that take place in ART procedures. Also, it will be helpful to properly discuss these embryological findings and their clinical significance with our patients. It is obviously not the same to have a large number of micronucleated embryos with several blastomeres involved versus a few binucleated embryos with less than 50 percent cell involvement.

Recently, Ciray et al. (35) reported that in their opinion, only embryos presenting blastomeres with three or more nuclei should qualify for the term embryo MNC as there is evidence that binucleated embryos could develop normally (36). This was challenged by Sundstrom (37), who claims that multinucleated blastomeres, whether having two or more nuclei, should be regarded as pathological (disarrangement of the chromosomes), and these early embryos should be avoided or not considered for transfer because of the low implantation potential.

We consider the classification proposed in this chapter an effort in the right direction, considering both the type of MNC present in a given embryo, as well as the percentage of the embryo involved with MNC. Some loopholes remain (mixed patterns, difference in the size of the nuclei), which may have to be corrected in the future as we gain more knowledge and experience in this area of clinical embryology.

There is a general agreement that if mononucleated embryos are available for transfer, those should be the one(s) selected, over those that present MNC, regardless of the pattern or type identified. As stated, binucleation does not seem to affect the rest of the embryo cohort not showing MNC, while the presence of micronucleation negatively affects (and repair is unlikely) the rest of the embryos, as reflected in the low – blastocyst formation potential as well as in the low incidence of ongoing pregnancies if those embryos are transferred.

An ethical dilemma is present if the patient only has multinucleated embryos for transfer. We believe that in this situation, if morphologically the embryos looked "transferable" based on established criteria, and binucleation was the MNC pattern identified, it seems reasonable to transfer those embryos. In contrast, if micronucleated embryos with acceptable morphology is all the patient has for transfer, appropriate counseling prior to performing the embryo transfer is mandatory, in order to share with the couple what we know about chromosomal anomalies in micronucleated embryos, the fact that pregnancy is unlikely to take place, and that a spontaneous miscarriage may be the end result if a pregnancy was established after transfer. A healthy newborn may result from transferring micronucleated embryos (31), but based on our limited knowledge about chromosomal defects (19) in micronucleated embryos, this seems an unlikely outcome.

From our preliminary data on embryo MNC in egg donation cycles, we conclude that if MNC is present in fewer than 50 percent of the embryo cohort, the overall incidence of implantation and clinical pregnancy rates do not seem to be affected. Yet, if MNC prevails among the embryos available for transfer, the clinical pregnancy rates and implantation rates are negatively affected (30).

In summary, the detection and pattern of embryo MNC should continue to be part of the morphological embryo-quality assessment in our search for the embryo(s) with the best implantation potential. Keeping data on binucleation and micronucleation separately seems prudent, given the different impact that each has on the rest of the embryo cohort.

Excluding multinucleated embryos from being transferred seems prudent at this time, in favor of those embryos without MNC, and understanding that the presence of micronucleation seems to affect the rest of the embryos, even those without MNC in their implantation potential.

Hopefully, future research will shed light and help improve our understanding on the etiology of embryo MNC, its triggering mechanisms, and how some multinucleated embryos self-correct and generate blastocysts with a full capacity to implant and produce a normal pregnancy. That is why, understanding the cellular pathway that operates in embryo MNC, as well as its biological and clinical significance, is one of the great challenges still present in reproductive biology.

KEY POINTS FOR CLINICAL PRACTICE

■ Embryo MNC is a common problem in ART and should serve as a morphological marker of embryo quality.

■ Binucleated embryos appear to have a better prognosis compared to micronucleated embryos in reaching blastocyst stage in vitro, or achieving a pregnancy if transferred.

■ The incidence of chromosomal anomalies in multinucleated blastomeres is increased, specially in those that are micronucleated.

■ In oocyte donation cycles MNC is also present, but the pregnancy rate is negatively affected only when the MNC prevails in the overall embryo cohort.

■ Multinucleated embryos should be excluded in embryo transfers, in favor of mononucleated embryos.

REFERENCES

1. Gerris J and Van Royen E. Avoiding multiple pregnancies in ART. A plea for single embryo transfer. *Hum Reprod* 2000; 15: 1884–1888.

2. Gleicher N and Barad D. The relative myth of elective single embryo transfer. *Hum Reprod* 2006; 21: 1337–1344.

3. Rizk B and Abdalla H. Controlled ovarian hyperstimulation for IVF. In: Rizk B, Abdalla H, Eds. *Assisted Reproductive Technology*, Chapter III.3. Oxford, UK: Health Press, 2007; pp. 180–183.

4. Veeck L. *An Atlas of Human Gametes and Conceptuses.* New York: Parthenon Publishing Group; pp. 178–183.

5. Nagy ZP, Dozortaev D, Diamond M et al. Pronuclear morphology evaluation with subsequent evaluation of embryo morphology significantly increases implantation rates. *Fertil Steril* 2003; 80: 67–74.

6. Sakkas D, Shoukir Y, Chardonnens D et al. Early cleavage of human embryos to the two cell stage after ICSI as an indicator of embryo viability. *Hum Reprod* 1998; 13: 182–187.

7. Salumets A, Hyden-Granskog C, Makinen S et al. Early cleavage predicts the viability of human embryos in elective single embryo transfer procedures. *Hum Reprod* 2003; 18: 821–825.

8. Van Montfoort AP, Dumoulin JC, Keater AD et al. Early cleavage is a valuable addition to existing embryo selection parameters: a study using single embryo transfers. *Hum Reprod* 2004; 19: 2103–2108.

9. Morikawi T, Suganuma N, Hayakawa M et al. Embryo evaluation by analysing blastomere nuclei. *Hum Reprod* 2004; 19: 152–156.

10. Tesarik J, Kopecny V, Plachot M et al. Ultrastructural and autoradiographic observations on multinucleated blastomeres of human cleaving embryos obtained by IVF. *Hum Reprod* 1987; 2: 127–136.

11. Sathananthan A, Wood C and Leeton J. Ultrastructural evaluation of 8–16 cell human embryos cultured in vitro. *Micron* 1982; 13: 193–203.

12. Lopata A, Kohlman D and Johnston I. The fine structure of normal and abnormal human embryos developed in culture. In: Beier HM, Lindner HR, eds. *Fertilization of the Human Egg In Vitro*. Springer-Verlag, Berlin, 1983; 211–221.

13. Trounson A and Sathananthan AH. The application of electron microscopy in the evaluation of two to four cell human embryos. *J In Vitro Fertil Embryo Transfer* 1984; 1: 153–165.

14. Morikawa T, Suganuma N, Hayakawa M et al. Embryo evaluation by analysing blastomere nuclei. *Hum Reprod* 2004; 19: 152–156.

15. Hardy K, Winston R and Handyside AH. Binucleate blastomeres in preimplantation human embryos in vitro: failure of cytokinesis during early cleavage. *J Reprod Fertil* 1993; 98: 549–558.

16. Munné S and Cohen J. Unsuitability of multinucleated blastomeres for PGD. *Hum Reprod* 1993; 7: 1120–1125.

17. Kligman I, Benadiva C, Alikani M et al. The presence of multinucleated blastomeres in human embryos is correlated with chromosomal abnormalities. *Hum Reprod* 1996; 11: 1492–1496.

18. Pelinck MJ, De Vos M, Dekens M et al. Embryos cultured in vitro with multinucleated blastomeres have poor implantation potential in human IVF-ET. *Hum Reprod* 1998; 13: 960–963.

19. Meriano J, Clark C, Cadesky K et al. Binucleated and micronucleated blastomeres in embryos derived from human assisted reproduction cycles. *Reprod Biomed Online* 2004; 9: 511–520.

20. Hnida C, Engenheiro E and Ziebe S. Computer-controlled multilevel morphometric analysis of blastomere size as biomarker of fragmentation and multinuclearity in human embryos. *Hum Reprod* 2004; 19: 288–293.

21. Rawe VY, Payne C and Schatten G. Profilin and actin related proteins regulate microfilaments dynamics during early mammalian embryogenesis. *Hum Reprod* 2006; 21: 1143–53.

22. Rizk B, Edwards RG, Nicolini U et al. (1991). Edwards syndrome after the replacement of cryopreserved thawed embryos. *Fertil Steril* 55(1): 208–210.

23. Munné S, Alikani M, Tomkin G et al. Embryo morphology, developmental rates and maternal age are correlated with chromosomal abnormalities. *Fertil Steril* 1995; 64: 382–391.

24. Kirsch-Volders K, Vanhauwert A, De Boeck M et al. Importance of detecting numerical versus structural chromosome aberrations. *Mutat Res* 2002; 504: 137–148.

25. Yakin K, Balaban B and Urban B. Impact of the presence of one or more multinucleated blastomeres on the developmental potential of the embryo to the blastocyst stage. *Fertil Steril* 2005; 83: 243–245.

26. Jackson KV, Ginsburg E, Hornstein M et al. Multinucleation in normally fertilized embryos is associated with an accelerated ovulation induction response and lower implantation and pregnancy rates in IVF-ET cycles. *Fertil Steril* 1998; 70: 60–66.

27. Park J, Kort J, Bodine R et al. Is blastomere multinucleation associated with poor growth and lower rates of blastocyst development? *Fertil Steril* 2005; 84 (Suppl. 1): S234.

28. Van Royen E, Mangelschots K, Vercruyssen M et al. Multinucleation in cleavage stage embryos. *Hum Reprod* 2003; 18: 1062–1069.

29. Glujovsky D, Fiszbajn G, Lipowicz R et al. Practice of sharing oocytes among several recipients. *Fertil Steril* 2006; 86: 1786–1788.

30. Lavolpe M, Nodar F, Fiszbajn G et al. Significance of embryo multinucleation in oocyte donation cycles. *Fertil Steril* 2006; 86 (Suppl. 3): S182.

31. Lavolpe M, Nodar F, Rawe VY et al. The transfer of micronucleated embryos resulted in a term pregnancy and healthy newborn. *Reproduccion* 2007, 22(2): 62–64.

32. Balakier H and Cadensky C. The frequency and developmental capability of human embryos containing multinucleated blastomeres. *Hum Reprod* 1997; 12: 800–804.

33. Pelinck MJ, De Vos M, Dekens M et al. Embryos cultured in vitro with multinucleated blastomeres have poor implantation potential in human IVF and ICSI. *Hum Reprod* 1998; 13: 960–963.

34. Hertig AT, Rock J and Adams EC. On the preimplantation stages of the human ovum: a description of four normal and four abnormal specimens ranging from the second to the fifth day of development. *Contrib Embryol* 1953; 35: 201–220.

35. Ciray HN, Karagenc L, Bener F et al. Early cleavage morphology affects the quality and implantation potential of day 3 embryos. *Fertil Steril* 2006; 85: 358–365.

36. Staessen LA and Van Steirteghem A. The genetic constitution of multinuclear blastomeres and their derivative daughter blastomeres. *Hum Reprod* 1998; 13: 1625–1631.

37. Sundstrom P. Interpretations of multinucleation—is it ever normal? *Fertil Steril* 2006; 86: 494.

58

QUALITY AND RISK MANAGEMENT IN THE IVF LABORATORY

David Mortimer, Sharon T. Mortimer

BACKGROUND

The rapid expansion of assisted reproduction during the past two decades, combined with the great media interest in the "mistakes" that can occur in IVF centers, has resulted in many governments introducing regulation to control the activities that underlie the provision of assisted conception treatment and various national professional and nongovernmental organizations implementing peer-based accreditation schemes. Concurrently, increasing numbers of IVF centers have sought certification under the ISO 9001:2000 standard for quality management (1,2).

While not wanting to denigrate the achievement of ISO9001:2000 certification, it must be remembered that this standard only looks at organizational systems and procedures; while it is the framework upon which any quality system must be built, it does not inherently *require* or *create* quality assurance or improvement aspects. Indeed, it has often been said that it would be quite conceivable for an IVF center to achieve ISO9001:2000 certification even if it had a zero pregnancy rate. For medical laboratories, there also exists a further ISO standard, 15189:2003 entitled *Medical laboratories – Particular requirements for quality and competence* that emphasizes quality assurance and improvement (3,4). Rather than focus on the ISO 9001:2000 standard, we have for many years espoused the concepts and principles of *Total Quality Management* (TQM), a holistic framework that integrates quality management, risk management, and process management to create a proactive organizational and operational philosophy of "best practice" for the entire team involved in providing infertility care (5).

In this way quality management is no longer seen as just additional, annoying, costly regulatory requirements that "don't help the patients get pregnant" – the provision of effective and safe IVF treatment depends on achieving improved standards of technical services and medical care. We have previously identified three features that characterize an IVF lab that is not "in control" (5):

1. Unpredictable and unexplained variations in outcomes and/or indicators, with a likely general downward trend in results. In extreme cases, things might deteriorate to such a state that the best description is that "the wheels have fallen off."
2. A generalized perception that the feeling of "comfort" that you had when things were running smoothly has faded, leading ultimately to a sense of unease, or even panic.
3. Everyone becomes "defensive," leading to faultfinding, "finger-pointing," the need to blame someone, and even seek retribution. Eventually, this can lead to a general "culture of fear" developing, and the lab (and probably the whole clinic) can become a "toxic workplace" (6).

Although the *terminology* specific to quality and risk management has been covered elsewhere (5), some basic definitions must be considered here, especially in order to clarify specific differences between terms that are often used more or less synonymously.

Regulations are legal requirements to which an organization or individual must conform in order to operate. *Compliance* is often verified by *inspection* (examination for individuals) and confirmed by the issuance of a *license*. Regulations are typically highly prescriptive as to what an organization or individual must/must not do in order to be compliant.

Accreditation is a collegial process based on a combination of both *self-assessment* and *peer-assessment*, whereby an authoritative body (usually a nongovernment organization) gives formal recognition that an organization is in voluntary compliance with *standards* set by the authoritative body. Unlike *licensing*, accreditation is based upon process rather than procedure, and the principles of quality improvement rather than strict obedience of regulations, so that it is not prescriptive in relation to technical procedures or rules. See also *accreditation*, below.

Licensing is the process whereby an organization (or individual) is identified as being compliant with required regulations. Licensing is a legal requirement under government regulations in order for an organization to be allowed to operate; for individuals, licensing is conferred to denote their competence to perform a given activity (e.g., driving a motor vehicle) in compliance with regulations.

Standards are published documents that contain technical specifications or criteria to be used consistently as rules, guidelines, or definitions of characteristics to ensure that materials, products, processes, and services are fit for their purpose (i.e., they are not synonymous with "minimum standards"). Unlike a regulation, a standard is a "living document" that describes a voluntary agreement between all stakeholders relevant to the product or service and encompasses everything that can have a profound influence on the product or service, especially its safety, reliability, and efficiency. Compliance with standards is ascertained through a process of peer assessment, for example, an accreditation *survey*, rather than by inspection.

QUALITY AND QUALITY MANAGEMENT

What is Quality?

While "quality" is often used to describe a product's superiority, it is not synonymous with luxury, which represents that products that are better than they need to be to serve their primary purpose (and hence typically more expensive). Therefore, from a basic product-manufacturing perspective, quality can be defined as *conformance to specifications* – specifications that are set by the manufacturer, based on the manufacturer's experience of customer wants. However, in service industries understanding the concept of quality is easier when it is defined as *fitness for use* – based on the customers' perceptions and opinions. In marketing terms, this change in perspective is a switch from being a "product-out" company to a "market-in" company, with quality now being seen as *conformance to customer requirements*.

In medicine, quality can also be defined as *duty of care* and has been equated to the achievement of *best practice*. Consequently, for an IVF lab, these definitions can be combined with *conformance to customer requirements* to establish a framework that embraces the provision of quality services that not only meet the customers' needs but also their expectations. From a holistic perspective, these services must also be effective, efficient, and safe, while protecting the rights and dignity of all parties involved – including the children who will result from successful treatment.

Quality Management

Quality management, which integrates quality control, quality assurance, and quality improvement into a management philosophy, had its roots in the rebirth of the Japanese manufacturing industry after World War II, where the philosophy of "total quality control" was taught by Deming and Juran (7,8). When the principles were embraced by Western companies and organizations in the 1980s and 1990s, it became known as "Total Quality Management" or TQM. For many experts, TQM is simply *the scientific way of doing business* – and therefore ideally suited to running an IVF lab (5).

In industry, quality control (QC) focuses on inspection and checking, its purpose is to reduce waste, and uses inspectors to check the work of others. In a laboratory, QC is about making sure each task is done correctly and typically equates to ensuring instruments were working properly (e.g., using calibrators) and making sure an assay was run properly (e.g., using reference standards), i.e., to verify that the results come out close to where they should. However, *quality assurance* ("QA") focuses on procedures and systems so that quality is designed into a process to increase the likelihood that the process will go exactly as planned, increasing consistency and overall performance, i.e., QA relates to the *way* in which work is done.

While the goal of "quality" is to satisfy requirements, these change with customers' increasing expectations, creating a commercial, as well as professional, need to optimize our IVF/ICSI fertilization rates, our embryo culture systems, and our cryopreservation techniques. In addition, within the context of the IVF center, services must be made more easily available and provided in a more pleasant environment with more personalized attention. Finally, the now more-effective services must be provided more efficiently. The part of the quality system that is focussed on continually increasing effectiveness and efficiency is referred to as *quality improvement* ("QI"), and usually involves application of the *quality cycle*. In the quality cycle (a.k.a. the "plan-do-check-act" or "PDCA cycle"; see Figure 58.1) process, an issue or problem is recognized, a solution identified and put into effect, and the outcome checked to ensure that the issue or problem has been resolved. Scientists will immediately recognize the PDCA cycle as a simple expression of fundamental scientific method. If an issue is complex, with several solutions to its component problems, the cycle can be repeated (also see *Troubleshooting*).

TQM is an all-encompassing quality system integrating QC, QA, and QI into a perpetual reiterative process based upon inspection and audit. This means that TQM is not a short-term project: like an accreditation scheme, it is not "finished" once the initial certification/accreditation has been awarded but rather is a never-ending process of continually seeking improvement via a continuum of quality cycle events punctuated by self-assessment exercises and peer-review surveys. So TQM must be seen as a long-term goal: there are no shortcuts or quick fixes for its implementation; there is no "magic fix" or panacea for all the problems and woes of an organization; no turn-key systems that can be plugged into an organization's preexisting management structure. From practical experience, achieving a "TQM-enabled" IVF center should not be expected to take less than two years.

Implementing TQM requires both sequential and parallel processes. In summary:

- Develop a clear, long-term approach that is integrated into all the organization's other business plans and strategies (e.g., operations, human resources, facility development, information management and technology, and fiscal planning).
- Create a comprehensive collection of policies addressing the needs of all areas within the organization. These policies form the basis of TQM implementation within the organization and will include goals, objectives, targets, specific projects, and resources. They must be developed in full consultation with those individuals who will have the responsibility for translating the policies into achievements.
- Deploy these policies through all levels of the organization's hierarchy and through all areas of the organization's activities.

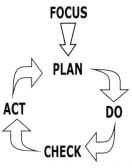

Figure 58.1. The quality cycle, also known as the PDCA Cycle. Reproduced from ref. 5 with permission.

- Conduct systems analysis and integrate of quality into all processes at the most fundamental levels.
- Develop prevention-based activities. This includes risk analysis and management and often a cultural shift from faultfinding and blame to recognizing "genuine" mistakes as opportunities for improvement (while not trivializing poor performance or ignoring incompetence).
- Educate *everyone* in the organization so that they embrace change. Creating a sense of "ownership" is essential in order to achieve "buy-in" from the organization's greatest asset – its people.
- Develop and introduce targeted quality assurance processes so that QI can take place. This is essential for the quality cycle.
- Develop the organization's management and infrastructure to support quality and QI activities. While some new positions are essential to achieving this, for example, the quality manager, this function must not be seen as a separate part of the organization's management; it must be tightly integrated into the normal business management structure.
- Continue to pursue standardization, systematization, and simplification of all work instructions, procedures and systems. This depends on process mapping and systems analysis.

Competent and effective management – and leadership – are essential (2,5,7,9). Senior management play a vital role in ensuring that TQM implementation does not stall, which would cause a major loss of faith in the process by personnel – and getting them to "buy back in" will be far more difficult. Common causes for an organization's failure in its implementation of a TQM program include:

- Insufficient or inappropriate human and/or financial resources.
- Lack of commitment by and/or support from the management ("hollow words").
- Active or passive resistance to change (see *Resistance to Change*).
- Insufficient knowledge and/or understanding of what was required (failure of education).
- Inadequate information management resources and/or systems (includes both documentation and data).
- Wrong attitudes or an inappropriate environment, for example, a culture of fear, faultfinding, blame, and retribution – see the *Toxic Workplace*).

Resistance to change stems from the intrinsic human fear of change. However, confident, competent people understand – or can learn – that change can be good and that the challenges it brings can lead to major professional, personal, and financial rewards. Resistance to change can be either *passive* (e.g., inertia or complacency) or *active* (where positive action is taken to block, undermine, or destroy changes). Both can be dealt with via team building – which is not always about being supportive and doing positive things; sometimes it requires the removal of apparently immovable obstacles.

A *toxic workplace* is characterized by one or more (or all) of the following features: no support for workers from management; no support between the workers themselves; lethargy; absenteeism; verbal and physical intimidation; an increased level of complaints; changes in employees' behavior including loss of confidence or initiative, declining interpersonal relationships, development of turf wars, incidences of "work rage," and/or avoidance of company social functions; and a culture of fear (6).

RISK AND RISK MANAGEMENT

Introduction

As in all areas of industry, reducing medical errors and enhancing patient and staff safety is a prime focus in modern medicine. But what is "risk"? Simplistically, it is any uncertainty about a future event that might threaten an organization's ability to accomplish its mission. Risk management was originally an engineering discipline dealing with the possibility that some future event might cause harm or "loss." It includes strategies and techniques for recognizing and confronting any such threat and provides a disciplined environment for proactive decision making for the purpose of assessing on a continuous basis what can go wrong, determining which risks need to be dealt with, and implementing strategies to deal with these risks (5,10–12).

Over the past twenty-five years, continued developments in reproductive biomedicine, combined with heightened regulatory requirements, have led to more unexpected, and often complex, risk issues for IVF centers (10–13). At its most basic, risk management asks – and answers – three basic questions:

1. "What can go wrong?"
2. "What will we do?" (both to prevent the harm from occurring and in the aftermath of an incident)
3. "If something happens, how will we resolve it, put things right and/or pay for it?"

In an effective risk management program, risks are continuously identified, analyzed, and minimized, mitigated, or eliminated and problems are prevented before they occur. In layman's terms, there is a cultural shift from "fire fighting" and "crisis management" to proactive decision making and planning. Again there is no "magic bullet" solution to implementing risk management – nor does it guarantee success (because there are many aspects to achieving success in an IVF center). However, *not* pursuing risk management means that (5)

- more resources will be expended to correct problems that could have been avoided,
- catastrophic problems will occur without warning,
- there will be no ability to respond rapidly to such "surprises" and recovery will be very difficult and/or costly, or even impossible,
- decisions will be made with incomplete information or inadequate knowledge of their possible future consequences,
- the overall probability of success will be reduced, and
- the organization will always be in a state of crisis.

Risk Management Tools

There are two main tools used in risk management: a proactive tool called failure modes and effects analysis or "FMEA" and a reactive tool called root cause analysis or "RCA" (5,8).

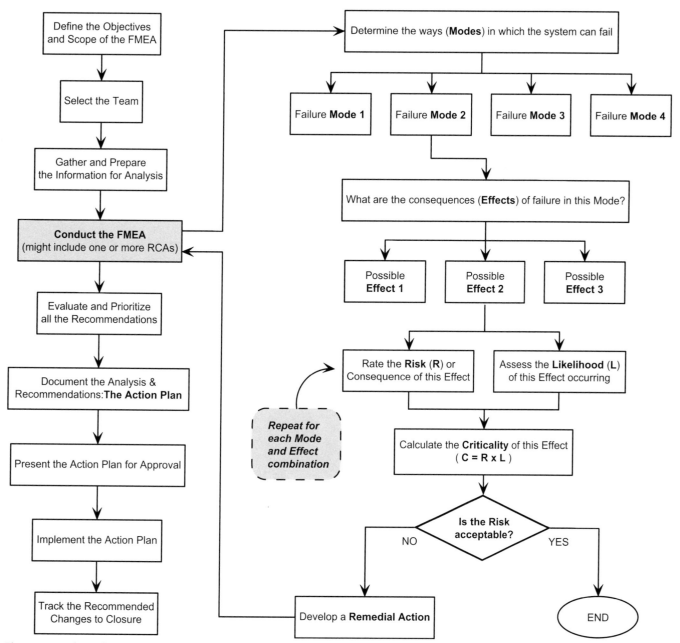

Figure 58.2. A basic flow chart describing the process for performing an FMEA. Reproduced from ref. 5 with permission.

While FMEA works toward the prevention of risk, RCA is used to deal with actual adverse events and troubleshooting. Both tools analyze systems and processes, so an understanding of process analysis and process mapping is a prerequisite to effective risk management (see *Process Management*).

Failure Modes and Effects Analysis

"FMEA" is a straightforward, powerful engineering quality management technique that helps identify and counter weaknesses in the design or manufacture of products or in the design and execution of processes. It uses a structured approach to identify process components that need improvement, based on relative ratings of their anticipated frequency of failure,

and on the severity of adverse effects or events. Its applicability has made it a widely used tool that can be used to improve processes in any organization.

Conducting an FMEA requires the team to follow a sequence of steps (summarized in Figure 58.2).

1. Examine and map the process: Identify all the functions that are expected to occur.
2. Identify *failure modes*: Identify the ways in which any of the functions might go wrong.
3. Determine the *effects*: Establish the consequences of each failure mode.
4. Identify *contributory factors*, that is, all the possible underlying causes for each failure mode.

Table 58.1: Suggested Lists of Likelihood Ratings for Failure Modes as well as of Consequences of Failure Effects for an FMEA Risk Analysis. Modified from Ref. 5.

Rating	Likelihood	Consequence
0	Impossible – can never happen, hence it is not a real risk	None – hence it cannot be considered as a real risk
1	Very unlikely, *e.g.*, a well-controlled or minimized risk, but which cannot be completely eliminated	Trivial, *i.e.*, in reality there is no measurable adverse risk
2	Unlikely, *e.g.*, the circumstances for such a risk's occurrence are all controlled as far as practically possible, but external factors remain which the organization cannot control	Minimal, *i.e.*, in reality the risk is more of a nuisance or inconvenience, with no identifiable impact on patient care
3	Somewhat possible	Quite minor, *e.g.*, impacts the organization's internal systems only
4	Possible	Minor, *e.g.*, a definite adverse effect on efficiency but without any measurable effect on treatment outcome
5	Very possible	Quite serious, *e.g.*, a definite risk of diminished treatment outcome
6	Likely	Serious, *e.g.*, a definite adverse effect on a patient's management or treatment outcome
7	Quite likely	Very serious, *e.g.*, one or more definite adverse impacts upon multiple patients' management or treatment outcomes or risk of injury to patients or staff
8	Very likely	Major, *e.g.*, loss of embryos, OHSS, infection of patients or staff, causes actual injury to patient(s) or staff
9	Extremely likely	Extreme, *e.g.*, loss of life, damage to facility (must be at least "very unlikely")
10	Certain, hence this situation should never exist in a real-world situation	Catastrophic, *e.g.*, loss of multiple lives, destruction of facility – in a real-world situation this should apply only to "acts of God," war or terrorism

5. Rate the *likelihood* (expected frequency) of each failure mode or contributory factor and the severity of its *consequence*, using standardized rating schemes (e.g., Table 58.1). Although many schemes employ scales of 1–5, we prefer the greater dynamic range of 1–10 scales for prioritizing the risks.

6. Calculate the *criticality* of each failure mode (i.e., each risk) as the product of the likelihood and consequence ranks. (Because of this step, FMEA is sometimes referred to as failure modes, effects, and *criticality* analysis or "FMECA.")

7. Tabulate the scores for each of the risks into a *risk matrix* and partition the criticality scores to allow them to be ranked (for example) as either no risk, low risk, medium risk, significant risk, or high risk.

8. Identify any existing controls: Analyze the process map, identify any monitoring or detection systems, mitigation systems, and so on, and assess their impact on the assigned criticality scores (this might result in modification of the risk matrix).

9. Prepare and implement an *action plan*: It is vital that there is a system for monitoring the effectiveness and efficacy for each change that is instituted within the action plan, as per the PDCA cycle.

Root Cause Analysis

"RCA" is a sequence of steps taken to identify the underlying causes (contributory factors) of an adverse event or outcome with the goal of preventing its recurrence. Clearly, an RCA has to be undertaken with the full support of upper management, or there is a risk of it being performed in a perfunctory manner for the sole purpose of meeting some regulatory requirement. Moreover, it must be understood that most errors result from faulty systems rather than human error: poorly designed processes put people in situations where errors are more likely to occur (see Figure 58.5, for a detailed discussion of this). Consequently, an RCA can only be effective if it is accepted throughout the organization that its goal is to aid

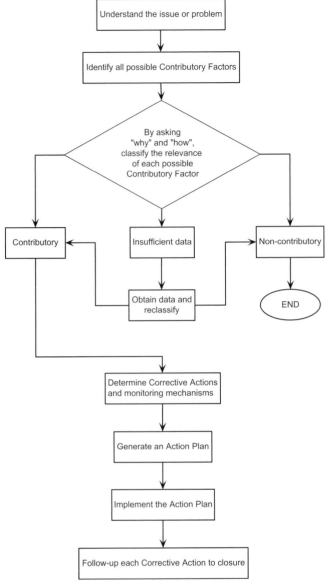

Figure 58.3. A basic flow chart describing the process for performing a root cause analysis (RCA). Reproduced from ref. 5 with permission.

improvement and not to assign blame (in keeping with the principles of continuous improvement intrinsic to TQM philosophy).

Undertaking an RCA (Figure 58.3) is essentially the same as an after-the-fact FMEA and has six stages:

1. Understand the issue: Discover everything possible about the incident, focusing on the systems and processes that could have contributed to the event happening.
2. Develop a diagram of the contributory factors: Ask "why?" or "how?" for each contributory factor so that it can be classified as either "insufficient data, "noncontributory," or "contributory."
3. Resolve items classified as "insufficient data": Obtain data for each of these real or potential contributory factors so that they can be definitively classified.
4. Generate an action plan: The action plan should include at least one corrective action or improvement for each

contributory factor identified. An RCA reporting table is developed for the action plan.
5. Implement the action plan: Implement the planned corrective actions and their monitoring processes.
6. Follow-up: Use the monitoring processes to assess the effectiveness of the corrective actions. If the problem is not fully resolved, then it might be necessary to revise and repeat the RCA process.

Again it is essential that everyone involved understands that the goal is to discover everything possible about the incident, with the focus on the systems and processes that could have contributed to the event happening and on the prevention of future recurrence. Every "contributory factor" that has no lower level derivative is considered to be a root cause (for psychological and legal reasons, contributory factor is used instead of "cause"). The RCA reporting table developed from an RCA has the following columns for each contributory factor:

■ Corrective action(s).
■ Person(s) responsible for implementing the corrective action(s). Unless there is someone specifically assigned to oversee each corrective action, not all will be pursued, and the expectations of successful outcome will be greatly reduced.
■ Action due date. This sets the timetable for each corrective action, which deters procrastination and gives a sense of the process being finite, as well as a date by which the problem will be resolved.
■ Measurement technique. There must be some way of determining whether the corrective action has had an effect.
■ Person(s) responsible for monitoring each corrective action. Again, unless someone is specifically assigned to oversee each corrective action, follow-through can drag on.
■ Follow-up date. This is the date by which everyone involved can expect significant progress to have been made.

PROCESS MANAGEMENT

Although the terms "process" and "system" might seem synonymous, they are not. A *process* is a series of continuous actions or tasks or a method by which something is done, whereas a *system* is a group of objects related or interacting so as to form a unity or a methodically arranged set of ideas, principles, methods, procedures, and so on. Hence, a system is more macro than a process and typically comprises a collection of processes that occur either sequentially or simultaneously with other processes, where the output of one is an input to another. Fundamentally, a process can be defined as a single, simple sequence that has inputs to which "something happens" in order to generate the output (Figure 58.4).

Systems analysis is the diagnosis, formulation, and solution of problems arising from the complex interactions of a system's components. In the IVF lab, systems analysis is used to guide decisions on issues such as planning laboratory operations,

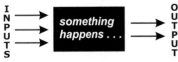

Figure 58.4. A generic process. Reproduced from ref. 5 with permission.

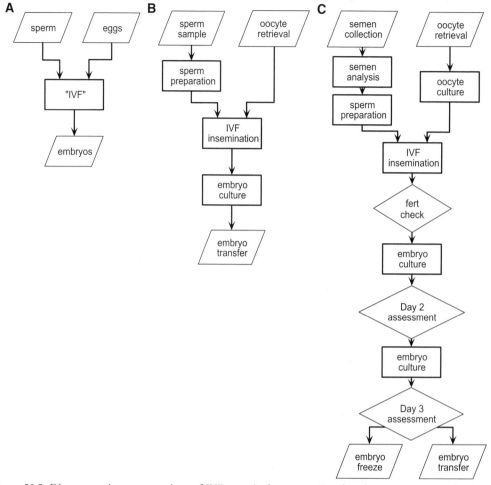

Figure 58.5. Diagrammatic representations of IVF as a single process. Panel A shows it at its simplest level, while panels B and C reveal progressively greater depths of detail in the sequence of generalized stages in the process. Reproduced from ref. 5 with permission.

resource use and staff/environment protection, research and development, implementing new methods, educational needs, and clinical service provision.

However, it is not possible to understand a whole system without knowing both the individual processes and all the extrinsic factors affecting each process. This analysis is often undertaken graphically, via *process mapping*, in which the system or "complex process" is drawn as a flowchart with every step or individual component process in the system identified. This requires the system to be reduced to its fundamental steps, with no lower level derivative processes, so that the factors acting on every component process can be identified and analyzed. For example, although the IVF lab system can be drawn as a simple process, it cannot be analyzed *in toto* due to the large numbers of component subprocesses (Figure 58.5). Indeed, the amount of detail present in the "IVF process" is vast and even Figure 58.6 only presents an overview of the actual steps involved. While these examples have been illustrated using the well-known process-mapping tool of *flowcharting*, there are many other, often more complex, tools, such as *swim lane analysis* or *top-down process mapping* (5,14) that are variously better suited to different types of analysis or scenarios. For example, a top-down process map is an excellent way to start developing a standard operating procedure (SOP) from scratch.

A successful process-mapping exercise will have the following outcomes:

◾ increased understanding of the process,
◾ increased consensus among those who created the map about what the process is and how it operates,
◾ increased buy-in to the need for change, and
◾ an environment where ideas for process improvement can be generated more rapidly.

When a process-mapping exercise is complete, knowledge that has been hidden away inside the heads of many individuals will have been unlocked and made available throughout the organization. Everyone feels empowered and more confident in their work, and corporate knowledge can be passed on to the next generation without any gaps or misconceptions.

Process analysis is the first step toward process control and depends on scientific methods and statistical techniques (5). The analysis of a process for either quality or risk management purposes requires prior knowledge of its normal parameters of operation, including reliable information on the process's historical performance and knowledge of its inherent variability. The identification of all the intrinsic and extrinsic factors affecting the process can then be made. *Intrinsic factors* are those

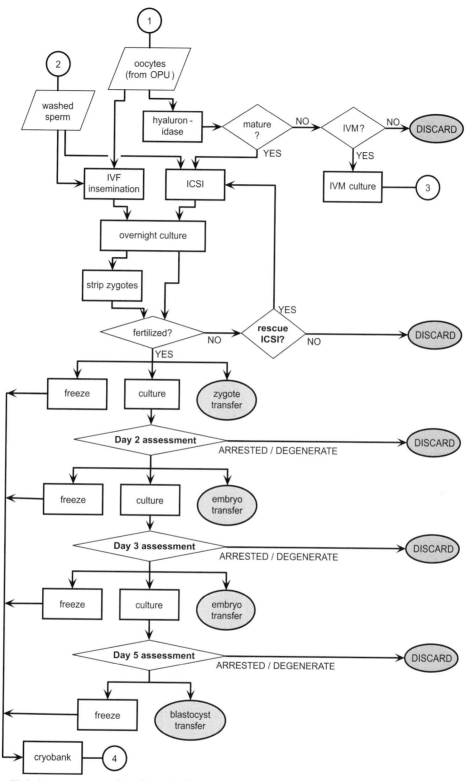

Figure 58.6. A process map of the "standard" IVF laboratory process. Off-page connectors relate to: ① the actual oocyte retrieval process; ② obtaining, analyzing, and preparing the sperm sample; ③ the ancillary process of in vitro maturation of oocytes; and ④ the process whereby specimens are transferred into the cryobank. Note that, even at this level of detail, there remain many lower level/subordinate processes in each step. Reproduced from ref. 5 with permission (figure created using SmartDraw software: SmartDraw.com, San Diego, CA, www.smartdraw.com).

inherent to the process, that is, they are the effects that cause or control the process (the most common intrinsic factors in IVF laboratory systems are those regulating temperature, pH, and humidity). *Extrinsic factors* are ones that are not inherently involved in the process, that is, uncontrolled sources of cooling, toxic vapors, and biological variation.

This is why the SOPs in lab manuals must include sufficient technical/procedural detail for anyone with basic biology lab competence to perform the procedure *in exactly the way it was intended*. This is especially important in procedures where variations in the technical method can result in reduced control over factors affecting the process or even allow the incursion of extrinsic factors that would otherwise have been excluded. Knowing exactly what must be specified in an SOP to achieve the necessary level of correct technique and standardization, as opposed to being unnecessarily picky, therefore requires that the SOP author understand not just how the process in question is regulated by biology, chemistry, and physics (and hence engineering) but also how it might be impacted by extrinsic factors, the lab environment, or ergonomics.

Knowing, or, perhaps better, understanding, why we do things in certain ways – and also perhaps why we do not do them in other ways – requires more than a simple technical ability to do the specific task. This is why a proper training program for anyone in an IVF lab must include both the "how" and the "why." Proper training is vital and must be provided within an encompassing framework of education; learning from history is paramount. In some labs, the unauthorized variation of methods is a persistent problem and is due to either poor training of new scientists or a failure to maintain control over staff. Although the problem typically arises either from a lab director who fails to (re)train new staff, or fails to recognize (and eradicate) sloppy or lazy behavior by a staff member, any scientist who will not respect and follow SOPs has no place in an IVF lab.

Process control is another technique taken from industry, where it was developed to monitor the performance of manufacturing processes (8). The measurement of interest is called an *indicator*; but in the IVF lab, rather than comparing the performance of a process in relation to some external reference or *benchmark*, we are often concerned with monitoring performance relative to the historical performance of our own implementation of a process. Basically, process control techniques allow us to know at any point in time, whether or not our systems are "under control" compared to our "normal" performance levels. The most frequently used tool for this is the process control chart (a.k.a. "Shewhart chart, after one of its early proponents; Figure 58.7).

As long as the periodic values in a process control chart remain within the control limits, the process is considered to be "in control." However, there are four scenarios that require further action:

1. The indicator crosses its control limit in the adverse direction: Immediate action is required to determine whether there is a genuine problem and, if verified, to seek its resolution.
2. The indicator crosses its warning limit in the adverse direction: Action is required to determine whether a problem might exist or be developing.
3. The indicator shows three consecutive changes in the adverse direction but does not cross the warning (or control) limit: Action is required to determine whether a problem might be developing.

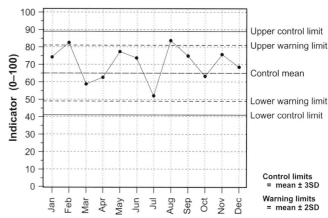

Figure 58.7. An example of a control chart for a generic process whose outcome is measured using an indicator that has a range of from 0 to 100 (e.g., percentage values). Baseline data on the performance of the process are required for a representative period of operation, for example, monthly average values for the indicator over the preceding six months. The mean and standard deviation (SD) of these six values are calculated, and these values used to establish the "control mean" and two types of operational limits: (a) "warning limits," defined as the mean ±2SD; and (b) "control limits," defined as the mean ±3SD. The number of prior data periods required to calculate the control limits for an indicator is not predetermined arbitrarily. The number used must be sufficient to give a good indication of the variability of the indicator, but at the same time not be so many that the SD is reduced to the extent that the control limits become too narrow, with the result that apparent control deviations frequently turn out to be random fluctuations in the indicator. Reproduced from ref. 5 with permission (figure created using MedCalc software: Mariakerke, Belgium; www.medcalc.be).

4. The indicator crosses its control limit in the beneficial direction: The system should be reviewed to see why it occurred and whether the improvement is real and sustained (Figure 58.8).

Indicators are crucial to the development and maintenance of a quality system: as the old maxim says "You can't control what you can't measure." Each indicator must reflect the process being monitored and needs to have the following characteristics:

Reliable: It must measure something useful, and the process to be monitored must be well defined.
Robust: The influence of extraneous effects must be minimized so that only the intended process is measured.
Routine: Data collection must not be arduous or involve a lot of extra work. If it does, then there will be resistance to determining indicators regularly, and the entire activity will become a chore, undermining its perceived value to the lab.

The regular determination of indicators eloquently demonstrates the crucial role of information/data systems in the well-run IVF lab, exemplifying the principle of "working smarter not harder." Even though the clinical pregnancy rate, or "take-home baby rate," is an important indicator of the overall performance of an IVF program, it is too "macroscale" for effective monitoring of individual lab processes. Consequently,

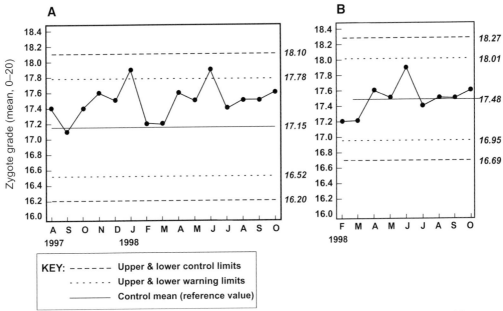

Figure 58.8. The control chart shows data for zygote grade (based on a score out of twenty). Monthly average values for the six months preceding the period shown in chart A (i.e., February to July 1997) were used to establish the control mean and the warning and control limits. However, the introduction of an improved IVF and embryo culture system in mid-August 1997 (13) resulted in all the values for subsequent months except one being above the control mean, necessitating recalculation of the control values, using the August 1997 to January 1998 monthly average values, as shown in chart B. The increased value for the control mean indicates a systematic improvement in zygote grade while the narrower control limits express the improved stability (i.e., reproducibility) of the new culture system. Reproduced from ref. 5 with permission.

for the IVF lab's purposes, *laboratory performance indicators* (LPIs) that each monitor a specific process via a control chart are required (5,16). Maintaining a comprehensive panel of LPIs allows an IVF lab to reply quickly to the seemingly perpetual question of "what's wrong in the lab?" – if all the LPIs are within their control limits, then the lab can conclusively state that everything is still the same as before, nothing has changed, and hence the questioner should seek an explanation elsewhere for the perceived decrease in whatever end point they are looking at. Of course, if a problem does arise, then the lab will recognize it early via the LPIs – presumably before it can manifest itself in any clinical end points. The lab will then be able to investigate it and either disregard it as a fluctuation unrelated to any change in operational performance or adverse factor(s) acting on one or more lab processes or identify the source of the problem and deal with it.

However, while the use of control charts to monitor lab processes via LPIs will have meaning to the lab manager or director, it must be recognized that, in the vast majority of IVF centers, this information will often seem uninformative, even pointless, to the physicians or other team members. While those other team members will understand what *program performance indicators* ("PPIs," e.g., pregnancy rate, clinical pregnancy rate, and implantation rate) mean for the IVF center, there is very often a "disconnect" in perceptions between lab operations and pregnancy rates. From the patients' perspective, apart from cost and location, a center's pregnancy rate and implantation rate are the most likely indicators that will be sought. It is important, therefore, that everyone in a center understands that PPIs summarize the center's performance as a whole, not just of the laboratory's performance. It is also important to realize that different

IVF programs may have (indeed, will likely have) different definitions for their PPIs – hence, it is essential that these definitions are known before any attempt at benchmarking is made, illustrating why the use of reference populations for reporting results is so important for effective benchmarking.

Benchmarking is, basically, the proof of what is possible. In a traditional business setting, benchmarking is the continuous process of measuring one's products or services against one's (strongest) competitors or those renowned as world leaders in the field (5). In its practical application for IVF Centers, benchmarking employs various PPIs and can be viewed at three levels:

- Internal benchmarking: comparisons between centers within a group or network.
- Competitive benchmarking: comparisons against the direct competition.
- Functional or generic benchmarking: comparisons against the "best-in-the-world" centers.

For an IVF laboratory, benchmarking can be used to verify that the laboratory outcomes (monitored by LPIs) are maintained, to monitor the implementation or amendment of processes to improve outcomes to match those of competing centers and to evaluate the development of better processes or technology to meet, or exceed, the performance of other centers. Benchmarking is an effective way of avoiding complacency.

TROUBLESHOOTING

Figure 58.9 illustrates a generic troubleshooting process, showing that the application of scientific method is fundamental to

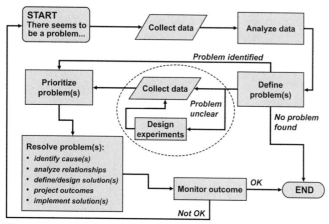

Figure 58.9. A basic flowchart illustrating the troubleshooting process, demonstrating its fundamental equivalence to RCA.

the process and, indeed, is essential for effective troubleshooting (5,12). For someone who has successfully learned scientific method, a structured approach to problem solving should have become intuitive – a good scientist will essentially go through all the steps of an RCA automatically, if subconsciously, whenever confronted by a problem. Formalizing the procedure allows less well-trained or less-experienced people to apply the same technique and it also provides the framework whereby it is documented.

An effective troubleshooter can be likened to a scientific detective (5) – and this is why it is so important when teaching someone a method that you take the time to explain "why" things are done the way they are (and perhaps why they are *not* done a certain way). Just describing the "how" cannot produce a truly competent scientists, and a lack of comprehensive knowledge will greatly compromise their ability to minimize or eliminate problems.

Essentially, the same troubleshooting approach can be applied to processes, methods, incidents, or even entire systems – once they have been mapped in sufficient detail.

ACCREDITATION

Regulation and licensing are nonoptional systems that are imposed on an organization. They are created and enforced via legislation and consequently vary widely between countries (and even between states in countries such as Australia and the United States). Licensing bodies (e.g., the Human Fertilisation and Embryology Authority, or HFEA, in the UK) typically issue a license after an inspection process to confirm that an organization is, indeed, operating in accordance with the law. While this process might create some minimum standard level to which a licensed IVF lab will operate, there is often no consideration of performance standards or quality within the terms of the licensing process. Interestingly, the recently introduced *European Tissues and Cells Directives* 2004/23/EC, 2006/17/EC and 2006/86/EC (17–19) combine a regulatory framework with the requirement for a quality management system. While there were grave initial concerns regarding the proposals that were mooted in draft of the original directive (20), the final directive that affects the operation of IVF labs (i.e., 2006/86/EC) will be highly beneficial in promoting the need for effective quality management in IVF labs.

In contrast, accreditation is a voluntary, collegial process based on self- and peer assessment to determine an organization's compliance with an agreed set of "standards" (4,5). Accreditation is based entirely on process and upon the principles of quality improvement rather than strict obedience of regulations. While an accreditation standard might contain technical specifications or criteria that must be applied consistently – whether as rules, guidelines, or definitions of characteristics – to ensure that materials, products, processes, and services are fit for their purpose, accreditation schemes are not prescriptive in relation to any technical procedures or rules. An accreditation standard describes a voluntary agreement between all parties involved in the product or service and encompasses all components or factors that might influence the product or service, especially its safety, reliability, and efficiency. It must be a "living document" because our understanding of the processes by which we create a product, or provide a service, grow with experience and hence standards must not be embodied within legislation that will take years to modify.

Effective accreditation schemes share the same three basic characteristics stages (summarized in Figure 58.10):

Stage 1: An initial *self-assessment* of all aspects of the organization's mission, programs, and services, necessarily involving individuals from all areas and levels, as well as its customers (patients) and, ideally, the public. Input from these stakeholders is used to create a detailed self-assessment that documents the organization's current status quo, with the major concomitant benefit of buy-in from everyone involved. The goals of the self-assessment process are

- to determine compliance with established accreditation criteria or "standards";
- to assess the organization's alignment with its own stated philosophies and goals, as well as with those imposed by any regulatory authority, in terms of patient care and service delivery;

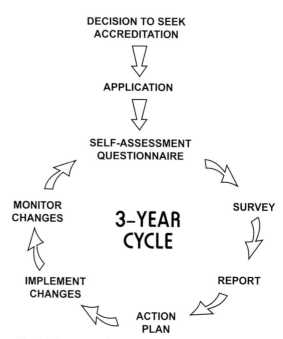

Figure 58.10. Diagrammatic representation of a generic accreditation process. Reproduced from ref. 5 with permission.

- to evaluate outcomes and effectiveness; and
- to identify, and prioritize, areas for improvement.

Stage 2: *External assessment* via a *survey* by a team of peers (not an "inspection" or "assessment" site visit). The survey team, comprising a group of objective professionals trained in performing surveys, views the premises, meets with management, conducts interviews with members of staff and (willing) patients, and examines data to assess the organization's compliance with the accrediting authority's established criteria or standards. The surveyors typically conduct an "exit interview" to present their findings and also perhaps the recommendations to be included in the written report.

Stage 3: *Report and recommendations*. The survey team's findings in relation to the self-assessment document are presented in a written report that focuses on the organization's strengths and weaknesses. Recommendations are made to help the organization develop plans to improve areas of weakness and also to maintain and expand areas of strength. The recommendations follow a standardized code of expression to facilitate their interpretation by the organization seeking accreditation.

Must or *shall* denote recommendations that are considered necessary for the organization to become compliant against a particular standard or alleviate a recognized problem.

Should denote recommendations that, in the light of the surveyors' experience, will either improve the organization's rating for a particular standard or are likely to provide significant benefit to the organization's operational standards or performance (although they might be subject to prioritization).

Could identify suggestions for changes that might, in light of the surveyors' experience and/or that of other similar organizations, improve the organization's operational standards or performance and would be expected to generate an improvement in the organization's rating according to a particular standard.

Unlike accreditation, quality is not a cyclical process. While the surveys might well run on a three-year cycle, quality must be an ongoing, perpetual process built upon the quality cycle. There should never be a need to "get back to" the quality management program: it should be tightly integrated into the daily functioning of every part of the clinic (*not* just the lab). Quality must be integral, it cannot be an add-on, and any organization that relaxes its commitment to quality and considers that it does not have to worry about "accreditation stuff" until the time comes around to prepare for the next self-assessment has simply failed to see the point of accreditation and will not reap the full benefit of everyone's hard work.

IDENTIFYING A "POOR QUALITY" OR "HIGH-RISK" IVF LAB

IVF is an area of rapidly advancing technology and so continual training and proficiency testing are imperative. But these tactics in isolation will neither ensure quality nor prevent potentially catastrophic errors, and the overall work environment must support, not obstruct, both technical training and improvements in operational systems. From experience, the following are the most likely areas where risk factors can be identified in an IVF lab (although this is by no means an exhaustive risk analysis of an IVF Lab) (5).

Inadequate Resources

Centers that insist on running with the minimum possible resources (physical, human, or financial) will be at greater risk. There must be sufficient capacity in critical equipment to deal with the busiest of times, for example, incubator space (so incubator doors are not opened too often) or controlled rate freezer capacity (so all patients' embryos can be frozen at the right time).

Insufficient Staff

A recent workload analysis revealed that more than 70 percent of IVF labs in the UK are understaffed (21). That study also confirmed our own earlier (unpublished) calculations that in an IVF laboratory operating to established quality standards, one full-time embryologist is required for each 125 stimulated treatment cycles per annum.

Overworking

Embryologists must be alert and not distracted by tiredness in order to perform all aspects of their jobs accurately and reliably, with the lowest possible risk of making mistakes. Any circumstances that contribute to overtiredness or exhaustion represent serious risk factors. Staffing levels must reflect the maximum caseload, with some slack in the system so that staff are not constantly working at maximum capacity.

The Need for Slack

Slack must be present in any organization to allow not only for the differential between the average and busiest activity levels but also to cope with "unpredictable" events such as an influenza epidemic. An allowance for slack time is essential for an organization to evolve (22).

Inexperienced Staff

Even with effective training programs, a high staff turnover increases the number of people who are less sure of the laboratory's systems, SOPs, and usual practices. Laboratories with a higher proportion of relatively inexperienced embryologists are less equipped to recognize and deal with operational problems as they arise.

Poorly Trained Staff

Comprehensive, formal programs are essential for training all embryologists in new techniques and procedures (i.e., novices and more junior staff), and for the orientation, and retraining as necessary, of embryologists coming from other laboratories. Unintentional failure by embryologists to complete all aspects of their assigned tasks is an expression of inadequate or incomplete training and should be remedied.

Not Accepting Professional Responsibility

This occurs when one or more members of a team do not take enough care to ensure that they have performed – and completed – all the tasks that were assigned to them. This can be either intentional or unintentional, but in all cases is unprofessional. The intentional omission of tasks will jeopardize outcomes unless others are prepared to take (or make) the time to ensure that the whole process is completed: effectively being the "safety net." All professionals must be prepared to work without a safety net; if someone cannot do this then, (s)he should not be working in an IVF lab.

Equipment Failure

All equipment must be included in a preventative maintenance program and all "mission critical" equipment must be monitored on a continual basis, for example, cryostorage tanks, incubators, CO_2 supply, and liquid nitrogen supply. In addition, an out-of-hours alarm system that can call or page a list of contact persons capable of resolving the issue is essential.

Power Failure

Continuity of electrical power supply to critical equipment must be ensured, while items sensitive to power fluctuations need to be protected by an uninterruptible power supply or "UPS."

Not Double Checking

Every time that something is labeled, or material (i.e., gametes or embryos), is moved from one container to another, identity checks must be followed strictly and verified either by a competent witness or some validated process or technological solution. In the UK, the HFEA introduced a requirement for "double witnessing" of all such events in October 2002 (23).

Inadequate SOPs

Incomplete, or poorly written, SOPs create opportunities for embryologists to make mistakes.

Unauthorized Changes in Methods

All staff must follow the laboratory's SOPs exactly. Any changes to documented SOPs must be authorized by the lab director to ensure that the changes would not be detrimental. Introduction of variations, shortcuts, or perceived "improvements" without authorization should be a disciplinary offence because of the enormous increase in risk.

Poor Documentation

Great care must be taken when completing all documentation (and everything must be documented) to ensure that all records (laboratory, medical, and government) are complete and accurate. Indicators of carelessness or lack of attention to detail (i.e., risk) include personnel not being aware of patients' appointments/procedures/management plan, mistakes in patient accounts, telephone calls being made to the wrong patient, and so on.

Omissions

Lack of a comprehensive, documented system of notifications and/or task lists to ensure that the laboratory staff know exactly what has to be done each day will increase the risk of critical tasks being forgotten.

Unrecognized Incidents

Unless a comprehensive system of incident reports ("nonconformity reports" in ISO 9001:2000 parlance) for all adverse events is in place, enforced, and employed constructively, many mistakes will never be recognized or remembered. In this context, an "adverse event" can be defined as any event that potentially or actually affects staff safety, patient safety, or the provision of treatment according to the patient's care plan or the expected outcome of their treatment.

Use of Nonapproved Products or Devices

Some IVF Centers use products or devices that are intended for veterinary use or that have not been approved for medical use by the appropriate regulatory authorities, for example, the Food and Drug Administration in the United States, CE marking in Europe, and so forth. A common example of this is the Tomcat catheter, a veterinary product that is still used in some centers for intrauterine insemination and even embryo transfer. Several studies have reported a detrimental effect of this catheter for embryo transfer (e.g., 24), and consequently, its continued use is not only a significant risk factor for decreased success rates but it must also be considered a risk for potential liability.

CONCLUSIONS

It has only been possible in this chapter to provide an overview of the tools and techniques that are the foundation for the three pillars that support TQM: process management, quality management, and risk management. Numerous reference texts for all these specialist areas exist in the business world, and the concepts can be readily applied in IVF once the fundamentals are understood. While the application of TQM cannot guarantee success, or even improved IVF success rates, it will ensure that the IVF lab systems will operate smoothly and efficiently. Well-controlled operational systems facilitate the identification of problems or problem areas, and TQM provides the tools for minimizing or eliminating the sources of such problems. It should also be apparent that risk management is the "alter ego" of quality management and that both operate in close harmony. Anyone who has been involved in the successful implementation of TQM – into any organization, not just in IVF – will attest to its many and multifaceted benefits to the organization, to its people, and to its customers.

REFERENCES

1. International Organization for Standardization. International Standard ISO 9001. Quality Management Systems – Requirements. Geneva, Switzerland: International Organization for Standardization, 2000.
2. Carson BE, Alper MM, Keck C. *Quality Management Systems for Assisted Reproductive Technology – ISO 9001:2000*. London, England: Taylor & Francis, 2004.
3. International Organization for Standardization. International Standard ISO 15189. Medical Laboratories – Particular Requirements for Quality and Competence. Geneva, Switzerland: International Organization for Standardization, 2003.
4. Burnett D. *A Practical Guide to Accreditation in Laboratory Medicine*. London, England: ACB Venture Publications, 2002.

5. Mortimer D, Mortimer ST. *Quality and Risk Management in the IVF Laboratory*. Cambridge, England: Cambridge University Press, 2005.

6. Coombs A. *The Living Workplace. Soul, Spirit and Success in the 21st Century*. Toronto, Canada: HarperCollins Publishers Ltd., 2001.

7. Dale B, McQuater R. *Managing Business Improvement and Quality. Implementing Key Tools and Techniques*. Oxford, UK: Blackwell Publishers, 1998.

8. Hutchison D. *Total Quality Management in the Clinical Laboratory*. Milwaukee: ASQC Quality Press, 1994.

9. Heller R, Hindle T. *Essential Manager's Manual*. New York: DK Publishing, 2003.

10. Kennedy CR. Risk management in assisted reproduction. *Clin Risk* 2004;10:169–175.

11. Kennedy CR, Mortimer D. Risk management in IVF. In: Edozien L, ed. *Risk Management in Obstetrics and Gynaecology*. Best Pract Res Clin Obstet Gynaecol 2007;21(4):691–712.

12. Mortimer D. Setting up risk management systems in IVF laboratories. *Clin Risk* 2004;10:128–137.

13. Keck C, Fischer R, Baukloh V, Sass P, Alper M. Quality management in reproductive medicine. In: Brinsden PR, ed. *A Textbook of In-Vitro Fertilization and Assisted Reproduction*, 3rd edn. London, UK: Taylor and Francis Medical Books, 2005: 501–520.

14. Grout JR. Process mapping. (accessed 29/12/2006 at http://campbell.berry.edu/faculty/jgrout/processmapping/).

15. Mortimer D, Henman MJ, Jansen RPS. *Development of an Improved Embryo Culture System for Clinical Human IVF*. Eight Mile Plains, Queensland, Australia: William A. Cook Australia, 2002.

16. Mayer JF, Jones EL, Dowling-Lacey D, Nehchiri F, Muasher S, Gibbons W, Oehninger S. Total quality improvement in the IVF laboratory: choosing indicators of quality. *Reprod Biomed Online* 2003;7:695–699.

17. European Union. Directive 2004/23/EC of the European Parliament and of the Council on setting standards of quality and safety for the donation, procurement, testing, processing, preservation, storage and distribution of human tissues and cells. Off J Eur Union, L102/48, 7.4.2004.

18. European Union. Commission Directive 2006/17/EC implementing Directive 2004/23/EC of the European Parliament and of the Council as regards certain technical requirements for the donation, procurement and testing of human tissues and cells. Off J Eur Union, L38/40, 9.2.2006.

19. European Union. Commission Directive 2006/86/EC implementing Directive 2004/23/EC of the European Parliament and of the Council as regards traceability requirements, notification of serious adverse reactions and events and certain technical requirements for the coding, processing, preservation, storage and distribution of human tissues and cells. Off J Eur Union, L294/32, 24.10.2006.

20. Mortimer D. A critical assessment of the impact of the European Union Tissues and Cells Directive (2004) on laboratory practices in assisted conception. *Reprod Biomed Online* 2005;11:162–176.

21. Harbottle S. Are you working too hard? Annual Meeting of the Association of Clinical Embryologists, *Glasgow (UK)*, 2003.

22. DeMarco T. *Slack: Getting Past Burnout, Busywork, and the Myth of Total Efficiency*. New York: Broadway Books, 2001.

23. Brison DR, Hooper M, Critchlow JD, Hunter HR, Arnesen R, Lloyd A, Horne G. Reducing risk in the IVF laboratory: implementation of a double-witnessing system. *Clin Risk* 2004;10:176–180.

24. McDonald JA, Norman RJ. A randomized controlled trial of a soft double lumen embryo transfer catheter versus a firm single lumen catheter: significant improvements in pregnancy rates. *Hum Reprod* 2002;17:1502–1506.

59

THE NURSE AND REI

Ruth Kennedy

INTRODUCTION

The world first heard about in vitro fertilization (IVF) with the miraculous birth of Louise Brown on July 25, 1978. The work of Dr. Patrick Steptoe and Dr. Robert Edwards of Bourn Hall at Cambridge, England, and gave the world its first glimpse of the newest obstetrics/gynecology (OB/GYN) branch – reproductive medicine (1). Louise's birth gave hope to millions of infertile couples – the dream of family now aided by science and medicine with real possibilities of success.

On the front lines of this emerging specialty was Jean Marion Purdy, the first IVF nurse. Jean Purdy was an operating room nurse and laboratory technician working at Bourn Hall, side by side with Dr. Steptoe and Dr. Edwards. She developed the first aspiration catheter, was the first person to provide a written description of the human blastocyst, and was the first nurse to work with urinary lutenizing hormones (1). She opened a door for a nursing role never before seen and one that has grown and evolved since its inception. Today, nurses have multiple opportunities in this still emerging field to fulfill a critical role, while also adding to its development. Jean Purdy's legacy challenges the reproductive endocrinology nurse.

Reproductive endocrinology and infertility (REI) both in academic and independent practice settings will continue to attract the best and the brightest in OB/GYN (2). Dr. Barbieri feels strongly that in the next fifty years, REI physicians in all settings will enjoy thriving practices because of the huge scientific and technical advances in assisted reproductive technology (ART) (2). These include intracytoplasmic sperm injection (ICSI), embryo and oocyte donation and cryopreservation, preimplantation genetic diagnosis (PGD), and embryonic stem cell biology. Also, in its infancy is cryopreservation of ovarian tissue for women undergoing chemotherapy, giving hope for future fertility to these patients. Dr. Barbieri passionately believes that an REI renaissance is at hand and invites the OB/GYN community to join the ranks (2).

So, where does the nurse fit in? In this "vibrant and growing field," nurses can find many exciting and profoundly fulfilling opportunities to reach their full potential, growing professionally and personally (2). If one is looking for an innovative and challenging professional landscape with both technical and interpersonal demands, reproductive medicine certainly offers it all.

THE NURSE

(For this text, "the nurse" will be referred to as "she," since the vast majority of nurses currently in this field are women.) Who is the REI nurse? To the couple, she is a link to the dream of family. It is the *nurse* the patient interacts with, at times, on a daily basis and it is from this professional that the couple receives most of their information and encouragement. What is the plan for today, how are my numbers, how is my cycle going, and how are my embryos? The information comes from multiple team members–physicians, embryologists, lab technicians, and ultrasonographers, to name a few, but the nurse is the main disseminator of information and orders to the patient. Patients "hang" on every word and nuance. It is one of the most intimate of nurse/patient relationships since so much information, both medical and personal, is exchanged during the course of treatment. There are multiple abilities needed to be an REI nurse, and indeed, this is being refined and redefined constantly as this field continues its technological and scientific growth. Since this is still a relatively young field for medicine and for nursing, the role is being developed daily by the nurses in their own practices, often without a template. Skills and knowledge can be acquired and learned and experience can be broadened, but the qualities that make a nurse *a nurse* are harder to teach. This especially applies to the REI nurse. According to Peplau, the nursing role is crucial in better enabling the patient to cope with the stressors of an illness and/or a perceived threat to health and well-being (3). The nurse is described as a primary ally and source of support. This alliance functions within a framework of knowledge and skill, art and science, and caring and compassion. Without this framework, the relationship is not completely effective. This especially applies to the REI nurse and the patient relationship. These nurses must come to this specialty armed with empathy, compassion, and an arsenal of interpersonal skills. She is a team leader and team player; she is a coordinator, traffic engineer, teacher, confidant, counselor, empathetic listener, and cheerleader; she must have tremendous patience, curiosity, and an appetite for knowledge. Peplau summarizes the concept of nursing as a significant, therapeutic, interpersonal process. It functions cooperatively with other human processes that make health possible for individuals in communities. She further believes nursing is an educative instrument, a maturing force that promotes forward movement of personality in the direction of creative, constructive, and productive personal and community living (3). The nurse transitions between the educative and therapeutic role, depending on the patient needs. These concepts say a great deal about nursing as a complex process and what is essential to put it into real practice.

HOW NURSES THINK

With today's challenging medical technology, the nurse needs to be a complex critical thinker and be fully engaged in the nursing process to manage a myriad of decisions and problems that come up every day, with every patient. This process consists of five steps: assessment, diagnosis, planning, implementation, and evaluation (4). It is a systematic approach for gathering, examining, and analyzing data and identifying patient response to a health problem; determining priorities, goals, and expected outcomes; taking appropriate action; and finally, evaluating the effectiveness of the action (5). Roper observes in her nursing text, "Even today many people consider nursing to be simply a series of tasks carried out by the nurse. Undoubtedly, observable tasks are a very important aspect of nursing, but this restrictive interpretation does not take into account the thinking processes which are involved before, during and after any observable task. Nor does it take into account the knowledge and attitudes which must be acquired to accompany the dexterous performance of a nursing activity which is only a part of a deliberate plan of care" (6). Effective clinical problem-solving skills must employ critical thinking. This is a cognitive process a nurse uses to make judgments, which span from basic levels to highly complex ones. The highest level of critical thinking is commitment (5). It involves forming conclusions, making decisions, drawing inferences, and reflecting (7). Successful critical thinkers employ independent thinking, fairness, responsibility and authority, discipline, perseverance, creativity, curiosity, and integrity, which result in confident decisions. It also assumes an intellectual humility. Whether she is a new graduate or a veteran, the responsible nurse is aware of what she *does not* know and will ask the appropriate questions in order to provide safe, quality care.

It is apparent that the REI nurse does more than simply consider alternatives to a problem. With so many variables and so many people involved, the thought process used to make multiple decisions must be creative, inclusive, and expansive. The REI nurse anticipates the need to make choices, is able to do so without the assistance from others, yet with personal consideration to those the decision effects, and takes responsibility for them. She selects an action or belief based on the alternatives available and holds herself accountable and approachable for the choice. With this commitment, attention is given to the results of the decision and the appropriateness of it (5). Another prized asset is intuition. Intuition is the understanding of a situation without conscious deliberation (8). It is that sixth sense that something *is so*. Intuition develops in a nurse as her clinical experience increases, triggering with its occurrence an analytical process leading to conscious collection of data and ensuing action. In REI, it is a pivotal tool in assessing the couple and their unique issues.

KNOWLEDGE AND PROFESSIONAL SUPPORT

Nursing is both art and science. A professional nurse delivers care with compassion, caring, and respect, considering each patient's dignity and humanity. Scientifically, nursing is based on a foundation of knowledge. While this body of knowledge serves as an underpinning for nursing, it is also ever changing – just as is REI. The integration of art, science, and experience provides a high level of quality care, benefiting the patient in many ways. While REI experience is always preferred in newly hired nurses, the reality is that this is not always the case. An REI practice needs seasoned registered nurses (RN) and/or nurse practitioners (NP) preferably grounded in a women's health. The nursing shortage is affecting all fields and newly hired nurses may have to be trained by the practice; training in the specifics of a fertility practice can be acquired if there is a solid base with which to start. It is also very important that nurses already working in the field continue to build on their existing knowledge and experience. The practice benefits from highly trained nurses, as do patients. Job satisfaction improves if the nurse feels valued. Provisions for continuing education and networking opportunities by the practice are a wise investment. It refreshes the staff and may encourage new approaches to patient care as nurses learn from each other. This interaction among nurses in the industry promotes confidence and lessens professional isolation. It also gives the nursing staff a signal that they are valued by the practice, promoting better job satisfaction and perhaps better retention. According to Denton, infertility nurses report a sense of isolation, likely caused by a lack of understanding from colleagues about the specific work they do. Many REI nurses are in small private practices that employ only one or two nurses. Meeting other colleagues in the field at training courses and meetings provides support as well as education (9).

INFORMED CONSENT

Informed consent in REI nursing warrants special consideration. While all centers have patients read and sign consent forms before treatment protocols begin, many patients often do not read or do not understand what the consent is saying, thus necessitating a review of the consent with the couple to ascertain if this is the case. With experience and knowledge, REI nurses are able to tackle concepts foreign to most patients and help them understand not just the treatment but the intended and unintended consequences of that treatment as well. The nurse's ability to understand complex protocols and their risks will enable her to put these into language to which the patient can understand and relate. For example, gaining true informed consent for cycle monitoring falls to both physician and nurse, with the nurse frequently re-explaining what the doctor just said. It becomes vital that the nurse herself understands the physician's rationales for continuation or cancellation of cycles, so patients can understand. Or patients sometimes have the idea that twins, or even triplets, are desirable and will give them a family all at once, enabling them to "stop trying." Patients sometimes see pregnancy, even multiples, in a rosy fantasy, a longed for dream, often unrealistically. In other cases, the goal of pregnancy has been such a driving focus for the couple that potential risks such as multiples, prematurity, fetal reduction, and ovarian hyperstimulation syndrome may not have been given thoughtful consideration by the potential parents, consent or not. Only when the couple understands the risks can they fully consent. As professionals, we need to be aware that consents could possibly be referred to at a future time, perhaps in a difficult situation. It is crucial that the consent was accurately and completely filled in by all parties and the implications discussed, understood, and agreed upon. Full documentation is important. As Muirhead and Kirkland observe in their textbook on IVF, "it could be argued that in no other field of medicine can consents have potentially such an influence on future generations" (10).

INTERPERSONAL AND COUNSELING SKILLS

A patient's infertility is not just a threat to her reproductive function but also to her psychological, emotional, and, in some cases, cognitive and spiritual stability. It strikes at the heart of many couple's ideal of relationship, marriage, and family. The stressors of a state of non–well-being (such as infertility) can lead to a situational crisis within the self and/or the couple causing a drain on resources and a failure of adaptive strategies (3).

Good interpersonal skills create a good nurse-patient relationship. This usually translates into daily and sometimes intense interactions with patients as cycles begin, progress, and finish and pregnancy tests are awaited or are completed. These skills will set the tone for rapport and trust with the nurse and the practice. The counseling done by the nurse in REI, in order to be effective and reassuring, hinges on well-honed, sensitive interpersonal skills. According to Muirhead and Kirkland, the counselor aspect of REI nursing can be broken down into at least four categories (10). With additional explanation they are:

1. Support counseling: Given to support emotional needs. This is rather a constant since patients experience varying levels of stress throughout a treatment cycle as well and have differing coping skills. Infertility couples find themselves riding on the infertility rollercoaster and most find it frustrating, frightening, and confusing. Since not all patients verbalize their needs, it is the nurse's experience and intuition that will tell her how much and what kind of support a particular patient needs.
2. Information counseling: Information is given to patients in all phases of treatment. It is meant to enhance their knowledge and improve compliance and their sense of control. Giving patients any feeling of personal control has proven to be especially useful to these patients who feel they now have very little. Information and support counseling are often used together.
3. Implication counseling: This helps couples to explore the choices and decisions placed before them for relevance and subsequent effects. This may include whether to continue treatment or stop, either temporarily or completely. It will involve informational counseling as their diagnosis will ultimately decide initial treatment plans or amendments to those plans. A diagnosis, for instance, of premature ovarian failure has a different implication for the couple than does a poor semen analysis or polycystic ovarian syndrome.
4. Therapeutic counseling: This is used to help individual patients and/or couples develop coping strategies for the myriad of issues that a diagnosis of infertility can bring. Marital strains may develop or worsen and financial distress may occur due to the great expense of the treatments and medications. Grief for the loss of the dream of a family – a dream that should have been much easier to achieve is very common. When some couples have a difficult time acknowledging and addressing the disappointment of a failed treatment or a pregnancy loss, this grief may be magnified. The invasive nature of infertility treatments along with the intensity of the experience contribute to

a loss of personal dignity and autonomy, which can be very difficult for most people to reconcile (10).

Additionally, referral to a support group (for example, RESOLVE) can be a Godsend for some couples. Finding other people who are struggling with the same issues and problems, someone who *really* understands can be immediately therapeutic. Lifelong friendships may develop and provide ongoing support for these couples throughout their lives, despite the pregnancy outcome. Many practices offer on-site support groups in order to ensure that their patients have professional leadership within the support group.

Some patients have better coping skills than others, and not all patients will require therapeutic counseling. This type of counseling may be done, at times, by a nurse as nurse/patient interactions do have a therapeutic arm. However, most people have finite emotional resources and not all couples share their feelings easily with each other. Men and women experience and define loss differently and often do not have the same coping mechanisms, causing distance, misunderstandings, and frustration within the relationship. Personal support systems may be nonexistent as friends and/or family may not be privy to the couple's pursuit of fertility treatment. It is important to be able to discern when a patient needs more than the doctor or nurse can realistically or safely provide and when it is time to refer the patient or couple to a professional counselor. Some practices have a psychologist or counselor on staff. In the United Kingdom, the Human Fertilization Embryology Act requires licensed fertility clinics to offer every patient an opportunity for counseling (11). In every fertility practice the nurse, as an advocate, is in a primary position to recommend this type of care and should be constantly alert for signals from patients who are in need of professional counseling services.

Since counseling is so integral to all that we do in REI, the correct intervention is vital to the patient to help preserve or reconstruct the person's sense of well-being and wholeness. Infertility often creates a feeling of brokenness within the individual and/or the couple. These patients have certain things in common: they are infertile, they are suffering, and they are looking for help. Understanding this, care should be taken with all encounters as patients may misinterpret even well-meaning "off-the-cuff" comments. Also common are feelings of anxiety, frustration, anger, guilt, isolation, and grief (12). It should be noted that patient counseling is not always a formal interaction; phone calls to deliver information to a patient often morphs into multiple layers as questions come up and patient reactions are expressed. During all interactions, patients must be treated gently and with respect. Stress manifests individually, and anger, born of frustration and fear, is not an uncommon reaction. The professional nurse knows that patient reactions are not to be taken personally. Greatly stressed individuals are more fragile, and confidence is eroded by failures of treatment and of physical and personal invasions. An appropriate sense of perspective and even humor should always be at the ready to help cope with these types of situations (10).

As with any situation, but particularly in REI nursing, thought must also be given to the meaning of the word "success." Initially, it would seem success here would culminate at the birth of a child. However, as patients proceed down the path of infertility, they will be faced with numerous choices, some extremely difficult and painful. The REI nurse is paramount in allowing the couple to integrate and make decisions based on

2. Demonstrate higher levels of clinical decision making.
3. Monitor and improve standards of care through supervision of practice.
4. Undertake clinical nursing audit and play a role in developing and leading the practice.
5. Contribute to research.
6. Teach and support professional colleagues (22).

The moral and ethical challenges provide even more complexity to fertility nursing. Some patients come in as innocents, never having been on the "infertility rollercoaster." Many of our patients come to us battle scarred, experiencing the four "Ds" – desperate, depressed, distraught, and demanding. They are also perpetually optimistic; for once they enter our doors, they are expressing hope. We as nursing caregivers need to meet these very special people with equal energy and enthusiasm for their hope of family. We, in effect, ride the rollercoaster with them. To accomplish this, we need dedicated, specialized nurses willing to grow in the REI field. This means defining the role in your own practice and becoming involved in a national organization such as the ASRM nursing group to help design and devise clear guidelines and protocols for such a specialty. Our patients deserve nothing less.

KEY POINTS

■ REI nursing is a growing, evolving, highly specialized field.
■ REI nursing requires high levels of critical thinking, clinical judgment, and acquisition of specialized skills and knowledge.
■ REI requires self-understanding of one's own moral and ethical values.
■ REI nursing care must be rendered in an empathetic, compassionate, and nonjudgmental framework.
■ The REI nurse as patient advocate must ensure real informed consent.
■ The REI patient should be treated as a whole human being, not merely an infertility patient.
■ The REI patient is really the couple, as both are invested in the outcome.
■ Success has a broader definition than pregnancy.
■ All options, including discontinuing treatment, and adoption must be considered and explored.

REFERENCES

1. Libraro J. The evolving roles of the ART nurse: a contemporary failure. In (Gardner DK, Howles CM, Weissman A, Shoham Z ed.), *Textbook Of Assisted Reproductive Techniques*, third edn., UK: Informa Healthcare, Chapter 69, 2004:891–900.
2. Barbieri R. A renaissance in reproductive endocrinology and infertility. *Fertil Steril* 2005;84:576–577.
3. Simpson H. *Peplau's Model in Action*. Palgrove Macmillan Education Ltd, 1991.
4. American Nurses Association. *Nursing's Social Policy Statement*. Washington, DC: The Association, 2003:6.
5. Kataoka-Yahiro M, Saylor C. A critical thinking model for nursing judgment. *J Nurs Educ* 1994;33(8):351.
6. Roper N. *The Elements of Nursing.* Churchill Livingstone, Inc, 1980.
7. Gordon M. *Nursing Diagnosis: Process and Application*, third edn. Saint Louis: Mosby, 1994.
8. Benner P, Wrubel J. *The Primacy of Caring*. Menlo Park: Addison-Wesley, 1989.
9. Denton J. The nurse's role in treating infertility problems. *Nurs Times* 1998;94(2):60–61.
10. Muirhead MA, Kirkland J. Nursing care in an assisted conception unit. In (Brinsden PR ed.), *Textbook of In Vitro Fertilization and Assisted Reproduction*, third edn. Volume 33. Nashville: Parthenon, 2005:557–569.
11. Code of Practice. *Human Ferilisation and Embryology Authority*, sixth edn. Part 7: Counselling. London: HFEA, 2003.
12. Mastroianni J. Evaluation of the infertile couple: Nurse practitioners play essential role. *Adv Nurse Pract* 2002;10(10):57–60.
13. Appleton T. The distress of infertility: impressions from 15 years of infertility counseling. In (Brinsden PR, ed.), *Textbook of In Vitro Fertilization and Reproduction*. Nashville, Tenn: Parthenon, 1999:401–406.
14. Jennings S. A lifeline offering support. *Prof Nurs* 1992;7(5): 539–542.
15. Kuczynski J. The holistic healthcare of couples undergoing IVF/ET. *Midwives Chron Nurs Notes* 1989;Jan:9–11.
16. Mocarski V. The nurse's role in helping infertile couples. *Am J Matern Child Nurs* 1977;2(4):264–266.
17. Ainsworth D. Coping with job burnout. http://www.berkeley.edu/news/berkeleyan/2001/04/25_burn.html 2001.
18. Burnout: signs, symptoms, and prevention. http://www.helpguide.org/mental/burnout_signs_symptoms.htm 2007:1–7.
19. Aguilera DC. *Crisis Intervention: Theory and Methodology*, eighth edn. St. Louis: Mosby, 1998.
20. Barber D. Research into the role of fertility nurses for the development of guidelines for clinical practice. *Hum Reprod Natl-Suppl JBFS 2(2)1997;12:195–197.
21. Castledine G, Brown R. A Survey of Specialist and Advanced Nursing Practice in England. *Br J Nurs* 1996 5(11):682–688.
22. United Kingdom Central Council for Nursing Midwifery and Health Visiting. The future of professional practice–the council's standards for education and practice following registration. London: UKCC, 1994.

60

Understanding Factors that Influence the Assessment of Outcomes in Assisted Reproductive Technologies

Brijinder S. Minhas, Barry A. Ripps

INTRODUCTION

Therapeutic intervention to alleviate infertility has steadily evolved since the initial success of in vitro fertilization in the late 1970s. The path to a desired outcome for many remains long, daunting, and uncertain. From the outset of assisted reproductive technologies (ART) applications, clinicians and patients held mutual desire for meaningful expression of its outcomes. The approaches to identifying such data have been diverse, controversial, at times contentious, and, as yet, continuously changing. Professional societies and government regulatory agencies have focused on deciphering parameters and collection of statistics that were substantive to clinicians and yet did not fail or mislead when viewed by the patient consumer. This effort has been in place in the United States and many other countries for a fair length of time. Recent legislation demanding compliance with and contribution to a national database has made reporting mandatory for ART clinics and laboratories within the United States. Debate exists as to whether adherence to a unified system has yielded recognizable improvements in the scientific or public understanding of ART outcomes. The following critical review may lead to the recognition that current methods of ART outcomes reporting and analysis offer no more certainty to clinicians than to the public for whose benefit the government-mandated reporting was imposed.

Despite disclaimers against the utility of direct comparison between practice-reported success rates, inherent and unavoidable human behavior, for both clinician and consumer, has created a very public and competitive environment. Has this improved patient care or impaired it? Prior to the evolution of this Internet-based consumers' market, motivations and incentives for ART success remained between the patient and physician with a tacit congruence of goals. Public access and direct comparison of outcomes have imposed new motivations to portray a practice with its highest numerical representation, but with dubious benefits to the now "well-informed" public.

Though there is a paucity of published research on this topic, this chapter reviews the current ART outcome analysis process in the United States to expand the reader's perspective and understanding of its complexity and intends to explore progress toward meaningful collection, analysis, and interpretation of ART outcomes by clinician and patient in the future.

HISTORICAL DEVELOPMENT OF ART CLINIC REPORTING IN THE UNITED STATES

Within the United States, ART clinics were mandated to report their outcome data to the Centers for Disease Control and prevention (CDC) with the passage and implementation of the Fertility Clinic Success Rate and Certification Act of 1992 (FCSRCA, also known as Wyden Act). The Society for Assisted Reproductive Technology (SART), an affiliate organization of the American Society for Reproductive Medicine (ASRM), worked with the CDC as the initial purveyor of data collection and publication, representing reproductive specialists and the majority of domestic ART practices. SART involved itself in outcomes data collection since 1985, prior to the Wyden Act. Since 2004, SART continued to collect member data, while the CDC contracted with a third party to collect, validate, and report ART outcomes. Membership in SART requires annual reporting to the CDC.

SART defines itself and its mission on the organization's Web site as, "SART is the primary organization of professionals dedicated to the practice of assisted reproductive technologies (ART) in the United States. Our organization includes over 392 member practices, representing over 85% of the ART clinics in our country. The mission of our organization is to set and help maintain the standards for ART in an effort to better serve our members and our patients" (1). SART also espouses its roles for consumer protection by setting advertising standards and as a governmental liaison for its members through ASRM Public Affairs Office, dealing with recent FDA guidelines on donor egg techniques. Thus, then and today SART has played a pivotal role in defining the criteria set for outcomes analysis. The motivations of the FCSRCA and the resulting impact on the public are not uniformly congruent. Whether SART has sought quality improvement or assistance with compliance or avoidance of additional federal regulatory intrusion, the impact of bureaucratic supervision has not been altogether positive as experienced in other countries (2).

CURRENT CRITERIA COLLECTED AND THEIR LIMITATIONS

Most putative factors that may impact ART outcomes have been identified, and those that are measurable have been added to the

■ Members of the scientific community should be prepared to avoid the emotional pitfalls faced by the public when evaluating ART outcomes by recognizing true limitations of current practices and reporting processes.

REFERENCES

1. Society for Assisted Reproductive Technologies. Internet Web address: www.sart.org.
2. Sharif K, Afnan M. The IVF league tables: time for a reality check. *Hum Reprod* 2003;18(3):483–5.
3. Katsoff B, Check JH, Choe JK, Wilson C. A novel method to evaluate pregnancy rates following in vitro fertilization to enable a better understanding of the true efficacy of the procedure. *Clin Exp Obstet Gynecol* 2005;32(4):213–16.
4. Stolwijk AM, Hamilton CJ, Hollanders JM, Bastiaans LA, Zielhuis GA. A more realistic approach to the cumulative pregnancy rate after in-vitro fertilization. *Hum Reprod* 1996;11(3):660–3.
5. Daya S. Life table (survival) analysis to generate cumulative pregnancy rates in assisted reproduction: are we overestimating our success rates? *Hum Reprod* 2005;20(5):1135–43.
6. Wilcox LS, Peterson HB, Haseltine FP, Martin MC. Defining and interpreting pregnancy success rates for in vitro fertilization. *Fertil Steril* 1993;60:18–25.
7. Ochsenkuhn R, Strowitzki T, Gurtner M, et al. Pregnancy complications, obstetric risks, and neonatal outcome in singleton and twin pregnancies after GIFT and IVF. *Arch Gynecol Obstet* 2003;268(4):256–61.
8. Zaib-un-Nisa S, Ghazal-Aswad S, Badrinath P. Outcome of twin pregnancies after assisted reproductive techniques—a comparative study. *Eur J Obstet Gynecol Reprod Biol* 2003;109(1):51–4.
9. Barlow P, Lejeune B, Puissant F, et al. Early pregnancy loss and obstetrical risk after in-vitro fertilization and embryo replacement. *Hum Reprod* 1988;3(5):671–5.
10. Soules MR. The in vitro fertilization pregnancy rate: let's be honest with one another. *Fertil Steril* 1985;43:511–13.
11. Deonandan R, Campbell MK, Ostbye T, Thummon I. Toward a more meaningful in vitro fertilization success rate. *J Assist Reprod Genet* 2000;17(9):498–503.
12. Marshal EC, Spiegelhalter DJ. Reliability of league tables of in vitro fertilization clinics: retrospective analysis of live birth rates. *BMJ* 1998;316:1701–4.
13. Dillner L. Infertility clinics show variation in success. *BMJ* 1995;311:1041.
14. Mohammed MA, Leary C. Analysing the performance of in vitro fertilization clinics in the United Kingdom. *Hum Fertil (Camb)* 2006;9(3):145–51.
15. Lu MC. Impact of "non-physician factors" on the "physician factor" of in vitro fertilization success: is it the broth, the cooks, or the statistics? *Fertil Steril* 1999;71(6):998–1000.
16. Deonandan R, Campbell MK, Ostbye T, Tummon I, Robertson J. IVF births and pregnancies: an exploration of two methods of assessment using life-table analysis. *J Assist Reprod Genet* 2001; 18(2):73–7.
17. Karande V, Morris R, Chapman C, Rinehart J, Gleicher N. Impact of the "physician factor" on pregnancy rates in a large assisted reproductive technology program: do too many cooks spoil the broth? *Fertil Steril* 1999;71:1001–9.
18. Rajkhowa M, McConnell A, Thomas GE. Reasons for discontinuation of IVF treatment: a questionnaire study. *Hum Reprod* 2006;21(2):358–63.
19. Collins J. Cost-effectiveness of in vitro fertilization. *Semin Reprod Med* 2001;19(3):279–89.
20. Hershlag A, Kaplan EH, Loy RA, DeCherney AH, Lavy G. Selection bias in in vitro fertilization programs. *Am J Obstet Gynecol* 1992;166:1–3.
21. Scott RT. Diminished ovarian reserve and access to care. *Fertil Steril* 2004;81:1489–92.
22. Legro RS, Shackleford DP, Moessner JM, et al. ART in women 40 and over. Is the cost worth it? *J Reprod Med* 1997;42:76–82.
23. Redshaw M, Hockley C, Davidson LL. A qualitative study of the experience of treatment for infertility among women who successfully became pregnant. *Hum Reprod* 2007;22(1): 295–304.
24. Collins J. An international survey of the health economics of IVF and ICSI. *Hum Reprod Update* 2002;8:265–77.
25. Robertson JA, Schneyer TJ. Professional self-regulation and shared-risk programs for in vitro fertilization. *J Law Med Ethics* 1997;25(4):283–91, 231.
26. The Ethics Committee of the American Society for Reproductive Medicine. Shared-risk or refund programs in assisted reproduction. Vol. 82, Suppl. 1, September 2004:S249–50.
27. Chambers GM, Ho MT, Sullivan EA. Assisted reproductive technology treatment costs of a live birth: an age-stratified cost-outcome study of treatment in Australia. *Med J Aust* 2006; 184(4):155–8.
28. Little SE, Ratcliffe J, Caughey. Cost of transferring one through five embryos per in vitro fertilization cycle from various payor perspectives. *Obstet Gynecol* 2006 108(3 Pt.1):593–601.
29. White C. Infertile couples to be given three shots at IVF. *BMJ* 2004;328:482.
30. Templeton A, Morris J, Parslow W. Factors that affect outcome of in vitro fertilization treatment. *Lancet* 1996;348:1402–6.
31. Centers for Disease Control for ART Practice Reporting in 2004. Web address: http://www.cdc.gov/ART/ART2004/sample.htm

61

The Revolution of Assisted Reproductive Technologies: How Traditional Chinese Medicine Impacted Reproductive Outcomes in the Treatment of Infertile Couples

Paul C. Magarelli, Diane K. Cridennda, Mel Cohen

Traditional Chinese Medicine (TCM) has gained a foothold in the Western medical modalities for pain, sports injuries skin conditions, anesthesia, and overall health maintenance (see WHO report; http://www.who.int/en/). Prior to 1990s, assisted reproductive technologies (ART or IVF – in vitro fertilization) depended on massive technical, pharmaceutical, and medical interventions to produce modest enhancements in expected outcomes (i.e., live births from treatments; see CDC at www.cdc.gov). The scope of the improvement was about 1 percent per year elevation in live births per embryo transfer from 1986 to 2000 (www.cdc.gov and Figure 61.1 SART data).

In 1996, a sentinel paper was published in human reproduction by Stener-Victorin et al. (1), which created a groundswell of interest by TCM practitioners in ways to assist IVF patients. She reported that acupuncture (Ac) in the form of electrostimulation (e-Stim) Ac increased uterine artery blood flow in IVF patients. This was quickly followed by another paper published in *Fertility and Sterility* (*F&S*) by Paulus et al. 2002 (2) that demonstrated enhanced pregnancy rates when Ac was used before and quickly after embryo transfer (ET). Although these studies provided important information, Western clinicians considered it far from proven, with editorials expressing condescension about premature adoption of TCM for IVF patients (3, 4).

Although the initial reaction by reproductive endocrinologists and infertility specialists was one of cautious resistance, persistence by D.K.C. in 1999 resulted in the first true collaboration of East and West research in this area. This chapter discusses our data, and we have diagrammed our approaches to answering the question (Figure 61.2): does adding Ac to IVF treatments improve outcomes and more importantly, how does it do this and what are the mechanisms? Outlined below are the scientific studies that form the basis for this chapter:

1. Ac and IVF poor responders: a cure? (5).
2. Ac and good-prognosis IVF patients: synergy (6).
3. Ac: impact on pregnancy outcomes in IVF patients (7).
4. Improvement of IVF outcomes by Ac: are egg and embryo qualities involved? (8).
5. Ac and IVF: does the number of treatments impact reproductive outcomes? (9).
6. Impact of Ac on prolactin and cortisol levels in IVF patients (10).
7. The demographics of Ac's impact on IVF outcomes: infertility diagnosis and SART/CDC age-groups (11).

We will also provide an overview of the world's literature on the role of TCM in ART. We review the criticisms of the current randomized controlled trials (RCT) and placebo controlled trials of Ac on IVF outcomes research as well as compare our studies with Western research.

INTRODUCTION

ART provides reproductive services to infertile couples throughout the world in the form of IVF. The process of IVF began with the birth of Louise Brown in 1978 by Edwards and Steptoe (12). The process has evolved into a technology rich in equipment, scientific jargon, steeped in tradition, and pregnant with innovation. Like the first heart transplant, IVF has gone from medical wonder to "standard of care." Unfortunately, this has also led to a somewhat depersonalized technology, which is the antithesis of what these desperate, injured, infertile couples need. Today more than 1,000,000 IVF cycles (13) are performed each year around the world for a population of six billion humans. Most estimates of infertility when calculated represent 15 percent of married/bonded couples. This would predict many more couples in need of reproductive care who are not receiving this gift of family building. What is happening?

Part of the problem is access and cost. Others include the depersonalization of the process and resistance factor on the part of the couples themselves! Fertility is a personal matter, which is publicly controlled. It is in the nature of a community to "require" reproduction for survival. This "resistance" to the existence of infertility leads most couples to believe the "urban legends" that our fertility is about 100 percent at age 15! This could not be further from the truth. Our fertility is best described by the graph in Figure 61.3.

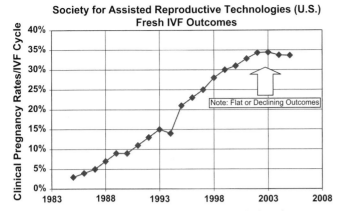

Figure 61.1. Clinical pregnancy rates per IVF cycle based on SART United States 1985–2005 (www.cdc.gov).

The peak of our fertility is at twenty-five years of age and allows humans a 25 percent chance to conceive each month. For most couples, it hovers at 10 percent since many couples do not even start thinking of having children until after education is complete, jobs are intact, and houses are purchased (Figure 61.3). By this time, the couples are nearing thirty years old and just beginning to consider having a baby (Figure 61.4) (14).

After months of trying to conceive, issues of personal identity, frustration, guilt, not to mention, losing faith in their body set in. Most couples lose a sense of freedom as they no longer have intercourse for the reasons of love and true intimacy. Sex now turns into a job, timed at best. Women are focusing on sticking the basal body thermometer under their tongues (instead of reaching for their husbands as they wake), peeing on sticks, checking for cervical mucous, focusing on bodily changes, and planning intercourse at just the right moment. These couples begin to lose sight of the reason for having a child together as they experience sorrow and frustration month after month when the menses occurs despite the vigorous attempts to achieve

a pregnancy. Technology has come to save the day, but in its wake, many couples remain disconnected and disaffected.

HISTORICAL PERSPECTIVE

In the United States, IVF programs started in the 1980s, proliferated during the mid- to late 90s, and have grown to represent more than 150,000 treatment cycles in the early part of the twenty-first century. In Figure 61.1, IVF programs have reported reproductive outcomes from 1986 to 2005. The average improvement each year represents 1–2 percent gain per treatment in positive outcomes, pregnancy, or babies, from 1985 to 2001. After 2001, we have not seen any improvement in outcomes; we have actually seen a modest decrease (34–33 percent, Figure 61.1)! Although the results are laudable, are we missing something that will enhance the rate of improvement? It was the latter issue that first drew one of the authors (D.K.C.) to challenge the Western treatments for IVF.

Stener-Victorin and Paulus (1, 2) were little known in the IVF community; however, TCM practitioners understandably were intrigued. In a gutsy move, D.K.C. contacted the IVF centers in Colorado regarding combining East and West for the enhancement of IVF outcomes. A tepid response ensued, however; D.K.C. is an accomplished triathlete so quitting was not an option! She met with Reproductive Medicine and Fertility Center's (RMFC) medical director (P.C.M.) and negotiated a plan. She would care for the worst candidates for IVF utilizing both the Stener-Victorin and Paulus protocols (1, 2). The reason for having access to the most difficult patients was that P.C.M. had exhausted his resources for helping these couples achieve a pregnancy and by this time he was convinced that Ac "couldn't hurt." What made them the "worst" candidates were their Western diagnoses: elevated follicle-stimulating hormone (FSH), a marker of ovarian follicular reserve; very poor sperm parameters (especially very large numbers of abnormally shaped sperm, called teratozoospermia); poor ovarian blood flow (called pulsatility indices, PI); and advanced maternal age (more than thirty-five). With

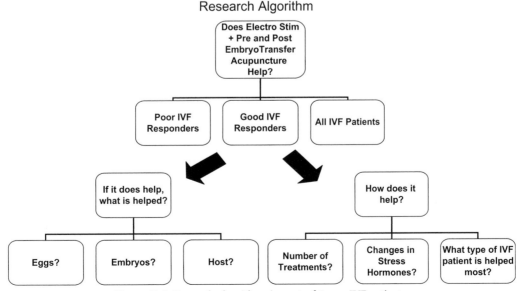

Figure 61.2. Research algorithm: impact of Ac on IVF patients.

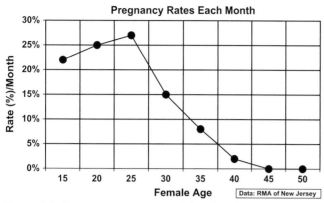

Figure 61.3. Pregnancy rates per month based on female age (Reproductive Medical Associates of New Jersey) based on natural and intrauterine insemination conceptions.

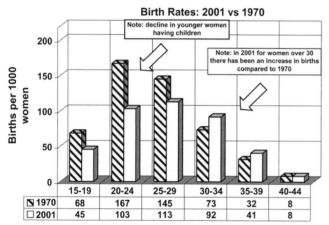

Figure 61.4. Birth rates by female age-group comparing 1970–1990 (14).

this foundation, a research protocol was developed. These research protocols form the basis for all subsequent studies we report herein. The key elements of the protocols are listed below:

1. Recruitment was prospective.
   a. Eliminates historical comparisons and strengthens study applicability.
2. Recruitment for Ac was hidden or "blinded" to the physician.
   a. Reduces physician bias.
3. IVF treatment protocols were hidden or "blinded" to the acupuncturist.
   a. Reduces acupuncturist bias.
4. Only "standardized" Ac treatments were allowed, that is, no differentiation of syndromes as a basis of treatments were done; each patient had same Ac protocols (much to the consternation of D.K.C.)!
   a. Eliminate treatment selection bias.
5. All data were collected by a third party, Mel Cohen (M.C.), and kept from the physician and acupuncturist for three years.
   a. Reduce investigator bias.
6. Contracts were written and signed by all TCM practitioners to follow the prescribed protocols for treatments to ensure

there were no variations or deviations from the protocol set forth.
   a. Eliminate treatment variability.
7. The TCM practitioners agreed to provide 24/7 coverage on an as-needed basis for patients in the study (many times the ET occurred on weekends and holidays); the patients had access to their acupuncturist at all times.
   a. Reduce timing/convenience bias.
8. Patients selected whether to participate or not and no coercion to participate was allowed, simple discussion by nurses to patients about the ability to have Ac was done.
   a. Does NOT eliminate selection bias.
      i. This is a weakness in most TCM studies.
9. No monetary gain was provided to participate.
   a. Reduces selection bias for monetary gains.
10. No reduction in IVF fees for participation in the study were given.
    a. Reduces treatment bias based on monetary gains.
11. No reduction in TCM treatment fees for participation in the study were given.
    a. Reduces treatment bias based on monetary gains.
12. Most study data collected from 1999 were reviewed in 2003, 2004, and 2005.
    a. Reduces impact of positive outcomes on choice to do Ac by patients.
13. The cortisol/prolactin study (2005 and 2006) was prospective in design.
    a. Although not randomized, the study was blinded to the acupuncturists, physicians, and statistician until analyzed.

The research protocol has remained in place since 1999, and we report herein the observations, results, and impact of our studies.

RESEARCH OVERVIEW

Patient Identification

Data collection occurred from 1999 to 2006. All females between the ages of twenty-two and forty-four years who were eligible for IVF (patients using their own eggs) were provided information regarding the permission to have Ac during their downregulation and stimulation medications, as well as just before and after ET. Total number of patients in our database to date is 801. Patient demographics were collected and used to determine similarities and differences between the control groups (IVF no Ac) and the treatment groups (IVF with Ac). The demographics collected and overall statistics are included in Tables 61.1, 61.4, 61.7, 61.10, and 61.13 that follow each subsection on experiments conducted. There are more than 377 parameters monitored by computer databases and patient populations in each of the study arms. Each had comparable demographics, Western medicine treatment protocols, and embryology results (except when study arms were designed to be different, see Poor Prognosis experiments, Table 61.1, ref. 5).

Treatment Groups

Our research algorithm (Figure 61.2) was designed to systematically determine the impact of defined Ac therapies

Table 61.1: Poor Prognosis: Demographic, Diagnosis, and Treatment Data

N = 128	Average prognosis controls Group A	PPr controls Group B	PPr Ac Group C	p value
Sample size, number (%)	64 (50)	18 (14)	46 (36)	
Cycle range	1–4	1–4	1–4	
Cycle average	1.32	1.38	1.65	
Patient age range (years)	23.0–42.9	22.2–41.5	25.1–41.2	
Patient age average (years)	34.3	37.8	34.5	
Partner age range (years)	23.0–55.3	22.1–54.0	23.5–59.8	
Partner age average (years)	36.1	38.9	36.6	
How long waiting, range	1–12	1–11	1–11	
How long waiting, average	3.2	3.8	2.7	
Male				
Count, average	79.5	73.1	74.6	
Motility, average	56.8	53.1	59.2	
Morphology, average	6.4*	5.5	3.1*	*$p < 0.05$
Fathered pregnancy	15 (23.4)	4 (22.2)	11 (23.9)	
Fathered this relationship	12 (18.8)	3 (16.7)	7 (15.2)	
Female				
FSH average	10.7	11.1	10.6	
FSH range	5.1–14.4	7.4–14.6	4.7–19.3	
Highest FSH average	**9.3*	13.1*	**15.2	*$p < 0.05$, **$p < 0.01$
Highest FSH range	5.1–13.9	12.0–16.4	4.7–19.8	
PI, average	1.94*	2.81	2.91	$p < 0.05$
PI, range	1–2.7	2.5–2.9	0.7–3.1	
Gravid, average	0.48	0.39	0.55	
Gravid, range	0–4	0–3	0–4	
Weight, average	156.6	154.7	157.8	
Weight, range	110–238	104–222	106–267	
Height, average	5.07	5.05	5.06	
Height, range	4.11–5.11	5.01–5.10	4.11–6.02	
BMI, average	35.8	34.9	35.6	
BMI, range	22.7–51.2	24.0–48.9	18–51	
Diagnostic				
PCOS	20 (31.2)	6 (33.4)	18 (39.1)	
Tubal	12 (18.8)	4 (22.2)	12 (26.0)	
Endometriosis	11 (17.2)	3 (16.7)	7 (15.2)	
Age more than thirty-five years	26 (40.6)	8 (44.4)	21 (45.6)	
Failed IUI	29 (45.3)	8 (44.4)	20 (43.7)	
Male factor	53 (82.8)	16 (88.9)	37 (88.1)	
Protocols				
Long	45 (54.9)	10 (55.6)	23 (50.0)	
MicroDose Flare	0 (0)	0 (0)	0 (0)	
Flare	6 (7.3)	2 (11.1)	3 (6.5)	

Poor prognosis defined as male factor, elevated day 3 FSH, and elevated average pulsatility index.

on IVF patients groups. These groups were indicated as follows:

1. Poor prognosis
2. Good prognosis
3. All IVF patients

Poor prognosis (PPr) is a general description of IVF patients who "should" require additional care and prolonged treatments before a successful outcome is achieved (i.e., a baby). We defined poor responders based on the following parameters:

■ years of trying to conceive,
■ age of female,
■ day 3 FSH serum levels,
■ severe male factor, that is, poor semen parameters
■ elevated PI of uterine artery.

Good prognosis (GP) were in reality any patient that was not a PPr (i.e. they were classified as a normal or potential good responder). We used GPs as the IVF controls (C) in our studies.

All IVF patients were defined as any patient who received Ac treatments and also received an IVF treatment.

Outcomes

In most IVF centers, positive outcomes are defined in one of three ways: biochemical pregnancy (positive serum hCG levels), clinical pregnancy (presence of a gestational and yolk sac), and ongoing pregnancy (presence of heart beat in fetus). For our studies, the authors consider biochemical pregnancy as our primary end point, but considered take-home baby (THB) as success. We also documented spontaneous abortions or miscarriages and ectopic pregnancies, which are pregnancies in a location other than the uterus. Finally, multiple pregnancies were defined as the presence of more than one gestational sac by ultrasound.

Biochemical Studies

We conducted a prospective study on serum cortisol and prolactin levels in patients who either received IVF alone or IVF plus Ac. Patients were prospectively consented to participate in this study. An Immulite AutoAnalyzer™ was used to detect serum levels of cortisol and prolactin.

STUDIES AND DESIGN

All Study Patients

Solicitation for Studies

All patients were educated on the option of adding Ac to their treatment options. This education was done by the nurses and was blinded to the physician (P.C.M.). The choice to participate in the study was voluntary.

Ac

Treatments during medication stimulation phase of IVF:

Modified Stener-Victorin protocol (1) (Table 61.18, Figure 61.5). The Ac treatment type was electrostimulation Ac or e-Stim (EA).

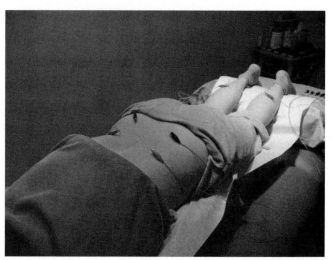

Figure 61.5. Picture of modified Stener-Victorin e-Stim protocol (EWA © 2000).

Treatments pre- and post-ET phase of IVF: Modified Paulus et al. protocol (2) (Table 61.19) and traditional/auricular Ac.

Ac Consortium

In order to isolate the Ac treatment *protocols*, rather than the *acupuncturist*, we created an Ac consortium to provide Ac treatments. This reduced or eliminated practitioner bias. Each participant in the Ac consortium agreed in writing to follow the Stener-Victorin (1) and Paulus (2) protocols (Tables 61.18, 61.19 and 61.20). They also agreed to report all data to one of the authors (D.K.C.). All acupuncturists were licensed and NCCAOM certified. All treatments took place in the acupuncturist's offices.

Inclusion Criteria for Patients

Inclusion criteria were all patients (Ac and controls) undergoing IVF must have FSH less than 20 mIU/mL (normal range <10.5), presence of sperm, and a normal uterus. Clinical indications for IVF included failed ovulation induction (OI) or failed OI/intrauterine insemination (IUI), male factor, endometriosis, and tubal factor. Patients usually fell into more than one category. Patients also had diagnoses consistent with polycystic ovarian syndrome (PCOS).

PI Monitoring

Stener-Victorin et al. (1) published the protocol for PI evaluation. This protocol was modified and used in our study: PI of the uterine arteries measured by transvaginal ultrasonography and pulsed Doppler curves (LOQIC 400 MD, GE Medical Systems, United States) were done at the initial new patient visit, utilizing a 7-MHz vaginal probe. The PI value for each artery was calculated electronically from a smooth curve fitted to the average waveform according to the formula: $P1 = (A - B)/mean$, where A is the peak systolic Doppler shift, B is the end diastolic shift frequency, and mean is the mean maximum Doppler shifted frequency over the cardiac cycle. A reduction in the value of PI is thought to indicate a reduction in impedance distal to the point of sampling (1). All measurements were done by one of the authors (P.C.M.) between 7 A.M. and 10 A.M. Stener-Victorin (1) used similar hours to reduce the risk that the PI measurements would be affected by the circadian rhythm in blood flow. We utilized an average PI greater than 3 as one of the criteria that the Ac population was in the PPr group.

Ac Treatment

Electrostimulation Acupuncture (EA)

A modified Stener-Victorin (1) protocol for the EA Ac treatment was used during gonadotropins stimulation. In their description of the protocol, they believed that the sympathetic outflow may be inhibited at the segmental level and the Ac points were selected in somatic segments according to the innervations of the uterus (thoracic 12 to lumbar 2, sacral 2–3). See table 61.21 for explantation by Traditional Chinese Medicine energetics of all acupuncture points used in this study. Table 61.22 describes the theoretical basis for the Ac points used in the Stener-Victorin protocol (1). Table 61.22 also describes the muscle innervations associated with these points.

PROCEDURE

Four needles [36 gauge (g) 1.5 inches, Korean DBC needles] were located bilaterally at the thoracolumbar and lumbosacral levels of the erector spinae (BL 23 and BL 28). Four needles were located bilaterally in the calf muscles BL 57 and SP 6. E-Stim (EA) was connected from BL 23 to BL 28 and SP 6 to BL 57. The AWQ D electro stimulator was set on direct current with variable frequency 0–100 Hz for thirty minutes. The intensity was sufficient to cause local muscle contractions (1). Once the eggs were retrieved, no further Stener-Victorin treatments were given.

Pre- and Post-ET Treatment (Modified Paulus et al. Protocol)

For this protocol, we used a modification of Paulus et al. protocol (2). In the Paulus et al. study, specific times were used for Ac treatment. Since this study was undertaken in an outpatient, private practice setting, it was impractical to give the Ac treatment in this manner due to location of Ac offices, schedules, and so on. There is a great deal of evidence in the complementary alternative medicine literature which supports a long-term affect of Ac treatments. We also supported our decision with Stener-Victorin (1) observation that reduction in PI lasted for more than two weeks.

Procedure

Per modified Paulus protocol (2): Ac needles were inserted within eighteen hours before and two hours after the ET. Sterile disposable stainless steel Korean DBC needles (32 g × 1.5 inches) were used. Needle reaction or *De Qi* was obtained and used as the end point for correct needle insertion. The depth of needle insertion was about 10 to 20 mm, depending on the region of the body undergoing treatment. After 10 minutes, the needles were rotated in order to obtain *De Qi* sensation again. Needle retention was twenty-five minutes per treatment. Before ET, the following Ac points were used: PC 6 (*Neiguan*), SP8 (*Diji*), LIV3 (*Taichong*), GV20 (*Baihui*), and ST29 (*Guilai*). Auricular needles (Vinco 7mm ND Detox) were used without rotation as follows: 1) right ear: shenmen, brain, 2) left ear: uterus, endocrine. After ET, we used the

following Ac points: ST36 (*Zusanli*), SP6 (*Sanyinjiao*), SP10 (*Xuehai*), and LI4 (*Hegu*). Auricular needles (Vinco 7mm ND Detox) right ear: uterus, endocrine, and left ear: shenmen, brain. Auricular needles were retained for twenty-five minutes during the treatment. After the treatment, auricular needles were removed and replaced with ear tacks following the same pattern (our modification). All treatments were given in the acupuncturist's clinic. Soft music, dimmed lights, and eye pillows were given to the patients and they were covered with a light silk scarf to keep them warm. In Tables 61.23 and 61.24 we present the theoretical basis for the Ac points used in the Paulus protocol (2). We also present auricular Ac points in Table 61.25.

IVF Protocols

Patients were downregulated with GnRHa in one of the following protocols: long (day 21 of menstrual cycle prior to IVF cycle) and flare or microdose flare (day 1 or 2 of menses of IVF cycle). Dosages and administration of rFSH and/or rFSH and HMG protocols were individualized and done according to established protocols (15). A generalized protocol would be day 2–3 cycle stimulation start with A.M. and P.M. administration of gonadotropins. Downregulation with Lupron™ (Luprolid acetate) injections were done in the evenings and hCG administration was done thirty-four to thirty-seven hours prior to oocyte retrieval. ET was predominately day 3 transfers. We have compared our day 5 blastocyst pregnancy outcomes with our day 3 outcomes, and they were the same (P.C.M. internal evaluation). Transfers were done under abdominal ultrasound guidance. All transfer patients received either 5 or 10 mg Diazepam thirty minutes prior to transfer. It was standard protocol in our IVF clinic to pretreat with Diazepam and based on a follow-up study by Paulus et al. (16), uterine motility was not found to be the mechanism of action of the Ac-treated patients' positive outcomes. Therefore, we believe would be an independent effect the Ac treatments.

All transfer catheters were flushed and the effluent examined for retained embryos prior to completing the ET procedure. Estradiol levels and progesterone levels were monitored throughout the stimulation cycle, and ultrasound confirmation of follicular growth was usually done on days 3, 5, 7, 8, 9, and 10 until day of hCG trigger shot. Supplemental progesterone was administered i.m. after oocyte retrieval in the pattern of twice a day at the 50-mg dose until results of pregnancy tests. These were continued for twelve weeks if the patient was pregnant. All patients received low-dose aspirin, 80 mg, per day at the beginning of their IVF treatment. Prenatal vitamins were encouraged for all patients. Fresh ejaculated sperm was used in all fertilization protocols. Only patients who had fresh IVF cycles with their own eggs were selected for this study. In both the Ac and control groups, the patients remained lying still for twenty-five minutes after ET and were encouraged to continue with modified bed rest for five days. Pregnancy tests were done ten to twelve days after transfer.

Statistical Analysis

The statistics used for this analysis included tests for normal distribution: chi-square test, Kolmogorov-Smirnov test, unpaired *t*-tests, stepwise multiple regression variance ratio test (F-test), one-way analysis of variance (ANOVA) with Student-Newman-Keuls (SNK) test for pairwise comparison of subgroups. Discrete multivariate analysis was also used. The studies reviewed above used the following high-level tools for the statistical analysis. The authors were provided guidance and analysis from Roger Lipker, Ph.D., Department of Mathematics, Colorado State University.

Legend: 1 = poor-prognosis, 2 = good-prognosis demographics, 3 = All IVF patients, 4 = embryology and eggs, 5 = stress study, 6 = demographics and outcomes

SUMMARY OF TRADITIONAL CHINESE

	1	2	3	4	5	6
Student t-test	Yes	Yes	Yes	Yes	Yes	No
Chi-square	Yes	Yes	Yes	Yes	Yes	No
Unpaired t-test	Yes	Yes	Yes	Yes	Yes	No
Stepwise multiple regression	Yes	Yes	Yes	Yes	No	No
Kolmogorov-Smirnov test	Yes	Yes	Yes	No	No	No
Variance ratio test	Yes	Yes	Yes	Yes	Yes	No
One-way ANOVA	Yes	Yes	Yes	Yes	Yes	No
Kaplan-meyer survival analysis	No	No	Yes	No	No	No
Mann-whitney U test	No	No	No	No	No	Yes
Log-rank	No	No	No	No	Yes	No

MEDICINE RESEARCH

Each research area is presented in the following format: abstract, pertinent tables and figures, discussion, and key points.

Patient Demographics and Diagnostic Data

For all studies, the controls and Ac-treated groups had parity in the following parameters (Tables 61.1, 61.4, 61.7, 61.10, and 61.13):

■ female age range
■ average female patient age
■ partner age range
■ average partner ages
■ female weight
■ female height
■ female percent body fat

Diagnostic categories and types of IVF protocols utilized were the same (Tables 61.1, 61.4, 61.7, 61.10, and 61.13). The types of gonadotropins used (recombinant and/or HMG) were the same (Tables 61.5, 61.7, and 61.10).

Male factor values were similar for semen average count, average motility and history of fathering a pregnancy, and fathering a pregnancy in this relationship (Tables 61.1, 61.4, 61.7, 61.10, and 61.13), except for the poor-prognosis research protocols (Table 61.1).

Endocrine values were also analyzed, and no significant differences were found in groups (Tables 61.1, 61.4, 61.7, 61.10, and 61.13), except for PPr experiment (Table 61.1).

Egg and embryo characteristics were similar between the groups, with no significant differences in the following parameters: number of eggs retrieved, average eggs retrieved, and average number transferred (Tables 61.2, 61.5, 61.8, 61.11, and 61.14).

RESEARCH, DATA, AND DISCUSSIONS SECTION

We will be presenting the data from the following studies: Magarelli P, Cridennda D. Ac and IVF poor responders: a cure? (5); Magarelli P, Cohen M, Cridennda, D. Ac and good prognosis IVF patients: synergy. (6); Magarelli P, Cohen M, Cridennda, D. Ac: impact on pregnancy outcomes in IVF patients. (7); Magarelli P, Cohen M, Cridennda, D. Improvement of IVF outcomes by Ac: are egg and embryo qualities involved? (8); Cridennda D, Magarelli P, Cohen M. Ac and in vitro fertilization: does the number of treatments impact reproductive outcomes? (9); Magarelli P, Cridennda D, Cohen M. Proposed mechanism of action of Ac on IVF outcomes. (10); Magarelli P, Cridennda D, Cohen M. The demographics of Ac's impact on IVF outcomes: infertility diagnosis and SART/CDC/age groups. (11).

1.0 Poor Prognosis (5)

Impact of Ac on Poor Prognosis IVF Patients

1.1 POOR PROGNOSIS: TABLES 61.1, 61.2, AND 61.3
AND FIGURE 61.6

1.2 POOR PROGNOSIS – DISCUSSION

This study was a prospective blinded cohort analysis of the impact of Ac on IVF outcomes in PPr patients; these results demonstrate important associations of Ac and true reproductive outcomes, that is, THB. This positive effect of Ac on IVF PPr patients occurred despite the fact that the average prognosis controls (Group A) had significantly lower peak day 3 FSH and significantly better male factor parameters as well as significantly lower PI (Table 61.1). These results occurred despite the fact that the Ac treatment groups were homogeneous for demographic, diagnostic, and therapeutic parameters (Table 61.1). What was most striking in the data was the huge improvement in reproductive outcomes, that is, THB, when Group C was compared to Group B (70 percent THB vs. 20 percent THB, Table 61.3). This represented a 50 percent improvement in THB for PPr patients treated with Ac. Overall, the improvements remained for ectopic pregnancy outcomes and THB rates per cycle or per ongoing pregnancy (data not shown with minimally $p < 0.05$) if the controls groups were combined (Group A plus Group B).

1.3 POOR PROGNOSIS: KEY POINTS

■ Improvements in reproductive outcomes were demonstrated when poor prognosis patients received Ac treatments before, during, and after their IVF treatments.
■ A "standardized" Ac treatment protocol in lieu of treatments utilizing differentiation of syndromes can be used to improve reproductive outcomes with positive end results, that is, THB.

Table 61.2: Poor Prognosis: IVF Cycle and Embryology Data

N = 128	Average prognosis controls: Group A	PPr controls: Group B	PPr Ac: Group C	p value
Sample size, number (%)	64 (50)	18 (14)	46 (36)	
Cycle and embryology				
E2, average	4,121	4,685	3,117	
E2, range	1,032–6,154	1,046–6,247	1,046–5,487	
P4, average	1.56	1.55	1.12	
P4, range	0.2–5.8	0.2–5.4	0.2–5.1	
Endometrial lining, average	11.4	11.4	10.3	
Endometrial lining, range	7.8–17.5	7.3–16.6	8.4–7.2	
No. of eggs retrieved, average	11.2	10.5	12.9	
No. of eggs retrieved, range	1–31	1–27	4–36	
No. of embryos transferred, average	2.2	2.8	2.2	
No. of embryos transferred, range	1–4	1–5	1–4	
Sample size, number	64 (50)	18 (14)	46 (36)	
ET data				
No. of day 3 transfers	64 (100)	18 (100)	46 (100)	
No. of day 5 transfers	0 (0)		0 (0)	
Fresh	64 (100)	18 (100)	46 (100)	
ICSI	60 (93.8)	17 (94.4)	45 (97.8)	

Table 61.3: Poor Prognosis: Reproductive Outcomes

N = 128	Average prognosis controls: Group A	PPr controls Group B	PPr Ac Group C	p value
Sample size, number (%)	64 (50)	18 (14)	46 (36)	
Outcomes				
Pregnancy	26 (41)	5 (27)	20 (43)	
SAB	4 (6)	0 (0)	3 (6)	
Ectopic	2/26 (8)	1/5 (20)	0 (0)	$p < 0.001$
Births overall	13 (20)	1 (15)*	13 (28)*	$p < 0.05$
Birth if pregnant	13/26 (50)*	1 (20)**	**14/20 (70)*	*$p < 0.01$, **$p < 0.05$

2.0 Good Prognosis (6)

Ac and Good-Prognosis IVF Patients: Synergy

2.1 GOOD PROGNOSIS: TABLES 61.4, 61.5, AND 61.6 AND FIGURE 61.7

2.2 GOOD PROGNOSIS: DISCUSSION

This study was a prospective blinded cohort analysis of the impact of Ac on IVF outcomes in good-prognosis patients; these results demonstrate important associations of Ac and true reproductive outcomes, that is, THB. This positive effect of Ac on IVF good prognosis patients occurred despite the fact that the pregnancy rates compared to controls were statistically the same (Table 61.6). These results occurred despite the fact that the Ac treatment groups were homogeneous for demographic, diagnostic, and therapeutic parameters (Table 61.4). What was most striking in the data was the huge improvement in reproductive outcomes, that is, THB, when the Ac group was compared to controls (Figure 61.7). This represented a 6 percent improvement in THB for good-prognosis patients treated with Ac. Overall there was significant improvements in ectopic pregnancy and miscarriage rates (SABs).

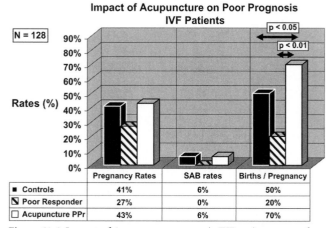

Figure 61.6. Impact of Ac on poor-prognosis IVF patients: reproductive outcomes.

2.3 GOOD PROGNOSIS: KEY POINTS

- *Pregnancy outcomes* were *equal* between the Ac group and the nonacupuncture group, not unlike poor prognosis study.
- *Birth outcomes* were *improved* between the Ac group and the nonacupuncture group.
- Improved pregnancy outcomes for all patients.
- Improved pregnancy outcomes for pregnant patients.
- Significantly fewer SABs.
- Significantly fewer ectopic pregnancies.

3.0 All IVF Patients (7)

Ac: Impact on Pregnancy Outcomes in IVF Patients

3.1 ALL IVF: TABLES 61.7, 61.8, AND 61.9 AND FIGURE 61.8

3.2 ALL IVF: DISCUSSION

Why pregnancy rates (PR) were equal, but birth rates improved? (PR are statistically better)

- TCM view
  - Ac points balance the kidney: in TCM, kidney and uterus are intimately related ... genitourinary system.
  - Reduce stress: relaxation; reduce cortisol?
  - Spleen 10 is noted invigorate blood/reduce abruptions?
  - DU 20 is used to "hold"; it brings Qi into balance lifts the yang Qi and the spirit.
- Western view
  - Better implantation due to improved blood flow to uterus.
  - Implantation is based on embryonic characteristics and uterine factors, whereas ongoing pregnancies depend on uterine factors. ... think gestational carriers!

3.3 ALL IVF: KEY POINTS

- Pregnancy outcomes were superior in the Ac group versus nonacupuncture group ($p < 0.05$).
  - Significantly more pregnancies at $p < 0.05$
  - Birth outcomes were improved between the Ac group and the nonacupuncture group
  - Improved pregnancy outcomes for pregnant patients

Table 61.4: Good Prognosis: Demographic, Diagnosis, and Treatment Data

$N = 131$	Ac	No Ac	p value
Sample size, number (%)	48 (37)	83 (63)	
Cycle range	1–4	1–4	
Cycle average	1.62	1.38	
Patient age range (years)	24.1–54.5	22.6–52.3	
Patient age average (years)	34.6	34.9	
Partner age range (years)	23.5–60.5	23.0–55.3	
Partner age average (years)	36.8	37.1	
How long waiting, range	1–11	1–12	
How long waiting, average	2.8	3.1	
Male			
Count, average	81.2	80.2	
Motility, average	56.3	54.2	
Morphology, average	12.9	13.2	
Fathered pregnancy	12 (25)	20 (24)	
Female			
FSH average	7.9	7.8	
FSH range	2.1–12.6	1.7–12.9	
Highest FSH average	7.2	7.4	
Highest FSH range	3.8–19.3	3.8–22.4	
PI, average	1.21	1.13	
Index, range	0.7–2.9	1–2.8	
Gravid, average	0.59	0.52	
Range	0–4	0–4	
Weight, average	163	166	
Weight, range	98–253	106–259	
Height, average	5.06	5.06	
Height, range	4.11–6.02	4.11–5.10	
% Body fat, average	33.3	34.5	
% Body fat, range	20–51	21–53	
Diagnostic			
PCOS	19 (40)	29 (32)	
Tubal	11 (23)	15 (18)	
Endometriosis	7 (15)	14 (17)	
Age more than thirty-five	20 (42)	38 (45)	
Failed Ol/or OI/IUI or IUI	18 (38)	35 (42)	
Male factor	29 (60)	47 (57)	

Table 61.5: Good Prognosis: IVF Cycle and Embryology Data

N = 131	Ac	No Ac	p value
Sample size	48 (37)	83 (63)	
Gonadotropins			
rFSH only	19 (40)	36 (43)	
rFSH and HMG	28 (58)	43 (52)	
HMG only	1 (2)	2 (3)	
Cycle and embryology			
E2, average	2,765	2,639	
Range	1,046–5,585	1,029–6,618	
P4, average	1.54	1.33	
Range	0.2–5.2	0.2–6.0	
Endo lining, average	10.2	11.1	
Range	8.3–17.4	7.9–18.8	
No. of eggs retrieved, average	12.8	11.8	
Range	4–36	1–32	
No. of embryos implanted, average	2.2	2.2	
Range	1–4	1–4	
No. of ET, average	1.6	1.7	
Range	1–3	1–3	
No. of embryos fertilized normally, average	7.9	7.7	
Range	1–22	1–21	
No. of embryos frozen, average	5.4	5.2	
Range	0–9	0–11	
No. of prior IVF cycles, average	1.4	1.5	
Range	0–4	0–4	

Table 61.6: Good Prognosis: Reproductive Outcomes Data

N = 131	Ac	No Ac	p value
Sample size	48	83	
Outcomes			
Pregnancy, n (%)	24 (50)	37 (45)	
SAB, n (%)	4 (8)	12 (14)	p < 0.05
Ectopic, n (%)	0 (0)	4 (5)	p < 0.01
Births overall, n (%)	29 (42)	29 (35)	p < 0.05

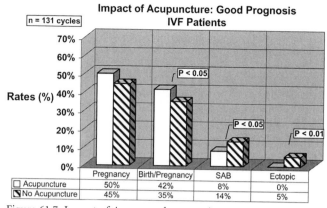

Figure 61.7. Impact of Ac on good-prognosis IVF patients.

- Fewer miscarriages
- Significantly fewer ectopic pregnancies ($p < 0.05$)
- Significantly fewer multiple pregnancies ($p < 0.05$)
  - Conclusion: Ac even if given to all-comers will benefit the IVF practice by improving reproductive outcomes.

4.0 Number of Treatments (9)

Ac and In Vitro Fertilization: Does the Number of Treatments Impact Reproductive Outcomes?

4.1 STATISTICAL SUMMARY

The population was stratified into pregnant and nonpregnant groups and then evaluated by Student t test and chi-square analysis for age, FSH levels, weight, BMI, and E-2 levels. The pregnant and nonpregnant groups were further subdivided into those who received or did not receive Ac and were analyzed by chi-square analysis. Since all patients received Ac consisting of modified Stener-Victorin e-Stim (1) and modified Paulus protocol (2), their distribution was analyzed utilizing Kaplan-Meier's survival analysis. Kaplan-Meier analysis is an actuarial survival curve. The test measures consecutive failures or successful end points (pregnancies) in a study. We analyzed the number of Ac treatments that would result in a pregnancy. The Kaplan-Meier analysis accumulated all patients at risk at the beginning (100 percent) and determined their pregnancy rate. As the number of patients at risk declined (i.e., did not achieve pregnancy), with each additional pregnancy, a curve was derived for that point resulting in a curve that when compared against those not becoming pregnant derived a statistical "sweet spot" for the minimum number of Ac treatments necessary to achieve pregnancy.

4.2 NUMBER OF TREATMENTS: FIGURE 61.9
4.3 NUMBER OF TREATMENTS: DISCUSSION

In TCM, only when Qi, Blood, Yin, and Yang are in a state of dynamic balance, will it function at its optimal level. In our study, patients who received more than eight Ac treatments received (Figure 61.9) the maximum benefit for IVF outcomes: pregnancy ($p < 0.05$). We also reviewed the independent effects of the Paulus protocol (16) that have been speculated to be a uterine muscle contraction phenomenon; however, due to small numbers, we could not perform the analyses. P.C.M. also utilized Valium™ (diazepam) for all ET. Subsequent research by Paulus et al. (16) elucidated the Ac effect. It was proven to not affect uterine contractions. Therefore, we do not believe that the diazepam interferes with the Ac effects.

Table 61.7: All IVF Patients: Demographic, Diagnosis, and Treatment Data

N = 130	Ac (%)	No Ac	p value
Sample size, number (%)	48 (36)	82 (64)	
Cycle, range	1–4	1–4	
Cycle, average	1.65	1.37	
Patient age, range	25.1–41.2	23.0–42.9	
Patient age, average	32.6	32.7	
Partner age, range	23.5–59.8	23.0–55.3	
Partner age, average	36.6	36.4	
How long waiting, range	1–11	1–12	
How long waiting, average	2.7	3.2	
Male			
Count, average	69	67	
Motility, average	48	53	
Morphology, average	6	7	
Female			
FSH average	5.5	6.4	
FSH range	4.7–19.3	5.1–14.6	
Highest FSH average	8.3	7.6	
Highest FSH range	4.7–19.8	5.1–16.4	
PI, average	1.4	1.3	
PI, range	0.7–3.1	1–2.9	
Gravid, average	0.55	0.48	
Gravid, range	0–4	0–4	
Weight, average	153.8	150.8	
Weight, range	106–267	100–240	
Height, average	5.06	5.06	
Height, range	4.11–6.02	4.11–5.10	
BMI, average	34.2	35.02	
BMI, range	18–51	22.5–51.3	
Diagnostic			
PCOS	18 (39.1)	26 (31.7)	
Tubal	12 (26.0)	16 (19.5)	
Endometriosis	7 (15.2)	14 (17.1)	
Age >35 years	21 (45.6)	36 (43.9)	
Failed IUI	20 (43.7)	37 (45.1)	
Male factor	37 (88.1)	70 (85.4)	
Protocols			
Long	23 (48)	45 (55)	
Microdose flare	0 (0)	0 (0)	

Table 61.7. (continued)

N = 130	Ac (%)	No Ac	p value
Flare	3 (6)	6 (7)	
pre–IVF HRT	2 (4)	3 (4)	
OCP	4 (8)	5 (6)	
GnRH antagonist	0 (0)	0 (0)	
Lupron	8 (17)	17 (20)	
FET	0 (0)	0 (0)	
Gonadotropins			
rFSH only	18 (39.1)	33 (40.2)	
rFSH and HMG	27 (58.7)	47 (57.3)	
HMG only	1 (2.1)	2 (2.4)	

Table 61.8: All IVF Patients: IVF Cycle and Embryology Data

N = 130	Ac	No Ac (%)	p value
Cycle and embryology			
E2, average	3,117	4,709	
E2, range	1,046–5,487	1,022–6,418	
P4, average	1.12	1.59	
P4, range	0.2–5.1	0.2–5.8	
Endometrial lining, average	10.3	11.7	
Endometrial lining, range	8.4–17.2	7.8–18.8	
No. of eggs retrieved, average	15	15	
No. of eggs retrieved, range	4–36	1–31	
No. of eggs normally fertilized, average	7.8	7.5	
No. of eggs normally fertilized, range	1–24	1–19	
No. of embryos frozen, average	5.4	5.2	
No. of embryos frozen, range	0–9	0–11	
No. of embryos transferred, average	2.2	2.2	
No. of embryos transferred, range	1–4	1–4	
No. of embryos implanted, average	0.7	0.6	
No. of embryos implanted, range	0–2	0–2	
No. of prior cycles, average	1.4	1.5	
No. of prior cycles, range	0–4	0–4	

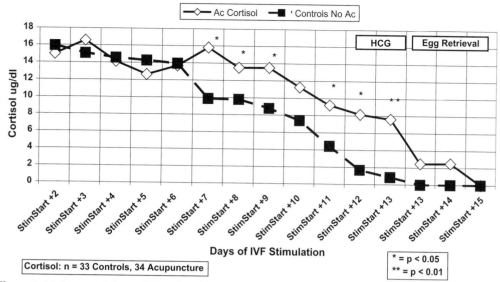

Figure 61.12. Impact of Ac on IVF patients' stress hormones during gonadotropin treatment: cortisol levels, Log rank comparison of lines, $p < 0.05$.

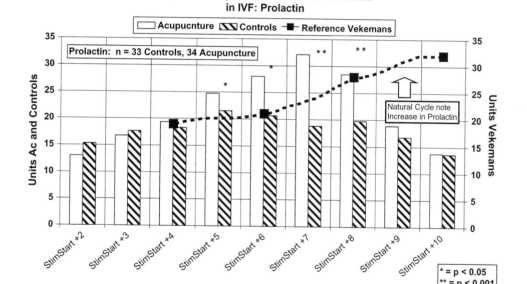

Figure 61.13. Impact of Ac on IVF patients' stress hormones during gonadotropin treatment compared with reported values for natural menstrual cycle: prolactin levels. Log rank comparison of bars, $p < 0.034$.

☐ Male factor

☐ Tubal factor

▪ Patients with the highest opportunity for success with IVF, younger, and with good prognosis may not be helped as much. This may represent selection bias in our population since the average age for IVF patients was 35 years old.

DISCUSSION

Although these studies were prospective blinded cohort clinical trials, the impact of Ac on IVF outcomes in these patients' repeatedly demonstrated positive effects of Ac equating to improved "true" reproductive outcomes, that is, THB. A 50 percent improvement in THB for PPr patients treated with Ac was observed. Overall, for all patients, the improvements for ectopic pregnancy outcomes and THB rates per cycle or per ongoing pregnancy were observed.

These studies do not eliminate the selection biases (*patient self-selected treatments*) and potential treatment biases (*nurse may have encouraged poor-prognosis patients more* strongly than those they perceived as good-prognosis patients). We believe this latter bias strengthens our conclusions rather than weaken it. One would have expected a lower pregnancy rate and certainly lower THB rates, when PPr was compared to the average prognosis controls (Figure 61.6). These outcomes were not observed, and in fact, all reproductive outcomes were better in the Ac

Table 61.18: Modified Stener-Victorin et al. Protocol (1)

- Average nine treatments before retrieval
- The patients were treated twice a week for an average of five weeks up to retrieval of eggs
- Point locations (all points are needled bilaterally) needles twirled to achieve DeQi sensation
  - □ UB 23 (black clip) to UB 28 (red clip, one lead)
  - □ SP 6 (black clip) to UB 57 ((red clip, one lead)
- Electrostimulation was set on direct current with variable frequency: 0
- –100 Hz for thirty minutes (this is our modification of the protocol)
  - □ (AWQ-104 D digital Electro Ac Stimulator)
- TDP lamp on the low back is optional for the patient (our variation)
- Needles
  - □ 36-g 1- to 1.5-inch needles

Patient has panic button in case e-Stim stops or gets too strong

Table 61.19: Treatments during Pre- and Post-ET Phase of IVF; Modified Paulus Protocol (2)

Pre-ET points:

- □ Du 20, PC 6, ST 29, SP 8, LIV 3

Auricular points:

- □ Right shenmen, brain left uterus, endocrine
- □ Press tacks were secured in each ear using the same pattern and the patients was asked to stimulate them during transfer

Post-ET points:

- □ Occurred within one hour after ET
- □ LI 4, SP 10, ST 36, SP 6

Auricular points:

- □ Right uterus, endocrine left shenmen, brain
- □ Press tacks were secured in each ear using the same pattern. Patients were instructed to remove the tacks in three days

Needles:

- □ 32-g 1.5-inch needles
- □ Stimulate to obtain "de Qi"
- □ Restimulate the needles after ten minutes; retain needles another fifteen minutes. Total needle retention twenty-five minutes

Note: Auricular point locations were taken from *Ac A Comprehensive Text.* Shanghai College of Traditional Medicine O'Connor and Bensky.

groups when compared to the average prognosis controls except for SAB, and these were equivalent (Table 61.9 and Figure 61.8).

Another area that strengthens the noted association of increased THB and Ac treatments was the fact that the results were observed despite the use of many different acupuncturists. This supports our premise that TCM treatments to "balance" patients are not practitioner specific (i.e., practitioner bias).

The lack of sham/placebo Ac treatments may also be a criticism of this study. Quintero (22) presented an abstract demonstrating a positive impact of Ac on IVF outcomes in a small prospective randomized placebo controlled crossover study. Although encouraging, these data palliate the Western perspective of CAM study design. Many CAM researchers have found that even the use of sham needles at the Ac points as well as the use of nonacupuncture points created a response, and therefore, it may be impossible to create a true sham study. Continued studies in the development and design of sham Ac treatments are needed.

In a MEDLINE computer review of the role of Ac in the treatment of infertility, Chang et al. (23) concluded "although the definitive role of Ac in the treatment of female infertility is yet to be established, its potential impact centrally on the hypothalamic-pituitary-ovarian axis and peripherally on the uterus needs to be systematically examined." The data presented in our studies provide clear clinical evidence of the impact of Ac on IVF patients.

Evolution of the Use of Ac with ART

In 1996, Stener-Victorin et al. (1) reported on improvement of uterine blood flow by lowering PI using e-Stim Ac. She demonstrated a decrease in PI after eight e-Stim Ac treatments on women with stimulated cycles. She hypothesized that the increase was caused by an increased chance of embryo implantation due to increase blood flow through the uterine artery.

It has been demonstrated in previous studies (24, 25) that uterine blood flow, as measured by PI, between 2.0 and 2.99 on the day of ET is optimal for implantation, so a PI greater than 3.0 is used by us as the poor-prognosis indicator. The next published study that received a lot of press was Paulus et al. (2). Paulus et al. reported on pregnancy rate in patients who underwent assisted reproduction therapy utilizing pre- and post-ET Ac treatments using an Ac protocol rather than using differential diagnosis according to TCM. He reported 16.2 percent increased rates of pregnancies in the Ac group. All women who had failed one previous cycle were removed from the study. Paulus repeated this study (26) using sham Ac (27) to rule out the possibility that Ac produces only psychological or psychosomatic effects. Two hundred women undergoing ICSI or IVF were included in this prospective, randomized, placebo controlled trial (placebo RCT). Paulus studies patients that exclusively had good embryo quality. The pre- and post-ET treatments were done precisely twenty-five minutes before the transfer and twenty-five minutes after the transfer ($n = 100$). Sham Ac was used on the same points without penetration of the needle within the same time frame. Chi-squared test was used for comparison of both groups. Clinical pregnancy was defined by the presence of a fetal sac at six to eight weeks with ultrasound exam. Clinical pregnancies in the Ac group were 43 percent compared to 37 percent in the placebo group, which were not statistical different. Paulus stated "Our placebo needle set induces an acupressure effect thus leading to a higher pregnancy rate than in our population without any

Table 61.20: Copy of Consortium Contract, ©EWA 1999

The Ac and RMFC Consortium Agreement ©EWA 1999

Diane Cridennda, L.Ac., Ac Coordinator

e-Mail eastwindstcm@earthlink.net

I _____ agree to abide by the following guidelines set forth for performing Ac on patients undergoing IVF cycles.

I agree to abide by the protocol set up this committee, based on the Wolfgang E. Paulus study Christian-Lauritzen Institute, Ulm, Germany for the pre-transfer and post transfer Ac treatments.

I agree to provide Diane Cridennda with a list of all patients treated and which protocol was done at the end of each cycle. This is for statistical purposes to determine success rates using Ac with patients refereed by RMFC.

The patient is required to sign the disclosure form set forth by the Ac and RMFC Consortium.

The patient will not be charged for broken appointments due to cancellation of their cycle.

After embryo transfer the patient will not sit in the waiting room or wait for more than ten to fifteen minutes for her treatment. If a treatment room is not immediately available, a reclining chair for the patient to lie on is acceptable.

* No Herbs are allowed during the patient's cycle

IVF Protocol

I agree to use the following IVF protocol when treating RMFC patients prior to their IVF cycles.

UB23 to UB 28; UB 57 to SP 6, The Electro Stimulator will be set on direct current with variable frequency 0–100 Hz for 30 minutes). Recommended treatment is two times a week for four weeks prior to egg retrieval for a total of NINE treatments, using 36g-1-11/2" needles.

Pre-Embryo Transfer

Right ear: brain, shenmen

Left ear: endocrine, uterus

Du 20, Stomach 29, Pericardium 6, Spleen 8, Liver 3

(after removing needles place ear tacks in the same pattern as ear needles and instruct patient to stimulate these during the transfer).

Post-Embryo Transfer

Right ear: endocrine, uterus

Left ear: brain, shenmen

Large Intestine 4, Stomach 36, Spleen 10 and Spleen 6

(after removing needles place ear tacks in the same pattern as ear needles and instruct patient to stimulate these a few times a day and remove tacks in 3 days)

20 x 25(32g 1.5 inch needles)

achieve De Qi sensation at the needle site, the re-stimulate the needles after 10 minutes, Total time of needle retention is 25 minutes.

Practitioner Signature _____
Date: _____

©East Winds Ac 1999

Table 61.21: Theoretical Basis Ac Points in Stener-Victorin Protocol (1)

- UB 23 (kidney shu point)
  a. Powerful point which tonifies and regulates the kidneys (yin and yang), affects the low back, regulates whole body
- UB 28 (bladder shu)
  a. Local points over the uterine arteries, regulates the uterus
- UB 57 (supporting mountain)
  a. Relaxes sinews, invigorates the blood
- SP 6 (three yin crossing or meeting of the yin)
  a. All female issues, affects kidneys, liver, and spleen

Table 61.22: Innervations and Muscle Localizations of the Ac Points Used in the Stener-Victorin Protocol (1)

Ac Points	Segmental innervations afferent muscle	Muscle localization
BL 23	L 1, 2, 3	Erector spinae thoracolumbar
BL 28	L4, 5 S1, 2, 3	Erector spinae lumbosacral
SP6	L4, 5 S2, 3	Tibialis posterior at the medial side
BL 57	S1, 2	Gastrocnemius and M. soleus at the dorsal side

Table 61.23: Theoretical Basis for the Ac Points in Paulus Protocol (2): Pre-ET

Pre-ET (2)

- DU 20 Hundred meetings
  - Any pre- and postpartum issues, prolapse of any kind, lifts the yang Qi and lifts the spirit
- PC 6 Inner gate
  - Calms and opens the heart, regulates Qi, regulates middle jiao
- SP 8 Earth mechanism
  - Regulates uterus
- ST 29 Coming back
  - Affects ovaries, vagina all female issues
- LIV 3 Bigger rushing
  - Calms the mind, regulates blood, pacifies liver, opens channel calms spasms

Table 61.24: Theoretical Basis for the Ac Points in Paulus Protocol (2): Post-ET

Post-ET (2)

- LI 4 Union of the Valleys
- Pain in uterus, tonifies and regulates Qi
- ST 36
  - Regulates Qi and blood, aids digestion, strengthens whole body, treats weak and deficient conditions
  - SP 10
  - Invigorates, cools, and tonifies the blood (a heparin like *effect*)
  - SP 6
  - Regulates the uterus, calms the mind by relationship to the heart, benefits kidney, liver and spleen. Nourishes yin and blood.

Table 61.25: Auricular Ac

Points

- Uterus
- Endocrine
- Shen Men
- Brain

** Vinco 7 mm ND: Detox needles were used

Note: Auricular point locations were taken from: O'Connor and Bensky. *Ac: A comprehensive Text.* Shanghai College of Traditional Medicine.

complementary treatment." [We based our Ac protocols on Stener-Victorin and Paulus et al. studies (1, 2).]

Our studies (5–11) repeatedly demonstrated improved pregnancy rates, fewer miscarriages, fewer ectopic pregnancies, as well as more THB in the Ac versus the nonacupuncture groups. We also noted that there were fewer multiple pregnancies in the Ac group (Figure 61.14, $p < 0.05$). This is the first report of lowering multiple pregnancy rates in IVF by incorporating Ac therapies.

Emmons (28) described improvements in numbers of follicles developed when IVF patients were treated with Ac as compared to their own historic data (mean 11.3 follicles vs. 3.9 follicles) in patients' cycles before Ac. They comment, "These cases have an obvious bias. The group was selected from those who responded poorly to gonadotropins therapy." We also would support the inclusion of such PPr patients. A possible mechanism for the improvement in reproductive outcomes with poorer prognosis IVF patients may well be explained as follows: in TCM, there is a strong connection between the penetrating vessel-blood-uterus and the kidneys. The penetrating vessel is the sea of blood, which arises from the uterus and pertains to the kidneys. Any deficiency or imbalance of the kidneys affects the uterus (which in turn stores blood). The penetrating or conception vessel originates from the space between the kidneys and plays a major role in not

Table 61.26: Impact of Ac on IVF Outcomes Based on the Demographics of Their Infertility Diagnosis

	n			Percent	
	232				
Acupuncture	172			74	
Nonacupuncture	60			26	
	Ac			*Nonacupuncture*	*p value*
	n	Pregnancy	%	n	Pregnancy	%	

Diseases	n	Pregnancy	%	n	Pregnancy	%	p value
PCOS	42	23	55	17	9	53	
Tubal Factor	27	13	48	16	2	12	$p < 0.05$
Endometriosis	14	8	57	8	4	50	
Over 35	73	22	30	23	8	34	
Failed IUI	24	15	63	12	9	75	$p < 0.05$
Male Factor	133	61	46	46	24	52	
PCOS and Tubal	2	2	100	2	0	0	
PCOS and endo	3	2	67	2	0	0	
PCOS and >35	8	3	38	4	2	50	
PCOS and IUI	7	4	57	4	4	100	
PCOS and male	35	20	57	14	7	50	$p < 0.05$
Tubal and endo	3	1	33	4	1	25	
Tubal and >35	11	2	18	7	1	14	
Tubal and IUI	4	4	100	1	0	0	
Tubal and male	18	7	39	12	5	41	
Endo and >35	3	2	67	3	0	0	
Endo and IUI	2	2	100	2	1	50	
Endo and male	9	6	67	5	2	40	
Tubal/>35/male	8	1	13	6	1	17	

Table 61.27: Impact of Ac on IVF outcomes Based on Age-Groups of Female Patients: Based on SART/CDC Categories

SART/CDC age groups	*Ac*			*Nonacupuncture*			
	n	Pregnancy	%	n	Pregnancy	%	p value
<35	90	49	54	35	20	57	
35–38	39	16	41	9	6	67	$p < 0.05$
38–40	18	3	17	7	2	28	
>40	25	8	32	9	2	22	$p < 0.05$

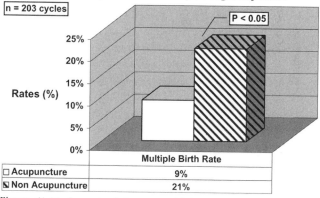

Figure 61.14. Impact of Ac on multiple pregnancy rates in IVF patients.

only follicle production but all aspects of fertility as well (29). TCM regulates the conception vessel and tonifies the kidney energy, thereby stimulating the production of follicles in the ovaries. This would imply that poor-prognosis patients would be the ideal candidates for Ac treatments. More studies need to be done to answer these questions.

Theoretical Basis for Ac's Impact on Fertility in IVF Patients

Modified Stener-Victorin Protocol

What is the theoretical basis or "biology of Ac"? Stener-Victorin used the following Ac points in their study, which reported on uterine blood flow:

- UB 23 (kidney shu point)
  □ Powerful point which tonifies and regulates the kidneys, affects the low back, and regulates whole body.
- UB 28 (bladder shu)
  □ Local points over the uterine arteries, regulates the uterus.
- UB 57 (supporting mountain)
  □ Relaxes sinews, invigorates the blood.
- SP 6 (three yin crossing or meeting of the yin)
  □ Enhances all female issues, affects kidneys, liver, and spleen.

Modified Paulus Protocol: Pre ET
- DU 20 Hundred meetings
  □ Any pre- and postpartum issues, prolapse of any kind, lifts yang Qi, lifts the spirit
- PC 6 Inner gate
  □ Calms and opens the heart, regulates Qi, regulates middle jiao
- SP 8 Earth mechanism
  □ Regulates uterus
- ST 29 Coming back
  □ Affects ovaries, vagina, all female issues
- LIV 3 Bigger rushing
  □ Calms the mind, regulates blood, pacifies liver, and opens channel calms spasms

Modified Paulus Protocol: Post-ET
- LI 4 Union of the Valleys
  □ Pain in uterus, tonifies and regulates Qi
- ST 36
  □ Regulates Qi and blood, aids digestion, strengthens whole body, treats any weak and deficient conditions.
- SP 10
  □ Invigorates, cools, and tonifies the blood (a heparin-like effect)
- SP 6
  □ Regulates the uterus, calms the mind by relationship to the heart, benefits kidney, liver and spleen, and nourishes yin and blood.

Stress Hormones in IVF: What Does Ac Have to Do with It?

Stress plays a major role in our every day existence. After years of trying to conceive, couples are at their wits end and have been in the "fight or flight" mode for quite some time. Stress increases the cortisol hormones as well as other neurochemicals. In prehistoric days, this flight or flight was our survival, when threatened by the saber-toothed tigers or wooly mammoths the adrenals would pump out adrenaline, blood was directed away from the endocrine, gastrointestinal, and reproductive systems. Large muscles in the legs would become engorged with blood to give us the ability to "survive" by running away. Now when faced with stress, we are sitting in front of our computers, in bumper to bumper traffic with no place to run, yet the adaptive mechanism remains in place. How does this affect our reproductive capacity when the key organs are not being nourished for reproduction? In Chinese medicine, we can compare stress with liver Qi stagnation, anger, resentment, and unfulfilled desires describe the emotional state of liver stagnation. Muscles become tight, blood vessels contract; hyperactive sympathetic nervous systems are in a constant state of hypervigilance with no mechanism to shut it off.

Recent studies have demonstrated how stress affects pregnancy rates. One such is by Gallinelli et al. (30). Forty infertile women were studied who were undergoing IVF-ET in a university hospital setting. Blood sampling was used. Gallinelli correlated stress and immunity with human fertility. Women with functional chronic anovulation have a higher serum cortisol and cerebrospinal fluid corticotrophin-releasing hormone concentrations than healthy controls. This cortisol hypersecretion has been reported in women undergoing IVF and ET who fail to achieve implantation. Moreover, a significant correlation between low adaptation to cognitive stress and poor outcomes has been reported in couples. Gallinelli (30) concluded that a prolonged condition of stress causes a decreased ability to adapt, and a transitory anxious state is associated with high proportion of activated T-cells in the peripheral blood and that such a condition reduces the embryo implantation rate. In another study, Smeenk et al. (31) examined urinary levels of stress hormones, adrenaline, noradrenaline, and cortisol during treatment with self-reported stress in order to investigate the mechanism for the previously observed negative association for anxiety and depression with the outcomes of IVF/ICSI. This was a prospective cohort study. Nocturnal urine samples were collected: pretreatment, preoocyte retrieval, and before ET. Two questionnaires were administered to measure anxiety and depression. There was a significant positive correlation between urinary adrenaline concentrations at baseline and ET and the scores on depression at baseline. Women who had successful treatment had a lower concentration of adrenaline at oocyte retrieval and lower concentrations of adrenaline and noradrenaline at ET compared to the unsuccessful women. He concluded that the association of adrenal hormone may be one of the links in the complex relationship between psychosocial stress and IVF outcomes. Klonoff-Cohen et al. (32) reported on the trauma associated with infertility. IVF contains a number of stressful aspects: daily injections, blood draws, ultrasound, laparoscopic surgery, and the possibility of failure at any of the various phases. He defined successful IVF as one gestational sac detected on the ultrasound. This cohort study consisted of 221 (151 completed the study) women undergoing IVF GIFT. Women completed two stress questionnaires, one at the first visit (baseline) and one at the time of their procedure. The baseline stressor: positive and negative effect scale and bipolar profile of moods states; the authors noted that there was a significant change in the perceived stress at baseline before and after hormone use. The women were categorized as having good levels of social support systems. Outcomes were interesting: for each unit, increase in a woman's chronic negative effect score on stress survey, a 2 percent decrease in the number of oocytes *retrieved*. Similarly, when a woman's chronic negative-effect score was high, one to two fewer embryos were *transferred*. Stress and anxiety had an effect on successful pregnancies and live births. A one-point increase in positive affect on the stress scale increased live birth delivery by 7 percent. Facchinetti et al. (33) demonstrated that an increased vulnerability to stress is associated with a poor outcome of IVF-ET treatment. We believe based on our preliminary data (Figures 61.12 and 61.13) that Ac may "correct" the depressive effects of IVF on prolactin and the nonsensitive adrenal response, and these effects may impact "stress" as perceived by the patient. In a recent unpublished review of over 586 IVF cycles in our database, 26% more pregnancies occurred when patients were treated with Ac and IVF. We believe these data represent the world's largest controlled trial measuring the impact of acupuncture on reproductive outcomes in patients treated with Assisted Reproductive Technologies.

Research Design: Placebo Effect or Real Phenomenon?

Major criticism of Ac research by Western physicians centers on appropriateness of the experimental design. In review, by utilizing prospective blinded cohort clinical trials, we have attempted to eliminate the following biases/deficiencies in our experiments:

1. Historical comparisons
   a) Recruitment was prospective.
2. Physician bias
   a) Recruitment for Ac was hidden or "blinded" to the physician.
3. Acupuncturist bias
   a) IVF treatment protocols were hidden or blinded to the acupuncturist.
4. Treatment selection bias
   a) Only "standardized" Ac treatments were allowed, that is, no differentiation of syndromes as a basis of treatments was done; all patients had the same Ac protocol (much to the consternation of D.K.C.)!

5. Investigator bias
   a) All data were collected by a third party, Mel Cohen (M.C.), and kept from the physician and acupuncturist for three years.
6. Treatment variability
   a) Contracts were written and signed by all TCM practitioners to follow the prescribed protocols for treatments to ensure there were no variations or deviations from the protocol set forth.
7. Timing/convenience bias
   a) The TCM practitioners agreed to provide 24/7 coverage on an as-needed basis for patients in the study since ETs, at times, occurred on weekends and holidays.
8. Patients selected whether to participate or not and no coercion to participate was allowed, simple discussion by nurses to patients about the ability to have Ac was done.
   a) Does NOT eliminate selection bias.
      i) This is a weakness of most TCM studies.
9. Selection bias for monetary gains
   a) No monetary gain was provided to participate.
10. Treatment bias based on monetary gains
    a) No reduction in IVF fees for participation in the study were given.
11. Treatment bias based on monetary gains
    a) No reduction in TCM treatment fees for participation in the study were given.
12. Placebo effect, that is, the impact of the knowledge of positive outcomes on the choice to do Ac by patients.
    a) Most study data collected from 1999 to 2003 were reviewed in 2003, 2004, and 2005.
13. Although not randomized, the cortisol/prolactin was blinded to the acupuncturists, physicians, and statistician until analyzed.
    a) The cortisol/prolactin study (2005 and 2006) was prospective in design.

Stener-Victorin stated that in her review of the role of experimental design in understanding Ac studies (34): "The lack of evidence of an effect does not equal evidence of the lack of effect." She reminds us that TCM has been used for at least 3,000 years, it is not exotic, nor is it a *new* method. She is quick to debate the fact that in fact historically Western medicine has not been rigorously tested either. In 1961, Greenblatt et al. was quoted in Dickey (35) to have stated "Although the mechanism of action of this compound (clomiphene citrate) is not clear at the present time, it is heartening to find a drug which holds much promise of inducing ovulatory type menses with considerable regularity in anovulatory women." The authors go on to state that in 1996, there were more than 5,400 studies on Clomid and "twenty five years after its introduction into clinical medicine, *less is known* about the effects of clomiphene on follicular development and steroid and gonadotropin concentration than is known about HMG and FSH . . . ." It would seem that Western-based physicians continually prescribe a medicine that remains somewhat enigmatic as to "how it works." Stener-Victorin (34) reminds us that "Once a treatment has been tested rigorously, it no longer matters whether it was considered alternative or not." If in fact it has been deemed safe and effective, it should be accepted. She readily admits that there are difficulties in designing Ac trials and that this hampers clinical investigation.

Table 61.28: Summary of Ac and IVF Studies: Pregnancy Outcomes

Study authors	n	Result reported	Control rate (%)	Ac Rx rate (%)	Percent difference	p value
Dieterle (21)	225	Ongoing pregnancy	14	28	15	$p < 0.05$
Magarelli poor prognosis (5)	128	Birth per pregnancy	50	70	20	$p < 0.05$
Magarelli good prognosis (6)	131	Birth per pregnancy	35	42	7	$p < 0.05$
Magarelli All IVF Pts (7)	130	Birth per pregnancy	82	88	6	N.S
Magarelli eggs and embryos (8)	208	Birth per pregnancy	82	88	0	N.S.
Magarelli stress hormones (10)	67	Birth per pregnancy	64	94	30	$p < 0.05$
Paulus (2)	160	Clinical pregnancy	26	43	16	$p < 0.03$

In a paper by Norman Latov (36), he writes about understanding evidence-based guidelines (EBGs). He supports evidence from biological experimentation based on work done by William Harvey, Louis Pasteur, and William Osler who most certainly did not make contributions based on controlled trials. He goes on to state, "The only evidence that can be considered in recommending a test, procedure, or treatment is that from blinded controlled trials. All other types of evidence including peer reviewed publication of uncontrolled trials, case report, or case series, which represent our collective experience are considered anecdotal and thus barred. Personal observations, experience, judgment or expert opinion are presumed biased and are disallowed." He makes a point that in clinical practice, physicians need to make recommendations based on the best available evidence; clinical experience as well as their own judgment. How many published research papers end with the statement "but more studies are needed to make any final conclusion"?

We believe the evidence presented in our experiments and other studies that have been published provide ample clinical evidence that Ac provides help to infertile patients without negative side effects. Under EBGs, therapies can only be definitively recommended, if they are based on evidence from rigorous blinded prospective controlled trials. Less rigorous trials can be used to justify a score of "may be considered" or should be considered but not recommended therapies. To us, EBGs appear to be an academic exercise designed for evaluating the quality of clinical trials with little thought given to what follows: controlled trials are designed only to compare one treatment option to another, they either work or they do not work. Yet, medical decision making is complex and requires consideration of many variables, including clinical presentation, severity, progression, coexisting conditions, genetic or biological variations, susceptibility to complications, and allergies to medications. It would be impossible to design trials that compare all the options. We need expertise as well as clinical judgment.

Traditionally, medical practices were proven through reproducibility and predictability rather than controlled trials, which are relatively new to Western medicine. A TCM physician would report a new observation, and if it was reproduced and confirmed by others, it would become general practice. This allowed rapid progress and dissemination of treatments demonstrated to "work." Latov (36) supports this point "Such anecdotal evidence is responsible for most human scientific progress, including discovery of the wheel, fire, rotation of the planets, gravity, anesthesia, penicillin and aseptic technique."

Summary of Studies

Commonality of reproductive outcomes based on the available IVF and Ac literature seems to suggest an overall 15 percent improvement in pregnancy/births (Table 61.28). We have summarized the Ac points used from the reported IVF studies in Table 61.29. Based on these results, it would seem that the following Ac points are common and "useful" or enhancing reproductive outcomes in IVF cycles:

■ PC 6
■ BL 23, 28, 57
■ SP 6, 8, 10
■ ST 36, 29
■ REN 3, 4'
■ DU 20
■ LI 4
■ LIV 3
■ Auricular points: shenmen, brain, uterus, endocrine

Issues Related to Placebo-Controlled Trials in Ac Studies

Defining a Placebo

Very few RCTs have been performed. The use of placebo RCTs were initially designed for pharmaceuticals to differentiate between real and placebo effects of specific medications. The issue of placebo studies has been raised in the literature and in conferences (personal observations) regarding the effects of Ac. The questions how does one navigate the placebo effect and how can one *pretend* to insert a needle through the patient's skin and is there then an acupressure effect as stated by Paulus (26) and Streitberger (27) studied the placebo Ac system; however, the placebo needle still gave the patient pricking sensation topically. One has to wonder if this (much like a Japanese-style needle technique) can actually affect the body.

Controls

With so much press now about Ac and IVF/ART, many patients are opting to NOT be in the control groups; we are thereby loosing our controls. For pharmaceutical trials designed to determine an effect of a "new medication," placebo

Table 61.29: Summary of Ac Points Used in IVF Studies (1, 2, 5–11, 19–22)

Study IVF	BL 23	Bl 25	BL 28	BL 40	BL 57	CV-4	DU 20	EAR	GB 20	GB 21	GB 31	GB 32	GB 34
Stener-Victorin (1)	X		X		X								
Paulus (2)								X					
Magarelli (5)	X		X		X			X					
Magarelli (6)	X		X		X			X					
Magarelli (7)	X		X		X			X					
Magarelli (8)	X		X		X			X					
Cridennda (9)	X		X		X			X					
Magarelli (10)	X		X		X			X					
Magarelli (11)	X		X		X			X					
Quintero (22)	X	X		X	X	X	X	X	X	X			
Smith (20)								X					
Dieterle (21)								X			X	X	X
Westergaard (19)													

Study IVF	REN 4	REN 12	REN 6	REN 3	SJ 9	SJ 12	SP 6	SP 9	SP 10
Stener-Victorin (1)							X		
Paulus (2)							X	X	X
Magarelli (5)							X	X	X
Magarelli (6)							X	X	X
Magarelli (7)							X	X	X
Magarelli (8)							X	X	X
Cridennda (9)							X	X	X
Magarelli (10)							X	X	X
Magarelli (11)							X	X	X
Quintero (22)	X	X	X				X	X	X
Smith (20)							X	X	X
Dieterle (21)	X		X		X	X	X	X	X
Westergaard (19)				X			X	X	X

Study IVF	GV 20	KD 3	LI 4	LI 11	LIV 3	PC 6	ST 25	ST 28	ST 29	ST 36
Stener-Victorin (1)										
Paulus (2)	X		X		X	X			X	X
Magarelli (5)	X		X		X	X			X	X
Magarelli (6)	X		X		X	X			X	X
Magarelli (7)	X		X		X	X			X	X
Magarelli (8)	X		X		X	X			X	X
Cridennda (9)	X		X		X	X			X	X
Magarelli (10)	X		X		X	X			X	X
Magarelli (11)	X		X		X	X			X	X

Society for Assisted Reproductive Technologies Fresh IVF Pregnancy Rates U.S. 1985 - 2006?

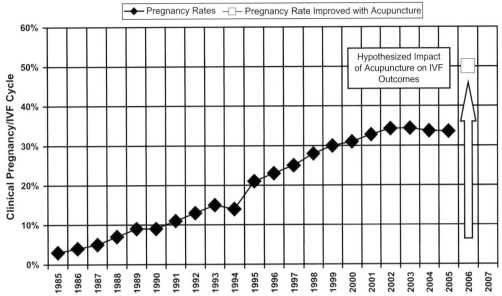

Figure 61.15. Hypothetical impact of Ac on U.S. IVF reproductive outcomes based on TCM by us and others, based on www.cdc.gov data.

randomized controlled studies are done and the investment by the pharmaceutical companies ranges in the tens of millions of dollars to complete them. Acupuncturists and needle supply companies do not have these kinds of funds for studies. This is not an excuse; it is a fact. Despite these problems, RCT and placebo-controlled RCTs have been performed (see following section).

Acupuncturists versus "Trained" Needle Inserters

Some studies are being performed in hospital settings, with nurses administering the Ac (19). To report negative or positive results from nonprofessional acupuncturists denigrates the 3,000-year tradition of TCM. It takes years to learn Ac techniques. We recommend only NCCAOM-certified acupuncturist provide these services to IVF patients.

Standard Protocols versus Differentiation of Syndromes

Should the studies be set up to use differentiation of syndrome complex, whereby each patient may have different acupoints or should a standard protocol be used (as in our studies, 5–11)? Although D.K.C. firmly believes that differentiation of syndromes "should" be more efficacious, Western designed studies (if we are going to mimic them) require that we use strict guidelines to ensure that each patient has the exact same Ac protocol using the same IVF protocols for all patients' outcomes. Given the overwhelming data supporting the use of Ac in IVF patients, we have "relaxed" our requirements for strict protocols, although we strongly recommend that the points used in our studies be considered and perhaps added to additional points based on differentiation of syndromes (DOS). Note: if patients required treatments using DOS, they were not included in any data presented in our studies (5–11).]

"Ideal" Ac Studies

Despite our protestations about designing prospective randomized placebo-controlled trials for Ac, we now present and review published RCTs. In May 2006, three well-designed papers were published in *F&S* (19–21). We outline each study below:

1. Westergaard et al. (19) (Denmark) published a study entitled Ac on the day of embryo transfer significantly improves the reproductive outcome in infertile women: a prospective, randomized trial. Key elements were:

■ Prospective RCT
■ *N* = 273
■ Demographics were similar is all three groups:
  □ Age
  □ BMI
  □ Previous IVF cycles
  □ Years of infertility
  □ Similar embryology
■ Control *N*-87 No Ac
■ Group 1, *N* = 95 Ac day of ET before and after utilizing the Paulus protocol
■ Group 2, *N* = 91 Ac day of ET Paulus plus two days post ET: DU 20, LI 4, REN 3, ST 29, SP 10, and SP 6
■ Ac administered by nurses; taught and supervised by acupuncturists.
■ In each case, two embryos were transferred.
■ Table 61.28 for pregnancy outcomes.

Results

■ Group 1 [Paulus pre-ET and post-ET (1)]
  □ Significantly more pregnancies and ongoing pregnancies.
■ Group 2 (day of ET and again three days later)
  □ Patients had numerically more pregnancies than control group but not statistically different.

■ Numerically, there were more early pregnancy losses in Group 2 (33 percent) than the control group (21 percent).

OUR VIEW

Contraindicated points were used – LI 4 and SP 6. We know that embryo implantation occurs within about twenty-four hours after transfer. Perhaps this is why the early pregnancy losses were noted in Group 2.

Smith et al. (20) (Australia) – Influence of Ac stimulation on pregnancy rates for women undergoing embryo transfer. Key elements were:

■ $N = 228$
■ Control as well as sham Ac patients were treated during Stim phase plus pre- and post-ET consisting of three treatments total, which took place within seven days of each other.
■ The first Ac treatment was on day 9 of IVF stimulation medication and second and third was pre- and post-ET.
■ Number of embryos transferred suggested two (but not clearly stated).
■ No differences in embryology characteristics between the groups.
■ Pregnancy was defined as fetal heart beat.
■ Ac Group A received true Ac based on Paulus (2) with point variation (not listed by authors) according to TCM differentiation of syndrome. Second and third Ac treatment was the modified Paulus pre- and post-ET protocol (modifications not listed by authors).
■ Sham with Streitberger placebo between meridians close to the acupoints with no penetration of the skin. The practitioner held the sham needle perpendicular to the skin and "stimulated" the needle with the other hand for three minutes.
■ Table 61.28 for pregnancy outcomes.

Results

The true Ac group had 31 percent pregnancy rate versus sham with 23 percent pregnancy rate, $p = 0.18$ (not statistically significantly different). When pregnancies were followed up to eighteen weeks, the results were 28 percent in the Ac group versus 18 percent for the placebo group, $p = 0.08$ (not statistically significantly different).

OUR VIEW:

An excellent study design with some details not explained (number of embryos transferred would greatly affect pregnancy outcomes, as well as which Ac points were used). We also note that placebo placement was "close to" acupoints. Paulus in his later study suggested that we cannot ignore an effect by placement of sham needles (19).

Dieterle et al (21) (Germany, China) – Effect of Ac on the outcome of in vitro fertilization and intracytoplasmic sperm injection: a randomized, prospective, controlled clinical study. Key elements were:

■ $N = 225$
■ Luteal phase Ac with ICSI
  □ Both groups treated thirty minutes post-ET and again in three days
■ Ear seeds used; shenmen, uterus, brain, and adrenal
  □ Caryophyllaceae seeds were left in place for two days
■ Average number of embryos transferred (2.6)
■ Pregnancy was measured by serum hCG two weeks after ET

■ Group 1 $N = 116$
  □ Patients received post-ET Ac using REN 4, REN 6, ST 29, PC 6, SP 10, and SP 8 plus ear seeds noted above.
  □ This group received Ac again three days post-ET using L I4, SP 6, ST 36, KD 3, and LIV 3 plus ear seeds noted above.
■ Group 2 $N = 109$
  □ Patients received Ac post-ET and again three days later using nonfertility points: SJ 9, SI 12, GB 31, GB 32, and GB 34 plus ear seeds different points.
  □ Placebo-controlled by placing needles at "nonfertility sites."
  □ Table 61.28 for pregnancy outcomes.

Results

Clinical and ongoing pregnancy rates were statistically significantly improved in Group 1 who had luteal phase Ac using fertility Ac points ($p < 0.05$). Group 1 Ac group had 33.6 percent clinical pregnancy versus Group 2 (nonfertility acupoints used) at 15.6 percent. When ongoing pregnancy rates were reported, the fertility Ac group had fewer miscarriages and more ongoing pregnancies compared to controls (28.4 versus 13.8, respectively, $p < 0.01$).

OUR VIEW

More rigor in the IVF protocol plus a larger study demonstrated a confirmation of results of the multitude of other non-RCT studies reported herein (5–11).

Controversy and Criticism of the RCTs

The goal of the *F&S* publication of these studies was to create a forum to discuss placebo effects (personal communication from editor). The TCM view was more that these studies reinforced and confirmed the role of Ac in IVF therapies. We would like to review the "invited" counterpoint authors published criticism of these studies:

■ Evan Myers, United States (37)
  □ Concerned that there were different points used in studies
    ■ Does not understand TCM
  □ Points not related to infertility were used
    ■ See comment above
  □ Does not rule out the effect of active treatment
    ■ Did this have detrimental affect on outcomes?
  □ Questioned possibility of placebo affect
  □ Did not share the opinion that placebo effects were balanced since it worked in some and did not work in others
  □ Providers of Ac were nurses
    ■ We agree
  □ Felt they should use live births as primary outcome
    ■ We agree
  □ Questioned the cost-effectiveness
    ■ This question will be discussed in later section.
■ Alice Domar, United States (38)
  □ Criticized the use of "Chinese DRUG" on the auricular points
    ■ Caryophyllaceae seeds were used not "drugs" (TCM practitioners utilize these seeds to physically stimulate the auricular points)
  □ Placebo effect/difficult to apply
    ■ We agree

□ Also the fact that nurses administered the Ac
  ■ We agree
□ Felt there was bias due to the fact it was not blinded
  ■ We agree
□ In a recent article in the LA Times "Ac for Fertility? Doctors say 'Why Not'" stated that Ms. Domar was going to be hiring an acupuncturist for her clinic and yet states that so far it has produced inconsistent proof.
  ■ We believe her position is not clear.
□ Also stated that it is difficult to do sham Ac as patient knows when they have been needled.
  ■ We believe this is a key issue and may be insurmountable.
■ John Collins, Canada (39)
□ Criticized that it was not blinded
  ■ We agree
□ Sample size did not meet the 250 per arm requirement for a "good" RCT to be valid.
  ■ Most medical studies published that are not phase III clinical trials do not meet this statistical power either.
□ Should try to figure out how many treatments would be needed
  ■ Based on our work (9), nine treatments provides minimally needed treatments for 50 percent pregnancy of experimental group studied.
□ Felt that adverse effects of Ac seem minimal.
  ■ We agree.

Utility of an Ac Consortium for Purposes of Research

Recent publications in *F&S* namely Westergaard et al. (19), Smith et al. (20), and Dieterle (21) reported on various protocols based on the Paulus publication (2), who reported on increased pregnancy rates in women who had pre- as well as post-ET Ac treatments. In Westergaard et al. study (19), the Ac was performed by "trained" nurses in a hospital setting. Ac is a skill that must be studied and practiced minimally for four years. A typical acupuncturist will have a soft, calming atmosphere, pleasing music, and nurturing energy in the office, which may contribute to the effectiveness of any given treatment. The ability for the patient to feel nurtured and cared for are so important for treatment outcomes. In all of our studies, we utilized NCCAOM-certified acupuncturist. An Ac consortium was developed to ensure the patient's had trained, experienced practitioners performing the Ac treatments. This not only provided 24/7 coverage but also ensured the patients had a nurturing experience versus a hospital setting experience.

Financial Considerations

There have been numerous articles published demonstrating effectiveness, as well as a financial benefit of Ac therapies when used in conjunction with Western treatments (40–43). A brief summary follows:

■ Ac treatment results in the avoidance of surgery
□ Christensen et al. (40) studied severe knee osteroarthrosis and found that of the twenty patients awaiting arthroplasty surgery, after randomization to Ac, resulted in seven not having to have the surgery.
  ■ Savings estimate: $9,000 per patient

■ Ac treatments result in fewer days in hospital or nursing home
□ Johansson et al. (41) studied stroke patients to determine if providing Ac resulted in quicker rehabilitation. After randomization, patients were given Ac and noted to recover faster spending 88 days/patient versus 161 days/patient in hospital or nursing homes.
  ■ Savings estimate: $26,000 per patient
■ Ac treatment results in quicker return to physical labor for patients suffering from low back pain.
□ Gunn et al. (42) studied workers in a workers compensation clinic who were randomized to receive physical therapy/occupational therapy/exercise (standard care) versus standard care plus Ac. If they received standard care, only four of twenty-seven returned to former occupation. If they received standard care plus Ac, eighteen of twenty-nine returned to their former occupation.
  ■ Savings estimate: not calculated.
■ Ac treatments of angina pectoris results in decreased number of in-hospital days, reduction in outpatient visits, and significant reduction in annual sick pay.
□ Ballegaard et al. (43) studied patient with angina pectoris who were treated with Ac plus shiatsu two times/day. He noted a decreased number of in-hospital days for all sixty-nine patients studied and reduced number of outpatient visits.
  ■ Savings estimate: $18,000/patient

We have therefore created the following table to estimate the impact of adding Ac to IVF treatments:

We project that for each 100 IVF cycles performed by an IVF practice, fifteen extra patients will achieve a pregnancy and THB, resulting in significant savings to the couple. More importantly, there will be better reproductive outcomes for the "integrated" IVF clinic, which translates to more patients and better profits. In the table above, we project what would happen if all the IVF programs in the United States converted to integrative medicine practices. If each of the 500 programs in the United State use Ac plus IVF and each demonstrates a "conservative" 10 percent improvement (the average benefit is closer to 15 percent, Table 61.28, and Figure 61.15), based on 100,000 cycles done each year in the United States, then 10,000 fewer cycles at $10,000 per cycle = savings of $100,000,000! Continued research into the mechanisms and modes of action of Ac in ART are needed. The next goal for research is male factor.

Proposed impact: THB (%)	Cost per IVF: $12,000/ cycle	Fewer cycles	Typical IVF		Total cost
			Practice	Cycles saved	savings
5		1 in 20	100 cycles/year	5	$60,000
10		1 in 10		10	$120,000
15		1.5 in 10		15	$180,000
20		2 in 10		20	$240,000

ACKNOWLEDGMENTS

None of this work would have been accomplished without the amazing, gifted, and compassionate clinical, laboratory, and administrative teams we have the privilege of working with. We especially thank Cecelia Roberts, R.N. M.P.H., Diane Polasky, D.O.M., Steve Chan, Ph.D., Ann Cohen, Cynde Tagg, R.N., Francis Byrn, M.D., and Tammie Parker for the unfailing support of this project. We extend our thanks to the Ac Consortium members . . . you guys rock!

REFERENCES

1. Stener-Victorin E, Waldenstrom U, Andersson SA, Wikland M. Reduction of blood flow impedance in the uterine arteries of infertile women with electro-acupuncture. *Hum Reprod* 1996; 11:1314–1317.
2. Paulus WE, Zhang M, Stehler E, El-Danasouri I, Sterzik K. Influence of acupuncture on the pregnancy rate in patients who undergo assisted reproduction therapy. *Fertil Steril* 2002; 77:721–724.
3. McDonough P. Editorial Comments. *Fertil Steril* 2004;78:4.
4. Opher C. Clinical decision-making when science is uncertain. *Fertil Steril* 2002;78:891.
5. Magarelli P, Cridennda D. Acupuncture and IVF poor responders: A cure? *Fertil Steril* 2004;81:S20.
6. Magarelli P, Cohen M, Cridennda D. Acupuncture and good prognosis IVF patients: synergy. *Fertil Steril* 2004;82:S80–S81.
7. Magarelli P, Cohen M, Cridennda, D. Acupuncture: impact on pregnancy outcomes in IVF patients. *12th World Congress on Human Reproduction*, Venice, Italy, March 2005.
8. Magarelli P, Cohen M, Cridennda D. Improvement of IVF outcomes by acupuncture: are egg and embryo qualities involved? *Fertil Steril* 2005;83:S9.
9. Cridennda D, Magarelli P, Cohen M. Acupuncture and in vitro fertilization: does the number of treatments impact reproductive outcomes? *Society for Acupuncture Research*, 2005.
10. Magarelli P, Cridennda D, Cohen M. Proposed mechanism of action of acupuncture on IVF outcomes. *Fertil Steril* 2006;86: S174–S175.
11. Magarelli P, Cridennda D, Cohen M. The Demographics of Acupuncture's Impact on IVF Outcomes: Infertility Diagnosis and SART/CDC /age Groups. *Fertil Steril* 2007;87:S10–S11.
12. Steptoe PC, Edwards RG. Birth after the reimplantation of a human embryo. *Lancet* 1978;2:366.
13. Horsey K. Progress Educational Trust 2006.3,000,000 IVF Babies Born Worldwide Since 1979. Presented at the annual conference of the European Society of Human Reproduction and Embryology (ESHRE) 2006.
14. Speroff L, Fritz M. *Clinical Gynecologic Endocrinology and Infertility*. 7th Edition. Lippincott Williams & Wilkins, 1013–1020.
15. Arslan M, Bocca S, Mirkin S, Barrososo G, Stadtmauer L, Oehninger S., Controlled ovarian hyperstimulation protocols for in vitro fertilization: two decades of experience after the birth of Elizabeth Carr. *Fertil Steril* 2005;84:555–569.
16. Paulus WE, Zhang M, Strehler E, Sterzik K. Motility of the endometrium after acupuncture treatment. *Fertil Steril* 2003; 80:S131.
17. Osaki T, Takahashi K, Kurioka H, Miyaki K. Influence of midluteal serum prolactin on outcome of pregnancy after IVF-ET: A preliminary study. *CAT.INIST.FR. Kuwer/Plenum publisher NY* 1992.
18. Keay SD, Harlow CR, Wood PJ, Jenkins JM, Cahill DJ. Higher cortisol:cortisone ratios in the preovulatory follicle of completely

unstimulated IVF cycles indicate oocytes with increased pregnancy potential. *Hum Reprod* 2002;17(9):2410–2414.
19. Westergaard LG, Mao Q, Krogslund M, Sandrini S, Lenz S, Grinsted J. Acupuncture on the day of embryo transfer significantly improves the reproductive outcome in infertile women: a prospective, randomized, trial. *Fertil Steril* 2006;85:1341–1346.
20. Smith C, Coyle M, Norman RJ. Influence of acupuncture stimulation on pregnancy rates for women undergoing embryo transfer. *Fertil Steril* 2006;85:1352–1358.
21. Dieterle S, Ying G, Hatzmann W, Neuer A. Effect of acupuncture on the outcome of in vitro fertilization and intracytoplasmic sperm injection: a randomized, prospective, controlled clinical study. *Fertil Steril* 2006;85:1347–1351.
22. Quintero R. A randomized, controlled, double-blind, cross-over study evaluating acupuncture as an adjunct to IVF. *Fertil Steril* 2004;81:S11–S12.
23. Chang R, Chung PH, Rosenwaks Z. Role of acupuncture in the treatment of female infertility. *Fertil Steril* 2002;78:1149–1153.
24. Tekay A, Martikainen H, Jouppila P. Blood flow changes in uterine and ovarian vasculature, and predictive value of transvaginal pulsed color Doppler ultrasonography in an in-vitro fertilization program. *Hum Reprod*, 1995;10:688–693.
25. Steer CV, Campbell S, Tan SL et al. Transvaginal colour flow imaging after in vitro fertilization to identify optimum uterine conditions before embryo transfer. *Fertil Steril* 1992;57: 372–376.
26. Paulus WE, Zhang M, Stehler E, Seybold B, Sterzik K. Placebo-controlled trial of acupuncture effects in assisted reproduction therapy.Letter to the Editor. *Fertil Steril* 2002;78: No. 4.
27. Streitberger K, Kleinhenz J. Introducing a placebo needle into acupuncture research. *Lancet* 1998;352:364–365.
28. Emmons SL, Patton P. Acupuncture treatment for infertile women undergoing intracytoplasmic sperm injection. Medical Acupuncture, A Journal For Physicians By Physicians Spring/ Summer 2000- Volume 12/Number 2.
29. Maciocia G. *Women's Pathology in Obstetrics and Gynecology in Chinese Medicine*. Churchill Livingstone, 1998; pp. 31–32.
30. Gallinelli A, Roncaglia R, Matteo M, Ciaccio I, Volpe A, Facchinetti F. Immunological changes and stress are associated with different implantation rates in patients undergoing in vitro fertilization-embryo transfer. *Fertil Steril* 2001;76:85–91.
31. Smeenk J, Verhaak C, Vingerhoets A, Sweep C, Merkus J, Willemsen S, van Minnen A, Straatman H, Braat D. Stress and outcome success in IVF: the role of self-reports and endocrine variables. *Hum Reprod* 2005;20(4):991–996.
32. Klonoff-Cohen H, Chu E, Natarajan L, Sieber W. A prospective study of stress among women undergoing in vitro fertilization or gamete intrafallopian transfer. *Fertil Steril* 2001;76:675–687.
33. Facchinetti M, Matteo M, Artini G, Volpe A, Genazzani A. An increased vulnerability to stress is associated with a poor outcome of in vitro fertilization-embryo transfer treatment. *Fertil Steril* 1997;67:309–314.
34. Stener-Victorin E, Wikland M, Waldenstrom U, Lundeberg T. Alternative treatments in reproductive medicine: much ado about nothing. Acupuncture – a method of treatment in reproductive medicine: lack of evidence of an effect does not equal evidence of the lack of effect. *Hum Reprod* 2002;17(8):1942–1946.
35. Dickey RP, Holtkamp D. Development, pharmacology and clinical experience with Clomiphene citrate. *Human Reprod Update* 1996;2(6):483–506.
36. Latov N. Evidence Based Guidelines: Not Recommended. *J Am Phys Surg* 2005; 10(1).

37. Meyers E. Acupuncture as adjunctive therapy in assisted repro-duction: *remaining uncertainties Fertil Steril* 2006;85:1362–1363.

38. Domar A. Acupuncture and infertility: we need to stick to good science. *Fertil Steril* 2006;85:1359–1361.

39. Collins J. The play of chance. *Fertil Steril* 2006;85:1364–1367.

40. Christensen BV et al. Acupuncture treatments of severe knee osteoarthritis; a long-term study. *Acta Anesthesiol Scandinavia* 1992;36:519–525.

41. Johansson K et al. Can sensory stimulation improve the func-tional outcome in stroke patients? *Neurology* 1994;43:2189–2192.

42. Gunn CC et al. Dry needling of muscle motor points for chronic low-back pain. *Spine* 1980;5:279–291.

43. Ballegaard et al. Acupuncture treatment results in avoidance of surgery, fewer hospital visits and greater return to employment. *Acupunct Electrother Res* 1996;21:187–197.

62

COMPLICATIONS OF ASSISTED
REPRODUCTIVE TECHNOLOGY

Gamal I. Serour

To date nearly two million babies were born as a result of ART which is widely used all over the world for virtually all forms of infertility. The world collaboration report on ART, for the year 2000, included 460,000 in vitro fertilization/intracytoplasmic sperm injection (IVF/ICSI) cycles from forty-nine countries and total number of babies conceived through ART was between 197,000 and 220,000 (1). It is estimated that the figures in the world IVF report represent only approximately two-thirds of ART cycles performed in the world. The European registers on ART for the year 2002 by ESHRE reported 324,238 treatment cycles, which represented 12 percent increase since year 2001. In thirteen countries where all clinics reported to the register, a total of 177,429 cycles were performed in a population of 193.7 million, corresponding to 916 cycles per million inhabitants. The percentage of infants born after ART ranged from 1.3 to 4.2 percent of the total number of live births in the country (2). The long-term health consequences of this widely used technique have yet to be determined. At every stage of the procedure there is a potential for complications, some of which are dangerous and may be life threatening. Considering the magnitude and the continuous increase in the number of ART cycles IVF, ICSI performed every year, complications of ART is a worldwide iatrogenic health problem. The ESHRE consensus meeting on risks and complications in ART in 2002 indicated that though ART is an efficacious treatment in subfertile couples, so far little attention had been paid to the safety of ART, that is, the adverse events and complications (3). Good clinical practice necessitates that reproductive medicine clinicians should pay great attention to prevention of these complications and establish the critical balance between efficacy and safety of ART (4).

INCIDENCE

The frequency of complications of ART varies among series and depending on whether the complications are reported in single treatment cycles or all treatment cycles. Bergh and Lunkvist surveyed twelve Scandinavian IVF clinics and received data on 10,125 cycles (5). The incidence of ovarian hyperstimulation syndrome (OHSS) and complications related to oocyte collection was 1.3 percent. Roest et al. reported an overall incidence of 2 percent for four major clinical complications in 2,495 transport IVF cycles, including severe and moderate OHSS, adnexal torsion, abdominal complications after oocyte collection, and ectopic pregnancy (6). Serour et al. in a series of 3,500 consecutive

IVF and ICSI cycles complications (including OHSS) occurred in 8.3 percent of cycles, with early pregnancy complications (including miscarriage) in 22.7 percent of pregnancies (7). Govaerts et al. reported a complication rate of 2.8 percent in 1,500 oocytee retrievals including OHSS in 1.8 percent, pelvic infections in 0.4 percent, intraperitoneal bleeding in 0.2 percent, and adnexal torsions in 0.13 percent, adnexal torsions during pregnancy in 0.18 percent and bowel endometriosis in 0.13 percent (8). The European register 2002 for ART reported 2,148 cases of OHSS in 224,327 cycles corresponding to a risk of 1.0 percent of all stimulated cycles. Other complications due to oocyte retrieval, bleeding, infection, and maternal death were reported in 1,156 (0.5 percent), 622 (0.25 percent), 227 (0.1 percent), and 2 (0.001 percent), respectively (2), which makes a total complication rate of 1.85 percent (2).

Klemetti et al. reported on complications of first treatment cycles and all treatment cycles (with an average of 3.3 cycles) in 9,175 IVF cycles in Finland. The complications rate per 1,000 women for one treatment cycle and all treatment cycles was 19 and 34.7 for OHSS, 1 and 2.4 for bleeding, 5.1 and 10.9 for infection, 41.9 and 93.1 for miscarriage, 9.3 and 20.9 for ectopic pregnancy, and 1.1 and 1.9 for other complications, respectively, which makes a total complication rate of 2.6 and 5 percent for first treatment and all treatment cycles, respectively. After all treatment cycles, 1,354 IVF (15 percent) women were hospitalized for complications. Of these hospital episodes, 10.5 percent of IVF women's episodes lasted for more than five days. Though there was a low risk of complications after each IVF treatment cycle, repeated attempts resulted in serious complications for many women (9) (Table 62.1).

Complications of ART are often underreported for various reasons. Centers in many parts of the world do not favor publishing their complication rates, particularly when there is a league table or a competing private market providing the service, which is often the case. Loss of follow-up of a large number of ART cycles and lack of recorded data are other important causes, which were clearly reflected in the 2000 IVF world report (1) and the ESHRE report (2). ART complications, particularly those related to OHSS are also underreported in reproductive medicine journals. A large number of these patients end up being admitted to the intensive care, general surgery, neurosurgery, vascular surgery, or pulmonary unit. A substantial number of publications on ART complications are published in medical journals of other specialties, and reproductive medicine physicians are often unaware of these publications.

Table 62.1: Incidence of Complication of ART

Author	Number of cycles	Overall incidence (%)
Berg and Lunckvist (4)	10,125	1.3
Roest et al. (6)	2,495	2
Serour et al. (6)	3,500	8.3
Govaerts et al. (8)	1,500	2.8
Klemetti et al. (7)	9,175	
First treatment cycle		2.6
All treatment cycle (average 3.3)		4.99
Anderson et al. (2)	224,327	1.85

In this chapter, the author considers each stage of ART and discusses its possible complications with options for prevention.

OVULATION INDUCTION

Ovarian Hyperstimulation Syndrome

The majority of ART cycles result in some degree of hyperstimulation. The iatrogenic condition of OHSS is the most important complication of ovulation induction and, in its severe form, is a potentially lethal disease (4,7,10). The prevalence of moderate-to-severe OHSS in the literature varies between 1 and 10 percent (4). Patients who are at risk of OHSS should be identified before scheduling them for ovarian hyperstimulation, during ovarian stimulation, and after oocyte pick up (OPU) (11).

Carcinoma

Ovarian Cancer

The first case report of invasive epithelial ovarian cancer following ovulation induction was by Bamford and Steele, in 1982 (12). Since then, cases have been published as case reports or as part of a review article or study (7,13,14). The implications of a possible link are important because ovarian cancer is the most frequent cause of death from gynecologic malignancy in the Western world, with a mortality in northwestern Europe and the United States of 7.3–13 per 100,000 women (15). Interpretation of studies to date has been fraught with difficulties of low numbers, retrospective incomplete data, a long lag time between treatment and disease as ovarian cancer is a relatively rare outcome and mostly occurs late in life, many years after normal childbearing age or infertility therapy, and the confounding effects of infertility and low parity on the incidence of ovarian cancer (4,16).

Three main hypotheses form the basis of the possible relation between ovarian stimulation and cancer. Fathalla's incessant ovulation hypothesis suggests that the cumulative effects of repetitive surface injury can lead to malignant transformation (17). Zajicek further proposed that epithelial inclusion cysts arising in association with ovulation on the surface of the ovary may initiate neoplastic change (18). The second hypothesis is that exogenous or endogenous gonadotropins or elevated level of E_2 act directly as carcinogens (19,20). The third hypothesis suggests that stimulation of production of chemical carcinogens by E_2 and gonadotropins within the local ovarian environment can lead to malignant transformation (21,22).

One of the first studies in this field was by Ron et al. in 1987, with a cohort of 2,632 women treated for infertility (23). No association was found between ovarian cancer and use of ovulation induction drugs in women with "hormonal" infertility, but a wide variety of drugs and regimens allowed no further conclusions. A Chinese study, in 1989, of 229 cases of ovarian cancer and population-based controls had similar flaws. It reported a nonsignificant association between the prior use of hormones to aid conception and the risk of developing ovarian cancer [relative risk (RR) = 2.1; 95 percent CI = 0.2–22.7] (24).

In 1992, Whittemore et al. and Harris et al. published the results from a combined analysis of twelve American case-control studies of ovarian cancer (25–27). In nulligravid women, there was an association between fertility drugs and invasive epithelial, borderline epithelial, and nonepithelial ovarian tumors (RR = 27.0; 95 percent CI = 2.3–315.6) caused much concern among clinicians and patients. However, the study has several weaknesses, including that only small numbers of women had used infertility drugs, lead-time bias may have allowed earlier diagnosis in infertile women, the cause of infertility was poorly reported, the duration and type of medication was not specified, criteria for diagnosis and tumor staging were poorly defined, and women with cancer may show recall bias. A causal link between fertility medications and ovarian cancer could not be confirmed.

A case-cohort study in 1994 by Rossing et al. of 3,837 infertile women used as cases and controls showed an increased risk of invasive and borderline ovarian tumors in nulligravid and gravid women after more than twelve months use of clomiphene citrate (CC) (RR = 11.1; 95 percent CI = 1.5–82.3) (28). This study has several strengths, including the use of an infertile cohort for cases and controls and data obtained from chart review before the diagnosis of cancer. However, a study in 1996 by Shushan et al. of 200 women with ovarian cancer failed to confirm this association, although a link was suggested between use of human menopausal gonadotropin (hMG) and borderline tumors (29). Another report by Venn et al. from Australia in 1995 looked at a cohort of 5,564 women exposed to ovarian stimulation for IVF and 4,794 referred for IVF but not receiving ovulation induction (30). Although there was no significantly increased risk of ovarian cancer with ovulation induction, low numbers of cases and variable follow-up (one to fifteen years) make firm conclusions difficult.

An Italian case-control study of 971 women with ovarian cancer published in 1997 by Parazzini et al. was reassuring in the absence of a strong association between fertility drugs and a subsequent risk of ovarian cancer (31). The authors admit the report's limitations in terms of statistical power and available information [only five cases (0.5 percent) reported use of fertility drugs]. A Danish study in 1997 by Mosgaard et al. with 684 cases and 1,721 age-matched population controls also found no association with infertility drugs in parous or nulliparous women, although the previously documented increased risk of ovarian cancer in nulliparous women or those with infertility (without medical treatment) was confirmed (32).

In a large-scale cohort study in the Netherlands, after a follow-up period of five to eight years, no increased risk of ovarian cancer was found in women who had undergone IVF as compared with subfertile women who had received no IVF (33). Klemetti et al. after an average follow-up period of 3.7 years reported no increase in the incidence of ovarian cancer in 9,175 IVF cycles compared with control (9).

Klip et al. identified papers published between 1966 and 1999 that examined fertility drugs (FDs) and specific causes of subfertility in relation to the risk of cancer of ovary, breast, endometrium, and thyroid and melanoma (33).

They reported that while positive findings in some studies on FDs and ovarian cancer risk have aroused serious concern, the associations observed in most of these reports appear to be due to bias or chance rather than being causal. The most important sources of bias are inadequate confounder control for both parity and causes of subfertility (33).

Mahdavi et al. recently critically reviewed the evidence in the medical literature, relating the effects of fertility drug use to ovarian risk (34). The studies that have adjusted for the effects of confounding factors such as duration of oral contraceptive use and number of pregnancies have noted an increased risk of ovarian cancer among infertile women who remain childless despite long periods of unprotected intercourse. Whether such women are at risk due to the primary basis for their infertility or factors such as ovulation-inducing drugs has been the basis of several studies. Overall, the findings on ovarian cancer (especially, invasive epithelial and nonepithelial) risk associated with fertility drug treatment are reassuring. However, a stronger association between FD use and borderline tumors of the ovary has been observed (34). They concluded that despite reassuring findings of the available studies, there is a strong need for well-designed clinical trials to understand the possible carcinogenic effects of ovulation-inducing drugs.

Until then, there is a need for careful clinical evaluation with ultrasound and a high index of suspicion in these high-risk patients. Women with infertility must be counseled and informed about the risks of treatment. The use of the lowest effective dose of ovulation stimulants, with close monitoring, is recommended.

Breast Cancer

One case of breast duct carcinoma was described by Serour et al. among 2,924 patients undergoing 3,500 cycles of ovarian stimulation (7). Klemetti et al. reported one case of breast cancer in 9,175 IVF cycles and three cases in the control group who did not receive ovulation induction after an average period of follow-up of 3.7 years (9). Klip et al. in a large-scale cohort study in the Netherlands, after a follow-up period of five to eight years, found no increased risk of breast cancer in women who had undergone IVF as compared with subfertile women who had received no IVF (33). Braga et al. reported no relation between fertility treatment and breast cancer risk in a multicenter case-control study in Italy in 2,569 women with breast cancer. However, they could not exclude completely the possibility that the use of specific drugs may be related to breast carcinogenesis (35).

Venn et al. examined the risk of breast cancer in 5,564 women having ovarian stimulation and 4,794 with no stimulation after referral for IVF (30). They observed a total of thirty-four cases of breast cancer and concluded that there was no increased risk of breast cancer in the treated women (RR = 1.11; 95 percent CI = 0.56–2.20), within the limits of the study.

In another cohort study of 29,700 women by Venn et al., 20,656 were exposed to fertility drugs and 9,044 were not. They found 143 breast cancers, 13 ovarian cancers, and 12 cancers of the uterus among these women. For breast and ovarian cancer, the incidence was no greater than expected standardized incidence ratio (SIR) 0.91 (95 percent C1 0.74–1.13) for breast cancer and 0.88 (0.42–1.84) for ovarian cancer in the exposed group and 0.95 (0.73–1.23) for breast cancer and 1.16 (0.52–2.59) for ovarian cancer in the unexposed group (36). They concluded that women who have been exposed to FD with IVF seem to have a transient increase in the risk of having breast cancer diagnosed in the first year after treatment, though the incidence overall is no greater than expected.

In a retrospective cohort study of 12,193 women evaluated for infertility between 1965 and 1988 at five clinical sites, Brinton et al. identified 292 in situ and invasive breast cancers in follow-up through 1999. SIR compared breast cancer risks with those of the general population. They found that infertile patients had a significantly higher breast cancer risk than the general population (SIR = 1.29; 95 percent CI 1.1–1.4). Analysis within the cohort showed adjusted RRs of 1.02 for clomiphene citrate and 1.07 for gonadotropins and no substantial relationships to dosage or cycles of use. Slight and nonsignificant elevations in risk were seen for both drugs after more than twenty years of follow-up. The risk associated with clomiphene for invasive breast cancers was statistically significant (37).

In conclusion, although there is no overall increase in breast cancer risk associated with use of ovulation stimulating drugs, long-term effects should continue to be monitored.

Other Malignancies

Johannes et al. raised the possibility that ovulation induction increases the risk of other hormonally sensitive tumors. They suggested that cancer of thyroid gland, endometrium, and melanoma should be considered as possible adverse outcomes of ovulation induction therapy (38). One case of choriocarcinoma of the fallopian tube (39), and one case of uterine and ovarian carcinoma (12) were also reported.

In a large-scale cohort study in the Netherlands, after a follow-up of five to eight years, an increased risk was observed for endometrial cancer in those exposed to IVF as well as in the unexposed group, suggesting a subfertility-related effect that needs further evaluation (33).

Other Complications of Ovarian Stimulation

There are few case reports in the literature of adverse reactions to hMG injection (40–42). A local urticarial reaction measuring 10×20 cm developing twenty-four hours, anaphylactic episodes in a woman with a history of atopy and delayed hypersensitivity to hMG were described.

Clomiphene citrate has been used for many years for ovulation induction and has several potential side effects, including hot flushes, abdominal discomfort, nausea, vomiting, depression, insomnia, breast tenderness, headache, intermenstrual spotting, menorrhagia, endometriosis, convulsions, weight gain, rashes, dizziness, and hair loss. Visual disturbances can occur and warrant withdrawal of the drug and initiation of an ophthalmological examination, as optic neuropathy has been reported (43).

Other unusual side effects of ovulation induction include bloody ascites in a woman with endometriosis and familial Mediterranean fever, pituitary hemorrhage after clomiphene citrate, and hypophyseal hypertrophy in pregnancy after bromocriptine treatment for prolactinoma. Acute intermittent porphyria was also reported following clomiphene citrate administration (44).

COMPLICATIONS OF OPU

The first report of IVF used a laparoscopic approach for the collection of oocytes (45). This has now been superseded by ultrasound-guided follicle aspiration. Several techniques of ultrasound-guided oocyte retrieval have been used, including transvaginal, transurethral, and percutaneous abdominal techniques. The transvaginal route became the preferred method, with its good yield of oocytes, decreased operating time, visualization of follicles without the need for a full bladder, and the possible avoidance of general anesthesia.

Transvaginal ultrasound-guided follicle aspiration (TVUGFA) was first described in the mid-1980s (46,47). Three main groups of complications can occur: hemorrhage, pelvic infection, and damage to pelvic structures such as the bowel or ureters.

Bleeding

Serour et al. reported vaginal bleeding in 0.09 percent of 3,500 oocyte retrievals (7). Anderson et al. reported an incidence of 0.25 percent in 224,327 cycles (2). In a prospective study of more than 1,000 cycles, Ludwig et al. reported vaginal bleeding from the puncture site in up to 2.8 percent of procedures (48). This is rarely a major problem, and there are no reports of bleeding heavy enough to warrant more than local pressure or oversewing (4,7,48). Intra-abdominal hemorrhage from the ovarian vessels, capsule puncture sites, or other pelvic vessels is a much more serious complication, with several reports of emergency laparotomy and transfusion being necessary life-saving procedures. The practice of visualizing a peripheral follicle in cross-section to differentiate it from a blood vessel is recommended as is the avoidance of overdistension of follicles during flushing and aspirating all follicles without withdrawing the needle tip from the ovary to avoid multiple punctures (7). If color Doppler is available, puncture of blood vessels can be avoided and this risk will be reduced to a great deal.

Infection

Several case reports have been published of patients with infective complications after TVUGFA, including pelvic abscess, ovarian abscess, or infected endometriotic cyst. The incidence of infection varies widely in different series between 0.1 and 3 percent, depending upon various factors including the technique of vaginal puncture, the presence or absence of pelvic infection or pelvic endometriosis, puncture of hydrosalpinx or bowel during the procedure, preoperative vaginal preparation by 10 percent povidone iodine or normal saline, and whether prophylactic antibiotics are used or not (12,4,7,49,50). There are four possible routes for pelvic infection after TVUGFA including reactivation of latent infection in patients with history of the disease, contamination after trauma to the bowel, direct inoculation of vaginal organisms, or puncture of a hydrosalpinx. In a prospective study of 1,058 oocyte retrievals, Ludwig et al. reported no case of pelvic infection but one case of unexplained fever was observed (48).

A uterine abscess after transcervical cryopreserved embryo transfer in a woman with previous pelvic infection was also reported (51).

Women with a history of pelvic infection should receive antibiotic prophylaxis before oocyte collection and possibly embryo transfer in cryopreserved cycles. While some authors recommended antibiotics for all vaginal oocyte collections (49), others feel the data do not support this practice (48). The use of cryopreservation and ET in a future cycle is suggested if signs of clinical infection occur before embryos are transferred.

Injury to Other Pelvic Structures

Patients also may present with acute abdominal symptoms necessitating laparotomy after ruptured endometriotic or dermoid cysts (52). A case of acute appendicitis with puncture holes in the appendix has been reported (6).

Trauma to the ureter has been described. A case of hydronephrosis, infection, and eventual nephrectomy after multiple oocyte collections, both laparoscopically and transvaginally, was reported (53). Patients with previous pelvic surgery and distorted pelvic anatomy developed a hematoma after transvaginal oocyte collection that obstructed the ureter, necessitating insertion of a stent (48,54). A ureteral lesion with secondary ureterovaginal fistula after oocyte collection was described by Coroleu et al. (55). Ureteral injury resulting in acute ureteral obstruction was also reported after TVUGFA in patients with normal pelvic anatomy (56).

Postoperative Pain

Although most patients tolerate OPU well, a prospective Cohort study of 1,058 OPU reported severe to very severe pain after OPU in 3 percent of patients and 2 percent of patients were still suffering from severe pain two days after the procedure. The pain level increased with the number of oocytes retrieved. About 0.7 percent of patients required hospitalization for pain treatment (48).

Other Rare Complications of OPU

Wong et al. reported rectus sheath hematoma after TVUGFA (57). Ayestran et al. (58) and Serour et al. (7) reported severe bradycardia and bradypnea following TVUGA due to a possible toxic effect of paracervical mepivacaine or deep abdominal pressure on enlarged ovaries, respectively. Azem et al. reported a massive retroperitoneal bleeding from the sacral vein requiring emergency laparotomy (59). Cho et al. reported vaginal perforation during TVUGFA in older patients with a history of repeated TVUGFA, particularly when the ovaries are difficult to visualize (60).

Almog et al. reported vertebral osteomyelitis, which resulted in severe low back pain, which was successfully treated with antibiotics (61). Wehner Caroli et al. reported anaphylactic reaction to bovine serum albumin after embryo transfer. The risk can be reduced substantially if a detailed medical history is obtained (62).

ART PREGNANCY COMPLICATIONS

Miscarriage

It has been widely reported that the incidence of miscarriage in pregnancies resulting from ART is higher than in spontaneous pregnancies (4). Serour et al., in a study of 702 ART pregnancies, reported a miscarriage rate of 20.6 percent (7).

Klemetti et al. (9) in a study of 9,175 IVF cycles found that more than 9 percent of the pregnant women received hospital care due to miscarriage. The number of miscarriages per 100 IVF births was 23, which suggests similar miscarriage rates found (15–23 percent) by several authors (7,63–65).

In one study from United States, the miscarriage rate was similar (15 percent) among ART women and the rest of the female population (64). However, in another study from United States, the risk of miscarriage slightly increased after ART (65). Whether this is a direct result of the procedure or simply reflects the population concerned presents some difficulties due to different definitions of miscarriage, use of highly sensitive assays for β-hCG, the close monitoring of women receiving ART treatment, and the knowledge that the embryos were transferred on a particular day. All these factors can give a false higher rate of miscarriage when compared to the general population. In contrast, the fertilization of postmature ova following long periods of anovulation, the luteal phase defect after hMG ovulation induction, and the possible adverse effects of handling the oocytes are some of the potential factors leading to an increased miscarriage risk in ART pregnancies (4).

Ectopic Pregnancy

The first pregnancy in an IVF program was an ectopic pregnancy (EP) (45). Since then, the rate of EP after ART has been quoted as between 2 and 11 percent (66,67). Figures from large studies tend to be at the lower end of the range. Serour et al. reported a rate of 1.9 percent in 702 ART pregnancies, (7) and Roest et al. found 2.1 percent of pregnancies to be EPs (6). In a recent Finish Study of 9,175 ART cycles, the rate of EPs per 100 IVF births was 5 percent, which is twice that of earlier studies in Finland (9). The frequency per initiated IVF cycle (0.8 percent) is also somewhat higher than in earlier studies of IVF treatments (5,7,66).

The association between EP and ovulation induction drugs is unclear. Although some earlier studies suggested a link, this conclusion was later contested. However, there is no doubt that the most significant risk factor for EP in patients undergoing ART is tubal pathology. This was illustrated by Dubuisson et al. (67), in a study of 556 pregnancies resulting from ART, who found an EP rate of 11.1 percent in patients with tubal factor, decreasing to 2.1 percent for women with endometriosis and 3.4 percent in unexplained infertility cases. Pathological examination of the specimens from all three groups showed preexisting tubal lesions. The type of stimulation protocol, E_2 level, number of embryos transferred, and type of luteal phase support did not significantly affect the EP rate. Asung et al. (68) analyzed total of 97,240 women who underwent 156,454 cycles resulting in 31,666 pregnancies of which 765 (2.4 percent) were ectopic. EP incidence was higher following IVF (2.8 percent) than ICSI (1.3 percent) $P < 0.001$. Within the IVF group, EP incidence was inversely correlated with maternal age. For those with tubal disease aged less than 25, 25–29, 30–34, 35–39, and more than 40 years, it was 6.1, 4.1, 3.9, 3.0, and 2 percent, respectively; a significant trend ($P < 0.004$). There was a small but significantly higher incidence when three embryos (2.6 percent) were transferred compared with two embryos (2.2 percent) $P < 0.036$. The indication for treatment appeared to be a risk factor: tubal disease (3.8 percent), endometriosis (2.3 percent), other or unexplained female factors (1.8 percent), and male factor (1.2 percent). Rebic-Pucelj et al. (69), in a study of 1,059 pregnancies, reported that forty-two of forty-four EPs were in patients with tubal factor infertility. They also found that type of ovarian stimulation, knee-chest, or lithotomy position at ET and the number of embryos transferred were not significant factors. Because of the importance of tubal disease in the etiology of EP, prophylactic salpingectomy before IVF has been suggested, but this would treat more than 89 percent of patients while removing any chance of normal spontaneous pregnancy and would not prevent interstitial pregnancies (69). Agarwal et al. reported that of twenty-six ectopic pregnancies after ET over seven years, seven were located in the cornual or tubal stump after prior salpingectomy (70). Arbab et al. described five cases of uterine rupture after cornual pregnancy following IVF in women with a history of salpingectomy (71). Two women needed a hysterectomy in this series, emphasizing the need for vigilance and a high index of suspicion for this serious complication.

EP also may occur in other unusual sites following ART. Reports include simultaneous bilateral tubal pregnancy, bilateral simultaneous interstitial sextuplets after salpingectomy, intramural, ovarian, and abdominal pregnancies. Cervical pregnancy has been reported, with a possible increased risk in ART pregnancies associated with reflux of embryos into the cervix after transfer or trauma to the cervix during ET. This risk is difficult to quantify with low numbers of cases, but early diagnosis is particularly important in cervical pregnancy, with the risk of severe hemorrhage increasing with advancing gestational age (4).

The early detection of EP can allow minimal access surgery or other treatment modalities. Highly sensitive β-hCG assay and vaginal ultrasound have had a great impact in this field (4). The usual algorithms may not apply in ART cases because more than one embryo usually is transferred, affecting the β-hCG level. Marcus et al. found that three β-hCG levels and a day 13 progesterone measurement combined with a history of pelvic inflammatory disease achieved a predictive value of up to 90 percent for EP after ART (72). Mol et al. suggested that a single β-hCG measurement nine days after ET of over 18 IU/L can be used as a cutoff value, justifying expectant management (in an asymptomatic patient) because the probability of EP is only 1 percent in these women (73).

Heterotopic Pregnancy

Coexistent intrauterine and ectopic gestation, or heterotopic pregnancy, is more common after ART. The reported incidence in spontaneous pregnancies varies from 1 in 2,600 to 1 in 30,000 pregnancies (74,75). The rate following ART is quoted in a review of 139 case reports as approximately 1 to 100 pregnancies (76). Other authors of more recent reviews on this subject reported an incidence of 0.1–0.3 percent heterotopic pregnancy (6,7,63,66,77). The increased risk of heterotopic pregnancy is the result of multiple ovulations and multiple ET in a population with tubal or pelvic disease. Transfer of four or more embryos gives an odds ratio of 10.0 for heterotopic pregnancy versus EP (78). Half of the cases studied by Tal et al. had one or more previous EPs, and 45 percent of women had previous pelvic surgery (76). The technique of ET, including the volume and viscosity of medium, deep or superficial insertion of the catheter, and the degree of difficulty of the procedure also has been proposed as an etiologic factor for heterotopic pregnancy, but the data at the present time are not adequate to draw firm conclusions.

Delayed diagnosis with rupture, hemorrhage, and emergency intervention was recorded, emphasizing the importance of prompt surgical treatment. However, there is a trend for earlier diagnosis, using ultrasonography, allowing the use of newer techniques, by laparoscopic removal, transvaginal ultrasonographically guided instillation of hyperosmolar glucose into the ectopic gestational sac of a heterotopic pregnancy, or potassium chloride injection with aspiration of the tubal sac (69,70).

Molar Pregnancy

Assessment of any potential increased risk of molar pregnancy associated with ART is difficult. Theoretically, the use of immature ova after ovulation induction or disruption of meiosis and loss of maternal chromosomes as a result of oocyte handling or degeneration could increase the risk of complete mole. Alternatively, postmature oocytes are more prone to polyspermy with resultant heterozygous complete or partial molar pregnancy. Few cases of recurrent molar pregnancies and choriocarcinoma were reported in the literature (4).

Further assessment of this complication is impossible without the collation of data from many centers. The use of modern molecular biology techniques, preimplantation diagnosis, and ICSI will provide further insights into this disease, with possible strategies for prevention in women with recurrent molar pregnancies.

Multiple Pregnancy

In natural conception, one in eighty pregnancies results in twins. However, in ART, rate of multiple pregnancy is more than one in five, even in countries where the number of embryos transferred is limited to three embryos. Serour et al., in a study of 702 pregnancies resulting from 3,500 IVF/ICSI cycles, reported a multiple pregnancy rate of 27.9 percent, with twins, triplets, and quadruplets being 19.8, 6, and 2.1 percent, respectively (7). The seventh world collaborative report on IVF, 2000, from forty-nine countries and six regions on 460,157 procedures reported a twin rates of 26.9 and 26.2 percent for conventional IVF and ICSI respectively, and triplet rates were 2.8 and 2.9 percent, respectively, for an estimated total of approximately 197,000–220,000 babies worldwide (1).

In ESHRE report 2006 on results of 324,238 treatment cycles of IVF/ICSI, the distribution of singleton, twin, and triplet deliveries for IVF and ICSI cycles combined was 75.5, 23.2, and 1.3 percent, respectively. A total multiple delivery rate was 24.5 percent compared with 25.5 percent in the year 2001 (2).

The overall contribution of ART to the multiple pregnancy rate in the population was assessed by several workers. Between 1972 and 1974 (before ART) and 1990 and 1991 (after ART), the rate of triplet and higher order multiple gestation infants per 100,000 white live births increased by 191 percent, with 38 percent attributable to ART and 30 percent to increased childbearing among older women (81). These authors suggested that

ovulation stimulation drugs may be responsible for the remaining third of this increase.

Multiple pregnancy appeals to many infertile couples undergoing ART who have unsuccessfully tried for long time to have a child as well as to some reproductive medicine physicians. In this regards, many would forget that, unlike other mammals, the human womb is designed to carry babies singly. It does less efficiently with multiples. While the majority, but not all, of twin pregnancies produce healthy children, this is less likely with higher order multiple pregnancies (HOMP) (7,82–84).

Multifetal pregnancies, and most notably triplet and HOMP, are associated with a significantly increased risk of adverse clinical outcomes, primarily owing to prematurity and its short-term and long-term sequelae. Neonatal mortality is four times as great among twins as it is among singletons, and twins are at increased risk for long-term disability, including cerebral palsy (85).

The stress associated with rearing children resulting from multiple pregnancies and HOMP and the greatly increased cost of prenatal and neonatal intensive care are also crucial health service issues (86).

The unacceptability of high rate of infertility treatment–related multiple pregnancies has been identified as the biggest threat to the future safety and success of ART (84,87). World Health Organization recognized multiple pregnancies as a major complication of ART treatment (88). The challenge for ART clinics is to reduce the risk of twins, triplets, and HOMP without jeopardizing the success rates. A balance between our ability to establish successful ART programs and pregnancy rate on one side and its safety on the other side had to be found. However, safety should come first. ART success rate should be measured as a singleton live birth rate and not as a pregnancy rate.

In most European countries, elective transfer of two embryos has substantially reduced triplets and HOMP but has had no impact on twin pregnancies (2). The only certain method of eliminating iatrogenic twin multiple pregnancies in ART is to transfer a single embryo in women who are at significant risk of multiple gestation. This includes women who are relatively young, who are in their first or second IVF cycles, and who have a number of good-quality embryos (87,89,90).

A meta-analysis of single embryo transfer versus double embryo transfer had shown that elective single embryo transfer significantly reduces the risk of multiple pregnancy but also reduces the chances of live birth in a fresh IVF cycle (91).

The data available today suggest that by using strict embryo selection criteria in specific groups of women, single embryo transfer can achieve an acceptable pregnancy rate of 30–40 percent per fresh treatment cycle and twin pregnancy virtually eliminated (92,93). The outcome is further enhanced by repeated transfer of thawed cryopreserved spare embryos, which can lead to a cumulative pregnancy rate comparable to that achieved by double embryo transfer, 47–53 percent (94). In women younger than thirty-six years, transferring one fresh embryo and then, if needed, one frozen-and-thawed embryo dramatically reduces the rate of multiple births while achieving a rate of live births that is not substantially lower than the rate that is achievable with a double embryo transfer (95). However, the trials performed so far have been small and the conclusions are not robust enough to catalyze a widely acceptable change in clinical practice. It is not surprising that the ESHRE report of ART 2002 indicated that of 203,877 embryo transfers performed only 13.7 percent were single, 54.8 percent double, 26.9

percent triple, and 4.7 percent transfers were 4+ embryos (2). We still need definitive trials comparing single embryo transfer versus double embryo transfer concerning clinical outcome, maternal and perinatal complications, cost-effectiveness, as well as acceptability.

Recent evidence suggests that singleton pregnancies from ART have significantly higher risks of very low birth weight and very preterm birth as compared with naturally conceived controls. Confounding factors such as maternal age and parity do not change this outcome (96). Factors such as social economic status, sex of the fetus, and delivery date and site also seem unable to explain the difference (96,97). A history of subfertility, irrespective of infertility treatment, has also been found to be associated with increased perinatal death in a case-control study (98).

Using data from a Dutch population–based historical cohort of women treated for subfertility comparing the perinatal outcome of singletons conceived after controlled ovarian hyperstimulation and IVF (IVF + COHS, $n = 2,239$) with perinatal outcome in subfertile women who conceived spontaneously (subfertile controls, $n = 6,343$) and in women who only received COHS (COHS only, $n = 84$), the poor perinatal outcome of IVF singletons could not be explained by subfertility and suggests that other factors may be important (99).

In ART, singleton pregnancies resulting from transfer of more than one embryo, crowdedness of embryos, and multiple suboptimal placentation may be responsible for this deleterious effect. Even in ART, pregnancies that progress as singleton abnormalities established early during placentation may adversely affect the outcome (100).

More recently, it had been shown that good-prognosis patients in whom single embryo transfer is applied do not only have a higher chance of conception but also do not have unfavorable outcome of their singleton baby when compared to spontaneous singletons (101).

Reducing the number of embryos transferred is often resisted by the patients and their reproductive medicine physicians alike. This is mostly based on the previously published data showing a lower pregnancy rate with the decrease in the number of embryos transferred (102). In these early studies, the embryos transferred were the only available embryos for those patients who are often poor-prognosis patients (103).

The essence when applying single embryo transfer is to be able to actively select or elect the right embryo in the right patient and in the right cycle. Various methods are available for embryo screening as aneuploidy screening, DNA finger printing, noninvasive technology as amino acid consumption of embryos, morphological selection, human leukocyte antigen-G (HLA-G) assessment, embryo cleavage rate, and the number of mononucleate blastomeres at six to eight cells' stage embryo. Clinicians need to individualize protocols for couples, based on their risk of MP (104).

With the published data on the results of multifetal pregnancy reduction (MFPR), some reproductive medicine physicians believe that it provides a satisfactory solution to the problem of MP and HOMP. MFPR does not address the problem of twins. MFPR for HOMP is surrounded with ethical dilemma and involves psychological trauma to the couple. It should never be considered as a standard line of management for prevention of MP and HOMP. It is only a rescue line of management if other methods fail in the prevention of MP and HOMP (104,105).

Tackling the problem of MP and HOMP should extend beyond providing medical solutions to the problem. Studies had shown that in some clinics, about 10 percent of couples seeking fertility treatments ask their clinics to help them to have twins, rather than have one baby at a time. Various reasons are given for this request including an instant family with just one pregnancy, minimizing disruption of women's career, twins are good because women would get their whole family out of the way, and women are too old to have a second pregnancy at a later date (104). In China, use of fertility drugs to beat china's one-child law is expanding. The number of twins born last year had doubled in a number of hospitals across China. Health education of couples and the society at large on the hazards of MP and HOMP to change the society's attitude toward MP is essential. Also the reproductive medicine physicians and practitioners should be convinced that MP and HOMP and its obstetrical, neonatal, developmental, and financial consequences represent the main iatrogenic complication of infertility treatment, and every measure should be taken for its prevention (104,105). A move in our emphasis from pregnancy rate per cycle in ART program to cumulative live birth per patient, as a measure of performance, will help to challenge current practices. Single embryo transfer should be introduced carefully and progressively in each ART program after careful tuning of both embryo and patient's characteristics relating to a high risk of MP. The combination of single embryo transfer with an optimized cryopreservation program should become the standard of care for routine IVF/ICSI treatment.

Reproductive medicine physicians should help their patients to minimize the potential for conflict. Policymakers should be informed about the consequences of MP particularly cost and the potential cost-effectiveness of infertility treatment aiming at singleton pregnancy.

MATERNAL AND FETAL COMPLICATIONS

Obstetric Complications

The incidence of first-trimester bleeding is high in ART pregnancies, varying between 29 and 36.2 percent (106–109). It has been shown that first-trimester bleeding is correlated with an increased risk for miscarriage both in spontaneous pregnancy (50 percent) (110) and in ART pregnancies (25–44 percent) (106–109). Sutter et al. analyzed data from their ART database (1993–2006) with 1,432 singleton ongoing pregnancies included in the study. Significantly, more singleton pregnancies resulted from a vanishing twin in the group with first-trimester bleeding (8.7 percent) than in the controls (4 percent) (111). A correlation was found between the incidence of first-trimester bleeding and the number of embryos transferred. First-trimester bleeding led to increased second-trimester (OR = 4.56, C1 2.76–7.56) and third-trimester bleeding rates (OR = 2.85, C1 = 1.42–5.73), PROM (OR = 2.44, C1 = 1.38–4.31), preterm contractions (OR 2.27, C1 1.48–3.47), and NICU admissions. It also increased the risk for preterm birth and extreme preterm birth.

In a case-control study, Tallo et al. reported IVF mothers had more pregnancy-induced hypertension compared with non-IVF control subjects (21 vs. 4 percent) (112). In a nation-wide population-based study of 845,384 pregnancies reported to the Medical Birth Registry of Norway between 1988 and 2002, the risk of placenta previa in 7,568 pregnancies conceived after ART was found to be sixfold higher in singleton pregnancies conceived by ART compared with naturally conceived pregnancies (adjusted OR 5.6, 95 percent CI 4.4–7.0). Among mothers who had conceived both naturally and after ART, the risk of placenta previa was nearly threefold higher in the pregnancy following ART (adjusted OR 2.9, 95 percent CI 1.4–6.1), compared with that in the naturally conceived pregnancy (113).

In a study of 702 pregnancies resulting from IVF/ICSI cycles, Serour et al. reported pregnancy-induced hypertension, preterm labor, low birth weight, and intrauterine death in 10, 21.5, 30.5, and 2 percent, respectively (7). Women with pregnancies conceived after ART are generally older and more often primiparous. They also are more likely to have a multiple pregnancy. These recognized risk factors play a large part in the increased incidence of obstetric complications seen in ART pregnancies (7,114–116). Higher levels of anxiety in both parents and clinicians in these precious pregnancies lead to a lower threshold for intervention. However, the question remains whether the ART process itself results in an increased risk of obstetric problems. Several case-control studies comparing ART-related and spontaneous singleton pregnancies have been conducted, some with analysis of outcomes controlling for maternal variables, such as age and parity (117–120). Findings include increased rate of pregnancy-induced hypertension, gestational diabetes, placenta previa, and cesarean section in ART pregnancies, although Reubinoff et al. only found increased risk of cesarean delivery in their population (119). The equivalent adverse outcomes in both IVF and ovulation induction patients suggest that a factor other than the IVF method is responsible for the increased risk (117). Further studies are necessary to assess the importance of specific infertility causes or treatments as predisposing factors for obstetric complications.

Perinatal Complications

The periantal outcomes of ART pregnancies are recorded in several studies, some of which are based on national data (7,121,125). The percentage of preterm infants varies from 21.5 to 37 percent of births overall (5.3–13.0 percent for singletons). Low birth weight (<2,500 g) is reported in 30.6–37.5 percent of all births (7.7–11.0 percent of singletons). The rates of stillbirth, perinatal mortality, and infant mortality are generally higher than the national averages in national registry series (121–125). Case-control studies that account for confounding variables do not always confirm this (126,127). Most of the impact of infertility treatment on neonatal morbidity seems to be mediated by multiplicity and prematurity (127).

In a national cohort study of twin and singleton births occurring in Denmark, Pinborg et al. found no major differences in physical health between IVF/ICSI twins and non–IVF/ICSI twins. Compared with IVF/ICSI singletons, more IVF/ICSI twins were admitted to NICU ($P < 0.01$) and more had surgical interventions ($P = 0.03$) and special needs ($P = 0.02$); moreover, they had poorer speech development ($P < 0.01$). All discrepancies between IVF/ICSI twins and singletons disappeared after stratification for birth weight except for NICU admissions and speech development (128).

In a Danish national cohort study of 3,438 IVF/ICSI and 10,362 non–IVF/ICSI twins born between 1995 and 2000, Pinborg et al. reported no differences in malformation or mortality rates between the two cohorts (129). Despite higher birth weight discordance and more NICU admissions among IVF/

ICSI twins, neonatal outcome in IVF/ICSI twins seem to be comparable with that of non–IVF/ICSI twins, when only dizygotic twins were considered in the comparison.

The growth and development of children born after in vitro maturation of oocytes was assessed at six, twelve, and twenty-four months by Soderstrom-Anttila et al. (130).

The prenatal outcome was good, and the mean birth weight of infants was normal. Major developmental delay was overexpressed at twelve months, but the development of the children was normal at two years (130).

Congenital Abnormality

Concern has been expressed about the health of children born after ART. Particularly, the risk of boys born to couples with male factor subfertility as in a substantial number of male factor cases, a genetic cause can be suspected. These include Y-chromosomal microdeletions, X-chromosomal and autosomal aberrations (i.e., Robertsonian translocations), syndromal disorders featuring infertility (i.e., Kallman's syndrome), and ultrastructural sperm defects with a genetic basis (Meschede et al. 2000) (131).

Some studies have reported an increase in the prevalence of neural tube defects, esophageal atresias, omphalocele, and hypospadias (after ICSI) among IVF children compared with spontaneously conceived controls (132,133). However, this increase in congenital malformation could be mainly explained by increased maternal age. Koivurova et al. in Finland in a large population-based study reported an excess of cardiac septal defects, but not of other congenital malformations, in the IVF children (134). While some follow-up studies of ART children have suggested that ART poses little risk to normal development and child health, other investigators have reported a twofold excess of major birth defects in ART children (135).

Infertile women are frequently of advanced age at the time of conception, and they may have a variety of causes for infertility. Furthermore, during the IVF procedure, the embryo is exposed to mechanical, thermal, and chemical alterations. Theoretically, these factors can increase the risk of congenital malformations.

The different percentages found in the published studies about major and minor congenital malformations cannot be compared for various reasons related to the design of these studies and the definition of major congenital malformation. Overall, the data in large and reliable surveys do not indicate a higher rate of malformation in ICSI children than in IVF or naturally conceived children (136,137). Also available data on ICSI fetal karyotypes revealed a slight increased risk of chromosomal anomalies, predominantly of the sex chromosomes, in comparison with a general neonatal population (138). With the increased use of ICSI for patients with azoospermia, in whom several workers had shown that their spermatozoa have an increased chromosomal aneuploidy rate (139–143), pregnancy outcome in these patients was studied by several workers (144–146). Ludwig et al. in 229 pregnancies in which testicular sperm was used found no additional risk of major malformations in children born after the use of testicular spermatozoa (145). The major malformation rate, up to eight weeks after birth, was 9 percent based on live-born and stillborn children and including spontaneous and induced abortions compared with 8.4 percent in ICSI with ejaculated spermatozoa. Bonduelle et al. (136) found no differences up to eight weeks after birth between ejaculated (3.4 percent n = 2,477) and testicular sperm (2.9 percent n = 206). Vernaeve et al. (146) found a major congenital malformation rate of 4 percent after the use of testicular sperm for nonobstructive azoospermia (NOA) patients and 3 percent after the use of testicular sperm for obstructive azoospermia (OA) patients (NS). Prenatal karyotypes showed 7 percent de novo abnormalities in the NOA group versus 1 percent in the OA group (NS).

Published series of small studies and case reports has suggested that births resulting from ART may have an increased risk of imprinting disorders such as Beckwith-Wiedemann syndrome, a disorder characterized by large tongue, organs, and body size, and Angelman syndrome (a neurological disorder once known as "happy puppet" because of the child's sunny outlook and jerky movements). However, the evidence is suggestive but not sufficient to conclude that ART is associated with malformations that occur with Angelman syndrome and Beckwith-Wiedemann syndrome (147). These congenital conditions sometimes occur due to errors in imprinting, a process by which certain genes from either the mother or father are normally switched off. Although such imprinting disorders may be shown to be only rare complications of ART, epigenetic errors might account for a much more wide spectrum of ART-related complications than is recognized currently (148).

Cryopreservation of embryos is used increasingly in ART, and several studies have assessed outcomes. Theoretically, there is concern that the important cellular changes in cryopreservation and thawing might have adverse effects. However, rates of minor congenital anomaly and major congenital malformation were normal in one study of children conceived from cryopreserved embryos, up to the age of four years (149), and no pathological features were found in a cohort of children aged one to nine years (150). A study of 270 infants by Wennerholm et al. concluded that the process did not adversely influence fetal development, and no increase in perinatal risk was observed (151). Vetrification, on ultrarapid cooling technique, offers a new perspective in attempts to develop an optimal cryopreservation procedure for human oocytes as well as embryos. A recent study of the outcome of vitrified oocytes reported fertilization rate, pregnancy rate, and implantation rate per embryo of 92.9, 32.5, and 13.2 percent, respectively, and babies born were healthy (152).

The use of frozen donor sperm was investigated in a study of 11,535 pregnancies, and no increase in nonchromosomal malformations or other adverse perinatal outcome was found (153). A slightly increased risk of trisomy 21 was recorded related to increased donor age, although further research is needed to clarify this.

PSYCHOLOGICAL COMPLICATIONS

Methodological and conceptual difficulties exist in researching this area including difficulty in matching controls, small sample sizes, debate on the validity of the various questionnaires used, and a tendency to positive self-reporting in couples undergoing ART (4). In retrospective studies, perception of the stress of treatment may be influenced by the impact of treatment failure. Generally, IVF participation is reported as very stressful with a negative impact on lifestyle and depression and diminished marital satisfaction after failure (154,155). A prospective study found significant increase in anxiety and depressive symptoms after a failed first cycle, with increased levels of mild and moderate depression, especially among women (156). A prospective longitudinal study of 144 couples found that at intake for IVF treatment, women were more anxious than their partners and comparative norms, but those who conceived were less depressed and more positive about their relationships (157).

IVF mothers are more anxious than matched controls about the survival and normality of their unborn babies, damage during birth, and postnatal separation. A study of forty-five couples during IVF treatment, pregnancy, and delivery reported the psychological burden of the treatment exceeded the physical burden, and pregnancy was more stressful than in controls with spontaneous conceptions (158). However, mothers experienced delivery, and fathers the pregnancy, as more exceptional than controls, and fathers enjoyed the pregnancy more than their control equivalents. The positive aspects of ART also were recorded by Boivin and Takefman, with higher levels of optimism (as well as more stress and changes to marital and social relationships) in women during a treatment cycle compared to a nontreatment cycle (159).

In a recent study by Colpin and Soenen, they reported that parenting and the children's psychological development do not differ significantly between IVF families and control families (160).

Pinborg et al. in a Danish National cohort study of 472 IVF/ICSI twins and 634 IVF/ICSI singletons reported the implications for families are stronger in IVF/ICSI twins compared with IVF/ICSI singletons (128).

Both IVF/ICSI and non–IVF/ICSI twin parents experienced more marital stress (OR 2.9, 95 percent CI 2.2–3.8) and twins had more impact on the mother's life (OR 1.7, 95 percent CI 1.2–2.4) compared with singleton (128).

The impact of HOMP has been reported by Garel and Blondel in series of articles assessing the psychological consequences of having triplets, up to four years after delivery (161,162). Only one of twelve pregnancies was spontaneous. At one year, a majority of mothers reported difficulties related to home help, social isolation, marital relationship, and relationships with the children. Eight of the twelve mothers expressed psychological difficulties, and three were treated for depression. By four years after birth, all mothers reported emotional distress (mainly fatigue and stress), four women had a high depression score and were on psychotropic medication, and four mothers spontaneously expressed regrets about having triplets (162).

The findings of increased psychological distress in couples undergoing infertility treatment necessitate counseling as an essential part of an ART program. Counseling compared to information alone did not lead to any enhanced reduction in levels of anxiety or depression. The challenge is to identify those individuals who may benefit from specific intervention at an early stage.

FINANCIAL IMPLICATIONS

Although the financial aspect of ART is not strictly a medical complication, for many couples it is of paramount importance. The implications at a personal, social, and political levels are great. Estimates vary as to the overall costs, depending on the place of treatment, order of pregnancy with subsequent neonatal care costs, and number of attempts needed to conceive per baby. Callahan et al. estimated the costs of IVF procedures, maternal, and neonatal costs as $9,845 for a singleton and $37,947 for twins. The maternal and neonatal costs alone were more than $109,000 for the average triplet pregnancy in 1994 (163).

In 1996, Goldfarb et al. quoted a cost of $39,000 for singleton or twin pregnancies and $340,000 for triplet or quadruplet pregnancies, including the maternal and neonatal expenses (164). The cost varied in the study by Neumann et al. from $66,667 for success in the first cycle to $800,000 for a woman older than forty years with accompanying male factor infertility and success in the fifth cycle (165).

The cost of ART treatment presents a great burden to couples seeking this modality of treatment in countries where the cost of service is not covered by the health authorities or insurance system, particularly in low-income and very low-income countries. In these countries, access to ART service becomes available only for the rich who can afford to pay for the service. This is of great ethical concern as it represents violation of the ethical principle of justice and equity. In a study by Serour et al., only 60 percent of couples seen at a private clinic who needed ART treatment could afford to have it done. Only 40 percent of those who did not get pregnant after the first trial could afford to have the procedure repeated for the second time (166).

In low-income countries where the procedure is not supported by the government, a mechanism had to be found to provide the service for the needy who cannot afford it. The application of soft stimulation protocols, natural cycles, and in vitro maturation of oocytes may present a hope for those patients in future.

A policy of transferring one embryo in selected patients may be more cost effective when compared to two-embryo transfer because of savings in maternal and neonatal expenditure, even if more treatment cycles are needed.

KEY POINTS OF CLINICAL PRACTICE (TABLE 62.2)

Table 62.2: Key Points of Clinical Practice – Guidelines for Reducing Complications of ART

Risk	Measures to reduce risk
General	BMI
	Blood tests
	Kidney function tests
	Liver function tests
	Blood sugar assessment
	FSH and E_2 assessment
	Abdominal and pelvic ultrasound scan
	Electrocardiogram in selected patients
	Mammography in selected patients
	Salpingectomy in selected patients
	Hysteroscopy in selected patients
OHSS and its complications	Please see other chapter on OHSS
OPU	Prophylactic use of antibiotics and antimycotics
	Avoidance of deep abdominal pressure on high ovaries
	Proper vaginal sterilization
	Minimal number of vaginal punctures
	Ultrasound visualization of peripheral follicles in a cross-section before puncture
	Use of color Doppler if available
	Gentle manipulation of the needle all through the procedure
	Proper visualization of tip of the needle all through the procedure
	Postoperative sedation if necessary
Pregnancy complications	Uterine cavity empty with positive BHCC exclude ectopic and heterotopic pregnancies
	Health education of patients on risks of MP
	Single embryo transfer in selected patients
	Multifetal pregnancy reduction for HOMP
Congenital of abnormalities	Proper genetic counseling of the couple
	Karyotyping of male partners before ICSI for severe oligoasthenospermia or NOA
	Cystic fibrosis testing in both partners before ICSI for CAVD
	PGD in some patients
Psychological and socioeconomic	Proper informative, implicative, and supporting counseling of the couple before, during, and after treatment
	Identification of those couples who need special attention

REFERENCES

1. Adamson GD, De Mouzon J, Lancaster P, Nygren KG, Sullivan E, Zegers-Hochs Child F. World collaborative report on in vitro fertilization, 2000. *Fertil Steril* 2006;85:6:1586–1622.
2. Anderson AN, Gianaroli L, Felberbaum R, Mouzon Jde, Nygren KG. Assisted reproductive technology in Europe, 2000. Results generated from European registers by ESHRE. *Hum Reprod* 2006;21:7:1680–1697.
3. Land JA, Evers JLH. Report of an ESHRE consensus meeting prepared. Risks and complications in assisted reproduction techniques. *Hum Reprod* 2003;18:2:455–457.
4. Serour GI, Rhodes C, Sattar MA, Aboulghar MA, Mansour R. Complications of assisted reproductive techniques. A review. *Assist Reprod* 1999;9:4:214–232.
5. Bergh T, Lundkvist O. Clinical complications during in-vitro fertilization treatment. *Hum Reprod* 1992;7:625–626.
6. Roest J. Mous HV, Zeilmaker GH, et al. The incidence of major complications in a Dutch transport IVF programme. *Hum Reprod Update* 1996;2:345–353.
7. Serour GI, Aboulghar M, Mansour R, et al. Complications of medically assisted conception in 3500 cycles. *Fertil Steril* 1998;70:638–642.

8. Govaerts F, Devreker F, Delbaere A, Revelard PH, Englert Y. Short-term medical complications of 1500 Oocyte retrievals for in vitro fertilization and embryo transfer. *Eur J Obstet Gynec and Reprod Biol* 1998;239–243.

9. Klemetti R, Sevon T, Gissler M, Hemminki E. Complication of IVF and ovulation induction. *Hum Reprod* 2005;20:12: 3293–300.

10. Broat D, Bernardus R, Gerris J. Anonymous reports of lethal cases of ovarian Hyperstimulation syndrome. In (Eds) Gerris J, Delvigne A, Olivennes F. *Ovarian Hyperstimulation Syndrome.* Informa Health Care, 2006;59–70.

11. Serour GI. Clinical manifestations of ovarian hyperstimulation syndrome. In (Eds) Gerris J, Delvigne A, Olivennes F. *Ovarian Hyperstimulation Syndrome.* Informa Health Care, 2006;25–40.

12. Bamford PM, Steele SJ. Uterine and ovarian carcinoma in a patient receiving gonadotropin therapy: a case report. *Obstet Gynecol* 1982;89:962–964.

13. Schenker JG, Ezra Y. Complications of assisted reproductive techniques. *Fertil Steril* 1994; 61:411–422.

14. Kaufman SC, Spirtas R, Alexander NJ. Do fertility drugs cause ovarian tumors? *J Women's Health* 1995;4:247–259.

15. Heintz AP, Hacker NF, Lagasse LD. Epidemiology and etiology of ovarian cancer: a review. *Obstet Gynecol* 1985;66: 127–135.

16. Nugent D, Salha O, Balen AH, et al. Ovarian neoplasis subfertility treatments. *Br J Obstet Gynecol* 1998;105:584–591.

17. Fathalla MF. Incessant ovulation: a factor in ovarian neoplasis? *Lancet* 1971;2:163.

18. Zajicek L. Prevention of ovarian cystomas by inhibition of ovulation: a new concept. *J Reprod Med* 1978;2:114.

19. Stadel BV. The etiology and prevention of ovarian cancer. *Am J Obstet Gynecol* 1975;123:772–774.

20. Daly MB. The epidemiology of ovarian cancer. *Hematol Oncol Clin North Am* 1992;6:729–738.

21. Bengtsson M, Rydstrom J. Regulation of carcinogen metabolism in the rat ovary by the estrous cycle and gonadotropin. *Science* 1983;219:1437–1438.

22. Bengtsson M, Hamberger L, Rydstrom J. Metabolism of 17,12-dimethyl-benz(a)anthracene by different types of cells in human ovary. *Xenobiotica* 1988;18:1255–1270.

23. Ron E, Lunenfeld B, Menczer J, et al. Cancer incidence in a cohort of infertile women. *Am J Epidemiol* 1987;125:780–790.

24. Shu XO, Brinton LA, Gao YT, et al. Population-based case-control study of ovarian cancer in Shanghai. *Cancer Res* 1989; 49:3670–3674.

25. Whittemore AS, Harris R, Itnyre J, et al. The Collaborative Ovarian Cancer Group. Characteristics relating to ovarian cancer risk: collaborative analysis of 12 U.S. case-control studies. I. *Methods. Am J Epidemiol* 1992;136:1175–1183.

26. Whittemore AS, Harris R, Itnyre J. The Collaborative Ovarian Cancer Group. Characteristics relating to ovarian cancer risk: collaborative analysis of 12 U.S. case-control studies. II. Invasive epithelial ovarian cancers in white women. *Am J Epidemiol* 1992;136:1184–1203.

27. Harris R, Whittemore AS, Itnyre J. The Collaborative Ovarian Cancer Group. Characteristics relating to ovarian cancer risk: collaborative analysis of 12 U.S. Case-control studies. III. Epithelial tumors of low malignant potential in white women. *Am J Epidemiol* 1992;136:1204–1211.

28. Rossing MA, Daling JR, Weiss NS, et al. Ovarian tumors in a cohort of infertile women. *N Engl J Med* 1994;331:771–776.

29. Shushan A, Paltiel O, Iscovich J, et al. Human menopausal gonadotropin and the risk of epithelial ovarian cancer. *Fertil Steril* 1996;65:13–18.

30. Venn A, Watson L, Lumley J, et al. Breast and ovarian cancer incidence after infertility and in vitro fertilization. *Lancet* 1995; 346:995–1000.

31. Parazzini F, Negri E, La Vecchia C, et al. treatment for infertility and risk of invasive epithelial cancer. *Hum Reprod* 1997; 12:2159–2161.

32. Mosgaard BJ, Lidegaard O, Kjaer SK, et al. Infertility, fertility drugs, and invasive ovarian cancer: a case-control study. *Fertil Steril* 1997;67:1005–1012.

33. Klip H, Burger CW, Kenemans P, Leeuween V. Cancer risk associated with subfertility and ovulation induction: a review. *Cancer Causes Control* 2000;11:319–344.

34. Mahdavi A, Pejovic T, Nezhat F. Induction of ovulation and ovarian cancer: A critical review of the literature. *Fertil Steril* 2006;85:4:819–826.

35. Braga C, Negri E, La Vecchia C, et al. Fertility treatment and risk of breast cancer. *Hum Reprod* 1996;11:300–303.

36. Venn A, Watson L, Bruinsma F, Giles G, Healy D. Risk of cancer after use of fertility drugs with in vitro fertilization. *Lancet* 1999;354:1586–1590.

37. Brinton L, Scoccia B, Moghissi KS, Westhoff CL, Althuis MD, Mabie JE, Lamb EJ. Breast cancer risk associated with ovulation stimulation drugs. *Hum Reprod* 2004;19(9):2005–2013.

38. Johannes CB, Caro JJ, Hartz SC, et al. Adverse effects of ovulatory stimulants – a review. *Assist Reprod Rev* 1993;3: 68–74.

39. Flam F, Lundstrom V, Lindstedt J, et al. Choriocarcinoma of the fallopian tube associated with induced superovulation in an IVF program: a case report. *Eur J Obstet Gynecol Reprod Biol* 1989;33:183–186.

40. Li TC, Hindle JE. Adverse local reaction to intramuscular injections of urinary-derived gonadotrophins. *Hum Reprod* 1993; 8:1835–1836.

41. Harika G, Gabriel R, Quereux C, et al. Hypersensitization to human menopausal gonadotropins with anaphylactic shock syndrome during a fifth in vitro fertilization cycle. *J Assist Reprod Genet* 1994;11:51–53.

42. Redfearn A, Hughes EG, O'Connor M, et al. Delayed-type hypersensitivity to human gonadotropin: case report. *Fertil Steril* 1995;64:855–856.

43. Lawton AW. Optic neuropathy associated with clomiphene citrate therapy. *Fertil Steril* 1994;61:390–391.

44. Wang JC, Guarnaccia M, Weiss SF, Sauer MV, Choi JM. Initial presentation of undiagnosed acute intermittent porphyria as a rare complication of ovulation induction. *Fertil Steril* 2006; 86:2:462–e1–e3.

45. Steptoe PC, Edwards RG. Reimplantation of a human embryo with subsequent tubal pregnancy. *Lancet* 1976;1:880–882.

46. Dellenbach P, Nisand I, Moreau L, et al. Transvaginal sonographically controlled ovarian follicle puncture for egg retrieval. *Lancet* 1984;1:1467.

47. Feichtinger W, Kemeter P. Laparoscopic or ultrasonically guided follicle aspiration for in vitro fertilization? *J In Vitro Fertil Embryo Transfer* 1984;1:244–249.

48. Ludwig AK, Glawatz M, Griesinger G, Diedrich K, Ludwig M. Perioperative and postoperative complications transvaginal ultrasound-guided oocyte retrieval. Prospective of study of >1000 oocyte retrievals. *Hum Reprod* 2006;21:12:3235–3240.

49. Howe RS, Wheeler C, Mastroianni L, et al. Pelvic infection after transvaginal ultrasound-guided ovum retrieval. *Fertil Steril* 1988;49:726–728.

50. Bennet SJ, Waterstone JJ, Cheng WC, et al. Complications of transvaginal ultrasound-directed follicle aspiration. A review

of 2670 consecutive procedures. *J Assist Reprod Genet* 1993;10: 72–77.

51. Scoccia B, Marcovici I, Brandt T. Uterine abscess after ultrasound guided ovum retrieval in an in vitro fertilization-embryo transfer program: case report and review of the literature. *J Assist Reprod Genet* 1992;9:285–289.

52. Coccia ME, Becattini C, Bracco GL, et al. Acute abdomen following dermoid cyst rupture during transvaginal ultrasonographically guided retrieval of oocytes. *Hum Reprod* 1996;11: 1897–1899.

53. Jones WR, Haines CJ, Matthews CD, et al. Traumatic ureteric obstruction secondary to oocyte recovery for in vitro fertilization: a case report. *J In Vitro Fertil Embryo Transfer* 1989;6: 186–187.

54. Neuwinger J, Todorow S, Wildt L. Ureteral obstruction: a complication of oocyte retrieval. *Fertil Steril* 1994;61:787 (Letter).

55. Coroleu B, Lopez Mourelle FL, Hereter L, et al. Ureteral lesion secondary to vaginal ultrasound follicular puncture for oocyte recovery in in-vitro fertilization. *Hum Reprod* 1997; 12:948–950.

56. Miller PB, Price T, Nichols JE Jr., Hill L. Acute ureteral obstruction following transvaginal oocyte retrieval for IVF. *Hum Reprod* 2002;17:1:137–138.

57. Wang JG, Huchko MJ, Kavic S, Sauer MV. Rectus sheath hematoma after transvaginal follicle aspiration: a rare complication of in vitro fertilization. *Fertil Steril* 2005;84(1): 217.e1–e3.

58. Ayestaran C, Matorras R, Gomez S, Arce D, Rodriguez-Escudero F. Severe bradycardia and bradypnea following vaginal oocyte retrieval: a possible toxic effect of paracervical mepivacaine. *Eur J Obstet Gynaecol Reprod Biol* 2000;91:71–73.

59. Azem F, Wolf Y, Botchan A, Amit A, Lessing JB, Kluger Y. Massive retroperitoneal bleeding: a complication of transvaginal ultrasonography-guided oocyte retrieval for in vitro fertilization-embryo transfer. *Fertil Steril* 2000;74:2:405–406.

60. Cho MM, McGovern PG, Colon JM. Vaginal perforation during transvaginal ultrasound-guided follicle aspiration in a woman undergoing multiple cycles of assisted reproduction. *Fertil Steril* 2004;81(6):1695–1696.

61. Almog B, Rimon E, Yovel I, Bar-Am A, Amit A, Azem F. Vertebral osteomyelitis: a rare complication of transvaginal ultrasound-guided oocyte retrieval. *Fertil Steril* 2000;73(6): 1250–1252.

62. Wehner-Caroli J, Schreiner T, Schippert W, Lischka G, Fierlbeck G, Rassner G. Anaphylactic reaction to bovine serum albumin after embryo transfer. *Fertil Steril* 1998;70:4:771–773.

63. Kupka MS, Dorn C, Richter O, Felderbaum R, Van Der Ven H. Impact of reproductive history on in vitro fertilization and intracytoplasmic sperm injection outcome: evidence from the German IVF Registry. *Fertil Steril* 2003;80:508–516.

64. Schieve LA, Tatham L, Peterson HB, Tones J, Jeng G. Spontaneous abortion among pregnancies conceived using assisted reproductive technology in the United States. *Obstet Gynecol* 2003;101:959–967.

65. Wang JX, Norman RJ, Wilcox AJ. Incidence of spontaneous abortion among pregnancies produced by assisted reproductive technology. *Hum Reprod* 2004;19:272–277.

66. Bryant J, Sullivan EA, Dean JH. Supplement to assisted reproductive technology in Australia and New Zealand. *Assist Reproductive Technology Series. Number 8.* Publication of AIHW National Perinatal Statistics Unit, no. PER 26, Sydney, Australia, 2004.

67. Dubuisson JB, Aubriot FX, Mathieu L, et al. Risk factors for ectopic pregnancy in 556 pregnancies after in vitro fertilization: implications for preventive management. *Fertil Steril* 1991; 56:686–690.

68. Asung E, Cuckle HS, Dirnfeld M, Grudzinskas GJ. *Ectopic pregnancy following IVF/ICSI-ET in the United Kingdom*, HFEA Register (1991–1999). Abstracts of the 19th Annual meeting of ESHRE, Madrid, Spain, 2003:xviii34–xviii35.

69. Rebic-Pucelj M, Tomazevic T, Vogler A, et al. Risk factors for ectopic pregnancy after in vitro fertilization and embryo transfer. *J Assist Reprod Genet* 1995;12:594–598.

70. Agarwal SK, Wisot AL, Garzo G, et al. Cornual pregnancies in patients with prior salpingectomy undergoing in vitro fertilization and embryo transfer. *Fertil Steril* 1996;65: 659–660.

71. Arbab F, Boulieu D, Bied V, et al. Uterine rupture in first or second trimester of pregnancy after in vitro fertilization and embryo transfer. *Hum Reprod* 1996;11:1120–1122.

72. Marcus SF, Macnamee M, Brinsden P. The prediction of ectopic pregnancy after in vitro fertilization and embryo transfer. *Hum Reprod* 1995;10:2165–2168.

73. Mol BWJ, Van der Venn F, Hajenius PJ, et al. Diagnosis of ectopic pregnancy after in vitro fertilization and embryo transfer. *Fertil Steril* 1997;68:1027–1032.

74. Dicken D, Goldman F, Felding D, et al. Heterotopic pregnancy after IVF-ET: report of a case and a review of the literature. *Hum Reprod* 1989;4:335–336.

75. De Vroe RW, Pratt JH. Simultaneous intrauterine and extrauterine pregnancy. *Am J Obstet Gynecol* 1948;56:1119–1123.

76. Tal J, Haddad S, Gordon N, et al. Heterotopic pregnancy after ovulation induction and assisted reproductive technologies: a literature review from 1971 to 1993. *Fertil Steril* 1996; 66:1–12.

77. Westergaard HB, Tranberg Johansen AE, Erb K, Nyboe Andersen A. Danish National IVF Registry 1994 and 1995. Treatment pregnancy outcome and complications during pregnancy. *Acta Obstet Gynecol Scand* 2000;79:384–389.

78. Tummon IS, Whitmore NA, Daniel SA, et al. Transferring more embryos increases risk of heterotopic pregnancy. *Fertil Steril* 1994;61:1065–1067.

79. Kasum M, Grizelj V, Simunic V. Simultaneous bilateral tubal pregnancy following in vitro-fertilization and embryo transfer. *Hum Reprod* 1998;13:465–467.

80. Chang C-C, Wu T-H, Tsai H-D, et al. Bilateral simultaneous tubal sextuples: pregnancy after in-vitro fertilization-embryo transfer following salpingectomy. *Hum Reprod* 1998;13: 762–765.

81. Wilcox LS, Kiely JL, Melvin CL, et al. Assisted reproduction technologies: estimates of their contribution to multiple births and newborn hospital days in the United States. *Fertil Steril* 1996;65:361–366.

82. Seoud MA, Toner JP, Kruithoff C, Muasher SJ. Outcome of twin, triple and quadruplet in in-vitro fertilization pregnancies: the Nor Folk experience. *Fertil Steril* 1992;57:825–834.

83. Yokoyama Y, Shimizu T, Hayakawa K. Incidence of handicaps in multiple births and associated factors. *Acta Genet Med Gemellol* 1995;44:81–91.

84. Bergh T, Ericson A, Hillensjo T, et al. Deliveries and children born after in-vitro fertilization in Sweden 1982-95: a retrospective cohort study. *Lancet* 1999;354:1579–1585.

85. Davis OK. Elective single-embryo transfer. Has its time arrived? *N Engl J Med* 2004;351:2440.

86. Goldfarb J, Kinzer DJ, Boyle M, Kurit D. Attitudes of in vitro fertilization and intrauterine insemination couples towards multiple gestation pregnancy and multifetal pregnancy reduction. *Fertil Steril* 1996;65:815–820.

87. ESHRE Campus Report. Prevention of twin pregnancies after IVF/ICSI by single embryo transfer. *Hum Reprod* 2001;16:4: 790–800.

88. Vayena E, Rowe P, Griffin P. *Current practices and controversies in assisted reproduction.* WHO Report of a meeting on Medical, Ethical and Social Aspects of Assisted Reproduction 17–21 September 2001. WHO, 2002, Geneva.

89. Templeton A. Avoiding multiple pregnancies in ART. Replace as many embryos as you like – one at a time. *Hum Reprod* 2000;15:8:1662–1665.

90. Hunault CC, Eijkemans MJC, Pieters MHEC, te Velde ER, Habbema JDF, Fasuer BCJM, Macklon N. A prediction model for selecting patients undergoing in vitro fertilization for elective single embryo transfer. *Fertil Steril* 2002;77(4): 725–732.

91. Panadian Z, Bhattacharya S, Ozturk O, Serour GI, Templeton A. Number of embryos for transfer following in-vitro fertilization or intracytoplasmic sperm injection. Cochrane Review 25/8/2004. *Human Reprod* 2005;20(10):2681–2687.

92. Gerris J, De Neubourg D, Mangelschots K, et al. Prevention of twin pregnancy after in-vitro fertilization or intracytoplasmic sperm injection based on strict embryo criteria: a prospective randomized clinical trial. *Hum Reprod* 1999;14:2581–2587.

93. Martikainen H, Tiitinen A, Candido T, et al. One versus two embryo transfer after IVF and ICSI: a randomised study. *Hum Reprod* 2001;16(9):1900–1903.

94. Tiitinen A, Halttunen M, Harkki P. Elective single embryo transfer: the value of cryopreservation. *Hum Reprod* 2001; 16(6):1140–1144.

95. Thurin A, et al. Elective single embryo transfer versus double-embryo transfer in vitro fertilization. *N Engl J Med* 2004;351: 2392.

96. Helmerhorst FM, Perquin DA, Donker D, Keirse MJ. Perinatal outcome of singletons and twins after assisted conception: a systematic review of controlled studies. *BMJ* 2004;328:261–265.

97. Jackson RA, Gibson KA, Wu YW, Croughan MS. Perinatal outcomes in singletons following in vitro fertilization: a meta-analysis. *Obstet Gynecol* 2004;103:551–563.

98. Draper ES, Kurinczuk JJ, Abrams KR, Clarke M. Assessment of separate contributions to perinatal mortality of infertility history and treatment: a case-control analysis. *Lancet* 1999;353: 1746–1749.

99. Kapiteijn K, Bruijn CS de, Boer E de, Craen AJM de, Burger CW, Leeuwen FE, Helmerhost FM. Does subfertility explain the risk of poor perinatal outcome after IVF and ovarian hyperstimulation? *Hum Reprod* 2006;21(12):3228–3234.

100. Rosen MP, Friedman BE, Shen S, Dobson AT, Shaline LK, Cedars MI. UCSF, San Francisco, CA. The effect of a vanishing twin on perinatal outcomes. *Fertil Steril* 2005;84(1):1–2.

101. De Neubourg D, Gerris J, Mangelschots K, Van Royen E, Vercruyssen M, Steylemans A, Elseviers M. The obstetrical and neonatal outcome of babies born after single-embryo transfer in IVF/ICSI compares favourably to spontaneously conceived babies. *Hum Reprod* 2006;21(4):1041–1046.

102. WHO. Recent advances in medically assisted conception. Report of WHO Scientific Group (Co-Rapporteur) Geneva (820). 1992.

103. Ludwig M, Schopper B, Katalinic A, et al. Experience with the elective transfer of two embryos under the conditions of the German embryo protection law: results of a retrospective data analysis of 2573 transfer cycles. *Hum Repord* 2000; 1(5):319–324.

104. Serour GI. Multiple pregnancy. An ongoing epidemic. What can we do about it? *Egyptian J Fertil Steril* 2006;10(2):1–4.

105. FIGO Ethics Committee guidelines. Ethical recommendations on multiple pregnancy and multifetal reduction. *Int J Gynecol Obstet* 2006;92(3):331–332.

106. Goldman JA, Ashkenazi J, Ben-David M, Feldberg D, Dicker D, Voliovitz I. First trimester bleeding in clinical IVF pregnancies. *Hum Reprod* 1988;3:807–809.

107. Dantas ZN, Singh AP, Karachalios P, Asch RH, Balmaceda JP, Stone SC. Vaginal bleeding and early pregnancy outcome in an infertile population. *J Assist Reprod Genet* 1996;13: 212–215.

108. Hofmann G, Gundrun C, Drake L, Bertsche A. Frequency and effect of vaginal bleeding in pregnancy outcome during the first 3 weeks after positive B-hCG test results following IVF-ET. *Fertil Steril* 2000;74:609–610.

109. Pezeshki K, Feldman J, Stein DE, Lobel SM, Grazi RV. Bleeding and spontaneous abortion after therapy for infertility. *Fertil Steril* 2000;74:504–508.

110. Everett C. Incidence and outcome of bleeding before the 20th week of pregnancy: prospective study from general practice. *BMJ* 1997;315:32.

111. Sutter PD, Bontinck J, Schutysers V, Elst J Van Der, Gerris J, Dhont M. First-trimester bleeding and pregnancy outcome in singletons after assisted reproduction. *Hum Reprod* 2006; 21(7):1907–1911.

112. Tallo CP, Vohr B, Oh W, Rubin LP, Seifer DB, Haning VR Jr. Maternal and neonatal morbidity associated with in vitro fertilization. *J Pediatr* 1995;127(5):794–800.

113. Romundstad LB, Romundstad PR, Sunde A, During VV, Skjaerven R, Vatten LJ. Increased risk of placenta previa in pregnancies following IVF/ICSI; a comparison of ART and non-ART pregnancies in the same mother. *Hum Reprod* 2006;21(9):2353–2358.

114. Tan SL, Doyle P, Campbell S, et al. Obstetric outcome of in vitro fertilization pregnancies compared with normally conceived pregnancies. *Am J Obstet Gynecol* 1992;167:778–784.

115. Brinsden PR, Rizk B. The obstetric outcome of assisted conception treatment. *Assist Reprod Rev* 1992;2:116–125.

116. Tallo CP, Vohr B, Oh W, et al. Maternal and neonatal morbidity associated with in vitro fertilization. *J Pediatr* 1995;127: 794–800.

117. Olivennes F, Rufat P, Andre B, et al. The increased risk of complication observed in singleton pregnancies resulting from in-vitro fertilization (IVF) does not seem to be related to the IVF method itself. *Hum Reprod* 1993;8:1297–1300.

118. Tanbo T, Dale PO, Lunde O, et al. Obstetric outcome in singleton pregnancies after assisted reproduction. *Obstet Gynecol* 1995;86:188–192.

119. Reubinoff BE, Samueloff A, Ben-Haim M, et al. Is the obstetric outcome of in vitro fertilize singleton gestation different from nature ones? A controlled study. *Fertil Steril* 1997;67:1077–1083.

120. Maman E, Lunenfeld E, Levy A, et al. Obstetric outcome of singleton pregnancies conceived by in vitro fertilization and ovulation induction compared with those conceived spontaneously. *Fertil Steril* 1998;70:240–245.

121. De Mouzon J, Lancaster P. International Working Group for Registers on Assisted Reproduction: World Collaborative Report on In Vitro Fertilization Preliminary data for 1995. *J Assist Reprod Genet* 1997;14 (Suppl):251S–265S.

122. Report of the Working Party on Children Conceived by In Vitro Fertilization. Births in Great Britain Resulting from Assisted Conception, 1978–87. *BMJ* 1990;300:1229–1233.

123. Doyle P, Beral V, Maconochie N. Preterm delivery, low birth weight and small-for-gestational-age in liveborn singleton

babies resulting from in vitro fertilization. *Hum Reprod* 1992; 7:425–428.

124. Rufat P, Olivennes F, de Mouzon J, et al. Task force report on the outcome of pregnancies and children conceived by in vitro fertilization (France: 1987 to 1989). *Fertil Steril* 1994; 61:324–330.

125. FIVNAT (French in Vitro National). Pregnancies and births resulting from in vitro fertilization: French national registry, analysis of data 1986 to 1990. Fertil Steril 1995;64:746–756.

126. Dhont De Nuebourg F, Van der Elst J, et al. Perinatal outcome of pregnancies after assisted reproduction: a case-control study. *J Assist Reprod Genet* 1997;14:575–580.

127. Addor V, Santos-Eggimann B, Fawer C-L, et al. Impact of infertility treatments on the health of newborns. *Fertil Steril* 1998;69:210–215.

128. Pinborg A, Loft A, Schmidt L, Andersen AN. Morbidity in a Danish National cohort of 472 IVF/ICSI twins, 1132 non-IVF/ICSI twins and 634 IVF/ICSI singletons: health-related and social implications for the children and their families. *Hum Reprod* 2003;18:6:1234–1243.

129. Pinborg A, Loft A, Rasmussen S, Schmidt L, Langhoff-Roos J, Greisen G, Andresen AN. Neonatal outcome in a Danish national cohort of 3438 IVF/ICSI and 10 362 non-IVF/ICSI twins born between 1995 and 2000. *Hum Reprod* 2004; 19:2:435–441.

130. Soderstrom-Anttila V, Salokorpi T, Pihlaja M, Serenius-Sirve S, Suikkari A-M. Obstetric and perinatal outcome and preliminary results of development of children born after in vitro maturation of oocytes. *Hum Reprod* 2006;21(6):1508–1513.

131. Meschede D, Lemcke B, Behre HM, De Greyer C, Nieschlag E, Horst J. Clustering of male factor infertility in the families of couples treated with intra cytoplasmic sperm injection. *Hum Reprod* 2000;15:1604–1608.

132. Bergh T, Ericson A, Hillensjo T, et al. Delivery and children born after in vitro fertilization in Sweden 1982-1995. *A retrospective cohort study. Lancet* 1999;1579–1585.

133. Ericson A, Kallen B. Congenital malformations in infants born after IVF: a population-based study. *Hum Reprod* 2001;16: 504–509.

134. Koivurova S, Hartikainen AL, Gissler M, Hemminki E, Sovio U, Jarvelin MR. Neonatal outcome and congenital malformations in children born after in-vitro fertilization. *Hum Reprod* 2002;17:5:1391–1398.

135. Hancen M, Kurinczuk JJ, Bower C, Webb S. The risk of major birth defects after intracytoplasmic sperm injection and in vitro fertilization. *N Engl J Med* 2002;346:725–730.

136. Bonduelle M, Liebaers I, Deketelaere V, Derde MP, Camus M, Devroey P, Van Steirteghem A. Neonatal Data on a cohort of 2889 infants born after ICSI (1991–1999) and of 2995 infants born after IVF (1983–1999). *Hum Reprod* 2002; 17:671–694.

137. Wennerholm U-B, Bergh C, Hamberger L, Lundin K, Nilsson L, Wikland M, Kallen B. Incidence of congenital malformation in children born after ICSI. *Hum Reprod* 2000;15:944–948.

138. Bonduelle M, Van Assche E, Joris H, Keymolen K, Devroey P, Van Steirteghem A, Liebaers I. Prenatal testing in ICSI pregnancies: incidence of chromosomal anomalies in 1586 karyotypes and relation to sperm parameters. *Hum Reprod* 2002; 17:2600–2614.

139. Bernardini L, Gianaroli L, Fortini D, Conte N, Magli C, Cavani S, Gaggero G, Tindiglia C, Ragni N, Venturini PL. Frequency of hyper-hypohaploidy and diploidy in ejaculated, epididymal and testicular germ cells of infertile patients. *Hum Reprod* 2000;15:2165–2172.

140. Aytoz A, Camus M, Tournaye H, Bonduelle M, Van Steirteghem A, Devroey P. Outcome of pregnancies after intracytoplasmic sperm injection and the effect of sperm origin and quality on this outcome. *Fertil Steril* 1998;70:5000–5005.

141. Levron J, Aviram-Goldring A, Madgar I, Raviv G, Barkai G, Dor J. Sperm chromosome abnormalities in men with severe male factor infertility who are undergoing in vitro fertilization with intracytoplasmic sperm injection. *Fertil Steril* 2001; 76:479–484.

142. Mateizel I, Verheyen G, Van Assche E, Tournaye H, Liebaers I, Van Steirtegheme A. FISH analysis of chromosome X, Y and 18 abnormalities in testicular sperm from azoospermic patients. *Hum Reprod* 2002;17:2249–2257.

143. Martin RH, Greene C, Rademaker A, Barclay L, Ko E, Chernos J. Chromosome analysis of spermatozoa extracted from tests of men with non-obstructive azoospermia. *Hum Reprod* 2000; 15:1121–1124.

144. Wennerholm U-B, Bergh C, Hamberger L, Westlander G, Wikland M, Wood M. Obstetric outcome of pregnancies following ICSI, classified according to sperm origin and quality. *Hum Reprod* 2000;15:1189–1194.

145. Ludwig M, Katalinic A. Malformation rate in fetuses and children conceived after ICSI: results of a prospective cohort study. *Reprod Biomed Online* 2002;5:171–178.

146. Vernaeve V, Bonduelle M, Tournaye H, Camus M, Van Steirteghem A, Devroey P. Pregnancy outcome and neonatal data of children born after ICSI using testicular sperm in obstructive and non-obstructive azoospermia. *Hum Reprod* 2003; 18(10):2093–2097.

147. Tracy Hampton B. Panel reviews health effects data for assisted reproductive technologies. *J Am Med Assoc* 2004;292(24): 2961–2962.

148. Maher ER, Afnan M, Barratt HL. Epigenetic risks related to assisted reproductive technologies: epigenetics, imprinting, ART and icebergs? *Hum Reprod* 2003;18(12):2508–2511.

149. Suteliffe AG, D'Souza SWD, Codman J, et al. Minor congenital anomalies, major congenital malformations and development in children conceived from cryopreserved embryos. *Hum Reprod* 1995;10:3332–3337.

150. Olivennes F, Schneider Z, Remy V, et al. Perinatal outcome and follow up of 82 children aged 1–9 years old conceived from cryopreserved embryos. *Hum Reprod* 1996;11: 1565–1568.

151. Wennerholm UB, Hamberger L, Nilson L, et al. Obstetric and perinatal outcome of children conceived from cryopreserved embryos. *Hum Reprod* 1997;12:1819–1825.

152. Antinori M, Licata E, Dani G, Cerusico F, Versaci C, Antinori S. Cryotop vetrification of human oocytes results in high survival rate and healthy deliveries. *RBM Online* 2007;14(1):72–79.

153. Thepot F, Mayaux MJ, Czylick F, et al. Incidence of birth details after artificial insemination with frozen donor spermatozoa: a collaborative study of the French CECOS Federation on 11.535 pregnancies. *Hum Reprod* 1996;11:2319–2323.

154. Mahlstedt PP, Macduff S, Bernstein L. Emotional factors and the in vitro fertilization and embryo transfer process. *J In Vitro Fertil Embryo Transfer* 1987;4:232–236.

155. Baram D, Tourtelot E, Muechler E, et al. Psychosocial adjustment following unsuccessful in vitro fertilization. *J Psychosom Obstet Gynaecol* 1988;9:181–190.

156. Newton CR, Hearn MT, Yuzpe AA. Psychological assessment and follow up after in vitro fertilization: assessing the impact of failure. *Fertil Steril* 1990;54:879–886.

157. Slade P, Emery J, Laeberman BA. A prospective, longitudinal study of emotions and relationships in vitro fertilization treatment. *Hum Reprod* 1997;12:183–190.

158. Van Balen F, Naaktgeboren N, Trimbos-Kemper TCM. In-vitro fertilization the experience of treatment, pregnancy and delivery. *Hum Reprod* 1996;11:95–98.

159. Boivin J, Taketman JE. Impact of the in-vitro fertilization process on emotional, physical and relational variables. *Hum Reprod* 1996;11:903–907.

160. Colpin H, Soenen S. Parenting and psychological development of IVF children: a follow up study. *Hum Reprod* 2002; 17(4):1116–1123.

161. Garel M, Blondel B. Assessment at one year of the psychological consequences of having triplets. *Hum Reprod* 1992;7:729–732.

162. Garel M, Salobir C, Blondel B. Psychological consequences of having triplets: a 4 year follow-up study. *Fertil Steril* 1997; 67:1162–1165.

163. Callahan TL, Hall JE, Ettner SL, et al. The economic impact of multiple-gestation pregnancies and the contribution of assisted-reproduction techniques to their incidence. *N Engl J Med* 1994;331:244–249.

164. Goldfarb JM, Austin C, Lisbona H, et al. Cost-effectiveness of in vitro fertilization. *Obstet Gynecol* 1996;87:18–21.

165. Neumann PJ, Gharib SD, Weinstein MC. The cost of a successful delivery with in vitro fertilization. *N Engl J Med* 1994; 331:239–243.

166. Serour GI, Aboulghar M, Mansour RT. In vitro fertilization and embryo transfer in Egypt. *Int J Obstet Gynaecol* 1991;36:49–53.

63

ECTOPIC AND HETEROTOPIC PREGNANCIES FOLLOWING IN VITRO FERTILIZATION

Ziad R. Hubayter, Suheil J. Muasher

INTRODUCTION

Ectopic pregnancy is defined as an abnormal implantation of the conceptus in a location outside the uterine cavity. Heterotopic pregnancy is when there are concomitant intrauterine and extrauterine pregnancies (1). Ectopic pregnancy is a life-threatening condition and is one of the leading causes of maternal mortality. It accounts for 9 percent of all pregnancy-related deaths and is the most common etiology of maternal deaths in the first trimester (2).

Assisted reproductive technologies (ART) are associated with several medical complications. These include ovarian hyperstimulation syndrome, bleeding, infections (ovarian abcess and endometritis), and a higher incidence of ectopic pregnancies. The incidence of ectopic pregnancies is increased in ART due to a higher number of embryos transferred and a higher prevalence of tubal disease in patients undergoing in vitro fertilization (IVF) (3).

Abulcasis was the first to describe an ectopic pregnancy in the tenth century AD. He was an Arabic writer and one of the first to perform and discuss different types of surgical procedures. He discussed a case where he was able to retrieve fetal parts from a draining abdominal wound (4). Riolan, in the early seventeenth century, described a woman who died at four months of gestation. She presented with acute abdominal pain and syncope. Later, a fetus was identified in one of her fallopian tubes (5). In 1708, Duverney described a heterotopic pregnancy on autopsy (4). In the late nineteenth century, Tait, a British surgeon, performed a laparotomy and a salpingectomy and saved a woman with a ruptured ectopic pregnancy (5). Since then, the traditional treatment of ectopic pregnancies had been primarily surgical. The first conception following IVF was an ectopic pregnancy (5). In recent decades, earlier diagnosis and better techniques and equipment have made conservative surgical approaches and medical management more applicable.

EPIDEMIOLOGY

The incidence of ectopic pregnancy in the general population is 19 per 1,000 pregnancies (2). Following IVF, the incidence of ectopic pregnancy varies among centers and studies (from 2 to 11 percent of pregnancies). In a recent Center of Disease Control and Prevention review of ART cycles done in the United States in 2002, the incidence of ectopic pregnancy was 0.7 percent of all total ART cycles or around 2 percent of all clinical pregnancies (6). The higher incidence with IVF may be explained by the fact that ectopic pregnancies as well as normal pregnancies are more diagnosed in ART programs due to more extensive monitoring (7–9). In a more recent analysis of 6,007 embryo transfers resulting in 38.7 percent clinical pregnancies, 4.05 percent were ectopic pregnancies. The majority of patients who had an ectopic pregnancy were undergoing IVF for tubal pathology (91.5 percent) (10). In a collaborative study involving 1,163 pregnancies following IVF, up to 5 percent of these were ectopic gestations (11). The incidence of heterotopic pregnancies in the general population is rare. It occurs in 1 out of 4,000 pregnancies (12). This rises to 1 percent in women undergoing ART as first highlighted by Rizk et al. 1991 and then several other series (3, 13).

The mortality rate from an ectopic pregnancy has been decreasing with the improvements made in the diagnostic and therapeutic interventions. In the late nineteenth century, when Tait first performed a salpingectomy, the mortality rate from ectopic pregnancy was around 72–90 percent. Currently, the case fatality rate of a tubal ectopic pregnancy is 0.14 percent (14). Conception implanting within the portion of the tube that is within the uterus is defined as an interstitial pregnancy. Unlike other ectopic tubal gestations, interstitial pregnancies are associated with a higher mortality. The case fatality rate is around 2 percent (14).

RISK FACTORS

There are several known risk factors for ectopic pregnancy following a natural conception. These include prior tubal surgery, prior ectopic pregnancies, in utero diethyl stilbestrol exposure, prior pelvic inflammatory diseases, and smoking (9). The risk of ectopic pregnancies in smokers is dose dependent. Smoking affects the immune system, leading to a higher risk of pelvic infections and subsequent tubal disease. It also can affect tubal motility (15). Women who undergo IVF tend to have a higher prevalence of these risk factors and are at risk of ectopic pregnancy even if they conceived naturally. In addition, there are other risks that apply particularly to women desiring fertility. Infertile women have a higher risk of ectopic pregnancy, even without tubal disease. Women receiving superovulation have a higher risk of extrauterine pregnancies. In a multicenter study, women undergoing ovulation induction with clomiphene citrate had a twofold increase in the incidence of ectopic pregnancy (11). Similarly, the incidence is higher with the use of gonadotropins. The rate of ectopic pregnancies was 2.7 percent (16).

Different ART procedures have different risks on the incidence of ectopic pregnancies. The rate of ectopic pregnancy in women undergoing IVF with transcervical transfer of fresh embryos is 2.2 percent. With donor oocytes, the risk is lower (1.6 percent). When the embryos are transferred to a gestational carrier, the risk is 0.9 percent. The risk of ectopic pregnancy is significantly increased (up to 3.6 percent) with zygote intrafallopian transfer (17). The incidence of ectopic pregnancy is also increased with assisted hatching. In a retrospective review of 623 pregnancies from IVF, the incidence of ectopic pregnancies in patients with assisted hatching was 5.5 percent (18).

In a retrospective cohort review by Strandell et al., the risk factors for ectopic pregnancy after assisted reproduction were evaluated. The most predictive risk factor to develop an ectopic pregnancy in women undergoing IVF was tubal factor infertility (up to 6.4 percent) (19). An embryo may reach the fallopian tube after a transfer. If already damaged, a fallopian tube may not be able to propel the embryo back into the uterine cavity (4). Fibroids and a history of myomectomy did not increase the risk, unless there is a concomitant tubal disease. In these women, the probability of ectopic pregnancy can be as high as 27 percent (19). Ectopic pregnancies rarely occur in IVF patients after bilateral salpingectomy. In these situations, heterotopic or interstitial pregnancies may be missed (19, 20). In women who underwent a unilateral salpingectomy, the incidence of ectopic pregnancy was higher in the contralateral tube (19). The presence of a hydrosalpinx was associated with a 9.2 percent risk of developing an ectopic gestation. Women without a hydrosalpinx and who undergo IVF had a risk of an ectopic pregnancy of only 3.4 percent (19). Prior salpingitis, prior abdominal surgery, and a prior ectopic pregnancy were also associated with a significantly higher risk of developing an ectopic pregnancy (19). In addition, patients with a known cause for their infertility had a 4.6 percent chance of an ectopic pregnancy compared with 0.9 percent in patients with unexplained infertility (19).

The number of oocytes retrieved, the number and quality of embryos transferred, and the day of embryo transfer did not affect the incidence of developing an ectopic pregnancy (19). There was no difference in the incidence comparing fresh or cryopreserved embryos. Similarly, there were no differences comparing different types of transfer catheters (19). However, the risk of ectopic pregnancy was higher when the catheter was introduced up to the fundus (3, 21, 22). Furthermore, a larger volume injected at transfer correlated with an increased incidence of ectopic pregnancy (23). Embryos transferred on day 3 and those on day 5 had similar rates of an ectopic pregnancy (24).

The incidence of heterotopic pregnancies increased with increasing number of embryos transferred (3, 25–27). Other associated findings identified in women who developed heterotopic gestations were high levels of serum estradiol and progesterone that are believed to impair the propulsion of embryos back into the uterine cavity after reaching the tubes. In addition, the volume and the viscosity of the transfer medium may cause a higher hydrostatic pressure and may push the embryos into the tubes. As mentioned before, the technique of embryo transfer may also increase the risk of heterotopic pregnancies (13).

There are some protective factors for ectopic pregnancies. In the general population, the use of contraception (including intrauterine devices) decreases the risk of an ectopic pregnancy by decreasing the total number of pregnancies. In the ART population, intracytoplasmic sperm injection (ICSI) is associated with a lower risk of ectopic pregnancy than conventional IVF (19). ICSI may have a protective role due to the fact that it is mainly used for male factor infertility rather than for tubal factor (19). Embryo transfers performed under ultrasound guidance did not reduce the rate of ectopic pregnancy with experienced physicians (28, 29). However, the ultrasound remains a useful and relatively inexpensive method to ensure miduterine position of the catheter tip during the transfer of the embryos, particularly for newly trained physicians.

LOCATION

Ectopic pregnancy occurs usually within the fallopian tubes. Most tubal pregnancies are within the ampullary portion. In a population-based study involving 1,800 ectopic pregnancies that were surgically removed, Bouyer et al. studied the sites of implantation of these ectopic pregnancies (30). In this report, 70 percent of the ectopic pregnancies were in the ampullary portion of the fallopian tube. Isthmic and fimbrial implantations occurred in 12 and 11 percent, respectively, while interstitial pregnancies were uncommon (2.4 percent of all ectopics).

As mentioned before, mural or interstitial pregnancy can occur in women who underwent a prior salpingectomy. They are often missed and can result in disastrous consequences. They can bleed within the uterine wall and may lead to uterine rupture, which is reported to occur in up to 20 percent of cases if undetected during the first trimester (14). Interstitial and cornual pregnancies are commonly used interchangeably. However, cornual pregnancy is defined as a pregnancy implanting in the endometrial cavity of a cornua, while interstitial pregnancy results when the implantation is within the tube embedded within the uterus (14).

Other sites may also be a milieu for an ectopic pregnancy implantation. Cervical pregnancy accounts for 0.15 percent of all ectopic gestations (4). Ovarian pregnancies occur in 3.2 percent of all ectopic pregnancies. They are usually difficult to diagnose, particularly in cases of heterotopics. They are often misdiagnosed initially as hemorrhagic cysts (31). Abdominal pregnancy is extremely rare with an incidence of 1 in 5,000 deliveries (32). In other reports, 1.3 percent of ectopic pregnancies were abdominal (30). The origin of these pregnancies may be the rupture of a fimbrial ectopic (30). These ectopics may be unrecognized, and the gestation may proceed into the second and even third trimesters. An ectopic pregnancy may also implant in the hysterotomy scar in women who had a prior cesarean delivery (33).

CLINICAL MANIFESTATIONS

Without tubal rupture, more than 50 percent of patients are asymptomatic. The clinical manifestations of those who develop symptoms occur at around six weeks of gestation. Abdominal pain is the most common presentation. It occurs in 90 percent of cases. Other symptoms and signs include vaginal spotting (80 percent), amenorrhea (80 percent), and a pelvic mass (50 percent) (34).

The rate of tubal rupture of ectopic pregnancies is 18 percent (35). In a population-based study conducted in France, risk factors for tubal rupture were assessed. Women who had never used contraception, had a history of tubal damage and

Table 63.1: Clinical Presentation and Ultrasonographic Diagnosis of 17 Heterotopic Pregnancies after IVF

| Patient No. | Clinical | Diagnosis | | | | | Duration of pregnancy at time of diagnosis | |
| | | Ultrasonographic findings | | | | | | |
		Type	Gest sac in utero	Fetal hearts in utero	Ectopic pregnancy	IUP	Ectopic
1	Abd. pain	Abd.	1	1	1	6	8
2	Abd. pain	Abd.	3	2	0	6	NO
3	Abd. pain	Abd.	1	0	0	5	NO
4	Abd. pain	Abd.	1	0	1	6	6
5	Abd. pain	Abd.	1	0	0	5	NO
6	Abd. pain	Abd.	1	0	1	7	7
7	Abd. pain and bleeding	Abd.	2	1	1	7	7
8	Abd. pain and bleeding	Abd.	1	0	0	7	NO
9	Abd. pain and bleeding	Abd.	1	0	1	8	8
10	Acute abd.	Abd.	1	0	0	5	NO
11	Acute abd.	Abd.	2	2	0	8	NO
12	Acute abd.	Abd.	1	1	0	6	NO
13	Asymptomatic	Abd.+vag	1	1	1	7	7
14	Asymptomatic	Abd.+vag	2	2	1	7	7
15	Asymptomatic	Abd.+vag	1	1	1	7	7
16	Asymptomatic	Abd.+vag	1	1	1	7	7
17	Asymptomatic	Abd.+vag	1	1	1	7	7

Reproduced with permission from Rizk et al. AJOG 1991 reference 3.

infertility, had undergone ovulation induction, or had a serum beta human chorionic gonadotropin (hCG) level higher than 10,000 mIU/mL were at a higher risk for rupture (35). In cases of ruptured ectopic pregnancies, the abdomen becomes severely tender and rigid, and the patient may develop orthostatic hypotension and tachycardia suggestive of hemodynamic instability. On pelvic examination, both adnexal and cervical motion tenderness, due to peritoneal irritation, may also be present.

DIAGNOSIS

Several decades ago, most ectopic pregnancies were diagnosed after rupture.

The recent advances in ultrasound technology and the higher expertise of sonographers have improved the early diagnosis of ectopic pregnancies. Earlier diagnosis resulted in a lower mortality rate from ectopic pregnancies. In the IVF population, due to a closer follow-up, along with serial ultrasounds as well as quantitative hCG assays, the diagnosis of ectopic pregnancy usually occurs before clinical symptoms develop. The higher number of embryos transferred and the risk of heterotopic pregnancies often complicate the diagnosis (Table 63.1).

Beta Human Chorionic Gonadotropin

The beta subunit of hCG has been used to differentiate a developing viable intrauterine pregnancy from an abnormal pregnancy (miscarriage or ectopic). The beta hCG is produced by the trophoblastic tissues. Initially, the rise is curvilinear until it plateaus at around ten weeks of gestation. In normal pregnancies, the serum level of hCG increases by more than 66 percent every forty-eight hours early in the pregnancy (36). The slowest rise in a normal viable intrauterine pregnancy (IUP) is a 53 percent increase in forty-eight hours (37). However, 15 percent of normal viable IUP will have a smaller rise in the level and 17 percent of ectopic pregnancies will have a doubling of the hCG (29). After seven weeks of gestation, the doubling of serum beta hCG becomes less reliable but an IUP should be identified on the transvaginal sonogram. In cases of spontaneous miscarriages, the hCG may decline. However, a decline of less than 21 percent after two days should raise the suspicion for either retained products or an ectopic pregnancy (38).

Several reports have assessed the value of a single discriminatory hCG value after IVF in predicting ectopic gestations. The aim of these studies is to decrease the need for serial hCG measurements and frequent office or laboratory visits. One study that evaluated the predictive value of beta hCG showed that a level higher than 265 mIU/mL on day 16 following an embryo transfer correlated with an intrauterine implantation with a probability of 90 percent (39). In another study, serum beta hCG level on day 9 after embryo transfer was analyzed. A level higher than 18 mIU/mL correlated with a viable IUP. An ultrasound was done at seven weeks of gestation to confirm the IUP. Women with an hCG level higher than 18 mIU/mL did not need an ultrasound before seven weeks of gestation. However, an ultrasound is needed earlier than seven weeks of gestation in cases where the hCG level is lower than 18 mIU/mL and in patients with vaginal bleeding or abdominal pain (40). In another study by Chen et al., serial early hCG levels to predict a normal pregnancy were found to be helpful. Women undergoing IVF had hCG levels drawn on days 15 and 22 after the embryo transfer. If the level on day 15 was higher than 150 mUI/mL then, the positive predictive value (PPV) for a normal pregnancy was 89 percent. However, the negative predictive value (NPV) was 51 percent. In those with a lower level on day 15, the ratio of hCG on day 22 to that on day 15 was used instead. If the ratio was higher than 15, then the rise was considered appropriate and the PPV for a normal pregnancy was 90 percent. If the ratio was less than 15, then the NPV was 84 percent (41).

Ultrasonography

In 1993, Rizk et al. studied the value of transvaginal ultrasound and hCG and the diagnosis of heterotopic pregnancies (42). Usually, the diagnosis of ectopic pregnancy is ruled out when an intrauterine gestation is identified, except in cases of heterotopic gestations. Transabdominal ultrasound should detect an intrauterine gestation once the serum hCG level is above 6,000 mIU/mL. The value of a transabdominal ultrasound is diminished with improvement and more experience with the transvaginal route. Using the later, an hCG level of as low as 1,000 mIU/mL may be enough to identify an IUP. At this hCG level, the nonvisualization of an intrauterine gestation is highly suggestive of an ectopic pregnancy. Unfortunately, due to multiple-embryo transfers, the hCG level could be erroneously high due to multiple gestations and rarely heterotopic pregnancies. In these cases, repeating the ultrasound few days later in an asymptomatic patient is recommended.

The in utero gestational sac is usually seen at around five weeks of gestation. The yolk sac is apparent at around five to six weeks. At six weeks, an embryo is usually visualized. Once the crown rump length measures 3–5 mm, a fetal heart is identified. These landmarks are important, especially in IVF, as the gestational age is accurately known (43). Visualization of an adnexal ring, a complex adnexal mass, and echogenic fluid are associated with an ectopic pregnancy (44). If an extrauterine gestational sac is seen with a living pregnancy or a yolk sac, the likelihood of an extrauterine pregnancy is extremely high. However, these findings have a lower sensitivity compared to a complex adnexal mass (45). Color Doppler flow was found to improve the sensitivity of the transvaginal sonogram in diagnosing an ectopic pregnancy (46). The invasion of the trophoblasts increases the blood flow in the affected tube (47).

In assisted reproduction, the incidence of heterotopic pregnancy is increased and the presence of an IUP cannot exclude with certainty an ectopic gestation. Careful examination of the adnexa is mandated (42). In a prospective study, transvaginal ultrasonography performed in women prior to surgery for sus-

pected ectopic pregnancies was able to accurately predict an ectopic pregnancy in 90.9 percent of cases (48).

In the IVF population, findings suggestive of an ectopic pregnancy may be difficult to assess. Cul de sac free fluid may be present with ascites in hyperstimulated patients. A hydrosalpinx may also be present in some patients. Patients typically will have enlarged ovaries that can be painful when pressure is applied with the probe, and this may limit accurate visualization. Enlarged ovaries and multiple corpora lutea may also mask an ectopic pregnancy (49).

In some cases where the ultrasound findings are indeterminate, magnetic resonance imaging (MRI), although more expensive, may be helpful (50, 51). Kataoka et al. evaluated thirty-seven patients prospectively and concluded that MRI with intravenous contrast can diagnose an ectopic pregnancy due to tubal wall enhancement and a developing hematoma (52). In another study, MRI and ultrasound with Doppler were similar in diagnosing early ectopic pregnancies (53).

Several case reports have shown a benefit from the adjunctive use of three-dimensional ultrasound in identifying the accurate location of an ectopic pregnancy, particularly in patients with prior surgery (myomectomy or salpingectomy) or in interstitial pregnancies (54).

Progesterone

In ART, the interpretation of serum progesterone is more complicated. Following superovulation, many corpora lutea are formed and progesterone supplementation is common. Although there are wide variations in the assays in the IVF population, serum progesterone is significantly lower in abnormal pregnancies. In a prospective study, progesterone levels on day 14 following embryo transfer after IVF/ICSI was significantly higher in those patients with a normal viable pregnancy (55). A serum progesterone level higher than 25 ng/mL is usually associated with a normal viable pregnancy in 99 percent of cases (56). A level lower than 5 ng/mL is usually associated with an abnormal pregnancy in 99.8 percent of cases (57). Unfortunately, most pregnancies tend to have a level in between these two values, thereby limiting the value of this assay as a single discriminatory test.

Others Tests

There are several other markers that are being evaluated for the diagnosis of an ectopic pregnancy. Vascular endothelial growth factor (VEGF) is elevated in ectopic pregnancies. Unlike other serum tests, VEGF levels can differentiate ectopic pregnancies from miscarriages. In the latter situations, the VEGF levels are low. The cutoff value used to differentiate an ectopic gestation from a miscarriage is 200 pg/mL (58). In a retrospective review, serum VEGF levels on day 11 after embryo transfer correlated with an ectopic pregnancy with a PPV of 64 percent and an NPV of 71 percent (59).

In a prospective study by Saha et al., serum creatine kinase levels were evaluated. Patients with an ectopic pregnancy had a higher value than those with a normal pregnancy. This could be due to damage of the tubal musculature. However, the test is not specific and may be elevated with other muscular pathology (60). Other serum markers evaluated include estradiol, relaxin, placental proteins, alpha fetoprotein, alkaline phosphatase, vascular cell adhesion molecule, fetal fibronectin, and CA 125.

MANAGEMENT

There are several methods of therapy for an ectopic pregnancy. Early diagnosis of an ectopic gestation allows the option of a more conservative management. Medical and surgical treatments will be discussed as well as expectant management.

Medical or Surgical Treatment

Early diagnosis and medical management of an ectopic pregnancy is associated with a lower cost and preservation of the fallopian tubes for future fertility (3, 27). An ectopic pregnancy may still rupture after the administration of methotrexate, and therefore, a reliable and compliant patient is mandatory. Surgical intervention is needed in cases where tubal rupture occurs and when medical therapy fails. The two commonly used protocols include the single-dose and the multidose methotrexate. The overall success rate following medical therapy in properly selected patients is above 90 percent for both regimens (61).

Predictors of failure of medical therapy include a history of a prior ectopic pregnancy, irrespective of the prior mode of treatment and pretreatment serum hCG levels. Women with a recurrent ectopic pregnancy have an 18.6 percent risk of failure with methotrexate treatment. The risk is significantly lower (6.8 percent) in those who have a first-time ectopic pregnancy (62). The higher the pretreatment serum hCG levels, the higher the chance of failure of medical therapy. In one study assessing methotrexate success, a level of beta hCG lower than 1,000 mIU/mL resulted in a 98 percent success rate. If values were lower than 5,000 mIU/mL, the success rate remains above 90 percent. This rate drops to 87 and 82 percent if the hCG level is between 5,000 and 9,999 mIU/mL and if it is between 10,000 and 14,999 mIU/mL, respectively. Ectopic pregnancies with an hCG level higher than 15,000 mIU/mL are successfully treated with methotrexate in only 68 percent of cases (63). This study also found a significant association between progesterone levels and fetal cardiac activity with success rates. A higher progesterone level and fetal cardiac activity were associated with a pregnancy that is more resistant to methotrexate. This could be indirectly related to a higher level of serum hCG. A higher hCG titer usually correlates with a higher progesterone level and with the presence of fetal cardiac activity (63). Free peritoneal fluid and size and volume of the ectopic gestation did not correlate significantly with success rates (63). Another useful sonographic finding that can predict failure is the presence of a yolk sac. In a retrospective review, a yolk sac was not seen in any ectopic pregnancy that was successfully medically treated compared to the presence of yolk sac in 88 percent of those that failed therapy (64).

In a randomized trial comparing single-dose methotrexate and surgical intervention, the medical therapy was less effective. However, if a repeat dose of methotrexate is given, in cases of suboptimal decline in hCG levels, the success rates became comparable (65). Patients who were treated medically had a better psychological perception of the treatment (65). Sowter et al. also evaluated the economic aspect of the treatment of ectopic pregnancy. Medical therapy was significantly associated with a lower cost compared to surgery (66).

Methotrexate

Methotrexate is an antineoplastic agent that affects primarily rapidly dividing cells. It is used for multiple purposes including cancer, rheumatoid arthritis, and psoriasis. Methotrexate is a folic acid antagonist that binds to the enzyme dihydrofolate reductase and leads to a reduction in tetrahydrofolate. The latter is needed for nucleic and amino acids formation. Methotrexate can be toxic to all rapidly dividing tissues such as malignant cells, fetal cells, bladder cells, bone marrow, buccal mucosa, and intestinal mucosa. The side effects are dependent on the dose and the duration of treatment. Patients may report nausea, vomiting, stomatitis, conjunctivitis, diarrhea, and dizziness. Rare complications include severe neutropenia, reversible alopecia, and pneumonitis. In the management of ectopic pregnancy, the dose used is typically much lower than in chemotherapy regimens and the side effects are transient and mild.

Candidates for medical therapy have to be hemodynamically stable and compliant. Unreliable or unstable patients are contraindications to medical treatment. Other contraindications include women who are breastfeeding, are immunosuppresed, have peptic ulcer disease, or have pulmonary, hepatic (alcoholism), renal, or hematological disorders. Prior allergic reaction is another contraindication (67). Relative contraindications are conditions associated with a lower success rate. A pretreatment hCG level higher than 5,000 mIU/mL, an ectopic pregnancy larger than 3.5 cm, and presence of fetal cardiac activity are the commonly cited relative contraindications.

Prior to the administration of methotrexate, patients should be informed of the increase in abdominal pain and in the quantitative serum hCG levels within the first few days. Patients may also have some vaginal bleeding. In those who fail medical therapy, the pain may persist and hCG levels may not decline appropriately. All patients should have a pretreatment quantitative serum hCG level, complete blood count, serum creatinine level, and liver function tests. The rhesus status should also be determined since Rh-negative patients need a Rhogam injection as well. Patients should also stop taking prenatal vitamins and folic acid.

There are several routes for administration of methotrexate. It can be given intravenously, intramuscularly (IM), orally, or locally. The most commonly used method of administration is the intramuscular method. Treatment can be given in single dose or in multidose regimens.

SINGLE-DOSE METHOTREXATE

The overall success rate is 91.5 percent with single-dose methotrexate (61). The dose of methotrexate is determined by the calculated body surface area, and 50 mg of methotrexate per m^2 is given in an intramuscular injection. Serum hCG levels may increase initially to a maximum value on day 4 following the injection. Treatment is considered successful if the hCG value on day 7 is at least 15 percent lower than that on day 4 (67). If an appropriate drop did not occur, a second dose may be given. Twenty percent of women will require another dose. Patients should be followed with weekly hCG levels, and it may take up to 109 days for the hCG level to become completely negative (61). Table 63.2 illustrates the single-dose protocol.

MULTIDOSE METHOTREXATE

In this regimen, 1 mg/kg is given IM on days 1, 3, 5, and 7. Rescue doses of 0.1 mg/kg of folinic acid should be given on days 2, 4, 6, and 8. The regimen may be repeated if the serum hCG did not fall appropriately. This regimen requires more

Table 63.2: Single-Dose Methotrexate Protocol

Pretreatment testing	hCG, CBC, BUN, creatinine, SGOT, SGPT, Rh status
Methotrexate dose	50 mg/m^2 on day 1
Leucovorin dose	None
hCG	Day 0, day 4, day 7, and then weekly until hCG level is negative
Frequency	Repeat on day 7 if hCG did not decline by 15 percent between day 4 and day 7 (up to four total doses)

Reproduced with permission from Rizk et al. 1991 reference 3.

Table 63.3: Multidose Methotrexate Protocol

Pretreatment testing	hCG, CBC, BUN, creatinine, SGOT, SGPT, Rh status
Methotrexate dose	1 mg/kg on days 1, 3, 5, 7
Leucovorin dose	0.1 mg/kg on days 2, 4, 6, 8
hCG	Day 0, day 1, day 3, day 5, and day 7 until hCG declines by 15 percent from prior value
Frequency	Repeat doses until hCG declines by 15 percent from prior hCG

Reproduced with permission from Rizk et al. 1991 reference 3.

frequent office visits and is more expensive than single therapy. Table 63.3 illustrates the multidose protocol.

In a meta-analysis reviewing data between 1966 and 2001, the multidose protocol was found to be more successful than the single-dose protocol. The latter was more commonly used and resulted in fewer side effects (68). More recently, a prospective randomized controlled trial by Alleyassin et al. compared single-dose and multidose regimens of methotrexate in the treatment of ectopic pregnancy. There were no significant differences in both success rates and side effects (69). Lipscomb et al. had similar findings when comparing these two regimens (70). Table 63.3 illustrates the multidose protocol.

ORAL METHOTREXATE

In one study by Lipscomb et al., oral methotrexate was compared to intramuscular injection. Methotrexate was given orally in two doses, two hours apart. The dose used was calculated to correspond to 60 mg/m^2. The success rate was 86 percent and was comparable to IM injection. Side effects were also similar. However, there are no clear indications when oral methotrexate treatment is preferable (71).

LOCAL METHOTREXATE

Methotrexate can be injected locally within the ectopic gestation. It can be performed under transvaginal ultrasound guidance or at the time of laparoscopy. In a prospective non-randomized study, transvaginal local injection of methotrexate resulted in up to 92.8 percent success rate in selected patients with hCG levels lower than 5,000 mIU/mL (72). In a random-

ized trial comparing local injection of methotrexate (1 mg/kg) and laparoscopic salpingostomy, the success rates were comparable in appropriately selected patients (73). In another study, advanced ectopic pregnancies were found to respond to higher doses of local methotrexate (100 mg). If fetal cardiac activity was present, potassium chloride injection was given in addition (74).

Local injection in lower doses has been used successfully in heterotopic pregnancy (75). However, systemic toxicity to the coexistent normal pregnancy may occur due to passage of the medication into the systemic circulation. This may be teratogenic to the normal fetus.

METHOTREXATE AND MIFEPRISTONE

In a randomized trial comparing methotrexate and placebo with methotrexate followed by 600 mg of mifepristone orally, there were no differences in success rates. However, in cases where the progesterone level was higher than 10 ng/mL, the administration of mifepristone along with methotrexate had a higher success rate (76).

Surgical Treatment

Surgery is recommended in hemodynamically unstable patients, tubal rupture, or failed medical therapy and in those who may be poorly compliant. It is also recommended in those who will not have access to a center capable of emergency surgery in case of tubal rupture. Ectopic pregnancies measuring larger than 3.5 cm, those with fetal cardiac activity, and those with hCG levels higher than 5,000 mIU/mL have a higher chance of failing medical therapy.

Rupture of an ectopic gestation has been reported even after forty-two days following administration of methotrexate (77). Signs of failing medical therapy and tubal rupture are worsening abdominal pain, hemodynamic instability, and inadequate fall, plateau, or rise of serum beta hCG.

Laparoscopy or Laparotomy

In two randomized trials, laparoscopy was found to be associated with a significantly lower blood loss, postoperative stay, and cost compared to laparotomy. The operative times were similar. Future fertility and rates of recurrent ectopic pregnancies were also comparable. The IUP were 56 and 58 percent following laparoscopy and laparotomy, respectively. As such, laparoscopy is a more appropriate first-line surgical intervention (78,79). In a Cochrane review by Hajenius et al., laparoscopy was found to be a better approach, although there was a higher risk of persistent trophoblastic tissue (80).

Salpingostomy or Salpingectomy

Salpingostomy is a conservative method of surgical management of an ectopic pregnancy. Salpingectomy is easier to perform and has a lesser risk of persistent trophoblastic tissue. For fertility preservation, most physicians tend to perform a linear salpingostomy in cases of unruptured ectopic pregnancies. The reproductive outcome for future IUP is comparable following either procedure. The recurrence of ectopic pregnancy is higher in those who undergo a conservative surgical approach (81). The rate of future IUP depends on the status of the contralateral fallopian tube. If a patient has history of tubal disease, the chances of normal pregnancies are reduced (82). Partial salpingectomy does not ensure absence of a future ectopic pregnancy. Extrauterine pregnancy may recur following a partial or a total salpingectomy. The rate of recurrence is around 10 percent, while it is around 15 percent in those who underwent a salpingostomy.

The location of the ectopic pregnancy within the tube is also an important factor to consider. Pregnancies in the ampullary portion typically grow out of the tube and salpingosotmy is recommended, whereas in cases of isthmic pregnancies, the conception grows in the tube and the tubal lumen gets severely damaged. In isthmic ectopic pregnancies, a partial salpingectomy may be preferable (83). Salpingectomy is preferable in cases of recurrent ectopic pregnancies in the same tube, a severely damaged tube, uncontrolled bleeding, large ectopic gestations (>5 cm), and in women not interested in future fertility (84).

To minimize blood loss during surgical intervention, a dilute solution of vasopressin can be injected in the mesosalpinx adjacent to the ectopic pregnancy. However, systemic toxicity, such as hypertension and bradycardia, can result from the injection of vasopressin.

Expectant Management

Observation can be an option in some cases. This will avoid the risks of surgery and side effects of methotrexate. Asymptomatic women with low serum hCG levels (<1,000 mIU/mL) can occasionally spontaneously abort. Without intervention, the success with expectant management is up to 88 percent in selected cases (85). Similarly, this approach may be appropriate in women with an early ectopic pregnancy and an already declining serum hGG levels. One-fifth of ectopic pregnancies present with falling hCG levels (86).

Management of Cervical Pregnancy

Cervical pregnancy is uncommon but can present with hemorrhage necessitating a hysterectomy. With earlier diagnosis, conservative management may be performed. Systemic methotrexate is the first-line therapy. Local injection of methotrexate along with potassium chloride when fetal cardiac activity is identified is another mode of therapy. Other approaches include embolization, foley catheter tamponade, curettage, and cervical cerclage. Success rate is around 80 percent (87). In cases where childbearing is complete, a simple hysterectomy may be performed.

Management of Interstitial Pregnancy

Interstitial pregnancy is difficult to diagnose. Once identified, either a laparotomy or laparoscopy may be performed to surgically evacuate the pregnancy. The bleeding may be reduced with injection of vasopressin into the myometrium or the use of endoloops or suture ligature. In a review of interstitial pregnancies by Lau et al., medical management is becoming an acceptable approach. Methotrexate injected locally or systemically has an overall success rate of 91 and 79 percent, respectively (14). Combined therapy involves instillation of methotrexate or potassium chloride after the aspiration of the conceptus.

Management of Abdominal Pregnancy

Abdominal pregnancies are difficult to diagnose and can reach the third trimester. The treatment is surgical. To avoid injury to involved organs, the placenta is left intact after the cord is clamped. Methotrexate is given concomitantly through

systemic IM injection. Rarely, arterial embolization may be necessary for control of bleeding.

Management of Heterotopic Pregnancy

Heterotopic pregnancy is usually treated surgically (3, 27). Partial or total salpingectomies are usually performed. This method will avoid the difficulty arising in following serum hCG levels later, particularly that persistent trophoblastic tissue can occur following salpingostomies. During these salpingectomies, electrocoagulation should be used cautiously to avoid compromise in blood supply to the remaining IUP.

In cases of heterotopic pregnancies involving an interstitial pregnancy, aspiration of the ectopic gestation and instillation of potassium chloride (KCl) may be performed. KCl is not toxic to the trophoblastic tissue but is lethal to pregnancies with fetal cardiac activity. In cases where the ectopic pregnancy does not have evidence of fetal cardiac activity, injection of lower doses of methotrexate may be used instead (49, 75). Local injections are performed under either ultrasound or laparoscopic guidance.

CONCLUSIONS

Ectopic pregnancy is a major health issue. Although the mortality rate is declining, it is the leading cause of maternal deaths in the first trimester. In assisted reproduction, due to a higher prevalence of tubal factor infertility and higher number of embryos transferred, the incidence of ectopic pregnancy may be increased. Reproductive endocrinologists and gynecologists need to be familiar with the diagnostic and therapeutic interventions. Although many studies have evaluated the role of single discriminatory tests to differentiate a normal viable from an ectopic pregnancy, clinical suspicion along with serial serum hCG levels and transvaginal ultrasonography remains the preferred method of diagnosis. Following superovulation and IVF, visualization of an IUP does not rule out an ectopic pregnancy. Heterotopic pregnancies are significantly higher in IVF patients and are difficult to diagnose before clinical symptoms occur. The optimal treatment of ectopic pregnancy in selected patients is conservative with methotrexate. When surgery is needed, laparoscopy rather than laparotomy is more appropriate, and salpingostomy is believed by many to preserve future fertility. Future research may reveal serum markers characteristic of an ectopic pregnancy. This will allow an even earlier diagnosis and more successful conservative medical treatments.

KEY POINTS

- Ectopic pregnancy is a life-threatening condition and accounts for 9 percent of all pregnancy-related deaths.
- Following IVF, the incidence of ectopic and heterotopic pregnancies is increased, mainly due to an increase in the number of embryo transferred and to the higher prevalence of tubal diseases in this population. Heterotopic pregnancy after IVF occurs in 1 percent of pregnancies.
- Knowledge of risk factors is helpful to follow more closely women predisposed to have an ectopic pregnancy. These risk factors include prior tubal surgeries, prior ectopic pregnancies, in utero exposure to DES, prior pelvic inflammatory diseases, smoking, superovulation, zygote intrafallopian transfer, assisted hatching, advancing the transfer

catheter up to the fundus, and tubal pathology. The latter is the most significant factor.

■ Mortality rate has significantly improved with the advances in diagnostic and therapeutic techniques. Ectopic pregnancy can be diagnosed at an early stage before tubal rupture.

■ The early diagnosis of ectopic pregnancy depends on serial hCG levels and sonographic findings. Future research involves identification of a serum marker for the abnormal implantation. Due to a higher incidence of heterotopic pregnancies, the adnexa should always be evaluated even after visualization of an intrauterine gestation. Sonographic findings suggestive of an ectopic pregnancy include adnexal ring, complex adnexal mass, echogenic fluid, and an extra-uterine gestation.

■ Conservative surgical or medical management have been comparable. Medical intervention with methotrexate, in appropriately selected patient, is more cost effective. The single-dose and multiple-dose protocols are associated with similar success rates and side effects.

■ When compared to laparotomy, laparoscopic surgery is considered to be less expensive, associated with lower blood loss and a shorter hospital stay. Conservative surgery is associated with higher persistent trophoblastic tissue.

■ In heterotopic pregnancies, the ectopic gestation is managed surgically to avoid methotrexate systemic toxicity to the IUP.

REFERENCES

1. Barbieri RL, Hornstein MD. Assisted reproduction. In: Strauss JF, Barbieri RL, eds. *Yen and Jaffe's Reproductive Endocrinology*. Fifth edn. Elsevier Saunders, Philadelphia, 2004: 839–73.

2. Ectopic pregnancy – United States, 1990-1992. *MMWR Morb Mortal Wkly Rep* 1995; 44: 46–8.

3. Rizk B, Tan SL, Morcos S, et al. Heterotopic pregnancies following in-vitro fertilization and embryo transfer. *Am J Obstet Gynecol.* 1991; 164(1): 161–4.

4. Abusheikha N, Marcus SF. Ectopic pregnancy following assisted reproductive technology. In: Brinsden PR, ed. *A Textbook of In Vitro Fertilization and Assisted Reproduction. The Bourn Hall Guide to Clinical and Laboratory Practice*, second edn. The Parthenon Publishing Group Inc., Pearl River, 1999: 333–42.

5. Jain A, Solima E, Luciano AA. Ectopic pregnancy. *J Am Assoc Gynecol Laparosc* 1997; 4: 513–31.

6. Department of Health and Human Services. CDC. 2002 Assisted Reproductive Technology (ART) Report, 2002. (Accessed December 1, 2006, at http://www.cdc.gov/ART/ART02/index.htm).

7. Rizk B, Morcos S, Avery S, et al. Rare ectopic pregnancies after in-vitro fertilization: one unilateral twin and four bilateral tubal pregnancies. *Hum Reprod* 1990; 5(8): 1025–28.

8. Rizk B, Lachelin GCL, Davies MC, et al. Ovarian pregnancy following in-vitro fertilization and embryo transfer. *Hum Reprod* 1990; 5(6): 763–4.

9. Dimitry ES, Rizk B. Ectopic pregnancy: epidemiology, advances in diagnosis and management. *Brit J Clin Pract* 1992; 46(1): 52–4.

10. Xiao HM, Gong F, Mao ZH, Zhang H, Lu GX. Analysis of 92 ectopic pregnancy patients after in vitro fertilization and embryo transfer. *Zhong Nan Da Xue Xue Bao Yi Xue Ban* 2006; 31: 584–7.

11. Cohen J, Mayaux MF, Guihard-Moscato ML, Schwartz D. In vitro fertilization and embryo transfer: a collaborative study of 1163 pregnancies on the incidence and risk factors of ectopic pregnancies. *Hum Reprod* 1986; 1: 255–8.

12. Seeber BE, Barnhart KT. Suspected ectopic pregnancy. *Obstet Gynecol* 2006; 107: 399–413.

13. Tal J, Haddad S, Gordon N, Timor-Tritsch I. Heterotopic pregnancy after ovulation induction and assisted reproductive technologies: a literature review from 1971 to 1993. *Fertil Steril* 1996; 66: 1–12.

14. Lau S, Tulandi T. Conservative medical and surgical management of interstitial ectopic pregnancy. *Fertil Steril* 1999; 72: 207–15.

15. Bouyer J, Coste J, Shojaei T, et al. Risk factors for ectopic pregnancy: a comprehensive analysis based on a large case-control, population based study in France. *Am J Epidemiol* 2003; 157: 185–94.

16. Gemzell C, Guillome J, Wang CF. Ectopic pregnancy following treatment with human chorionic gonadotropins. *Am J Obstet Gynecol* 1982; 143: 761–5.

17. Clayton HB, Schieve LA, Peterson HB, Jamieson DJ, Reynolds MA, Wright VC. Ectopic pregnancy risk with assisted reproductive technology procedures. *Obstet Gynecol* 2006; 107: 595–604.

18. Jun SH, Milki AA. Assisted hatching is associated with a higher ectopic pregnancy rate. *Fertil Steril* 2004; 81: 1701–3.

19. Strandell A, Thorburn J, Hamberger L. Risk factors for ectopic pregnancy in assisted reproduction. *Fertil Steril* 1999; 71: 282–6.

20. Dumesic DA, Damario MA, Session DR. Interstitial heterotopic pregnancy in a woman conceiving by in vitro fertilization after bilateral salpingectomy. *Mayo Clin Proc* 2001; 76: 90–2.

21. Yovich JL, Turner S, Murphy A. Embryo transfer technique as a cause of ectopic pregnancies in in vitro fertilization. *Fertil Steril* 1985; 44: 318–21.

22. Knutzen V, Stratton CJ, Shee G, McNamee PI, Huang TT, Soto-Albors C. Mock embryo transfer in early luteal phase, the cycle before in vitro fertilization and embryo transfer: a descriptive study. *Fertil Steril* 1992; 57: 156–62.

23. Marcus S, Brinsden P. Analysis of the incidence and risk factors associated with ectopic pregnancy following in vitro fertilization embryo transfer. *Hum Reprod* 1995; 10: 199–203.

24. Milki AA, Jun SH. Ectopic pregnancy rates with day 3 versus day 5 embryo transfer: a retrospective analysis. *BMC Pregnancy Childbirth* 2003; 3: 7.

25. Dor J, Seidman DS, Levran D, Ben-Rafael, Ben-Shlomo I, Mashiach S. The incidence of combined intrauterine and extrauterine pregnancy after in vitro fertilization and embryo transfer. *Fertil Steril* 1991; 55: 833–4.

26. Rizk B, Dimitry ES, Morcos S, Edwards RG, et al. *A multicenter study on combined intrauterine and extrauterine pregnancy after IVF.* 2nd joint meeting of ESHRE and European Sterility Congress Organization, Milan, Italy. August. *Reproduction* 1990; Abstract No. 377: 113–4.

27. Rizk B, Tan SL, Riddle A, et al. Heterotopic pregnancy and IVF. *British Fertility Society Annual Meeting, The London Hospital*, London, England, 1989.

28. Tang OS, Ng EH, So WW, Ho PC. Ultrasound-guided embryo transfer: a prospective randomized controlled trial. *Hum Reprod* 2001; 16: 2310–15.

29. Sallam HN, Sadek SS. Ultrasound-guided embryo transfer: a meta-analysis of randomized controlled trials. *Fertil Steril* 2003; 80: 1042–6.

30. Bouyer J, Coste J, Fernandez H, et al. Sites of ectopic pregnancy: a 10 year population based study of 1800 cases. *Hum Reprod* 2002; 17: 3224–30.

31. Comstock C, Huston K, Lee W. The ultrasonographic appearance of ovarian ectopic pregnancies. *Obstet Gynecol* 2005; 105: 42–45.

32. Martin JN Jr., Sessums JK, Marin RW, et al. Abdominal pregnancy: current concepts of management. *Obstet Gynecol* 1988; 71: 549–57.

33. Maymon R, Halperin R, Mendlovic S. Ectopic pregnancies in Caesarean section scars: the 8 year experience of one medical centre. *Hum Reprod* 2004; 19: 278–84.

34. Pisarska MD, Carson SA, et al. Ectopic pregnancy. *Lancet* 1998; 351: 1115–20.

35. Job-Spira N, Fernandez H, Bouyer J, et al. Ruptured tubal ectopic pregnancy: risk factors and reproductive outcome: results of a population-based study in France. *Am J Obstet Gynecol* 1999; 180: 938–44.

36. Kadar N, Caldwell BV, Romero R. A method of screening for ectopic pregnancy and its indications. *Obstet Gynecol* 1981; 58: 162–6.

37. Barnhart K, Sammel MD, Rinaudo PF, Zhou L, Hummel AC, Guo W. Symptomatic patients with an early viable intrauterine pregnancy: hCG curves redefined. *Obstet Gynecol* 2004; 104: 50–5.

38. Barnhart K, Sammel MD, Chung K, Zhou L, Hummel AC, Guo W. Decline of serum human chorionic gonadotropin and spontaneous complete abortion: defining the normal curve. *Obstet Gynecol* 2004; 104: 975–81.

39. Glastein IZ, Hornstein MD, Kahana MJ, et al. The predictive value of discriminatory human chorionic gonadotropin levels in the diagnosis of implantation outcome in in vitro fertilization cycles. *Fertil Steril* 1995; 63: 350–6.

40. Mol BW, Veen VF, Hajenius JP, et al. Diagnosis of ectopic pregnancy after in vitro fertilization and embryo transfer. *Fertil Steril* 1997; 68: 1027–32.

41. Chen CD, Ho HN, Wu MY, Chao KH, Chen SU, Yang YS. Paired human chorionic gonadotropin determination for the prediction of pregnancy outcome in assisted reproduction. *Hum Reprod* 12: 2538–41.

42. Rizk B, Marcus S, Fountain S, et al. The value of transvaginal sonography and hCG in the diagnosis of heterotopic pregnancy. 9th Annual meeting of the ESHRE, Thessaloniki, June. *Hum Reprod* 1993; Abstract No. 102.

43. Levi CS, Lyons EA, Lindsay DJ. Ultrasound in the first trimester. *Radiol Clin North Am* 1990; 28: 19–38.

44. Tongsong T, Pongsatha S. Transvaginal sonographic features in diagnosis of ectopic pregnancy. *Int J Gynaecol Obstet* 1993; 43: 277–83.

45. Brown DL, Doubilet PM. Transvaginal sonography for diagnosing ectopic pregnancy: positivity criteria and performance characteristics. *J Ultrasound Med* 1994; 13: 259–66.

46. Pellerito JS, Taylor KJ, Quedens-case C, et al. Ectopic pregnancy: evaluation with endovaginal color flow imaging. *Radiology* 1992; 183: 407–11.

47. Kirchler HC, Seebarcher S, Alge AA, Muller-Holzner E, Fessler S, Kolle D. *Obstet Gynecol* 1993; 82: 561–5.

48. Condous G, Okaro E, Khalid A, et al. The accuracy of transvaginal ultrasonography for the diagnosis of ectopic pregnancy prior to surgery. *Fertil Steril* 2005; 20: 1404–9.

49. Fernandez H, Gervaise A. Ectopic pregnancies after infertility treatment: modern diagnosis and therapeutic strategy. *Hum Reprod Update* 2004; 10: 503–13.

50. Bassil S, Gordts S, Nisolle M, Van Beers B, Donnez J. A magnetic resonance imaging approach for the diagnosis of a triplet corneal pregnancy. *Fertil Steril* 1995; 64(5): 1029–31.

51. Ginsburg ES, Frates MC, Rein MS, Fox JH, Hornstein MD, Friedman AJ. Early diagnosis and treatment of cervical pregnancy in an in vitro fertilization program. *Fertil Steril* 1994; 61: 966–9.

52. Kataoka ML, Togashi K, Kobayashi H, Inoue T, Fuji S, Konishi J. Evaluation of ectopic pregnancy by magnetic resonance imaging. *Hum Reprod* 1999; 14: 2644–50.

53. Takeuchi K, Yamada T, Oomori S, Ideta K, Moriyama T, Maruo T. Comparison of magnetic resonance imaging and ultrasonography in the early diagnosis of interstitial pregnancy. *J Reprod Med* 1999; 44: 265–8.

54. Izquierdo LA, Nicholas MC. Three-dimensional transvaginal sonography of interstitial pregnancy. *J Clin Ultrasound* 2003; 31: 484–7.

55. Ioannidis G, Sacks G, Reddy N, et al. Day 14 maternal serum progesterone levels predict pregnancy outcome in IVF/ICSI treatment cycles: a prospective study. *Hum Reprod* 2005; 20: 741–6.

56. Mol BW, Lijmer JG, Ankum WM, et al. The accuracy of single serum progesterone measurement in the diagnosis of ectopic pregnancy: a meta-analysis. *Hum Reprod* 1998; 13: 3220–7.

57. McCord ML, Muram D, Buster JE, et al. Single serum progesterone as a screen for ectopic pregnancy: exchanging specificity and sensitivity to obtain optimal test performance. *Fertil Steril* 1996; 66: 513–16.

58. Daniel Y, Geva E, Lerner-Geva L, et al. Levels of vascular endothelial growth factor are elevated in patients with ectopic pregnancy: is this a novel marker? *Fertil Steril* 1999; 72: 1013–17.

59. Fasouliotis SJ, Spandorfer SD, Witkin SS, Liu HC, Roberts JE, Rosenwaks Z. Maternal serum vascular endothelial growth factor levels in early ectopic and intrauterine pregnancies after in vitro fertilization treatment. *Feril Steril* 2004; 82: 309–13.

60. Saha PK, Gupta I, Ganguly NK. Evaluation of serum creatine kinase as a diagnostic marker for tubal pregnancy. *Aust NZ J Obstet Gynaecol* 1999; 39: 366–7.

61. Lipscomb GH, Bran D, McCord ML, Portera JC, Ling FW. Analysis of three hundred fifteen ectopic pregnancies treated with single-dose methotrexate. *Am J Obstet Gynecol* 1998; 178: 1354–8.

62. Lipscomb GH, Givens VA, Meyer NL, Bran D. Previous ectopic pregnancy as a predictor of failure of systemic methotrexate therapy. *Fertil Steril* 2004; 81: 1221–4.

63. Lipscomb GH, McCord ML, Stovall TG, Huff G, Portera G, Ling FW. Predictors of success of methotrexate treatment in women with tubal ectopic pregnancies. *N Engl J Med* 1999; 341: 1974–8.

64. Bixby S, Tello R, Kuligowska E. Presence of yolk sac on transvaginal sonography is the most reliable predictor of single-dose methotrexate treatment failure in ectopic pregnancy. *J Ultrasound Med* 2005; 24: 591–8.

65. Sowter MC, Farquhar CM, Petrie KJ, Gudex G. A randomised trial comparing single dose systemic methotrexate and laparoscopic surgery for the treatment of unruptured tubal pregnancy. *Br J Obstet Gynecol* 2001; 108: 192–203.

66. Sowter MC, Farquhar CM, Gudex G. An economic evaluation of single dose systemic methotrexate and laparoscopic surgery for the treatment of unruptured ectopic pregnancy. *Br J Obstet Gynecol* 2001; 108: 204–12.

67. Medical management of tubal pregnancy. ACOG Practice bulletin #3. American College of Obstetricians and Gynecologists, 1998.

68. Barnhart KT, Gosman G, Ashby R, Sammel M. The medical management of ectopic pregnancy: a meta-analysis comparing "single dose" and "multidose" regimens. *Obstet Gynecol* 2003; 101: 778–84.

69. Alleyassin A, Khademi A, Aghahosseini M, Safdarian L, Badenoosh B, Hamed EA. Comparison of success rates in the medical management of ectopic pregnancy with single dose and multiple dose administration of methotrexate: a prospective, randomized clinical trial. *Fertil Steril* 2006; 85: 1661–6.

70. Lipscomb GH, Givens VM, Meyer NL, Bran D. Comparison of multidose and single dose methotrexate protocols for the

treatment of ectopic pregnancy. *Am J Obstet Gynecol* 2005; 192: 1844–7.

71. Lipscomb GH, Meyer NL, Flynn DE, Peterson M, Ling FW. Oral methotrexate for treatment of ectopic pregnancy. *Am J Obstet Gynecol* 2002; 186: 1192–5.

72. Fernandez H, Benifla JL, Lelaidier C, Baton C, Frydman R. Methotrexate treatment of ectopic pregnancy: 100 cases treated by primary transvaginal injection under sonographic control. *Fertil Steril* 1993; 59: 773–7.

73. Fernandez H, Yves Vincent SC, Pauthier S, et al. Randomized trial of conservative laparoscopic treatment and methotrexate administration in ectopic pregnancy and subsequent fertility. *Hum Reprod* 1998; 13: 3239–43.

74. Tzafettas JM, Stephanatos A, Loufopoulos A, et al. Single high dose of local methotrexate for the management of relatively advanced ectopic pregnancies. *Fertil Steril* 1999; 71: 1010–13.

75. Oyawoye S, Chander B, Pavlovic B, Hunter J, Abdel Gadir A. Heterotopic pregnancy with aspiration of corneal/interstitial gestational sac and instillation of small dose of methotrexate. *Fetal diagn ther* 2003; 18: 1–4.

76. Rozenberg P, Chevret S, Camus E, et al. Medical treatment of ectopic pregnancies: a randomized clinical trial comparing methotrexate-mifepristone and methotrexate-placebo. *Hum Reprod* 2003; 18: 1802–8.

77. Lipscomb GH, Stovall TG, Ling FW. Nonsurgical treatment of ectopic pregnancy. *N Engl J Med* 2000; 343: 1325–9.

78. Murphy AA, Kettel LM, Nager CW, et al. Operative laparoscopy versus laparotomy for the management of ectopic pregnancy: a prospective trial. *Fertil Steril* 1992; 57: 1180–5.

79. Vermesh M, Silva PD, Rosen GF, et al. Management of unruptured ectopic gestation by linear salpingostomy: a prospective, randomized clinical trial of laparoscopy versus laparotomy. *Obstet Gynecol* 1989; 73: 400–4.

80. Hajenius PJ, Mol BW, Bossuyt PM, Ankum WM, Van Der Veen F. Interventions for tubal ectopic pregnancy. *Cochrane Database Syst Rev* 2000; (2):CD000324.

81. Silva PD, Schaper AM, Rooney B. Reproductive outcome after 143 laparoscopic procedures for ectopic pregnancy. *Obstet Gynecol* 1993; 81: 710–15.

82. Dubuisson JB, Morice P, Chapron C, De Gayffier A, Mouelhi T. Salpingectomy—the laparoscopic surgical choice for ectopic pregnancy. *Hum Reprod* 1996; 11: 1199–203.

83. Mueller MD. Ectopic pregnancy. In: Lebovic DI, Gordon JD, Taylor RN, Eds. *Reproductive Endocrinology and Infertility – Handbook for Clinicians.* First edn. Scrub Hill Press, Inc., Arlington, 2005: 113–23.

84. Tulandi T. *Surgical treatment of ectopic pregnancy and prognosis for subsequent fertility.* In: Rose BD ed. UpToDate. Waltham, MA, 2006.

85. Trio D, Stoblet N, Picciolo C, et al. Prognostic factors for successful expectant management of ectopic pregnancy. *Fertil Steril* 1995; 63: 15–19.

86. Shalev E, Peleg D, Tsabari A, et al. Spontaneous resolution of ectopic tubal pregnancy: natural history. *Fertil Steril* 1995; 63: 469–72.

87. Lemus JF. Ectopic pregnancy: an update. *Curr Opin Obstet Gynecol* 2000; 12: 369–75.

64

The Impact of Oxidative Stress on Female Reproduction and ART: An Evidence-Based Review

Sajal Gupta, Lucky Sekhon, Nabil Aziz, Ashok Agarwal

INTRODUCTION

Aerobic metabolism is associated with the generation of pro-oxidant molecules called free radicals or reactive oxygen species (ROS) that include the hydroxyl radicals, superoxide anion, hydrogen peroxide, and nitric oxide. There is a complex interaction of the pro-oxidants and antioxidants, resulting in the maintenance of the intracellular homeostasis. Whenever there is an imbalance between the pro-oxidants and antioxidants, a state of oxidative stress (OS) is initiated.

OVERVIEW OF OS AND ROS

Under normal conditions, paired electrons create stable bonds in biomolecules. However, if the bond is weak, it might break, leading to the formation of free radicals. Free radicals are defined as any species with one or more unpaired electrons in the outer orbit that include ROS such as superoxide, hydrogen peroxide, hydroxyl, and singlet oxygen radicals. They are generally very small molecules and are highly reactive due to the presence of unpaired valence shell electrons, initiating a cascade of reactions of more free radicals leading to uncontrolled chain reactions (1). Free radicals such as the superoxide radical are formed when high-energy electrons leak from the electron transport chain. The dismutation of superoxide results in the formation of hydrogen peroxide. The hydroxyl ion is a major type of ROS that is highly reactive, having the ability to modify purine and pyrimidines and cause damaging DNA strand breaks (2,3).

ROS are formed endogenously as a natural byproduct of aerobic metabolism and through the activity of various metabolic pathways and enzymes of oocytes and embryos. ROS may originate directly from the embryos or their surroundings. Exogenous factors such as oxygen consumption, metallic cations, visible light, amine oxidase, and spermatozoa can inflate the amount of ROS produced by embryos (3,4). Phagocytes, leukocytes, parenchymal steroidogenic cells, and endothelial cells are potential sources of ROS. Enzymes known to generate ROS include plasma membrane NADPH oxidase in phagocytes; oxidases of mitochondrial, microsomal, and peroxisomal origin; and cytosolic xanthine oxidase in the endothelial cells (5).

While controlled production of ROS is necessary for certain physiological functions, higher levels of ROS may overwhelm antioxidant capacity and cause OS to occur (6). Oxygen-free radicals may be produced normally, as a part of cellular metabolism, or as a part of the body's defense mechanisms. There is a complex interplay of cytokines, hormones, and other stressors that affects cellular generation of free radicals. Free radicals then further act through the modulation of gene expression and transcription factors. ROS have important roles in mediating tissue remodeling, hormone signaling, oocyte maturation, folliculogenesis, tubal function, ovarian steroidogenesis, cyclical endometrial changes, and germ cell function (2,3,7). However, during times of environmental stress, ROS levels can increase dramatically, leading to significant damage to cell structures. There is an assortment of antioxidants that hinder ROS production, scavenge ROS, and repair the cell damage they inflict (8,9). Nonenzymatic antioxidants consist of vitamin C, taurine, hypotaurine, cysteamine, and glutathione. Enzymatic antioxidants include superoxide dismutase, catalase, glutathione peroxidase, and glutaredoxin (6). Intracellular homeostasis is maintained as a result of the complex interaction between pro-oxidants and antioxidants.

OS is caused by the relentless formation of free radicals within an environment lacking proper antioxidant balance, resulting in pathological changes in cells. OS is thought to have cytotoxic effects by instigating the peroxidation of membrane phospholipids and altering most types of cellular molecules such as lipids, proteins, and nucleic acids. Subsequently, these changes could lead to an increase in membrane permeability, loss of membrane integrity, enzyme inactivation, structural damage to DNA, mitochondrial alterations, adenosine triphosphate depletion, and apoptosis (4,6,10). Free radicals can influence the oocyte, sperm, and embryos in their follicular fluid, tubal fluid, and peritoneal fluid microenvironments, thus influencing reproductive outcome (3).

PHYSIOLOGICAL ROLE OF ROS IN FEMALE REPRODUCTION

Various biomarkers of OS have been studied in the female reproductive tract. ROS and the transcripts of the various antioxidant enzymes have been localized and different studies have confirmed their presence in the female reproductive tract. ROS may act as important mediators in hormone signaling, oocyte maturation, ovarian steroidogenesis, ovulation, luteolysis, luteal maintenance in pregnancy, implantation, compaction, blastocyst development, germ cell function, and corpus luteum formation (2,6).

ROS and Folliculogenesis

ROS are thought to play a regulatory role in oocyte maturation, folliculogenesis, ovarian steroidogenesis, and luteolysis. Folliculogenesis refers to the maturation of the ovarian follicle, a densely packed shell of somatic cells that contains an immature oocyte. The developmental process entails the progression of a number of small primordial follicles into large preovulatory follicles. Follicular fluid ROS levels may represent the physiological ranges of ROS required for the normal development of the oocyte and the subsequent embryo (5). Controlled OS is thought to play a pivotal role in ovulation. Inflammatory-like modifications first occur in the theca interna and granulose layers of follicles in response to hCG during luteinization. The final stages of oocyte maturation before follicle rupture are orchestrated with the production of various cytokines, kinins, prostaglandins, proteolytic enzymes, nitric oxide, and steroids. These events have been demonstrated to influence blood flow in the ovaries during the periovulatory period (11).

The follicular fluid environment surrounding the oocytes may play a critical role in fertilization and embryo development, influencing IVF outcome parameters such as fertilization, embryo cleavage, and pregnancy rates (6). In addition to granulosa cells, growth factors, and steroid hormones, the follicular fluid environment contains leukocytes, macrophages, and cytokines, which can all produce ROS (5). Ovarian folliculogenesis also involves local autocrine and paracrine factors, such as the nitric oxide (NO) radical. Follicular NO is thought to be produced by either endothelial NO synthase or inducible NO synthase. NO exerts its effects through the activation of various iron-containing enzymes (12). Some studies have shown a relationship between NO concentrations and follicular growth and programmed follicular cell death, implicating the involvement of the free radical in both of these processes (13,14). Low concentrations of NO may prevent apoptosis, whereas at higher concentrations the effects of NO may be pathological, promoting cell death by peroxynitrite generation. Cells involved in steroidogenesis such as theca cells, granulose lutein cells, and hilus cells show stronger oxidative enzyme activity, suggesting an association between OS and ovarian steroidogenesis.

The expression of various markers of OS has been demonstrated in normally cycling ovaries (15,16). The concentrations of various OS markers have been demonstrated to be lower in the follicular fluid than in the serum, suggesting that follicular fluid contains high concentrations of antioxidant systems, which help protect an oocyte from oxidative damage (17). Primordial, primary, preantral, nondominant antral follicles in follicular phase, dominant follicles, and atretic follicles have been studied for superoxide dismutase (SOD) expression as a representative of enzymatic antioxidant (18) SOD is a metal-containing antioxidant enzyme that catalyzes the decomposition of superoxide into hydrogen peroxide and oxygen, protecting the cells from harmful free radicals of oxygen. SOD was found to be present in the ovary, particularly in the theca interna cells in the antral follicles (18). Therefore, theca interna cells may act as important protectors of the oocyte from OS during oocyte maturation. The preovulatory follicle has a potent antioxidant defense, which can be exhausted by intense peroxidation (19). Transferrin, a blood plasma glycoprotein that binds iron, is known to suppress ROS generation and has been proven an important factor for the successful development of follicles (20). The antioxidant factor, ascorbic acid can be depleted both by oxidant scavenging and impaired cellular recycling of vitamin C. Ascorbic acid deficiency characteristically results in ovarian atrophy, extensive follicular atresia, and the premature resumption of meiosis, illustrating the importance of its protective role against OS. Other antioxidant enzymes, such as catalase and other nonenzymatic antioxidants such as vitamin E, the peroxidase cofactor–reduced glutathione, and the carotenoid lutein have been suggested to protect the oocyte and the embryo from OS by detoxifying and neutralizing ROS production (5).

ROS and the Endometrial Cycle

OS is involved in the modulation of cyclical changes in the endometrium. Fluctuations in the expression of SOD in the endometrium have been investigated. Altered SOD and ROS levels have been demonstrated in the endometrium during the late-secretory phase, just before menstruation (21). An elevated lipid peroxide concentration and decreased SOD concentrations have been reported in human endometrium in the late-secretory phase, and these changes may be responsible for the breakdown of the endometrium, implicating the involvement of OS in the process of menstruation (21). The expression of endothelial NO synthase (NOS) and inducible NOS have been demonstrated in the human endometrium and the endometrial vessels (12,22). Endothelial NOS is distributed in glandular surface epithelial cells in the human endometrium (23). NO is thought to regulate the microvasculature of the endometrium. Expression of endothelial NOS mRNA has been detected in the midsecretory phase and late-secretory phase, indicating its involvement in the decidualization of the endometrium and menstruation. Endothelial NOS is also thought to bring about changes that prepare the endometrium for implantation. Recent studies exploring the underlying mechanisms of endometrial shedding have established that estrogen and progesterone withdrawal in endometrial cells cultured in vitro leads to a decrease in SOD activity, thereby increasing ROS concentrations. In turn, ROS may activate nuclear factor kappa B, which stimulates increased cyclooxygenase-2 mRNA expression and prostaglandin F2α synthesis, facilitating the physiological changes required for endometrial shedding and/or implantation to occur (21).

VEGF and Ang-2 are key regulators of endometrial angiogenesis. VEGF and Ang-2 are induced by hypoxia and ROS (24) and have been observed to be upregulated in the endometria of patients taking long-term progestin-only contraceptives. The changes in VEGF and Ang-2 expression are thought to play an integral role in producing the abnormally distended, fragile vessels that are the cause of abnormal uterine bleeding associated with long-term progestin-only contraceptives use. The later induces the abnormal angiogenesis by decreasing endometrial blood flow, inducing hypoxia (25). In vitro, hypoxia was demonstrated to increase OS by inducing the expression of nitrotyrosine, a marker of peroxinitrite anion generation in cultured endometrial microvascular endothelial cells. OS is thus implicated in the genesis of endometrial pathophysiology seen in long-term progestin-only contraceptives users (25).

ROLE OF OS IN FEMALE INFERTILITY

OS induces infertility in women through a variety of mechanisms. We have discussed how ovarian follicles experiencing OS can lead to direct damage to oocytes. Oocytes and spermatozoa can also experience direct damage, which can lead to impaired fertilization due to an environment of OS in the peritoneal cavity. Even when fertilization occurs, apoptosis leading to embryo fragmentation, implantation failure, abortion, or congenital abnormalities in offspring can occur. OS in the fallopian tubes can cause direct adverse effects on the embryo. Defects in the endometrium, which normally supports the embryo and its development, can arise when there is an ROS-antioxidant imbalance in the female reproductive tract (26). ROS-antioxidant imbalance is also implicated in luteal regression and insufficient luteal hormonal support for the continuation of a pregnancy (8). OS has been implicated in many other causes of infertility, such as endometriosis, hydrosalpinx, polycystic ovarian disease, unexplained infertility, and recurrent pregnancy loss (27).

OS and Endometriosis

The association between endometriosis and infertility remains a highly controversial topic of debate. Severe cases of infertility associated with endometriosis are thought to possibly result from mechanical blockage of the sperm-egg union by endometriomata, adhesions, and pelvic anatomy malformations. However, the pathogenesis of infertility experienced by patients with mild to moderate endometriosis and with no anatomical distortions is poorly understood.

Women with endometriosis have been reported to have an increased volume of peritoneal fluid, containing increased concentrations of peritoneal macrophages, cytokines, and prostaglandins. Activated peritoneal macrophages have been implicated in the pathology of endometriosis as they may be responsible for increased production of ROS (28). It has been suggested that ROS may increase growth and adhesion of endometrial cells in the peritoneal cavity, promoting endometriosis adhesions and infertility (29).

There are several hypotheses as to why OS may occur in relation to endometriosis. There is considerable evidence that suggests that menstrual reflux transplants cell debris into the peritoneal cavity and is associated with the development of endometriosis. Erythrocytes release hemoglobin and hem, which act as proinflammatory factors. Hem contains the redox-generating iron molecule (30). The presence of iron, (31), macrophages (32), and/or environmental contaminants such as polychlorinated biphenyls (33) in the peritoneal fluid may disturb the balance between ROS and antioxidants, resulting in endometriosis and tissue growth. Circulating levels of OS from other sources may also contribute to the pathogenesis of disease. A definitive conclusion about the association between OS and endometriosis is difficult to reach as most of the research studies investigating this relationship differ greatly in many regards including the selection of the control population, eligibility criteria, markers of OS and antioxidant status, and the biological medium in which OS was measured (1).

An increase in ROS production by peritoneal fluid macrophages, with increased lipid peroxidation, has been demonstrated in endometriosis patients (34), whereas other researchers have reported contrary findings (10). Epitopes produced as a result of lipid peroxidation have been demonstrated in macrophage-enriched areas of both the endometrium and endometriosis implants. Jackson et al. reported a weak association between the thiobarbituric acid reactive substances, a measure of overall OS and endometriosis, after adjusting for confounding factors such as age, BMI, gravidity, serum vitamin E, and serum lipid levels (35). Women with idiopathic infertility and endometriosis have been seen to have higher peritoneal fluid concentrations of ROS than tubal ligation control patients (10). However, this effect has not been observed to correlate with the severity of endometriosis and was not observed to be significant, suggesting that in patients with the disease, peritoneal fluid ROS may not directly cause infertility. OS may contribute to angiogenesis in ectopic endometrial implants and aids the progression of endometriosis by increasing VEGF production (24). This effect is partly mediated by glycodelin, a glycoprotein whose expression is increased by OS. Glycodelin may act as an autocrine factor within ectopic endometrial tissue by augmenting VEGF expression (24).

Greater amounts of NO and NOS have been detectable in the endometrium of women with endometriosis (1). Increased expression of inducible NOS and increased levels of endothelial NOS in the glandular endometrium have been reported in patients with endometriosis. Variations in the expression of the endothelial NOS gene may be involved in endometrial angiogenesis, thus modulating the process of endometriosis. These changes in NOS expression could also alter endometrial receptivity and impair embryo implantation. Some studies have found the peritoneal fluid from patients with endometriosis to contain increased concentrations of NO. Elevated concentrations of NO, such as those produced by activated macrophages, can hinder infertility in a myriad of ways, including changing the composition of the peritoneal fluid environment that hosts the processes of ovulation, gamete transport, sperm-oocyte interaction, fertilization, and early embryonic development (1).

Endometriosis patients have exhibited increased lipid-protein complex modification in the endometrium. Lipid peroxide concentrations have been demonstrated to be the highest among patients with endometriosis. The peritoneal fluid of women with endometriosis has been observed to have insufficient antioxidant defense, having a lower total antioxidant capacity (TAC) and significantly reduced levels of the individual antioxidant enzymes such as SOD (36,37). The concentrations of SOD have been demonstrated at statistically significant lower concentrations in infertile women with endometriosis compared with fertile controls.

Various studies have failed to demonstrate a difference in ROS, NO, lipid peroxide, and antioxidant levels in the peritoneal fluid of women with endometriosis compared to fertile women (38,10). This might be explained by the fact that only persistent markers of OS, such as enzymes or stable byproducts of oxidative reactions, may still be detected at the time endometriosis is diagnosed. Another possible reason might be that OS occurs only locally and therefore would not result in an increase in total peritoneal fluid ROS concentrations.

OS may contribute to the pathogenesis of endometriosis via molecular genetic pathways. Investigation of endometriotic tissue has yielded results showing gene deletion of mitochondrial

DNA resulting in its rearrangement. Differences in gene expression levels in ectopic and eutopic endometria have been elucidated, including 904 differentially expressed genes and the differential expression of the glutathione-S-transferase gene family, which are implicated in the metabolism of the potent antioxidant glutathione. The cellular responses to OS, which include cell proliferation and angiogenesis, may also be determined by differential gene expression (39).

An imbalance between ROS and antioxidant levels may play an important role in the pathogenesis of endometriosis-associated infertility. Increased concentrations of ROS in the oviductal fluid could have adverse effects on oocyte and spermatozoa viability and the process of fertilization and embryo transport in the oviduct. Also, the associated presence of activated neutrophils and macrophages and proinflammatory factors in the oviductal fluid could significantly amplify ROS production by foci of endometriosis (29). A significant increase in ROS production could result in oxidative damage to the sperm plasma and acrosomal membranes, leading to a loss of motility and the ability of spermatozoa to bind and penetrate the oocyte, respectively. OS resulting in DNA damage may lead to failed fertilization, reduced embryo quality, pregnancy failure, and spontaneous abortion.

Therapies for autoimmune diseases, which share many similarities with endometriosis, may be useful in treating endometriosis. Pathological levels of tumor necrosis factor alpha (TNF-α) may be present in the female reproductive tract in women with endometriosis. In the female endometrium, TNF-α plays a role in the normal physiology of endometrial proliferation and shedding and also in the pathogenesis of endometriosis (40). Abnormally high levels of TNF-α have been demonstrated in the peritoneal fluid of women with endometriosis, and an increase in its levels appears to be positively correlated with the stage of endometriosis (40,41).

It has been shown in an in vitro experiment that spermatozoa quality declined following incubation with TNF-α in a dose-dependent and time-dependent manner (42). This may offer some explanation for the endometriosis-associated infertility. In the same experiment, sperm motility and membrane and chromatin integrities were higher in the samples incubated with TNF-α plus infliximab (a monoclonal antibody that binds both soluble and membrane forms of TNF-α, neutralizing its toxic effects) than in the samples treated with TNF-α only. It has been suggested that infliximab could potentially be used to help treat female infertility caused by endometriosis in those with elevated levels of TNF-α in their peritoneal fluid.

Another drug being investigated for its potential use in the treatment of endometriosis-associated infertility is pentoxifylline, a $3',5'$-nucleotide phosphodiesterase inhibitor. Pentoxifylline has potent immunomodulatory properties and has been shown to significantly reduce the embryotoxic effects of hydrogen peroxide (43).

OS and Hydrosalpinx

Although IVF is considered to be the best fertility treatment for hydrosalpinx, some investigations have shown the presence of a hydrosalpinx to decrease the success rates of IVF. Fluid within the hydrosalpinx appears to reduce embryo implantation rates and increase the risk of miscarriage, motivating some physicians to advise removing the tube or separating it from the uterus prior to undergoing IVF. The adverse effect of hydro-

salpinges has been shown to be reversible by salpingectomy prior to IVF (44).

The exact mechanism by which hydrosalpingeal fluid (HSF) induces its embryotoxic effect is unknown, but it is hypothesized that an OS-mediated mechanism may be involved in this phenomenon. Lab studies have demonstrated the presence of ROS, antioxidants, and lipid peroxidation products in hydrosalpingeal fluid. At low levels, ROS in the tubal fluid has been shown to be positively correlated with blastocyst development. Low levels of ROS, beneath a threshold for being deleterious to embryos, may represent normal ROS generation by a functional endosalpinx, whereas extensive endosalpingeal damage may yield nondetectable levels of ROS in the HSF. Therefore, detection of ROS at low concentrations might serve as a marker of normal tubal secretory function. Levels of IL-6 in the HSF were found to be positively correlated with blastocyst development rates, suggesting its contribution in preventing some tubal fluid samples from becoming embryotoxic (Bedaiwy et al., 2005). IL-1b, which is known to inhibit ovarian follicular cell apoptosis, was also found in all tubal fluid samples tested and may be a marker of normal tubal secretory function (45).

Fluid leaking from Fallopian tubes enlarged with hydrosalpinx has been shown to exert a concentration-dependent embryotoxic effect (46). The presence of toxic substances, at high concentrations, in HSF is thought to mediate its negative effects. HSF has also been shown to reduce endometrial integrins, which may facilitate implantation. HSF flow into the endometrial cavity may lead to mechanical flushing of the embryos from the uterus. Excision of hydrosalpinges is suggested to restore integrins to normal and improve implantation rates. The tubal epithelium may secrete cytokines, leukotrienes, or prostaglandins into the sequestered fluid that could directly alter endometrial function. Cytokines, associated with inflammatory processes and involved in embryotoxic effects, have been implicated in the poor outcome of IVF-ET in women with distally occluded fallopian tubes. Bedaiwy et al. (2005) studied the biochemical nature of HSF and found TNF-α in 100 percent of all HSF samples. TNF-α is a cytotoxic, angiogenic cytokine, produced by macrophages and many other types of cells.

OS and Unexplained Infertility

It is hypothesized that elevated levels of ROS disturb the pro-oxidant/antioxidant balance in peritoneal fluid and may be the cause of infertility in women who do not have any other obvious cause. Elevated levels can damage the ovum after its release from the ovary, the zygote/embryo, and the spermatozoa, which are very sensitive to OS (8). Studies comparing ROS levels in peritoneal fluid between women undergoing laparoscopy for infertility evaluation and fertile women undergoing tubal ligation have shown levels of peritoneal fluid ROS to be significantly higher in patients with unexplained infertility compared with the fertile women (10). Elevated ROS levels in patients with unexplained infertility imply reduced levels of antioxidants such as vitamin E and glutathione, resulting in a reduced ability to scavenge ROS and neutralize its toxic effects (10). This was demonstrated in a study where concentrations of antioxidants in patients with unexplained infertility have been shown to be significantly lower than in fertile patients, suggesting a potential use for antioxidant supplementation to treat the high levels of ROS in patients with idiopathic infertility.

AGE-RELATED FERTILITY DECLINE, MENOPAUSE, AND ROS

The fertility potential of the average woman begins to decline appreciably at the age of thirty-five years and begins to decline dramatically beyond the age of forty years. ROS may play a role in age-related decrease in estrogen production. SOD and glutathione peroxidase expression decreases in the ovary from the premenopausal to menopausal period (47). SOD and glutathione peroxidase levels are significantly and positively correlated with aromatase enzyme activity.

Higher levels of OS have been demonstrated in women of advanced reproductive age undergoing IVF (48). Ovarian senescence is thought to result from increased OS in the follicular fluid. Free radical–induced damage may be implicated, at least partly, for the age-related decline in quantity and quality of follicle reserves (49). This process may involve oxidative damage to mitochondrial DNA, proteins, and lipids. ROS are known to significantly perturb the intracellular calcium (Ca) homeostasis in the oocytes and cause aging of the oocytes (50). IVF patients of advanced reproductive age may exhibit a reduced expression of genes mainly involved in the neutralization of ROS (48) such as decrease in the expression of SOD1, SOD2, and catalase mRNA content, representing the first evidence that reproductive aging can downregulate the gene expression of granulosa cells (51). This downregulation of genes involved in the front-line defense against ROS was associated with the accumulation of oxidative damage mainly affecting mitochondria. Age-related changes that have adverse consequences in granulosa cells may be one of the mechanisms by which advanced reproductive aging causes a reduction in the developmental competence of oocytes. These changes may lead to effects often seen in pregnancies in older women, which include damaged cytoskeleton fibers, causing degeneration or apoptosis. In addition, impaired fertilization and poor-quality embryos, most of which are aneuploid, result from the aging process.

OS AND MALE GAMETES

The paternal genome is of paramount importance in normal embryo and fetal development. ROS-induced sperm damage during sperm transport through the seminiferous tubules and epididymis is one of the most important mechanisms leading to sperm DNA damage (52–57). These result in single- and double-stranded DNA fragmentation (primary damage) and the generation of secondary DNA damage of the 8-OH-2′-deoxyguanosine type. Fertilization of the oocyte by a spermatozoon with unrepaired primary or secondary DNA damage may result in implantation failure, embryo development arrest, pregnancy loss, or birth defects (58–61). In addition, recent studies suggest that sperm DNA fragmentation may be associated with an increase in sperm aneuploidy (61,62). Sperm aneuploidy is mainly the result of meiotic alterations during spermatogenesis (63). ROS- and/or caspase or endonuclease-induced DNA fragmentation may be increased in aneuploid sperm during passage through the epididymis (57). Therefore, couples diagnosed with recurrent pregnancy loss may benefit from testing of sperm DNA fragmentation.

OS AND ITS IMPACT ON ART

OS has an important role in ovulation process. We discussed above how follicular fluid microenvironment has a crucial role in determining the quality of the oocyte. The oocyte quality in turn impacts the fertilization rate and the embryo quality. OS markers have been localized in the follicular fluid in patients undergoing IVF/embryo transfer (5,64–66).

Low intrafollicular oxygenation has been associated with decreased oocyte developmental potential as reflected by increasing frequency of oocyte cytoplasmic defects, impaired cleavage, and abnormal chromosomal segregation in oocytes from poorly vascularized follicles (67). ROS may be responsible for causing increased embryo fragmentation, resulting from increasing apoptosis (68) (refer Figure 64.1). Thus, increasing ROS levels are not conducive to embryo growth and result in impaired development. Current studies are focusing on the ability of growth factors to protect embryos cultured in vitro from the detrimental effects of ROS such as apoptosis. These growth factors are normally found in the fallopian tubes and endometrium. The factors being investigated are insulin growth factor, and epidermal growth factor in mouse embryos, which in many respects are similar to human embryos (69).

The effects of follicular OS on oocyte maturation, fertilization, and pregnancy have also been studied (66). Follicular fluid ROS and lipid peroxidation levels may be markers for success with IVF. Patients who became pregnant following IVF or ICSI had higher lipid peroxidation levels and TAC in follicular fluid. However, both markers were unable to predict embryo quality. Pregnancy rates and levels of lipid peroxidation and TAC demonstrated a positive correlation. Levels of follicular fluid ROS were reported to be significantly lower in patients who did not become pregnant compared with those who became pregnant (5). Thus, intrafollicular ROS levels may be viewed as a potential marker for predicting success with IVF. OS in follicular fluid from women undergoing IVF was inversely correlated with the women's age (48). Using a thermochemiluminescence assay, the slope was found to positively correlate with maximal serum estradiol levels, number of mature oocytes, and number of cleaved embryos and inversely with the number of gonadotrophin ampoules used. The pregnancy rate achieved was 28 percent, and all pregnancies occurred when the thermochemiluminescence amplitude was small. This is in agreement with another study that reported minimal levels of OS were necessary for achieving pregnancy (66). A recent large study in 156 couples undergoing ART demonstrated high follicular fluid levels of homocysteine and their inverse association with embryo quality in women with endometriosis (70). Elevated homocysteine levels are caused by heightened OS and lead to poor oocyte and embryo quality in women with endometriosis. However, the view that low levels of ROS in follicular fluid have beneficial effects on IVF outcomes (4) is not universally held. Recent studies have reported that high levels of ROS in follicular fluid lead to decreased fertilization potential of the oocytes in ART cycles (71).

Other OS markers such as thiobarbituric acid–reactive substances, conjugated dienes, and lipid hydroperoxides have been studied in the preovulatory follicular fluid (17). No correlation was seen between these markers and IVF outcome (fertilization rates or biochemical pregnancies) (17).

8-Hydroxy-2-deoxyguanosine is a reliable indicator of DNA damage caused by OS. This compound is an indicator of OS in

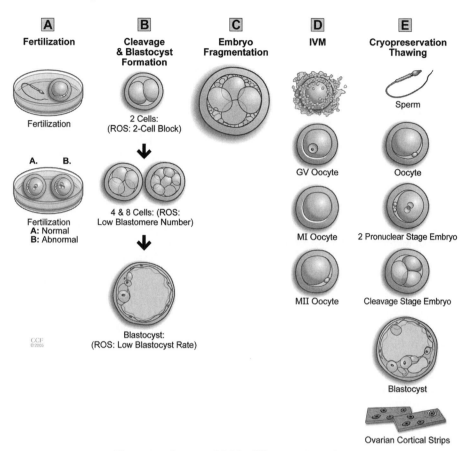

Figure 64.1. Impact of OS in different ART settings.

various other disease processes such as renal carcinogenesis and diabetes mellitus. Higher levels of 8-hydroxy 2-deoxyguanosine were associated with lower fertilization rates and poor embryo quality (72). High levels of 8-hydroxy 2-deoxyguanosine are also found in granulosa cells of patients with endometriosis, and this may impair the quality of oocytes.

Bedaiwy et al. in a study from our group reported that slow early embryo development (seven cells on day 3), high fragmentation (10 percent), and reduced formation of morphologically normal blastocysts may be associated with increased levels of ROS in the culture media on day 1. Moreover, high day 1 ROS levels in culture media had no relationship with the fertilization rate (FR) in conventional IVF cycles but were significantly related to higher FRs and blastocyst development rates with ICSI cycles (46).

Literature reports have shown that women who became pregnant after IVF therapy had a tendency toward higher levels of TAC in their follicular fluid compared to those who did not achieve pregnancy (66). The mean TAC in fluid from follicles that yielded oocytes that were successfully fertilized was significantly greater than the mean TAC from follicular fluid associated with oocytes that were not. Similarly, mean glutathione peroxidase levels were increased, in follicles yielding oocytes that were subsequently fertilized (73). Conversely, the mean TAC of fluid from follicles whose oocyte gave rise to an embryo that survived till time of transfer was reported to be significantly lower than the mean TAC in follicular fluid associated with oocytes that gave rise to nonviable embryos (64). TAC levels in day 1 culture media appear to be an additional biochemical marker reflecting the OS status during early embryonic growth. Day 1 TAC levels signif-

icantly correlated with the clinical pregnancy rates in ICSI cycles (74). On a different front, high TAC level has been reported as a marker for poor response to ovulation induction in women with polycystic ovarian syndrome (75).

Levels of selenium in follicular fluid of women with unexplained infertility were found to be lower than those in women with tubal factor or male factor infertility (73). Higher levels of SOD activity were present in fluid from follicles whose oocytes did not fertilize compared with those that did (76). These discrepancies may be due to the fact that the studies measured different parameters.

Smoking has been associated with prolonged and dose-dependent adverse effects on ovarian function (77). According to a meta-analysis, the overall value of the odds ratio for the risk of infertility associated with smoking was 1.60 [95 percent confidence interval (CI) 1.34–1.91]. ARTs, including IVF, are further shedding light on the effects smoking has on follicular health. Intrafollicular exposure to cotinine increases lipid peroxidation in the follicle.

Further large studies need to determine the correlation between ROS activity levels and TAC levels in the follicular fluid on ovulation process, oocyte quality, developmental competence, and fertilization potential of oocytes, as ROS may be having differing effects at different stages of ART.

REDOX AND EMBRYO DEVELOPMENT

Physiological levels of redox may be important for embryogenesis (refer Figure 64.2). Overproduction of ROS is detrimental

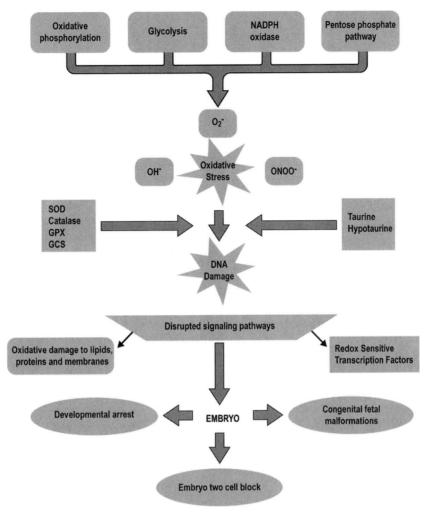

Figure 64.2. Redox and embryo development.

for the embryo, resulting from impaired intracellular milieu and disturbed metabolism (78,79). OS can be generated in the sperms and leucocytes and on sperm-mediated oocyte activation and on the activation of the embryonic genome. Oxidative phosphorylation, NADPH oxidase, and xanthine oxidase are predominant sources of ROS generation in oocytes and embryos. Oxidative phosphorylation is a process necessary for the generation of ATP in order to meet embryo energy requirements, and it results in ROS production. Electrons leak from the electron transport chain at the inner mitochondrial membranes. These electrons are transferred to the oxygen molecule, resulting in an unpaired electron in the orbit. This leads to the generation of the superoxide molecule. The other points of generation of ROS are the cytoplasmic NADPH oxidase, cytochrome p450 enzymes, and the xanthine oxidoreductase enzymes. Excessive OS can have deleterious effects on the cellular milieu and can result in impaired cellular growth in the embryo or apoptosis resulting in embryo fragmentation. Thus, OS-mediated damage of macromolecules plays a role in fetal embryopathies. Thioredoxins are a widely distributed group of small proteins with strong reducing activities, and their expression was found to be essential for early differentiation and morphogenesis of the mouse embryo (80).

Deficient folate levels in the mother result in elevated homocysteine levels. The homocysteine-induced OS has been proposed as a potential factor for causing apoptosis and disrupting palate development and causing cleft palate (81). OS-mediated damage of the macromolecules has been proposed as a mechanism of thalidomide-induced embryopathy (82,83). Hyperglycemia/diabetes-induced downregulation of cycloxygenase-2 gene expression in the embryo results in low PGE2 levels and diabetic embryopathy (84).

Preimplantation embryos are not a static entity as demonstrated by sequential culture. Embryos pass through many hurdles during their developmental process and have ever-changing needs. Preimplantation embryonic development is associated with a change in preference of energy metabolism pathways. Embryos possess inherent energy requirements that are met by ATP generation from oxidative phosphorylation and glycolysis. Blastocyst development is accompanied by a shift in pathway of ATP generation from oxidative phosphorylation to an increasing dependence on ATP generation from glycolysis. Increased glucose uptake in the postcompaction stage meets the increased energy demands of an embryo. Blastocyst development from the two-cell-stage embryo is modulated by the ratio of pyruvate to lactate in the culture medium as this in turn affects the intracellular pyruvate to lactate ratio. Excessive generation of ROS occurs at certain critical points accompanied by increased energy demands such as embryonic genome activation, embryonic compaction, and hatching (85). Minimal levels of ROS may play a role during the critical points of embryogenesis. Excessive levels of ROS have adverse impacts on embryo quality and competence (6,78,86). The literature reports that a reduction in OS levels leads to better ART outcomes (87,88).

In the ART setting, a majority of retrieved mature oocytes fertilize, but of these only up to 70 percent undergo the first three cleavage divisions during the first three days in culture (89). Less than 50 percent of the cleaved embryos undergo cavitation and proceed to blastocyst formation by day 5 in culture (90,91). Similarly, only approximately 30 percent of day 3 embryos will progress to develop into morphologically normal blastocysts. OS has been implicated as a causative factor associated with the poor fertility outcomes in ART.

During the first trimester, an embryo grows best under low oxygen concentrations as documented in maternofetal oxygen diffusion studies (92). In human embryos, elevated blastulation rates have been reported by decreasing the oxygen tension (5 percent O_2) and maintaining low illumination levels throughout the embryo manipulation period (93). High O_2 concentrations during in vitro cultures lead to an increase in hydrogen peroxide (H_2O_2) levels, DNA fragmentation, and reduction in embryo development competency. ROS such as H_2O_2 are responsible for programmed cell death, also known as apoptosis, and may cause the failure of blastocyst development and preimplantation embryo death. An animal study has emphasized the protective role of the enzyme G6PD (glucose 6-phosphate dehydrogenase) against OS. The protection of the embryos against OS prevented the embryopathies (94).

Early embryo development in mammals, from fertilization through differentiation of principal organ systems, occurs in a low-oxygen environment (83). A marginal improvement in preimplantation embryonic viability has been reported under low oxygen concentrations in patients undergoing IVF and ICSI (95). Lower concentrations of oxygen in in vitro culture of porcine embryos decreased the H_2O_2 content and resulted in reduced DNA fragmentation, which thereby improved developmental ability (96). The higher oxygen concentrations of 20 percent have been associated with lower developmental competence. Accelerated development was seen under low (5 percent) oxygen concentrations.

OS AND GAMETE CRYOPRESERVATION

ROS are generated from the semen cells during the cooling process (97). Cryopreservation enhances lipid peroxidation, as ROS-induced membrane lipid damage, DNA damage, and apoptosis have been demonstrated in frozen spermatozoa (97). Reduction of antioxidant defenses also adversely affects cryopreserved spermatozoa. Supplementation of the thawing media with antioxidants such as glutathione helps improve spermatozoa function and in vitro fertilizing capabilities (98). Cryopreserved oocytes because of oxidative toxicity were reported to show DNA damage on comet assay (99).

Ovarian transplantation and oocyte cryopreservation continue to have poor outcomes, which have been proposed to be caused by ischemia and resultant OS. Ischemia time strongly correlates with the ovarian tissue damage, and treatment with

the antioxidant vitamin C reduces the stromal tissue apoptosis and damage (100).

STRATEGIES TO OVERCOME OS IN ASSISTED REPRODUCTION

ROS may originate from the male or female gamete or the embryo or indirectly from the surroundings, which includes the cumulus cells, leucocytes, and culture media (refer Figure 64.1). In human IVF/ICSI procedures, the clinical pregnancy rates have remained unchanged at 30–40 percent (101). It is hypothesized that the altered redox state in in vitro conditions may play a role in poor ART outcomes, and controlling OS may improve ART outcomes (68,78). Fertilization and embryo development in vivo occur in an environment of low oxygen tension (83). It has been noted that blastocyst development in vitro always lags behind blastocyst development in vivo as there is a variation in the ability of IVF media and its components to scavenge ROS and prevent DNA damage and apoptosis (102).

During ART procedures, it is important to emulate in vivo conditions by avoiding conditions that promote ROS generation. Achieving that has been shown to lead to a reduction in blastocyst degeneration, increased blastocyst development rates, increased hatching of blastocysts, and reduction in embryo apoptosis, and other degenerative pro-oxidant influence has been reported (78). The available strategies include the following.

1. Ensuring in vitro culture under low–oxygen tension conditions: During culture, low–oxygen tension conditions improve the implantation and pregnancy rate better than high oxygen tension (103).
2. Metal ion culture media supplementation: It has been shown that metal ions may enhance the production of oxidants. As a result, it was suggested that it may be useful to add metal ion–chelating agents to culture media to decrease the production of oxidants (103).
3. Enzymatic and nonenzymatic antioxidant culture media supplementation: Higher implantation and clinical pregnancy rates are reported when antioxidant-supplemented media is used rather than standard media without antioxidants. Various nonenzymatic antioxidants including beta-mercaptoethanol (104), protein (102), vitamin E (96), vitamin C (105,106), cysteamine (107,108), cysteine (109), taurine and hypotaurine (110), and thiols (111) added to the culture media with the purpose of improving the developmental ability of the embryos by reducing the effects of ROS.

Also, the addition of the enzymatic antioxidant, for example, SOD to the culture media prevented the deleterious effects of OS on sperm viability and on the embryo development both in vivo and in vitro (112). This was demonstrated by increased development of the two-cell-stage embryos to the expanded blastocyst stage in the SOD-supplemented media. Mechanical removal of ROS in IVF/ET has been studied as a method to improve IVF outcome (113). The rinsing of cumulus oophorus has been shown to overcome the deleterious effects of ROS in patients with ovarian endometriosis (113).

4. Control of sperm ROS production and sperm chromatin damage: Spermatozoa are particularly susceptible to ROS-induced damage because their plasma membranes contain

large quantities of polyunsaturated fatty acids and their cytoplasm contains low concentrations of the scavenging enzymes (114). The seminal plasma is rich in antioxidants and protects the spermatozoa from DNA damage and lipid peroxidation (115). Sperm preparation techniques such as density gradient centrifugation and glass wool separation reduce the ROS formation by removing the leucocytes, cellular debris, and immotile spermatozoa. It has been shown that sperm preparation methods affect ART outcomes. Sperm preparation by centrifugation may be associated with generation of ROS. Taurine, an essential amino acid, is an antioxidant that has been shown to improve spermatozoa motility, capacitation, and fertilization and support early embryonic development (116). Also many antioxidant (vitamins C and E, glutathione and beta-carotene, pentoxifylline, etc.) supplementation of sperm preparation media have been shown to improve sperm motility and acrosome reaction (117,118). Supplementation of IVF media with N-tert-butyl hydroxylamine and SOD/catalase mimetics was reported to block the breakdown of sperm chromatin (119). Standard sperm preparation media are supplemented with human serum albumin, polyvinylpyrrolidine, and HEPES, which are DNA protectors (120). Adding ascorbate during cryopreservation reduces the levels of hydrogen peroxide and thus the OS in mammalian embryos (89). As a consequence, embryo development improved with enhanced blastocyst development rates.

5. Reducing sperm-oocyte coincubation time: Reports suggest that a prolonged sperm-oocyte coincubation time (sixteen to twenty hours) increases the generation of ROS. Two prospective randomized controlled studies have advocated using a shorter sperm-oocyte coincubation time (121,122). Coincubation times of one to two hours resulted in better quality embryos and significantly improved fertilization and implantation rates (123).

TROPHOBLASTIC OS AND PREGNANCY: ROLE IN ABORTIONS, HYDATIDIFORM MOLE, AND PREECLAMPSIA

Although oxygen is essential for sustaining life in cells, it undergoes extensive metabolism that can result in the production of toxic derivatives. This metabolism is mainly confined to the electron transport chain in the mitochondria that ultimately results in the generation of ATP, which supports cell metabolism. The end products of oxygen metabolism may include molecules in an activated electronic state that have unpaired electrons and are highly reactive with molecules found in biological systems. Collectively, these activated molecular species derived from oxygen metabolism are designated as ROS (124). ROS extensively damage cellular organelles including the mitochondria, nuclear and mitochondrial DNA, and cell membrane, ultimately leading to cellular demise (125–127).

Normal human placentation is determined for the most part by the proper invasion of the uterine spiral arteries by a genomically normal trophoblast. This invasion governs the changes in the anatomy of the placental vasculature to ensure optimum perfusion by the maternal vessels. Definite metabolic changes occur in embryos during the transition from first to second trimester. It is evident that during the period of embryonic organogenesis, the prevailing oxygen tension is low and metabolism is largely anaerobic (128). Thus, the production of

ROS is reduced perhaps to prevent DNA damage induced by oxidants. This is also supported by animal research that shows increased blastocyst rate at low oxygen tension (129). At the end of the first trimester, there occurs a definite rise in oxygen tension in the intervillous space from less than 20 mmHg to more than 50 mmHg (130,131), leading to a burst in OS. Studies show that lower oxygen tension in the first trimester stimulates the invasive capacity of the trophoblast (132). This is probably due to increased activity of integrins that help trophoblast cells to proliferate. Persistent low oxygen tension also diminishes placental proliferation and invasion, and hence increased oxygen tension enables persistence of cytotrophoblast proliferation (133). It is suggested that impaired placental development or degeneration of syncytiotrophoblast in early pregnancy may be an effect of placental OS that may lead to complications such as recurrent abortions, preeclampsia, and congenital anomalies in diabetes (83). Several biomarkers have been associated with preeclampsia and increased OS, and some of the primary culprits are NOS-1, an isoform of NADPH oxidase, and endothelin 1 (134). It is possible that some of these factors may play an inhibitory role in cell proliferation and maturation and trigger OS in the human placenta by altering the balance between oxidant (increased MDA levels) and antioxidants (decreased GSH, GSSG, and AA). This can result in cell apoptosis leading to derangements in placental invasion and early abortion. In one study, the placental circulation was investigated using immunohistochemical analysis for heat shock protein (HSP 70i), a marker for cellular stress such as nitrotyrosine residues, and hydroxynonenal, as markers of protein and lipid oxidative damage, respectively (135). In this case-control study in normal pregnancies, intervillous blood flow increased with gestational age, being detected in nine of twenty-five cases at eight to nine weeks but in eighteen of twenty at twelve to thirteen weeks.

OS AND ITS RELATIONSHIP TO IVM OF OOCYTES

Follicle development and maturation of the oocyte is a dynamic process with high levels of metabolic activity. In vitro maturation of oocytes constitutes the in vitro advancement from diplotene stage of prophase I to metaphase II oocyte, along with cytoplasmic maturation, which is essential for the fertilization and early development of the embryo. The free radicals generated during this phase are numerous. Whenever the balance between the pro- and antioxidants in the cell is disturbed, OS results. Preserving fertility and treatment of infertility has merged in the recent years, thus introducing the concepts of in vitro maturation of immature oocytes that otherwise would have been lost in the physiological process. There are many scientific reports in the literature that analyze the potential correlation between the various markers of OS and the antioxidant protection with oocyte quality, developmental competence, fertilization capability, and blastocyst development. Various challenges hinder the selection of in vitro maturation of oocyte as an established mode of assisted reproduction in spite of the advantages of absent hyperstimulation syndrome and low cost. It is evident that the quality of in vitro mature oocytes are suboptimal since embryos derived from them have increased cleavage blocks. A well-documented fact that may be responsible for varied effects on cells is the generation of OS within cell culture media. It is evident that increased OS generated in the in vitro media may have varied effects on ART outcomes (78). The generation of ROS being an invariable phenomenon in external culture may also influence follicular and oocyte development in vitro. The oxidative insult on developing oocytes might be a responsible factor for low outcomes in IVM or may be responsible for aneuploidy in the fertilized oocytes (136). This phenomenon has led researchers to find methods to prevent such cell damage due to OS, but the final consensus for supplementing media with antioxidants in order to enhance oocyte development and quality is yet to be achieved though empirical usage seems to be feasible.

ROLE OF THERAPEUTIC ANTIOXIDANT SUPPLEMENTATION

Antioxidant supplementation of sperm preparation and gamete culture media was discussed in detail above. In this section, the preconceptional therapeutic use of antioxidants is discussed. It has been shown that OS results in luteolysis and that oral antioxidant supplementation, for example, vitamin C and vitamin E, have beneficial effects in preventing luteal phase deficiency and resulting in higher pregnancy rate (137,138). Other studies failed to demonstrate this favorable effect of antioxidant supplementation (139). A meta-analysis investigating the effect of vitamin C supplementation on pregnancy outcome was inconclusive (140). Another meta-analysis that used the fixed effects' model for women taking any of the vitamin supplements starting prior to twenty weeks gestation revealed no reduction in total fetal losses or in early and late miscarriage (141). Improved pregnancy rates were also reported with combination oral therapy with the antioxidants pentoxifylline and vitamin E supplementation for six months in patients with thin endometrium, undergoing IVF with oocyte donation because of history of radiotherapy (142).

Since OS can induce sperm dysfunction, many recent literature reports have emphasized the importance of the beneficial antioxidant effects of folate and zinc in male subfertility. Nutritional factors such as folate, zinc, and thiols may lead to fertility enhancement through their antiapoptotic effect and by prevention of DNA damage (143). Although many advances are being made in the field of antioxidants therapy, the data are still debatable and need further controlled evaluations in larger population.

CONCLUSIONS

ROS plays an essential role in the pathogenesis of many reproductive processes. In male factor infertility, OS attacks the fluidity of the sperm plasma membrane and the integrity of DNA in the sperm nucleus. ROS-induced DNA damage may accelerate the process of germ cell apoptosis, leading to the decline in sperm counts associated with male infertility. OS modulates a range of physiological functions and plays a role in pathological processes affecting female reproductive life span and even thereafter, that is, menopause. ROS-mediated female fertility disorders share many pathogenic similarities with the ones on the male side. The role of OS is becoming increasingly important as there is newer evidence of its role in conditions such as polycystic ovarian disease, abortions, preeclampsia, hydatidiform mole, fetal embryopathies, preterm labor, and intrauterine growth retardation. It is important to further elucidate the role of OS in unexplained infertility and recurrent early pregnancy losses and therefore devise strategies to overcome its adverse effects. There are, for example, ongoing trials with antioxidant supplementation, which will provide evidence on the safety and effectiveness of antioxidants and if they could improve the maternal and fetal outcomes. High follicular fluid ROS levels are associated with negative IVF outcomes, particularly in smokers. Successful management of infertility in the ART scenario depends on overcoming OS in the in vitro conditions.

KEY POINTS

■ OS has been implicated in different reproductive scenarios such as endometriosis, folliculogenesis, oocyte maturation, and sperm DNA damage and is detrimental to both natural and assisted fertility.

■ Many extrinsic and intrinsic conditions exist in ART setting that can be modified to reduce the toxic effects of ROS.

■ ART laboratory personnel should avoid procedures that are known to be deleterious, especially when safer procedures preventing OS can be used.

■ Although nutritional factors folate, zinc, and thiols may lead to fertility enhancement, the data are debatable and need evaluation in controlled studies on large population.

REFERENCES

1. Gupta S, Agarwal A, Krajcir N, Alvarez JG. Role of oxidative stress in endometriosis. *Reprod Biomed Online* 2006;13(1):126–34.
2. Agarwal A, Gupta S, Sharma R. Oxidative stress and its implications in female infertility — a clinician's perspective. *Reprod Biomed Online* 2005;11(5):641–50.
3. Agarwal A, Gupta S, Sharma RK. Role of oxidative stress in female reproduction. *Reprod Biol Endocrinol* 2005;3:28.
4. Wang X, Falcone T, Attaran M, Goldberg JM, Agarwal A, Sharma RK. Vitamin C and vitamin E supplementation reduce oxidative stress-induced embryo toxicity and improve the blastocyst development rate. *Fertil Steril* 2002;78(6):1272–7.
5. Attaran M, Pasqualotto E, Falcone T, et al. The effect of follicular fluid reactive oxygen species on the outcome of in vitro fertilization. *Int J Fertil Womens Med* 2000;45(5):314–20.
6. Agarwal A, Saleh RA, Bedaiwy MA. Role of reactive oxygen species in the pathophysiology of human reproduction. *Fertil Steril* 2003;79(4):829–43.
7. Sharma A. Role of reactive oxygen species in gynecologic diseases. *Reprod Med Biol* 2004;3:177–99.
8. Agarwal A, Allamaneni SS. Role of free radicals in female reproductive diseases and assisted reproduction. *Reprod Biomed Online* 2004;9(3):338–47.
9. Agarwal A, Gupta S, Sikka S. The role of free radicals and antioxidants in reproduction. *Curr Opin Obstet Gynecol* 2006;18(3):325–32.
10. Wang Y, Sharma RK, Falcone T, Goldberg J, Agarwal A. Importance of reactive oxygen species in the peritoneal fluid of women with endometriosis or idiopathic infertility. *Fertil Steril* 1997;68(5):826–30.
11. Du B, Takahashi K, Ishida GM, Nakahara K, Saito H, Kurachi H. Usefulness of intraovarian artery pulsatility and resistance indices measurement on the day of follicle aspiration for the assessment of oocyte quality. *Fertil Steril* 2006;85(2):366–70.
12. Rosselli M, Keller PJ, Dubey RK. Role of nitric oxide in the biology, physiology and pathophysiology of reproduction. *Hum Reprod Update* 1998;4(1):3–24.

13. Lee TH, Wu MY, Chen MJ, Chao KH, Ho HN, Yang YS. Nitric oxide is associated with poor embryo quality and pregnancy outcome in in vitro fertilization cycles. *Fertil Steril* 2004;82(1):126–31.

14. Manau D, Balasch J, Jimenez W, et al. Follicular fluid concentrations of adrenomedullin, vascular endothelial growth factor and nitric oxide in IVF cycles: relationship to ovarian response. *Hum Reprod* 2000;15(6):1295–9.

15. Suzuki T, Sugino N, Fukaya T, et al. Superoxide dismutase in normal cycling human ovaries: immunohistochemical localization and characterization. *Fertil Steril* 1999;72(4):720–6.

16. Tamate K, Sengoku K, Ishikawa M. The role of superoxide dismutase in the human ovary and fallopian tube. *J Obstet Gynaecol* 1995;21(4):401–9.

17. Jozwik M, Wolczynski S, Szamatowicz M. Oxidative stress markers in preovulatory follicular fluid in humans. *Mol Hum Reprod* 1999;5(5):409–13.

18. Sugino N, Takiguchi S, Kashida S, Karube A, Nakamura Y, Kato H. Superoxide dismutase expression in the human corpus luteum during the menstrual cycle and in early pregnancy. *Mol Hum Reprod* 2000;6(1):19–25.

19. Aten RF, Duarte KM, Behrman HR. Regulation of ovarian antioxidant vitamins, reduced glutathione, and lipid peroxidation by luteinizing hormone and prostaglandin F2 alpha. *Biol Reprod* 1992;46(3):401–7.

20. Briggs DA, Sharp DJ, Miller D, Gosden RG. Transferrin in the developing ovarian follicle: evidence for de-novo expression by granulosa cells. *Mol Hum Reprod* 1999;5(12):1107–14.

21. Sugino N, Karube-Harada A, Taketani T, Sakata A, Nakamura Y. Withdrawal of ovarian steroids stimulates prostaglandin F2alpha production through nuclear factor-kappaB activation via oxygen radicals in human endometrial stromal cells: potential relevance to menstruation. *J Reprod Dev* 2004;50(2):215–25.

22. Ota H, Igarashi S, Hatazawa J, Tanaka T. Endothelial nitric oxide synthase in the endometrium during the menstrual cycle in patients with endometriosis and adenomyosis. *Fertil Steril* 1998;69(2):303–8.

23. Tseng L, Zhang J, Peresleni T, Goligorsky MS. Cyclic expression of endothelial nitric oxide synthase mRNA in the epithelial glands of human endometrium. *J Soc Gynecol Investig* 1996;3(1):33–8.

24. Park JK, Song M, Dominguez CE, et al. Glycodelin mediates the increase in vascular endothelial growth factor in response to oxidative stress in the endometrium. *Am J Obstet Gynecol* 2006;195(6):1772–7.

25. Hickey M, Krikun G, Kodaman P, Schatz F, Carati C, Lockwood CJ. Long-term progestin-only contraceptives result in reduced endometrial blood flow and oxidative stress. *J Clin Endocrinol Metab* 2006;91(9):3633–8.

26. Iborra A, Palacio JR, Martinez P. Oxidative stress and autoimmune response in the infertile woman. *Chem Immunol Allergy* 2005;88:150–62.

27. Agarwal A, Said TM, Bedaiwy MA, Banerjee J, Alvarez JG. Oxidative stress in an assisted reproductive techniques setting. *Fertil Steril* 2006;86(3):503–12.

28. Zeller JM, Henig I, Radwanska E, Dmowski WP. Enhancement of human monocyte and peritoneal macrophage chemiluminescence activities in women with endometriosis. *Am J Reprod Immunol Microbiol* 1987;13(3):78–82.

29. Alpay Z, Saed GM, Diamond MP. Female infertility and free radicals: potential role in adhesions and endometriosis. *J Soc Gynecol Investig* 2006;13(6):390–8.

30. Reubinoff BE, Har-El R, Kitrossky N, et al. Increased levels of redox-active iron in follicular fluid: a possible cause of free radical-mediated infertility in beta-thalassemia major. *Am J Obstet Gynecol* 1996;174(3):914–18.

31. Arumugam K, Yip YC. De novo formation of adhesions in endometriosis: the role of iron and free radical reactions. *Fertil Steril* 1995;64(1):62–4.

32. Murphy AA, Palinski W, Rankin S, Morales AJ, Parthasarathy S. Evidence for oxidatively modified lipid-protein complexes in endometrium and endometriosis. *Fertil Steril* 1998;69(6):1092–4.

33. Donnez J, Van Langendonckt A, Casanas-Roux F, et al. Current thinking on the pathogenesis of endometriosis. *Gynecol Obstet Invest* 2002;54 (Suppl. 1):52–8; discussion 9–62.

34. Murphy AA, Palinski W, Rankin S, Morales AJ, Parthasarathy S. Macrophage scavenger receptor(s) and oxidatively modified proteins in endometriosis. *Fertil Steril* 1998;69(6):1085–91.

35. Jackson LW, Schisterman EF, Dey-Rao R, Browne R, Armstrong D. Oxidative stress and endometriosis. *Hum Reprod* 2005;20(7):2014–20.

36. Polak G, Koziol-Montewka M, Gogacz M, Blaszkowska I, Kotarski J. Total antioxidant status of peritoneal fluid in infertile women. *Eur J Obstet Gynecol Reprod Biol* 2001;94(2):261–3.

37. Szczepanska M, Kozlik J, Skrzypczak J, Mikolajczyk M. Oxidative stress may be a piece in the endometriosis puzzle. *Fertil Steril* 2003;79(6):1288–93.

38. Ho HN, Wu MY, Chen SU, Chao KH, Chen CD, Yang YS. Total antioxidant status and nitric oxide do not increase in peritoneal fluids from women with endometriosis. *Hum Reprod* 1997;12(12):2810–15.

39. Wu Y, Kajdacsy-Balla A, Strawn E, et al. Transcriptional characterizations of differences between eutopic and ectopic endometrium. *Endocrinology* 2006;147(1):232–46.

40. Bedaiwy MA, Falcone T, Sharma RK, et al. Prediction of endometriosis with serum and peritoneal fluid markers: a prospective controlled trial. *Hum Reprod* 2002;17(2):426–31.

41. Bedaiwy MA, Falcone T. Peritoneal fluid environment in endometriosis. Clinicopathological implications. *Minerva Ginecol* 2003;55(4):333–45.

42. Said TM, Agarwal A, Falcone T, Sharma RK, Bedaiwy MA, Li L. Infliximab may reverse the toxic effects induced by tumor necrosis factor alpha in human spermatozoa: an in vitro model. *Fertil Steril* 2005;83(6):1665–73.

43. Zhang X, Sharma RK, Agarwal A, Falcone T. Effect of pentoxifylline in reducing oxidative stress-induced embryotoxicity. *J Assist Reprod Genet* 2005;22(11–12):415–17.

44. Strandell A, Lindhard A, Waldenstrom U, Thorburn J. Hydrosalpinx and IVF outcome: cumulative results after salpingectomy in a randomized controlled trial. *Hum Reprod* 2001;16(11):2403–10.

45. Strandell A, Lindhard A. Why does hydrosalpinx reduce fertility? The importance of hydrosalpinx fluid. *Hum Reprod* 2002;17(5):1141–5.

46. Bedaiwy MA, Falcone T, Mohamed MS, et al. Differential growth of human embryos in vitro: role of reactive oxygen species. *Fertil Steril* 2004;82(3):593–600.

47. Okatani Y, Morioka N, Wakatsuki A, Nakano Y, Sagara Y. Role of the free radical-scavenger system in aromatase activity of the human ovary. *Horm Res* 1993;39 (Suppl. 1):22–7.

48. Wiener-Megnazi Z, Vardi L, Lissak A, et al. Oxidative stress indices in follicular fluid as measured by the thermochemiluminescence assay correlate with outcome parameters in in vitro fertilization. *Fertil Steril* 2004;82 (Suppl. 3):1171–6.

49. Tarin JJ. Potential effects of age-associated oxidative stress on mammalian oocytes/embryos. *Mol Hum Reprod* 1996;2(10):717–24.

50. Takahashi T, Takahashi E, Igarashi H, Tezuka N, Kurachi H. Impact of oxidative stress in aged mouse oocytes on calcium oscillations at fertilization. *Mol Reprod Dev* 2003;66(2):143–52.

51. Tatone C, Carbone MC, Falone S, et al. Age-dependent changes in the expression of superoxide dismutases and catalase are associated with ultrastructural modifications in human granulosa cells. *Mol Hum Reprod* 2006;12(11):655–60.

52. Steele EK, McClure N, Maxwell RJ, Lewis SE. A comparison of DNA damage in testicular and proximal epididymal spermatozoa in obstructive azoospermia. *Mol Hum Reprod* 1999;5(9):831–5.

53. Ollero M, Gil-Guzman E, Lopez MC, et al. Characterization of subsets of human spermatozoa at different stages of maturation: implications in the diagnosis and treatment of male infertility. *Hum Reprod* 2001;16(9):1912–21.

54. Dalzell LH, McVicar CM, McClure N, Lutton D, Lewis SE. Effects of short and long incubations on DNA fragmentation of testicular sperm. *Fertil Steril* 2004;82(5):1443–5.

55. Alvarez JG. Efficient treatment of infertility due to sperm DNA damage by ICSI with testicular sperm. *Hum Reprod* 2005;20(7):2031–2; author reply 2–3.

56. Alvarez JG. The predictive value of sperm chromatin structure assay. *Hum Reprod* 2005;20(8):2365–7.

57. Suganuma R, Yanagimachi R, Meistrich ML. Decline in fertility of mouse sperm with abnormal chromatin during epididymal passage as revealed by ICSI. *Hum Reprod* 2005;20(11):3101–8.

58. Fraga CG, Motchnik PA, Shigenaga MK, Helbock HJ, Jacob RA, Ames BN. Ascorbic acid protects against endogenous oxidative DNA damage in human sperm. *Proc Natl Acad Sci USA* 1991;88(24):11003–6.

59. Carrell DT, Liu L, Peterson CM, et al. Sperm DNA fragmentation is increased in couples with unexplained recurrent pregnancy loss. *Arch Androl* 2003;49(1):49–55.

60. Alvarez JG. DNA fragmentation in human spermatozoa: significance in the diagnosis and treatment of infertility. *Minerva Ginecol* 2003;55(3):233–9.

61. Rubes J, Selevan SG, Evenson DP, et al. Episodic air pollution is associated with increased DNA fragmentation in human sperm without other changes in semen quality. *Hum Reprod* 2005;20(10):2776–83.

62. Young TW, Mei FC, Yang G, Thompson-Lanza JA, Liu J, Cheng X. Activation of antioxidant pathways in ras-mediated oncogenic transformation of human surface ovarian epithelial cells revealed by functional proteomics and mass spectrometry. *Cancer Res* 2004;64(13):4577–84.

63. Egozcue J, Sarrate Z, Codina-Pascual M, et al. Meiotic abnormalities in infertile males. *Cytogenet Genome Res* 2005;111(3–4):337–42.

64. Oyawoye O, Abdel Gadir A, Garner A, Constantinovici N, Perrett C, Hardiman P. Antioxidants and reactive oxygen species in follicular fluid of women undergoing IVF: relationship to outcome. *Hum Reprod* 2003;18(11):2270–4.

65. Paszkowski T, Clarke RN, Hornstein MD. Smoking induces oxidative stress inside the Graafian follicle. *Hum Reprod* 2002;17(4):921–5.

66. Pasqualotto EB, Agarwal A, Sharma RK, et al. Effect of oxidative stress in follicular fluid on the outcome of assisted reproductive procedures. *Fertil Steril* 2004;81(4):973–6.

67. Van Blerkom J, Antczak M, Schrader R. The developmental potential of the human oocyte is related to the dissolved oxygen content of follicular fluid: association with vascular endothelial growth factor levels and perifollicular blood flow characteristics. *Hum Reprod* 1997;12(5):1047–55.

68. Yang HW, Hwang KJ, Kwon HC, Kim HS, Choi KW, Oh KS. Detection of reactive oxygen species (ROS) and apoptosis in human fragmented embryos. *Hum Reprod* 1998;13(4):998–1002.

69. Kurzawa R, Glabowski W, Baczkowski T, Wiszniewska B, Marchlewicz M. Growth factors protect in vitro cultured embryos from the consequences of oxidative stress. *Zygote* 2004;12(3):231–40.

70. Ebisch IM, Peters WH, Thomas CM, Wetzels AM, Peer PG, Steegers-Theunissen RP. Homocysteine, glutathione and related thiols affect fertility parameters in the (sub)fertile couple. *Hum Reprod* 2006;21(7):1725–33.

71. Das S, Chattopadhyay R, Ghosh S, et al. Reactive oxygen species level in follicular fluid — embryo quality marker in IVF? *Hum Reprod* 2006;21(9):2403–7.

72. Seino T, Saito H, Kaneko T, Takahashi T, Kawachiya S, Kurachi H. Eight-hydroxy-2'-deoxyguanosine in granulosa cells is correlated with the quality of oocytes and embryos in an in vitro fertilization-embryo transfer program. *Fertil Steril* 2002;77(6):1184–90.

73. Paszkowski T, Traub AI, Robinson SY, McMaster D. Selenium dependent glutathione peroxidase activity in human follicular fluid. *Clin Chim Acta* 1995;236(2):173–80.

74. Bedaiwy M, Agarwal A, Said TM, et al. Role of total antioxidant capacity in the differential growth of human embryos in vitro. *Fertil Steril* 2006;86(2):304–9.

75. Ferda Verit F, Erel O, Kocyigit A. Association of increased total antioxidant capacity and anovulation in nonobese infertile patients with clomiphene citrate-resistant polycystic ovary syndrome. *Fertil Steril* 2007.

76. Sabatini L, Wilson C, Lower A, Al-Shawaf T, Grudzinskas JG. Superoxide dismutase activity in human follicular fluid after controlled ovarian hyperstimulation in women undergoing in vitro fertilization. *Fertil Steril* 1999;72(6):1027–34.

77. Shiverick KT, Salafia C. Cigarette smoking and pregnancy I: ovarian, uterine and placental effects. *Placenta* 1999;20(4):265–72.

78. Guerin P, El Mouatassim S, Menezo Y. Oxidative stress and protection against reactive oxygen species in the pre-implantation embryo and its surroundings. *Hum Reprod Update* 2001;7(2):175–89.

79. Harvey AJ, Kind KL, Thompson JG. REDOX regulation of early embryo development. *Reproduction* 2002;123(4):479–86.

80. Matsui M, Oshima M, Oshima H, et al. Early embryonic lethality caused by targeted disruption of the mouse thioredoxin gene. *Dev Biol* 1996;178(1):179–85.

81. Knott L, Hartridge T, Brown NL, Mansell JP, Sandy JR. Homocysteine oxidation and apoptosis: a potential cause of cleft palate. *In Vitro Cell Dev Biol Anim* 2003;39(1–2):98–105.

82. Parman T, Wiley MJ, Wells PG. Free radical-mediated oxidative DNA damage in the mechanism of thalidomide teratogenicity. *Nat Med* 1999;5(5):582–5.

83. Burton GJ, Hempstock J, Jauniaux E. Oxygen, early embryonic metabolism and free radical-mediated embryopathies. *Reprod Biomed Online* 2003;6(1):84–96.

84. Wentzel P, Welsh N, Eriksson UJ. Developmental damage, increased lipid peroxidation, diminished cyclooxygenase-2 gene expression, and lowered prostaglandin E2 levels in rat embryos exposed to a diabetic environment. *Diabetes* 1999;48(4):813–20.

85. Gott AL, Hardy K, Winston RM, Leese HJ. Non-invasive measurement of pyruvate and glucose uptake and lactate production by single human preimplantation embryos. *Hum Reprod* 1990;5(1):104–8.

86. Warren JS, Johnson KJ, Ward PA. Oxygen radicals in cell injury and cell death. *Pathol Immunopathol Res* 1987;6(5–6):301–15.

87. Buhimschi IA, Kramer WB, Buhimschi CS, Thompson LP, Weiner CP. Reduction-oxidation (redox) state regulation of matrix metalloproteinase activity in human fetal membranes. *Am J Obstet Gynecol* 2000;182(2):458–64.

88. Machaty Z, Thompson JG, Abeydeera LR, Day BN, Prather RS. Inhibitors of mitochondrial ATP production at the time of

compaction improve development of in vitro produced porcine embryos. *Mol Reprod Dev* 2001;58(1):39–44.

89. Lane M, Maybach JM, Gardner DK. Addition of ascorbate during cryopreservation stimulates subsequent embryo development. *Hum Reprod* 2002;17(10):2686–93.

90. Lighten AD, Moore GE, Winston RM, Hardy K. Routine addition of human insulin-like growth factor-I ligand could benefit clinical in-vitro fertilization culture. *Hum Reprod* 1998;13(11):3144–50.

91. Racowsky C, Jackson KV, Cekleniak NA, Fox JH, Hornstein MD, Ginsburg ES. The number of eight-cell embryos is a key determinant for selecting day 3 or day 5 transfer. *Fertil Steril* 2000;73(3):558–64.

92. Jauniaux E, Gulbis B, Burton GJ. Physiological implications of the materno-fetal oxygen gradient in human early pregnancy. *Reprod Biomed Online* 2003;7(2):250–3.

93. Noda Y, Goto Y, Umaoka Y, Shiotani M, Nakayama T, Mori T. Culture of human embryos in alpha modification of Eagle's medium under low oxygen tension and low illumination. *Fertil Steril* 1994;62(5):1022–7.

94. Nicol CJ, Zielenski J, Tsui LC, Wells PG. An embryoprotective role for glucose-6-phosphate dehydrogenase in developmental oxidative stress and chemical teratogenesis. *FASEB J* 2000; 14(1):111–27.

95. Dumoulin JC, Meijers CJ, Bras M, Coonen E, Geraedts JP, Evers JL. Effect of oxygen concentration on human in-vitro fertilization and embryo culture. *Hum Reprod* 1999;14(2):465–9.

96. Kitagawa Y, Suzuki K, Yoneda A, Watanabe T. Effects of oxygen concentration and antioxidants on the in vitro developmental ability, production of reactive oxygen species (ROS), and DNA fragmentation in porcine embryos. *Theriogenology* 2004;62(7): 1186–97.

97. Wang AW, Zhang H, Ikemoto I, Anderson DJ, Loughlin KR. Reactive oxygen species generation by seminal cells during cryopreservation. *Urology* 1997;49(6):921–5.

98. Gadea J, Gumbao D, Matas C, Romar R. Supplementation of the thawing media with reduced glutathione improves function and the in vitro fertilizing ability of boar spermatozoa after cryopreservation. *J Androl* 2005;26(6):749–56.

99. Chan PJ, Calinisan JH, Corselli JU, Patton WC, King A. Updating quality control assays in the assisted reproductive technologies laboratory with a cryopreserved hamster oocyte DNA cytogenotoxic assay. *J Assist Reprod Genet* 2001;18(3):129–34.

100. Kim SS, Yang HW, Kang HG, et al. Quantitative assessment of ischemic tissue damage in ovarian cortical tissue with or without antioxidant (ascorbic acid) treatment. *Fertil Steril* 2004;82(3):679–85.

101. Speroff L GR, Kase NG. *Assisted Reproduction Clinical Gynecologic Endocrinology and Infertility*, 6th edn. Philadelphia: Lippincott Williams & Wilkins, 1999:643–724.

102. Esfandiari N, Falcone T, Agarwal A, Attaran M, Nelson DR, Sharma RK. Protein supplementation and the incidence of apoptosis and oxidative stress in mouse embryos. *Obstet Gynecol* 2005;105(3):653–60.

103. Catt JW, Henman M. Toxic effects of oxygen on human embryo development. *Hum Reprod* 2000;15 (Suppl. 2):199–206.

104. Feugang JM, de Roover R, Moens A, Leonard S, Dessy F, Donnay I. Addition of beta-mercaptoethanol or Trolox at the morula/blastocyst stage improves the quality of bovine blastocysts and prevents induction of apoptosis and degeneration by prooxidant agents. *Theriogenology* 2004;61(1):71–90.

105. Tatemoto H, Ootaki K, Shigeta K, Muto N. Enhancement of developmental competence after in vitro fertilization of porcine oocytes by treatment with ascorbic acid 2-O-alpha-glucoside during in vitro maturation. *Biol Reprod* 2001;65(6):1800–6.

106. Dalvit G, Llanes SP, Descalzo A, Insani M, Beconi M, Cetica P. Effect of alpha-tocopherol and ascorbic acid on bovine oocyte in vitro maturation. *Reprod Domest Anim* 2005;40(2):93–7.

107. Oyamada T, Fukui Y. Oxygen tension and medium supplements for in vitro maturation of bovine oocytes cultured individually in a chemically defined medium. *J Reprod Dev* 2004;50(1):107–17.

108. de Matos DG, Furnus CC, Moses DF. Glutathione synthesis during in vitro maturation of bovine oocytes: role of cumulus cells. *Biol Reprod* 1997;57(6):1420–5.

109. Ali AA, Bilodeau JF, Sirard MA. Antioxidant requirements for bovine oocytes varies during in vitro maturation, fertilization and development. *Theriogenology* 2003;59(3–4):939–49.

110. Guerin P, Guillaud J, Menezo Y. Hypotaurine in spermatozoa and genital secretions and its production by oviduct epithelial cells in vitro. *Hum Reprod* 1995;10(4):866–72.

111. Takahashi M, Nagai T, Hamano S, Kuwayama M, Okamura N, Okano A. Effect of thiol compounds on in vitro development and intracellular glutathione content of bovine embryos. *Biol Reprod* 1993;49(2):228–32.

112. Nonogaki T, Noda Y, Narimoto K, Umaoka Y, Mori T. Effects of superoxide dismutase on mouse in vitro fertilization and embryo culture system. *J Assist Reprod Genet* 1992;9(3):274–80.

113. Lornage J. [Biological aspects of endometriosis in vitro fertilization]. *J Gynecol Obstet Biol Reprod (Paris)* 2003;32(8 Pt. 2): S48–50.

114. Saleh RA, Agarwal A. Oxidative stress and male infertility: from research bench to clinical practice. *J Androl* 2002;23(6):737–52.

115. Potts RJ, Notarianni LJ, Jefferies TM. Seminal plasma reduces exogenous oxidative damage to human sperm, determined by the measurement of DNA strand breaks and lipid peroxidation. *Mutat Res* 2000;447(2):249–56.

116. Bidri M, Choay P. [Taurine: a particular aminoacid with multiple functions]. *Ann Pharm Fr* 2003;61(6):385–91.

117. Henkel RR, Schill WB. Sperm preparation for ART. *Reprod Biol Endocrinol* 2003;1:108.

118. Paul M, Sumpter JP, Lindsay KS. Factors affecting pentoxifylline stimulation of sperm kinematics in suspensions. *Hum Reprod* 1996;11(9):1929–35.

119. Lamond S, Watkinson M, Rutherford T, et al. Gene-specific chromatin damage in human spermatozoa can be blocked by antioxidants that target mitochondria. *Reprod Biomed Online* 2003;7(4):407–18.

120. Ermilov A, Diamond MP, Sacco AG, Dozortsev DD. Culture media and their components differ in their ability to scavenge reactive oxygen species in the plasmid relaxation assay. *Fertil Steril* 1999;72(1):154–7.

121. Kattera S, Chen C. Short coincubation of gametes in in vitro fertilization improves implantation and pregnancy rates: a prospective, randomized, controlled study. *Fertil Steril* 2003;80(4): 1017–21.

122. Gianaroli L, Fiorentino A, Magli MC, Ferraretti AP, Montanaro N. Prolonged sperm-oocyte exposure and high sperm concentration affect human embryo viability and pregnancy rate. *Hum Reprod* 1996;11(11):2507–11.

123. Dirnfeld M, Shiloh H, Bider D, et al. A prospective randomized controlled study of the effect of short coincubation of gametes during insemination on zona pellucida thickness. *Gynecol Endocrinol* 2003;17(5):397–403.

124. Halliwell B, Gutteridge JM. Free radicals and antioxidant protection: mechanisms and significance in toxicology and disease. *Hum Toxicol* 1988;7(1):7–13.

125. Kowaltowski AJ, Vercesi AE. Mitochondrial damage induced by conditions of oxidative stress. *Free Radic Biol Med* 1999; 26(3–4):463–71.

126. Ronnenberg AG, Goldman MB, Chen D, et al. Preconception folate and vitamin B(6) status and clinical spontaneous abortion in Chinese women. *Obstet Gynecol* 2002;100(1):107–13.

127. Pierce JD, Cackler AB, Arnett MG. Why should you care about free radicals? *RN* 2004;67(1):38–42; quiz 3.

128. Jauniaux E, Watson A, Burton G. Evaluation of respiratory gases and acid-base gradients in human fetal fluids and utero-placental tissue between 7 and 16 weeks' gestation. *Am J Obstet Gynecol* 2001;184(5):998–1003.

129. Quinn P, Harlow GM. The effect of oxygen on the development of preimplantation mouse embryos in vitro. *J Exp Zool* 1978; 206(1):73–80.

130. Jauniaux E, Watson AL, Hempstock J, Bao YP, Skepper JN, Burton GJ. Onset of maternal arterial blood flow and placental oxidative stress. A possible factor in human early pregnancy failure. *Am J Pathol* 2000;157(6):2111–22.

131. Rodesch F, Simon P, Donner C, Jauniaux E. Oxygen measurements in endometrial and trophoblastic tissues during early pregnancy. *Obstet Gynecol* 1992;80(2):283–5.

132. Barrionuevo MJ, Schwandt RA, Rao PS, Graham LB, Maisel LP, Yeko TR. Nitric oxide (NO) and interleukin-1beta (IL-1beta) in follicular fluid and their correlation with fertilization and embryo cleavage. *Am J Reprod Immunol* 2000;44(6): 359–64.

133. Caniggia I, Mostachfi H, Winter J, et al. Hypoxia-inducible factor-1 mediates the biological effects of oxygen on human trophoblast differentiation through TGFbeta(3). *J Clin Invest* 2000;105(5):577–87.

134. Myatt L, Cui X. Oxidative stress in the placenta. *Histochem Cell Biol* 2004;122(4):369–82.

135. Jauniaux E, Hempstock J, Greenwold N, Burton GJ. Trophoblastic oxidative stress in relation to temporal and regional differences in maternal placental blood flow in normal and abnormal early pregnancies. *Am J Pathol* 2003;162(1):115–25.

136. W. Choi JB, Agarwal A, Falcone T, Sharma RK. Can vitamin C supplementation reduce oxidative stress induced cytoskeleton damage of mouse oocyte. *Fertil Steril* 2005;84 (Suppl. 1):S452.

137. Henmi H, Endo T, Kitajima Y, Manase K, Hata H, Kudo R. Effects of ascorbic acid supplementation on serum progesterone levels in patients with a luteal phase defect. *Fertil Steril* 2003;80(2):459–61.

138. Crha I, Hruba D, Ventruba P, Fiala J, Totusek J, Visnova H. Ascorbic acid and infertility treatment. *Cent Eur J Public Health* 2003;11(2):63–7.

139. Griesinger G, Franke K, Kinast C, et al. Ascorbic acid supplement during luteal phase in IVF. *J Assist Reprod Genet* 2002; 19(4):164–8.

140. Rumbold A, Crowther CA. Vitamin C supplementation in pregnancy. *Cochrane Database Syst Rev* 2005(2):CD004072.

141. Rumbold A, Middleton P, Crowther CA. Vitamin supplementation for preventing miscarriage. *Cochrane Database Syst Rev* 2005(2):CD004073.

142. Ledee-Bataille N, Olivennes F, Lefaix JL, Chaouat G, Frydman R, Delanian S. Combined treatment by pentoxifylline and tocopherol for recipient women with a thin endometrium enrolled in an oocyte donation programme. *Hum Reprod* 2002;17(5):1249–53.

143. Ebisch IM, Thomas CM, Peters WH, Braat DD, Steegers-Theunissen RP. The importance of folate, zinc and antioxidants in the pathogenesis and prevention of subfertility. *Hum Reprod Update* 2007;13(2):163–74.

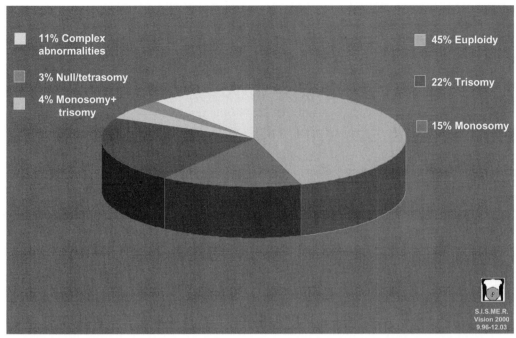

Figure 65.1. Distribution of the chromosomal status of 3,937 oocytes tested by FISH analysis of the first polar body.

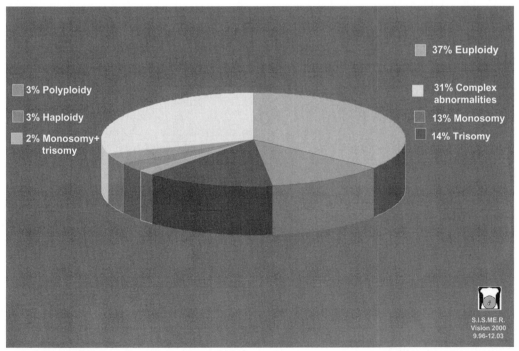

Figure 65.2. Distribution of the chromosomal status of 5,217 in vitro generated embryos tested by FISH analysis of one blastomere.

meiosis II errors (13). Eleven per cent of the eggs showed aneuploidy in two or more chromosomes (complex abnormalities).

On embryos, complex abnormalities (involving more than three of the tested chromosomes) were the most frequently observed (46 percent of the total anomalies), while monosomy and trisomy showed a lower incidence (23–25 percent). Chromosomes mostly involved in embryo aneuploidy were found to be, in order, chromosome 22, 16, 15, and 21. In addition to

aneuploidy, postmeiotic errors can account for several abnormalities in early-cleavage embryos. The majority of the detected defects were incompatible with live or even implantation, but 967 embryos (18 percent) were carrying monosomy (X, 21) or trisomy (21, 22, 16, 13, 15, 18) with the potential to implant.

According to several other studies (18–21), our observations on blastocysts showed that significantly less aneuploid embryos are able to reach the blastocyst stage compared to euploid embryos

(22 vs. 40 percent), but still high levels of monosomy, trisomy, and even complex abnormalities can be detected on blastocysts (22). Haploid and polyploid embryos had a very low potential (<5 percent) to develop to blastocysts, but still these abnormalities can be detected at the blastocyst stage and it is known that polyploid pregnancies can reach first trimester and beyond.

Before entering in the analysis of the main factors affecting aneuploidy, it is necessary to remember that the material analyzed belongs to a population (infertile couples undergoing ART) that cannot be completely representative of the general population. In addition, the majority of the couples selected for PGD-AS were poor-prognosis patients and all underwent ovarian stimulation with gonatotropins. Whether the rates of aneuploidy detected were "natural" or partially influenced by gonadotropins is unknown; no reports comparing natural and stimulated cycles are presents in the literature.

Nevertheless, still the figures are impressive and the current reality is that, in humans, the chromosomal defects detected at the postimplantation level are just the "tip of the iceberg" of the wastage determined by meiotic and early mitotic errors in the preimplantation stage.

Factors Related to Gametes and Embryos Aneuploidy

Maternal Age

The maternal origin of aneuploidy is prevalent in abnormal human conceptuses, and reproductive maternal aging is the most important factor affecting the frequency of aneuploidy (23). The association between maternal age and Down's syndrome was recognized as early as 1933, and today the link is incontrovertibly well documented (3, 24).

Very young women (less than twenty-eight years) show low risk of aneuploidy both in oocytes (<25 percent) and embryos (<35 percent) (25). Unlikely, both in vivo and in vitro reproduction is today postponed to later age. Demographic studies clearly show that the mean age of women at birth is thirty years (3, 26), and the ICMART data indicate that almost 50 percent of ART treatments in the world are performed in women aged thirty-five years or more (27).

Figure 65.3 shows the mean frequency of first meiosis errors and the mean percentage of abnormal embryos depending on maternal age. In the tested population, a clear increase is constantly observed with aging. A statistically significant difference is present between women aged less than or equal to thirty-five years and women older than forty years ($p < 0.01$); but it is important to stress that even women considered in the youngest reproductive age by means of ART (thirty to thirty-four years) can produce up to more than 50 percent of aneuploid embryos under certain circumstances. In women older than forty-two, two oocytes out of three show first meiosis errors and four embryos out of five are carrying chromosomal defects in their very early stage of development. It is not surprising that all data collections (national, regional, and worldwide) report a very low implantation rate (2–4 percent) in those aged patients.

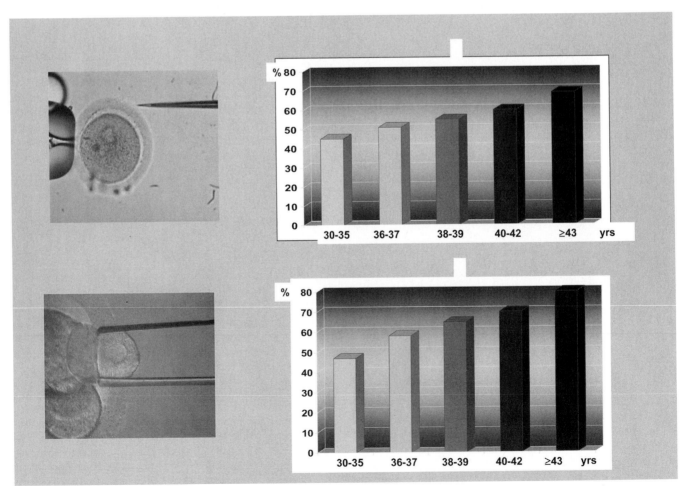

Figure 65.3. Incidence of chromosomal anomalies on oocytes (upper) and embryos (bottom) in relation to maternal age.

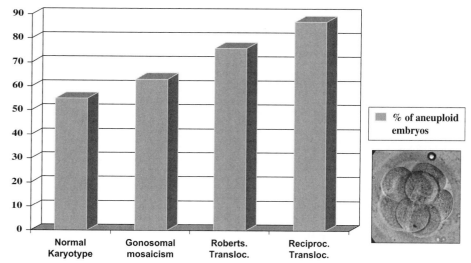

Figure 65.4. Incidence of embryo's chromosomal anomalies in relation to the parental peripheral karyotype.

As expected, chromosomes 15, 21, and 22 exhibit significantly higher frequencies of aneuploidy with increasing maternal age both in oocytes and embryos, followed by chromosomes 13 and 16. Chromosomes 1, 14, 17, 18, X, and Y show similar aneuploidy rates irrespective of age. While monosomies and trisomies are increasing with age, complex abnormalities, haploidy, and polyploidy are not affected by maternal aging, inverting the ratio between these types of abnormalities.

Abnormal Karyotype

Balanced translocations occur in 0.6–0.9 percent of infertile couples and are well known to be responsible for recurrent postimplantation pregnancy wastage (28).

Figure 65.4 shows the frequency of preimplantation aneuploidies in young patients (age less than thirty-eight years) carrying an altered karyotype in peripheral blood: women with low-level gonosomic mosaicism and couples with one partner carrying chromosomal translocations (Robertsonian or reciprocal). Compared to similar-aged patients with normal karyotype, the frequency of embryo aneuploidy resulted significantly higher, reaching an incidence of 88 percent, in reciprocal translocation. The study of the detected abnormalities suggested that an interchromosomal effect could influence the behaviour at meiosis of chromosomes other than those involved in translocation (29). Among the abnormalities observed, the most frequent resulted complex abnormalities (45 percent) and monosomy and trisomy (43 percent).

Recurrent Pregnancy Loss

Previous history of spontaneous abortions is a risk factor of pregnancy loss even in patients with normal karyotype. Excluding other factors such as uterine malformation or thrombophilia predisposition, young women with spontaneous RPL undergoing chromosomal analysis in ART cycles demonstrated a high risk of producing aneuploid oocytes (54 percent) and aneuploid embryos (68 percent). The most frequent abnormalities detected were monosomy and trisomy involving chromosomes 15 and 16.

Poor Response

Repeated poor response to COH in young women can be the first clinical sign of premature ovarian aging. When compared to normal responders, these patients not only show a lower probability of pregnancy per started cycle but also the implantation rate of the transferred embryos is reduced.

Definition of poor response is a controversial issue and actually each centre is using its own identification criteria (30). SISMER Centres define as "real" poor responders those women younger than thirty-eight years who produced less than or equal to three oocytes after high doses (>3,500 total IU) of FSH.

Testing those patients by PGD and PB1 analysis, the incidence of oocytes and embryo aneuploidies resulted, respectively, 60 and 68 percent, significantly higher than those observed in equal-aged normal responders (50 and 56 percent). Similar to women older than forty, the most frequent abnormalities were monosomy and trisomy, confirming a biological aging of the ovary but, interestingly, only chromosomes 15 and 13 (and no. chromosomes 22 and 21) showed higher incidence of nondisjunction defects.

Repeated Implantation Failure in Conventional IVF/ICSI Cycles

ART treatment registered a substantial improvement in the past decade, offering young women a high cumulative pregnancy rate (50–70 percent) in the first three cycles (31). However, still a relevant percentage of relatively young (less than thirty-eight years) normal responders women able to produce in vitro morphologically normal embryos repeatedly fail to achieve a pregnancy. Those patients are classified as having a poor prognosis. The results obtained by PB1 biopsy in this category of patients give 50 percent mean incidence of aneuploidy; the mean percentage of aneuploid embryos by PGD-AS was 59 percent (32). But the interesting finding was that patients generating only aneuploid embryos in their first PGD-AS cycle maintained a similar chromosomal performance in following cycle: more than 90 percent of their embryos repeatedly were carrying aneuploidies even if deriving from different cohorts of collected oocytes (33).

The distribution of chromosomal abnormalities was significantly different from that characterizing the maternal age factor: monosomy and trisomy accounted only for 35 percent of total abnormalities versus 44 percent detected in older women

($p < 0.005$). Other defects such as haploidy, polyploidy, and complex abnormalities had the highest incidence, evoking a dysfunction in the processes or structures entering cell division.

Paternal Contribution

Numerical and structural abnormalities in sperm increase somewhat with aging, but since the increase starts over forty and is initially very slow, sperm aneuploidies are not clinically relevant in the fertile male population (34, 35). However, gonosomic aneuploidy and trisomy 21 have been demonstrated to have a possible paternal origin (36).

Among the infertile population entering ART treatment, a male factor is frequently involved. Almost 30–40 percent of men suffer of some degree of OAT and 5–8 percent need to use sperm extracted from the testis because of nonobstructive azoospermia (TESE) or from the epidydimus because of obstructive azoospermia (MESA).

Studies applying FISH in human sperm start to show a higher frequency of aneuploidy in OAT patients and in TESE sample compared to normospermic (37), but still some concerns are present regarding the reliability of the test and its clinical relevance.

The data obtained with the protocol designed in our center for FISH sperm analysis (14) demonstrated that very few (<2 percent) normospermic men had semen samples with a high percentage of abnormal chromosomal complement, while the same figure ranged from 12 percent (moderate OAT) to 89 percent (testicular samples) in the infertile male population. The mean percentage of aneuploid spermatozoon was 1.27 percent in normospermic samples, 4.02 percent in severe OAT, and 13.7 percent in TESE, clearly showing that testicular sperm are significantly more prone to aneuploidy

than ejaculated sperm. In OAT patients, the aneuploid rates for gonosomes and for chromosomes 13, 21, and 22 were significantly higher compared to the rates for chromosomes 15, 16, and 18, and to the incidence reported in the normal population. A similar figure was detected in testicular sperms, with the addition of chromosome 15 in the most frequently involved in aneuploidies.

Figure 65.5 shows the frequency of chromosomal anomalies in embryos generated by ICSI, depending on the severity of the male factor: severe OAT and nonobstructive TESE spermatozoa generate a significantly higher incidence of aneuploid embryos compared to other groups, strongly suggesting a paternal contribution to embryonic aneuploidies when severe infertile samples are used for ICSI. Gonosomic aneuplodies and complex abnormalities resulted, the most frequent detected in those embryos.

Embryo Morphology and Development

Besides the fact that any type of chromosomically abnormal embryos can reach blastocyst stage and several are still compatible with implantation and detected in first-trimester abortions, same recent reviews clearly show a correlation between the chromosomal complement and the morphological and developmental variants of the cleavage-stage embryos (38, 39).

To analyze the data supporting this evidence would require fully dedicated chapter, but a summary has to be made for its clinical relevance in ART.

■ Fragmentation, multinucleation, and asymmetric blastomere cleavage increase the change of an embryo to be chromosomally abnormal. What increases with dysmorphism is not aneuploidy but postmeiotic abnormalities, such as mosaicism, polyploidy, haploidy, and chaotic embryos.

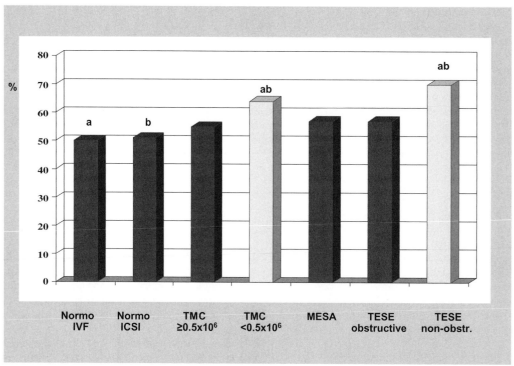

Figure 65.5. Incidence of embryo's chromosomal anomalies in relation to the characteristics of the semen samples utilized for insemination (TMC = total motile count).

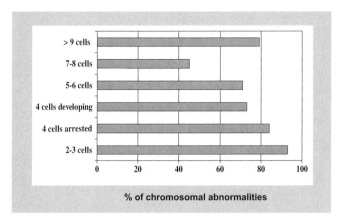

Figure 65.6. Incidence of embryo's chromosomal anomalies in relation to the cellular stage observed sixty-two hours after insemination.

■ According to the rate of cleavage, the number of cells observed after three days of culture is significantly related with the risk of an embryo being abnormal (Figure 65.6). The "perfect" embryos (seven to eight cells) carry the lowest rate of abnormalities, while more than 80 percent of arrested and very slow embryos have chromosomal defects. Based on conventional criteria, those embryos are not transferred, but even embryos with five to six cells or embryo with more than nine cells (that can be chosen for transfer in the absence of perfect embryos) have a 75 percent risk to carry chromosomal abnormalities. Postmeiotic abnormalities are most common in arrested and slow embryos, while trisomies are most frequently detected in accelerate embryos.

Based on these observational studies and assuming that good IVF centers practice proper morphological and developmental embryonic selection, careful evaluation under powerful inverted microscope is able to select and discharge a fraction of chromosomally abnormal embryos but still does not allow to select against the majority of aneuploidies (and some postmeiotic abnormalities), which occur with a frequency of 30–40 percent in apparently morphologically normal embryos. This rate increases to about 60–70 percent in women aged more than forty years.

Culture to blastocyst stage, often considered the major indicator for embryos resulting in offspring, can further select against some chromosomal abnormalities. However, the most selected abnormalities are those almost incompatible with implantation, still leaving a clinically relevant risk of transferring monosomic and trisomic blastocysts. In addition, this approach may easily discharge slow embryos that are chromosomally normal but not able to survive so long in culture when, in fact, could implant.

More recently, a new morphological criteria assessed at the precleavage stage (pronuclear morphology) has been proposed as a scoring system for the prediction of embryo development and implantation (40). In a recent study (41), the pronuclear morphology of zygotes generated from euploid oocytes (diagnosed by PB1 biopsy) was compared with the configuration observed in chromosomally normal embryos (diagnosed by blastomere biopsy) and with their potential to implant. The results clearly showed that some configurations of the pronuclear stage are associated with the highest proportion of euploidy and live births, confirming the validity of this scoring system to select embryos for transfer.

Clinical Application of Preimplantation Genetic Screening in ART

Rationale

If 50 percent or more embryos are chromosomally abnormal, and this frequency is much higher than that reported in spontaneous abortions, this indicates that a sizable part of chromosomally abnormal embryos are eliminated before clinical recognition (42). Such loss of embryos could account for the low implantation potential of ART embryos and a selection was hypothesized to reverse this trend. Thus, selecting against chromosome abnormalities and replacing only normal embryos should significantly increase implantation rates and reduce both chromosomally abnormal conceptions and spontaneous abortions, which in turn should result in higher take-home baby rates.

After more than ten years, this issue still raises several controversies. Reviewing the literature there have been two starkly different conclusions: a first group of investigators represent and support the hypothesis that PGD-AS for infertility improves implantation and reduces miscarriage rates, resulting in higher take-home baby rates (43–45); a second group was not able to demonstrate any significant differences between control and PGD-AS patients (46, 47).

The lack of positive results in these studies may have been due to inappropriate methodology. The latest authors biopsied two cells instead of one, tested insufficient number of chromosomes, and used fixation methods prone to error and poor embryo selection. One study in which only one cell was biopsied also used a restrictive set of chromosomes (43), and here implantation rates did not increase, yet the incidence of miscarriage was diminished and the take-home baby rate increased. Other studies using a single-cell biopsy technique and nine-chromosome probes, all demonstrated an acceptable efficiency of FISH for detecting aneuploidy and improved implantation rates (44, 45). Sample size was not appropriate to determine an improvement in pregnancy rate.

Today, the scientific community is divided: for one half, the additional intrusive and expensive embryo biopsy can be justified only if a marked improvement in the pregnancy rate is achieved (48) and still PGD-AS should be considered an experimental procedure being not enough evidence of its efficacy in the literature; the other half is supporting PGD-AS as an added selection tool to improve implantation rate and to reduce spontaneous abortions, provided that is properly performed. However, even the latter admit that the clinical results are less spectacular than previously expected.

The aim of the second part of this chapter is to demonstrate that, on ensuring its safety and evaluating its efficiency, PGD-AS should be ethically and clinically acceptable as it gives several benefits on the management of infertile couples undergoing ART, beside its direct effect on the cycle outcome.

Safety of Oocytes and Embryo Biopsy

Data from the first 1,000 children born in the world demonstrated that PGD babies are not exposed to greater risk of having neonatal pathologies or malformations than ICSI babies

(9). Other reviews confirm these preliminary observations. Data from babies born in our centre after embryo biopsy ($n = 170$) report three major congenital malformations and one minor, giving a malformation rate (2.35 percent) similar to the incidence observed in IVF/ICSI babies ($63/2333 = 2.7$ percent).

Of course, the data available so far are too small to draw final conclusions and the careful follow-up of the babies born is still an ethical obligation as well as the information to patients about "potential" unknown long-term consequence.

Regarding the risk that biopsy may negatively affect the implantation potential of the embryos, data on polar bodies' removal demonstrate that fertilization, cleavage, and blastocyst formation are not decreased (49). PBs are not involved in embryo development, and their removal theoretically should not affect implantation rate. On the contrary, embryo biopsy could potentially affect subsequent embryo development. Human studies have shown that the biopsy of one cell at the eight-cell-stage embryo is not detrimental for embryo development to blastocyst stage (50), but the removal of two cells, as well as the removal of one-fourth of a four-cell embryo seem to reduce the ratio between inner cell mass and trophectoderm (51). The interpretation of these experiments is not consistent, and biomass reduction is often discussed in the context of a superfluous cell number with totipotency. In its clinical application, PGD has been shown to not negatively affect implantation rates but in some studies the contrary has been clearly demonstrated (43–45). However, as previously underlined, the increase in implantation obtained in these studies is less spectacular than previously thought and is not confirmed by other studies. A reason for this could be the embryo itself; but the assumption that biopsy has little effect on the embryo simply remains unproven. So far, to obtain the best results, the recommendation is to perform one-cell biopsy in embryo at the eight-cell stage.

Efficiency of FISH Technique

FISH procedure to analyze oocytes or embryos still suffers because of technical limitations (unsuitable probe hybridization, signal overlapping, and micronuclei loss during fixation) that can give rise to misdiagnosis with clinical and ethical relevance (47, 52).

The risk of PGD-AS false negative (transfer of embryos carrying aneuploidy) is evaluated to be 3–4 percent. In IVF couples, the clinical consequence of this misdiagnosis can be more devastating than the failure to achieve the pregnancy.

The risk of false positive (discharge of normal embryos) is reported to be 4–5 percent. In our centers, the reanalysis of all the blastomeres from 853 aneuploid embryos by one-cell FISH has shown that thirty-two discharged embryos were actually normal, giving a false-positive risk of 3.7%.

People who believe that the embryo is a "person" cannot justify even one single embryo discharged. For most of the others, it can be ethically acceptable whether important human interests are sufficiently strong to meet the demands of special respect for embryos (53).

The risk of misdiagnosis of oocyte's chromosomal complement by PB product FISH analysis have been estimated to be approximately 10 percent (13). Handling such a small amount of genetic material and obtaining good quality preparation can be more difficult than handling and processing a blastomere, but ethical interests have minor relevance in discarding eggs

rather then embryos. The reanalysis of seventy-five oocytes performed in our center showed a 2 percent misdiagnosis, significantly lower than those reported in the literature.

New evolving technologies will be able to significantly increase the sensitivity of PGD and reduce the diagnostic errors. Despite technological advances, this issue will not be solved because misdiagnosis can be even due to biological events as mosaicism, postzygotes aneuploides, and trisomic rescue.

MOSAICISM

Thirty percent of the embryos are mosaics (54). Depending on the type of mosaic, the risk of misdiagnosis and the outcome of the misdiagnosis can be different. Mosaic embryos with more than three abnormal cells out of eight are probably unable to implant. Those with lower number of abnormal cells are benign mosaics and the full development of the embryo can result mostly in normally developing fetuses. The chance of misdiagnosis produced by mosaicism is 5.6 percent, where the false positive (discharge of mostly normal embryos) is 1.3 percent and the false negative (transfer of embryos with detrimental mosaic) accomplish for a 4.3 percent. Most, but not all, of these embryos do not reach the blastocyst stage (55).

POST ZYGOTES ANEUPLOIDES

Twenty-five percent of the mosaics are produced by mitotic nondisjunction (23). Earlier, if the postzygote error occurs, more detrimental effects can be produced in the embryos. When the errors occur before the six- to eight-cell stage, misdiagnosis (both false positive and false negative) is high, but the embryos have low probability to further develop because of detrimental mosaics.

In case of latter errors, after the stage in which PGD-AS is performed, mosaic embryos can be transferred (false negative) but most of them would carry benign mosaicisms.

TRISOMIC RESCUE

Trimosic rescue is a described phenomenon, which occurs when the zygote is initially trisomic for a particular chromosome but subsequently loses the extrachromosome. In two third of the cases, the lost chromosome, which contributes the extrachromosome (56), is of parental origin. In this case, PGD-AS can lead to the discharge of an almost normal embryo only if embryos would be able to rescue trisomy in more than 40 percent of mitosis after the six-to eight-cell stage. No data are available on the evidence and frequency of this phenomenon. In a third of the cases, the trisomic rescue can result in two copies of a chromosome from the same parent (UPD, uniparental disomy). UPD can involve both autosome and sex chromosomes and can be responsible for non-Mendelian transmission of genetic diseases and has also been implicated in both Prader Willi and Angelman syndromes. UPD cannot be detected by conventional PGD-AS (false negative).

A similar hypothetical mechanism of aneuploidy rescue has been suggested for oocytes. Since a significant proportion of oocytes display both segregation errors in first and second polar bodies, balanced zygotes can be formed through sequential errors in the meiosis I and II female division.

Based on these data, PGD-AS can be considered as a safe and efficient tool for screening several preimplantation chromosomal defects but not yet as an alternative to prenatal genetic diagnosis. Patients have to be informed on the risk of

Table 65.2: Cumulative PGD-AS Results Compared to Conventional Cycles (Pre-Law Period)

	PGD-AS cycles	Conventional IFV/ICSI cycles
No. of egg retrievals	971	2,636
Female age	37.3 ± 4.5	35.1 ± 7.3
No. of analyzed embryos	4,898	—
FISH normal	1,554 (32%)	—
No. of transferred cycles (mean embryos/transfer)	665 (1.7 ± 0.8)	1,926 (1.8 ± 0.6)
No. of clinical pregnancies	201 (30%)	675 (35%)
Implantation rate	21	22
No. of miscarriages	30 (15%)	90 (13%)

misdiagnosis and be recommended to undergo prenatal diagnosis to confirm the PGD results.

PGD-AS Indications and Clinical Outcome

As previously described, PGD-AS has been performed in our centre from September 1996 to March 2004 in infertile couples with a high risk of producing aneuploid embryos: advanced maternal age, repeated previous IVF failures, altered karyotype, and RPL without clear etiology. On the evidence that male with severe defects can produce high proportion of aneuploid sperm (57), PGD-AS has been also proposed when testicular spermatozoa (TESE) were used after at least one failure with conventional ICSI cycle.

Table 65.2 shows the cumulative outcome of 971 PGD-AS cycles performed in a population aged 37 ± 4.5 years. The data are compared to the results obtained in the same period (1997–2003) in conventional IVF/ICSI cycles performed in younger patients without PGD-AS indications and, therefore, considered having a good prognosis. In the PGD-AS group, 4,898 morphologically normal embryos were analyzed by FISH (5.2 ± 2.1 per cycle) and 68 percent were chromosally abnormal. Thanks to PGD-AS selection before transfer, the implantation rate obtained in poor-prognosis patients was very similar to those observed in "typical" patients (21 vs. 22 percent), as well as the early miscarriage rate (15 vs. 13 percent). The live birth rate was 26 percent.

The data have to be analyzed and discussed by indication because of the different reproductive potential of the studied groups (Table 65.3).

The first three groups (RPL, gonosomic mosaicism, and translocation) are, by definition, patients with preserved embryo implantation potential but high risk of postimplantation wastage because of aneuploidy. Indeed, the in vitro fecundity measured as IR was similar to the in vivo fecundity reported per similar age. This is, in our opinion, a clear biological index that embryo manipulation for PGD-AS does not affect further development and implantation potential.

The combination of probes (13, 15, 16, 18, 21, 22, X, and Y) used in our PGD-AS programme was able to detect close to 80 percent of all chromosally abnormal embryos at risk of causing a miscarriage. In eighty-one cycles (equal to 31 percent), no euploid embryos were available for transfer and those

patients were avoided of a high risk of miscarriage because of the high implantation potential of their embryos, although abnormal. The transferred patients experienced a total of sixty-six clinical pregnancies with a miscarriage rate substantially lower than expected (58): 17 versus 37 percent.

After PGD-AS, fifty-five patients delivered a baby. The previous reproductive history of these patients accounted for a total of fifty-one abortions out of fifty-seven spontaneous pregnancies. The take-home baby after PGD-AS was significantly higher.

The benefits of PGD-AS in these groups of patients with high risk of chromosomal miscarriage have been confirmed in a multicenter study (59). Nevertheless, some concern still arises (60).

The patients with an indication of advanced maternal age and repeated failures are more representative of the poor-prognosis infertile population treated by ART. Female aging is the most important factor in the decline of ART efficacy (27). Sharma et al. (31) clearly showed that in young normal responders the delivery rate per cycle is maintained the same during the first three attempts but is dramatically reduced afterward. Focusing on the role of PGD-AS in these categories of patients, a debate is present in the literature.

The most frequent argument against the efficacy of PGD-AS is the fact that very few and small-size prospective studies (15, 43–45) were able to demonstrate a higher implantation and/or live birth rates compared to control in these groups of infertile patients undergoing ART. The largest set of data are published in a retrospective fashion. However, one can argue that prospective studies showing no benefits of PGD-AS were not properly applying the technique (46, 47). A large controlled prospective study performed in programs with expertise in PGD, using one-cell biopsy, eight or more chromosomes analysis, and with dubious results retested is still needed.

A second argument is that PDG-AS, even showing in some condition to increase the PR per transferred cycle, is not able to produce more pregnancies per started cycle compared to control and, therefore, is not efficient for the ART system (61).

The randomized controlled study performed in our center in the first 127 cycles and published in 1999 (12) showed an immediate impact of PGD-AS on the implantation and on the ongoing implantation rates. The tendency was maintained during the ten years of activity, as evident in the cumulative data presented in Table 65.3: women aged more than thirty-eight years have been exposed to a 26 percent PR and to a risk of miscarriage lower than expected; young women with three or more previous failures maintained 38 percent PR per transferred cycle even in subsequent attempts.

Beside its direct effect on the end points normally utilized to measure ART efficiency, the implementation of ART procedure by PGD-AS offered to our program clear additional benefits in the management of infertile couples:

1. Even developing morphologically normal embryos, 32 percent of the patients who underwent PGD-AS were not transferred because no one-euploid embryo was available. These couples were avoided not only the luteal phase support but also, more important, an expectation of pregnancy and delivery that could have never been achieved.
2. The patients transferred after PGD-AS selection received a mean number of 1.8 ± 0.8 embryos.

Table 65.3: PGD-AS Results Depending on Indication

Indication	Repeated pregnancy loss	Sex-chromosomes mosaicism	Translocations	Advanced female age	Repeated previous failures	TESE
No. of cycles	110	66	84	529	120	62
Female age	37.8 ± 1.8	34.4 ± 3.6	34.9 ± 4.5	39.8 ± 2.1	32.6 ± 2.4	35.2 ± 4.4
No. of analyzed embryos	589	350	415	2,656	626	262
FISH normal, n (%)	187 (32)	128 (37)	77 (18)	813 (31)	261 (42)	88 (34)
FISH abnormal, n (%)	402 (68)	222 (63)	338 (82)	1,843 (69)	365 (58)	174 (66)
No. of transferred cycles	79 (72)	49 (74)	51 (61)	348 (66)	96 (80)	42 (68)
No. of transferred embryos (M ± SD)	1.6 ± 0.7	2 ± 0.1	1.4 ± 0.5	1.7 ± 0.8	1.9 ± 0.8	1.6 ± 0.7
No. of clinical pregnancies, n (%)	23 (29)	25 (51)	18 (35)	91 (26)	37 (38)	7 (17)
Implantation rate, %	22	36	35	18	27	13
No. of miscarriages, n (%)	3 (13)	2 (8)	6 (33)	15 (16)	3 (8)	1 (14)

In the past years, the whole international infertility community was recommended to reduce the number of multiple births associated with infertility treatments (62). No more than two embryos should be transferred, and the single embryo transfer has to be encouraged (63). However, poor-prognosis patients are often considered an exception to this limitation and more embryos are transferred in order to increase their chances of pregnancy (64). Thanks to PGD-AS selection, since 1998 no more than two embryos were always transferred in our center even in the poor-prognosis patients, and no triplets occurred due to the clinical need to transfer more embryos.

Embryo culture to the blastocyst stage for a better selection has also been proposed as an alternative for these patients. Compared to this approach, PGD-AS has the advantage to select chromosomal abnormalities compatible with normal development to blastocyst and implantation (monosomy, trisomy, unbalanced translocation, and, in some cases, even more complex abnormalities), increasing the probability of transferring chromosomal normal embryos.

3. When the apparently homogeneous population of poor-prognosis patients was tested with PGD-AS, two clear different subgroups were identified. The patients who develop only aneuploid embryos in the first PGD-AS cycle showed a clear tendency to the same performance in subsequent treatments. Out of 419 embryos screened in fifty-four additional cycles, only 35 (8.3 percent) were chromosomally normal. Accordingly, the prognosis of a term pregnancy was very poor: 8.5 percent. Conversely, when euploid embryos were detected in the first PGD cycle, the prognosis was still highly favorable for the patients: 33 percent per stared cycle and 70 percent of cumulative term pregnancy with additional three cycles (33).

PGD-AS can be regarded as a tool for estimating the ability of each couple to generate euploid embryos and for predicting the outcome in subsequent cycles. In addition to select embryos, PGD-AS can select patients by recognizing the subpopulation(s) for which further attempts are still recommended.

Patients could be supported to persist in their quest for children or to be assisted in the difficult decision of refraining from further attempts.

4. As described in the first part of the chapter, the analysis of the chromosomal abnormalities detected showed a different distribution between women with advanced reproductive age and young women experiencing repeated implantation failures. In our aged infertile population, the increase in the abnormalities with aging was due to monosomy and trisomy as physiologically occurs in the normal female population, suggesting no additional factors in determining chromosomal defects. Differently, haploidy, polyploidy, and complex abnormalities were the most common defects found in the second group, suggesting that processes or structures entering cell division could be for these couples an additional factor affecting the in vivo and in vitro reproductive performance. These information can have fundamental relevance in revisiting classical infertility's diagnosis and classification.

The last indication, *severe male factor,* involved sixty-two couples undergoing ICSI with sperms surgically extracted by the testis who failed at least one previous conventional cycle. The percentage of aneuploid embryos reached almost 70 percent, but even transferring only euploid embryos selected by PGD-AS, the PR and the IR were very poor. Probably, embryo competence to implant was affected by other factors than chromosomal defects or by defects in different chromosomes from those tested. Further studies are needed to offer those patients better chance of pregnancy. However, on the light that ICSI babies seem to be exposed to higher incidence of de novo abnormalities, TESE can be evaluated as an indication for PGD-AS (63).

FIRST–POLAR BODY BIOPSY AS A TOOL TO PRESELECT OOCYTES FOR INSEMINATION

As previously explained, first–polar body analysis as a procedure to select oocytes for insemination was applied as a consequence of the limits imposed by law in Italy.

Table 65.4: First Polar Body Analysis to Preselect Oocytes Compared to Conventional IVF/ICSI (Post-Law Period)

	PB1 cycles	Conventional IVF/ICSI cycles
No. of egg retrievals	266	254
No. of transferred cycles (mean embryos/transfer)	227 (1.7)	224 (1.8)
No. of clinical pregnancies, n (%)	52 (23)	56 (25)
Implantation rate, %	15.5	17.3
No. of miscarriages, n (%)*	6 (11.5)	16 (28.5)

*$p < 0.05$.

Although PBs FISH analysis is an established technique used as an alternative to embryo biopsy for aneuploidies prevention, to our knowledge it has never been tested for oocyte preselection because no other contexts impose by law a limit to the number of inseminated oocytes. Further, no one of the criteria available for embryo selection (embryo grading, 2PN morphology, blastocyst culture, and blastomere FISH analysis) can be applied according to law and all embryos generated have to be transferred.

As expected, a decline in the treatment's efficiency was observed in our center after the approval of the law. Comparing the results obtained in the past year before the law (648 cycles) to those registered in the first year after the law (534 cycles) in similar-aged patients, the pregnancy rate decreased from 33 to 24 percent, the implantation rate from 22 to 14 percent, and the miscarriage rate increased from 15 to 23 percent.

Safety and efficacy of PB1 biopsy were evaluated in a prospective controlled study as a tool to overcome the law limitation, preselecting competent oocytes for insemination and to increase the chance of transferring viable embryos. As described in Materials and Methods, soon after collection, MII oocytes were tested for six chromosomes (13, 15, 16, 18, 21, and 22) by PB1 analysis having the chromosomal results in time for correct insemination (within three hours).

The results of the study performed in 266 cycles versus 244 controls (conventional IVF/ICSI of three mature oocytes) are presented in Table 65.4.

No differences were found in the age of the patients, in the number of collected oocytes, in the fertilization and cleavage rates, and in the mean number of embryos transferred. The pregnancy and implantation rates were similar between the groups, while a significant lower miscarriage rate was observed in the PB1 group. A lower risk of abortion was registered in all age-group patients after PB1 selection compared to controls (Table 65.5).

These preliminary data led for the first time to same observations: 1) early PB1 biopsy do not affect fertilization, embryo development, and implantation potential as demonstrated by the similar rates obtained in the controls; 2) PB1 screening of first meiosis errors that can permit development to blastocyst and first-trimester pregnancy can decrease the risk of transferring normally cleaved aneuploid embryos with implantation potential, as demonstrated by the lower abortion rate in the study group; and 3) the technical and biological limits of this procedure does not allow to select against the abnormalities most involved in embryo preimplantation failure, and therefore, no more clinical pregnancies were registered after PB1 analysis. These limits would be partially overcome in the future by the implementation of the procedure or by new techniques able to fully karyotype the cell in a short time.

CONCLUSIONS

In vitro generated embryos are always selected before transfer by visual examination of development and morphology. These criteria are able to select against some chromosomal abnormalities, but even after observational selection, more than 50 percent of normally developing cleavage-stage embryos and 30 percent of blastocysts are chromosomally abnormal. PGD-AS is a tool to improve grounds for this selection and does not implicate ethical concerns about risk of eugenetics. In humans, the majority (98 percent) of aneuploidies are not compatible with life or even with embryo implantation.

The data generated by PGD-AS technique provide direct and valuable information on chromosomal anomalies that occur at the preimplantation stage, contributing to our understanding of the whole process in humans (Figure 65.7).

Further technical improvements are needed to increase the accuracy of single-cell genetic analysis and to avoid technical errors.

The current follow-up of children born after PGD-AS (65) indicates no detrimental effect of the biopsy as no differences have been reported when compared with conventional ICSI cycles. However, the number of the babies born is still limited and no final conclusion can be drawn at present.

By measuring the efficacy through the classical end points (implantation, pregnancy, and live birth rates) utilized for testing new IFV/ICSI protocols or techniques, results are still controversial and not enough evidence is present in the literature to determine the current value of PGD-AS (66). Anyway, this is not new in the ART system; despite several studies and meta-analysis, several questions are still open, that is, the efficacy of rFSH versus uFSH, the need of LH supplementation, the blastocyst transfer versus day 3 transfer (just to mention some!).

Table 65.5: PB1 Cycle's Outcome Divided by Age in the Study and Control Groups

Age-groups oocyte's selection	≤34 Years PB1	≤34 Years conventional	35–37 Years PB1	35–37 Years conventional	38–43 Years PB1	38–43 Years conventional
Clinical pregnancies rate (%)	33	36	30	18	15	24
Implantation rate (%)	22	23	19	10	10	15
Miscarriage rate (%)	6	21	12	50	18	33

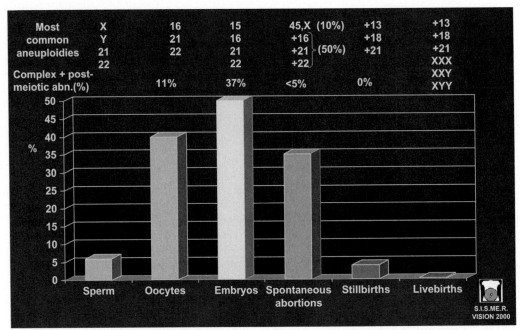

Figure 65.7. Frequency of chromosomal anomalies in different stages of the human reproductive process.

Our ten years' experience supports the evidence that PGD-AS can be justified at present not only because it is able to improve the probability of term pregnancy in selected groups of patients but also because it can produce other clinical benefits in the management of difficult couples.

With the view that efficiency can be significantly improved in the near future, PGD-AS has to be considered as a tool to implement ART procedure and as a tool to better understand the mechanisms of embryo development and implantation.

At present, PGD-AS requires specialized equipment, methodology, experienced, and dedicated professionals and has to be properly performed to obtain the best results.

KEY POINTS FOR CLINICAL PRACTICE

■ Human reproduction is largely affected by chromosomal defects. The in vitro generated embryo can be more prone to errors both because it is generated by an infertile population and because of the ART procedure itself.

■ As in natural conception, maternal aging is the major factor affecting aneuploidy frequency, but some infertility conditions seem to express higher incidence than expected.

■ The analysis of preimplantation gametes and embryos revealed that each chromosome originates aneuploidies at a different rate and that distribution of abnormalities differs depending on patient characteristics.

■ Also not yet perfectly efficient for technical and biological events, PGD-AS is a safe and established procedure to identify preimplantation abnormalities and could therefore be an added tool to select in vitro generated embryos for transfer and to increase their probability to produce an ongoing pregnancy.

■ Patients have to be informed on the risk of misdiagnosis and be recommended to undergo prenatal diagnosis to confirm the PGD results.

■ Clinical data on the beneficial effects of PGD-AS in the infertile population undergoing ART are still controversial. According to some authors, there is insufficient evidence to implement this procedure in a routine basis. According to others, PGD-AS has already demonstrated to be an important tool in the management of some categories of patients, provided that is properly performed.

■ Further randomized trials, together with the improvement of the technique, are needed to clearly establish the usefulness of PGD-AS. Preselection of aneuploidy-free embryos has to have an impact on the reproductive outcome, considering that human reproductive process is well known to be affected by meiotic errors.

REFERENCES

1. Menken J, Trussel J, Larsen U. Age and infertility. *Science* 1986; 233:1389–94.
2. Inge GB, Brinsden PR, Elder KT. Oocyte number per live birth in IVF: were Steptoe and Edwards less wasteful? *Hum Reprod* 2005; 20:588–92.
3. Baird DT, Collins J, Egozcue, et al. Fertility and ageing (Eshre Capri Workshop Group). *Hum Reprod Update* 2005; 11:261–76.
4. Eiben B, Bartels I, Bahr-Porsch S, et al. Cytogenetic analysis of 750 spontaneous abortions with the direct-preparation method of chorionic villi and its implications for studying genetic causes of pregnancy wastage. *Am J Hum Genet* 1990; 47:656–63.
5. Handyside AH, Kontoganni E, Hardy K, Winston R., Pregnancies from biopsied human preimplantation embryos sexed by Y-specific DNA amplification. *Nature* 1990; 344:768–70.
6. Griffin DK, Wilton LJ, Handyside AH, Winston RMK, Delhanty JDA. Dual fluorescent in situ hybridisation for simultaneous detection of X and Y chromosome-specific probes for the sexing of human preimplantation embryonic nuclei. *Hum Genet* 1992; 89:18–22.

7. Munné S, Lee A, Rosenwaks Z, Grifo J, Cohen J., Diagnosis of major chromosome aneuploidies in human preimplantation embryos. *Hum Reprod* 1993; 8:2185–91.

8. The Practice Committee of the American Society for Reproductive Medicine and the Practice Committee of the Society for Assisted Reproductive Technology. Preimplantation genetic diagnosis. *Fertil Steril* 2006; 86 (Suppl. 4):257–8.

9. Harper JC, Boelaert K, Geraedts J, et al. ESHRE PGD Consortium data collection V: cycles from January to December 2002 with pregnancy follow-up to October 2003. *Hum Reprod 2006*; 21:3–21.

10. Gianaroli L, Magli MC, Fiorentino F, Baldi M, Ferraretti AP. Clinical value of preimplantation genetic diagnosis. *Placenta* 2003; 24:77–83.

11. Benagiani G, Gianaroli L. The new Italian IVF legislation. *RBM Online* 2004; 9:117–25.

12. Verlinsky Y, Cieslkak J, Ivanhnenko V, et al. Prevention of age-related aneuploidies by polar body testing of oocytes. *J Assist Reprod Genet* 1999; 16:165–9.

13. Pellestor F, Anahory T, Hamamah S. The chromosomal analysis of human oocytes. An overview of established procedures. *Hum Reprod* 2005; 11:15–32.

14. Gianaroli L, Magli MC, Cavallini G, et al. Frequency of aneuploidy in spermatozoa from patients with extremely severe male factor infertility. *Hum Reprod* 2005; 20:2140–52.

15. Gianaroli L, Magli C, Ferraretti AP, Munné S. Preimplantation diagnosis for aneuploidies in patients undergoing in vitro fertilization with a poor prognosis: identification of the categories for which it should be proposed. *Fertil Steril* 1999; 72: 837–44.

16. Magli MC, Ferraretti AP, Crippa A, Lappi M, Feliciani E, Gianaroli L. First meiosis errors in immature oocytes generated by stimulated cycles. *Fertil Steril* 2006; 86:629–35.

17. Gianaroli L, Magli MC, Ferraretti AP. Sperm and blastomere aneuploidy detection in reproductive genetics and medicine. *J Histochem Cytochem* 2005; 53:261–8.

18. Sandalinas M, Sadowy S, Alikani M, Calderon G, Cohen J, Munné S. Developmental ability of chromosomally abnormal human embryos to develop to the blastocyst stage. *Hum Reprod* 2001; 16:1954–8.

19. Bielanska M, Tan SL, Ao A. chromosomal mosaicism throughout human preimplantation development in vitro: incidence, type, and relevance to embryo outcome. *Hum Reprod* 2002; 17:413–19.

20. Veiga A, Gil Y, Boada M, et al. Confirmation of diagnosis in preimplantation genetic diagnosis (PGD) through blastocyst culture: preliminary experience. *Prenat Diagn* 1999; 19:1242–7.

21. Clouston HJ, Herbert M, Fenwick J, Murdoch AP, Wolstenholme J. Cytogenetic analysis of human blastocysts. *Prenat Diagn* 2002; 22:1143–52.

22. Magli MC, Jones GM, Gras L, Gianaroli L, Korman I, Trounson AO. Chromosome mosaicism in day-3 aneuploid embryos that develop to morphologically normal blastocysts in vitro. *Hum Reprod* 2000; 15:1781–6.

23. Nicolaidis P, Peterson MB. Origin and mechanisms of non-disjunction in human autosomas trisomies. *Hum Reprod* 1998; 13:313–19.

24. Hassold T, Chiu D. Maternal-age specific rates of numerical chromosome abnormalities with special reference to trisomy. *Hum Genet* 1995; 70:11–17.

25. Plachot M. Genetic analysis of oocyte – a review. Placenta 24 (Suppl. B) 2003;S66–9.

26. Daguet F. *Un siecle de fecondité francaise: 1901–1999.* INSEE, Paris 2002.

27. Adamson GD, de Mouzon J, Lancaster P, Nygren K-G, Sullivan E, Zegers-Hochschild F. World collaborative report on in vitro fertilization, 2000. *Fertil Steril* 2006; 85:1586–622.

28. Munné S, Sandalina M, Escudero T, Fung J, Gianaroli L, Cohen J, Outcome of preimplantation genetic diagnosis of translocations. *Fertil Steril* 2000; 73:1209–18.

29. Gianaroli L, Magli MC, Ferraretti AP, et al. Possible interchromosomal effect in embryos generated by gametes from translocation carriers. *Hum Reprod* 2002; 17:3201–7.

30. Tarlatzis BC. Clinical management of low ovarian response to stimulation for IVF: a systematic review. *Hum Reprod* 2003; 9:61–76.

31. Sharma V, Allagar V, Rajkhowa M. Factors influencing the cumulative conception rate and discontinuation of in vitro fertilization treatment for infertility. *Fertil Steril* 2002; 78:40–6.

32. Gianaroli L, Magli MC, Ferraretti AP, et al. Gonadal activity and chromosomal constitution of in vitro generated embryos. *Mol Cell Endocrinol* 2000; 161:111–16.

33. Ferraretti AP, Magli MC, Kopcow L, Gianaroli L. Prognostic role of preimplantation genetic diagnosis for aneuploidy in assisted reproduction technology outcome. *Hum Reprod* 2004; 19:694–9.

34. Sloter ED, Lowe X, Moore II DH, Nath J, Wyrobek AJ. Multicolor FISH analysis of chromosomal breaks, duplications, deletions, and numerical abnormalities in the sperm of healthy men. *Am J Hum Genet* 2000; 67:862–72.

35. McInnes M, Rademarker AW, Martin RH. Donor age and the frequency of disomy for chromosomes 1, 13, 21 and structural abnormalities in human spermatozoa using multicolour fluorescence in-situ hybridization. *Hum Reprod* 1998; 13:2489–94.

36. Kühnert B, Nieschlag E. Reproductive functions of the ageing male. *Hum Reprod Update* 2004; 10:327–39.

37. Egozcue S, Blanco J, Anton E, Egozcue S, Serrate Z, Vidal F. Genetic analysis of sperm and implications of severe male infertility – a review. *Placenta* 2003; 24:62S–5.

38. Magli MC, Gianaroli L, Ferraretti AP, Lappi M, Ruberti A, Farfalli V. Embryo morphology and development is dependent on the chromosomal complement. *Fertil Steril* 2007; in press.

39. Munné S. Chromosome abnormalities and their relationship to morphology and development of human embryos. *RBM Online* 2006; 12:234–53.

40. Scott L, Alvero R, Leondires M, Bradley M. The morphology of human pronuclear embryos is positively related to blastocyst development and implantation. *Hum Reprod* 2000; 15: 2394–403.

41. Gianaroli L, Magli Mc, Ferraretti AP, Lappi M, Borghi E, Ermini B. Oocyte euploidy, pronuclear zygote morphology and embryo chromosomal complement. *Hum Reprod* 2007; in press.

42. Munné S, Chen S, Fischer J, et al. Preimplantation genetic diagnosis reduces pregnancy loss in women 35 and older with a history of recurrent miscarriages. *Fertil Steril* 2005; 84:331–5.

43. Munné S, Magli C, Cohen J, et al. Positive outcome after preimplantation diagnosis of aneuploidy in human embryos. *Hum Reprod* 1999; 14:2191–9.

44. Gianaroli L, Magli MC, Munné S, Fortini D, Ferraretti AP. Advantages of day 4 embryo transfer in patients undergoing preimplantation genetic diagnosis of aneuploidy. *J Assist Reprod Genet* 1999; 16:170–5.

45. Munné S, Sandalinas M, Escudero T, et al. Improved implantation after preimplantation genetic diagnosis of aneuploidy. *RBM Online* 2003; 7:91–7.

46. Platteau P, Staessen C, Michiels A, Van Steirteghem A, Liebaers I, Devroey P., Preimplantation genetic diagnosis for aneuploidy

screening in patients with unexplained recurrent miscarriages. *Fertil Steril* 2005; 83:393–7.

47. Staessen C, Platteau P, Van Assche E, et al. Comparison of blastocyst transfer with or without preimplantation genetic diagnosis for aneuploidy screening in couples with advanced maternal age: a prospective randomized controlled trial. *Hum Reprod* 2004; 19:2849–58.

48. Robertson JA. Extending preimplantation genetic diagnosis: the ethical debate. Ethical issues in new uses of preimplantation genetic diagnosis. *Hum Reprod* 2003; 18:465–71.

49. Verlinsky Y, Kuliev AM (Eds.). *Preimplantation diagnosis of genetic diseases: a new technique in assisted reproduction*. New York: Wiley-Liss, 1993.

50. Hardy K, Martin KL, Leese HJ, Winston RML, Handyside AH. Human preimplantation development in vitro is not adversely affected by biopsy at the 8-cell stage. *Hum Reprod* 1990; 5: 708–14.

51. Tarin JJ, Conaghan J, Winston RML, Handyside AH. Human embryo biopsy on the 2nd day after insemination for preimplantation diagnosis: removal of a quarter of embryo retards cleavage. *Fertil Steril* 1992; 58:970–6.

52. Gianaroli L, Magli MC, Ferraretti AP. The in vivo and in vitro efficiency and efficacy of PGD for aneuploidy. *Mol Cell Endocrinol* 2001; 183:13–18.

53. Shenfield F, Pennings G, Devroey P, et al. ESHRE Ethics Task Force 5: preimplantation genetic diagnosis. *Hum Reprod* 2003; 18:649–51.

54. Munné S, Sandalinas M, Escudero T, Marquez C, Cohen J. Chromosome mosaicism in cleavage stage human embryos: evidence of a maternal age effect. *RBM Online* 2002; 4:223–32.

55. Evsikov S, Verlinsky Y. Mosaicism in the inner cell mass of human blastocysts. *Hum Reprod* 1998; 11:3151–55.

56. Yaron Y, Orr-Urtreger A. New genetic principles. *Clin Obstet Gynaecol* 2002; 45:593–604.

57. Bernardini L, Gianaroli L, Fortini D, et al. Frequency of hyper-, hypohaploid and diploidy in ejaculate, epididymal and testicular germ cells of infertile patients. *Hum Reprod* 2000; 15:2165–72.

58. Brigham SA, Colon C, Farquharson RG. A longitudinal study of pregnancy outcome following idiopathic recurrent miscarriage. *Hum Reprod* 1999; 14:2868–71.

59. Munné S, Fischer J, Warner A, Chen S, Zouves C, Cohen J, and referring centers PGD group. Preimplantation genetic diagnosis significantly reduces pregnancy loss in infertile couples: A Multi-Center Study. *Fertil Steril* 2006; 85:326–332.

60. Ogasawara M, Suzumori K. Can implantation genetic diagnosis improve success rates in recurrent aborters with translocations? *Hum Reprod* 2005; 20:3267–70.

61. Shahine LK, Cedars MI. Preimplantation genetic diagnosis does not increase pregnancy rates in patients at risk for aneuploidy. *Fertil Steril* 2006; 85:51–6.

62. Infertility therapy-associated multiple pregnancies (births): an ongoing epidemic. Proceeding of an expert meeting in New York, USA. April 12–13 2003. *RBM Online* 7 (Suppl. 2).

63. World Health Organization. Current Practises and Controversies in Assisted Reproduction, Report of a Meeting on Medical, Ethical and Social Aspects of Assisted Reproduction held ad WHO Headquarters in Geneva, Switzerland, 17–21 September 2001. Vayena E, Rowe PJ, Griffin PD (Eds.), 2002.

64. Azem F, Yaron Y, Amit A, et al. Transfer of six or more embryos improves success rates in patients with repeated in vitro fertilization failures. *Fertil Steril* 1995; 63:1043–6.

65. Verlinsky Y, Cohen J, Munnè S, Gianaroli L, et al. Over a decade of experience with preimplantation genetic diagnosis: a multicenter report. *Fertil Steril* 2004; 82:292–4.

66. Donoso P, Staessen C, Fauser BCJM, et al. Current value of preimplantation genetic aneuplody screening in IVF. *Hum Reprod Update* 2007; 13:15–25.

66

PREIMPLANTATION GENETIC DIAGNOSIS FOR SINGLE-GENE DISORDERS

Hany F. Moustafa, Botros R. M. B. Rizk, Zsolt Peter Nagy

Although preimplantation genetic diagnosis (PGD) was first reported more than thirty years ago by Robert G. Edwards and his colleagues when they managed to identify the sex of rabbit blastocysts, it was not until later in the 1980s when PGD of human embryos was extensively investigated. In 1990, Alan Handyside reported the birth of healthy females after sex selection using polymerase chain reaction (PCR) to amplify a Y chromosome repeat sequence to exclude male embryos (1).

Further advancements in the arena of IVF, micromanipulation, and DNA technology led to remarkable progress in the field of PGD. It is now an established clinical option in reproductive medicine and has already helped couples all over the world to conceive healthy children. Based on the 186 responses from IVF centers in the United States to a survey by the Genetics and Public Policy Center at Johns Hopkins University in 2006, PGD was reported to be provided by nearly three-quarters of these IVF clinics and it is estimated that 4–6 percent of all their IVF cycles include PGD (2). Many international bodies have strived to come up with evidence-based protocols for the procedure, including the American Society of Reproductive Medicine, the European Society for Human Reproduction and Embryology, and the PGD International Society. In the absence of wide, randomized controlled trials, most of the recommendations that these international bodies came up with are considered general guidelines based on clinical experience and published data (3–8).

Currently, the common indications for PGD include carriers of Mendelian disorders, human leukocyte antigen (HLA) typing, translocation carriers, recurrent pregnancy loss, recurrent implantation failure and advanced maternal age. Less solid indications for PGD include certain categories of infertile couples as poor responders and TESE patients (8, 9).

Recently, the term PGS (preimplantation genetic screening) was designated to refer to a certain group of low-risk patients who may need PGD. This includes IVF patients who have suffered from repeated implantation failure, recurrent miscarriages or simply those with advanced age. This group is considered a low-risk group and evidence shows that they may benefit from genetic screening of their embryo prior to transfer and hence the term PGS. The term preimplantation genetic diagnosis for aneuploidy screening (PGD-AS) is used interchangeably with PGS. The use of the term "screening" has been criticized by some authorities since the results obtained from the preimplantation genetic testing are

considered diagnostic and are literally used to choose or determine which embryos to be transferred. Others believe that the term screening is more "legally" appropriate based on the suboptimal accuracy of some of the tests, which calls for further confirmation through prenatal testing (Verlinsky, personal communication). It is currently estimated that two-thirds of the PGD cycles in the United States are done for aneuploidy screening. Patients who are known to carry a genetic disorder or a chromosomal structural abnormality (balanced translocation) are at high risk of transmitting the condition to their offspring, so they are considered a higher risk group and they require PGD (10).

PGD FOR SINGLE-GENE DISORDERS

There is a wide range of single-gene disorders that could be screened for using PGD. The number of such diseases has been growing exponentially in the past few years. These mostly include Mendelian disorders like autosomal or X-linked disorders, whether recessive or dominant. According to the latest ESHRE PGD consortium data (9), the most common autosomal recessive diseases for which PGD is done are cystic fibrosis, β-thalassemia, and spinal muscular dystrophy. The most common autosomal dominant diseases include myotonic dystrophy, Huntington disease, neurofibromatosis, and adenomatous polyposis coli. While the most common X-linked diseases are fragile X syndrome, Duchenne and Becker muscular dystrophy, and hemophilia. With the use of some of the novel techniques in PGD testing, as will be detailed later, screening for several genes is possible in one setting, which will further allow screening for disorders that could be polygenic in nature or associated with genetic heterogeneity. Also PGD could be performed for conditions for which a specific mutation has not been determined as long as informative linkage analysis for that condition could be established. Table 66.1 shows a list of the most common genetic diseases that could be screened for using PGD. PGD can also be used for screening of late-onset genetic diseases like cancer, Huntington disease, and Alzheimer disease, which were not considered for testing before through prenatal diagnosis (11–13).

Another unique use, although a source of a big ethical debate, is combining PGD with HLA typing. This was first reported by Verlinsky et al. in 2001 for Fanconi anemia (14).

Adding HLA typing offers not only the chance of conceiving a healthy offspring but also the possibility to conceive an

Table 66.1: List of the Most Common Genetic Diseases That Could be Screened for by Using PGD

21-Hydroxylase deficiency	Fanconi anemia E	Neurofibromatosis
Achondroplasia; ACH	Fanconi anemia F (and HLA)	N-acetylglutamate synthase deficiency
Acyl-CoA dehydrogenase, medium-chain, deficiency	Fanconi anemia J (and HLA)	Neonatal epileptic encephalopathy (PNPO gene)
Acyl-CoA dehydrogenase, very long-chain; ACADVL	Fanconi anaemia, complementation group C; FANCC	Neurofibromatosis, type I; NF1
Adadenosine deaminase deficiency; ADA	Fanconi anaemia, complementation group E; FANCE	Neurofibromatosis, type II; NF2
Adenine deaminase dificiency	Fanconi anaemia, complementation group F; FANCF	Neuropathy, hereditary sensory and autonomic, type III; HSAN3
Adenomatous polyposis of the colon; APC	Fanconi anaemia, complementation group G	Niemann-Pick disease
Adenosine aminohydrolase (ADA) deficiency	Fanconi anaemia, complementation group J	Norrie disease
Adrenoleukodystrophy; ALD	Fanconi anaemia, complementation group A; FANCA	Norrie disease; NDP
Adrenoleukodystrophy; X-linked ALD	FG syndrome	Oculocutaneous albinism, type I; OCA1
Adult polycystic kidney disease	Fragile site, folic acid type, rare, FRA(X)(q28); FRAXE	Oculocutaneous albinism, type II; OCA2
Agammaglobulinaemia	Fragile site mental retardation I	Omenn syndrome
Albinism, ocular, type I; OA1	Fragile-X A syndromes (FMR1)	Optic atrophy
Alopecia, congenital	Fragile-X E syndromes	Optic atrophy I; OPA1
Alopecia universalis congenita; ALUNC	Fragile X syndrome	Opitz-Kaveggia
Alpers diffuse degeneration of cerebral gray matter with hepatic cirrhosis	Friedreich ataxia	Oral-facial-digital syndrome type 1
Alpers syndrome	Friedreich ataxia 1, FRDA	Ornithine carbamoyltransferase (OTC) deficiency
Alpha-1-antitrypsin deficiency (AAT)	Gaucher's disease	Ornithine transcarbamylase deficiency
Alport syndrome, X-linked; ATS	Galactosaemia	Osteogenesis imperfecta coli A1 and coli A2 Mutations
Alzheimer's disease	Gangliodidosis type 1 (GM1)	Osteogenesis imperfecta congenita; OIC
Amyloidosis I, hereditary neuropathic	Gangliosidosis, generalized GM1, type 1	Osteogenesis imperfecta types I and IV
Androgen insensitivity syndrome	Gaucher disease, type 1	Osteopetrosis, autosomal recessive
Androgen receptor; AR (testicular feminization; spinal and bulbar muscular atrophy; Kennedy disease)	Glucose-6-phosphatase deficiency	Osteopetrosis, malignant, autosomal recessive
Aneploidies by STR genotyping	Glomuvenous malformation (GVM)	Pancreatitis, hereditary; PCTT
Angioedema, hereditary; HAE	Glutaric acidaemia I	P53 mutations
Ataxia-telangiectasia; AT	Glutaric aciduria type 1	PDH deficiency
Autism	Glutaric aciduria type 2	Pelizaeus-Merzbacher disease
Barth syndrome	Glycogen storage disease type VI	Pelizaeus-Merzbacher-like disease; PMLD
Basal cell nevus syndrome; BCNS (Gorlin syndrome)	Golabi-Rosen syndrome	Peutz-Jeghers syndrome; PJS
Becker muscular dystrophy	Goltz syndrome	Phenylketonuria
Blepharophimosis	Gorlin syndrome	Plakophilin deficiency
Blepharophimosis, ptosis, and epicanthus inversus; BPES	Granulomatous Disease	Polycystic kidney disease

(continued)

Table 66.1. *(continued)*

Blood group-Kell-Cellano system	Haemoglobin-alpha locus 1; HBA1	Polycystic kidney disease 1; PKD1
Brachydactyly	Haemoglobin-alpha locus 2; HBA 2	Polycystic kidney disease 2; PKD2
Brachydactyly, Type B1; BDB1	Haemoglobin-beta locus; HBB	Polycystic kidney disease autosomal dominant type 1
Brain tumour, posterior fossa of infancy, familial	Haemophilia A and B	Polycystic kidney disease autosomal dominant type 2
Breast cancer, familial	Hemophagocytic lymphohistiocytosis, familia, 2	Polycystic kidney disease, autosomal recessive; ARPKD
BRCA1	Hemophilia A	Popliteal pterygium syndrome; PPS
Bruton agammaglobulinaemia tyrosine kinase; BTK	Hemophilia B	Prader-Willi syndrome
Canavan disease	Hereditary nonpolyposis colorectal cancer	Proliferative disease
Carbohydrate deficient glycoprotein syndrome type 1A	Hereditary breast/Ovarian Cancer (BRCA1)	Propionic acidaemia
Central core disease	HLA matching genotyping	Recurrent hydatidiform mole
Ceroid lipofuscionosis, neuronal 2, lae infantile; CLN2 (batten disease)	HLA typing	Renal agenesis
Charcot-Marie-Tooth disease, axonal, type 2E	Holoprosencephaly	Retinitis pigmentosa
Charcot-Marie-Tooth disease, demyelinating, type 1A; CMT1A	Homocystinuria due to deficiency of N(5,10)-methylenetetraphydrofolate reductase activity	Retinitis pigmentosa 3; RP3
Charcot-Marie-Tooth disease, demyelinating, type 1B; CMT1B	Hoyeraal-Hreidarsson syndrome; HHS	Retinoblastoma; RB1
Charcot-Marie-Tooth disease type 1a and 2a	Hunter's disease	Retinoschisis
Charcot-Marie-Tooth disease, X-linked, 1; CMTX1	Hunter's syndrome	Rett syndrome; RTT
Cholestasis, progressive familial intrahepatic 2	Hunter syndrome (mucopolysaccharidosis type II)	Rhesus blood group, CcEe antigens; RHCE
Chondrodysplasia punctata 1, X-linked recessive; CDPX1	Huntington chorea	Rhesus blood group, D antigen; RHD
Chondrodysplasia punctata, X-linked, CMTX1	Huntington's disease; HD	Rhesus factor compatibility (RH factor)
Chondrodysplasia punctata, X-linked	Hurler syndrome	RhD sensitization
Choroideraemia; CHM	Hurler syndrome (MPS 1, Alpha-L-Iduronidase deficiency (IDUA))	Rhizomelic chondro dysplasia punctata
Chronic granulomatous disease	Hydrocephalus, X-linked; L1CAM	Sandhoff disease
Citrullinaemia, classic	Hyperinsulinaemic	Severe combined immunodeficiency
Coffin-Lowy syndrome	Hyperinsulinemic hypoglycaemia, familial, 1; HHF1	Sex chromosome mosaicism
Collagen, type IV, alpha-5; COL4A5	Hypoglycaemia	Sickle cell anaemia
Colorectal cancer, hereditary non-polyposis, type 1; HNPCC1	Hypohidrotic ectodermal dysplasia	Sickle cell anemia (hemoglobin SS and SC disease)
Colorectal cancer, hereditary non-polyposis, type 2; HNPCC2	Hypophosphatasia, infantile	Sickle cell disease
Complex IV deficiency (Leigh syndrome dysostosis)	Hypophosphatasia X-linked	Skewed X inactivation
Congenital adrenal hyperplasia (CAH)	Hypophosphatasia rickets, X-linked dominant	Skin fragility syndrome

Connexin 26 (Autosomal recessive non-syndromic sensoneural deafness)

Craniofacial dysostosis, type I; (CFDI)

Crouzon syndrome (Craniofacial dysostosis)

Currarino syndrome

Currarino triad

Cutis laxa, autosomal recessive, type 1

Crouzon syndrome

Cycles without indications

Cystic fibrosis; CF

Cystinosis

Cystinosis, nephropathic; CTNS

Darier-White disease; DAR

Deafness, neurosensory, autosomal recessive 1; DFNB1

Diamond-Blacfan anaemia; DBA

Duchenne muscular dystrophy

Dysautonomia, familial

Early-onset familial Alzheimer disease

Ectodermal dysplasia 1, anhidrotic; ED1

Ectodermal dysplasia, anhidrotic, ED1 (X-linked)

Ectodermal dysplasia, anhidrotic

Ectodermal dysplasia, anhidrotic (autosomal recessive)

Ectrodactyly, ectodermal dysplasia, and cleft lip/palate syndrome 1; EEC1

Emery-Dreifuss muscular dystrophy, autosomal recessive; EDMD3

Emery-Dreifuss muscular dystrophy (Dominant, recessive, & X-linked)

Emery-Dreifuss muscular dystrophy, X-linked; EDMD

Epidermolysis bullosa

Epidermolysis bullosa dystrophica, Pasini type

Epidermolysis bullosa (PLEG1, LAMB3, COL7A1)

Epidermolysis bullosa lethalis

Epidermolysis bullosa simplex and limb-girdle muscular dystrophy

Epilepsy

Epiphyseal dysplasia, multiple

Hypospadias

Immunodeficiency with hyper-IgM, type1; HIGMI

Incontinentia pigmenti; IP

Infantile neuronal ceroid lipofuscinosis

Inversion X

Isovaleric acidaemia; IVA

Junctional epidermolysis bullosa

Kallman syndrome

Kell blood group compatibility

Kennedy disease

Lesch-Nyhan disease

Lesch-Nyhan syndrome

Leukoencephalopathy with vanishing white matter; VWM

LHON mitochondrial

Li-Fraumeni syndrome 1; LFS1

Li-Fraumeni syndrome(mutations in P53 gene)

Loeys-Dietz syndrome; LDS

Long-chain 3-hydroxyacyl-CoA dehydrogenase deficiency; HADHA

Long-chain hydroxylacyl-CoA dehydrogenase deficiency (LCHAD)

Lowe syndrome

Machado-Joseph disease; MJD

Marfan syndrome; MFS

Meckle-Gruber syndrome

Medium chain acyl-CoA dehydrogenase deficiency (MCAD)

MELAS

Menkes' disease

Metachromatic leukodystrophy

Metaphyseal dysplasia

Metaphyseal chondrodysplasia, schmid type; MCDS

Methylenetetrahydrofolate reductase deficiecy (MTHFR)

Methylmalonic aciduria and homocystinuria (MMACHC)

Microcoria-congenital nephrosis syndrome

Smith-Lemli-Opitz syndrome; SLOS

Sonic hedgehog; SHH

Spinal and bulbar muscular atrophy

Spinal muscular atrophy (SMA)

Spinal muscular atrophy, type I; SMA1

Spinocerebellar ataxia 1; SCA1

Spinocerebellar ataxia 2; SCA2

Spinocerebellar ataxia 3 (SCA3)

Spinocerebellar atacia 6; SCA6

Spinocerebellar ataxia 7 (SCA7)

Stickler syndrome

Sticker syndrome, type I; STL1

Succinic semialdehyde dehydrogenase deficiency

Sulphatidosis

Symphalangism, proximal; SYM1

Tay-Sachs disease; TSD

Thalassaemia

Thalassaemia alpha

Thalassaemia beta

Torsion dystonia (DYT1)

Torsion dystonia 1, autosomal dominant; DYT1

Treacher collins syndrome

Treacher Collins-Franceschetti syndrome; TCOF

Trifunctional protein deficiency

Tuberous sclerosis

Tuberous sclerosis type 1

Tuberous sclerosis type 2

Tyrosinaemia

Tyrosinaemia, type 1

Ulnar-mammary syndrome; UMS

Vanishing white matter disease

Very long chain Acyl-CoA dehydrognase deficiency (VLCAD)

(continued)

Table 66.1. (*continued*)

Epiphyseal dysplasia, multiple, 1; EDM1	Microcoria-congenital nephrosis syndrome (LAMB 2)	Vitamin D resistant rickets
Exep macrosom males	Migraine, familial hemiplegic, 1; FHM1	Von Hippel-Lindau syndrome; VHL
Exostoses, multiple, type I	Morquio syndrome, non-keratosulfate-excreting type	Waardenburg syndrome
Fabry disease	Mucopolysaccharidosis type II (Hunter) Hunter-McAlpine craniosynostosis syndrome	Wiskott-Aldrich syndrome; WAS
Facioscapulohumeral muscular dystrophy (FSHMDIA)	Multiple acyl-CoA dehydrogenase deficiency; MADD	X-linked
Facioscapulohumeral muscular dystrophy 1A; FSHMDIA	Multiple endocrine neoplasia type I (MEN1)	X-linked chondrodysplasia
Falizaeus-Merzbacher	Multiple endocrine neoplasia, type IIA; MEN2A	X-linked haemophagocytic
Familial adenomatous polyposis	Multiple exostoses	X-linked mental retardation
Familial adenomatous polyposis coli (Gardner syndrome)	Muscular dystrophy, Becker type; BMD	X-linked Myotublar
Familial amyloid polyneuropathy	Muscular dystrophy, Duchenne type; DMD	X-linked ocular albinism
Familial dysautonomia (Riley-day syndrome, DYS)	Myotonic dystrophy (DMI)	X-linked retinoschisis
Fanconi anaemia	Myotubular myopathy	Y deletion
Fanconi anemia C (and HLA)	Myotublular myopathy X-linked	Zellweger syndrome; ZS
Fanconi anemia C (and HLA)	Myotubular myopathy 1; MTM1	Zellweger syndrome (PEX1 AND PEX 2)
		ZFX/ZFY for sexing only

HLA-compatible cord blood donor to treat older siblings with congenital or acquired bone marrow diseases. The cord blood, which is usually otherwise discarded, is obtained after the delivery of the HLA-matched child for stem cell culture and transplantation to the affected sibling (6).

GENETIC COUNSELING

The aim of genetic counseling is to enable couples and families with genetic disadvantages to live and reproduce as normally as possible. Most couples wishing to have PGD have already experienced a genetic condition in one of their family members and wish to avoid having an affected child. Typically, the counseling process begins when the couples are referred to the clinical geneticist by their general practitioner. The genetic condition should be identified after discussions with the couples and possibly some of their relatives. Once the clinical condition is identified, the plan for diagnostic confirmation should be further discussed. At this point, it might be prudent to offer genetic testing for other family members as well. If available, identification of closely linked genetic markers should be done since it improves the diagnostic accuracy of PGD as will be detailed later in the chapter (15). Once the diagnosis is confirmed, risk assessment and recurrence risk should be done by an experienced genetic counselor who should also discuss the nature, severity, and the implications of the disease. He should also explain other alternatives to PGD that can help them to have healthy offspring. These alternatives include different forms of prenatal diagnosis, gamete donation, adoption, or simply accepting the risk without doing any testing. For couples who wish to remain childless, it is important to counsel them about the chances of naturally conceiving an affected child and to provide them with the appropriate method of contraception.

The cost, feasibility, pregnancy rate, risks, adverse outcomes (including multiple pregnancies and other risks related to ovarian stimulation), and limitations of all procedures should be discussed with the couple to help in choosing the most suitable option. It is currently estimated that the cost of a single PGD cycle ranges between $3,000 and $5,000 USD, in addition to the cost of the IVF/ICSI cycle. The reliability of PGD and chances of a misdiagnosis should be also thoroughly discussed (16, 17). Currently, there are validated figures for the accuracy and the error rates encountered during different types of PGD, and these should be used during the counseling process. Because the error rate associated with single-cell genetic testing is not negligible, prenatal diagnosis should always be recommended to confirm the results of PGD (3, 6, 18).

Fertile couples should be informed that pregnancy rates are expected to be lower after PGD when compared to natural cycles. Although part of this decline is due to the use of ICSI, the nature of the genetic condition remains the main determinant of the pregnancy rate. For example, if both parents are carriers of an autosomal recessive condition like cystic fibrosis, it is estimated that 25 percent of the embryos will be homozygous for cystic fibrosis gene, leaving only 75 percent of the embryos amenable for transfer (including both heterozygous and homozygous normal). In contrast, with an autosomal dominant condition, usually 50 percent of the embryos would be affected, thus reducing the number of sound embryos to be transferred to half. Also when PGD is done for HLA typing, it is expected that only 25 percent will be available for transfer. For autosomal recessive conditions, the decision should be made with the couple regarding the transfer of carrier embryos (heterozygous embryos) as opposed to homozygous normal embryos. In some cases, the couple would choose to eliminate the disease from their families and thus refuse transferring carrier embryos. During counseling, it is very important to use a nondirective style to ensure maximum patient autonomy. It is important to realize that although PGD may be seen as the most reasonable option to some, others may still consider it unethical based upon their religious or cultural beliefs.

ELIGIBILITY CRITERIA FOR PGD/PGS

There is a considerable debate regarding the conditions for which PGD should be offered. As highlighted earlier, there are no current regulations in the United States concerning the eligibility criteria for PGD testing, which is usually left to the discretion of its providers. In other countries, legislation varies considerably. For example, France limits the provision of PGD services only to certain conditions and Italy only allows PGD to be performed on polar bodies but not on blastomeres while Germany has totally banned the whole procedure. Other countries like Greece have not yet developed a legal framework that regulates PGD (19, 20).

The following are general guidelines that should be considered while offering the service.

The Genetic Condition

Generally, PGD should only be offered for genetic conditions that could be diagnosed using techniques with a reliability of more than 90 percent. PGD should not be offered if no precise diagnosis of the genetic condition was made, if the mode of inheritance was not determined, or when the condition is caused by genetic heterogeneity. The genetic conditions should have a high recurrence rate (e.g., more than 10 percent for chromosomal rearrangement or 25 percent for monogenic disorders). When PGD is done for HLA typing in order to conceive a potential stem cell donor baby, the condition in the sibling child should be likely to be cured after stem cell transplantation or at least the life expectancy is expected to be prolonged. Consideration should be also given with regard to the time frame required for PGD testing, pregnancy, and the delivery of an HLA-matched sibling, especially in situations where the child is terminally ill and has a short life expectancy (6).

The Couple

Couples who should be considered for PGS include those with recurrent miscarriages (more than two miscarriages), repeated implantation failure (those who had three embryo transfers of high quality or more than ten embryos in multiple transfers), and women with advanced maternal age (more than thirty-seven years).

It is not recommended to provide PGD/PGS to women between forty and forty-five years of age, especially those with poor ovarian reserve (less than seven antral follicles) or with high basal FSH levels (greater than 15 IU/L). It is also not recommended to offer PGD/PGS to patients who have contraindications to IVF/ICSI or have poor embryo quality (6).

PATIENT PREPARATION

One of the important prerequisites for a successful PGD cycle is appropriate ovarian stimulation to ensure retrieval of the highest number of mature oocytes, and consequently an adequate number of embryos for testing. ESHRE data show that the average number of retrieved oocytes in PGD cycles is fifteen (21). Some authors propose that if less than nine cumulus-oocyte complexes are expected to be recovered, the couple should be counseled that the prognosis is poor and that the PGD cycle should be canceled if less than six oocytes are expected to be retrieved (22). Retrospective analysis of data showed that patients who had ten mature oocytes, eight normally fertilized oocytes, and six embryos for biopsy had a 90 percent probability of having an embryo transfer (23). More aggressive stimulation protocols are usually used during PGD/PGS cycles to ensure higher pregnancy rates. Ovarian hyperstimulation syndrome (OHSS) is one of the serious complications that should not be overlooked or underestimated if aggressive stimulation protocols are employed (24). Recently, there has been a growing concern that although increased gonadotropin dosage positively correlates with the number of retrieved oocytes, it may correlate negatively with the number of euploid embryos, suggesting that ovarian stimulation may lead to an increased aneuploidy rate. Some studies implicate certain ovarian stimulation protocols more than others, but no solid conclusion can be drawn at this point (25). For example, a recent study by Weghofer and his colleagues showed that LH-containing ovarian stimulation protocols are associated with lower aneuploidy rates in the tested embryos when compared to recombinant FSH stimulation, and that this observation may explain higher IVF pregnancy rates reported for hMG stimulation in some studies (26). It was thus recommended by some authors that future ovarian stimulation strategies should avoid maximizing oocyte yield, but rather aim at generating a sufficient number of chromosomally normal embryos by reduced interference with ovarian physiology (26).

Couples undergoing PGD should be advised to have protected intercourse or to abstain from sex to avoid the risk of spontaneous pregnancy during that cycle. Also, all patients should be counseled regarding all possible risks related to IVF/ICSI/PGD, including the risk of premature birth, low birth weight, OHSS, multiple pregnancy, abortion, and so on (27).

INSEMINATION AND EMBRYO CULTURE

ICSI should be performed when PCR is to be used during PGD. This is to avoid any possible contamination by other sperms that might remain embedded in the zona if in vitro fertilization is used. If FISH is to be used, either ICSI or IVF could be an alternative for insemination (21, 28).

Embryo culture should proceed according to the standard protocols employed by the IVF laboratory (29). After biopsy, the embryos must be rinsed to remove any residues of acid or biopsy media. Each embryo should be cultured and identified separately either in individual drops or in dishes to ensure proper tracking of blastomeres.

EMBRYO BIOPSY

Generally, the biopsy could be performed during three stages: polar body, cleavage stage (day 3), or blastocyst stage (days 5–6) (30–32). Polar body biopsy is also known as preconception or pre fertilization biopsy, and in some countries, it is the only form of PGD that is legally approved. The first polar body biopsy is usually performed after the retrieval of the oocytes (approximately, thirty-six to forty-two hours after hCG injection) (33). The second polar body is obtained when the embryos are at the pronucleate zygote stage. For aneuploidy screening using FISH, both polar bodies could be removed simultaneously or sequentially (31, 33, 34), while in PGD for single-gene disorder, they have to be removed sequentially and tested separately (35). Polar body biopsy is more suitable for aneuploidy screening since more than 70 percent of aneuploidies are of maternal origin and arise from either the first or the second meiotic divisions or both (33) (Figure 66.2). This biopsy procedure is not very useful in PGD for single-gene disorders, except in maternally derived autosomal dominant disorders, as it does not allow testing of the paternal genetic element (36, 37). Embryo biopsy is performed in most facilities during the cleavage stage, or on day 3, when the embryo is at about eight-cell stage (6).

Some authors recommend doing both polar body biopsy and blastomere biopsy to increase the validity of the results when testing for aneuploidies. This is based on the fact that some aneuploidies that occur during the first and the second meiotic divisions may correct themselves (a condition known as a trisomic rescue) yielding euploid blastomeres, except that these embryos usually start to show evidence of mosaicism later in development, and frequently fail to implant.

Embryo biopsy dishes should contain drops of biopsy media and rinse media of appropriate volume to maintain the temperature, pH, and osmolality throughout the procedure.

The biopsy process is achieved through two phases: the first involves breaching the zona pelucida and the second involves the removal of the polar body or blastomere. The procedure is done under an inverted microscope with the use of a micromanipulator (Figure 66.1). Breaching the zona could be done mechanically, chemically (by using acid solution, e.g. acid Tyrode's) or by laser. Non contact laser is becoming the tool of choice for biopsy and is gradually taking the upper hand over acid Tyrode's. Based on the latest ESHRE data, laser drilling was more commonly used during PGD for monogenic diseases (in 64 percent of biopsy cycles) (12). It is worth noting here that it is preferable to avoid the use of acid Tyrode's while breaching the zona to obtain polar body biopsy as it may adversely affect the mitotic spindle (38).

Every effort must be made to make a single, average-size zonal opening in the shortest possible time. Ideally the opening

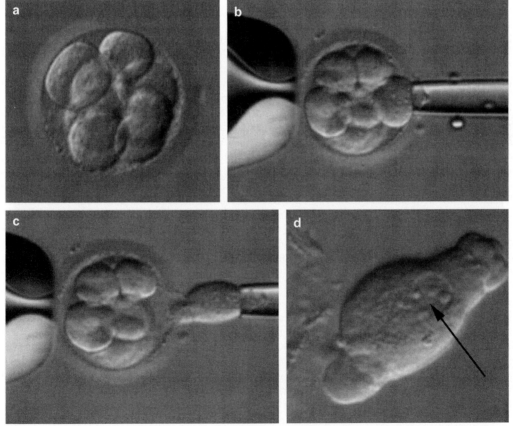

Figure 66.1. Blastomere biopsy of a human cleavage-stage embryo. (a) Eight-cell embryo, day 3 post fertilization; (b) embryo on holding pipette (left), with biopsy pipette (right) breaching the zona pellucida; (c) blastomere removal by suction; (d) biopsied blastomere with a clearly visible single nucleus (indicated by arrow). [Yacoub Khalaf (2007). Preimplantation genetic diagnosis. *Obstetrics, Gynecology and Reproductive Medicine* 17:1.]

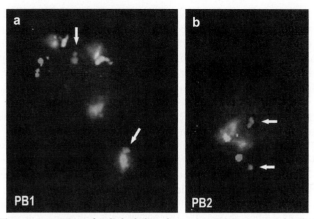

Figure 66.2. PGD of X-linked disorders using FISH. Two nuclei that have been hybridized with probes that are complementary to sequences on chromosomes X (green), Y (red), and 18 (blue). (a) A nucleus from the blastomere of a normal female embryo has two green and two blue signals, whereas (b) a nucleus from a normal male has one red, one green, and two blue signals. [Yacoub Khalaf (2007). Preimplantation genetic diagnosis. *Obstetrics, Gynecology and Reproductive Medicine* 17:1.]

should not be more that 60 μm and the biopsy time should not exceed one to two minutes. Also the duration where the oocytes or the embryos are out side the incubators should be kept to the minimum.

Once the zona is opened, micropipettes are used to manipulate the embryo and aspirate the polar bodies or blastomeres. Every effort must be made to select the most normal, regular, and mononucleate blastomere during biopsy (38). Unfortunately, embryo compaction may adversely affect the biopsy outcome.

Different techniques have been described for the removal of blastomeres including extrusion or displacement in case of cleavage embryo or herniation combined with laser or mechanical excision of the trophoectoderm in case of blastocysts embryos (32, 39–41). The procedure is not technically difficult and is usually successful in 97 percent of cases (42). One of the main problems that can arise during the process is lysis of blastomeres with subsequent loss of the genetic material. Using media deprived of divalent cations (Ca++ Mg ++-free media) during the embryo biopsy helps in reducing this complication (43).

After biopsy, single embryo culture is compulsory. Special attention should be made to proper identification of the obtained blastomeres or polar bodies and their corresponding dishes.

The effect of biopsy on subsequent embryo development has been clearly demonstrated. Most published data indicate that the biopsy of one cell from a cleavage embryo (six to eight cells) has no detrimental effect on embryo development (30). In contrast, the removal of two cells or even the removal of one cell from a four-cell-stage embryo seems to affect its development, although results are inconsistent with regard to this matter (39, 44). The biopsy of two cells is justified when there is doubt about the reliability and accuracy of the diagnostic test. Re-biopsy of the same embryo may be done in the case of failure to make a diagnosis or in the case of a loss of the genetic material. In this case, the same opening in the zona that was used during the first biopsy should be used as a portal to access the second blastomere.

GENETIC TESTING

Unlike prenatal diagnosis, genetic testing during PGD is more challenging due to the small amount of genetic material available for testing, usually obtained from one or maximum two cells, which in turn calls for the use of more sensitive tests. Both FISH and PCR are used in PGD for single-gene disorders. FISH is only useful in X-linked conditions.

FISH

Fluorescent in situ hybridization involves the use of fluorescent-tagged DNA probes that bind to their complementary DNA sequences on the chromosome with a high degree of specificity. These probes are labeled with different fluorochromes that emit fluorescent signals, thus helping in identifying each chromosome. FISH is particularly useful when examining interphase nuclei, as with blastomeres. Routine karyotyping is not efficient due to the clumping of chromosomes seen on interphase spread (45). Currently, FISH allows for the examination of a limited number of chromosomes at one time (five chromosomes in each round), due to the limited number of available fluorochromes. Accordingly, the use of more probes entails performing a second or even a third round of hybridization. Unfortunately, there is always a compromise between the number of FISH rounds and the hybridization efficiency. The hybridization efficiency can decrease significantly with repeated rounds. Some authors even reported a drop in the hybridization efficiency below 80% by the third hybridization round. One of the other limitations of FISH is that specific probes are not available for all chromosomes (46–49).

Most of the currently used probes are CEP (chromosome enumeration) or LSI (loci specific) probes. CEP probes are also known as centromeric probes which bind to satellite DNA sequences that are usually located near the centromeres, for example, CEP 16 that binds to satellite II D16Z3 and CEP 18 that binds to alpha satellite D18Z1 . Locus-specific probes consist of DNA probe sequences that bind to specific regions on each chromosome, for example, LSI 13 (13q14) and LSI 22 (22q11.2). CEP probes emit the strongest fluorescent signals but there is the problem of cross-hybridization, which may occur due to considerable sequence homology between the centromeres of certain chromosomes especially between Ch13/Ch21 or Ch14/Ch22 (50). Another form of probe is the telomeric probe, which is a repeat-sequence probe. These probes bind to the telomeres which are areas of repetitive DNA sequences found at the ends of eukaryotic chromosomes, thus they are useful for detecting chromosomal rearrangement as in translocations (50).

When PGD is performed for aneuploidy screening, most facilities use the five-set probes for chromosomes 13, 16, 18, 21 and 22, which has been shown to identify approximately 80 percent of all abnormal embryos. Those five chromosomes are responsible for the most common aneuploidies detected in 70 percent of spontaneous abortion (46). If the results from this round are normal, further testing of chromosomes X, Y, 15, and 17 should be done in a second round. This usually helps to detect another 15 percent of abnormal embryos. Some studies reported that screening for another four chromosomes (namely 2, 3, 4, and 11) in a third round can identify another 3 percent of abnormal embryos that could be missed during the first two rounds (51). Obviously, the yield of this third round is low compared to the cost and the effort. Currently, these eight chromosomes (13, 15, 16, 17, 18, 21, 22, and XY) are the most commonly recommended for screening. This is not only because these chromosomes are the most involved in aneuploidy but also because other chromosome aneuploidies tend to occur along with aneuploidies involving these eight chromosomes. These data were further confirmed by CGH studies (52–56).

For translocations, the appropriate combination of probes should be tested first on the carrier's lymphocytes to verify the ability to detect unbalanced rearrangements (3, 56, 57).

For sex selection, it is recommended to use a probe set containing at least one probe specific to each of the sex chromosomes along with another probe for an autosome (preferably Ch18)

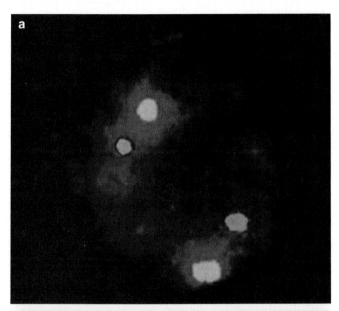

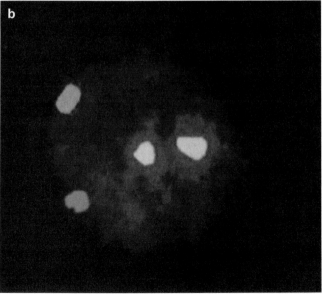

Figure 66.3. Polar body biopsy showing meiosis II error leading to monosomy 13. In PB1, there are two red signals for chromosome 13 (one of them is split). In PB2, there are two signals for chromosome 13 indicating monosomy in the oocyte. (Verlinsky Y and Anver Kuliev. Preimplantation diagnosis for aneuploidies. In Verlinsky Y and Anver Kuliev, eds. Atlas of preimplantation genetic diagnosis. Taylor and Francis, Abingdon, UK, 2005; pp. 156).

(Figure 66.3) (59). In fact, the first application for FISH in PGD was done in 1991 for sex selection, using probes for X and Y chromosomes (60). Occasionally, a pre-cycle workup might be required when using certain probes that have been shown to be associated with high polymorphism rate in their region, that is, DYZ1. In these cases, examination of the male interphase nuclei is warranted before doing FISH on the blastomeres.

FISH probes are commercially available and could be also homemade. The former is more reliable as they usually come with quality control and validation. Still, it is recommended to test all vials before the actual clinical application using lymphocytes, fibroblast cells, or even previously biopsied and fixed blastomeres to ensure the specificity of probes to each chromosome and to assess the signal brightness and discreteness. Currently, most available probes are directly labeled DNA probes for which the immunochemical detection step that was needed earlier while using the indirectly labeled probes is negated. Also the hybridization time is much lower (three versus seven hours) (50, 61).

Although FISH is mainly used for PGS and for chromosomal rearrangement, it is also useful for sex selection in X-linked diseases (60–65), which are estimated now to be more than 400 diseases and account for 6–7 percent of single-gene defects (66).

According to ESHRE PGD consortium data I–V, out of 613 PGD cycles that were done for sexing, 545 were done using FISH, leaving only 68 cases that were diagnosed using PCR (12).

It is currently recommended to use FISH when PGD is done for a sex-linked disease rather than using PCR as it possesses many advantages. First, FISH does not require the time or effort needed for PCR, not to mention the lower chances of contamination, as will be discussed later (28, 42, 67). Second, FISH can be used when dealing with an X-linked disease for which the exact location and nature of the genetic mutation has not been determined and particularly when linkage analysis is not possible. Third, FISH also offers the advantage of providing information about the number of sex chromosome copies that cannot be obtained by standard PCR (i.e., PCR cannot distinguish XX from XO, or XXY from XY). This lowers or almost eliminates the chances of transferring XO females, which are observed in 1 percent of embryos during PGD and which would be otherwise diagnosed as normal females if PCR was used. Therefore, only embryos that show two X chromosome signals should be transferred when using FISH for sexing (68).

Fixation

After obtaining the blastomere biopsy, the cells should be fixed on glass slides. Fixation is a very important step during FISH analysis. The main aim of fixation is to remove as much cytoplasm as possible, leaving nuclear DNA accessible to the hybridization probes. An ideal fixation technique should completely remove the cytoplasmic proteins that interfere with probe binding to the nucleus, leaving only the chromosomal DNA and proteins intact. In short, the presence of cytoplasm increases the misdiagnosis rate and the number of noninformative cells.

Different fixation techniques have been described, including the use of 1) acetic acid/methanol (Carnoy method), 2) Tween 20 HCl, or 3) Tween 20-HCl and acetic acid/methanol (61, 69–71). Based on number of cells lost after fixation, average rate of informative cells, rate of signal overlaps, and FISH errors, Carnoy is the most efficient of all these methods as it gives the best nuclear quality for PGD analysis. The other two methods involving the use of Tween 20 or Tween 20 plus Carnoy solution are technically easier but do not achieve as big nuclear diameter as the Carnoy method (72).

The process of fixation should be done under a dissecting microscope and the presence and location of fixed nuclei can be confirmed using a phase-contrast microscope. It is important to ensure that the humidity and the temperature ranges remain within the acceptable limits throughout all the steps.

Hybridization

The specific probes for the targeted chromosomes to be tested are available in a premixed solution from the manufacturer or could be mixed together in the lab. The slides containing the fixed polar bodies or blastomeres should be dehydrated using 70, 85, and 100 percent ethanol, then the hybridization solution is applied and the slides are covered with cover slips. The slides are then covered by a parafilm or the edges of the cover slip are sealed by rubber cement before heating to DNA melt temperature and subsequent incubation. The available automated systems such as the HYBrite (Vysis) or ThermoBrite (Abbott) have programs that allow both steps (melting and incubation) to be carried out in the same chamber. Typically, the hybridization time should be at least three hours. Extending the time of hybridization to four hours is recommended, as it seems to produce clearer and brighter signals. After the hybridization, the rubber cement and the cover slips are removed, the slides are washed in 0.7× sodium chloride/sodium citrate (SSC)/0.3% NP-40 at 71–73 °C, then again in 2× SSC/0.1% NP-40, pH 7.4 at room temperature. Finally, the slides are mounted with DAPI counterstain in antifade solution and covered with a cover slip. Some labs prefer not to use DAPI as it may obfuscate the spectrum blue-labeled probe signal. The slides are then ready for analysis.

FISH slides should be analyzed using a fluorescent microscope, equipped with the optimum filter sets. Occasionally, digital computer imaging is necessary for analysis and image storage. Some labs use the triple-band pass filter set, while others use the single-band pass filter sets. The latter is available for each of the fluorescent-labeled probes and they usually provide the brightest fluorescent intensities and lower background noise. When using single-band pass filters, the more sensitive fluorophores should be viewed first to avoid photo-bleaching. Thus, the spectrum blue probe signal should be viewed first followed by the aqua, then the green, yellow, and finally the red.

FISH results should be analyzed by two independent observers. Based on unpublished results from Reprogenetics, this helps to decrease the error rate in interpretation from 10.25 percent (in case of one observer) to 4.7 percent (in case of two observers). If there are any discrepancies, a third observer's scoring might be needed.

After the analysis of the first set of probes, the slides should be washed in 0.7× SSC at room temperature until the cover slips fall off and dipped in distilled water at 71°C for 10 seconds. The slides should be then dehydrated using 70, 85, and 100 percent ethanol, for two minutes each. The next steps should proceed in the same sequence mentioned earlier.

In some cases, when no conclusive results are obtained during interpretation, the use of alternative locus probes is recommended to resolve the doubt. This process is known as no-result rescue, which was shown to decrease the no results rate from 7.5 to 3.2 percent and decrease the false-positive error rate from 7.2 to 4.7 percent (73, 74). Slides can be stored at 4 °C (75, 76). In cases where biopsy and FISH diagnosis are performed at different locations, slides can be shipped at ambient temperature before FISH is performed.

Errors During FISH Analysis

It is estimated that the overall FISH error rate is 8–15 percent, consequently, all patients are recommended to undergo prenatal diagnosis should pregnancy be initiated.

Errors in FISH usually result from inappropriate fixation, signal overlap, signal splitting, or mosaicism. Inappropriate fixation can yield nuclei covered with cytoplasm, which cause the hybridization signals to appear too weak and blurred or can result in too small and condensed nuclei leading to overlaps of signals leading to false-negative results. In contrast, too much spreading can lead to loss of micronuclei, also leading to false-negative results.

Occasionally, a single signal can split into two signals and produce erroneous results. This has many causes such as the type of probes used (some probes are associated with splitting more than others, i.e. α satellite probe for chromosome 18 and satellite III probe for chromosome Y). Also the cellular stage at which fixation was done could be a source of signal splitting (double-dotted signals may represent two sister chromatids after reduplication).

Errors caused by overlaps between signals of different targets are less common than errors produced by signal splitting. This is because attention to signal size and shape can detect most overlaps between two signals of different targets, especially when they do not overlap completely.

During FISH analysis, two types of errors could occur. The first, which is the most serious, is known often as type 1, and refers to false-positive and false-negative errors. This occurs when an embryo is diagnosed as normal by PGD, when in fact it was abnormal, or when the embryo is diagnosed as abnormal when in fact it was normal. The second type of error is known as type 2 and occurs when an embryo is classified as having a specific abnormality, but then found to have a different abnormality after re-analysis. Obviously, this type of error is less serious than the first one as it poses no effect on the pregnancy outcome, and usually it accounts for almost two thirds of the overall FISH errors.

Most of the published data show that the highest percentage of errors are those of type II followed by type I false positive (when the embryo is diagnosed as abnormal when in fact it was normal), with the chances of false-negative type I error being around 6 percent. While this ratio is not acceptable by some, this means that 94 percent of trisomies would be detected, therefore decreasing the probability that women aged forty or older would have a trisomic pregnancy to the levels found in women aged thirty-four or younger.

One problem that will always remain a cause of FISH errors is mosaicism. The error rate due to mosaicism is estimated to be around 5–7 percent (46, 51).

PCR

PCR stands for polymerase chain reaction, which involves the amplification of a specific DNA fragment from a DNA strand to a level where it can be further analyzed. This analysis is done either by restriction enzyme digestion and evaluation of the DNA fragments produced based on their size, or by using mutation detection techniques. These techniques are either simple tests to detect a specific mutation or more advanced scanning methods that allow for the detection of a heterogeneous spectrum of mutations (17, 77). Due to the limited quantity of genetic material available for PCR during PGD, every effort must be made to optimize the reaction conditions in order to increase the diagnostic reliability. One of the challenges encountered during single-cell PCR is the amplification efficiency, which is normally around 100 percent when dealing with larger DNA samples but falls to 90–95 percent in single-cell PCR (78). Possible reasons include the loss of the genetic material during biopsy, the biopsy of an anucleate cell, or degenerate cell (79, 80).

To improve the results of amplification, various techniques have been advocated during cell lysis, including the use of alkaline lysis buffers and buffers containing proteinase K/SDS (potassium/sodium dodecyl suphate).

In addition to amplification failure, there are two other important limitations while using PGD-PCR, which are contamination and allele dropout. Contamination is a commonly encountered problem in any PCR reaction, although it becomes more pronounced during single-cell PCR due to the use of a larger number of PCR cycles that can easily amplify the contaminant fragments (78). This should be avoided through applying strict laboratory protocols to avoid any source of contamination. The source of contamination may be the biopsy material itself due to the inadvertent presence of a paternal sperm or maternal cumulus cells. Contamination should be avoided by using ICSI and proper washing of the blastomere prior to transfer to the PCR tube. Another form of contamination is known as "carry-over" contamination, which occurs due to the accidental amplification of DNA material from a previous experiment. For that reason, it is very important that all the equipment and reagents used for PGD-PCR should be reserved only for that purpose (77).

In order to ensure the absence of any contaminant DNA, each case sample should be accompanied by negative controls of the cell free wash and reagents. Positive controls of homozygous normal, homozygous abnormal, and heterozygous DNA should be included in the test. After obtaining the blastomere biopsy, the cells should be washed at least twice before the transfer to PCR tubes preferably under microscopic visualization.

It is crucial that all reagents, solutions, and buffers used during the process should be carefully tested prior to the clinical application. The use of filtration, ultraviolet light, and restriction enzymes can also help in the process of decontamination. To avoid any other sources of contamination, the PCR room should be separated from the rest of the laboratory and constantly kept under positive pressure. Recently, the use of nested PCR was shown to decrease the risk of misdiagnosis due to carry-over contamination (Figure 66.4). This procedure comprises two sequential PCR reactions where the first aims at generating a larger DNA fragment that encompasses the mutation site while the second reaction amplifies a smaller DNA fragment of the mutation itself, within the first amplicon. Such amplification of smaller fragments possesses a lessened risk of carry-over contamination in subsequent reactions, especially that these smaller fragments cannot be amplified by the first set of primers (81).

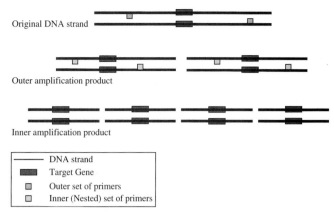

Figure 66.4. Nested PCR.

The other important challenge that could be encountered during PGD-PCR is allele dropout (ADO). ADO occurs when one of the alleles in a heterozygous embryo fails to amplify, giving a false impression that the embryo is homozygous. It has been estimated that ADO occurs in 5–20 percent of single-cell amplifications, although it was reported to occur in up to 30 percent of single-cell PCR by some laboratories (82, 83).

The exact cause of ADO remains vague, although it seems that ADO occurs with a higher frequency in some cells than others, including blastomeres (Figure 66.5) (84). Other factors that were implicated as a cause of ADO are cell lysis and less than perfect PCR conditions. Some authors consider ADO to be a form of extreme preferential amplification (PA), where there is an extreme discrepancy between the amplified DNA from the two alleles, with one of the alleles only producing very small amount of PCR products that cannot be easily visualized. It is estimated that preferential amplifications occur in as many as 25 percent of single-cell PCR. To avoid false-negative results due to ADO, two techniques are recommended. These include the use of highly polymorphic linked markers during the PCR reaction, or the use of fluorescent PCR (Figure 66.6) (85).

Highly polymorphic linked markers are short tandem repeats that are present within the gene it self or closely linked

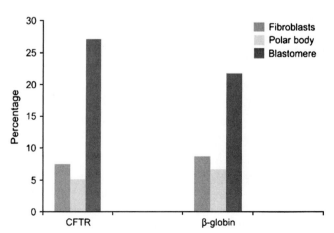

Figure 66.5. Allele dropout in different types of single cells. (Verlinsky Y and Anver Kuliev. Preimplantation diagnosis for single-gene disorders. In Verlinsky Y and Anver Kuliev, eds. Atlas of preimplantation genetic diagnosis. Taylor and Francis, Abingdon, UK, 2005; pp. 233).

to it. The choice of the appropriate markers to be incorporated in the test differs from case to case. Linked markers analysis requires preliminary work up on DNA samples from the couple, their families, other affected siblings, and possibly from the paternal sperms. The latter is known as single-sperm typing and is important in establishing paternal haplotyping, especially in paternally derived dominant conditions and de-novo mutations. Approximately three to five markers should be used for each tested gene. A lower number of markers is needed if real-time PCR is used. These markers are simultaneously amplified with the tested gene in the same PCR reaction (Multiplex PCR), which increases the diagnostic accuracy and helps in detecting cases of ADO (86, 87) (Figure 66.6).

Multiplex PCR simply refers to the possibility of amplifying multiple loci simultaneously during the same PCR reaction, by using a combination of unrelated primers. This is useful when more than one gene needs to be tested, if HLA typing is needed along with the mutation analysis or as pointed out earlier when using linked markers (88–90).

Multiplex PCR is also very useful to test for aneuploidy while testing for single-gene disorders to allow selection of euploid embryos from among those embryos that tested negative for the mutation. This is achieved through the use of primers for chromosome-specific microsatellite markers during the multiplex reaction.

Another type of PCR is fluorescent PCR, which was shown to decrease the incidence of ADO at least by fourfold. In this technique, fluorescent primers are used instead of the regular radioactively labeled primers. Fluorescent PCR has the advantage of producing products that can be easily detected using a laser analysis system, even when they are too small to be visualized using the traditional techniques. Consequently, it can detect cases of PA or ADO where one of the allele products is markedly underrepresented (88). The sensitivity of product detection of fluorescent PCR is over a thousand times greater than the standard PCR. Since only a small amount of PCR products are necessary for visualization, only thirty-five to forty cycles of PCR are required for diagnosis, which dramatically decreases the diagnostic time (78, 91).

Fluorescent PCR was also proven to be highly effective in the diagnosis of single-gene disorders where the mutation site is too small to be clearly differentiated from the normal allele. Because of the high precision of the fragment analysis laser system used in fluorescent PCR (which allows for sizing of the produced amplicon to single-nucleotide accuracy), these conditions could be easily diagnosed without the need of heteroduplex analysis.

Other measures that were shown to decrease the rate of ADO include increasing the denaturation temperature from 90°C to 96°C (92), and the proper choice of DNA polymerase, primers, and lyses buffers (alkaline lysis buffer or those containing proteinase and detergent) (84, 93, 94). Also, the use of two blastomeres during PCR helps in detecting ADO since there is a very low chance that the same allele will fail to amplify in both cells. A more efficient approach, especially in maternally derived mutations, is to do sequential first and second polar analysis along with the blastomere analysis. For example, if PB1 is homozygous for the mutant allele and PB2 is hemizygous normal, this means that the corresponding oocyte carries the normal allele. Also, if PB1 is heterozygous for the mutant and normal allele (due to cross over) and PB2 shows the mutant allele, this means that the corresponding oocyte is normal. If the scenario is different in the latter example and PB2 shows the normal allele, this means that the corresponding oocyte carries the mutant allele (87). Figure 66.7 shows the incidence of ADO with the use of different types of PCR.

ADO is good proof that it is best not to rely on negative results in determining the genotype of the affected cell. In fact, this was the reason behind the reported failure during the first clinical applications of PCR by Alan Handyside in 1999.

A recently introduced technique known as multiple displacement amplification is used to substantially expand the available genetic material for testing, which decreases the chance of misdiagnosis due to amplification failure (78).

PCR Pre-Assay Validation

Assay validation before the clinical application is crucial to assess the amplification efficiency, ADO rate, and contamination.

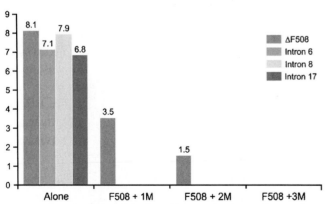

Figure 66.6. ADO rate with the addition of polymorphic markers. Simultaneous analysis of two linked loci decrease the rate of ADO to 3.5 percent, while simultaneous analysis of three loci decrease that rate to 1.5 percent. (Verlinsky Y and Anver Kuliev. Preimplantation diagnosis for single-gene disorders. In Verlinsky Y and Anver Kuliev, eds. Atlas of preimplantation genetic diagnosis. Taylor and Francis, Abingdon, UK, 2005; pp. 233).

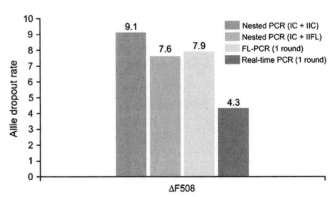

Figure 66.7. ADO rates in the analysis of F508 mutation in the CFTR gene following different types of PCR. The red bar indicates nested conventional PCR, the blue bar nested combined PCR (first round is conventional and the second round fluorescent), the yellow bar fluorescent PCR, and the green bar real-time PCR, which is the most sensitive. (Verlinsky Y and Anver Kuliev. Preimplantation diagnosis for single-gene disorders. In Verlinsky Y and Anver Kuliev, eds. Atlas of preimplantation genetic diagnosis. Taylor and Francis, Abingdon, UK, 2005; pp. 234).

This should be done both on affected and unaffected DNA samples (17). The number of cells to be used for validation is variable, depending on the cell type. Generally, it is recommended to use at least fifty cells when using lymphocytes or lymphoblastoid cells and a minimum of ten when using blastomeres. To test for contamination, a similar number of cell wash blanks should be included in the run. The amplification efficiency should be at least 90 percent and the ADO rate should not exceed 10 percent. The contamination rate should be zero but values up to 5 percent are acceptable. Higher ADO rates could be acceptable in autosomal recessive but not in autosomal dominant.

EMBRYO SELECTION AND TRANSFER

The selection of embryos for transfer should be primarily based on an unaffected diagnosis and, secondarily, on morphology. The pre- and post biopsy embryo morphologies along with active cell division are important criteria that should be considered during selection. The transfer of carrier embryos (autosomal recessive and females with X-linked recessive conditions) depends on the nature of the disease as some of the recessive traits may be associated with a milder form of the disease. Under any circumstances, it is not acceptable to transfer affected embryos even when there are no unaffected embryos for transfer. These embryos might be used for quality control and quality assurance of the procedure since they provide the staff and prospective PGD patients with a reliable misdiagnosis rate in that facility (3).

It is not recommended to transfer undiagnosed embryos, especially if PGD was employed for the diagnosis of a monogenic disorder; but, when insisted upon by the couple and if approved by the facility's ethical committee, this transfer could be carried out provided that the couple will be offered prenatal diagnosis (6). As pointed earlier in the counseling section, all these issues should be discussed in detail with the couple prior to transfer.

In PGD, embryo transfer could be carried out starting from day 3 up to day 6 post fertilization (95, 96). Delayed transfer on day 5 or 6 entail that the IVF team should be familiar with extended embryo culture protocols. Although delayed transfer allows more time for diagnosis and relieves stress on the staff, the number of embryos available for transfer is expected to be lower. There are also a number of factors that can influence the number of embryos available for transfer. Perhaps the most important of which in a case of PGD is the nature of the genetic condition under screening. For example, in autosomal dominant disorders, only 50 percent of embryos are expected to be suitable for transfer, while in HLA typing, only 25 percent of the embryos may be suitable for transfer. The latter figure drops down to 18.8 percent when HLA typing is combined with PGD for an autosomal recessive disorder and further drops down to 12.5 percent when combined with sexing for an X-lined disorder (6, 41). Based on ESHRE data of PGD cycles for monogenic disorders, embryo transfer is usually achieved in 75–77 percent of cycles that reach the stage of oocyte retrieval (9, 12).

The number of embryos to be transferred should be discussed with the couple prior to the transfer session. There are number of factors that should be considered while deciding upon this matter including the female's age, embryo quality, the number of previous transfers, and the presence of medical conditions in the female partner that may increase the risk of multiple pregnancy. Based on the data from the PGD consortium, it is estimated that the pregnancy rate is around 13, 15, 34, 35, or 50 percent when one, two, three, four, or five embryos are transferred, respectively. It was also shown that 22 percent of PGD cycles started did not result in a transfer (42). Generally, it is recommended not to transfer more than two embryos in favorable prognosis patients (age less than thirty-seven, normal ovarian response, good fertilization rate, good embryo quality, and history of IVF success) (6). Surplus unaffected embryos could be cryopreserved for future transfer, although currently available data regarding the results of the post-thaw survival of biopsied embryos are not impressive. Also, success rates of cryopreservation of the embryos in cleavage stage versus blastocyst stage are inconsistent (56, 97–100).

Currently, there are no recommendations regarding a specific type of transfer media or transfer catheters that should be used for PGD embryos. It is recommended though to use ultrasonographic guidance during transfer as it was shown to increase the pregnancy rates.

SAFETY OF PGD

Over the past decade, PGD has been applied in more than 30,000 cycles for various indications and resulted in the birth of thousands of healthy babies (8). Preliminary reports confirm that PGD does not impart a higher risk of congenital malformations. Most published studies reported a rate of 2.3–4 percent, which is very comparable to the rate of malformations associated with ICSI. Currently, the biopsy of one-cell at eight-cell stage is considered the safest and has the least detrimental effect on the embryo (30). Also the removal polar bodies was showed to have no effect on subsequent embryo development (101). Multiple micromanipulation to combine polar body biopsy with blastomere biopsy was also shown to be safe and has no deleterious effect on future embryo development (102, 103). The removal of two cells and performing the technique during an earlier stage of development might affect embryonic development, presumably as a result of disrupting the trophoectoderm and the inner cell mass. Because PGD is always combined with IVF/ICSI, there is also increased risk of low birth weight, premature delivery, and higher perinatal mortality (27).

THE VALIDITY OF PGD RESULTS AND POTENTIAL FOR MISDIAGNOSIS

The effectiveness of PGD for single-gene disorders has been accepted despite the lack of randomized control trials because its success in reducing the transmission of a genetic condition is self-evident. Unfortunately, misdiagnosis is frequently reported during PGD, which usually carries significant medical, psychological, and economic implications. For single-gene somatic disorders, diagnosis is usually made in 86 percent of the successfully biopsied embryos, while in PGD for X-linked disorders, diagnosis is made in 92 percent of the successfully biopsied embryos (12). False-negative results occur in less than 1 percent of cases, and this can only be discovered by testing the fetus or newborn (10). For that reason, almost all IVF-PGD clinics recommend confirmatory prenatal diagnosis once pregnancy is established. Common causes of misdiagnosis include embryo mosiacism, amplification failure, ADO, contamination, improper FISH signal interpretation due to splitting or overlap, mislabeling/identification error, or unprotected sex. The exact cause and rate of misdiagnosis depends upon the nature of the test being employed. For example, the error rate if FISH was used for diagnosis is estimated to be 15 percent (46).

Mosaicism remains one of the main obstacles during PGD. The central idea of PGD is that the biopsied cell is representative of the whole embryo; this is not the case in mosaicism, which is not uncommon in preimplantation embryos. When the ratio between abnormal to normal cells is more than 3/8, the embryo should be diagnosed as mosaic. Mosaicism is the most common abnormality found in cleavage embryos as it represents two-thirds of all chromosomal abnormalities. It is estimated that mosaicism affects 40–50 percent of all embryos, and could originate either from meiotic or post zygotic mitotic errors. It is estimated that half of the mosaic embryos originate at the first mitotic division, one quarter at the second division, and one quarter at the third division. Mosaicism may not affect embryo development, especially if the abnormal cells do not contribute in the formation of the embryo itself. Generally, the earlier the stage at which mosaicism occurs, the more harmful the effect on the embryos. Different types of mosaicism have been described, including polyploid, haploid, aneuploid, split, and chaotic mosaics. Misdiagnosis due to mosaicism seems to be particularly important in autosomal dominant conditions as it will lead to failure to diagnose affected embryos. Equally important is the effect of mosaicism in the diagnosis of aneuploidies like monosomies and trisomies. The effect of mosaicism during embryo sexing and autosomal recessive disorders is less significant. The analysis of two cells dramatically decreases the diagnosis error due to mosaicism (104, 105).

Other measures that were shown to decrease the potential of misdiagnosis include the use of nested PCR, fluorescent PCR, multiplex PCR, and the incorporation of polymorphic markers. It is also hoped that the validity of PGD results will continue to increase in the future through the use of some new techniques as will be detailed later.

PREGNANCY RATES AFTER PGD

Unfortunately, the pregnancy rates after PGD remains disappointingly low. This is mainly due to the low pregnancy rates after IVF, which also remained around 20–35 percent despite the various attempts over the past few years to improve the procedure. As detailed earlier, the pregnancy rates after PGD depend to a great extent on the reason for testing. Cumulative ESHRE data show that the overall fertilization rate of oocytes collected in PGD cycles performed for single-gene disorders was 71 percent. Also in these cycles, diagnostic results were obtained in 88 percent of the biopsied embryos of which only 52 percent were transferable. Embryo transfer was achieved in 77 percent of cycles that reached oocyte retrieval, giving an implantation rate of 16 percent. The overall pregnancy rate was 20 percent per oocyte retrieval and 26 percent per embryo transfer (9). Table 66.2 shows the different pregnancy rates according to the indication of PGD. The best results of PGD were obtained when at least two sound embryos of good morphology were available for transfer. Other prognostic factors include:

- Female age.
- Previous IVF success.
- Response to ovulation induction.

Table 66.2: Pregnancy Rates according to the Indication of PGD

	Autosomal disorder	X-Lined disease	Social sexing	PGS
Pregnancy rate per oocyte retrieval	20	22	19	18
Pregnancy rate per embryo transfer	27	30	32	24

- Number of retrieved oocytes.
- Pre- and post biopsy embryo quality.
- Number of available embryos for transfer (12, 64).

THE EFFICACY OF PGD FOR ANEUPLOIDY SCREENING IN ORDER TO IMPROVE IVF PREGNANCY RATES

Many studies and reports were published about the role of PGD for aneuploidy screening in improving IVF outcomes in certain groups of IVF patients, like those with advanced maternal age, repeated unexplained miscarriages, implantation failure, or TESE patients. Poor IVF results in these groups are thought to result from higher rates of aneuploidies, which were observed in up to 73 percent of embryos in some studies. Based on the latest ESHRE PGD consortium data, 529 out of 1,182 cycles of PGD were done for aneuploidies screening, and this number is steadily increasing (10). Although many studies and reports conducted by well-known centers showed significant improvement in implantation rates and clinical pregnancy rates after PGS, none of them were randomized controlled trials and their results still cannot be regarded as the best evidence-based data (48, 106). Furthermore, most of these studies used the implantation rate and the clinical pregnancy rate as a primary outcome, while in fact, the live birth rate is a more valid primary outcome in these kinds of studies. To date, there have been only three randomized clinical trials about the role of PGS in improving IVF outcome in patients with advanced maternal age (107). Two of these clinical trials did not show that PGS improves IVF outcome in these patients and the third even pointed to the detrimental effect of PGS in terms of reducing the implantation rate and clinical pregnancy rate (48, 108, 109). Unfortunately, all of these three studies did not use the live birth rate as a primary outcome in their study design. Also, each of them could be criticized for different reasons as will be detailed later. These trials triggered a considerable debate regarding the role and efficacy of PGD for aneuploidies screening in improving IVF outcomes.

The most recently published study by Mastenbroeck et al. in 2007 showed that PGS was not only ineffective but also significantly reduces the live birth rate (108). This large multicenter randomized double-blinded trial showed that live birth ate was 24 percent in the PGS group as opposed to 35 percent in the control group with no PGS. Based on these results, the authors concluded that PGS appears to do no more than to interfere with the natural selection process. They also pointed to the fact that such lower rates of implantation could be explained by the failure to transfer positively tested embryos that may have had a mosaic pattern that could self-correct.

This study triggered a huge controversy and was strongly criticized by many PGD experts. The criticism focused on the substandard embryo biopsy techniques used in the study, the exclusion of two key chromosomes from testing (CH15 and CH22), along with the failure of the test in a large percentage of the embryos (20 percent as opposed to the generally accepted range which is 5–10 percent). The substandard biopsy techniques were possibly the cause of the discrepancy of implantation rates between the control group and a subset of the PGD group where undiagnosed embryos were transferred (14.7 percent in the control group vs. 6 percent in the undiagnosed PGD group) (110).

Another randomized clinical trial conducted by Staessen et al. in 2004 showed that PGD screening did not result in any significant increase in the outgoing pregnancy rates despite increasing the implantation rate from 11.5 to 17.1 percent. Still, the results of this study should be interpreted cautiously since two cells were biopsied from the PGD group, which could have affected subsequent embryo development (48). The third clinical trail was conducted by Stevens et al. in 2004 and reported on only thirty-nine patients, thus the results were of poor statistical power (109).

This huge debate regarding PGD screening calls for optimized, adequately powered randomized trials with standardized biopsy and testing techniques to document the efficacy of PGS not only for AMA but also for other indications for which PGS is currently used.

FUTURE PERSPECTIVES

There are many novel techniques that are expected to increase the efficiency of PGD/PGS. Most of these techniques seek to maximize the information that could be obtained from a single cell. One of these advances is the whole genomic amplification (WGA), which aims to amplify the entire genome of a single cell rather than amplifying multiple fragments as in multiplex PCR (111, 112). This is particularly useful if large numbers of genes need to be analyzed as in conditions caused by polygenic disorders. WGA also provides a source of DNA that could be stored for further testing at a later stage. The two principle methods currently used in WGA are primer extension pre-amplification and degenerate oligonucleotide-primed PCR (113).

Another technique that increases the efficiency of chromosomal analysis is interphase chromosome conversion, which is expected to be particularly useful for age-related aneuploidy screening and in translocation patients. It has long been known that interphase FISH is not as efficient as metaphase FISH; interphase chromosome conversion aims at arresting the nuclei in metaphase making it possible to examine each chromosome individually (114). This is usually achieved by fusing the polar bodies or the blastomeres into oocytes or zygotes to induce metaphase formation. It is believed that factors in the cytoplasm induce them to enter metaphase (115, 116). Other substances like okadaic acid could also be used to ensure premature chromosome condensation. Having achieved this stage, each of the chromosomes could be examined either by G-banding or by other techniques such as SKY (spectral karyotyping) or multi-fluorochrome karyotyping (83). In the latter two techniques, chromosome-specific paint probes labeled with different combinations of fluorochromes allows the analysis of all

chromosomes at one time. It should be noted though that interphase chromosome conversion is a labor-intensive procedure (117–119).

One of the novel techniques, which is extensively researched in the field of PGD, is comparative genomic hybridization (CGH). CGH allows the determination of the copy number of every chromosomal region to be assessed in a single hybridization step (120). This is achieved by hybridizing the tested DNA with another DNA sample that was previously determined to have normal karyotype. Since each of the DNA samples are labeled with a different fluorescent tag, the presence of any chromosomal imbalance could be easily detected. This is achieved through the use of computer analysis software, which allows precise calculations of the fluorescent signals ratio along the length of each chromosome. Unfortunately, one of the main drawbacks of this procedure is the long time necessary before achieving results (three or four days). This means that if a biopsy was obtained on day 3, the transfer will not be possible before day 7. Current research is attempting to reduce the time frame of the procedure (112, 121, 122).

One promising technique, which has been rapidly evolving in the past few years and was recently successfully applied in PGD, is the use of DNA microarray (or chip). DNA microarray allows the detection of thousands of possible sequence variances in previously defined genes (83). This can be achieved in different ways. In its simplest form, short oligonucleotide probes, complimentary to known mutations are arrayed on to the chip and allowed to hybridize with the tested DNA. The presence of a hybridization signal indicates the presence of that mutation. Certain variances of DNA microarray tests can also allow the determination of copy number of all chromosomes along with the possibility of the detection of common microdeletions (123).

Some recent studies showed that the combination of WGA and DNA microarray can provide alternative solutions to FISH-based screening for PGD. One study showed that single-nucleotide polymorphism – based microarray after WGA can provide an accurate single-cell 23 chromosome aneuploidy screening with 100 percent accuracy and 93 percent overall reliability (124).

The uses of the previously mentioned techniques are still experimental in the field of PGD, and more data are necessary before considering them in clinical application.

ETHICAL CONSIDERATIONS

PGD provoked considerable media attention and continues to be a source of controversy especially to the medical community, to governments, and to the public in general. Possibly because of the eugenic potential of PGD and the fear that its use will gradually shift from screening for serious genetic conditions to the creation of designer babies where children will be regarded as made-to-order consumer product (125). These concerns may be understandable especially since PGD has already been used for nonmedical reasons like sex selection for social reasons (126, 127). It is estimated that almost half of the IVF clinics in the United States that provide PGD service are offering nonmedical sex selection (2).

Unfortunately, PGD can be used for morally ambiguous procedures, for example, HLA typing for the sake of conceiving a tissue-matched child or a compatible stem cell donor (13, 113). These situations may create an ethical dilemma and it is recommended in these cases to obtain an advice from a specialized committee concerned with ethics of clinical practice, especially if there is no national legislation or a legal frame work that controls PGD practice. HLA typing has raised many ethical and social concerns lately, which led some PGD centers to deny any parental request for HLA typing unless it is combined with genetic testing of embryos. This is based on the notion that the welfare of the child being selected must be considered first and foremost and takes precedence over the desires of the parents in determining the ethical acceptability of PGD. In other words, it is generally agreed that the new baby should not be regarded as merely instrumental in the process of healing an already existing sick child.

To further complicate the debate, PGD is currently not only offered to screen for serious fatal genetic conditions but it is additionally being offered to screen for late-onset diseases (e.g., early-onset Alzheimer's, Huntington disease, and inherited cancers).

While such uses of PGD could be regarded as a logical extension of the original goal, there are growing concerns that PGD may go far beyond ethical boundaries. This is especially true with the rapidly evolving research in the field of molecular biology and cytogenetics, which will soon allow for the simultaneous testing of hundreds of genes in a single step and hence the assessment of complex polygenic traits (skin color, IQ, etc.) (128). Although from the practical point of view, this is a remote possibility since there would probably be no suitable embryos for transfer, this highlights the need for oversight, laws, or regulations in PGD testing (125). Such laws or regulations should be a subset of ethical positions that reflect sufficient public agreement.

Fortunately, many countries have already provided a legal frame work for PGD research and practice while regrettably many countries have enacted laws that restrict or oppress PGD. Interestingly, some of these countries will allow prenatal diagnosis and the termination of the fetus but not PGD, which seems very illogical (129).

One of the main opponents of PGD are disability rights activists who argue that the use of PGD to select against certain conditions imply that those living with those conditions should not have been born. It is important to distinguish between the disability and people with disabilities, in that selecting embryos without disability does not mean that the lives of those with disabilities are less valuable or less meaningful.

PGD usually involves the collaboration of many teams like clinical geneticists, molecular biologists, fertility clinicians, and embryology scientists. Patient confidentiality is crucial and every effort should be made not to breach any ethical or legal boundaries especially when such a large multidisciplinary approach is used (130–131).

THE PGD FACILITY

The PGD services could be provided at IVF centers (in house) or in independent facilities. The latter is usually known as satellite PGD. A recent survey of the IVF clinics in the United States showed that PGD is performed in satellite facilities in more than 86 percent of cases. Both FISH and PCR tests can be performed in satellite PGD centers, although with PCR extra caution should be given to avoid any possible contamination. The satellite PGD facility should have certain laboratory protocols for the referring IVF centers regarding sample

processing and shipment. The PGD facility should also verify that these protocols were strictly followed upon receiving the samples to ensure proper hybridization in case of FISH samples and proper amplification efficiency and low risk of contamination in case of PCR samples. In the majority of IVF clinics (69 percent), the biopsy is taken by IVF clinic personnel. The IVF lab will usually send the slides containing the fixed cells (in case of FISH) or the centrifuge tubes containing lysed or unlysed cells (in case of PCR). It is recommended that the referring IVF centers should send a dry run to their reference laboratory before sending the actual samples for testing. This dry run in case of PCR consists of a number of PCR tubes with positive and negative controls. This is important to verify the absence of DNA contamination and ensure proper amplification efficiency. In case of FISH, a dry run of fixed cells should be sent to the laboratory to determine the quality of fixation. Some satellite PGD centers will only accept samples that have been biopsied and prepared by personnel that they have deemed proficient in training situations.

KEY POINTS

- It is currently estimated that 4–6 percent of all IVF cycles in the United states include PGD.
- As opposed to PGD, the term PGD-AS, or PGS, is used to refer to the genetic screening of lower risk groups including those with repeated implantation failure, recurrent miscarriages, and advanced maternal age.
- PGD for single-gene disorders is mainly used to screen for early fatal congenital diseases but can also be used for the screening of late-onset genetic diseases like Huntington disease, Alzheimer, inherited cancers, along with HLA typing. Currently, there are more than 400 diseases that could be screened for.
- PGD should be only offered to conditions that could be diagnosed using currently available techniques with a reliability of diagnosis of more than 90 percent. Such conditions should have high recurrence rate (e.g., >10 percent for chromosomal rearrangement or 25 percent for monogenic disorders).
- There are no current regulations in the United States concerning the eligibility criteria for PGD testing, while in other countries, legislations vary considerably.
- In preparing patients for PGD, more aggressive ovarian stimulation might be needed to ensure the retrieval of the highest number of mature oocytes.
- ICSI should be performed when PCR is to be used during PGD. This is to avoid any possible contamination by other sperms that might remain embedded in the zona. If FISH is to be used, either ICSI or IVF can be used for insemination.
- The majority of PGD centers perform an embryo biopsy during the cleavage stage, or day 3, when the embryo is about eight-cell stage. The biopsy of one cell from a cleavage embryo (six to eight cells) has no detrimental effect on embryo development, while the effects of the removal of two cells are still controversial.
- Breaching the zona could be done mechanically, chemically, or by non contact laser.
- FISH is mainly used for PGS, although it is currently recommended to use FISH when PGD is done for a sex-linked disease rather than using PCR as it possesses many advantages over PCR.

- In FISH, up to nine chromosomes could be tested in two consecutive rounds to screen for the most common aneuploidies present in spontaneous abortions (13, 15, 16, 17, 18, 21, 22, X, and Y).

- PCR is the main test used for the diagnosis of single-gene disorders. The limitations of the test include amplification failure, contamination, and ADO. The use of nested PCR, fluorescent PCR, and multiplex PCR decrease the likelihood of these limitations.

- Embryo transfer can be done starting from day 3 up to day 6 post fertilization. Selection of embryos for transfer should be primarily based on an unaffected diagnosis and, secondarily, the pre- and post biopsy embryo morphology along with active cell division.

- Preliminary reports confirm that PGD does not impose a higher risk of congenital malformations more than that associated with ICSI.

- Currently, there is extensive research in the field of WGA, interphase chromosome conversion, CGH, and DNA microarray, which is expected to revolutionize the clinical applications of PGD.

REFERENCES

1. Handyside AH, Kontogianni EH, Hardy K, Winston RML. Pregnancies from biopsied human preimplantation embryos sexed by Y-specific DNA amplification. *Nature* 1990;344:768–70.
2. Baruch S, Kaufman D, Hudson KL. Genetic testing of embryos: practices and perspectives of US in vitro fertilization clinics. *Fertil Steril* (published online 20 September 2006).
3. Gleicher N, Weghofer A, Barad D. Preimplantation genetic screening: "established" and ready for prime time? *Fertil Steril* 2008 Apr;89(4):780–8.
4. American Society of Reproductive Medicine and Society for Assisted Reproductive Technology (2001) Practice Committee Report. Preimplantation Genetic Diagnosis. Released June 2001.
5. American Society for Reproductive Medicine and Society for Assisted Reproduction Technology Practice Committees. Preimplantation genetic diagnosis. *Fertil Steril* 2004;82:120–2.
6. ESHRE PGD Consortium 'Best practice guidelines for clinical preimplantation genetic diagnosis (PGD) and preimplantation genetic screening (PGS)'. Hum Reprod 2005;20(1):35–48.
7. Simpson JL, Rebar R, Carson SA. Professional self-regulation for preimplantation genetic diagnosis: experience of the American Society for Reproductive Medicine and other professional societies. *Fertil Steril* 2006;85(6):1653.
8. Preimplantation Genetic Diagnosis International Society. The Preimplantation Genetic Diagnosis International Society (PGDIS): Guidelines for good practice in PGD. *Reprod Biomed Online* 2004 Oct;9(4):430–4.
9. Harper JC, de Die-Smulders C, Goossens V, Harton G, Moutou C, Repping S, Scriven PN, SenGupta S, Traeger-Synodinos J, Van Rij MC, Viville S, Wilton L, Sermon KD. ESHRE PGD consortium data collection VII: cycles from January to December 2004 with pregnancy follow-up to October 2005. *Hum Reprod.* 2008 Apr;23(4):741–55.
10. Sermon KD, Michiel A, Harton G, Moutou C, Repping S, Scriven PN, SenGupta S, Traeger-Synodino J, Vesela K, Viville S, Wilton L, Harper JC. ESHRE PGD Consortium data collection VI: cycles from January to December 2003 with pregnancy follow-up to October 2004. *Hum Reprod* 2007;22(2): 323–36.
11. ESHRE PGD Consortium data collection V: cycles from January to December 2002 with pregnancy follow-up to October 2003. *Hum Reprod* 2006;21(1):3–21.
12. ESHRE PGD Consortium data collection VI: cycles from January to December 2003 with pregnancy follow-up to October 2004. *Hum Reprod* 2007;22(2):323–36.
13. Sermon K, Goossens V, Seneca S et al. Preimplantation diagnosis of Huntington's disease (HD): clinical application and analysis of the HD expansion in affected embryos. *Prenat Diagn* 1998;18(13):1427–36.
14. Verlinsky Y, Rechitsky S, Schoolcraft W, Strom C, Kuliev A. Preimplantation diagnosis for Fanconi anemia combined with HLA matching. *JAMA* 2001;285(24):3130–3.
15. Verlinsky Y, Kuliev A. *An Atlas of Preimplantation Genetic Diagnosis*. Parthenon Publishing Group, New York, 2000.
16. Rechitsky S, Verlinsky O, Amet T et al. Reliability of preimplantation diagnosis for single gene disorders. *Mol Cell Endocrinol* 2001;183:S65–8.
17. Sermon K. Current concepts in preimplantation genetic diagnosis (PGD): a molecular biologist's view. *Hum Reprod Update* 2002;8:11–20.
18. Renwick P, Ogilvie CM. Preimplantation genetic diagnosis for monogenic diseases: overview and emerging issues. *Expert Rev Mol Diagn* 2007;7(1):33–43.
19. Viville S, Nisand I. Legal aspects of human embryos research and preimplantation genetic diagnosis in France. *Hum Reprod* 1997;12(11):2341–2.
20. Fiddler M, Pergament D, Pergament E. The role of the preimplantation geneticist in human cloning. *Prenat Diagn* 1999;19: 1200–5.
21. ESHRE PGD Consortium data collection IV: May-December 2001. *Hum Reprod* 2005;20(1):19–34.
22. Vandervorst M, Liebaers I, Sermon K, Staessen C, De Vos A, Van de Velde H, Van Assche E, Joris H, Van Steirteghem A, Devroey P. Successful preimplantation genetic diagnosis is related to the number of available cumulus–oocyte complexes. *Hum Reprod* 1998;13:3169–76.
23. Platteau P, Staessen C, Michiels A, Van Steirteghem A, Liebaers I, Devroey P. Which patients with recurrent implantation failure after IVF benefit from PGD for aneuploidy screening? *Reprod Biomed Online* 2006;12(3):334–9.
24. Rizk B. Epidemiology of ovarian hyperstimulation syndrome: iatrogenic and spontaneous. In Rizk B (ed), *Ovarian Hyperstimulation Syndrome*. Cambridge, New York: Cambridge University Press, 2006.
25. Weghofer A, Munne S, Brannath W, Chen S, Cohen J, Gleicher N. The quantitative and qualitative impact of gonadotropin stimulation on human preimplantation embryos: a preliminary study. *Fertil Steril* 2006; 86 (Suppl. 2):O-137.
26. Weghofer A, Munné S, Brannath W, Chen S, Tomkin G, Cekleniak N, Garrisi M, Barad D, Cohen J, Gleicher N. The impact of LH-containing gonadotropins on diploidy rates in preimplantation embryos: long protocol stimulation. *Hum Reprod* 2008 Mar;23(3):499–503.
27. Baart EB, Martini E, Eijkemans MJ, Van Opstal D, Beckers NG, Verhoeff A, Macklon NS, Fauser BC. Milder ovarian stimulation for in-vitro fertilization reduces aneuploidy in the human preimplantation embryo: a randomized controlled trial. *Hum Reprod* 2007;22(4):980–8.
28. ESHRE PGD Consortium Steering Committee. ESHRE Preimplantation Genetic Diagnosis (PGD) Consortium: Data collection III (May 2001). *Hum Reprod* 2002;17:233–46.

29. Gianaroli L, Plachot M, van Kooij R, Al-Hasani S, Dawson K, DeVos A, Magli MC, Mandelbaum J, Selva J, van Inzen W. ESHRE guidelines for good practice in IVF laboratories. Committee of the Special Interest Group on Embryology of the European Society of Human Reproduction and Embryology. *Hum Reprod* 2000;15:2241–6.

30. Hardy K, Martin KL, Leese HJ, Winston RML, Handyside AH. Human preimplantation development in vitro is not adversely affected by biopsy at the 8-cell stage. *Hum Reprod* 1990;5:708–14.

31. Verlinsky Y, Rechitsky S, Cieslak J, Ivakhnenko V, Wolf G, Lifchez A, Kaplan B, Moise J, Walle J, White M et al. Preimplantation diagnosis of single gene disorders by two-step oocyte genetic analysis using first and second polar body. *Biochem Mol Med* 1997;62:182–7.

32. De Boer KA, Catt JW, Jansen RPS et al. Moving to blastocyst biopsy for preimplantation genetic diagnosis and single embryo transfer at Sydney IVF. *Fertil Steril* 2004;82:295–8.

33. Verlinsky Y, Ginsberg N, Lifchez A, Valle J, Moise J, Strom CM. Analysis of the first polar body: preconception genetic diagnosis. *Hum Reprod* 1990;5:826–9.

34. Verlinsky Y, Cieslak J, Ivakhnenko V, Evsikov S, Wolf G, White M, Lifchez A, Kaplan B, Moise J, Valle J et al. Preimplantation diagnosis of common aneuploidies by the first- and second-polar body FISH analysis. *J Assist Reprod Genet* 1998;15:285–9.

35. Strom CM, Ginsberg N, Rechitsky S, Cieslak J, Ivakhenko V, Wolf G, Lifchez A, Moise J, Valle J, Kaplan B et al. Three births after preimplantation genetic diagnosis for cystic fibrosis with sequential first and second polar body analysis. *Am J Obstet Gynecol* 1998;178:1298–306.

36. Harper J, Thornhill AR. Embryo biopsy. In Harper J, Delhanty JDA, Handyside AH (eds.), *Preimplantation Genetic Diagnosis*. John Wiley and Sons, Chichester, UK, 2001; pp. 141–163.

37. Harper JC, Doshi A. Micromanipulation: biopsy. In Gardner DK, Lane M, Watson AJ (eds.), *Laboratory Guide to the Mammalian Embryo*. Oxford University Press, 2003.

38. Munné S, Cohen J. Unsuitability of multinucleated human blastomeres for preimplantation genetic diagnosis. *Hum Reprod* 1993;8:1120–5.

39. Dokras A, Sargent IL, Ross C, Gardner RL, Barlow DH. Trophectoderm biopsy in human blastocysts. *Hum Reprod* 1990;5:821–5.

40. Pierce KE, Michalopoulos J, Kiessling AA, Seibel MM, Zilberstein M. Preimplantation development of mouse and human embryos biopsied at cleavage stages using a modified displacement technique. *Hum Reprod* 1997;12:351–6.

41. De Boer K, MacArthur S, Murray C, Jansen R. First live birth following blastocyst biopsy and PGD analysis. *Reprod Biomed Online* 2002;4:35.

42. ESHRE PGD Consortium Steering Committee. ESHRE Preimplantation Genetic Diagnosis (PGD) Consortium: preliminary assessment of data from January 1997 to September 1998. *Hum Reprod* 1999;14:3138–48.

43. Dumoulin JC, Bras M, Coonen E, Dreesen J, Geraedts JP, Evers JL. Effect of Ca2þ/Mg2þ-free medium on the biopsy procedure for preimplantation genetic diagnosis and further development of human embryos. *Hum Reprod* 1998;13:2880–3.

44. Van de Velde H, De Vos A, Sermon K, Staessen C, De Rycke M, Van Assche E, Lissens W, Vandervorst M, Van Ranst H, Liebaers I et al. Embryo implantation after biopsy of one or two cells from cleavage-stage embryos with a view to preimplantation genetic diagnosis. *Prenat Diagn* 2000;20:1030–37.

45. Jamieson ME, Coutts JRT, Connor JM. The chromosome constitution of human embryos fertilized in vitro. *Hum Reprod* 1994;9:709–15.

46. Munne S, Magli C, Bahce M et al. Preimplantation diagnosis of the aneuploidies most commonly found in spontaneous abortions and live births, XY, 13, 14, 15, 16, 18, 21, 22. *Prenat Diagn* 1998;18:1459–66.

47. Gianaroli L, Magli MC, Ferraretti AP, Munne S. Preimplantation diagnosis for aneuploidies in patients undergoing in vitro fertilization with a poor prognosis: identification of the categories for which it should be proposed. *Fertil Steril* 1999;72:837–44.

48. Staessen C, Platteau P, Van Assche E et al. Comparison of blastocyst transfer with or without preimplantation genetic diagnosis for aneuploidy screening in couples with advanced maternal age: a prospective randomized controlled trial. *Hum Reprod* 2004;19:2849–58.

49. Hopman AHN, Raemakers FCS, Reap AK, Beck JLM, Devilee P, Ploeg van der M, Vooijis GP. In-situ hybridisation as a tool to study numerical chromosome aberrations in solid bladder tumors. *Histochemistry* 1988;89:307–16.

50. Harper JC, Wilton L. FISH and embryo sexing to avoid X-linked disease. In Harper JC, Delhanty J, Handyside A (eds.), *Preimplantation Genetic Diagnosis*. John Wiley & Sons, Ltd., 2001.

51. Abdelhadi I, Colls P, Sandalinas M, Escudero T, Munne S. Preimplantation genetic diagnosis of numerical abnormalities for 13 chromosomes. *Reprod Biomed Online* 2003;4(2):226–31.

52. -Verlinsky Y and Anver Kuliev. Preimplantation diagnosis for aneuploidies. In Verlinsky Y and Anver Kuliev (eds.). *Atlas of Preimplantation Genetic Diagnosis*. Taylor and Francis, Abingdon, UK, 2005; pp. 49–61

53. Munné S, Magli C, Cohen J, Morton P, Sadowy S, Gianaroli L, Tucker M, Marquez C, Sable D, Ferraretti A et al. Positive outcome after preimplantation diagnosis of aneuploidy in human embryos. *Hum Reprod* 1999;14:2191–9.

54. Jobanputra V, Sobrino A, Kinney A et al. Multiplex interphase FISH as screen for common aneuploidies in spontaneous abortions. *Hum Reprod* 2002;17:1166–70.

55. Wilton L. Preimplantation genetic diagnosis for aneuploidy screening in early human embryos: a review. *Prenat Diagn* 2002; 22:1–7.

56. Voullaire L, Wilton L, McBain J, Callaghan T, Williamson R. Chromosome abnormalities identified by comparative genomic hybridization in embryos from women with repeated implantation failure. *Mol Hum Reprod* 2002;8:1035–41.

57. Gianoroli L, Magli MC, Ferraretti AP et al. Possible interchromosomal effect in embryos generated by gametes from translocation carriers. *Hum Reprod* 2002;17:3201–7.

58. Munné S. Preimplantation genetic diagnosis of numerical and structural chromosome abnormalities. *Reprod BioMed Online* 2002;4:183–96.

59. Staessen C, Van Assche E, Joris H, Bonduelle M, Vandervorst M, Liebaers I, Van Steirteghem A. Clinical experience of sex determination by fluorescent in-situ hybridization for preimplantation genetic diagnosis. *Mol Hum Reprod* 1999;5:382–9.

60. Griffin DK, Handyside AH, Penketh RJA, Winston RML, Delhanty JDA. Fluorescent in situ hybridisation to interphase nuclei of human pre-implantation embryos with X and Y chromosome specific probes. *Hum Reprod* 1991;6:101–5.

61. Harper JC, Coonen E, Ramaekers FCS, Delhanty JDA, Handyside AH, Winston RM, Hopman AHN. Identification of the sex of human preimplantation embryos in two hours using an improved spreading technique and fluorescent in-situ hybridization (FISH) using directly labeled probes. *Hum Reprod* 1994;9:721–4.

62. Griffin DK, Wilton LJ, Handyside AH, Winston RML, Delhanty JDA. Dual fluorescent in situ hybridisation for the simultaneous detection of X and Y chromosome specific probes for the sexing

of human preimplantation embryonic nuclei. *Hum Genet* 1992;89:18–22.

63. Griffin DK, Wilton LJ, Handyside AH, Atkinson GHG, Winston RML, Delhanty JDA. Diagnosis of sex in preimplantation embryos by fluorescent in situ hybridisation. *BMJ* 1993;306:1382.

64. Griffin DK, Handyside AH, Harper JC et al. Clinical experience with preimplantation diagnosis of sex by dual fluorescent in situ hybridisation. *J Assist Reprod Genet* 1994;11:132–43.

65. Verlinsky Y, Handyside A, Grifo J et al. Preimplantation diagnosis of genetic and chromosomal disorders. *J Assist Reprod Genet* 1994;11:236–41.

66. McKusick V. *Mendelian Inheritance in Man*, 11th edn. John Hopkins University Press, Baltimore, MD, 1994.

67. ESHRE PGD Consortium Steering Committee. ESHRE Preimplantation Genetic Diagnosis (PGD) Consortium: Data collection II (May 2000). *Hum Reprod* 2000;15:2673–83.

68. Delhanty JDA, Harper JC, Ao A, Handyside AH, Winston RML. Multicolour FISH detects frequent chromosomal mosaicism and chaotic division in normal preimplantation embryos from fertile patients. *Hum Genet* 1997;99:755–60.

69. Coonen E, Dumoulin JCM, Ramaekers FCS, Hopman AHN. Optimal preparation of preimplantation embryo interphase nuclei for analysis by fluorescence in situ hybridization. *Hum Reprod* 1994;9:533–7.

70. Dozortsev DI, McGinnis KT. An improved fixation technique for fluorescence in situ hybridization for preimplantation genetic diagnosis. *Fertil Steril* 2001;76:186–8.

71. Baart EB, Van Opstal D, Los FJ, Fauser BCJM, Martini EM. Fluorescence in situ hybridization analysis of two blastomeres from day 3 frozen–thawed embryos followed by analysis of the remaining embryo on day 5. *Hum Reprod* 2004;19:685–93.

72. Velilla E, Escudero T, Munné S. Blastomere fixation techniques and risk of misdiagnosis for preimplantation genetic diagnosis of aneuploidy. *Reprod Biomed Online* 2002;4(3):210–17.

73. Colls P, Escudero T, Cekleniak N, Sadowy S, Cohen J, Munné S. Increased efficiency of preimplantation genetic diagnosis for infertility using "no result rescue". *Fertil Steril* 2007;88(1):53–61.

74. Magli MC, Sandalinas M, Escudero T, Morrison L, Ferraretti AP, Gianaroli L, Munné S. Double locus analysis of chromosome 21 for preimplantation genetic diagnosis of aneuploidy. *Prenat Diagn* 2001 Dec;21(12):1080–5.

75. Munné S, Márquez C, Magli MC et al. Scoring criteria for preimplantation genetic diagnosis of numerical abnormalities for chromosomes XY, 13, 16, 18 and 21. *Mol Hum Reprod* 1998;4:863–70.

76. Magli MC, Sandalinas M, Escudero T et al. Double locus analysis of chromosome 21 for preimplantation genetic diagnosis of aneuploidy. *Prenat Diagn* 2001;21:1080–5.

77. Thornhill AR, Snow K. Molecular diagnostics in preimplantation genetic diagnosis. *J Mol Diagn* 2002;4:11–29.

78. Wells D, Sherlock J. Diagnosis of single gene disorders. In Harper J, Delhanty JC, Handyside A (eds.), *Preimplantation Genetic Diagnosis*. John Wiley & Sons Ltd., 2001.

79. Ray PF, Ao A, Taylor DM, Winston RML, Handyside AH. Assessment of the reliability of single blastomere analysis for preimplantation diagnosis of the AF508 deletion causing cystic fibrosis in clinical practice. *Prenat Diagn* 1998;18(13):1402–12.

80. Cui KH, Matthews CD. Nuclear structural conditions and PCR amplification in human preimplantation diagnosis. *Mol Hum Reprod* 1996;2(1):63–71.

81. Stern HJ, Harton GL, Sisson ME, Jones SL, Fallon LA, Thorsell LP, Getlinger ME, Black SH, Schulman JD. Non-disclosing preimplantation genetic diagnosis for Huntington disease. *Prenat Diagn* 2002;22:503–7.

82. Ray PF, Handyside AH. Increasing the denaturation temperature during the first cycles of amplification reduces allele dropout from single cells for preimplantation genetic diagnosis. *Mol Hum Reprod* 1996;2(3):213–18.

83. Harper JC, Wells D. Future developments in PGD. In Harper J, Delhanty J, Handyside A (eds.), *Preimplantation Genetic Diagnosis*. John Wiley & Sons Ltd., 2001.

84. Rechitsky S, Strom C, Verlinsky O, Amet T, Ivakhnenko V, Kukharenko V, Kuliev A, Verlinsky Y. Allele dropout in polar bodies and blastomeres. *J Assist Reprod Genet* 1998;15:253–7.

85. Hattori M, Yoshioka K, Sakaki Y. High-sensitive fluorescent DNA sequencing and its application for detection and mass-screening of point mutations. *Electrophoreses* 1992;13(8):560–5.

86. Fiorentino F, Biricik A, Nuccitelli A, De Palma R, Kahraman S, Iacobelli M, Trengia V, Caserta D, Bonu MA, Borini A, Baldi M. Strategies and clinical outcome of 250 cycles of Preimplantation Genetic Diagnosis for single gene disorders. *Hum Reprod* 2006 Mar;21(3):670–84.

87. Verlinsky Y and Anver Kuliev. Preimplantation diagnosis for single-gene disorders. In Verlinsky Y and Kuliev Anver (eds.). *Atlas of Preimplantation Genetic Diagnosis*. Taylor and Francis, Abingdon, UK, 2005; pp. 29–40

88. Sherlock J, Cirigliano V, Petrou M, Tutschek B, Adinolfi M. Assessment of quantitative fluorescent multiplex PCR performed on single cells. *Ann Hum Genet* 1998;62(1):9–23.

89. Eggerding FA, Lovannisci DM, Brinson E, Grossman P, Winn-Deen ES. Fluorescence-based oligonucleotide ligation assay for analysis of cystic fibrosis transmembrane conductance regulator gene mutations. *Hum Mutat* 1995;5(2):153–65.

90. Pertl B, Weitgasser U, Kopp S, Kroisel PM, Sherlock J, Adinolfi M. Rapid detection of trisomy 21 and 18 and sexing with quantitative fluorescent multiplex PCR. *Hum Genet* 98:55–9.

91. Sermon K, De Vos A, Van de Velde H et al. Fluorescent PCR and automated fragment analysis for the clinical application of preimplantation genetic diagnosis of myotonic dystrophy (Steinert's disease). *Mol Hum Reprod* 1998;4(8):791–6.

92. Piyamongkol W, Bermudez MG, Harper JC, Wells D. Detailed investigation of factors influencing amplification efficiency and allele dropout in single cell PCR: implications for preimplantation genetic diagnosis. *Mol Hum Reprod* 2003;9:411–20.

93. Thornhill AR, McGrath JA, Braude P, Eady R, Handyside AH. Comparison of different lysis buffers to assess allele dropout from single cells for preimplantation genetic diagnosis. *Prenat Diagn* 21:490–7.

94. El-Hashemite N, Delhanty JDA. A technique for eliminating allele specific amplification failure during DNA amplification of heterozygous cells for preimplantation diagnosis. *Mol Hum Reprod* 2001;3:975–8.

95. Grifo JA, Giatras K, Tang YX, Krey LC. Successful outcome with day 4 embryo transfer after preimplantation diagnosis for genetically transmitted diseases. *Hum Reprod* 1998;13:1656–9.

96. Gardner DK, Lane M. Blastocyst transfer. *Clin Obstet Gynecol* 2003;46:231–8.

97. Joris H, Van Den Abbeel E, Vos AD. Reduced survival after human embryo biopsy and subsequent cryopreservation. *Hum Reprod* 1999;14:2833–7.

98. Magli MC, Gianaroli L, Fortini D et al. Impact of blastomere biopsy and cryopreservation techniques on human embryo viability. *Hum Reprod* 1999;14:770–3.

99. Jericho H, Wilton L, Gook DA et al. A modified cryopreservation method increases the survival of human biopsied cleavage stage embryos. *Hum Reprod* 2003;18:568–71.

100. McArthur SJ, Leigh D, Marshall JT, de Boer KA, Jansen RP. Pregnancies and live births after trophectoderm biopsy and preimplantation genetic testing of human blastocysts. *Fertil Steril* 2005 Dec;84(6):1628–36.

101. Lee M, Munné S. Pregnancy after polar body biopsy and freezing and thawing of human embryos. *Fertil Steril* 2000;73(3):645–7.

102. Cieslak-Janzen J, Tur-Kaspa I, Ilkevitch Y, Bernal A, Morris R, Verlinsky Y. Multiple micromanipulations for preimplantation genetic diagnosis do not affect embryo development to the blastocyst stage. *Fertil Steril* 2006;85(6):1826–9.

103. Magli MC, Gianaroli L, Ferraretti AP, Toschi M, Esposito F, Fasolino MC. The combination of polar body and embryo biopsy does not affect embryo viability. *Hum Reprod* 2004;19(5): 1163–9.

104. Munné S, Cohen J. Chromosome abnormalities in human embryos. *Hum Reprod Update.* 1998 Nov-Dec;4(6):842–55.

105. International Working Group on Preimplantation Genetics. Tenth anniversary of preimplantation genetic diagnosis. *J Assist Reprod Genet* 2001 Feb;18(2):64–70.

106. Munné S, Sandalinas M, Escudero T, Velilla E, Walmsley R, Sadowy S, Cohen J, Sable D. Improved implantation after preimplantation genetic diagnosis of aneuploidy. *Reprod Biomed Online* 2003;7(1):91–7.

107. Harper J, Sermon K, Geraedts J, Vesela K, Harton G, Thornhill A, Pehlivan T, Fiorentino F, SenGupta S, de Die-Smulders C, Magli C, Moutou C, Wilton L. What next for preimplantation genetic screening? *Hum Reprod.* 2008 Mar;23(3):478–80.

108. Mastenbroek S, Twisk M, van Echten-Arends J et al. In vitro fertilization with preimplantation genetic screening. *N Engl J Med* 2007;357:9–17.

109. Stevens J, Wale P, Surrey ES, Schoolcraft WB. Is aneuploidy screening for patients aged 35 or over beneficial? A prospective randomized trial. *Fertil Steril* 2004;82(Suppl. 2):249.

110. Munné S, Gianaroli L, Tur-Kaspa I, Magli C, Sandalinas M, Grifo J, Cram D, Kahraman S, Verlinsky Y, Simpson JL. Substandard application of preimplantation genetic screening may interfere with its clinical success. *Fertil Steril* 2007;88(4):781–4.

111. Zhang L, Cui X, Schmitt K, Hubert R, Navidi W, Arnheim N. Whole genome amplification form a single cell – implications for genetic-analysis. *Proc Natl Acad Sci USA* 1992;89:5847–51.

112. Wells D, Sherlock JK, Handyside AH, Delhanty JDA. Detailed chromosomal and molecular genetic analysis of single cells by whole genome amplification and comparative genomic hybridisation (CGH). *Nucleic Acids Res* 1999;27(4):1214–18.

113. Ao A, Wells D, Handyside AH, Winston RM, Delhanty JDA. Reimplantation genetic diagnosis of inherited cancer: familial adenomatous polyposis coli. *J Assist Reprod Genet* 1998;15(3): 140–4.

114. Ruangvutilert P, Delhanty JDA, Rodeck C, Harper JC. Relative efficiency of FISH on metaphase and interphase nuclei from non-mosaic trisomic or triploid fibroblast cultures. *Prenat Diagn* 2000;20:159–62.

115. Evsikov S, Verlinsky Y. Visualization of chromosomes in single human blastomeres. *J Assist Reprod Genet* 1999;16(3):133–7.

116. Willadsen S, Levron Munne S, Schimmel T, Marquez C, Scott R, Cohen J. Rapid visualization of metaphase chromosomes in single human blastomeres after fusion with in-vitro matured bovine eggs. *Hum Reprod* 1999;14(2):470–5.

117. Schrock E, S du Manoir, Veldman T et al. Multicolor spectral karyotyping of human chromosomes. *Science* 1996;273:494–7.

118. Speicher MR, Ballard SG, Ward DC. Karyotyping human chromosomes by combinatorial multi-fluor FISH. *Nat Genet* 1996;12:368–75.

119. Marquez C, Cohen J, Munne S. Chromosome identification in human ocytes and polar bodies by spectral karyotyping. *Cytogenet Cell Genet* 1998;81:254–8.

120. Kallioniemi A, Kallioniemi OP, Sudar D, Rutovitz D, Gray JW, Waldman F, Pinkel D. Comparative genomic hybridization for molecular cytogenetic analysis of solid tumors. *Science* 1992;258(5083):818–21.

121. Wells D, Delhanty JDA. Comprehensive chromosome analysis of human pre-implantation embryos using WGA and single cell CGH. *Mol Hum Reprod* 2000;6:1055–62.

122. Vouliare L, Slater H, Williamson R, Wilton L. Chromosome analysis of blastomeres from human embryos by using. *Coll Hum Genet* 2000;105:210–17.

123. Pinkel D, Segraves R, Sudar D et al. High resolution analysis of DNA copy number variation using comparative genomic hybridization to microarrays. *Nat Genet* 1998;20(2):207–11.

124. Treff NR, Su J, Mavrianos J, Bergh PA, Miller AK, Scott RT. Accurate 23 chromosome aneuploidy screening in human blastomeres using single nucleotide polymorphism (SNP) microarrays. *Fertil Steril* 2007;88:S1, Q1.

125. Viville S, Pergament D, Fiddler M. Ethical perspectives and regulation of preimplantation genetic diagnostic practice. In Harper JC, Delhanty J, Handyside A (eds.), *Preimplantation Genetic Diagnosis.* John Wiley & Sons, 2001.

126. Nagy A-M, De Man X, Anibal N, Lints FA. Scientific and ethical issues of preimplantation diagnosis. *Ann Med* 1998;30:1–6.

127. Berkowitz JM. Sexism and racism in preconceptive trait selection. *Fertil Steril* 1999;71:415–17.

128. King DS. Preimplantation genetic diagnosis and the 'new' eugenics. *J Med Genet* 1999;25:176–82.

129. Viville S, Pergament D. Results of a survey of the legal status and attitudes towards preimplantation genetic diagnosis and conducted in 13 different countries. *Prenat Diagn* 1998; 180(3):1374–80.

130. Geraedts JP, Harper J, Braude P, Sermon K, Veiga A, Gianaroli L, Agan N, Munne S, Gitlin S, Blenow E et al. Preimplantation genetic diagnosis (PGD), a collaborative activity of clinical genetic departments and IVF centres. *Prenat Diagn* 2001;21: 1086–92.

131. Kuliev A, Verlinsky Y. Thirteen years experience of preimplantation diagnosis. *Reprod BioMed Online* 2004;8:229–35.

67

EPIGENETICS AND ART

Martine De Rycke

SAFETY OF ART

Assisted reproductive technologies (ART) are increasingly used worldwide to overcome infertility problems, and it has been estimated that more than one million children have been born relying on these techniques. ART births now account for 1–3 percent of all births in developed countries. ART have considerably evolved since the beginning, and now they include controlled ovarian stimulation, (immature) gamete retrieval and manipulation, standard in vitro fertilization (IVF), intracytoplasmic sperm injection (ICSI), (extended) embryo culture, freezing/thawing of embryos, embryo biopsy in cases of preimplantation genetic diagnosis, and more recently in vitro maturation of oocytes and techniques of cryopreservation of testicular/ovarian tissues. There has been concern about the health of the children conceived ever since the birth of the first IVF baby in 1978 (1) and certainly after the introduction of the more invasive ICSI procedure in the early 1990s. The safety aspect has been addressed in various epidemiological studies of children conceived by ART as well as experimental studies. The follow-up studies including a review by Rizk et al. of the major congenital anomalies in the first 1,000 babies conceived by IVF have shown that generally ART-conceived children are as healthy as naturally conceived children (1), except that ART may increase the risk of a few outcomes. There is accumulating evidence of an increase in chromosomal abnormalities in ICSI children, as well as evidence for an increase in malformation rate and in the number of singleton children with a low birth weight in the IVF/ICSI population compared to the general population. It is, however, not clear whether these findings are related to the parental infertility problems or to the infertility treatment.

Recently, syndromes involving epigenetic defects have been reported in animals and humans after ART. The large offspring syndrome has been described in sheep and cattle, while in humans rare imprinting disorders have been reported.

The first part of this chapter provides background information about basic epigenetic mechanisms, the phenomenon of genomic imprinting, and human imprinting syndromes. An overview of the epigenetic reprogramming events during gametogenesis and in the early embryo is presented as well. The second part reviews epidemiological data on epigenetic risk in ART children and discusses the significance and implications of these findings.

WHAT IS EPIGENETICS?

The term "epigenetics" has over time been used in various senses. The root term "epigenesis" goes back to Aristotle and describes embryonic development as a series of events where new structures and functions appear with increasing complexity. The developmental biologist Conrad Waddington introduced the term "epigenetics" in 1942 as the study of the processes by which genotype gives rise to phenotype. In his book *Organisers and Genes* published in 1940, he proposed the idea of "the epigenetic landscape," in which he visualized embryonic development as a ball (the embryo) rolling down a sloping surface with branching valleys representing the choices of developmental pathways for an embryonic cell. The current definition of epigenetics has been narrowed to a molecular one.

Epigenetics is defined as the study of reversible changes in gene expression that occur without changes in the DNA code and that do not follow Mendelian laws. This includes the study of how gene expression patterns are inherited through DNA replication and cell division (mitosis and meiosis), how gene expression patterns change during differentiation, and how they can be influenced by environmental factors. The epigenome refers to the overall epigenetic state of a cell at a specific time and stage: hence, one genome can correspond to many epigenomes.

The field of epigenetics is relatively new as researchers only started to learn its molecular basis in the 1990s. Eukaryotic DNA is compacted with histones into chromatin. The basic unit of chromatin, the nucleosome, consists of an octamer of core histones (two copies of each histone H2A, H2B, H3, and H4) around which 147 bp of DNA is wrapped. Further folding of this nucleosomal array gives higher order structures. Chromatin is organized into either highly condensed or open domains, called "heterochromatin" and "euchromatin," respectively. Heterochromatin is transcriptionally repressed and late replicating, while euchromatin is transcriptionally active and early replicating. Chromatin structure and function are regulated by epigenetic modifications including DNA methylation at CpG dinucleotides, the covalent modification of histone (phosphorylation, acetylation, methylation, and ubiquitination), chromatin remodeling, and noncoding RNAs. Modifications of DNA or associated histones will modulate the interactions between histones, DNA, RNA, and non-histone proteins, whereas chromatin-remodeling complexes may displace nucleosomes. This will change the overall chromatin structure and influence DNA accessibility, thereby regulating gene expression as well as other cellular processes such as replication, recombination, repair, and chromosome segregation (2).

BASIC EPIGENETIC MECHANISMS

DNA Methylation

DNA methylation can be found in almost all living organisms. In eukaryotes, it mainly involves the covalent addition of a methyl group to a cytosine at CpG dinucleotides. The establishment and the maintenance of methylation patterns depend on at least three different DNA methyltransferases, one "maintenance" methyltransferase, Dnmt1, which prefers hemimethylated DNA as a substrate, and two "de novo" methyltransferases, Dnmt3A and Dnmt3B, which act preferentially on nonmethylated DNA. Mice lacking either one of these methyltransferases die pre- or postnatally (2).

It has been well established that mammalian DNA methylation is essential for embryonic development, genome stability, X chromosome inactivation, and genomic imprinting. DNA methylation plays a pivotal role in gene silencing. Some genomic regions like the repetitive sequences and transposons are hypermethylated and silenced; other regions such as the CpG islands in the promoters of housekeeping genes are hypomethylated and are transcriptionally active. The methylation levels of differentiated cells are relatively stable through mitosis. Nevertheless, it remains a reversible modification that may be susceptible to environmental changes. With age, specific genes become hypermethylated, while repeated sequences loose their methylation patterns. Aberrant DNA methylation patterns have been associated with cancer, methylation at transposons is lost, oncogenes are activated due to global hypomethylation, and tumor suppressor genes are inactivated because of CpG island hypermethylation, leading to an overall picture of changes in gene expression and chromatin structure along with genome instability.

Histone Modifications and Chromatin Remodeling

The posttranslational modifications of specific amino acids (AA) within the NH_2-terminal histone tails have been known for a long time. Modifications within the globular histone cores at the histone-DNA interface have been mapped only recently (3). Some modifications like acetylation and phosphorylation have a high turnover rate and are linked with inducible gene expression patterns; others like methylation are very stable and are linked with long-term expression patterns. Several classes of chromatin remodeling and histone modification complexes have been identified. Histone acetyl transferase enzymes (HATs) transfer an acetyl group from the cofactor acetyl CoA to lysines. The reverse reaction is catalyzed by histone deacetylases (HDACs). Both HATs and HDACs are often part of transcription regulatory protein complexes. Histone methylation is catalyzed by histone methyl transferases, which use S-adenosylmethionine as a cofactor in a relatively irreversible reaction. Another family of protein complexes are the ATP-dependent chromatin remodeling complexes that are capable of (re)positioning nucleosomes using the energy of ATP hydrolysis.

The idea of the histone code hypothesis is that histone modifications, alone or in various combinations, will influence chromatin structure and determine whether the underlying genetic information is active or not. Modifications at the histone-DNA interface may have a direct impact on chromatin, whereas modifications in the histone tails may alter chromatin structure indirectly by recruitment of chromatin-associated proteins that will modulate chromatin structure. The methyl modification of lysine 9 in H3 has been shown to recruit chromodomain proteins that will induce heterochromatin assembly and epigenetic silencing. Proteins with bromodomains are attracted to acetylated lysines and this has been linked with transcriptional activation. The acetyl modification reduces the histone-DNA interactions within nucleosomes and recruits transcriptional coactivators. Similarly, phosphorylation and ubiquitination "marks" form binding sites for specific chromatin-associated proteins. The findings that the various histone modifications can work antagonistically or synergistically and that the core histones can be replaced with specialized histone variants add further complexity to the system.

GENOMIC IMPRINTING

The vast majority of autosomal genes undergo biallelic expression. The two copies of such genes, one from each parent, have identical function. Genomic imprinting is an epigenetic form of gene regulation, which involves the monoallelic expression of one of the two parental alleles in a parent-of-origin specific manner.

The phenomenon of genomic imprinting was discovered in the early 1980s. Pronuclear transplantation studies in mice showed that gynogenetic embryos containing two maternal genomes and androgenetic embryos with two paternal genomes were arrested early in development. The gynogenetic embryos showed a relatively normal embryo but poor extraembryonic growth, whereas there were mainly extraembryonic tissues and poor embryonic development in the androgenetic embryos. These experiments demonstrated that certain genes are preferentially expressed from only one parental genome and that both paternal and maternal genomes are required for normal embryonic development (4, 5). The generation of mice with uniparental disomy (UPD) for a specific chromosome or chromosomal region allowed the identification of imprinting clusters in chromosomal regions displaying parent-of-origin effects on the phenotype (6). Again, opposite phenotypes, reduced growth versus overgrowth, were found for specific maternal versus paternal UPDs.

Imprinting is only found in placental mammals and in marsupials, which have limited placentation. There is no evidence for genomic imprinting in the egg-laying monotremes, the earliest offshoot of the mammalian lineage, suggesting that imprinting arose during mammalian evolution in association with placentation. About eighty imprinted genes have been identified in humans and mouse so far, with the total number estimated to lie between 100 and 600 genes. About half of the identified genes are preferentially expressed from the maternal chromosome, the paternal allele being silenced. The other half shows paternal expression and maternal silencing. Imprinted genes have a crucial role in embryonic growth and placental function. Maternally expressed genes tend to inhibit growth, whereas most paternally expressed genes enhance embryonic growth. Imprinted genes also influence brain function and behavioral development, and they are involved in carcinogenesis (2).

Imprinted genes are usually located in clusters with paternally and maternally expressed genes, imprinted noncoding RNAs and nonimprinted genes. An imprinting center (IC), a DNA element of a few kb, controls the imprints and imprinted expression in the cluster. The underlying mechanisms are not completely clear but the findings that IC elements may act as chromatin insulators (insulators can block interactions between enhancers and gene promoters as well as block the spreading of chromatin modifications) and also contain promoters for noncoding RNAs are important factors in the control mechanisms. The parental alleles of the IC element are differentially marked or "imprinted" in the parental germ lines when the two genomes are separate (imprint resetting) (Figure 67.1). These germ-line imprints, present in all ICs, are maintained in the zygote and further through somatic cell divisions (imprint maintenance). They will lead to monoallelic expression in the embryo and in the adult. The imprints are reset in the germ line according to the sex of the embryo. The differential epigenetic marking involves allele-specific histone modifications, differential DNA methylation, and allelic differences in chromatin structure. Imprinting is a reversible process: an imprinted gene that has been inactivated after passage through the maternal germ line will be reactivated after passage through the paternal germ line and vice versa.

Several human syndromes such as Angelman syndrome (AS) (OMIM 105830) and Beckwith-Wiedemann syndrome (BWS) (OMIM 130650) are associated with defective imprinting. These imprinting disorders do not follow Mendelian inheritance patterns. AS is a rare neurological disorder. The syndrome has an incidence of one in 15,000 newborns and is clinically characterized by severe mental retardation, delayed motor development, absence of speech, jerky movements, and a happy disposition. Most cases are sporadic and the underlying cause is deregulation of an imprinted region on chromosome 15q11–13, which leads to loss of function of *UBE3A*, a gene showing monoallelic expression in the brain. The majority of cases are due to genetic defects (uniparental disomy, translocations, large chromosomal deletions, microdeletions, and point mutations), and only a minority of cases, less than 5 percent, are caused by epigenetic defects (7).

BWS, another rare imprinting disorder with an incidence of 1 in 14,000, is due to genetic or epigenetic defects in an imprinted cluster with two imprint control elements (IC1 and IC2) on chromosome 11p15.5. BWS patients present with pre- and/or postnatal overgrowth, macroglossia, abdominal wall defects, and ear abnormalities and are predisposed to embryonic tumors such as Wilms' tumors. Most cases are sporadic although 10–15 percent are familial cases. About 50–60 percent of cases involve an epigenetic alteration, namely loss of maternal methylation at IC2 of the BWS imprinted region (8).

EPIGENETIC REPROGRAMMING DURING THE MAMMALIAN LIFE CYCLE

Major epigenetic reprogramming takes place during gametogenesis and in the early embryo. Epigenetic patterns are imposed on the genome during embryonic development and differentiation through predetermined programs (genetic or intrinsic factors). The establishment of the appropriate gene expression patterns in space and time is essential for further development. Epigenetic systems also allow the early as well as the mature organism to modulate gene expression patterns in response to environmental changes (hormones, growth factors, etc.) without changing the genetic code. In addition to intrinsic and environmental factors, it seems that the epigenetic state of some genomic regions is determined stochastically (9).

Epigenetic reprogramming in the germ line starts with complete erasure of existing modifications in imprinted and nonimprinted genes to ensure genetic totipotency in the future embryo. Later during gametogenesis, de novo methylation and chromatin remodeling take place in the whole genome, whereas allele-specific marks are established at imprinted loci (imprint resetting). This reprogramming provides the genome in the gametes with molecular programs for oocyte activation, zygotic gene activation, and embryonic development.

The male imprint is acquired at an earlier stage of gametogenesis than the female one. Mouse studies showed that paternal imprints are completed by the round spermatid stage. Extrapolation of these data to the human implies that imprint resetting has been completed in immature sperm cells, which are sometimes used during ICSI, and that the risk for defective imprinting will be small. The findings in humans of complete imprint resetting at the IC1 of the BWS region and the presence of paternal imprints at the IC of the AS region at the stage of round spermatids indicate similarities in the timing of imprint establishment between mouse and human (10).

The female imprints in mouse are established asynchronously at different loci between the diplotene and the metaphase II stage. This time window coincides with the time window of hormonal stimulation, in vitro manipulation, culture, and maturation of oocytes during ART. Hormonal stimulation and/or in vitro culture/maturation may interfere with female imprint establishment. Mouse experiments showed abnormal imprints in oocytes that had been matured in vitro for several days (11). Aberrant methylation patterns at the IC1 of the BWS region were detected in human oocytes after in vitro maturation (12).

The gametes that come together at fertilization are epigenetically quite different. Both genomes are highly methylated and transcriptionally repressive. The oocyte chromatin structure that is packed with highly methylated histones is much more repressive than that of sperm, which is packed with protamines. After fertilization, stored ooplasmic factors as well as other factors modify the epigenetic status of the parental

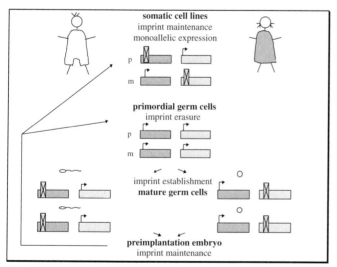

Figure 67.1. Imprint resetting and imprint maintenance during the mammalian life cycle. The imprints are erased in the primordial germ cells. Later during gametogenesis, new, sex-specific imprints are established. After fertilization, the imprints inherited from the gametes are maintained through somatic cell divisions and they lead to monoallelic expression.

Table 67.1: Overview of Studies of BWS after ART

No. of ART cases/cohort	Study	No. of LOM/ No. of tested	No. of ICSI/ No. of IVF	RR	Country	References
4	Retrospective	5/6	5/2	X6	USA	DeBaun et al. (21)
3/65*	Prospective					
6/149	Retrospective	2/2	3/3	X4	UK	Maher et al. (22)
6/149	Retrospective	6/6	2/4	X3	France	Gicquel et al. (23)
4/37	Retrospective case-control	3/3	1/3	X9	Australia	Halliday et al. (24)
19/341	Retrospective		5/5		USA	Chang et al. (25)

LOM, loss of maternal methylation; RR, relative risk.

genomes. The extent and timing of the epigenetic reprogramming in the early embryo may vary from species to species, but a similar sequence of remodeling steps is usually present. In mouse, the paternal chromosomes decondense and a rapid remodeling occurs: protamines are substituted with maternal, highly acetylated histones and the DNA undergoes active demethylation before replication. Only paternally methylated imprinted genes escape from this. The maternal genome, except for the maternally methylated imprinted genes, is passively demethylated after the first cell division. This general passive loss of methylation relates to the exclusion of Dnmt1 from the nucleus in oocytes and in the early cleavage stages. The mechanism of methylation maintenance at specific sequences (imprinted genes, pericentromeric regions, and IAP retrotransposons) has not been elucidated yet. Paternal and maternal genomes reach about equivalent DNA methylation levels in the eight-cell stage. At the time of implantation, a genome-wide DNA methylation takes place preferentially in the inner cell mass compared to the trophectoderm. Imprinted genes resist this global wave of de novo methylation (imprint maintenance), and their allele-specific methylation patterns are stably inherited through somatic cell divisions (10). Epigenetic reprogramming in the early embryo is required for accurate gene expression and differentiation. Various factors may adversely influence the epigenetic remodeling during embryonic development or/and during gametogenesis.

ANALYSIS OF DATA FROM ANIMAL STUDIES

There has been accumulating evidence from animal studies for an association between embryo culture conditions and epigenetic deregulation of imprinted and nonimprinted genes. These epigenetic changes during early development may lead to altered phenotypes later in life. For instance, Khosla et al. (13) have shown that the culture of mouse embryos in medium with serum influenced imprinted gene expression and resulted in a lower birth weight. The mechanisms by which culture media induce epigenetic alterations are unknown so far. It can be argued that the currently applied culture conditions in human ART centers have been carefully optimized and do not resemble the suboptimal animal culture conditions shown to induce altered gene expression and imprinting. In this way, the report of Gardner et al. (14) demonstrated normal imprinting in mouse blastocysts cultured in a sequential medium from human IVF centers.

The remarkable phenotype of LOS, observed in cattle and sheep born after cloning and in vitro embryo production, is characterized by fetal and postnatal overgrowth and developmental abnormalities. The syndrome is reminiscent of BWS in humans. It was shown that LOS in sheep after embryo culture is associated with a reduced maternal methylation and reduced IGF2R expression (15).

ANALYSIS OF HUMAN EPIDEMIOLOGICAL DATA

Data on AS

A possible association between ART and AS was considered after two case reports about three ICSI children with AS (16, 17). Further molecular genetic testing showed an epigenetic defect in these patients. Three AS children with epimutations are predicted to occur with a chance of 1 in 900,000. Assuming that about one million children have been born after ART (18) and that a complete ascertainment of AS children after ART is unlikely, then these three cases already point to a link between AS and ART, although they do not give proof of a causal link. More recently, a German retrospective AS cohort study, investigating the correlation between infertility treatment and imprinting defects, found that sixteen out of seventy-nine children had been born to subfertile couples, where subfertility had been defined as a time to pregnancy (TTP) longer than two years or/and infertility treatment (19). The relative risk for imprinting defects for subfertile couples without treatment was 6.25, which was similar to the relative risk of couples that had hormone treatment or ICSI, indicating that subfertile couples seem to be predisposed to epigenetic defects. A relative risk of 12.5 was seen for couples that had a TTP more than two years and underwent treatment, suggesting that the infertility-associated risk is somehow further increased by infertility treatment.

Data on BWS

A number of studies in different countries (United States, France, UK, and Australia) compared the prevalence of ART in a BWS registry with the prevalence in the general population (Table 67.1). DeBaun et al. (20) reported a total of seven children with BWS after ART, four from an initial study and three out of sixty-five in the prospective part of the study. Five children had been conceived after ICSI, two after regular IVF. Molecular analysis showed that five of the six children studied had a specific epigenetic defect. The retrospective studies of the British and French BWS registries reported similar figures: 6 out of 149 BWS patients had been born after ART. The six patients (three IVF and three ICSI) described by Maher et al. (21) represent a fourfold increase in prevalence of ART. Epigenetic defects were found in both patients for which genetic testing was carried out. The BWS patients in the American and British studies had been clinically diagnosed, while in the French registry, patients had been molecularly diagnosed with BWS (22). The six patients (two ICSI and four IVF) from the French registry all showed loss of maternal methylation at IC2. The risk of BWS after ART in this study was calculated to be three times higher than in the general population (4 vs. 1.3 percent).

A critical remark on these studies is that the frequency of ART cases in the general population was estimated and not measured and that the frequency of ART cases in the registries may be underestimated since a detailed reproductive history was not always available. Other limitations were the lack of appropriate control groups and the small size of the groups, yielding large confidence intervals.

Part of these limitations was circumvented in a retrospective Australian study. Halliday et al. (23) designed a case-control study of BWS patients from a single genetic clinic. They found four BWS children born after ART (one ICSI and three IVF) (4 in 14,894 babies) compared to thirty-seven born after natural conception (37 in 1,316,500 births), yielding a risk for BWS that was nine times higher in the ART population than in the general population. The confidence interval was rather large (1.8–432.9) due to the small size of the study. Again, an epigenetic deregulation was found in the three children that could be molecularly analyzed.

More recently, Chang et al. (24) reviewed the reproductive endocrine records of mothers of twelve BWS patients born after ART, in order to detect which factor(s) contributed to the epigenetic abnormalities. However, the only common factor for all women was the hormonal stimulation. The sample size of the study was too small to exclude further factors.

Despite the different methodologies used and other limitations of the studies, the epidemiological data indicate an association between ART and BWS. Further evidence is given by the overrepresentation of a specific epigenetic defect, loss of maternal methylation, in BWS cases after ART, compared to the numerous genetic and epigenetic defects involved in naturally conceived BWS patients. These results are consistent with the epimutations found in the ART-conceived AS cases (loss of maternal methylation at the IC of the *SNRPN* gene at chr15q11-13) and the LOS phenotype in sheep (loss of maternal methylation of *IGF2R*).

Taking all the data together, it seems that only a higher incidence of AS and BWS has been reported in children born after ART. The absolute risk, based on the highest relative risk reported from the epidemiological data, is estimated at 1/3,000 for BWS and 1/20,000 for AS, which is too low to set up routine screening of all ART children born.

CAUSES OF EPIGENETIC DEREGULATION AFTER ART

It is not yet known which specific factor or mechanism is responsible for the reported epigenetic defects, but it has been suggested that in vitro embryo culture may interfere with the maintenance of maternal methylation patterns at imprinted loci in preimplantation embryos or with maternal imprint resetting in case of genes that are only reset during late oogenesis (i.e., later than the germinal vesicle stage). There has been ample evidence from animal studies that support this hypothesis. Another hypothesis is that the hormonal stimulation of the ovaries interferes with maternal imprint resetting. Using a mouse embryo donation model, it has been shown that ovarian stimulation appears to impair oocyte/embryo quality as well as the uterine milieu (25) and leads to a reduced implantation and fetal development. Another study comparing the incidence of abnormal overall DNA methylation patterns in mice found a twofold increase in superovulated mice versus naturally ovulated mice (26). To our knowledge, there are currently no data on possible effects of hormonal stimulation on epigenetic reprogramming in human gametes and preimplantation embryos. The third hypothesis is that the epigenetic defects after ART are not caused by the techniques but are related to the infertility problems of the couples. Supporting evidence for this hypothesis comes from a study showing incomplete establishment of imprints (incomplete methylation) in spermatozoa from men with fertility problems (27).

An important question is whether the epigenetic deregulation is restricted to a few sensitive loci such as the functionally haploid imprinted loci or whether epigenetic defects occur at various genomic loci. According to this latter hypothesis, called the iceberg theory, imprinting disorders only represent the tip of the iceberg (28). AS and BWS are congenital syndromes with a relatively clear phenotype and a known molecular cause for which genetic analysis can be carried out. Epigenetic deregulation may cause a broader spectrum of phenotypes that may be more difficult to diagnose, the molecular basis may be complex and not completely understood, and testing may not be available or may only be carried out later in life. As loss of imprinting and overall epigenetic deregulation contributes to the initiation or progression of tumor development, an expected phenotype is an increased cancer risk. So far, follow-up studies on childhood cancer did not find any significant increased risk, although some small studies have reported an increased risk of specific cancers (29–32). A Dutch registry – based study of Moll et al. (33) reported an increased risk for retinoblastoma (Rb), a rare tumor of the eye, in children born after ART. The majority of Rb cases are caused by genetic defects, and only a minority of cases is due to an epigenetic defect. A genetic mutation was identified in two of the five children from the Dutch study. Further molecular testing is required to see whether epigenetic defects are present in the other children. Another study in the UK found no increased risk for Rb; they found no cases of Rb in a group of 176 IVF children, while 24 cases were detected in a control group of 358,094 children (34). The conclusion of a recent study of Lidegaard et al. (35) is not in favor of the iceberg theory. This Danish study involved a systematic follow-up of 6,052 ART singletons versus a control group of 442,349 naturally conceived children. The incidence rate of childhood cancer, mental diseases, congenital syndromes, and developmental disturbances was similar in both groups.

CONCLUSIONS

In conclusion, evidence from human epidemiological data indicates a higher incidence of imprinting disorders after

ART; however, the evidence is limited. In order to better quantify the risk and to learn about the underlying cause, it will be necessary to organize large-scale studies to detect risks for low-frequency events with sufficient statistical power. Prospective case-control studies with aggregation of data from multiple centers are a good option to collect reliable data at large scale since such studies have a high detection rate of problems. Yet, they are expensive, and the selection of a good control group is difficult. When considering epigenetic risks, long-term continuous follow-up of ART children is necessary, with assessment of the neonatal outcome as well as monitoring of imprinting disorders, cancer incidence, and neurobehavioral development. Data collection should include records of IVF cycles (infertility history, culture media, hormone stimulation, etc.) in order to identify the contributing factor(s). In addition to the follow-up studies, it is also necessary to continue basic research on epigenetic reprogramming in animal models and in humans.

KEY POINTS

■ The field of epigenetics, involving the study of gene regulation through DNA methylation, histone modifications, and chromatin remodeling, is relatively new and the unravelling of mechanisms has just started.

■ Imprinting is a special epigenetic mechanism and imprinted genes have a key role during embryonic development.

■ ART may interfere with the process of imprinting and epigenetic reprogramming in gametes and preimplantation embryos and lead to epigenetic defects.

■ Data from animal studies and human epidemiological studies suggest a higher incidence of imprinting defects after ART, but this is still controversial.

■ Long-term, continuous follow-up of ART children must be performed, together with fundamental research in this field.

REFERENCES

1. Rizk B, Doyle P, Tan SL et al. Perinatal outcome and congenital malformations in in-vitro fertilization babies from the Bourn-Hallam group. *Hum Reprod* 1991;6(9):1259–64.

2. Viewpoints and reviews on epigenetics. *Science* 2001;293:1063–103.

3. Cosgrove MS, Boeke JD, Wolberger C. Regulated nucleosome mobility and the histone code. *Struct Mol Biol* 2004;11:1037–43.

4. McGrath J, Solter D. Inability of mouse blastomere nuclei transferred to enucleated zygotes to support development in vitro. *Science* 1984;226:1317–19.

5. Barton SC, Surani MA, Norris ML. Role of paternal and maternal genomes in mouse development. *Nature* 1984;311:374–6.

6. Cattanach BM, Kirk M. Differential activity of maternally and paternally derived chromosome regions in mice. *Nature* 1985;315:496–8.

7. Horsthemke B, Buiting K. Imprinting defects on human chromosome 15. *Cytogenet Genome Res* 2006;113:292–9.

8. Weksberg R, Shuman C, Smith AC. Beckwith-Wiedemann syndrome. *Am J Med Genet C Semin Med Genet* 2005;137:12–23.

9. Jaenisch R, Bird A. Epigenetic regulation of gene expression: how the genome integrates intrinsic and environmental signals. *Nat Gen* 2003;33:245–54.

10. Lucifero D, Chaillet JR, Trasler JM. Potential significance of genomic imprinting defects for reproduction and assisted reproductive technology. *Hum Reprod Update* 2004;10:3–18.

11. Kerjean A, Couvert P, Heams T et al. In vitro follicular growth affects oocyte imprinting establishment in mice. *Eur J Hum Genet* 2003;11:493–6.

12. Borghol N, Lornage J, Blachere T, Sophie Garret A, Lefevre A. Epigenetic status of the H19 locus in human oocytes following in vitro maturation. *Genomics* 2006;87:417–26.

13. Khosla S, Dean W, Reik W, Feil R. Culture of preimplantation embryos and its long-term effects on gene expression and phenotype. *Hum Reprod Update* 2001;7:419–27.

14. Gardner DK, Hewitt EA, Lane M. Sequential media used in human IVF do not affect imprinting of the H19 gene in mouse blastocysts. *Fertil Steril* 2003;80 (Suppl. 3):S256.

15. Young LE, Fernandes K, McEvoy TG, Butterwith SC, Gutierrez CG, Carolan C, Broadbent PJ, Robinson JJ, Wilmut I, Sinclair KD. Epigenetic change in IGF2R is associated with fetal overgrowth after sheep embryo culture. *Nat Genet* 2001;27:153–4.

16. Cox GF, Burger J, Lip V, Mau UA, Sperling K, Wu BL, Horsthemke B. Intracytoplasmic sperm injection may increase the risk of imprinting defects. *Am J Hum Genet* 2002;71:162–4.

17. Orstavik KH, Eiklid K, van der Hagen CB, Spetalen S, Kierulf K, Skjeldal O, Buiting K. Another case of imprinting defect in a girl with Angelman syndrome who was conceived by intracytoplasmic semen injection. *Am J Hum Genet* 2003;72:218–19.

18. Schultz RM, Williams CJ. The science of ART. *Science* 2002;296:2188–90.

19. Ludwig M, Katalinic A, Gross S, Sutcliffe A, Varon R, Horsthemke B. Increased prevalence of imprinting defects in patients with Angelman syndrome born to subfertile couples. *J Med Genet* 2005;42:289–91.

20. DeBaun MR, Niemitz EL, Feinberg AP. Association of in vitro fertilization with Beckwith-Wiedemann syndrome and epigenetic alterations of LIT1 and H19. *Am J Hum Genet* 2003;72:156–60.

21. Maher ER, Brueton LA, Bowdin SC, Luharia A, Cooper W, Cole TR, Macdonald F, Sampson JR, Barratt CL, Reik W, Hawkins MM. Beckwith-Wiedemann syndrome and assisted reproduction technology (ART). *J Med Genet* 2003;40:62–64.

22. Gicquel C, Gaston V, Mandelbaum J, Siffroi JP, Flahault A, Le Bouc Y. In vitro fertilization may increase the risk of Beckwith-Wiedemann syndrome related to the abnormal imprinting of the KCN1OT gene. *Am J Hum Genet* 2003;72:1338–41.

23. Halliday J, Oke K, Breheny S, Algar E, J Amor D. Beckwith-Wiedemann syndrome and IVF: a case-control study. *Am J Hum Genet* 2004;75:526–8.

24. Chang AS, Moley KH, Wangler M, Feinberg AP, Debaun MR. Association between Beckwith-Wiedemann syndrome and assisted reproductive technology: a case series of 19 patients. *Fertil Steril* 2005;83:349–54.

25. Ertzeid G, Storeng R. The impact of ovarian stimulation on implantation and fetal development in mice. *Hum Reprod* 2001;16:221–5.

26. Shi W, Haaf T. Aberrant methylation patterns at the two-cell stage as an indicator of early developmental failure. *Mol Reprod Dev* 2002;63:329–34.

27. Marques CJ, Carvalho F, Sousa M, Barros A. Genomic imprinting in disruptive spermatogenesis. *Lancet* 2004;363:1700–02.

28. Gosden R, Trasler J, Lucifero D, Faddy M. Rare congenital disorders, imprinted genes, and assisted reproductive technology. *Lancet* 2003;361:1975–7.

29. Doyle P, Bunch KJ, Beral V, Draper GJ. Cancer incidence in children conceived with assisted reproduction technology. *Lancet* 1998;352:452–3.

30. Bruinsma F, Venn A, Lancaster P, Speirs A, Healy D. Incidence of cancer in children born after in-vitro fertilization. *Hum Reprod* 2000;15:604–7.

31. Klip H, Burger CW, de Kraker J, van Leeuwen FE; OMEGA-project group. Risk of cancer in the offspring of women who underwent ovarian stimulation for IVF. *Hum Reprod* 2001;16: 2451–8.

32. Lerner-Geva L, Toren A, Chetrit A, Modan B, Mandel M, Rechavi G, Dor J. The risk for cancer among children of women who underwent in vitro fertilization. *Cancer* 2000;88: 2845–7.

33. Moll AC, Imhof SM, Schouten-van Meeteren AY, van Leeuwen FE. In-vitro fertilisation and retinoblastoma. *Lancet* 2003;361: 1392.

34. Bradbury BD, Jick H. In vitro fertilization and childhood retinoblastoma. *Br J Clin Pharmacol* 2004;58:209–11.

35. Lidegaard O, Pinborg A, Andersen AN. Imprinting diseases and IVF: Danish National IVF cohort study. *Hum Reprod* 2005;20: 950–4.

68

CONGENITAL ANOMALIES AND ASSISTED REPRODUCTIVE TECHNOLOGY

Amutha Anpananthar, Alastair Sutcliffe

INTRODUCTION

Assisted reproductive technology (ART) has become the standard of care for the treatment for many types of infertility. In Denmark, 4 percent of all infants are born after in vitro fertilization (IVF) or intracytoplasmic sperm injection (ICSI). It is well established that children born after ART have poorer outcomes than spontaneously conceived children mainly due to the high rate of multiple births and the associated perinatal mortality, preterm birth, and low birth weights. The evidence relating to ART and congenital anomalies will be discussed in this chapter.

Lancaster's study from the late 1980s was the first to report a higher prevalence of neural tube defects and transposition of the great vessels among IVF children (1). Though ART is considered to be relatively safe, recent evidence has shown an increase in the order of 30–40 percent in birth defects among children conceived by ART compared to infants conceived spontaneously (2–4). This enforces the importance of counseling prospective patients effectively.

Many congenital anomalies are noted at birth and some become apparent later in life. Some malformations are incompatible with life, some can be corrected with surgery, and others are compatible with continued life but cannot be corrected with treatment (5). Some malformations are related to prematurity (e.g., patent ductus arteriosus), some to multiple births, and some to infertility itself.

Relatively little is known about the cause of most congenital anomalies. Estimates suggest that approximately 14 percent are due to single mutant genes and major chromosomal abnormalities, about 5 percent are due to environmental factors (such as infections and toxins, e.g. drugs, alcohol), and a further 20 percent are due to the combined effects of environmental and genetic factors, but the cause of the remaining 60 percent or more of malformations remains unknown (5). Other reasons that may be considered as a risk for congenital anomalies are ovarian stimulation, with the possibility of changes in follicle milieu and oocyte structure, sperm preparation with the theoretical possibility of exposure to substances that might change their natural function, the manipulation of oocytes in IVF and ICSI cycles by oocyte pick-up, and further processing and the use of sperm from subfertile men with the possibility of more genetic abnormalities or abnormal imprinting (6).

Congenital anomalies can be:

1. Mutagenic, with the fetus inheriting a gene defect or chromosomal anomaly through their affected family or through a new mutation;
2. At conception, including most noninherited chromosomal anomalies; and
3. Postconception, including teratogenic agents with nonheritable effects. The effect of any teratogen will depend on when in the pregnancy it acted, the strength of the dose, and the fetal genetic susceptibility to that teratogen.

The theoretical risks to which all children conceived with ART are exposed to are illustrated in Figure 68.1.

As with all studies, there are limitations in interpreting and comparing the results of pregnancies and children born after ART including precise definition of terms, the comparability of the cohorts, and other epidemiological problems with these cohorts. The risk of "major malformation" is difficult to estimate since the percentage of affected children will vary considerably depending on:

– whether only liveborns, spontaneous abortions, induced abortions, and stillbirths are included;
– whether the children/fetuses are examined by an obstetrician directly after delivery or by an experienced neonatologist or geneticist during the first days or weeks of life;
– whether the examination is done only by physical procedures or also includes more costly procedures including ultrasound of the kidneys, the hips, or the skull or echocardiography; and
– how major malformation is defined and whether the same criteria for all these items are used for both the study and the control cohort (6).

When analyzing major birth defects alone, an increased risk of birth defects is noted as major defects are less subjected to problems of definition and under reporting than minor defects (2). For rare problems, such as imprinting disorders, large enough prospective studies are too expensive, thus registry-based studies are more useful. Population-based registry studies of malformations have the clear advantage of large sample sizes, enabling cross-linkage research; they do not require patient contact and minimize losses to follow-up. Taking the

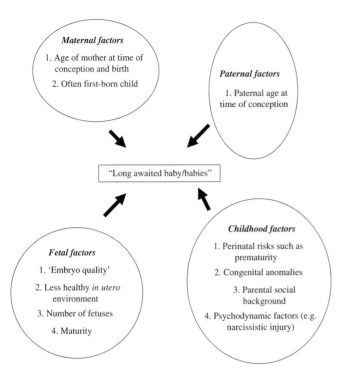

Maternal factors
1. Age of mother at time of conception and birth
2. Often first-born child

Paternal factors
1. Paternal age at time of conception

"Long awaited baby/babies"

Fetal factors
1. 'Embryo quality'
2. Less healthy *in utero* environment
3. Number of fetuses
4. Maturity

Childhood factors
1. Perinatal risks such as prematurity
2. Congenital anomalies
3. Parental social background
4. Psychodynamic factors (e.g. narcissistic injury)

Figure 68.1. Consideration of Some of the potential factors, which may have a bearing on the well-being of ART children.

above into consideration, many recent meta-analyses of ART studies have shown an increased risk of congenital anomalies compared with spontaneously conceived babies (2,7–9).

ART consists of a variety of techniques, and a few are briefly discussed below.

IVF is widely accepted as a treatment for unexplained infertility (NICE 2004, RCOG 1998) (10,11). The first child conceived after IVF was born in the United Kingdom in 1978 (12). More than two million babies have now been born after IVF worldwide (13). The usage of IVF has increased, and its efficacy has risen over time especially with the introduction of embryo cryopreservation and ICSI (14).

IVF involves harvesting oocytes from the mother to be, after treatment for ovulation induction. Recent advances advocate natural-cycle IVF to avoid exposure of the mother to known short-term complications (such as ovarian hyperstimulation syndrome) and the unknown long-term side effects of these hormones. The fresh ejaculated sperm, or in some cases freeze-thawed sperm, is then "mixed" with the oocytes after sperm preparation. If normal fertilization occurs, up to three of the resulting embryos are transferred to the uterus forty-eight hours after egg collection. The techniques involved in IVF have become more refined since its original inception.

IVF is considered to be an effective treatment as it circumvents most of the causes of unexplained infertility, including ovarian dysfunction, cervical factors, sperm and egg transport, and problems with sperm-egg interaction. However, IVF is expensive and invasive and is associated with a number of complications, including multiple pregnancies and ovarian hyperstimulation syndrome. The increase in concerns of these complications has led to the effectiveness of other treatment options for this group of patients being evaluated.

A recent Cochrane review (15) concluded that there is insufficient evidence at present to suggest that IVF is more effective than the other treatment options available for unexplained infertility. Adverse events and the costs associated with the interventions compared have not been adequately assessed. Until more evidence is available, IVF may not be the preferred first line of treatment for these couples and it might be appropriate to continue with less invasive options (15). Although IVF with fresh embryo transfer has resulted in successful treatment for a number of infertile couples, it fails to be effective in cases of primary male infertility. In addition, embryo transfer was initially performed immediately after fertilization, but if the procedure was successful and more than three embryos were created, these additional embryos would often be destroyed.

The use of other techniques, such as *embryo cryopreservation* and subsequent thawing, is important if the mother is thought to be developing ovarian hyperstimulation syndrome following embryo replacement. This condition can be fatal and is known to be exacerbated by pregnancy. Freezing the embryo will defer embryo transfer until a later cycle. Embryo cryopreservation also allows clinics to "quarantine embryos" while screening egg or sperm donors for infectious diseases. Cryopreservation of oocytes is a technique developed to preserve oocytes of patients undergoing cancer treatment or for oocyte donors. Cryopreserved oocytes require ICSI for fertilization (after defrosting) because the cryopreservation process brings about changes in the zona pellucida, preventing sperm penetration (5).

Table 68.1 summarizes some of the recent studies with regard to congenital anomaly risk and IVF. Hansen et al. (2005) reviewed twenty-five papers originating from Europe, Middle East, Australia, and United States from 1989 to 2003 (2). However, only seven of these were deemed appropriate for inclusion in the meta-analysis. Of these, the majority were population-based studies with a clear definition of a birth defect and most had a large sample size. All seven included data adjusted or matched for maternal age and parity. Others were excluded due to serious methodological limitations, and many were not designed to assess birth defect risk. The odds ratio for the seven reviewer-selected studies was 1.40 (95 percent CI 1.28–1.53), indicating a significantly increased risk of birth defects in children born following ART.

Examples of congenital anomalies with ART include anencephaly, spina bifida, cardiovascular defects, orofacial clefts, and alimentary tract atresia. Increases in risk have been found for most categories of defects (2). Anencephaly and hydrocephaly have been associated with higher rates of multiple births, and the general increased risk of congenital anomalies with ART could be to a large extent due to parental characteristics. (8) A four fold increase in the incidence of heart malformations, specifically septal defects, was found in an IVF group compared with the spontaneously conceived group by Koivurova et al. (22). Congenital heart malformations are due to multifactorial genetic and environmental causes and few arise from recognized chromosomal aberrations and mutations of single genes. It was noted that some mothers of children with ventricular septal defects (VSD) had a worse reproductive history than mothers without a child with VSD, and from this, it was concluded that reproductive ability with differing maternal hormones may be inversely related to the risk of VSD (29). An association of ovarian stimulation and the birth of infants with orofacial clefts and with neural tube defects has been described (30). The possibility of increased risks of neural tube defects with IVF has been observed (31). An increased prevalence

Table 68.1: A Summary of Recent Studies of IVF Children and the Risk of Congenital Anomalies

Author	Number of IVF children	Type	Country	Risk of congenital anomaly in IVF versus naturally conceived children ± odds ratio (OR)
Zhu et al. (3)	1,483	Population-based study	Denmark	6.6% (hazard ratio 1.20)
Bonduelle et al. (13)	540	Population-based study	Denmark	OR 1.80
Kallen et al. (8)	16,280	Population-based registry	Sweden	5% versus 4% (relative risk 1.26)
Klemetti et al. (16)	4,559	Population-based registry	Finland	OR 1.3
Merlob et al. (17)	278	Population-based registry	Israel	9.35% versus 4.05%
Olson et al. (18)	1,462	Population-based registry	Iowa	6.2% versus 4.4%
Anthony et al. (19)	4,224	Population-based registry	The Netherlands	OR 1.20
Hansen et al. (20)	837	Population-based registry	Australia	9% versus 4.2% (OR 2.0)
Isaksson et al. (21)	92	Case-control study	Finland	7.2% versus 3.5% in singletons
Koivurova et al. (22)	304	Population-based registry	Finland	6.6% versus 4.4% (OR 1.53)
Ericson and kallen (23)	9,111 (estimated)	Population-based study	Sweden	OR 0.89
Koudstaal et al. (24)	307	Clinic	The Netherlands	2.3% (OR 1.0)
Bergh et al. (25)	5,856	Population-based study	Sweden	5.4% versus 3.9%*
Bowen et al. (26)	84	Case-control study	Australia	3.6% versus 5% No significant difference#
D'Souza et al. (27)	278	Case-control study	USA	2.5% versus 0%
Sutcliffe et al. (28)	91	Clinic	UK	OR 1.4

*Difficult to interpret as terminations due to malformations not included on registry.
#Increased risk among singleton boys and decreased risk among multiple girls.

only of genital organ malformations has been associated with singletons born of infertile couples, which may be explained by the use of ovulation-inducing drugs, common to most courses of infertility treatment (3).

ICSI was first described by Palermo and colleagues in Belgium. In ICSI, a single spermatozoa is injected directly into the cytoplasm of the (harvested) egg using a fine glass needle and is thus a more invasive technique than IVF. The sperm can be ejaculated, aspirated from the epididymis (transepididymal sperm aspiration, TESA), or collected directly from the testis (the latter two techniques requiring general anesthesia). For affected men who suffer from low sperm counts, poor-quality sperm, and/or poor sperm motility, ICSI is used to overcome a variety of severe male factor infertility, including genetic causes such as Kleinefelters syndrome and carriers of cystic fibrosis.

As the oocyte membrane is mechanically pierced with ICSI, appearing to bypass all biological and genetic selection, there have been a number of reports suggesting an increased incidence of chromosomal anomalies, congenital abnormalities, and perinatal hazards in offspring conceived with this technique. There are also ICSI procedure-independent risks, and both types of risks are summarized below (32).

The risk related to the ICSI procedure itself may be due to the:

– physical and/or biochemical disturbance of the ooplasm or of the meiotic spindle,

– errors in selection of the injection site (due to variability of the location of the metaphase II spindle leading to the selection of a damaging site),
– the injection of biochemical contaminants, and
– the injection of foreign, sperm-associated exogenous DNA.

The ICSI procedure-independent risks include:

– the microinjection of sperm carrying a chromosomal anomaly (e.g., an aneuploidy or structural defect),
– the transmission of a genetic defect that is often the origin of male factor infertility,
– male gamete structural defect,
– anomalies of sperm-activating factors,
– potential for incorporating sperm mitochondrial DNA,
– female gamete anomalies (oocyte age-related).

Although most children conceived by ICSI are healthy and develop normally, there is an increased risk of mild delays in development at one year when compared with children conceived by routine IVF or conceived naturally (26). These findings support the need for ongoing developmental follow-up of children conceived by ICSI to see whether they are at increased risk of intellectual impairment or learning difficulties at school age.

Studies suggest an increase of chromosomal anomalies, mainly sex chromosomes after ICSI (33). This slight increase in de novo chromosomal aberrations and the higher frequency of transmitted chromosomal aberrations are probably linked

Table 68.2: A Summary of Recent Studies of ICSI Children and the Risk of Congenital Anomalies

Author	Number of ICSI children	Type	Country	Risk of congenital anomaly in IVF versus naturally conceived children ± odds ratio (OR)
Zhu et al. (3)	398	Population based study	Denmark	8.8% (hazard ratio 1.39)
Bonduelle et al. (13)	540	Population based study	Denmark	4.6% OR 2.7
Katalinic et al. (34)	3,372	Tertiary infertility centre	Germany	8.7 versus 6.1% OR 1.24%
Hansen et al. (20)	301	Population based study	Australia	8.6 versus 4.2% OR 2
Ludwig et al. (35)	3,372	Population based study	Germany	8.6 versus 6.9% RR 1.25
Sutcliffe et al. (36)	208	Case-control study	UK	4.8 versus 4.5% OR 1.06
Wennerholm et al. (37)	1,139	Population based study	Sweden	7.6% OR 1.75
Bowen et al. (26)	89	Case-control study	Australia	4.5 versus 5% - no significant difference
Bonduelle et al. (33)	877	Population based study	Belgium	2.6% (within normal range)*
Sutcliffe et al. (28)	56	Fertility centre	Australia	OR 0.67

*But suggestion of increased sex chromosome anomalies.

directly to the characteristics of the infertile men treated rather than to the ICSI procedure itself. Table 68.2 summarizes the risk of congenital anomalies with ICSI from recent studies.

Recent meta-analyses concluded that there were no additional risks of major birth defects in children conceived by ICSI compared with children conceived by other IVF methods (7,8,32). However, the specific malformation that appears to occur in excess in ICSI babies is hypospadias, which may be related to paternal subfertility (8,37). An increased occurrence of testicular anomalies had been described in fathers of boys with hypospadias in 1974 (38), but no conclusive results have been obtained yet. A possible explanation is the transfer from father to son of a gene that causes testicular impairment as early as fetal stages, resulting in an increased risk for hypospadias. In the father, the same gene may cause subfertility.

Clomiphene citrate has a small beneficial effect on pregnancy rates, as compared to placebo or no treatment (39), but there have not been many trials comparing the effectiveness of clomiphene citrate with IVF.

Intrauterine insemination (IUI), with or without the use of gonadotrophins, is widespread in the treatment of infertility (RCOG 1998) (11). The sperm is directly injected into the uterine cavity through a small catheter passed through the cervix, thus increasing the number of motile spermatozoa that reach the uterus and Fallopian tubes by bypassing the cervical barrier. There is a threefold increase in pregnancy rates with IUI alone, with a further increase with concomitant ovarian stimulation, in couples with unexplained infertility (40). The likelihood of pregnancy was also increased for treatment with IUI compared to timed intercourse, both in stimulated cycles. There is insufficient data on multiple pregnancies and other adverse events for treatment with ovarian hyperstimulation (41).

Gamete intrafallopian transfer (GIFT) involves controlled ovarian stimulation; oocyte retrieval and replacement with sperm into the tubal ampulla at laparoscopy has been found to be effective in the treatment of unexplained infertility (RCOG 1998) (11). There are mixed conclusions on comparing the effectiveness of GIFT versus IUI, and IVF may be preferred because of the additional diagnostic information it provides

and also because it avoids laparoscopy and possibly general anesthesia (42).

IMPRINTING DISORDERS

In addition to the well-established risks of multiple gestations, recent reports have suggested a link between ART and rare disorders of imprinting. Imprinting disorders are caused by meiotically or mitotically heritable changes in gene function, which cannot be explained by the DNA sequence. Imprinted genes are expressed in a nonrandom parent-of-origin specific manner.

The syndromes and cancers that are already known to be caused by genes that are imprinted (but not necessarily linked to ART) include Prader-Willi syndrome, Angelman syndrome, Russell-silver syndrome, and Beckwith Weidemann syndrome and the cancers are bilateral retinoblastoma, Wilm's tumor, osteosarcoma, and rhabdomyosarcoma.

There is increasing evidence that genetic factors in infertile couples as well as environmental factors (hormones and culture media) can have adverse effects on epigenetic processes controlling implantation, placentation, organ formation, and fetal growth (43). In addition, loss of epigenetic control may expose hidden genetic variation. These epimutations are more likely to occur in an abnormal environment such as in vitro (although every effort has been made to make the IVF media as physiological as possible).

As imprinting disorders are rare, patient-based studies are more feasible than large follow-up studies. For example, Beckwith-Wiedemann syndrome occurs in approximately 1 in 14,500 births (5). Imprinting disorders examined with regard to IVF/ICSI conception are Angelman syndrome and Beckwith-Wiedemann syndrome, and recent reports have suggested a higher risk of these specific disorders after ART (43,44).

It has been suggested that imprinting defects and subfertility can have a common, possibly genetic cause and that superovulation rather than ICSI may further increase the risk of conceiving a child with an imprinting defect (43,45). No association was found with other imprinting disorders such as Prader-Willi syndrome or transient neonatal diabetes mellitus (44).

TWINS VERSUS SINGLETONS

Multiple births continue to be the major risk for couples needing fertility treatment. Women receiving IVF treatment face a twentyfold increased risk of twins and a 400-fold increased risk of higher order births (triplet or more) (46). The higher frequency of multiple pregnancies goes in hand with higher perinatal risks, including higher prematurity rate and lower birth weight, which are themselves responsible for various health problems, childhood illnesses and chronic illnesses (6,47), and increased health costs.

It is clear that the babies born after ART are more likely to be born before their due date, and this is mainly as a result of there being more multiple births; but even with singleton births it is shown that these are likely to be born earlier (may be only by a few days on average). Compared with singletons conceived spontaneously, singleton ART infants have around a twofold increase in risk of perinatal mortality, low birth weight, and preterm birth, about a 50 percent increase in small for gestational age and a 30–35 percent increase in birth defects (48,49). These facts are unlikely to be due to ART itself, but more with the maternal characteristics. As an example, older maternity has higher risks of placental insufficiency, thus a risk of poorer fetal growth and subsequently a lower birth weight child.

In another study, similar poor perinatal outcome for singleton pregnancies from assisted reproduction compared with spontaneously conceived singleton pregnancies suggested this is less so for twin pregnancies (50). Helmerhost suggested perinatal mortality is about 40 percent *lower* in twin pregnancies after assisted compared with natural conception. Overall, the reviews indicate few differences between outcomes in ART twins compared with twins conceived spontaneously (49). Compared with twins born of fertile couples, twins born after infertility treatment have not shown a higher prevalence of congenital malformations (3,9). The presence of multiple births alone is not an added cause for increase in birth defects (2).

Multiple births are also a risk for the mother including increased rates of maternal hypertension, preeclampsia, spontaneous abortion, and cesarean delivery. The short- and long-term complications of prematurity itself should be discussed with prospective parents. Premature babies need to be helped to grow into mature babies in neonatal units and will face problems with warmth, feeding, infection, jaundice, neurological complications depending on gestation such as cerebral palsy, developmental delay, and, as detailed in the EPICURE study (51), the possibility of extreme premature birth and the neurological and developmental disabilities associated with it. Overall, the IVF children appear to survive the neonatal period worse than the general population group (22).

Some studies have observed an increased risk of neurological problems with ART children compared to spontaneously conceived children, especially cerebral palsy, but this can be largely explained by the higher frequency of twins born by low birth weight, intrauterine growth restriction, and low gestational age, but what cannot be excluded is the effect of IVF itself, the parents' infertility, or other factors (6). A fortyfold increased risk of cerebral palsy in a twin surviving death of the other twin in utero (mainly in the third trimester) has been observed. With the suggestion of 30 percent of all twin pregnancies ultimately resulting in singletons, this has led to discussions of whether vanishing twins could contribute to the increase risk of cerebral palsy found in singletons after IVF (6,42). However, the risk of cerebral palsy in vanishing twins due to death in first or second trimester has not been assessed.

After exclusion of patent ductus arteriosus, a population-based study in Denmark concluded there was no significant difference in malformation rates in singletons and twins conceived with ART (52); however, it is generally accepted that congenital anomalies are more common in twins than singletons, especially monozygotic twins.

A large observational study demonstrated that the elective transfer of two embryo resulted in a significant reduction of triplet rates without compromising live birth rates (53), and as a result, two embryo transfer policy is now common in most European centers. The risk of twins remains high at 24 percent even with two embryo transfer (54). *Single embryo transfer* significantly reduces the risk of multiple pregnancy but also decreases the chance of live birth in a fresh IVF cycle. Subsequent replacement of a single frozen embryo achieves a live birth rate comparable with double embryo transfer (15) and is also more cost-efficient if long-term morbidity is taken into account. It will, therefore, implicitly mean a reduction in ART-"induced" congenital abnormalities as there is known to be a doubling of overall congenital abnormality risk after twins versus singletons.

Sills et al. (2000) suggested monozygotic twinning is increased after IVF (55). Assisted hatching of the human blastocyst in its various forms has been observed to be associated with a higher rate of *monozygotic twins* (56). A rise in monozygotic (identical) twinning is more important than dizygotic twinning. Most difficulties arise in monozygotic twins during pregnancy as a result of a condition called twin-twin transfusion syndrome. In this condition, there is abnormal exchange of blood between twins so one becomes a net donor and the other becomes a net recipient. The donor twin becomes anemic, hypoxic, and growth retarded, and the recipient twin becomes edematous and can progress into heart failure. Untreated severe cases have 100 percent mortality. Almost all monozygotic twin pregnancies have some degree of this process going on. Several treatments have been introduced to try to improve pregnancy outcome including selective feticide, cord ligation, and repeated amniodrainage, with recent advances in fetoscopic laser ablation of the intercommunicating vessels. An association between monozygotic twinning and alimentary canal atresia has been suggested (57), and this could be due to a very early disturbance in embryonic development.

ART COUPLES

The rise in number of children born after ART reflects the increase in number of couples using infertility treatments. There is a need to differentiate between preconceptional causes associated with the underlying subfertility and risk factors associated with the type of fertility treatment. Much evidence suggests that infertility itself might be a risk factor, and further long-term follow-up studies involving different possible control groups will help determine whether these abnormalities are directly related to treatment.

Couples who have assisted reproduction are on average about five years older than those who conceive spontaneously (34), and more frequently have risk factors associated with a higher spontaneous abortion risk including thyroid disorders or polycystic ovarian syndrome. Advanced maternal age is associated with increased risk of pregnancy loss and liveborn aneuploidy, whereas advanced paternal age is associated with fresh Mendelian mutations (5). Paternal age is also increased. Various data have suggested that infertility, especially female infertility, is likely to be the most important factor in congenital anomalies after infertility treatment (48).

In male factor subfertility, an association between certain sperm abnormalities and numerical or structural chromosome abnormalities have been recognized. A higher rate of de novo chromosomal abnormalities have been observed in ICSI offspring, relating mainly to a higher number of sex chromosomal anomalies and partly to a higher number of autosomal structural anomalies (58). Park et al. have commented on the possible genetic causes of subfertility in a parent that are associated with congenital anomalies in a baby, and the need for future research to focus on establishing the mechanisms of these associations and then to provide risk assessment when counseling parents. Constitutional chromosomal rearrangements, including reciprocal and Robertsonian translocations, and inversions are all well-known causes of reduced fertility, miscarriages, and a whole spectrum of birth defects in offspring that inherit a chromosomal imbalance (48).

To address whether infertility itself is a cause for increased risk of congenital anomalies, an appropriate comparison group for infants born following ART treatment would include children born to infertile couples who do conceive spontaneously without IVF treatment (59). Practically, this comparison group would be difficult to identify, but an alternative group would be couples seeking ART treatment following failed vasectomy reversal or tubal ligation reversal since these couples are not infertile due to underlying disease process (2).

A Swedish study from 1991 analyzed a cohort of 384,589 children from Sweden 1983–1986. The result showed 7.8 percent with subfertility, defined by a time to conception of more than twelve months. No IVF/ICSI treatment was included, but 24 percent had used chlomiphene citrate. The risk of major malformations was higher, depending on time to pregnancy, with OR 1.18 after five years or more to pregnancy as compared to less time (60).

A 2006 Danish longitudinal study found that singletons born of infertile couples who conceived naturally or after treatment had a higher prevalence of congenital malformations compared with singletons born of fertile couples (hazard ratios 1.20 and 1.39, respectively) (3). The infertile couples who conceived naturally with no treatment were defined as all couples with a time to pregnancy of more than twelve months and no infertility treatment. It was also noted that the prevalence of congenital malformations increased with increasing time to pregnancy. The authors show that when the women who took more than twelve months to conceive naturally are compared with women who did receive infertility treatment, many of the apparent associations between assisted reproductive technologies and congenital abnormalities are lost (3,48).

Advances in ART occur continuously. *Preimplantation genetic diagnosis* (PGD) involves removing one or two cells from an embryo conceived with IVF and ICSI at the eight- to ten-cell stage of early human development. A typical family who may benefit from PGD would be one to experience the tragedy of loss of a previous child who had a lethal genetic disease. This allows the couple, when they conceive again, to be able to be screened for that particular disease. PGD involves the embryo, which has already undergone IVF/ICSI fertilization, being exposed to additional unknown risks, including chemicals, physical effects, removal of one or two blastomeres (used

for specific gene probing or fluorescent in situ hybridization (FISH) screening for chromosomal aneuploidy), and direct embryo damage from culture media secondary to zona drilling (5).

Its use is rapidly increasing in the early diagnostic testing of rare genetic diseases in high-risk populations (e.g., older mothers) and at-risk groups of families. PGD is ever evolving with FISH for sexing, aneuploidy screening, and structural chromosomal abnormalities and fluorescent and multiplex PCR as the most recent developments for monogenic diseases (61). Apart from this report, nothing is known about children post-PGD beyond birth. It would be ironic if a technique developed to enable couples to have healthy children itself harmed these children.

SUMMARY

Although many reviews and meta-analyses have suggested that infants born following ART treatment are at increased risk of birth defects, compared to spontaneously conceived infants, few studies have accounted for confounding factors such as maternal exposure to toxins and socioeconomic status (2). However, it has been suggested that women undertaking ART treatment are likely to have lower exposure to toxins such as alcohol and cigarettes and to be of higher socioeconomic status, than the general population of pregnant women (5).

When counseling patients, clinicians should mention a 30–40 percent increased risk of birth defects compared to the baseline birth defect prevalence for their population (2). An increased risk of congenital malformations provides another reason for recommending that any pregnancy in subfertile couples, whether achieved naturally or through infertility treatment, is carefully monitored by a fetal medicine specialist, with detailed antenatal imaging. Children born with ART are healthy and develop similar to children born after spontaneous conception. Regarding general health, growth, and mental and psychomotor development, IVF children do not differ from spontaneously conceived children, but lower birth weight and prematurity may contribute to some health problems (6).

Developments in ART continue apace. Careful thought needs to go into this area of protocol development as can be seen by the above discussion that highlights a variety of ways in which risks arise.

KEY POINTS FOR CLINICAL PRACTICE

- Children conceived by ART are more likely to have congenital anomalies compared to children conceived spontaneously.
- There are no additional risks of major birth defects in children conceived by ICSI compared with children conceived by other IVF methods (though hypospadias occurs in excess with ICSI).
- ART is probably associated with a higher risk of imprinting disorders, especially Angelman syndrome and Beckwith-Wiedemann syndrome.
- Twins born after infertility treatment have not shown a higher prevalence of congenital malformations than twins born of fertile couples.
- An increase in monozygotic twinning results in many associated problems.
- Infertility itself is likely to be an important factor in congenital anomalies after ART.

REFERENCES

1. Lancaster PA. Obstetric outcome. *Clin Obstet Gynaecol* 1985; 12(4):847–64.

2. Hansen M, Bower C, Milne E, de KN, Kurinczuk JJ. Assisted reproductive technologies and the risk of birth defects – a systematic review. *Hum Reprod* 2005; 20(2):328–38.

3. Zhu JL, Basso O, Obel C, Bille C, Olsen J. Infertility, infertility treatment, and congenital malformations: Danish national birth cohort. *BMJ* 2006; 333(7570):679.

4. Kurinczuk JJ, Hansen M, Bower C. The risk of birth defects in children born after assisted reproductive technologies. *Curr Opin Obstet Gynecol* 2004; 16(3):201–9.

5. Sutcliffe AG. *Health and welfare of ART children*. London: Taylor & Francis; 2006.

6. Ludwig AK, Sutcliffe AG, Diedrich K, Ludwig M. Post-neonatal health and development of children born after assisted reproduction: a systematic review of controlled studies. *Eur J Obstet Gynecol Reprod Biol* 2006; 127(1):3–25.

7. Lie RT, Lyngstadas A, Orstavik KH, Bakketeig LS, Jacobsen G. Birth defects in children conceived by ICSI with children conceived by other IVF-methods; a meta-analysis. *Int J Epidemiol* 2005; 34:696–701.

8. Kallen B, Finnstrom O, Nygren KG, Olausson PO. In vitro fertilization (IVF) in Sweden: infant outcome after different IVF fertilization methods. *Fertil Steril* 2005; 84(3):611–17.

9. Rimm AA, Katayama AC, Diaz M, Katayama KP. A meta-analysis of controlled studies comparing major malformation rates in IVF and ICSI infants with naturally conceived children. *J Assist Reprod Genet* 2004; 21(12):437–43.

10. NICE. National Collaborating Centre for Women's and Children's Health. *Fertility: Assessment and treatment for people with fertility problems. Clinical Guideline*. London: RCOG Press; 2004.

11. RCOG. RCOG Infertility Guideline Group. *The management of infertility in secondary care*. London: RCOG; 1998.

12. Steptoe PC, Edwards RG. Birth after the reimplantation of a human embryo [Letter]. *Lancet* 1978; 2(8085):366.

13. Bonduelle M, Wennerholm UB, Loft A et al. A multi-centre cohort study of the physical health of 5-year-old children conceived after intracytoplasmic sperm injection, in vitro fertilization and natural conception. *Hum Reprod* 2005; 20(2):413–19.

14. Palermo G, Joris H, Devroey P, Van Steirteghem AC. Pregnancies after intracytoplasmic injection of single spermatozoon into an oocyte. *Lancet* 1992; 340:17–18.

15. Pandian Z, Templeton A, Serour G, Bhattacharya S. Number of embryos for transfer after IVF and ICSI: a Cochrane review. *Hum Reprod* 2005; 20(10):2681–7.

16. Klemetti R, Gissler M, Sevon T, Koivurova S, Ritvanen A, Hemminki E. Children born after assisted fertilization have an increased rate of major congenital anomalies. *Fertil Steril* 2005; 84(5):1300–7.

17. Merlob P, Sapir O, Sulkes J, Fisch B. The prevalence of major congenital malformations during two periods of time, 1986-1994 and 1995-2002 in newborns conceived by assisted reproduction technology. *Eur J Med Genet* 2005; 48(1):5–11.

18. Olson CK, Keppler-Noreuil KM, Romitti PA et al. In vitro fertilization is associated with an increase in major birth defects. *Fertil Steril* 2005; 84(5):1308–15.

19. Anthony S, Buitendijk SE, Dorrepaal CA, Lindner K, Braat DD, den Ouden AL. Congenital malformations in 4224 children conceived after IVF. *Hum Reprod* 2002; 17(8):2089–95.

20. Hansen M, Kurinczuk JJ, Bower C, Webb S. The risk of major birth defects after intracytoplasmic sperm injection and in vitro fertilization. *N Engl J Med* 2002; 346(10):725–30.

21. Isaksson R, Gissler M, Tiitinen A. Obstetric outcome among women with unexplained infertility after IVF: a matched case-control study. *Hum Reprod* 2002; 17(7):1755–61.

22. Koivurova S, Hartikainen AL, Gissler M, Hemminki E, Sovio U, Jarvelin MR. Neonatal outcome and congenital malformations in children born after in-vitro fertilization. *Hum Reprod* 2002; 17(5):1391–8.

23. Ericson A, Kallen B. Congenital malformations in infants born after IVF: a population-based study. *Hum Reprod* 2001; 16(3):504–9.

24. Koudstaal J, Braat DD, Bruinse HW, Naaktgeboren N, Vermeiden JP, Visser GH. Obstetric outcome of singleton pregnancies after IVF: a matched control study in four Dutch university hospitals. *Hum Reprod* 2000; 15(8):1819–1825.

25. Bergh T, Ericson A, Hillensjo T, Nygren KG, Wennerholm UB. Deliveries and children born after in-vitro fertilisation in Sweden 1982-95: a retrospective cohort study. *Lancet* 1999; 354(9190): 1579–85.

26. Bowen JR, Gibson FL, Leslie GI, Saunders DM. Medical and developmental outcome at 1 year for children conceived by intracytoplasmic sperm injection. *Lancet* 1998; 351(9115):1529–34.

27. D'Souza SW, Rivlin E, Cadman J, Richards B, Buck P, Lieberman BA. Children conceived by in vitro fertilisation after fresh embryo transfer. *Arch Dis Child Fetal Neonatal Ed* 1997; 76(2): F70–4.

28. Sutcliffe AG, D'Souza SW, Cadman J, Richards B, McKinlay IA, Lieberman B. Minor congenital anomalies, major congenital malformations and development in children conceived from cryopreserved embryos. *Hum Reprod* 1995; 10(12):3332–7.

29. Sands AJ, Casey FA, Craig BG, Dornan JC, Rogers J, Mulholland HC. Incidence and risk factors for ventricular septal defect in "low risk" neonates. *Arch Dis Child Fetal Neonatal*Ed 1999; 81(1):F61–3.

30. Greenland S, Ackerman DL. Clomiphene citrate and neural tube defects: a pooled analysis of controlled epidemiologic studies and recommendations for future studies. *Fertil Steril* 1995; 64(5):936–41.

31. Lancaster PAL, Hurst T, Shafir E. Congenital malformations and other pregnancy outcome after microinsemination. *Reprod Toxicol* 2000; 14:74.

32. Bonduelle M, Liebaers I, Deketelaere V et al. Neonatal data on a cohort of 2889 infants born after ICSI (1991-1999) and of 2995 infants born after IVF (1983-1999). *Hum Reprod* 2002; 17(3): 671–94.

33. Bonduelle M, Wilikens A, Buysse A et al. Prospective follow-up study of 877 children born after intracytoplasmic sperm injection (ICSI), with ejaculated epididymal and testicular spermatozoa and after replacement of cryopreserved embryos obtained after ICSI. *Hum Reprod* 1996; 11 (Suppl. 4):131–55.

34. Katalinic A, Rösch C, Ludwig M. Pregnancy course and outcome after intracytoplasmic sperm injection (ICSI) – a controlled, prospective cohort study. *Fertil Steril* 2004; 81:1604–16.

35. Ludwig M, Katalinic A. Malformation rate in fetuses and children conceived after ICSI: results of a prospective cohort study. *Reprod Biomed Online* 2002; 5(2):171–8.

36. Sutcliffe AG, Taylor B, Saunders K, Thornton S, Lieberman BA, Grudzinskas JG. Outcome in the second year of life after in-vitro fertilisation by intracytoplasmic sperm injection: a UK case-control study. *Lancet* 2001; 357(9274):2080–4.

37. Wennerholm UB, Bergh C, Hamberger L et al. Incidence of congenital malformations in children born after ICSI. *Hum Reprod* 2000; 15(4):944–8.

38. Sweet RA, Schrott HG, Kurland R, Culp OS. Study of the incidence of hypospadias in Rochester, Minnesota, 1940-1970, and

a case-control comparison of possible etiologic factors. *Mayo Clin Proc* 1974; 49(1):52–8.

39. Hughes E, Collins J, Vandekerckhove P. Clomiphene citrate for unexplained subfertility in women. *Cochrane Database Syst Rev* 2000;(2):CD000057.

40. Hughes EG. The effectiveness of ovulation induction and intra-uterine insemination in the treatment of persistent infertility: a meta-analysis. *Hum Reprod* 1997; 12(9):1865–72.

41. Verhulst SM, Cohlen BJ, Hughes E, Te VE, Heineman MJ. Intra-uterine insemination for unexplained subfertility. *Cochrane Database Syst Rev* 2006;(4):CD001838.

42. Pandian Z, Bhattacharya S, Vale L, Templeton A. In vitro fertil-isation for unexplained subfertility. *Cochrane Database Syst Rev* 2005;(2):CD003357.

43. Horsthemke B, Ludwig M. Assisted reproduction: the epigenetic perspective. *Hum Reprod Update* 2005; 11(5):473–82.

44. Sutcliffe AG, Peters CJ, Bowdin S et al. Assisted reproductive therapies and imprinting disorders – a preliminary British sur-vey. *Hum Reprod* 2006; 21(4):1009–11.

45. Chang AS, Moley KH, Wangler M, Feinberg AP, Debaun MR. Association between Beckwith-Wiedemann syndrome and assis-ted reproductive technology: a case series of 19 patients. *Fertil Steril* 2005; 83(2):349–54.

46. Martin BM, Welch HG. Probabilities for singleton and multiple pregnancies after in vitro fertilization. *Fertil Steril* 1998; 70(3):478–81.

47. Ludwig AK, Sutcliffe AG, Diedrich K, Ludwig M. Post-neonatal health and development of children born after assisted repro-duction: a systematic review of controlled studies. *Eur J Obstet Gynecol Reprod Biol* 2006; 127(1):3–25.

48. Park SM, Mathur R, Smith GC. Congenital anomalies after treat-ment for infertility. *BMJ* 2006; 333(7570):665–66.

49. Bower C, Hansen M. Assisted reproductive technologies and birth outcomes: overview of recent systematic reviews. *Reprod Fertil Dev* 2005; 17(3):329–33.

50. Helmerhorst FM, Perquin DA, Donker D, Keirse MJ. Perinatal outcome of singletons and twins after assisted conception: a systematic review of controlled studies. *BMJ* 2004; 328(7434): 261.

51. Wood NS, Costeloe K, Gibson AT, Hennessy EM, Marlow N, Wilkinson AR. The EPICure study: associations and antecedents of neurological and developmental disability at 30 months of age following extremely preterm birth. *Arch Dis Child Fetal Neonatal Ed* 2005; 90(2):F134–40.

52. Pinborg A, Loft A, Nyboe AA. Neonatal outcome in a Danish national cohort of 8602 children born after in vitro fertilization or intracytoplasmic sperm injection: the role of twin pregnancy. *Acta Obstet Gynecol Scand* 2004; 83(11):1071–8.

53. Templeton A, Morris JK. Reducing the risk of multiple births by transfer of two embryos after in vitro fertilization. *N Engl J Med* 1998; 339(9):573–7.

54. Nyboe AA, Gianaroli L, Felderbaum R, de Mouzon J, Nygre KG. Assisted reproductive technology in Europe, 2001: results gen-erated from European registers by ESHRE. *Hum Reprod* 2005; 20:1158–76.

55. Sills ES, Moomjy M, Zaninovic N et al. Human zona pellucida micromanipulation and monozygotic twinning frequency after IVF. *Hum Reprod* 2000; 15(4):890–5.

56. Cohen J. Assisted hatching of human embryos. *J In Vitro Fert Embryo Transf* 1991; 8(4):179–90.

57. Harris J, Kallen B, Robert E. Descriptive epidemiology of ali-mentary tract atresia. *Teratology* 1995; 52(1):15–29.

58. Jacobs PA, Browne C, Gregson N, Joyce C, White H. Estimates of the frequency of chromosome abnormalities detectable in un-selected newborns using moderate levels of banding. *J Med Genet* 1992; 29(2):103–8.

59. Kovalevsky G, Rinuado P, Coutifaris C. Do assisted reproductive technologies cause adverse fetal outcomes? *Fertil Steril* 2003; 79(6):1270–2.

60. Ghazi HA, Spielberger C, Kallen B. Delivery outcome after infertility—a registry study. *Fertil Steril* 1991; 55(4):726–32.

61. Harper JC, Boelaert K, Geraedts J et al. ESHRE PGD Consortium data collection V: cycles from January to December 2002 with preg-nancy follow-up to October 2003. *Hum Reprod* 2006; 21(1):3–21.

PART IV

ETHICAL DILEMMAS IN FERTILITY AND ASSISTED REPRODUCTION

69

Stem Cell Research

M. E. Poo, Carlos Simón

ABSTRACT

Nowadays, stem cell represents one of the most promising research areas in regenerative medicine. They are defined by two basic properties: the ability to proliferate by a process of self-renewal and the potential to differentiate into specialized cell types. According to their origin, they can be classified as embryonic or adult stem cells.

Human embryonic stem cells (hESCs) are pluripotent cell lines derived from the inner cell mass (ICM) of human blastocyst. The differentiation potential of these cells to the three embryonic germ layers make them an attractive research tool for the study of early human developmental process as well as a potential therapeutic tool for various human diseases. hESCs are also invaluable research tools to study embryonic development and can serve as a platform to develop and test new therapies.

INTRODUCTION

The discovery and characterization of hESCs have revolutionized the scientific community due to the potential therapeutic use of these pluripotent cells. At the same time, research with hESCs is an extremely controversial and politicized issue in our society.

Reports on embryonic stem cells were first introduced by Cole et al. in the early sixties using rabbit blastocysts (1,2). Mouse embryonic stem cells (mESC) were isolated from ICM of murine preimplantation embryos (3,4). mESC are capable of proliferating indefinitely in an undifferentiated state and are pluripotent, making them a perfect vehicle for genetic manipulations in mice.

Since 1998, when the first report on the derivation of hESCs was published (5), it has become increasingly clear that the development of regenerative therapies using these cells is one of the major scientific challenges of this century. These cells possess unlimited self-renewal capacity and development potential to differentiate into virtually any cell type of the organism. They could also provide a unique model to study early human development, congenital anomalies, or other promising fields like tissue engineering or in vitro models for gene therapies in genetic diseases.

Many researchers are currently studying existing hESC lines. However, due to legal, ethical, and technical reasons, only a few of groups are active in the derivation of new hESC lines. Guhr et al. reported the number of currently existing hESC lines based on the consultation of verifiable public sources.

They estimated that 414 hESC lines are available and have been established in at least twenty countries. This study reveals that although this number appears be quite impressive, the data published on their characterization are quite limited. Only 49.2 percent of all cell lines have been published in peer-reviewed journals (6).

Given that both research and therapeutic applications involving hESC will require a considerable amount of stem cell lines, the pace of derivation needs to increase dramatically. It has been estimated that the number of hESC would be needed in the future to cover the major population requirements. Taylor et al. estimated that 150 donor cell lines are needed for HLA matching in UK population, considering them as homozygous lines for common HLA types (7). However, another study reveals that no homozygous line for all HLA loci has been derived in United States, suggesting that the lower estimates for the number of cell lines required is not supported by existing lines (8).

In this chapter, we present an overview of the progress that has been made in the methods used toward hESC derivation, maintenance, and differentiation, preparing the field for future clinical applications.

DERIVATION OF hESC

The human embryo at the blastocyst stage is composed by two defined tissue types named as 1) ICM, which will give rise to the embryo and its extraembryonic structures, and 2) the trophoectoderm, from where the different structures of the placenta originate (9). In vivo, cells of the ICM display the ability to proliferate and undergo self-replacement for a transient period, before progressively becoming restricted to more specific and committed cell progenitors. It is during this time that pluripotent ESC lines can be derived. The methodology for deriving ESC remains similar since their original description in 1981 (3,10). The immunosurgical isolation of ICM (11) has become a common practice in most of the laboratories working with hESC derivation. The expanded blastocyst is first treated with pronase to dissolve the zona pellucida (ZP). The ZP-free blastocyst is then treated with anti-human whole serum antibody and guinea pig complement. The blastocyst, with its lysed trophectoderm, is rinsed in fresh culture medium, and the ICM isolated and cultured on a layer of mitotically inactivated feeder cells in a gelatin-coated tissue culture dish. The first reported derivations of hESCs were performed using immunosurgery (5,12), and this methodology has been used for the majority of other reports (13,14).

Successful derivation of hESC lines using direct mechanical isolation has also been reported (15). The ICM is mechanically isolated from the surrounding trophoblast and then transferred to a feeder layer. Following a brief period of expansion, cells from the resulting outgrowth are dissociated and replated onto fresh feeder layers. More recently, the use of the whole blastocyst on an inactivated feeder layer was shown to be an alternative method for the isolation of human ICM (16). Using this method, the trophoectodem is immersed within the feeder layer and ceases to proliferate, while the ICM clump flourishes continuously (Figure 69.1).

The main sources of embryos for hESC derivation are those obtained from assisted reproductive techniques at the in vitro fertilization (IVF) clinics. Patients, following the successful completion of an IVF cycle, donate their surplus embryos. The general legislative framework in the majority of European countries and United States allows for these embryos to be donated for research, to another couple (embryo adoption), cryopreserved, or discarded.

Supernumerary frozen embryos have been successfully used for the generation of hESC lines (5). The pitfall of this source is that few of the cryopreserved embryos are available for research (17–19). Furthermore, the quality of most of them tends to be poor because higher quality embryos are used in fresh IVF cycles and the cryopreservation process itself damages the embryos significantly, reducing their potential for further development (18). In addition, the law in many countries allows hESC to be derived only from embryos that have been frozen for at least five years. This legal requirement imposes a limitation on the derivation process since, five years ago, the technology available for freezing embryos was not as advanced or as efficient as it is now, and therefore, the quality of embryos from that time is comparatively poor (20). Derivation efficacy is between 10 and 20 percent and seems higher in fresh versus frozen embryos, although there are examples of the opposite results (21).

Few reports provide information on the quality or grade of the embryos used to derive hESC (22,23). Some authors suggest that higher quality embryos result in a greater efficiency (20,24). However, it is possible to generate stable hESC lines from embryos deemed to have little or no potential of culminating in the birth of a live baby (22). At the moment, it is unclear whether the long-term genetic stability of lines obtained from poorer quality embryos differs from those derived from high-quality blastocysts. hESC lines have been derived from day 3 human embryos that have been discarded due to low morphological scores (25), from morula-stage embryos (26), and even from later stage blastocysts (seven to eight days) (27). Thus, existing hESC lines have been derived from embryos at different stages, morphological characteristics, and methods.

The debate over stem cell research is mainly based on the fact that hESC derivation deprives embryos of any further potential to develop into a human being. A novel method for generating mESC and hESC maintaining embryo viability represent an attempt to avoid this burden. The report, by Robert Lanza's group from the biotech company advanced cell technology, shows that single blastomeres can be extracted from mouse and human eight-cell embryos, aggregated with preexisting ESC lines, and then developed into independent ESC lines (28). They demonstrate in the murine model that the biopsied embryo is capable to implant and develop until birth. Similar embryo biopsy technique is already routinely carried out for preimplantation genetic diagnosis of human embryos (29). Recently, the same group reported successful derivation of two hESC lines from human embryo blastomere (30). In this important study, blastomeres from each embryo were separated and therefore did not allow the normal development of biopsied embryo; however, they prove the concept that hESC lines can be derived from human blastomeres. Further studies must be done in order to improve the efficiency of the procedure described avoiding the embryo destruction.

The derivation of hESC by nuclear transfer holds great promise for research and therapy but technically is not feasible yet. Altered nuclear transfer (ANT) has been proposed as a variation of the nuclear transfer technique to produce embryos that are inherently unable to implant into the uterus but would be capable of generating customized ESCs (31). ANT proposes to modify genetically the somatic cell nucleus in such a way that the product of the nuclear transfer is an embryo incapable to implant but still capable of producing pluripotent stem cells.

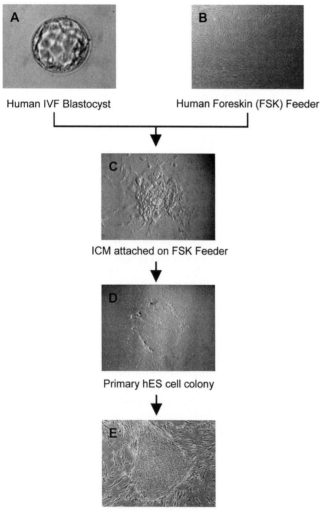

Figure 69.1. Derivation of hESC. Day 6 blastocyst (A) is treated with tyrode acid in order to remove the ZP. The ZP-free blastocyst is plated on a layer mitotically inactivated feeder cells (B), and in a few days, the trophectoderm ceases to proliferate while the ICM clump flourishes continuously (C), thereby generating hESC line. Sixteen-day-old primary hESC colony grown on human foreskin feeder (D). Undifferentiated hESC colony (E). Original magnifications: A: 200×; B, C, D, E: 100×.

To assess the experimental validity of this concept, Jaenisch's group used nuclear transfer to derive mouse blastocysts from donor fibroblasts that carried a short hairpin RNA construct targeting Cdx2, a gene critical for formation of the trophectoderm (32). The authors demonstrated that ANT products generated with Cdx2 knockdown somatic nuclei were morphologically abnormal and fail to implant into the uterus. Importantly, they also generate ESCs from the ANT product. After establishment of the ESC line, the anti-Cdx2 shoRNA can be removed by Cre recombinase, resulting in "normal" ESCs capable of pluripotent differentiation in multiple assays.

Despite these technical attempts, neither proposal has been fully embraced by those opposed to the use of human embryos for the generation of stem cells. The Lanza method still involves in vitro manipulation of human embryos, considered morally wrong by some. Jaenisch's work has been controversial too. Thus, it appears that the two reports have not yet solved, to everyone's satisfaction, the question of whether ESC can be made without destroying embryos.

MAINTENANCE OF hESC

hESCs are immortal cells, capable of self-renewal in culture while maintaining undifferentiated phenotype and normal karyotype. It is crucial to establish optimal growth conditions for hESCs considering the future therapeutic applications. The techniques used have evolved from the methods used for culture of mESC.

Initially, hESCs were cultured on a feeder layer of mouse embryonic fibroblasts (MEF), after these feeder cells have been irradiated or treated with mitomycin to prevent them from dividing (5). Feeder cells provide an ideal environment for the growth and maintenance of hESC because the feeder cells produce extracellular matrix, detoxify culture medium, and secrete many unique proteins that facilitate cell growth and undifferentiation (33). The initial cultured medium employed consisted of Dulbecco's modified Eagle's medium supplemented with 20 percent fetal bovine serum, 1 mM glutamine, 0.1 mM β-mercaptoethanol, and 1 percent nonessential amino acids. This culture medium composition has been adopted as the basic hESCs culture formula, and it is the most widely used. However, although these culture conditions are sufficient to maintain the hESCs in an undifferentiated state at some degree, spontaneous differentiation has also been observed during their routine culture (5,12).

hESC differs from mESC in the growth factors required to maintain their undifferentiated state. The cytokine leukemia inhibitory factor (LIF) can be used to maintain the undifferentiated state of mESCs (34,35). However, human LIF has not been found to prevent hESC from differentiating (5,12).

To develop optimal culture conditions, it is important to identify the growth factors that are required to maintain the undifferentiated cell state. It can be attained when cultured on human fibronectin in the presence of basic fibroblast growth factor and tumor growth factor β1 (TGFβ1) (36). It has recently been suggested that TGFβ1 signaling may be a prerequisite for the maintenance of hESCs in their undifferentiated state (37). The inhibition of bone morphogenetic protein signaling, as well as bFGF treatment, may also be important for the self-renewal activity of hESCs (38).

The majority of hESC have been isolated and maintained using fetal calf serum (xenoproteins) and MEFs as feeder layers

(xenosupports) or as a source of conditioned medium for cell propagation in an undifferentiated state (39). Recently, researchers have identified a potential drawback of using mouse feeder cells or mouse fibroblast–conditioned media. A foreign sugar molecule was detected on the surface of hESC grown with mouse feeders. hESC can incorporate the non-human sialic acid Neu5Gc from the mouse feeder layer and/or the medium, leading to an immune response to Neu5Gc mediated by natural antibodies that are present in most humans (40). There are also other potential implications for the incorporation of Neu5Gc with regard to general hESC biology. Many of the characteristic markers of hESC (SSEA-3, SSEA-4, TRA-1-60, and TRA-1-81) are glycolipids or glycoproteins, many of which can carry sialic acids (5). As sialic acids are involved in self-recognition events, the presence of Neu5Gc instead of Neu5Ac (the primary sialic acid in humans) could lead to unexpected impairment of cell function and tissue development (41).

The vast majority of the currently derived hESC lines have flaws in the context of their future therapeutic applications, due primarily to their reliance on serum, feeder cells, and chemicals from animal sources. Therefore, research is focused on the replacement of materials originated from non-human sources due to the possibility of zoonosis. Progress has been made toward the use of human components in hESC derivation and culture. Completely animal-free culture systems have been established with the use of human-originated feeders and medium compounds. So far, it has been possible to maintain hESCs in an undifferentiated state using fetal and adult muscle and skin, fallopian tube epithelium, glandular endometrium, stromal endometrium, marrow estromal, and foreskin cells (42,43). Richards et al. successfully grew and maintained undifferentiated hESC, which had initially been derived on MEFs, using feeder layers obtained from human fetal muscle and skin and human adult fallopian tube epithelial feeder layers. In fact, this group was responsible for the first derivation of hESC using human fetal muscle feeder layer and human serum (42). However, growth of the hESC lines on fetal muscle, fetal skin, and adult fallopian tube was slower than that on MEF cells. Also, the limited availability of fetal cells from human abortuses and the ethical concerns surrounding their use constituted a handicap. The same authors were able to grow hESC using feeder layers composed of fibroblasts from adult tissues (44).

An alternative xenobiotic-free feeder system for the growth of hESCs involves their growth on human foreskin cells obtained from newborn males following circumcision (46). A major advantage of using foreskin cell lines as feeder cells is their ability to be propagated for more than forty-two passages before undergoing senescence, while maintaining the ability to be frozen and subsequently thawed at any passage without losing the ability to support ESC growth in an undifferentiated state. Hovatta et al. derived hESC lines using commercially available human foreskin fibroblasts, but in the presence of fetal calf serum (13). More recently, the same group has successfully obtained hESC using the same human feeders but in the presence of serum replacement, thereby avoiding the use of animal serum (46). Serum replacement is now used by most groups that culture hESCs, but these serum replacement media also contain animal proteins, when ideally they should contain only human proteins. Interestingly, studies undertaken by Koivisto et al. have shown that the proliferation of hESC is higher in the presence of serum replacement than in human serum or fetal calf serum (47). Recently, our group reported the successful derivation, identification, and characterization of three new lines (VAL-3, VAL-4, and VAL-5) at the Valencia Stem Cell Bank using long-term cryopreserved embryos over irradiated, microbiologically tested, commercially available, human foreskin fibroblast, using techniques and products designed to minimize contact with xenocomponents (48).

Since in vivo undifferentiated hESCs are surrounded by the trophoectoderm during development, the use of human placental fibroblast lines as a feeder layer in the hESC derivation process is an approximation to the in vivo stem cell environment (20,49). In this context, two reports have shown that early-gestation placental fibroblasts can be used as feeders to propagate established hESC lines and derive new ones such as UCSF1-2 (49) and VAL-1-2 (20). In these reports, the derivation process was also designed to minimize contact with animal cells/products/proteins. The ZP was removed using acid Tyrode's solution rather than pronase, and without performing immunosurgery, thereby eliminating exposure to animal antibodies and complement factors. The derivation and culture processes took place in serum replacement rather than calf serum. As the placental fibroblasts were screened for animal and human pathogens, and no serum was used during the derivation process, the risk of zoonosis was greatly reduced, and thus a therapeutic grade line was approached. However, it is important to note that animal components were used in the establishment and propagation of the human placental fibroblast feeders, making necessary further experiments to derive both feeders and hESCs in the absence of serum and animal proteins (20,50). Besides, experience with organ and tissue allotransplantation has shown that human immunodeficiency virus HIV-1, HIV-2, Creutzfeld-Jakob disease, hepatitis B or C viruses, and other infectious agents can be transmitted from human donor cells to the recipient (50). In Table 69.1, representative hESCs are listed, specifying the different fibroblast feeder and serum sources employed to derivate and to maintain them.

Nevertheless, the use of feeder cells limits their medical application, as allogeneic feeders carry the risk of interspecies virus transfer (13,42,51). For this reason, the approach of using fibroblast-like cells differentiated from hESC as feeder cells has been put forward (52,53). However, it has to be considered that differentiation to fibroblasts may not be definitive and dedifferentiation might occur again, leading to a mix of colonies from different cell lines.

A feeder-free culture system in chemically defined medium would allow simplifying the conditions required. In addition, it is necessary for the genetic manipulation of hESC in gene therapy studies (54,55). Many groups have attempted to develop feeder-free systems using different sources. Most of them use extracellular matrix (ECM) extracted from murine or human sources supplemented with conditioned medium from feeders and/or additional growth factors. The ECM provides structural support in a multicellular layer, as well as important regulatory signals governing cell growth, metabolism, and differentiation (56).

Xu et al. (39) were the first to establish a feeder-free protocol, which constitutes the basis for many study groups (39,57–60). They have demonstrated that the bone morphogenetic protein antagonist noggin is critical in preventing differentiation of hESC in culture. In fact, the combination of noggin

and bFGF appears to maintain the prolonged growth while retaining all hESC features. However, the use of low levels of bFGF has been found to activate ectodermal and mesodermal markers in certain hESC (61).

In this context, three promising reports have been recently published. In the first, Klimanskaya et al. obtained an hESC line in the absence of cellular support or culture medium containing animal derivatives. They eliminate the risk of transmitting animal pathogens to hESC in order to validate the use of these cells in therapy. The use of an extracellular matrix minimizes the possibility of pathogen transmission; however, in this case, the matrix was prepared from MEFs and so the problem of xenocomponent immunogenicity remains (62). In the second report, Stojkovic's group demonstrates that hESCs can be grown and maintained, keeping their characteristic properties, on human serum as matrix and conditioned media from spontaneously differentiated fibroblast-like cells from hESC. However, conditioned media include, among their limitations, the presence of several undefined components necessary to control for proper hESC propagation (63). In the third, researchers have worked in the development of feeder-independent hESC culture that includes protein components solely derived from recombinant sources or purified from human material; the medium optimization included modifications to the physicochemical environment, growth factor supplements, and matrix components, and the resulting medium (TeSR1) was capable to support long-term proliferation of hESC on a combination of collagen IV, fibronectin, laminin, and vitronectin as a human matrix (64).

According to new EU directives (2003/94/EC and 2004/24/EC), hESCs for transplantation must be cultured using conditions of good manufacturing practice (GMP) in order to guarantee the safety and quality of the cells (22,44). Incorporating GMPs implies impeccable record keeping, qualified personnel, high sanitary standards, equipment verification, validation of processes, and complaint management. The task is demanding but understandable as the safety of cell transplantation recipients must be a priority. Culture with GMP is now an important challenge for those wishing to derive clinical-grade human embryonic stem cell lines.

DIFFERENTIATION OF hESC

The development of systems that permit to direct the differentiation of ESCs into specific lineages in vitro is required for the provision of cell types applicable to drug development, cell replacement therapeutics, and gene delivery systems. Several systems have been devised, but the production of embryoid bodies (Ebs) is the most powerful model system (Figure 69.2). In this method, ESCs are removed from the feeder layer and cultivated into 3D aggregates in suspension, termed Ebs. This aggregation step is required for the differentiation of most cell lineages (except neurogenesis), and it is believed that the cell interactions within the 3D structure are important for the differentiation process. Human Eb formation can be acquired by culturing hESC aggregates in suspension (i.e., using a nonadherent dish) or within hanging drops followed by their cultivation in Petri dishes (15). These Ebs characteristically express embryonic regional markers specific to different lineages of ectodermal, mesodermal, and endodermal origin (66). Although human Eb formation has failed to induce uniform

15. Amit M and Itskovitz-Eldor J. Derivation and spontaneous differentiation of human embryonic stem cells. *J Anat* 2002;200: 225–32.

16. Suss-Toby E, Gerecht-Nir S, Amit M, Manor D and Itskovitz-Eldor J. Derivation of a diploid human embryonic stem cell line from a mononuclear zygote. *Hum Reprod* 2004;19:670–5.

17. Elford K, Lawrence C and Leader A. Research implications of embryo cryopreservation choices made by patients undergoing in vitro fertilization. *Fertil Steril* 2004;81:1154–5.

18. Hoffman DI, Zellman GL, Fair CC, et al. Cryopreserved embryos in the United States and their availability for research. *Fertil Steril* 2003;79:1063–9.

19. McMahon CA, Gibson FL, Leslie GI, Saunders DM, Porter KA and Tennant CC. Embryo donation for medical research: attitudes and concerns of potential donors. *Hum Reprod* 2003;18:871–7.

20. Simon C, Escobedo C, Valbuena D, et al. A. First derivation in Spain of human embryonic stem cell lines: use of long-term cryopreserved embryos and animal-free conditions. *Fertil Steril* 2005;83:246–9.

21. Sjogren A, Hardarson T, Andersson K, et al. Human blastocysts for the development of embryonic stem cells. *Reprod Biomed Online* 2004;9:330–7.

22. Cowan CA, Klimanskaya I, McMahon J, et al. Derivation of embryonic stem-cell lines from human blastocysts. *N Engl J Med* 2004;350:1353–6.

23. Mitalipova M, Calhoun J, Shin S, et al. Human embryonic stem cell lines derived from discarded embryos. *Stem Cells* 2003;21:521–6.

24. Park SP, Lee YJ, Lee KS, et al. Establishment of human embryonic stem cell lines from frozen-thawed blastocysts using STO cell feeder layers. *Hum Reprod* 2004;19:676–84.

25. Chen H, Qian K, Hu J, et al. The derivation of two additional human embryonic stem cell lines from day 3 embryos with low morphological scores. *Hum Reprod* 2005;20:2201–6.

26. Strelchenko N, Verlinsky O, Kukharenko V and Verlinsky Y. Morula-derived human embryonic stem cells. *Reprod Biomed Online* 2004;9:623–9.

27. Stojkovic M, Lako M, Stojkovic P, et al. Derivation of human embryonic stem cells from day-8 blastocysts recovered after three-step in vitro culture. *Stem Cells* 2004;22:790–7.

28. Chung Y, Klimanskaya I, Becker S, et al. Embryonic and extra-embryonic stem cell lines derived from single mouse blastomeres. *Nature* 2006;439:216–19.

29. Magli MC, Gianaroli L, Fortini D, Ferraretti AP and Munne S. Impact of blastomere biopsy and cryopreservation techniques on human embryo viability. *Hum Reprod* 1999;14:770–3.

30. Klimanskaya I, Chung Y, Becker S, Lu S-J and Lanza R. Human embryonic stem cell lines derived from single blastomeres. *Nature* (AOP Aug.23, 2006); doi:10.1038/nature05412.

31. Hurlbut WB. Altered nuclear transfer as a morally acceptable means for the procurement of human embryonic stem cells. *Perspect Biol Med* 2005;48:211–28.

32. Meissner A and Jaenisch R. Generation of nuclear transfer-derived pluripotent ES cells from cloned Cdx2-deficient blastocysts. *Nature* 2006;439:212–15.

33. Lim JW and Bodnar A. Proteome analysis of conditioned medium from mouse embryonic fibroblast feeder layers which support the growth of human embryonic stem cells. *Proteomics* 2002;2:1187–203.

34. Smith AG, Heath JK, Donaldson DD, et al. Inhibition of pluripotential embryonic stem cell differentiation by purifed polypeptides. *Nature* 1988;336:688–90.

35. Williams RL, Hilton DJ, Pease S, et al. Myeloid leukaemia inhibitory factor maintains the developmental potential of embryonic stem cells. *Nature* 1988;336:684–7.

36. Amit M, Sharki C, Margulets V and Itskovitz-Eldor J. Feeder layer- and serum-free culture of human embryonic stem cells. *Biol Reprod* 2004;70:837–45.

37. James D, Levine AJ, Besser D and Hemmati-Brivanlou A. TGFbeta/activin/nodal signalling is necessary for the maintenance of pluripotency in human embryonic stem cells. *Development* 2005;132:1273–82.

38. Xu RH, Peck RM, Li DS, Feng X, Ludwig T and Thomson JA. Basic FGF and suppression of BMP signalling sustain undifferentiated proliferation of human ES cells. *Nat Methods* 2005b;2: 185–90.

39. Xu C, Inokuma MS, Denham J, et al. Feeder-free growth of undifferentiated human embryonic stem cells. *Nat Biotechnol* 2001;19:971–4.

40. Martin MJ, Muotri A, Gage F and Varki A. Human embryonic stem cells express an immunogenic nonhuman sialic acid. *Nat Med* 2005;11:228–32.

41. Varki A. Loss of N-glycolylneuraminic acid in humans: mechanisms, consequences, and implications for hominid evolution. *Am J Phys Anthropol Suppl* 2001;33:54–69.

42. Richards M, Fong CY, Chan WK, Wong PC and Bongso A. Human feeders support prolonged undifferentiated growth of human inner cell masses and embryonic stem cells. *Nat Biotechnol* 2002;20:933–6.

43. Cheng L, Hammond H, Ye Z, Zhan X and Dravid G. Human adult marrow cells support prolonged expansion of human embryonic stem cells in culture. *Stem Cells* 2003;21:131–42.

44. Richards M, Tan S, Fong CY, Biswas A, Chan WK and Bongso A. Comparative evaluation of various human feeders for prolonged undifferentiated growth of human embryonic stem cells. *Stem Cells* 2003;21:546–56.

45. Amit M, Margulets V, Segev H, et al. Human feeder layers for human embryonic stem cells. *Biol Reprod* 2003;68:2150–6.

46. Inzunza J, Gertow K, Stromberg MA, et al. Derivation of human embryonic stem cell lines in serum replacement medium using postnatal human fibroblasts as feeder cells. *Stem Cells* 2005;23: 544–9.

47. Koivisto H, Hyvarinen M, Stromberg AM, et al. Cultures of human embryonic stem cells: serum replacement medium or serum-containing media and the effect of basic fibroblast growth factor. *Reprod Biomed Online* 2004;9:330–7.

48. Valbuena D, Galan A, Sanchez E, et al. Derivation, characterization and differentiation of three new human embryonic stem cell lines (VAL-3, -4 and -5) on human feeder and serum-free conditions in Spain. *Reprod Biomed Online* 2006; 13(6): 875–86.

49. Genbacev O, Krtolica A, Zdravkovic T, et al. Serum-free derivation of human embryonic stem cell lines on human placental fibroblast feeders. *Fertil Steril* 2005;83:1517–29.

50. Rodríguez CI, Galan A, Valbuena D and Simon C. Derivation of clinical-grade human embryonic stem cells. *Reprod Biomed Online* 2006;12:112–18.

51. Gearhart J. New human embryonic stem cell lines-more is better. *N Engl J Med* 2004;350:1275–6.

52. Stojkovic P, Lako M, Stewart R, et al. An autogeneic feeder cell system that efficiently supports growth of undifferentiated human embryonic stem cells. *Stem Cells* 2005b;23:306–14.

53. Wang Q, Fang Z, Jin F, Lu Y, Gai H and Sheng HZ. Derivation and growing human embryonic stem cells on feeders derived from themselves. *Stem Cells* 2005b;239:1221–7.

54. Zwaka TP and Thomson JA. Homologous recombination in human embryonic stem cells. *Nat Biotechnol* 2003;21:319–21.

55. Ponsaerts P, Van der Sar S, Van Tenedlo VF, Jorens PG, Berneman ZN and Singh PB. Highly efficient mRNA-based gene

transfer in feeder-free cultured H9 human embryonic stem cells. *Cloning Stem cells* 2004;6:211–16.

56. Mecham RP. Extracellular Matrix. In: Bonifacino JS, Dasso M, Harford JB, Lippincott-Schwartz J, Yamada KM, eds. *Current Protocols in Cell Biology*. NJ, USA: John Wiley & Sons Inc., 2004:2:10.1.1.

57. Brimble SN, Zeng X, Weiler DA, et al. Karyotypic stability, genotyping, differentiation, feeder-free maintenance, and gene expression sampling in three human embryonic stem cell lines derived prior to August 9, 2001. *Stem Cells Dev* 2004;13:585–97.

58. Rosler ES, Fisk GJ, Ares X, et al. Long-term culture of human embryonic stem cells in feeder-free conditions. *Dev Dyn* 2004;229:259–74.

59. Wang G, Zhang H, Zhao Y, et al. Noggin and bFGF cooperate to maintain the pluripotency of human embryonic stem cells in the absence of feeder layers. *Biochem Biophys Res Commun* 2005a; 330:934–42.

60. Xu C, Rosler E, Jiang J, et al. Basic fibroblast growth factor supports undifferentiated human embryonic stem cell growth without conditioned medium. *Stem Cells* 2005a;23:315–23.

61. Schuldiner M, Yanuka O, Itskovitz-Eldor J, Melton DA and Benvenisty N. Effects of eight growth factors on the differentiation of cell derived from human embryonic stem cells. *Proc Natl Acad Sci USA* 2000;97:11307–12.

62. Klimanskaya I, Chung Y, Meisner L, Johnson J, West MD and Lanza R. Human embryonic stem cells derived without feeder cells. *Lancet* 2005;365:1636–41.

63. Stojkovic P, Lako M, Przyborski S, et al. Human-serum matrix supports undifferentiated growth of human embryonic stem cells. *Stem Cells* 2005a;23:895–902.

64. Ludwig TE, Levenstein ME, Jones JM, et al. Derivation of human embryonic stem cells in defined conditions. *Nature Biotech* 2006;24:185–7.

65. Tzukerman M, Rosenberg T, Ravel Y, Reiter I, Coleman R and Skorecki K. An experimental platform for studying growth and invasiveness of tumour cells within teratomas derived from human embryonic stem cells. *Proc Natl Acad Sci USA* 2003;100: 13507–12.

66. Itskoviz-Eldor J, Schuldiner M, Karsenti D, et al. Differentiation of human embryonic stem cells into embryoid bodies compromising the three embryonic germ layers. *Mol Med* 2000;6:88–95.

67. Reubinoff BE, Itsykson P, Turetsky T, et al. Neural progenitors from human embryonic stem cells. *Nat Biotechnol* 2001;19:1134–40.

68. Schuldiner M, Eiges R, Eden A, et al. Induced neuronal differentiation of human embryonic stem cells. *Brain Res* 2001;913: 201–5.

69. Zhang SC, Wernig M, Duncan ID, Brustle O and Thomson JA. In vitro differentiation of transplantable neural precursors from human embryonic stem cells. *Nat Biotechnol* 2001;19:1129–33.

70. Kehat I, Kenyagin-Karsenti D, Snir M, et al. Human embryonic stem cells can differentiate into myocytes with structural and functional properties of cardiomyocytes. *J Clin Invest* 2001;108:407–14.

71. Assady S, Maor G, Amit M, Itskovitz-Eldor J, Skorecki KL and Tzukerman M. Insulin production by human embryonic stem cells. *Diabetes* 2001;50:1691–7.

72. Chadwick K, Wang L, Menendez P, Murdoch B, Rouleau A and Bhatia M. Cytokines and BMP-4 promote hematopoietic differentiation of human embryonic stem cells. *Blood* 2003;102:906–15.

73. Zhan X, Dravid G, Ye Z, et al. Functional antigen-presenting leucocytes derived from human embryonic stem cells in vitro. *Lancet* 2004;364:163–71.

74. Levenberg S, Golub JS, Amit M, Itskovitz-Eldor J and Langer R. Endothelial cells derived from human embryonic stem cells. *Proc Natl Acad Sci USA* 2002;99:4391–6.

75. Gerecht-Nir S, Osenberg S, Nevo O, Ziskind A, Coleman R and Itskovitz-Eldor J. Vascular development in early human embryos and in teratomas derived from human embryonic stem cells. *Biol Reprod* 2004;71:2029–36.

76. Xu RH, Chen X, Li DS, et al. BMP4 initiates human embryonic stem cell differentiation to trophoblast. *Nat Biotechnol* 2002;20: 1261–4.

77. Clark AT, Bodnar MS, Fox M, et al. Spontaneous differentiation of germ cells from human embryonic stem cells in vitro. *Hum Mol Genet* 2004;13:727–39.

78. Verlinsky Y, Strelchenko N, Kukharenko V, et al. Human embryonic stem cell lines with genetic disorders. *Reprod Biomed Online* 2005;10:105–10.

79. Pickering SJ, Minger SL, Minger SL, et al. Generation of a human embryonic stem cell line encoding the cystic fibrosis mutation deltaF508, using preimplantation genetic diagnosis. *Reprod Biomed Online* 2005;10:390–7.

80. Soria B, Roche E, Berna G, Leon-Quinto T, Reig JA and Martin F. Insulin-secreting cells derived from embryonic stem cells normalized glycemia in streptozotocin-induced diabetic mice. *Diabetes* 2000;49:157–62.

81. Zang W, Lee WH and Triarhou LC. Grafted cerebellar cells in a mouse model of hereditary ataxia express IGF-I system genes and partially restore behavorial function. *Nat Med* 1996;2:65–71.

82. Kim JH, Auerbach JM, Rodriguez-Gomez JA, et al. Dopamine neurons derived from embryonic stem cells function in an animal model of Parkinson's disease. *Nature* 2002;418:50–6.

83. Klug MG, Soonpaa MH, Koh GY and Field LJ. Genetically selected cardiomyocytes from differentiating embryonic stem cells from stable intracardiac grafts. *J Clin Invest* 1996;98:216–24.

84. Li M, Pevny L, Lovell-Badge R and Smith A. Generation of purified neural precursors from embryonic stem cells by lineage selection. *Curr Biol* 1998;8:971–4.

85. Muller M, Fleischmann BK, Selbert S, et al. Selection of ventricular-like cardiomyocytes from ES cells in vitro. *FASEB J* 2000; 14:2540–8.

86. Galán A, Escobedo C, Valbuena D, Berna A and Simón C. From animal free to feeder free conditions. The desired derivation process for human embryonic stem cells. In: Grier EV, eds. *Embryonic Stem Cell Research*. NY, USA: Nova Science Publishers, Inc., 2006: 123–41.

87. Gepstein L. Derivation and potential applications of human embryonic stem cells. *Circulation Research* 2002;91:866–76.

88. Drukker M, Katz G, Urbach A, et al. Characterization of the expression of MCH proteins in human embryonic stem cells. *Proc Natl Acad Sci USA* 2002;99:9864–9.

89. Grusby MJ, Auchincloss H Jr, Lee R, et al. Mice lacking major histocompatibility complex class I and class II molecules. *Proc Natl Acad Sci USA* 1993;90:3913–17.

90. Hardy RR and Malissen B. Lymphocyte development: the (knock-) ins and outs of lymphoid development. *Curr Opin Immunol* 1998;10:155–7.

91. Harlan DM and Kirk AD. The future of organ and tissue transplantation: can T-cell costimulatory pathway modifiers revolutionize the prevention of graft rejection? *JAMA* 1999;282: 1076–82.

92. Lanza RP, Chung HY, Yoo JJ, et al. Generation of histocompatible tissues using nuclear transplantation. *Nat Biotech* 2002;20:689–96.

93. Chen Y, He ZX, Liu A, et al. Embryonic stem cells generated by nuclear transfer of human somatic nuclei into rabbit oocytes. *Cell Res* 2003;134:251–63.

94. Magnus D and Cho MK. Ethics. Issues in oocyte donation for stem cell research. *Science* 2005;308:1747–8.

95. Hübner K, Furhmann G, Christenson L, et al. Derivation of oocytes from mouse embryonic stem cells. *Science* 2003;300: 1251–6.

96. Dyce P, Wen L and Li J. In vitro germline potential of stem cells derived from fetal porcine skin. *Nat Cell Biol* 2006;8:384–90.

97. Cowan CA, Atienza J, Melton DA and Eggan K. Nuclear reprogramming of somatic cells after fusion with human embryonic stem cells. *Science* 2005;309:1369–73.

98. Raucy JL, Mueller L, Duan K, Allen SW, Strom S and Lasker JM. Expression and induction of CYP2C P450 enzymes in primary cultures of hepatocytes. *J Pharmacol Exp Ther* 2002;302:475–82.

99. Lamba JK, Lin YS, Thummel K, et al. Common allelic variants of cytochrome P4503A4 and their prevalence in different populations. *Pharmacogenetics* 2002;12:121–32.

100. Davila JC, Cezar GG, Thiede M, Strom S, Miki T and Trosko J. Use and application of stem cell in Toxicology. *Toxicol Sci* 2004;79:214–23.

101. Rohwedel J, Guan K, Hegert C and Wobus AM. Embryonic stem cells as an in vitro model for mutagenicity, cytotoxicity and embryotoxicity studies: present state and future prospects. *Toxicol In Vitro* 2001;15:741–53.

102. Lerou PH and Daley GQ. Therapeutic potential of embryonic stem cells. *Blood Rev* 2005;19:321–31.

103. Abe Y, Kouyama K, Tomita Y, et al. Analysis of neurons created from wild-type and Alzheimer's mutation knock-in embryonic stem cells by a highly efficient differentiation protocol. *J Neurosci* 2003;23:8513–25.

104. Ricordi C and Strom TB. Clinical islet transplantation: advances and immunological challenges. *Nat Rev Immunol* 2004;4: 259–68.

105. Aldhous P. Stem-cell research: after the gold rush. *Nature* 2005;434:94–6.

106. Ilic D. Going offshore: shady or shiny? *Regenerative Med* 2006;1:1–4.

107. Lanzendorf SE, Boyd CA, Wright DL, Muasher S, Oehninger S and Hodgen GD. Use of human gametes obtained from anonymous donors for the production of human embryonic stem cell lines. *Fertil Steril* 2001;76:132–7.

108. Lee JB, Lee JE, Park JH, et al. Establishment and maintenance of human embryonic stem cell lines on human feeder cells derived from uterine endometrium under serum-free condition. *Biol Reprod* 2005;72:42–9.

70

FERTILITY PRESERVATION IN FEMALE AND MALE CANCER PATIENTS

Mohamed A. Bedaiwy, Tommaso Falcone

INTRODUCTION

Female cancer patients between the ages of fifteen and forty-nine years are expected to not only survive their disease but also lead normal lives, mainly because of newer, more effective cancer therapies such as sterilizing chemotherapy and/or radiotherapy. Consequently, fertility preservation has become an important quality-of-life issue. Problems with fertility and obstetric disorders such as early pregnancy loss, premature labor, and low birth weight have all been described after cancer treatment (1).

Recent achievements in assisted reproductive technologies such as novel ovulation induction remedies, oocyte cryopreservation, and ovarian tissue cryopreservation and transplantation have further expanded the options for fertility preservation in women scheduled to receive chemotherapy and/or radiotherapy. However, most of the potential fertility preservation strategies do not have long-term follow-up data. The latest committee report of the American Society of Reproductive Medicine (ASRM) states that embryo cryopreservation is the only option for these patients with sufficient evidence of clinical utility. The remaining options, including orthotopic transplantation of cryopreserved ovarian tissue, are either experimental or without enough evidence to be proposed to patients at this stage.

We will review the recent evidence on the pathophysiology of chemotherapy/radiotherapy-induced gonadal toxicity and the recent data on the indications and the outcomes of techniques used for fertility preservation in female cancer patients.

BASIC OOCYTE BIOLOGY

In humans, primordial germ cells arrive in the gonadal ridge from the yolk sac endoderm by the seventh week of gestation. These germ cells become oogonia, which proliferate by mitosis before differentiating into primary oocytes. Some oogonia begin their transformation into primary oocytes and enter the first stages of meiosis at approximately eleven to twelve weeks of gestation. At twenty weeks gestation, the total germ cell number peaks at six to seven million primordial follicles. Meiosis arrests in the prophase I and only resumes around the time of ovulation. These arrested oocytes are referred to as primary oocytes. After this time, the rate of oogonial division declines. The postnatal germ cells do not undergo mitosis. This is contrary to spermatogenesis where mitosis occurs postnatally as well.

Primordial follicle formation begins around midgestation, when a single flattened layer of granulosa cells surround each oocyte and continues until just after birth (2). After oocytes are surrounded within the primordial follicles, they remain arrested in the dictyate stage of meiosis I. From a peak of six to seven million at twenty weeks gestation, the oocyte number falls dramatically so that at birth, there are only 300,000–400,000 remaining (2,3). The number of oocytes continues to fall throughout puberty so that only 200,000 follicles remain by age of puberty.

The fate of each ovarian follicle is determined by endocrine, paracrine, and autocrine factors (4). The follicles develop through primordial, primary, and secondary stages before acquiring an antral cavity. Some books refer to antral follicles as tertiary follicles. By the antral stage, most follicles have already undergone atresia and a few of them reach the preovulatory stage under the cyclic gonadotropin stimulation that occurs after puberty (4). The mature Graafian follicles are the main source of the cyclic secretion of ovarian estrogens in women of reproductive age. In response to preovulatory gonadotropin surges during each reproductive cycle, the dominant Graafian follicle ovulates to release the mature oocyte for fertilization, whereas the remaining theca and granulosa cells transform into the corpus luteum (5). The oocyte pool in the mammalian ovary becomes fixed early in life; thus, any factors affecting the follicular pool will lead to an early exhaustion and premature ovarian failure (POF).

Primordial follicles remain dormant under the continuous inhibitory influences of systemic and/or local origin (6). Acceleration of preantral and antral follicular growth depends on gonadotrophin stimulation. Follicle-stimulating hormone (FSH) is capable of accelerating the development of preantral follicles. However, FSH and luteinizing hormone (LH) are unlikely to exert direct actions on primordial follicles because they have not yet developed functional gonadotropin receptors (7).

Many genes, proteins, hormones, and factors are involved in the process of folliculogenesis. The most significant factors involved are summarized in Table 70.1 with their respective functions. Although follicles do not develop functional FSH receptors until the secondary stage, pregranulosa cells and primordial follicles respond to activators of the cAMP pathways by increasing expression of aromatase and FSH receptors (8). Factors involved in oocyte-granulosa cell communication in early follicles have also been proposed to have a role in initial recruitment. This interaction could also explain why if one cell

Table 70.1: Regulatory Genes of Oogenesis and Folliculogenesis

Gene/proteins	Pattern of ovarian expression	Developmental role
Bmp family	PGCs	Formation
Smad family		Migration
SCf		Proliferation
C-kit		Colonization of the forming gonads
Integrin-B		Survival
Scp family	Meiotic prophase 1 oocytes	Preleptotene-DNA replication
Mih family		Search and pairing of homologous chromosomes and synapses
Msh family		Crossing over, recombination, and DNA mismatch repair
		Meiotic arrest
Fig alpha	Primordial follicle	Maintenance of primordial follicles
Nobox	Primary follicle	Transition from the primordial and primary follicle
Connexins	Preantral follicles	Oocytes-granulosa cells' interactions
Gdf9, Bmp 15		Granulosa cell proliferation
		Theca precursor formation
FSH/FSHR	Antral/Graafian follicles	Antrum formation
LH/LHR		Follicular recruitment
ER-α/β		Preovulatory changes
PGE2, Cox2		Corpus luteum formation
		Ovulation

Bmp, bone morphogenic protein; ER-α/β, estrogen receptor alpha and beta; FSH/FSHR, follicle stimulating hormone and receptor; LH/LHR, luteinizing hormone and receptor; Mih and Msh, mismatch recognition and repair proteins; PGCs, primordial germ cells; PGE2, prostaglandin E2 and cyclo-oxygenase 2; Scf, stem cell factor; Scp, synaptonemal complex protein; Smad, *C. elegans* gene Sma and Drosophila gene mad.

dies due to cancer therapy or other cause, it leads to the death of another.

The kit ligand is expressed by granulosa cells of growing follicles, whereas c-kit, a tyrosine kinase receptor of the platelet-derived growth factor receptor family, is located on oocytes and theca cells. Mutations in mice that prevent the production of the soluble form of the kit ligand lead to failure of follicular growth beyond the primary stage. Mutations affecting the function of c-kit in humans, however, do not seem to affect female fertility (9).

The potential role of the oocyte in early follicle development was introduced by studies of a member of the transforming growth factor-β (TGF-β)/activin family called the growth differentiation factor-9 (GDF-9). It signals via serine-threonine kinase receptors and is produced by human oocytes (10) in primary and larger follicles but is absent in primordial follicles. In mutant mice, disruption of the GDF-9 gene prevents follicle development beyond the primary stage (11) and is associated with the absence of thecal cell markers and eventually oocyte death (12). Because kit ligand and GDF-9 are highly expressed in secondary follicles, they also are likely to play important roles in preantral follicle development. A homolog to GDF-9, named bone morphogenic protein BMP-15 (13), has also been identified, and it could exert similar functions. It is possible that multiple paracrine factors are involved in communication between oocyte and somatic cells during early follicle development.

A basic biological doctrine is that during the life of a female, there neither is nor can be any increase in the number of primary oocytes beyond those originally laid down when the ovary was formed. Although this dogma has persisted for more than fifty years, recent studies have shown that production of oocytes (oogenesis) in mice and their enclosure within somatic cells (folliculogenesis) persists in juvenile and adult life (14). Johnson et al. concluded that gonadal stem cells reside in the surface epithelium of mouse ovaries and are active throughout life (14). However, the same group modified this hypothesis by proposing that the bone marrow is a source of gonadal stem cells (15); this was done in response to several valuable critical comments (16,17). However, many leading experts in the field of reproductive physiology expressed concerns about their second hypothesis regarding the putative role of bone marrow cells in reproduction (18). These hypotheses await independent confirmation.

Although these genes and their products provide an insight into the growth process of very early follicles, the exact mechanisms by which the primordial follicles leave the resting pool remain unknown. With the secrets surrounding early folliculogenesis unraveling, new reproductive techniques could be developed. For instance, understanding the relationship between granulosa cells and oocytes could allow us to develop techniques that could put both cells in a dormant state at the time of sterilizing radiotherapy and/or chemotherapy in order to limit the degree of damage. However, more studies are needed to reveal potential factors involved in the initial stage of follicle recruitment.

CHEMOTHERAPY/RADIOTHERAPY-INDUCED OVARIAN FAILURE

Chemotherapy-Induced POF

Chemotherapy-induced POF has been documented in many publications (19). The exact incidence of POF following chemotherapy is difficult to establish since many factors contribute to ovarian failure. The most important parameters are the patient's age at the time of treatment, the drug type, and cumulative dose. The risk of gonadal damage increases with age. This is most likely due to the presence of fewer oocytes with increasing age. Cytotoxic chemotherapeutic agents are not equally gonadotoxic. Cell cycle–nonspecific chemotherapeutic agents are more gonadotoxic than cell cycle–specific ones.

Chemotherapeutic regimens that include a cell cycle–nonspecific alkylating agent are particularly gonadotoxic (Figure 70.1). Cyclophosphamide is the most gonadotoxic member of this category. It is commonly used in breast cancer treatment and consequently represents the most frequent chemotherapy-inducing ovarian failure agent. Manger et al. reported that in lupus patients treated with cyclophosphamide, 60 percent suffered from POF and hypergonadotropic amenorrhea. The POF rate was less than 50 percent in women younger than thirty years of age and 60 percent in women between the ages of thirty and forty years. The cumulative dose of cyclophosphamide also strongly influences the POF rate (19). Similar reports by many other investigators have documented the variable effects of different regimens on ovarian functions (20,21).

Consequently, not all patients receiving multiagent chemotherapy have the same risk for developing POF. Those at highest risk for POF after treatment for cancer include women who have received either high-dose alkylating agent therapy or pelvic or total body irradiation. Most young patients with Hodgkin's disease treated with multiagent chemotherapy and radiation to a field that does not include the ovaries will remain fertile, albeit with a shorter fertility window than age-matched controls (22). A recent case report documented a spontaneous conception in a young woman with POF after fourteen courses of ifosfamide chemotherapy combined with pelvic irradiation for Ewing's sarcoma of the pelvis (23).

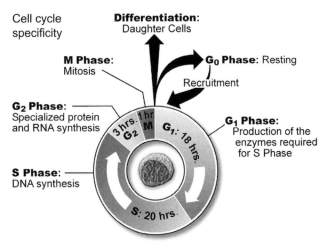

Figure 70.1. Schematic representation of the cell cycle. The relative gonadotoxicity and cell cycle specificity of the different chemotherapeutic agents are agents with phase specificity: *M phase*: A, podophyllotoxins as etoposide and teniposide; B, taxanes as docetaxel and paclitaxel; C, vinca alkaloids as vinblastine and vincristine. *G2 phase*: bleomycin. *S phase*: A, antimetabolites as A, antifolates: methotrexate, antipurines: mercaptopurine, thioguanine; B, antipyrimidines: cytarabine, fluorouracil, and azacitidine; and C, miscellaneous: hydroxyurea, procarbazine, cisplatin, and carboplatin. *G0 phase*: nitrosoureas as carmustine, lomustine, and semustine. *G1 phase*: asparaginase as diglycoaldehyde and steroids. Agents without phase specificity: A, alkylating agents as bulsulfan, chlorambucil, cyclophosphamide, mechlorethamine, and melphalan; B, anthracycline antibiotics as doxorubicin, daunomycin, rubidazone, and dactinomycin; C, miscellaneous: DTIC, cisplatin, and carboplatin; and D, nitrosoureas – also acts in G0.

Radiotherapy-Induced POF

Pelvic radiotherapy can damage both the ovaries and uterus. Several reproductive-age malignancies afflicting pelvic organs can be cured with radiotherapy. These include cervical, vaginal, and anorectal carcinomas; some germ cell tumors; Hodgkin's disease; and central nervous system tumors. Like chemotherapy, the degree and persistence of POF is related to the patient's age and the dose of radiation to the ovaries. The fractionation of the total dose plays an important role in determining the extent of ovarian damage because irradiation is more toxic when given as a single dose (24).

Two studies reported that the break point for radiation-induced ovarian failure is around 300 cGy to the ovaries. Only 11–13 percent of women experienced ovarian failure below 300 cGy versus 60–63 percent above that threshold value (25). The radiation doses to the ovaries with standard pelvic radiation therapy will uniformly induce ovarian failure. The addition of chemotherapy increases the risk of POF (26,27).

Ovarian follicles are remarkably vulnerable to DNA damage from ionizing radiation. Irradiation results in ovarian atrophy and reduced follicle stores (28). On the cellular level, oocytes show rapid onset of pyknosis, chromosome condensation, disruption of the nuclear envelope, and cytoplasmic vacuolization. Serum levels of FSH and LH rise progressively within four to eight weeks following radiation exposure, while serum E2 levels fall. A dose-dependant reduction in the primordial follicle pool was noted upon exposing the ovary to radiotherapy (29). It is estimated that less than 2 Gy is enough to destroy 50 percent of the oocyte population (LDL_{50} < 2 Gy) (30).

DIAGNOSIS AND PREDICTION OF POF

Prediction of POF in cancer survivors is not only of diagnostic importance but also of prognostic value. So far, no ideal marker has been developed to predict chemotherapy/radiotherapy-induced POF. Bath et al. showed that serum FSH levels were elevated in cancer survivors with regular menstrual cycles, while anti-Mullerian hormone (AMH) levels were lower than those of the controls. Despite smaller ovarian volumes in cancer survivors than controls, antral follicle counts (AFC) were similar (31). In addition, cancer chemotherapy is associated with a transient suppression of inhibin B in prepubertal girls. Consequently, inhibin B, together with sensitive measurements of FSH, was proposed as a potential marker of the gonadotoxic effects of cancer chemotherapy in prepubertal girls (32). Basal AFC is another test of ovarian reserve that has been used extensively either alone or with other markers.

Contrary to the majority of hormonal biomarkers that are dependent on the stage of the follicle development, specifically more mature stages, AMH is produced by the granulosa cells of a wide range of follicles from primary to the early antral stages. AMH seems to be independent of FSH, LH, and inhibin levels. AMH has been shown to have a stronger relationship with AFC than with other parameters. Given the fact that peripheral AMH concentrations decline during ovarian stimulation, growing follicles progressively lose their ability to produce AMH. Accumulating evidence suggests that the measurement of AMH levels could be a quantitative and possibly qualitative marker of granulosa cell activity and health (33). It may also be a good marker of ovarian function in prepubertal girls undergoing sterilizing cancer therapy; no other markers are available for this group at risk.

INDICATIONS OF FERTILITY PRESERVATION STRATEGIES

Breast cancer is currently the most common malignancy in reproductive-age women that requires immediate fertility intervention (34). Fifteen percent of all breast cancer cases are estimated to occur in women younger than forty years (35). Cervical cancer is another common malignancy in women of reproductive age that may require fertility-preserving intervention. The anatomic location renders fertility preservation even more challenging.

The indication list for fertility preservation is expanding and currently includes gonadotoxic chemotherapy/radiotherapy not only for malignancies but also for the treatment of other systemic diseases, including systemic lupus erythematosus acute glomerulonephritis, and Behcet's disease. In addition, a wide variety of cancer patients are candidates for fertility preservation including those with musculoskeletal cancers such as Ewing's sarcoma and osteosarcoma, hematopoietic cancers such as leukemias and lymphomas, neuroblastomas, and Wilm's tumor. Chemotherapy in the context of bone marrow transplantation and umbilical cord stem cell transplantation could also be a possible indication as well. Patients with nongynecologic cancers including colorectal carcinoma, lymphomas, and sarcomas are candidates for fertility preservation as well.

FERTILITY PRESERVATION OPTIONS

A wide variety of strategies have been assessed for fertility preservation. However, none of them has been tested in a prospective randomized controlled trial. Many of the available techniques are promising but are still highly experimental techniques.

Chemoprotection

Pretreatment with a gonadotropin-releasing hormone (GnRH) agonist has been attempted based on the observation that premenarchal female gonads appear to be less sensitive to cytotoxic drugs (36,37). The goal with the use of this agent is to keep the ovaries in a prepubertal quiescent state during chemotherapy treatment. This approach has also been tried with a variety of other medication that suppresses the hypothalamic pituitary ovarian access. The few noncontrolled observational studies that have been reported on this topic have produced conflicting conclusions regarding the effectiveness of this method.

Blumenfeld et al. reported on the largest group of females thus far (more than 90) who were exposed to both cytotoxic drugs and GnRH-a. The rate of POF was 5 percent in the chemotherapy-only group versus 55 percent in the GnRH-a/chemotherapy (38). However, the retrospective nature of the control group and the shorter follow-up in the group treated with the agonist makes the study less robust. Similar results were reported by Pereyra Pacheco (39) and Fox et al. (40). The only prospective controlled study showed that GnRH analogues were not effective in the prevention of POF. However, only eighteen women were enrolled in this study (41).

Criticism of this approach is also derived from the fact that if the mechanism of action is primarily through hypothalamic pituitary suppression, this should not protect early follicle damage that is gonadotropin independent. However, a direct gonadal effect is possible.

Given the poor evidence available, a prospective randomized study with sufficient power is needed to appropriately evaluate the effectiveness of GnRH analogue as a potential strategy for fertility preservation. However, this method is quite popular with patients and oncologists alike. The patients find it simple to initiate and can focus their energy on their life-saving medical treatment. It is appealing to oncologists because it allows no delay in proceeding to medical therapy compared with the time required for assisted reproductive technology. Suppressive therapy with a variety of suppressive agents such as oral contraceptives or progestins have not been shown to be effective in preventing damage from chemotherapy or radiation therapy.

Ovariopexy

Moving the ovaries out of the field of irradiation can help maintain ovarian function in patients scheduled to undergo gonadotoxic radiotherapy. This significantly reduces ovarian radiation exposure in patients who receive pelvic irradiation such as those with Hodgkin's disease or genitourinary or low intestinal malignancies. For instance, the ovarian dose following transposition is reduced to approximately 5–10 percent of the in situ ovaries (42). The dose to each transposed ovary is 126 cGy for intracavitary radiation, 135–190 cGy for external radiation therapy when the initial dose is 4,500 cGy, and 230–310 cGy with the addition of para-aortic node irradiation (4,500 cGy) (43).

The initial experience with medial transposition, which was accomplished by suturing the ovaries posterior to the uterus and shielding them during treatment, showed that it was generally ineffective. Lateral transposition appears to be more effective (44,45).

Lateral ovarian transposition is typically performed by laparotomy. This approach is used at the time of radical hysterectomy for cervical cancer and was used during staging laparotomy for Hodgkin's disease (46). Staging laparotomy for Hodgkin's is uncommon today. Ovarian transposition should be performed laparoscopically just prior to the initiation of radiation therapy. An important advantage of laparoscopic ovarian transposition is that radiation therapy can be initiated immediately postoperatively; this will help prevent POF in ovaries that have migrated back to the irradiation field (27,47,48). In cases of vaginal or cervical cancers being treated by brachytherapy, laparoscopic ovarian transposition can be performed under the same anesthetic that is used for inserting the brachytherapy device (49).

Since staging laparotomy and splenectomy are no longer required for stage I and stage II Hodgkin's disease, ovarian transposition can be performed laparoscopically as an outpatient procedure, leading to a more rapid recovery, less discomfort, better cosmesis, and lower cost. Nearly all women with stage I and stage II Hodgkin's disease treated with radiation alone or with minimal chemotherapy following laparoscopic ovarian transposition retain their ovarian function and fertility (27).

Ovarian failure may occur if the ovaries are not moved far enough out of the radiation field or if they migrate back to their original position. The latter situation may occur if absorbable sutures are used. Ovarian failure following transposition may also occur if the ovarian vessels were compromised by the surgical technique or if radiation injured the vascular pedicle (50).

Another concern with ovarian transposition is the development of symptomatic ovarian cysts. The mechanism causing the cysts is unknown, but they can be suppressed with oral contraceptives (51).

Assisted Reproductive Technologies

Assisted reproductive technology is probably the most used modality in patients that wish to proceed to fertility preservation. As was stated, the ASRM recognizes that there is sufficient evidence to recommend embryo cryopreservation as a routine clinical care compared with other therapeutic strategies.

Oocyte Cryopreservation

In women without a partner, freezing mature or immature oocytes may be the only practical option. The main factor that may influence the outcome in oocyte cryopreservation is its structural complexity. Oocyte subcellular organelles are far more complex, and perhaps more sensitive, to thermal injury than preimplantation embryos (52,53). A detailed review of oocyte cryopreservation is given in other chapters of this book.

Porcu et al. cryopreserved the oocytes of eighteen patients awaiting chemotherapy and radiotherapy for neoplastic disease. They found that the duration of oocyte storage did not seem to interfere with oocyte survival, as pregnancies occurred even after several years of gamete cryopreservation in liquid nitrogen (54). Pregnancy rates per vitrified-thawed oocyte are still quite low.

Given these recent laboratory modifications resulting in improved oocyte survival, oocyte fertilization, and pregnancy rates from frozen-thawed oocytes in IVF, the practice committee of the ASRM has recently evaluated the available current evidence. They concluded that despite the limited number of established pregnancies and deliveries resulting from cryopreserved oocytes, no increase in chromosomal abnormalities, birth defects, or developmental deficits have been noted in the children born from cryopreserved oocytes to date. Therefore, they recommend that the option of oocyte cryopreservation should be considered as an experimental technique only to be performed under investigational protocol under the auspices of an internal review board (55). Oocyte cryopreservation can be used as an adjunct to conventional IVF and as an option for fertile women as well as those at risk of losing their fertility.

Recent reports indicate that pregnancy rates are getting better, whether slow-freeze or vitrification methods are used (56). Larger prospective trials are needed to determine the efficacy and the long-term safety of oocyte cryopreservation. Until a sufficient number of births are reached and adequate outcome data are collected, oocyte cryopreservation should continue to be considered experimental and to be performed under the oversight of an institutional review board (57).

Embryo Cryopreservation

Embryo cryopreservation is the only fertility preservation option recommended by the ASRM. It is probably the most efficient technique that offers a reasonable opportunity for success for women who have a partner and can undergo ovarian stimulation regimens for IVF. According to Society for Assisted Reproduction Technology (58), the delivery rate per embryo transfer utilizing cryopreserved embryos is 31.8 percent for those younger than thirty-five years. The post-thaw survival rate of embryos ranges between 35 and 90 percent. Implantation rates between 8 and 30 percent have been reported, and cumulative pregnancy rates can reach more than 60 percent (59,60). This is the option with the best outcome for the patient. However, it may not be acceptable to prepubertal and adolescent females and women without a partner. If this option is acceptable to the patient, long-term data are available about the outcome of children born from these procedures that demonstrate developmental safety of the offspring.

The use of IVF may be problematic for patients with estrogen-sensitive tumors such as breast cancer because it results in extremely high estradiol levels. Typically, there is an interval of six weeks between the surgery and initiation of chemotherapy for breast cancer. Rather than using the standard protocol, a short flare protocol is used, which usually requires less time to achieve follicle recruitment (61). Conventional controlled ovarian hyperstimulation (COH) is associated with a significant rise in serum estrogen, which might affect the overall prognosis (62). For this reason, some centers offer natural-cycle (unstimulated) IVF. With this process, a single oocyte is aspirated. However, cancellation rates are high, and pregnancy rates are very low (7.2 percent per cycle and 15.8 percent per embryo transfer) (63,64). The nonsteroidal antiestrogen, tamoxifen (64), and the aromatase P450 inhibitor, letrozole (65), were introduced as possible ovulation induction agents for patients with breast cancer. Oktay et al. compared tamoxifen and letrozole for ovarian stimulation in breast cancer patients using a prospective controlled study design. They noted that when combined with low-dose FSH, both drugs have a better outcome than when tamoxifen is used alone. However, letrozole is preferred because it is associated with lower peak serum estradiol levels (65). Further evidence on the safety and success of ovarian stimulation with letrozole and tamoxifen in breast cancer patients undergoing IVF to cryopreserve their embryos for fertility preservation was provided by Oktay et al. The cancer recurrence rates were similar between those who underwent COH and those who did not (66).

Cryopreservation and Transplantation of Ovarian Tissue

Ovarian tissue cryopreservation and transplantation are other experimental procedures for preserving fertility in women with threatened reproductive damage. The concept is related to the principle of autotransplantation rather than transplantation between two genetically distinct humans. For this reason, cryopreservation of ovarian tissue is a critical component so that the extirpated germ cells can be replaced after completion of medical therapy for their primary medical disorder requiring gonadotoxic drugs. Autotransplantation will not require immunosuppressant medication. Transplantation of reproductive organs between genetically distinct humans will require immunosuppressant agents. Because cryopreservation of germ cells is an integral part of the potential autotransplantation procedure, it is expected that better survival will occur from primordial follicles in ovarian cortical strips because of their smaller size and lack of follicular fluid (67).

Animal models have provided useful information regarding transfer methods. Using sheep ovaries, which provide a reliable tool, Gosden et al. established the sheep model for ovarian tissue cryopreservation and transplantation. Using cryopreserved-thawed ovarian cortical strips, they showed follicular survival and endocrine function as well as pregnancy and delivery after transplantation of cryopreserved-thawed ovarian cortical strips (68,69).

TRANSPLANTATION: PREVENTION OF ISCHEMIC DAMAGE

The limited longevity of ovarian function in some human ovarian transplant cases using nonvascularized grafts may be partially due to the initial ischemic injury (Oktay, 2001 No. 9; Oktay, 2001 No. 10; Radford, 2001 No. 11). Immediate revascularization and ischemia time reduction may be essential for prolonging the functions of the grafts (Aubard, 1999 No. 12).

Almodin et al. proposed a technique to minimize ischemic damage in which frozen-thawed fragments of one ovary are injected into the cortex of the remaining sterile ovary. They administered radiotherapy to ewes to induce infertility on the remaining ovary, while the fragments of the other ovary were frozen. Subsequently, the thawed fragments of the frozen ovary were injected inside the cortex of the irradiated remaining ovary in a "sowing" procedure that eliminated the need for sutures. Six months following the grafting, they used rams to impregnate the ewes. They concluded that intracortical grafting of the germinative tissue could prevent ischemic damage (70).

Another approach to preventing initial ischemic damage to oocytes is transplantation into angiogenic granulation tissue created during wound healing. This approach shortened the ischemic period by twenty-four hours and significantly increased the pool of healthy primordial follicles and the perfused area of the transplanted grafts. The authors were able to detect functional blood vessels within the grafts as early as two days after transplantation. They were also able to demonstrate the functionality of the graft (71).

VASCULAR GRAFTS: ANIMAL MODELS

In our center, we studied the use of vascularized grafts as a possible solution to prevent ischemia to the graft. The potential for immediate revascularization of tissue makes this approach appealing. However, two major problems needed to be worked out. First was the technical difficulty in anastomosing small caliber vessels. However, the plastic surgery literature has an extensive experience with microsurgery of small vessels. More challenging was the cryopreservation of an entire organ and its vascular pedicle.

In a first series of experiments, we tried to assess if the time required for an anastomosis, referred to as the ischemia time, would cause damage to ovarian tissue; we demonstrated that large ovarian cortical strips can withstand ischemia for variable durations (72) without changing the histological architecture or inducing molecular damage (73). We also demonstrated that an intact fresh ovary could be transplanted with its vascular pedicle using microvascular anastomosis. If the vascular graft was technically successful, the ovarian graft survived (74). In the last set of experiments, we demonstrated that transplantation of a cryopreserved intact sheep ovary with its vascular pedicle could restore ovarian function (75).

We concluded that transplantation of fresh as well as cryopreserved-thawed intact ovaries to heterotopic sites is technically feasible with easy accessibility and a shorter operative time. A detailed technique for orthotopic autotransplantation of an intact frozen-thawed ovary together with the upper genital tract using microvascular anastomosis in rats has been described (76). We also provided a detailed description of the different techniques of autotransplantation of an intact fresh

Table 70.2: Potential Uses of Cryopreserved Ovarian Tissue

- Xenografting
- In vitro maturation of primordial follicles
- Autotransplantation

or frozen-thawed ovary together with its vascular pedicle using microvascular anastomosis in animal models. With these techniques, it is necessary to identify heterotopic locations that contain blood vessels that can be used to vascularize human ovarian grafts (77).

Recently, a study evaluated contralateral orthotopic autotransplantation of cryopreserved whole ovaries with microanastomosis of the ovarian vascular pedicle. The results are very encouraging, which shows that this entire concept is feasible. Four sheep showed postoperative luteal function, and one sheep conceived after spontaneous intercourse and delivered a healthy lamb 545 days after transplantation. However, histological examination of the ovaries eighteen to nineteen months after transplantation showed that the follicular survival rate in the grafted ovaries was only 1.7–7.6 percent (78). These data suggest that these grafts have limited survival even with a vascular anastomosis and that fertility may not be restored for a normal length of time. Nonetheless, the concept of whole-organ cryopreservation is gaining more popularity, and a recent model for cryopreservation of an intact uterus (79) as well as whole rabbit ovary has been proposed (80).

HUMAN TRIALS

All human trials of cryopreserved autotransplanted tissue have been with cortical strips. This concept was developed from previous work in animal models that have used cryopreserved-thawed ovarian cortical strips and reported follicular survival and endocrine function as well as restoration of fertility after transplantation of cryopreserved-thawed ovarian cortical strips (68,69).

There are several potential uses of cryopreserved ovarian tissue: transplantation back into the host, in vitro maturation of primordial follicles, and xenografting into a host animal (Table 70.2). The tissue can be transplanted back into patient. The potential for reintroduction of a cancer nidus may limit this use in malignancies that are known to have a predilection for the ovaries such as leukemias and potentially breast cancer. Using present techniques, ovarian tissue strips are removed from the patient prior to chemotherapy. They are frozen in small strips. When the patient is ready for pregnancy, they are transplanted back into the patient in a heterotopic or orthotopic site. Since this is an avascular graft, ischemic injury to the transplanted tissue results in the loss of virtually the entire growing follicle population and a significant number of primordial follicles.

Oktay et al. developed three different surgical techniques of ovarian cortical strips transplantation: orthotopic transplant into the pelvis and heterotopic transplant into the arm or abdominal wall. The orthotopic transplant ceased to function within the first nine months (81), whereas the heterotopic transplant resulted in the generation of a four-cell embryo that was transferred, but no pregnancy occurred (82). This one embryo was obtained after multiple cycles of ovarian stimulation.

More recently, a thirty-two-year-old Belgian woman gave birth to a healthy baby seven years after banking her ovarian tissue before starting chemotherapy for Hodgkin's lymphoma. Although she became infertile as a result of the chemotherapy, reimplantation of her ovarian tissue restarted ovulation five months later. She became pregnant eleven months after retransplantation by natural fertilization. This is the first case of a human live birth after successful orthotopic autotransplantation of cryopreserved ovarian tissue in a patient from whom tissue was collected and cryopreserved before chemotherapy was initiated (83).

Another pregnancy was reported after a modified IVF cycle following orthotopic autotransplantation of cryopreserved-thawed ovarian cortical strips in a woman with non-Hodgkins' lymphoma (84). The fact that the tissue was transplanted to the native ovary does not exclude the possibility of resumption of native ovarian functions. With increasing reports of documented spontaneous pregnancies in women with POF after prolonged courses of gonadotoxic chemotherapy/radiotherapy, one should be cautious about the exact site of origin of the oocytes that led to both pregnancies in the aforementioned reports (23).

One of the potential limitations of ovarian tissue cryopreservation and transplantation is loss of a large fraction of follicles during the initial ischemia after transplantation. Previous work indicated that whereas the loss due to freezing is relatively small (69,85,86), up to two-thirds of follicles are lost after transplantation. Given this limitation, it has been recommended that ovarian tissue freezing (81) should be restricted to patients younger than thirty-five years.

Research should focus on refining the cryopreservation protocols, cryoprotectants, and transplantation techniques that decrease ischemia, particularly the use of vascularized grafts (74–76). Selection of the transplantation site should consider an easy, a simple, and a minimally invasive surgical technique. Moreover, ample blood supply to the recipient site is important for graft establishment, survival, and long-term function.

OVARIAN TRANSPLANTATION FROM ONE PERSON TO ANOTHER

Silber et al. have reported this work in identical twins. They reported on monozygotic twenty-four-year-old twins presented with discordant ovarian function. One had had premature ovarian failure at the age of fourteen years, whereas her sister had normal ovaries and three naturally conceived children. The sterile twin received a transplant of ovarian cortical tissue from her sister by means of a minilaparotomy. Within three months after transplantation, the recipient's cycles resumed and serum gonadotropin levels fell to the normal range. During the second cycle, she conceived, and her pregnancy progressed uneventfully. At thirty-eight weeks' gestation, she delivered a healthy-appearing female infant (87).

This work should be seen as a proof that the concept of transplantation of large segments of ovarian tissue can be successfully adopted. In these cases of identical twins, no immunosuppressive drugs are necessary. A recent report in the media (newscientist.com) by Silber et al. also have shown that transplantation into a genetically different person is possible. In that case, the patient had received a bone marrow transplant from

her sister before the whole ovary transplant. In this way, she may avoid long-term use of immunosuppressive medication. This paradigm is not the most common one, and in the vast majority of patients, there will be the potential of acute rejection and risks of long-term immunosuppressive complications on the mother such as infection and obstetrical complications may limit its use.

Given the fact that ovarian function has been documented in a small number of cases following both orthotopic and heterotopic transplantation of thawed ovarian cortical strips, the ASRM practice committee recommended that ovarian tissue cryopreservation or transplantation procedures can be performed, but only as experimental procedures under the guidelines of an internal review board (55).

In the context of a multiorgan procurement surgery that took place in approximate 150 bodies, nine specifically consented for the uterus retrieval. Del Priore et al. performed uterine extirpation during a multiorgan retrieval from a cadaver. This group demonstrated the technical feasibility in eight donors. Pedicles used included the ovarian, uterine, or internal iliac vessels. After retrieval, serial histology sections throughout the period of cold ischemia, taken every fifteen to thirty minutes, showed no signs of change over twelve hours of cold ischemia. They concluded that the human uterus can be obtained from local organ donor networks using existing protocols (88). Research for human uterus transplantation is in its infancy. Numerous methodological and technical aspects should be solved before this option could be considered.

In Vitro Maturation (IVM)

IVM of primordial follicles obtained from the frozen-thawed ovarian cortical strips is a possibility, but it is not one that will be available in the near future. Results from transplantation studies in (severe combined immune deficiency mice) SCID mice clearly show follicle maturation and completion of meiosis I in preparation for ovulation and potential fertilization (89). Concerns regarding viral infections as well as general ethical reservations may limit the use of this option in clinical practice.

To avoid seeding of malignant cells, ovarian tissue culture with in vitro follicle maturation is desirable. Isolated follicle culture from the primordial stage is an attractive option because these cells represent more than 90 percent of the total follicular reserve and can withstand cryoinjury (90). Unfortunately, isolated primordial follicles do not mature properly in culture (91), and further studies are needed to identify the factors required to sustain proper follicular growth and maturation and the role of supporting theca and granulosa cells to these processes.

IVM of antral follicles has met with some limited success. Although principally reported with patients that have polycystic ovary syndrome, it may have applications for cancer patients. Given the fact that IVM of oocytes is a safe and an effective treatment offered in some fertility centers for assisted reproduction, it could be proposed as a fertility preservation strategy as well. It avoids ovarian stimulation with expensive gonadotropins, side effects of the medications, and risks such as ovarian hyperstimulation syndrome. The spectrum of IVM indications is increasing. The candidates initially considered were women with polycystic ovaries having multiple antral follicles, but the indications are widening to include women with primarily poor-quality embryos in repeated cycles and poor responders to stimulation. The two new applications IVM are for oocyte donors and for fertility preservation, especially in women with cancer who are undergoing gonadotoxic therapy. In young women without partners needing this treatment for fertility preservation, it is combined with vitrification of the oocytes. The clinical pregnancy rate per cycle in women having IVM is close to 38 percent for infertility treatment up to the age of thirty years, and around 50 percent clinical pregnancy rate per cycle in recipients of IVM egg donation. However, the clinical usefulness of IVM as a fertility preservation strategy is yet to be determined (92,93).

FERTILITY PRESERVATION IN MALE PATIENTS

Introduction

Similarly, there is greater success in cancer therapy for males suffering from a wide variety of cancers. This particular advance in cancer therapy was associated with an increasing need to neutralize the treatment-related quality-of-life issues including fertility. Many options have been proposed to preserve the fertility of those at risk.

Fertility Preservation Option

Chemoprotection

PROPER SELECTION OF CHEMOTHERAPEUTIC REGIMENS

Not all chemotherapeutic agents are equally gonadotoxic. Deciding about the treatment protocols should account for their potential gonadotoxicity. Wherever possible, less gonadotoxic chemotherapeutic agents should be used instead. For patients in the reproductive age-group, agents that are minimally toxic but still offer maximum therapeutic effect should be selected. As in women, alkylating agents are the most gonadotoxic agents in men. The vast majority of men receiving procarbazine-containing regimens for the treatment of lymphomas are rendered permanently infertile. On the other side, treatment with doxorubicin hydrochloride (Adriamycin), bleomycin, vinblastine, and dacarbazine appears to have a significant advantage, with a return to normal fertility in the vast majority of patients. Similarly, cisplatin-based chemotherapy for testicular cancer results in temporary azoospermia in most men, with a recovery of spermatogenesis in about 50 percent of the patients after two years and 80 percent after five years (94).

HORMONAL COTREATMENT

In rat animal model, the spermatogenesis and fertility lost following treatment with radiation or some chemotherapeutic agents can be restored by suppressing testosterone with GnRH agonists or antagonists, either before or after the cytotoxic insult. The applicability of this procedure to humans is still unknown. Clinical trials should focus on treating patients with hormones during or soon after anticancer treatment. The hormone regimen should involve suppression of testosterone production with minimum androgen supplementation. This strategy is not supported by enough evidence to be used clinically (95).

Testicular Shielding

The testicular epithelium is sensitive to radiation-induced damage, with changes to spermatogonia following as little as 0.2 Gy of irradiation. Testicular doses of less than 0.2 Gy had no

significant effect on FSH levels or sperm counts, whereas doses between 0.2 and 0.7 Gy caused a transient dose-dependent increase in FSH and reduction in sperm concentration, with a return to normal values within one to two years. However, no radiation dose threshold has been defined above which permanent azoospermia is inevitable. There is increasing evidence in the literature that doses of 1.2 Gy and above are likely to be associated with a reduced risk of recovery of spermatogenesis; the time to recovery, if it is to occur, is also likely to be dose dependent (94).

Keeping the testicles outside the field of radiation or being shielded has been shown to be an effective strategy to prevent radiation-induced testicular damage. Recently, testicular shielding to irradiation has been shown to be effective in protecting testicular growth and function in long-term survivors of bone marrow transplantation during childhood or adolescence (96).

Assisted Reproductive Technologies

SEMEN CRYOPRESERVATION

Semen cryopreservation is considered to be the oldest and the most successful option ever for fertility preservation in male cancer survivors. It is a very reliable, an easy to use, and a risk-free option associated with reasonable pregnancy rate. It has been documented that cryopreserved semen from patients with a variety of malignancies as well as systemic disorders survived the freeze-thawing insults efficiently in a similar fashion to frozen sperm of normal males (42). It is always advisable to cryopreserve sperm before chemotherapy or radiotherapy to avoid any added insults to the sperm quality. The main concern in these patients is the delay in consulting the andrology lab. These males are often quite ill and have poor semen parameters. However, even in these patients, they can achieve pregnancy after thawing with assisted reproductive technology.

TESTICULAR TISSUE CRYOPRESERVATION

Besides obtaining spermatozoa from cryopreserved testicular tissues, germ cells could be autotransplanted into the patient's own testis to restore natural fertility or matured in vitro with subsequent ICSI to achieve pregnancies. However, the latest two modalities are still experimental until effective transplantation and IVM protocol could be developed. Testicular stem cell transplantation of frozen-thawed testicular cells would be of particular importance for prepubertal boys undergoing sterilizing treatment because of the fact that spermatogenesis is not active yet and the nonfeasibility of sperm cryopreservation.

CONCLUSIONS

Fertility preservation options in women are increasing but are still mostly experimental. The main determinants of selecting any given strategy include patient age, type of cancer, and type of cytotoxic chemotherapy. Embryo cryopreservation is currently the most accepted option and the only one recommended by the ASRM. Oocyte and ovarian tissue cryopreservation are currently experimental but are promising future options. Despite the emotional vulnerability of cancer patients at the time of diagnosis, there is an ethical obligation to advise them regarding the available options for fertility preservation.

Given the desire of many individuals to preserve fertility after cancer, chronic illness, iatrogenic complications of treatment, or simply with advancing age, the ESHRE Task Force on Ethics and Law considered ethical questions and specific dilemmas surrounding the cryopreservation of gametes and reproductive tissue. In view of the transition time during which research becomes therapy, the taskforce stops short of giving recommendations in anticipation of the availability of new evidence, specifically in the case of cryopreservation of reproductive tissues, IVM, and in vitro follicle culture. Consent needs to be obtained within a research context rather than for therapy or preservation of fertility per se.

Sperm cryopreservation represents the most widely accepted method for fertility preservation in male cancer patients. Other procedures, which are currently being developed, are expected to make significant contribution in these cases.

KEY POINTS FOR CLINICAL PRACTICE

■ Fertility preservation options should be offered to candidates subjected to gonadotoxic therapy for the treatment of a variety of malignant and nonmalignant conditions.

■ Chemotherapy-induced premature ovarian failure is affected mainly by the age of the patient, the drug class, cell cycle specificity, and cumulative dose of the drug.

■ Radiotherapy-induced premature ovarian failure is determined by the patient age and cumulative dose of irradiation.

■ Day 3 serum FSH, inhibin B, AMH, and basal AFC are the currently available options for ovarian reserve screening for patients at risk.

■ Embryo cryopreservation is the only established option with the best outcome for patients with a partner. However, it is not acceptable to prepubertal, adolescent girls and women without a partner.

■ For patients with estrogen-sensitive tumors, modified ovarian stimulation protocols are frequently needed to avoid supraphysiological rise of serum estradiole levels, which could be detrimental to the overall prognosis of those patient.

■ Oocyte cryopreservation presently should be considered an experimental technique only to be performed under investigational protocol under the auspices of an IRB.

■ Ovarian tissue cryopreservation or transplantation procedures should be performed only as experimental procedures under IRB guidelines.

■ Ovarian transposition could be performed laparoscopically prior to the initiation of radiotherapy.

■ Sperm cryopreservation represents the most widely accepted method for fertility preservation in male cancer patients.

REFERENCES

1. Green DM, Whitton JA, Stovall M, et al. Pregnancy outcome of female survivors of childhood cancer: a report from the Childhood Cancer Survivor Study. *Am J Obstet Gynecol* 2002; **187**(4):1070–80.

2. Block E. A quantitative morphological investigation of the follicular system in newborn female infants. *Acta Anat (Basel)* 1953; **17**(3):201–6.

3. Forabosco A, Sforza C, De Pol A, Vizzotto L, Marzona L, Ferrario VF. Morphometric study of the human neonatal ovary. *Anat Rec* 1991;**231**(2):201–8.

4. Gougeon A. Regulation of ovarian follicular development in primates: facts and hypotheses. *Endocr Rev* 1996;**17**(2):121–55.

5. Fauser BC, Van Heusden AM. Manipulation of human ovarian function: physiological concepts and clinical consequences. *Endocr Rev* 1997;**18**(1):71–106.

6. Wandji SA, Srsen V, Voss AK, Eppig JJ, Fortune JE. Initiation in vitro of growth of bovine primordial follicles. *Biol Reprod* 1996;**55**(5):942–8.

7. Oktay K, Briggs D, Gosden RG. Ontogeny of follicle-stimulating hormone receptor gene expression in isolated human ovarian follicles. *J Clin Endocrinol Metab* 1997;**82**(11):3748–51.

8. Ahmed CE, Dees WL, Ojeda SR. The immature rat ovary is innervated by vasoactive intestinal peptide (VIP)-containing fibers and responds to VIP with steroid secretion. *Endocrinology* 1986;**118**(4):1682–9.

9. Ezoe K, Holmes SA, Ho L, et al. Novel mutations and deletions of the KIT (steel factor receptor) gene in human piebaldism. *Am J Hum Genet* 1995;**56**(1):58–66.

10. Elvin JA, Clark AT, Wang P, Wolfman NM, Matzuk MM. Paracrine actions of growth differentiation factor-9 in the mammalian ovary. *Mol Endocrinol* 1999;**13**(6):1035–48.

11. Dong J, Albertini DF, Nishimori K, Kumar TR, Lu N, Matzuk MM. Growth differentiation factor-9 is required during early ovarian folliculogenesis. *Nature* 1996;**383**(6600):531–5.

12. Elvin JA, Yan C, Wang P, Nishimori K, Matzuk MM. Molecular characterization of the follicle defects in the growth differentiation factor 9-deficient ovary. *Mol Endocrinol* 1999;**13**(6):1018–34.

13. Dube JL, Wang P, Elvin J, Lyons KM, Celeste AJ, Matzuk MM. The bone morphogenetic protein 15 gene is X-linked and expressed in oocytes. *Mol Endocrinol* 1998;**12**(12):1809–17.

14. Johnson J, Canning J, Kaneko T, Pru JK, Tilly JL. Germline stem cells and follicular renewal in the postnatal mammalian ovary. *Nature* 2004;**428**(6979):145–50.

15. Johnson J, Bagley J, Skaznik-Wikiel M, et al. Oocyte generation in adult mammalian ovaries by putative germ cells in bone marrow and peripheral blood. *Cell* 2005;**122**(2):303–15.

16. Gosden RG. Germline stem cells in the postnatal ovary: is the ovary more like a testis? *Hum Reprod Update* 2004;**10**(3):193–5.

17. Telfer EE. Germline stem cells in the postnatal mammalian ovary: a phenomenon of prosimian primates and mice? *Reprod Biol Endocrinol* 2004;**2**:24.

18. Telfer EE, Gosden RG, Byskov AG, et al. On regenerating the ovary and generating controversy. *Cell* 2005;**122**(6):821–2.

19. Manger K, Wildt L, Kalden JR, Manger B. Prevention of gonadal toxicity and preservation of gonadal function and fertility in young women with systemic lupus erythematosus treated by cyclophosphamide: the PREGO-Study. *Autoimmun Rev* 2006; **5**(4):269–72.

20. Schilsky RL, Sherins RJ, Hubbard SM, Wesley MN, Young RC, DeVita VT. Long-term follow up of ovarian function in women treated with MOPP chemotherapy for Hodgkin's disease. *Am J Med* 1981;**71**(4):552–6.

21. Blumenfeld Z, Avivi I, Linn S, Epelbaum R, Ben-Shahar M, Haim N. Prevention of irreversible chemotherapy-induced ovarian damage in young women with lymphoma by a gonadotrophin-releasing hormone agonist in parallel to chemotherapy. *Hum Reprod* 1996;**11**(8):1620–6.

22. BFS. MWGcbt. A strategy for fertility services for survivors of childhood cancer. Hum Fertil 2003;**6**:A1–40.

23. Bath LE, Tydeman G, Critchley HO, Anderson RA, Baird DT, Wallace WH. Spontaneous conception in a young woman who had ovarian cortical tissue cryopreserved before chemotherapy and radiotherapy for a Ewing's sarcoma of the pelvis: case report. *Hum Reprod* 2004;**19**(11):2569–72.

24. Meirow D, Nugent D. The effects of radiotherapy and chemotherapy on female reproduction. *Hum Reprod Update* 2001;7(6):535–43.

25. Husseinzadeh N, Nahhas WA, Velkley DE, Whitney CW, Mortel R. The preservation of ovarian function in young women undergoing pelvic radiation therapy. *Gynecol Oncol* 1984;18(3): 373–9.

26. Gaetini A, De Simone M, Urgesi A, et al. Lateral high abdominal ovariopexy: an original surgical technique for protection of the ovaries during curative radiotherapy for Hodgkin's disease. *J Surg Oncol* 1988;39(1):22–8.

27. Williams RS, Littell RD, Mendenhall NP. Laparoscopic oophoropexy and ovarian function in the treatment of Hodgkin disease. *Cancer* 1999;86(10):2138–42.

28. Meirow D, Schenker JG, Rosler A. Ovarian hyperstimulation syndrome with low oestradiol in non-classical 17 alpha-hydroxylase, 17,20-lyase deficiency: what is the role of oestrogens? *Hum Reprod* 1996;11(10):2119–21.

29. Gosden RG, Wade JC, Fraser HM, Sandow J, Faddy MJ. Impact of congenital or experimental hypogonadotrophism on the radiation sensitivity of the mouse ovary. *Hum Reprod* 1997;12(11): 2483–8.

30. Wallace WH, Thomson AB, Kelsey TW. The radiosensitivity of the human oocyte. *Hum Reprod* 2003;18(1):117–21.

31. Bath LE, Wallace WH, Shaw MP, Fitzpatrick C, Anderson RA. Depletion of ovarian reserve in young women after treatment for cancer in childhood: detection by anti-Mullerian hormone, inhibin B and ovarian ultrasound. *Hum Reprod* 2003;18(11): 2368–74.

32. Crofton PM, Thomson AB, Evans AE, et al. Is inhibin B a potential marker of gonadotoxicity in prepubertal children treated for cancer? *Clin Endocrinol (Oxf)* 2003;58(3):296–301.

33. Feyereisen E, Mendez Lozano DH, Taieb J, Hesters L, Frydman R, Fanchin R. Anti-Mullerian hormone: clinical insights into a promising biomarker of ovarian follicular status. *Reprod Biomed Online* 2006;12(6):695–703.

34. Weir HK, Thun MJ, Hankey BF, et al. Annual report to the nation on the status of cancer, 1975-2000, featuring the uses of surveillance data for cancer prevention and control. *J Natl Cancer Inst* 2003;95(17):1276–99.

35. Jemal A, Murray T, Samuels A, Ghafoor A, Ward E, Thun MJ. Cancer statistics, 2003. *CA Cancer J Clin* 2003;53(1):5–26.

36. Chiarelli AM, Marrett LD, Darlington G. Early menopause and infertility in females after treatment for childhood cancer diagnosed in 1964-1988 in Ontario, Canada. *Am J Epidemiol* 1999; 150(3):245–54.

37. Tangir J, Zelterman D, Ma W, Schwartz PE. Reproductive function after conservative surgery and chemotherapy for malignant germ cell tumors of the ovary. *Obstet Gynecol* 2003;101(2): 251–7.

38. Blumenfeld Z, Dann E, Avivi I, Epelbaum R, Rowe JM. Fertility after treatment for Hodgkin's disease. *Ann Oncol* 2002;13(Suppl. 1):138–47.

39. Pereyra Pacheco B, Mendez Ribas JM, Milone G, et al. Use of GnRH analogs for functional protection of the ovary and preservation of fertility during cancer treatment in adolescents: a preliminary report. *Gynecol Oncol* 2001;81(3):391–7.

40. Fox KR BJ, Mik R, Moore HC. Prevention of chemotherapy-associated amenorrhea (CRA) with leuprolide in young women with early stage breast cancer (Abstract). *Proc Ann Soc Clin Oncol* 2001(20):25a.

41. Waxman JH, Ahmed R, Smith D, et al. Failure to preserve fertility in patients with Hodgkin's disease. *Cancer Chemother Pharmacol* 1987;19(2):159–62.

42. Howell SJ, Shalet SM. Fertility preservation and management of gonadal failure associated with lymphoma therapy. *Curr Oncol Rep* 2002;4(5):443–52.

43. Covens AL, van der Putten HW, Fyles AW, et al. Laparoscopic ovarian transposition. *Eur J Gynaecol Oncol* 1996;17(3):177–82.

44. Hadar H, Loven D, Herskovitz P, Bairey O, Yagoda A, Levavi H. An evaluation of lateral and medial transposition of the ovaries out of radiation fields. *Cancer* 1994;74(2):774–9.

45. Howard FM. Laparoscopic lateral ovarian transposition before radiation treatment of Hodgkin disease. *J Am Assoc Gynecol Laparosc* 1997;4(5):601–4.

46. Anderson B, LaPolla J, Turner D, Chapman G, Buller R. Ovarian transposition in cervical cancer. *Gynecol Oncol* 1993;49(2): 206–14.

47. Treissman MJ, Miller D, McComb PF. Laparoscopic lateral ovarian transposition. *Fertil Steril* 1996;65(6):1229–31.

48. Yarali H, Demirol A, Bukulmez O, Coskun F, Gurgan T. Laparoscopic high lateral transposition of both ovaries before pelvic irradiation. *J Am Assoc Gynecol Laparosc* 2000;7(2):237–9.

49. Clough KB, Goffinet F, Labib A, et al. Laparoscopic unilateral ovarian transposition prior to irradiation: prospective study of 20 cases. *Cancer* 1996;77(12):2638–45.

50. Feeney DD, Moore DH, Look KY, Stehman FB, Sutton GP. The fate of the ovaries after radical hysterectomy and ovarian transposition. *Gynecol Oncol* 1995;56(1):3–7.

51. Chambers SK, Chambers JT, Holm C, Peschel RE, Schwartz PE. Sequelae of lateral ovarian transposition in unirradiated cervical cancer patients. *Gynecol Oncol* 1990;39(2):155–9.

52. Magistrini M, Szollosi D. Effects of cold and of isopropyl-N-phenylcarbamate on the second meiotic spindle of mouse oocytes. *Eur J Cell Biol* 1980;22(2):699–707.

53. Stachecki JJ, Cohen J, Willadsen S. Detrimental effects of sodium during mouse oocyte cryopreservation. *Biol Reprod* 1998;59(2): 395–400.

54. Porcu E, Fabbri R, Damiano G, Fratto R, Giunchi S, Venturoli S. Oocyte cryopreservation in oncological patients. *Eur J Obstet Gynecol Reprod Biol* 2004;113 (Suppl. 1):S14–16.

55. Ovarian tissue and oocyte cryopreservation. *Fertil Steril* 2004;82(4):993–8.

56. Oktay K, Cil AP, Bang H. Efficiency of oocyte cryopreservation: a meta-analysis. *Fertil Steril* 2006;86(1):70–80.

57. Jain JK, Paulson RJ. Oocyte cryopreservation. *Fertil Steril* 2006;86 (Suppl. 4):1037–46.

58. Assisted reproductive technology in the United States: 1998 results generated from the American Society for Reproductive Medicine/Society for Assisted Reproductive Technology Registry. *Fertil Steril* 2002;77(1):18–31.

59. Wang JX, Yap YY, Matthews CD. Frozen-thawed embryo transfer: influence of clinical factors on implantation rate and risk of multiple conception. *Hum Reprod* 2001;16(11):2316–19.

60. Son WY, Yoon SH, Yoon HJ, Lee SM, Lim JH. Pregnancy outcome following transfer of human blastocysts vitrified on electron microscopy grids after induced collapse of the blastocoele. *Hum Reprod* 2003;18(1):137–9.

61. Meniru GI, Craft I. In vitro fertilization and embryo cryopreservation prior to hysterectomy for cervical cancer. *Int J Gynaecol Obstet* 1997;56(1):69–70.

62. Pena JE, Chang PL, Chan LK, Zeitoun K, Thornton MH2nd, Sauer MV. Supraphysiological estradiol levels do not affect oocyte and embryo quality in oocyte donation cycles. *Hum Reprod* 2002;17(1):83–7.

63. Pelinck MJ, Hoek A, Simons AH, Heineman MJ. Efficacy of natural cycle IVF: a review of the literature. *Hum Reprod Update* 2002;8(2):129–39.

64. Oktay K, Buyuk E, Davis O, Yermakova I, Veeck L, Rosenwaks Z. Fertility preservation in breast cancer patients: IVF and embryo cryopreservation after ovarian stimulation with tamoxifen. *Hum Reprod* 2003;**18**(1):90–5.

65. Oktay K, Buyuk E, Akar Z, Rosenwaks N, Libertella N. Fertility preservation in breast cancer patients: a prospective controlled comparison of ovarian stimulation with tamoxifen and letrozole for embryo cryopreservation. *Fertil Steril* 2004;**82**(2):s1(Abstract).

66. Oktay K. Further evidence on the safety and success of ovarian stimulation with letrozole and tamoxifen in breast cancer patients undergoing in vitro fertilization to cryopreserve their embryos for fertility preservation. *J Clin Oncol* 2005;**23**(16):3858–9.

67. Mazur P. The role of intracellular freezing in the death of cells cooled at supraoptimal rates. *Cryobiology* 1977;**14**(3):251–72.

68. Gosden RG, Baird DT, Wade JC, Webb R. Restoration of fertility to oophorectomized sheep by ovarian autografts stored at -196 degrees C. *Hum Reprod* 1994;**9**(4):597–603.

69. Baird DT, Webb R, Campbell BK, Harkness LM, Gosden RG. Long-term ovarian function in sheep after ovariectomy and transplantation of autografts stored at −196 C. *Endocrinology* 1999;**140**(1):462–71.

70. Almodin CG, Minguetti-Camara VC, Meister H, Ceschin AP, Kriger E, Ferreira JO. Recovery of natural fertility after grafting of cryopreserved germinative tissue in ewes subjected to radiotherapy. *Fertil Steril* 2004;**81**(1):160–4.

71. Israely T, Nevo N, Harmelin A, Neeman M, Tsafriri A. Reducing ischaemic damage in rodent ovarian xenografts transplanted into granulation tissue. *Hum Reprod* 2006;**21**(6):1368–79.

72. Jeremias E, Bedaiwy MA, Nelson D, Biscotti CV, Falcone T. Assessment of tissue injury in cryopreserved ovarian tissue. *Fertil Steril* 2003;**79**(3):651–3.

73. Hussein MR, Bedaiwy MA, Falcone T. Analysis of apoptotic cell death, Bcl-2, and p53 protein expression in freshly fixed and cryopreserved ovarian tissue after exposure to warm ischemia. *Fertil Steril* 2006;**85** (Suppl. 1):1082–92.

74. Jeremias E, Bedaiwy MA, Gurunluoglu R, Biscotti CV, Siemionow M, Falcone T. Heterotopic autotransplantation of the ovary with microvascular anastomosis: a novel surgical technique. *Fertil Steril* 2002;**77**(6):1278–82.

75. Bedaiwy MA, Jeremias E, Gurunluoglu R, et al. Restoration of ovarian function after autotransplantation of intact frozen-thawed sheep ovaries with microvascular anastomosis. *Fertil Steril* 2003;**79**(3):594–602.

76. Wang X, Chen H, Yin H, Kim SS, Lin Tan S, Gosden RG. Fertility after intact ovary transplantation. *Nature* 2002;**415**(6870):385.

77. Bedaiwy MA, Falcone T. Harvesting and autotransplantation of vascularized ovarian grafts: approaches and techniques. *RBM Online* 2007;**14**(3):360–71.

78. Imhof M, Bergmeister H, Lipovac M, Rudas M, Hofstetter G, Huber J. Orthotopic microvascular reanastomosis of whole cryopreserved ovine ovaries resulting in pregnancy and live birth. *Fertil Steril* 2006;**85**(Suppl. 1):1208–15.

79. Dittrich R, Maltaris T, Mueller A, et al. Successful uterus cryopreservation in an animal model. *Horm Metab Res* 2006;**38**(3):141–5.

80. Chen CH, Chen SG, Wu GJ, Wang J, Yu CP, Liu JY. Autologous heterotopic transplantation of intact rabbit ovary after frozen banking at −196 degrees C. *Fertil Steril* 2006;**86**(Suppl. 4):1059–66.

81. Sonmezer M, Oktay K. Fertility preservation in female patients. *Hum Reprod Update* 2004;**10**(3):251–66.

82. Oktay K, Buyuk E, Veeck L, et al. Embryo development after heterotopic transplantation of cryopreserved ovarian tissue. *Lancet* 2004;**363**(9412):837–40.

83. Donnez J, Dolmans MM, Demylle D, et al. Livebirth after orthotopic transplantation of cryopreserved ovarian tissue. *Lancet* 2004;**364**(9443):1405–10.

84. Meirow D, Levron J, Eldar-Geva T, et al. Pregnancy after transplantation of cryopreserved ovarian tissue in a patient with ovarian failure after chemotherapy. *N Engl J Med* 2005;**353**(3):318–21.

85. Oktay K, Nugent D, Newton H, Salha O, Chatterjee P, Gosden RG. Isolation and characterization of primordial follicles from fresh and cryopreserved human ovarian tissue. *Fertil Steril* 1997;**67**(3):481–6.

86. Aubard Y. Ovarian tissue graft: from animal experiment to practice in the human. *Eur J Obstet Gynecol Reprod Biol* 1999;**86**(1):1–3.

87. Silber SJ, Lenahan KM, Levine DJ, et al. Ovarian transplantation between monozygotic twins discordant for premature ovarian failure. *N Engl J Med* 2005;**353**(1):58–63.

88. Del Priore G, Stega J, Sieunarine K, Ungar L, Smith JR. Human uterus retrieval from a multi-organ donor. *Obstet Gynecol* 2007;**109**(1):101–4.

89. Gook DA, Edgar DH, Borg J, Archer J, Lutjen PJ, McBain JC. Oocyte maturation, follicle rupture and luteinization in human cryopreserved ovarian tissue following xenografting. *Hum Reprod* 2003;**18**(9):1772–81.

90. Smitz JE, Cortvrindt RG. The earliest stages of folliculogenesis in vitro. *Reproduction* 2002;**123**(2):185–202.

91. Abir R, Fisch B, Nitke S, Okon E, Raz A, Ben Rafael Z. Morphological study of fully and partially isolated early human follicles. *Fertil Steril* 2001;**75**(1):141–6.

92. Rao GD, Chian RC, Son WS, Gilbert L, Tan SL. Fertility preservation in women undergoing cancer treatment. *Lancet* 2004;**363**(9423):1829–30.

93. Rao GD, Tan SL. In vitro maturation of oocytes. *Semin Reprod Med* 2005;**23**(3):242–7.

94. Howell SJ, Shalet SM. Spermatogenesis after cancer treatment: damage and recovery. *J Natl Cancer Inst Monogr* 2005(34):12–17.

95. Meistrich ML, Shetty G. Suppression of testosterone stimulates recovery of spermatogenesis after cancer treatment. *Int J Androl* 2003;**26**(3):141–6.

96. Ishiguro H, Yasuda Y, Tomita Y, et al. Gonadal shielding to irradiation is effective in protecting testicular growth and function in long-term survivors of bone marrow transplantation during childhood or adolescence. *Bone Marrow Transplant* 2007.

71

ETHICAL DILEMMAS IN ART: CURRENT ISSUES

Françoise Shenfield

Most treatments in assisted reproduction raise ethical issues, and it is difficult to be exhaustive and detailed. Nevertheless, the aim of this chapter was to highlight the main ethical concerns that have been discussed since the inception of the complex, although now routine, technique of IVF. That the human embryo could be observed outside the body captured the world's imagination, in a different way than, for instance, the less technically taxing but older techniques of sperm donation. This had also led to many debates, and so do eternal themes, which return only because of the use of more modern technology like social sex selection. This chapter will cover gametes donation for reproduction and research, including embryo research and the newer issues around stem cell research, a subject of major current interest, rekindled by the therapeutic hopes from the possible use of embryonic stem cells, with or without somatic cell nuclear transfer technology (SCNT). Furthermore, the complex choices to be made in the use of preimplantation genetic diagnosis (1) are also the matter for ethical debate, and finally, one should not avoid the international concerns about sex selection for social reasons, an issue that has implications far outside the specialist field of ART. Other more specialized issues, from the cryopreservation of reproductive tissues (2) to the use of posthumous gametes (3), have been included in previous publications.

Thus, the choice of emphasis in this chapter is necessarily eclectic, but one should start with an issue relevant to care in general, in particular, access to treatments and justice. Access to fertility treatments is far from equitable worldwide as some countries will only provide private or restricted treatments. Restricted access to IVF, however, occurs not only in resource-poor countries but also in some wealthy countries. One may thus contrast France and the UK, with their number of IVF cycles and funding policies vastly differing (4), and certainly, the UK postcode access to IVF treatment, with its double pronged iniquity (5), is an example that is still now relevant to daily practice.

GAMETE DONATION

Two main issues surround gamete donation: the traditional and more recently questioned anonymity of the gamete donor, which must be put in the context of the sense of identity of the offspring in relation to that of his/her intended (or psychosocial) parents and to his/her origins and; the other issue, older still, but often rekindled especially when donation becomes scarcer – should donors be paid, an oxymoron (6), or compensated for their donation and what is fair compensation?

Furthermore, the fact that sperm donation has been used for many years means that we have more evidence about the follow-up of children born from this method than for the offspring of oocyte (or embryo) donation, two techniques requiring the use of IVF. But before analyzing what is relevant to knowing one's origins, mention must be made of the issue of payment or compensation of the donors.

It seems obvious, at least from a semantic point of view (7), that a gift should be free. Indeed, the fact is that if society intends to pay gametes donors, the term "donation" itself should be changed to "sale" of gametes and embryos.

However, in most countries where gamete donation is used as a means of solving infertility problems, those who recruit the donors have difficulties matching the supply to the demand, especially in the case of oocytes. Thus, it has been argued that pragmatism should prevail in a scarce supply environment and that some type of financial inducement should certainly not be forbidden. In the UK, this, of course, must be within the frame of English law, which states that "no money or other kind of benefit shall be given or received in respect of any supply of gametes or embryos unless authorised by directions" (8). The notion of gifting is also enshrined, among others, in the law in France and Spain, although there compensation is given as a lump sum to egg donors.

With the conviction that the human body and its parts and products should remain outside commerce, one can attempt a rational argument in the realm of ethics, in order to outline the theoretical basis to altruistic donation. The special respect due to the person was most cogently articulated more than 200 years ago by Immanuel Kant. It stems from the observance of the second formulation of the categorical imperative, "to treat all humanity always at the same time as an end and never merely as a means," and is understood in modern terms as a prohibition of commercialization of the human body and its products.

The opposite utilitarian attitude has proposed that in a scarce-supply environment, one might choose to pay donors. But negative consequences identified by Titmuss about the payment for blood donation can be applied to gametes donation: this may deter genuine altruistic donors (9) and there may be an increased risk of transmitting disease by donors motivated by gain only and willing to falsify information and, especially, the risk of potential exploitation of the weakest socioeconomic groups of society (10). This very argument of potential coercion is that used by opponents to egg sharing, a pragmatic approach used in the UK to increase oocyte donation, and indeed the only possible way to donate oocyte in Denmark, in order to protect women from taking the risks of stimulation and egg retrieval they would not otherwise ensue. The HFE Act 1990 allowed benefits for female donors (those allowed being treatment services and sterilization), and the debate can be thus summed up: is this a form of coercion to donate or a form of payment or is it an acceptable "exchange"? An objection to the practice has been that it may compromise the chance of success of the donor, but her selection (young, with polycystic ovaries, and a male problem, for instance) may obviate this. Therefore, a perhaps even harsher dilemma involves the potential egg sharer who is refused because she is too old or has a prejudiced ovarian reserve, especially if she finds the cost of the procedure difficult to bear. It goes without saying that the counseling in such cases is even more complex, time consuming, and essential, as recommended in the UK by the HFEA code of Practice (11). But the main objection remains this intrinsic to the fact that the practice may be regarded as payment (12): indeed, there is now some evidence from Belgium about the degree of financial necessity, if not coercion, that may apply (13) as the number of women volunteering to share declined sharply after Belgium insurance became more generous of reimbursment of cycles.

Concerning the theme of anonymity, a recent change in UK law highlights the complexities involved: since 2005, similarly to Sweden from 1985, all new gamete donors must undertake to give their name at the offspring majority (14). Whether this will deter new donors, especially egg sharers who would find out eighteen years later that their recipient was successful, and if they were not, time only will tell, although national figures collated by the HFEA already show a decrease in number of donors in 2005.

New studies concerning children who have been told of their origins will offer evidence on the lack of secrecy of the procedure of gamete donation, but we may have to wait a long time before being able to observe the effects of known donation on children. The question is the meaning of knowing one's origins, a matter of importance to each and everyone of us, but one that has many different meanings, historical, psychological, and anthropological, while arguably the meaning of genetic origins is newer to humans than that of kinship in general.

Powerful voices of anger and distress of some children of sperm donation have been heard (15), arguing that they have been deprived of specific knowledge, the identity of the genetic sperm provider (avoiding the legal and emotional term father), information without which they do not find their sense of identity complete. We know, however, that in most cases, the interests of children and parents seem to coincide as several studies have already shown that children conceived by "assisted reproduction" fare very well in several measured personal and social criteria, when compared to children conceived "naturally" or adopted (16). Another argument used is that of "the right of the child" to know his/her "origins" and the potentially divisive role of secrets in families. When one enters the area of rights and finds a conflict of interests between those claiming rights, it is difficult to ascertain which one of them might take precedence. In this particular case, do we, for instance, prioritize the "right to privacy" of the parents and donors or the "right to know" of the prospective child. Thus, balancing parental choice, which is generally assumed to be benevolent to the offspring until proved otherwise, and children's interests, the European Society of Human Reproduction and Embryology (ESHRE) taskforce

recommendations (17) upheld the double-gate system, recently rescinded in the Netherlands. This system enabled parents and donors to choose or not choose the disclosure of identity later and to match thus prospective parents and donors. The fact that we have no evidence that the outcome is not generally at least as good as that of naturally conceived offspring is reassuring, but we must not forget our (ethical) responsibility to these children as a profession and indeed our (legal) duty of care, whether general or specific, as it is in UK law. It is indeed our duty to look prospectively and reflect on different approaches. For the time being, it seems that democratic openness to different approaches in families and the respect of their privacy favors a double-strand approach (18), with all the consequences for the children for whom we are jointly responsible.

PGD, WITH OR WITHOUT HLA MATCHING TO CHOOSE A SAVIOR SIBLING

Ever since it was first practiced, preimplantation genetic diagnosis (PGD) has evoked the fear of potential genetic manipulation and been criticized as a step on the slippery slope to criminal eugenics (19). If eugenics is defined as a practice imposed on a population and not in terms of individual couples' choice to avert possible serious disease (cystic fibrosis, for instance), this accusation can be refuted (20). Other fears voiced were whether it would lead couples to expect the assurance of a "perfect" baby, while all they wish for is a normal child, not affected by grave familial disease. But most questions are similar to those encountered in antenatal practice, when screening, and it may be argued that PGD could be called "pregravid diagnosis," enabling couples with serious genetic disease to avoid the suffering of deciding to terminate an affected pregnancy, while also taking on the burden of going through IVF when they are most often fertile. Their decision is enabled through information, including genetic counseling, a key to their autonomy. The aim of an unaffected pregnancy takes into account the welfare of the future child, an essential criterion in our specialty (21).

A newer dilemma is that of choosing by PGD an embryo free of a disease to facilitate the birth of a savior sibling, a child who would be an HLA match for a very sick older sibling (22).

The main argument against this kind of request by the parents is the instrumentalization of the future child. This dilemma is illustrated by two different cases that originated in the UK: either the child conceived by PGD and embryo transfer (ET) is also at risk of the genetic disease affecting the older sibling, as for the Hashmi family, or this future child has no such risk and PGD is solely performed for HLA typing, as for the Whittaker family.

In the UK, each PGD case must be licensed by the HFEA, and the Hashmis' request was accepted as they wished for an embryo to be matched to their seriously ill son with thalassemia, for whom all other treatment had become ineffective. However, the Whitakers' was refused because their sick child suffered from Diamond-Blackfan anemia, a disease that is mostly nongenetic, and thus the future planned child was not at risk of this condition and would be planned perhaps "merely" to save the older sibling. After much public debate, and a successful PGD in Chicago resulting in the birth of a savior sibling, the HFEA stated the following year that further similar cases would be licensed in the UK. Thus, the danger to the life of the existing sibling serves as the compelling reason to accept the technique. Even from the point of view of the future child, it may be seen as beneficial to be able to save its sibling as a matter of solidarity and seems acceptable if the future child's operation involves minimal risk (e.g., cord blood or bone marrow donation). Practical issues inform the consent obtained from the parents, like the fact that cord blood donation is only possible if the affected child weighs less than 25 kg and the fact that the technique is less likely to give results if the woman's age is thirty-eight years or more (23). In all cases, counseling may help the parents to foresee difficult events, as the failure of the initial aim, for instance: what if there is no embryo to match the sick child and what if the planned child does not save the life of the elder sibling?

Another problem concerns the acceptability of the motive for the selection of embryos: there the "postnatal" test is useful as it states (22) that it is ethically acceptable to enable the birth of a child by PGD/HLA who can be used for a certain goal if it is acceptable to use an existing child for the same goal (i.e., if it is acceptable to volunteer an existing child for stem cell donation to a sibling and if it is acceptable to enable this birth by PGD/HLA). But the creation of a child for the purpose of harvesting non regenerating organs seems extremely difficult to justify in view of the risks involved for the donor child, and adults' self-interest is unacceptable (i.e., not for parents themselves).

Finally, some have specified that this solution is morally acceptable if the use as a donor is not the only motive for the parents to have the child; but parental motivation is particularly difficult to assess (23), and thus, the postnatal test is preferred, as long as the parents "intend to love and care for this child to the same extent as they love and care for the affected child."

CLONING AND THE USE OF EMBRYO'S STEM CELLS

Let us first dispose of the issue of human reproductive cloning: in articles and comments (mostly) condemning reproductive cloning, words like dignity, identity, sameness, and the moral sense of "self" have been analyzed at length (24), not withstanding the fact that the technique is far from safe, which provides the main and overwhelming objection. One may also object on the grounds that reproductive cloning would threaten the autonomy of the future cloned person who may be treated by society as somewhat predetermined, entailing as it does an increase in (genetic) determinism even if relative as the clone is born into another environment than the person replicated. Safety and the psychological arguments seem to be the only arguments worth opposing the proponents of reproductive cloning: the narcissistic venture of the parent(s) may well threaten the building of the identity of the child, mostly by decreasing the possibility of separation from the initial model and thus his/her autonomy.

It is with this in mind that the ESHRE issued a statement "to continue the ban on reproductive cloning," after a five-year voluntary moratorium on reproductive cloning in 1999, when it became clear that technical advances arising from cloning animals could theoretically result in an attempt to clone a human.

Fortunately, the repulsion caused almost universally by reproductive cloning has not been universally matched by the same feelings or arguments concerning the use of stem cells from human embryos. Indeed, UK was the first state to allow therapeutic cloning (25): embryo research has been licensed under strict conditions since the HFE Act 1990, permitting only research linked to reproduction. After a democratic process involving a report by the chief medical officer and a vote in both chambers, new categories were added to statute January 31, 2001, allowing this time "research for serious disease." In all cases, though, the vexed question of the status of the human embryo has been rekindled.

Thus, aware of the potential exploitation of semantic games when discussing embryo research in general, the ESHRE task-force defined the preimplantation embryo in its first ethics consideration on behalf of the society (26). The taskforce stressed that this term was descriptive, meaning the embryo out of the body before it is given a chance of becoming a fetus and then a legal person by ET. But such a descriptive term does not imply a lesser quality.

Meanwhile, specific issues arise from the possible application of stem cells animal research to the human embryo.

Many fundamental ethical questions in this field are far from new. Indeed, consent must be obtained for research, reflecting the principle of autonomy. But the taskforce stresses "in view of the special nature of stem cells and their longevity, it should be specifically mentioned that the embryos will be used for research into the establishment of cell lines which can be kept indefinitely, may eventually be used for therapeutic purposes, and will never be replaced into a uterus. It should also be made clear whether the cells may be used for commercial and/or clinical purposes," making consent more specific than general.

There are also specific ethical considerations according to source of cells and especially regarding the creation of embryos specifically for research. Indeed, this question of the creation of embryos for research is especially vexed. While article 18 of the European Convention on Human Rights and Biomedicine (27) specifically forbids this, in the UK, the HFEA is charged with overseeing embryo research within the legal limits, by a licensing system: the creation of embryos de novo for research is not unlawful, but its "necessity" must be demonstrated, ensuring that embryos are not created for futile reasons, that indeed this creation de novo is licensed only if the information cannot be obtained by research on supernumerary zygotes.

Furthermore, in practice, the source of oocytes used for any embryos created (especially by SCNT) is a major problem, for two reasons. First, the already well-documented imbalance between needs and supply in the case of egg donation for reproductive purpose. But of special concern is the potential abuse of vulnerable women who might be enticed to sell their oocytes. Indeed, recent publications (28) have questioned the conditions of oocyte donation for research and the pressure put on women to take risks when "compensated" for their "gift". Interestingly, however, there was little mention of the compensation to women giving oocytes for reproduction, when this is sometimes far beyond this recommended by the ASRM ethics committee (29). This could be called the oocyte paradox, where value seems to vary according to the use to which oocytes will be put. It is possible that the concern of payment in this case reflects the fundamentalist stance on the status of the embryo, expressed by those opposed to the creation of embryos for research in general, rather than a concern for the women involved.

Several statements (30, 31) already highlight the issues that came to public notice with a vengeance when it was realized that the Korean experiments were not only faked but also breached the autonomy of women who had been coerced into giving their oocytes in the project, cumulating most possible sins to be performed in research (32).

Furthermore, as transborder iniquities may be worse than national ones (mostly for reason of sometimes great economic disparity), avoiding recruiting women abroad for egg donation might be a solution, even partial, to this problem (31).

SEX SELECTION FOR SOCIAL REASONS

The matter of gender social selection, which we discuss here within the frame of ART, is not novel in historical terms: baby girls have been exposed on the hill side to die from time immemorial and female and adolescent children submitted to negative discrimination in health and education of old in many societies. But the availability of technology, whether low key (sperm selection) or complex and intensive (PGD), has rendered the efficacy of sex selection more accurate and therefore less innocuous than the old mythology of having sex at a certain time or ingesting a special regime at conception in order to achieve the desired effect.

The facts are still that at the worldwide level, the practice of gender selection is more often to favor the birth of a son rather than a daughter (33, 34) and is, therefore, a women's rights issue. But in order to be nondiscriminatory against either sex, this debate is placed within the Human Rights context. This framework stresses its political connotation, as well as the ethical aspects, within the context of a universal rule and against cultural relativism.

The background is that of gender inequality worldwide, and as the social anthropologist M. Strathern said in 1993 "it is worth asking whether making (sex selection) acceptable to select one sex in preference to another at the moment of conception will make it easier or harder to promote anti-discriminatory measures in other areas of life" (35).

Indeed, gender discrimination is common worldwide and can have many guises. The obvious imbalance of sex ratio observed in areas of India (34) and China (36) is one extreme piece of evidence of its occurrence. In India, where A. Sen recently concludes that "reduction in female mortality has been counterbalanced by sex selective abortions," evidence has been surmised from a survey of births in 1.1 million households (37), concluding that the imbalanced ratio stems from the use of prenatal ultrasound gender diagnosis followed by TOP [Sheth (38)], although India passed in January 1996 the Pre-Natal Diagnostic Techniques (Regulation and Prevention of Misuse) Act. This had little effect, till recent years, as only 300 practitioners have been sued in India, with the medical profession accused of "arrogance." However, the jailing of Anil Sabhani in the state of Haryana may, represent a turning point (39). We know that worldwide, prenatal sex determination is performed with a view to terminate a pregnancy of the "wrong" sex merely for social reasons; this is actually in most legislations an illegal abortion. For instance, the Canadian example shows, however, how some women (mostly of Indian origin) cross the border to the United States to have fetal sex determination and return for a TOP in Canada, if the child is of the unwanted sex, when this is still acceptable within legal limits for "distress" (40).

China faces similar bias in some regions (36), but dissenting voices are coming from the National Institute of Philosophy, which declared in June 2004 that it was time to act and

recommended, in particular, the licensing and monitoring of the use of ultrasound machines and especially the application of existing laws against gender discrimination.

Till recently, some European countries were allowing by defect the seemingly innocuous methods of sperm sorting for couples to choose the sex of their offspring because only ART methods were covered by legislation. In such countries, discrimination is measured in general by educational and economic analysis rather than by sheer number of men and women but is nevertheless still a sizeable problem. However, recent national debates in Belgium and the UK have resulted in the banning of social sex selection, and the advice that evensperm sorting by flow cytometry should be subject to regulations (41), confirming that moral appraisal of such a grave issue does not depend on the method used. This contradicts the "gradualist" view that gender selection by PGD, or termination of pregnancy, is worse morally than if performed by a simple technique like sperm sorting. The logic there is that discarding an embryo for being of the wrong sex is a lesser evil than a TOP as the fetus is even nearer achieving its potential (at least legal) personhood and itself less serious than sperm sorting.

Over the Atlantic, although the American Society for Reproductive Medicine Ethics Committee found highly problematic the use of gender selection, it did not strictly condemn the principle.

But a comment by the advocate of reproductive rights demonstrates uneasiness: Robertson says that techniques for sex selection (42) although not to be "legally prohibited" or "morally condemned" should be "not encouraged" or even, in some cases, "actively discouraged" and concludes that only gender balancing is acceptable (43). This compromise (44) that allows choosing the sex of the second (or more) child only providing it is different to this of the first, interalia, was also presented in the ESHRE ethics taskforce on PGD (21), with the alternative of the totally disapproving and strict Human Rights view. To accept family balancing, however, implies that sex selection is not sexist per se or that the social consequences (in the sense described by M. Strathern) do not warrant such a sacrifice to procreative liberty.

Therefore, we would like here to stick to the strict view, holding that any kind of selection, whether called balancing or not, is inherently sexist; furthermore, a family of only boys or girls is not imbalanced, a negative qualification by comparison with the supposedly ideal boy and girl "balanced" family.

Indeed, some arguments trying to justify sex selection as a reproductive choice are worse than others. For instance, the known imbalance of sexes already existing in some societies has led to comments that this would lead to an increased "value" of females, a demeaning attitude for whichever gender becomes thus of "scarcity value." This terminology of the market place reduces further the status of women (in practice rather than men) to mere chattels.

Furthermore, one may argue even further that the issue is too important to reduce it to national boundaries: to the question, "does the practice of social sex selection in India justify prohibiting social sex selection in the UK?" (45), the answer is a resounding yes because the very value of Human Rights reside in their universal/international application (46).

Indeed, the whole history of human rights has been one of political reaction against injustice by discrimination on grounds of sex (as well as religion or phenotype), toward agents or groups (represented here by women as a group).

Finally, one must add that if any method, whether of low or high technology (sperm sorting versus PGD) is used to prevent disease or suffering, as in X-linked genetic disease, to be of the "wrong" gender in the eyes of one's family or of society, whether male or female, cannot be defined as a disease.

Without pointing out the obvious (a child knowing of the method used for his/her conception may have the feeling of "being conditionally wanted" and/or feel even more intense pressure than usual in her/his society to fulfill to a gender stereotype in behavior, profession, and private life) and without raising the specter of eugenics and the worn slippery slopes' warning, one may also feel that children would benefit to be born in a society where acceptance rather than rejection of any difference (of phenotype, gender, or disabilities) is the norm. It would be ideal to live in societies where the protection offered by Human Rights has become redundant, but there is no evidence as yet that this ideal is within reach.

So in practice, what can be done to slow if not stop this discrimination, which even starts before the birth of the female, as (47) "gender (is not) a serious handicap worthy of termination or selection." One may be hopeful after the case in India, and also hope that for China, the program "Action of Care for Girls," will be applied, especially in rural areas, as stated by the Institute of Philosophy.

Indeed, regardless of personal or cultural motivations, the message sex selection for nonmedical reasons ("including balancing") sends to broader society and the world at large is the suboptimal worth of women. The stakes are too high to allow any compromise till equality of opportunity (lack of discrimination) between the sexes is shown to be really implemented as demanded by Human Rights declarations. Maybe then, and only then, might one reconsider the possibility of gender balancing in families, although it is doubtful that by then many families will still be interested.

CONCLUSIONS

The discussion of these few dilemmas has implications at national and international levels, as do many others in our specialty. However, the individual dimension is often the most poignant, and this is the one practitioners certainly face in their daily practice. Nevertheless, international comparisons with the study of different sociocultural approaches help us to challenge dogma, a very sane attitude when one keeps in mind Wittgenstein's definition of philosophy, applicable to ethics ("philosophy is not a doctrine, but an activity with the aim to logically clarify one's thinking").

The interdisciplinary approach also allows us to best take into account the welfare of the future child, with the invaluable help of psychologists and counselors, especially those specialized in family dynamics.

Finally, a word about the law. According to Bernard Dickens, "Ethics frames the law within which law is voluntarily obeyed" (48). This is a final plea for debate and information before legislation is passed without bias or prejudice in all field related to ART.

REFERENCES

1. De Wert G, Geraedts J. Preimplantation genetic diagnosis for hereditary disorders which do not show a simple Mendelian pattern: an ethical exploration. In: Shenfield F, Sureau C, eds. *Contemporary Ethical Dilemmas in Assisted Reproduction*. UK: Informa Healthcare, 2006; 85–98.

2. Shenfield F, Davies MC, Spoudeas H. Attempts to preserve the reproductive capacity of minors with cancer: who should give consent? In: Shenfield, Sureau, eds. *Ethical Dilemmas in Human Reproduction*. Parthenon, 2002; 21–34.

3. Bahadur G. Till death do us part: to be or not to be a parent after one's death. In: Shenfield F, Sureau C, eds. *Contemporary Ethical Dilemmas in Assisted Reproduction*. UK: Informa Healthcare, 2006;29–42.

4. The European IVF monitoring (EIM) for ESHRE. Assisted reproductive technology in Europe, 2002. Results generated from European registers by ESHRE. *Hum Reprod* 2006; 21(7): 1680–97.

5. Shenfield F. Justice and access to fertility treatments. In: Shenfield F, Sureau C, eds. *Ethical Dilemmas in Assisted Reproduction*. Carnforth, UK: Parthenon Publishing, 1997;7–14.

6. Shenfield F. Too late for change, too early to judge, but an oxymoron will not solve the problem. *Reprod Biomed Online* 2005; 10(4): 433–5.

7. Shenfield F, Steele SJ. A gift is a gift is a gift, or why gametes donors should not be paid. *Hum Reprod* 1995; 10(2): 253–5.

8. HFE Act 1990. www.opsi.gov.uk/acts

9. Titmuss R. *The Gift Relationship: From Human Blood to Social Policy*. London: Allen and Unwin, 1971.

10. Rodrigez del Pozo P. Paying donors and the ethics of blood supply. *J Med Ethics* 1994; 20: 31–5.

11. Human Fertilisation and Embryology. 6th Code of Practice, HFEA. 2005. www.gov.hfea.uk

12. FIGO Ethical guidelines on the sale of gametes and embryos, (1997). In: *Ethical Issues in Obstetrics and Gynaecology by the Figo Committee for the Study of Ethical Aspects of Human Reproduction and Women's Health*. FIGO house, 2006. www.FIGO.org

13. Pennings G, Devroey P. Subsidized in-vitro fertilization treatment and the effect on the number of egg sharers. *Reprod Biomed Online* 2006; 13(1): 8–10.

14. Human Fertilisation and Embryology Authority (Disclosure of donor information) Regulations 2004 no 1511.

15. Gollancz D. Donor insemination: a question of rights. *Hum Fertil* 2001; 4: 164–7.

16. Golombock S, Breaways A, Cook R, Giavazzi MT, Guerra D, Mantovani A, van Hall E Crossignani PG, Dexeus S. The European study of assisted reproduction families: family functioning and child development. *Hum Reprod* 1996; 11: 2324–31.

17. ESHRE taskforce on law and ethics 3. Gametes and embryo donation. *Hum Reprod* 2002; 17(5).

18. Pennings G. The double track policy for donor anonymity. *Hum Reprod* 1997; 12: 2839–44.

19. Testard J, Sele B. Towards an efficient medical eugenics: is the desirable always the feasible? *Hum Reprod* 1995; 11: 3086–90.

20. Milliez J, Sureau C. PGD and the eugenic debate: our responsibility to future generations. In: Shenfield, Sureau eds. *Ethical Dilemmas in Assisted Reproduction*. Parthenon, 1997;51–6.

21. ESHRE taskforce 5; Shenfield F, Pennings G, Devroey P, Sureau C, Tarlatzis B, Cohen J. ESHRE Ethics Task Force: Preimplantation genetic diagnosis. *Hum Reprod* 2003; 18(3): 649–51.

22. ESHRE taskforce 9; Shenfield F, Pennings G, Cohen J, Devroey P, Tarlatzis B. The application of preimplantation genetic diagnosis for human leukocyte antigen typing of embryos. *Hum Reprod* 2005; 20(4): 845–7.

23. Pennings G, Liebaers I. Creating a child to save another: HLA matching of siblings by means of preimplantation diagnosis. In: Shenfield, Sureau, eds. *Ethical Dilemmas in Human Reproduction*. Parthenon, 2002;51–66.

24. CCNE, Reponse au President de la Republique au sujet du clonage reproductif, cahiers du CCNE, Paris, 1997.

25. The Human Reproductive Cloning Act 2001. www.legislation. Hmso.gov.uk/acts 20010023.

26. ESHRE Taskforce for Ethics and Law 1; Shenfield F, Pennings G, Sureau C, Cohen J, Devroey P, Tarlatzis B. European Society of Human Reproduction and Embryology Task Force on Ethics and Law. I. The moral status of the pre-implantation embryo. *Hum Reprod* 2001; 16(5): 1046–8.

27. Council of Europe Strasbourg. *Convention for the Protection of Human Rights and Dignity of the Human Being with Regard to the Application of Biology and Medicine*, 1997. www.coe.int

28. Check E. Special report ethicists and biologists ponder the price of eggs. *Nature* 2006; 442: 606–7.

29. Luket al. Evaluation of compliance and range of fees by ASRM-listed egg donor and surrogacy agencies (Oral Presentation). *ASRM*, 2006; P–156.

30. FIGO Ethical guidelines on embryo research (2005). In: *Ethical Issues in Obstetrics and Gynaecology by the FIGO Committee for the Study of Ethical Aspects of Human reproduction and Women's Health*. FIGO house, 2006. www.FIGO.org

31. ESHRE Taskforce for Law and Ethics 12. Oocyte donation for non reproductive purpose. *Hum Reprod* 2007; 22(5): 1210–13.

32. Edwards RG. Cloning and cheating. *Reprod Biomed Online* 2006; 12(2): 141.

33. Sen A. More than 100 million women are missing. In: *New York Review of Books*. 1990.

34. Sen A. Missing women-revisited. *Br Med J*; 327: 1297–8.

35. Strathern M. British Medical Association debate on sex selection. 1993.

36. Wu Z et al. Perinatal mortality in rural China: retrospective cohort study. *Br Med J* 2003; 327: 1319–22.

37. Prabath J et al. Low male to female sex ratio of children born in India: national survey of 1.1 million households. *Lancet* 2006; 367: 211–8.

38. Sheth S. Missing female births in India. *Lancet* 2006; 367(9506): 185–6.

39. Ganapar M. Doctors in India prosecuted for sex determination, but few selected. *Br Med J* 2006; 332: 257.

40. Nisker J, Jones M. The ethics of sex selection. In: Shenfield, Sureau eds. *Ethical Dilemmas in Assisted Reproduction*. Parthenon, 1997.

41. HFEA. Sex selection: options for regulation. Choice and responsibility in human reproduction. 2004. www.hfea.gov.uk

42. Ethics committee of ASRM. Preconception gender selection for non medical reasons. *Fertil Steril* 2001; 75: 861–4.

43. Robertson J. Sex selection: final word from the ASRM Ethics Committee on the use of PGD. *Hastings Cent Rep* 2002; 32(2): 6.

44. Pennings G. Ethics of sex selection for family balancing: family balancing as a morally acceptable application of sex selection. *Hum Reprod* 1996; 11: 2339–43.

45. Dahl E. No country is an island. Comment on the House of Commons Report. *RBM Online* 2005; 11: 10–11.

46. Shenfield F. Procreative liberty, or collective responsibility? A comment on the select committee on the Commons' Science and technology 5th report "Human reproductive technology and the law", and on Dahl's response. *RBM*.

47. Shenfield F. Sex selection, why not. *Hum Reprod* 1994; 9: 142.

48. Dickens B. Interfaces of assisted reproduction, ethics and law. In: Shenfield F, Sureau C, eds. *Ethical Dilemmas in Assisted reproduction*. Parthenon, 1997; 77–82.

72

Infertility Treatment in Perimenopausal Women: Ethical Considerations

Hyacinth N. Browne, Alicia Armstrong, Alan DeCherney

The number of women seeking treatment for infertility continues to grow. It is estimated that approximately 1 in 136 or two million people in United States are infertile (1). These numbers are explained, in part, by an age-related decline in fertility that is well documented in the medical literature. Despite the availability of new technologies such as in vitro fertilization (IVF), this age-related loss of fertility cannot be overcome by the use of assisted reproductive technologies (ART), if donor oocytes are not used (2–10).

ART has been viewed as a panacea for perimenopausal women seeking motherhood late in their reproductive lives. According to the 2003 CDC Assisted Reproductive Technology Report (11), 20 percent of women seeking ART were of the age of forty and older. Most women in this age-group either delayed childbearing to pursue higher education and careers, or are part of the large cohort of women born during the "baby boom" (1946–1964) period. Although these women can have spontaneous pregnancies, the likelihood of pregnancy and live birth is less than 1–2 percent in those older than forty-three (11), and the time to conception can be prolonged.

Age is the most important factor affecting the chance of a live birth when a woman uses her own eggs. Among women in their twenties, pregnancy and live birth rates are relatively stable; and decline steadily from the mid-thirties onward (11). The live birth rate for infertile women is 37 percent for women younger than thirty-five years, 30 percent at ages thirty-five to thirty-seven, 20 percent at ages thirty-eight to forty, and 4 percent after age forty (11). ART success rates also differ for women who are forty and older and declines with each year of age using fresh nondonor eggs or embryos (7). The average chance for pregnancy is nearly 23 percent for women aged forty, and the live birth rate is about 16 percent. For women aged forty-three and older, the live birth rates are less than 1–2 percent (11) (Figure 72.1).

The dramatic decline in female fertility, over the age of forty, characterizes the perimenopause. It occurs approximately ten years prior to menopause despite regular menses. It is the period with variations in menstrual cycle length in a woman who has a monotropic follicle-stimulating hormone rise and ends with the final menstrual period (12). Elevations of FSH and estradiol and a decrease in inhibin B levels represent the most clinically significant hormonal alterations in perimenopausal women (4, 6, 8, 13), and represents diminished ovarian reserve and impending ovarian failure.

Even when faced with the remote prospect of a live birth with ART, many women in this age-group often elect to continue their efforts to reproduce. They view ART as a realistic and viable option despite their age and medical evidence. These women often refuse to objectively consider the likelihood of achieving a live birth and are willing to accept a 1 percent chance of getting pregnant. They do not want to stop treatment, and seek alternative clinics and providers that will offer them additional IVF cycles (14). As a result, they demand utilization of reproductive technologies that is of little or no benefit to them. The difficulty for the physician lies in offering treatment to perimenopausal women knowing that the likelihood of success is low (14).

This chapter will review the literature on the effects of age on fertility in the perimenopausal woman. We will also look at the appropriateness and ethical implications of using ART to extend the reproductive lives of perimenopausal women despite their low likelihood of having a live birth. We will conclude the chapter by presenting potential clinical guidelines for age in perimenopausal women using their own oocytes.

REVIEW OF THE LITERATURE

The effect of age on female fertility is difficult to assess because of confounding variables such as coital frequency and other biological causes associated with infertility (2), the use of contraception and the social and economical constraints that limit family size (8). Cultures that prohibit the use of contraception are a useful model for examining the impact of age on fertility. Tietze (15) created fertility curves for a religious sect (Hutterites) living in the Dakotas and Montana that do not practice birth control or receive economic incentives to limit their family size. Three and a half percent of Hutterite women less than twenty-five years old were sterile, and the sterility rate increased markedly beyond ages thirty-five to forty. Eighty-seven percent of the Hutterite women older than forty were sterile, and all were sterile over the age of forty-five. Tietze also showed that with increasing age of the mother, there was a marked increase in the average duration of the interval between pregnancies.

Even though fertility rates vary between populations, consistent age-related trends are noted. A slow decline in fertility rates become more significant through the middle of the fourth decade of life followed by a much steeper decline thereafter (8). However, some authors (8) suggest that studies of "natural populations" overestimate the effect of aging on reproductive

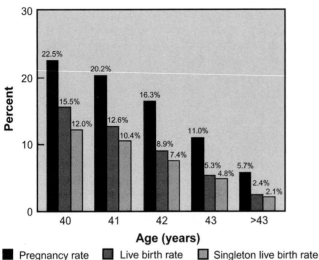

Figure 72.1. Pregnancy rates, live birth rates, and singleton live birth rates for ART cycles using fresh nondonor eggs or embryos among women aged forty and older, 2003.

potential because other biological causes associated with female infertility increase in frequency with age, and the frequency of coitus in older couples may decrease, thus decreasing the fecundity rate.

To control for coital frequency and the influences of male fecundity with age, Schwartz et al. (16) analyzed cumulative pregnancy rates for fertile women with azoospermic husbands undergoing insemination with donor sperm for twelve cycles. This was a prospective study of 2,193 fecund women. Women were divided into four age-groups, and the cumulative success rate after twelve cycles of insemination was 73 percent for those younger than twenty-five years, 74.1 percent for the twenty-six to thirty age-group, 61.5 percent for the thirty-one to thirty-five age-group, and 53.6 percent for the group older than thirty-five years. The curve of the cumulative success rate for women younger than twenty-five years was similar to that for women twenty-six to thirty years old. However, both pregnancy curves differed from the curves for the two older groups ($p < 0.001$, in comparison to the age-group over thirty-five; and $p < 0.03$, in comparison to the age-group of thirty-one to thirty-five). This study showed that there is a slight decrease in fecundability after thirty years of age and is marked after thirty-five years.

Although fertility decreases with age, not all perimenopausal women are infertile. This is because age is just one predictor of female fecundity, albeit a very important one. As a result, we are always seeking markers of ovarian reserve and responsiveness to predict female fecundability before stimulation. Before markers were available, many women in their forties were being excluded from IVF programs (17) since there had been no practical way to identify the subset with a better prognosis. Markers of ovarian reserve provide insight into ovarian responsiveness that age does not (18).

While they may predict a lower pregnancy rate, abnormal ovarian reserve test results do not preclude the possibility of pregnancy and should not be presented to patients as absolute (19). Likewise, ovarian reserve testing alone may yield falsely reassuring results as advanced maternal age and ovarian reserve test results are independent predictors of infertility (3, 19). There is a poor negative predictive value of a normal test result

in women older than forty years and emphasizes that these tests are quite specific but have limited sensitivity.

Basal FSH levels have been shown to provide more information than any other single static predictor of ovarian reserve (including age, LH, and E2) (17). Although markers of ovarian reserve are not very sensitive in predicting response, they are pretty consistent of poor fertility outcomes in older women (3, 17–18). Thus, "ovarian screening" may identify patients who should consider oocyte donation rather than traditional IVF.

Pearlstone et al. (3) conducted a prospective, observational study of 402 cycles in eighty-five infertile couples in whom the female partner was forty years or older and referred for ovulation induction therapy. Pregnancy and live birth rates were lower in this group. Women with a basal FSH less than 25 IU/L and age less than forty-four years had a clinical PR of 5.2 percent per cycle compared with a 0.0 percent per cycle in cases in which either basal FSH was 25 IU/L or higher or age was forty-four or more ($p < 0.005$). They concluded that basal FSH and chronological age are accurate predictors of reproductive outcomes in these couples, and both should be used in counseling patients about their chances for success.

To further substantiate the utility of FSH to predict ovarian responsiveness, Toner et al. (18) performed a prospective study of 1,478 consecutive IVF cycles to ascertain whether FSH was a better predictor of IVF performance than age. They showed that total and term pregnancy rates declined as age and FSH values increased ($p < 0.0001$). However, pregnancy rates (total and ongoing) per attempt steadily declined as basal FSH increased, whereby no decline in the slope of pregnancy rates with age was detected. Furthermore, there was no relationship between cancellation risk and age but with increasing FSH values. They concluded that basal day 3 FSH levels provided better predictive values for both IVF pregnancy and cancellation rates than age, but both need to be considered simultaneously for optimal prediction of ovarian reserve.

Moreover, the clomiphene citrate challenge test (CCCT) has been shown to be a better predictor of ovarian reserve than day 3 FSH. Scott et al. (20) did a prospective CCCT screening in women from the general infertility population. Approximately 10 percent of the 236 patients who were evaluated and followed for a minimum of one year had an abnormal CCCT. The incidence of an abnormal test rose with age (three percent at less than thirty years of age, 7 percent at thirty to thirty-four years, 10 percent at thirty-five to thirty-nine years, and 26 percent for women older than forty years). Most importantly, the pregnancy rates in patients with diminished ovarian reserve were markedly lower (9 percent) than those with adequate reserve. Even after controlling for age, the pregnancy rates were still significantly decreased. Only seven of twenty-three patients with an abnormal test had an elevated day 3 FSH level, again suggesting that the CCCT may be more sensitive than screening with day 3 samples alone.

Even with a normal CCCT, the authors (20) showed that age is a better predictor of pregnancy outcomes in older women. Two out of ninety-two women aged forty years or more, who had a normal CCCT, became pregnant compared to 34/92 women less than thirty years of age with a normal clomiphene challenge test. This further supports the notion that age trumps current hormonal markers in predicting ovarian function in perimenopausal women.

In all, a combination of markers of ovarian reserve and age are the best modalities to predict the likelihood of success or poor outcomes in older women. The aggressive use of fertility drugs and standard assisted reproductive techniques in older patients may be of limited value, especially if they have abnormal ovarian function testing (3, 5, 17, 20). These patients may benefit from egg donation to achieve pregnancy. The ability to identify individuals with diminished reproductive potential or "ovarian reserve" is therefore of practical value (8). The predictability of a normal test, in contrast, is more limited. It seems reasonable to offer standard IVF to women (forty to forty-two years of age) without laboratory evidence of compromised ovarian reserve, because although their chances of achieving a live birth are very low, they are not nonexistent (14).

AGE-RELATED OBSTETRICAL CONCERNS

So far, our discussion has been limited to the effects of advanced age on reproductive outcomes for perimenopausal woman. What about the obstetrical complications associated with advanced maternal age? Gestational diabetes, preeclampsia, abnormal placentation, labor dystocia requiring operative deliveries, and preterm delivery are dramatically increased in women older than forty (21). The risk of spontaneous abortion also increases with female age (4, 10). According to the 2003 CDC Assisted Reproductive Technology Report (11), miscarriage rates were below 13 percent among women younger than thirty-four. The rate increased among women in their mid-to-late thirties and continued to increase with age, reaching 29 percent at age forty and 48 percent at age forty-three. The age-associated decline in female fecundity and increased risk of spontaneous abortion are largely attributable to abnormalities in the oocyte (22–24).

EFFECTIVE ART TREATMENT FOR PERIMENOPAUSAL WOMEN

The most effective treatment for women older than forty years is oocyte donation. Although the resulting child will not be biologically related to the birth mother, oocyte donation yields the highest live birth rate of any ART treatment (19). Women older than forty have a 50 percent chance of live birth per transfer when fresh donor eggs are used (11) (Figure 72.2).

Miscarriage rates are significantly reduced from the rate normally seen in older mothers with donor eggs. The combined effect of higher implantation rates and lower miscarriage rates has made this method a more successful alternative for treating infertility in perimenopausal women.

ETHICAL CONSIDERATIONS

Infertility treatment in the perimenopausal woman raises many ethical questions. What constitutes poor prognosis or futile treatment? If a woman can afford treatment that is associated with less than 5 percent chance of success should it be offered? Does a patient's right to autonomy guarantee the right to futile or inappropriate care? Does a patient's desire and request for treatment oblige a physician to provide that care? What processes and procedures are necessary to address requests for ineffective, futile, or medically inappropriate medical care?

Turning to the first question, how do we define very poor prognosis and futility as it relates to infertility treatment, specifically IVF? Multiple authors in a variety of medical specialties

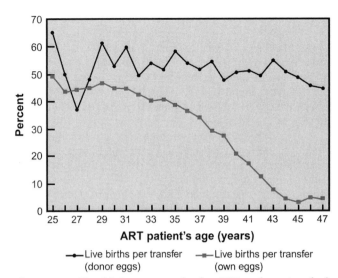

Figure 72.2. Live births per transfer for ART cycles using fresh embryos from own and donor eggs, by ART patient's age, 2003.

have defined futility, sometimes using case examples to illustrate the meaning of this term in a medical context. In one example, the family of an eighty-five-year old woman demanded medical treatment that the attending physician considered futile. The issue was further complicated by the fact that the husband was an attorney, and the funding of care was not an issue (25, 26). Many of the discussions involve treatment decisions in terminally ill patients. There are, however, several publications that address ethical issues that are germane to obstetrics and gynecology patients. In a committee opinion from the American College of Obstetricians and Gynecologists (27), one proposed definition of futile treatment required one or more of five elements:

1. Lethal diagnosis or prognosis of imminent death.
2. Suggested therapy cannot achieve its physiological goal.
3. Suggested therapy will not or cannot achieve the patient's or family's stated goals.
4. The suggested therapy will not or cannot extend the patient's life span.
5. The suggested therapy will not or cannot enhance the patient's quality of life.

Perhaps the most relevant answer to the question of fertility treatments in women older than forty years old comes from the Ethics Committee of the American Society for Reproductive Medicine (14). Futility was defined as a 0 or 1 percent or less chance of achieving a live birth, while "very poor prognosis" was used to describe very low but not nonexistent odds of achieving a live birth (>1 percent but about < 5 percent per cycle).

Moreover, if a patient can afford ineffective care, should it be offered? Ironically, the women who can best afford infertility treatment are often those women who have a poorer prognosis as a result of their age (28). This question was debated within both the hospital and the court system in the case of a patient receiving respirator support in spite of a dismal prognosis. It is clear that we cannot afford a universal health care system based on the desires and demands of every patient. In contrast, should financial resources enable a wealthy elderly dialysis patient with a poor prognosis and limited life expectancy to be able to "purchase" a kidney, while more appropriate candidates remain on a waiting list? In this and similar cases, it would appear that the principle of "ethical stewardship" should be considered. Physicians must exercise appropriate stewardship in their counseling of patients and their refusal to deny inappropriate and ineffectual treatment (25, 29, 30). This is true even when the treatment has minimal risk to the patient, as in the case of IVF.

In recent years, patient autonomy has also become an increasingly important consideration. However, respect for the patient's right to autonomy does not require physicians to provide treatment that is futile. At the same time, physicians should retain some flexibility in developing policies for initiating or continuing fertility treatments in patients with poor prognoses keeping in mind circumstances or emotional needs of individual patients (14).

Most physicians would not be reticent to offer fertility treatment to older women if they knew that the outcome would be successful. The difficulty for the physician lies in offering treatment to patients knowing that the likelihood of success is low or futile. For the patient, it is knowing when to stop seeking further treatment or to look for alternatives to obtain an end to a means. But how do we counsel women who are willing to accept that less than 1 percent chance of getting pregnant?

Furthermore, what should be done to create a happy medium for both the physician, who does not want to dispense futile reproductive treatments to perimenopausal women, and the patient, who views it as her reproductive right to bear children with assistance despite age? One way to address this ethical dilemma is to establish clinical guidelines for treatment of perimenopausal women using their own eggs (14). This would allow for consistency in practice, establish evidence-based policies, and enable us to better counsel our patients. This would prove to be a win-win situation for both the physician and patient. Physicians would be guided by evidence-based data enabling them to avoid futile treatment efforts and maintain their professional integrity. While the patient with a very low prognosis of having a live birth may still have a reasonable chance of achieving a pregnancy that results in a live birth with reproductive assistance.

The ASRM ethics committee (14) has issued such guidelines. In cases of very poor prognosis, the ethics committee stated that that it is ethical to treat, if the patient is fully informed of the prognosis and still wants to proceed. However, physicians may ethically refuse to accept or provide further treatment to patients with very poor prognoses provided that they follow evidence-based policies and the rules of their fertility centers, and avoid arbitrary decisions. All fertility centers should establish guidelines based on the literature and their success rates to appropriately counsel patients about the likelihood of live birth based on age. These policies should be discussed at the initial visit, and should guide decisions about initiating or stopping treatment.

KEY POINTS FOR CLINICAL PRACTICE

■ In conclusion, no fertility treatment, with the exception of oocyte donation, has been associated with a live birth rate of more than 15 percent in perimenopausal women. However, when older women decide to pursue ART with their own eggs, the decision making of proceeding with treat-

ment for the physician and patient becomes difficult. The concepts of futility and very poor prognosis of treatment must be entertained in every case, before a decision to treat is made while respecting patient autonomy. By establishing evidence-based guidelines using data in the literature and generated by each center, we are better able to counsel patients about the futility of treatment and when to consider seeking alternatives to achieve their goal of a live birth. These guidelines would also allow both the physician and the patient to justify treatment in those cases when the odds of success are low but are not nonexistent.

ACKNOWLEDGMENTS

We thank the Centers for Disease Control and Prevention; American Society for Reproductive Medicine; Society for Assisted Reproductive Technology, 2003; Assisted Reproductive Technology Success Rates: National Summary and Fertility Clinic Reports, Atlanta; and Centers for Disease Control and Prevention, 2006, for allowing us to use their figures.

This research is supported in part by the Program in Reproductive and Adult Endocrinology of the National Institute of Child Health and Human Development, NIH.

REFERENCES

1. www.wrongdiagnosis.com/f/female_infertility/prevalence.htm. (No author is listed.)
2. DeCherney AH, Berkowitz GS. Female fecundity and age. *The New England Journal of Medicine* 1982;306(7):424–6.
3. Pearlstone AC, Fournet N, Gambone JC, Pang SC, Buyalos RP. Ovulation induction in women age 40 and older: the importance of basal follicle-stimulating hormone level and chronological age. *Fertility and Sterility* 1992;58(4):674–9.
4. Gindoff PR, Jewelewicz R. Reproductive potential in the older woman. *Fertility and Sterility* 1986;46(6):989–1001.
5. Toner JP. Ovarian reserve, female age and the chance for successful pregnancy. *Minerva Ginecologica* 2003;55(5):399–406.
6. Speroff L. The effect of aging on fertility. *Current Opinion in Obstetrics and Gynecology* 1994;6(2):115–20.
7. Ron-El R, Raziel A, Strassburger D, Schachter M, Kasterstein E, Friedler S. Outcome of assisted reproductive technology in women over the age of 41. *Fertility and Sterility* 2000;74(3):471–5.
8. Klein J, Sauer MV. Assessing fertility in women of advanced reproductive age. *American Journal of Obstetrics and Gynecology* 2001;185(3):758–70.
9. Levi AJ, Raynault MF, Bergh PA, Drews MR, Miller BT, Scott RT, Jr. Reproductive outcome in patients with diminished ovarian reserve. *Fertility and Sterility* 2001;76(4):666–9.
10. Rowe T. Fertility and a woman's age. *The Journal of Reproductive Medicine* 2006;51(3):157–63.
11. www.cdc.gov/art/art2003/section2a.htm. (No author is listed.)
12. Soules MR, Sherman S, Parrott E, et al. Executive summary: Stages of Reproductive Aging Workshop (STRAW). *Fertility and Sterility* 2001;76(5):874–8.
13. Santoro N, Brown JR, Adel T, Skurnick JH. Characterization of reproductive hormonal dynamics in the perimenopause. *The Journal of Clinical Endocrinology and Metabolism* 1996;81(4): 1495–501.
14. Fertility treatment when the prognosis is very poor or futile. Ethics Committee, American Society for Reproductive Medicine. *Fertility and Sterility* 2004;82(4):806–10.

15. Tietze C. Reproductive span and rate of reproduction among Hutterite women. *Fertility and Sterility* 1957;8(1):89–97.

16. Schwartz D, Mayaux MJ. Female fecundity as a function of age: results of artificial insemination in 2193 nulliparous women with azoospermic husbands. Federation CECOS. *The New England Journal of Medicine* 1982;306(7):404–6.

17. Toner JP. The significance of elevated FSH for reproductive function. *Bailliere's Clinical Obstetrics and Gynaecology* 1993;7(2): 283–95.

18. Toner JP, Philput CB, Jones GS, Muasher SJ. Basal follicle-stimulating hormone level is a better predictor of in vitro fertilization performance than age. *Fertility and Sterility* 1991;55(4): 784–91.

19. Aging and infertility in women. Practice Committee, American Society for Reproductive Medicine. *Fertility and Sterility* 2006;82 (Suppl 5):S248–52.

20. Scott RT, Leonardi MR, Hofmann GE, Illions EH, Neal GS, Navot D. A prospective evaluation of clomiphene citrate challenge test screening of the general infertility population. *Obstetrics and Gynecology* 1993;82(4 Pt. 1):539–44.

21. Gilbert WM, Nesbitt TS, Danielsen B. Childbearing beyond age 40: pregnancy outcome in 24,032 cases. *Obstetrics and Gynecology* 1999;93(1):9–14.

22. Angell RR. Aneuploidy in older women. Higher rates of aneuploidy in oocytes from older women. *Human Reproduction (Oxford, England)* 1994;9(7):1199–200.

23. Lim AS, Tsakok MF. Age-related decline in fertility: a link to degenerative oocytes? *Fertility and Sterility* 1997;68(2): 265–71.

24. Hassold T, Hunt P. To err (meiotically) is human: the genesis of human aneuploidy. *Nature Reviews* 2001;2(4):280–91.

25. Miles SH. Informed demand for "non-beneficial" medical treatment. *The New England Journal of Medicine* 1991;325(7): 512–15.

26. Schneiderman LJ, Jecker NS, Jonsen AR. Medical futility: its meaning and ethical implications. *Annals of Internal Medicine* 1990;112(12):949–54.

27. ACOG Committee Opinion No.362: Medical Futility. Obstetrics and Gynecology 2007;109(3):791–4.

28. Rome N. Childless: Some by chance, some by choice. *The Washington Post*, November 28, 2006.

29. Lantos JD, Singer PA, Walker RM, et al. The illusion of futility in clinical practice. *The American Journal of Medicine* 1989;87(1): 81–4.

30. Jecker NS, Schneiderman LJ. Medical futility: the duty not to treat. *Cambridge Q Healthcare Ethics* 1993;2(2):151–9.

73

Religious Perspectives of Ethical Issues in Infertility and ART

Botros R. M. B. Rizk, Sherman J. Silber, Gamal I. Serour, Michel Abou Abdallah

This chapter was based upon the presentations of a symposium at the 59th American Society for Reproductive Medicine (ASRM) annual meeting in San Antonio October 2003. This was the ASRM/MEFS cultural exchange session and I was asked to put together presentations that represented the views of the main religions. The Jewish, Christian, and Islamic views were presented by Sherman Silber, Botros R. M. B. Rizk, Pier G. Crosignianni, and Gamal I Serour. This symposium was very stimulating and generated interesting discussions and published by the *Middle East Fertility Society Journal* in 2005, Volume (10), third issue. This chapter is produced with the permission of the journal with minor updating of my section. This led to another session at the ASRM 60th Annual Meeting in 2004 where presentations covered some more focused topics as stem cell and cord blood. Three presentations were given by Joe Leigh Simpson, Robert Casper, and Botros R. M. B. Rizk.

Religious Perspectives of Ethical Issues in ART. *Middle East Fertility Society Journal* 2005;10 (3): 185–204.

Infertility, IVF and Judaism

Sherman J. Silber, M.D.

Infertility Center of St. Louis, St. Luke's Hospital, Missouri, USA

Different Branches of Judaism

For most Jews, Judaism is not well defined. There are three main branches to Judaism: "Orthodox," "Conservative," and "Reformed." Only about 10% of Jews worldwide are Orthodox, and only Orthodox Judaism is quite well defined. Approximately 85 percent of Jews worldwide are "Reformed," and these Jews are, for the most part, secular. About 5 percent of Jews are "Conservative," which is a sort of a hybrid between Orthodox and Reformed Judaism. Thus, with the exception of Orthodox Jews (10 percent), most Jews would have a very difficult time defining their belief system. In fact, Orthodox Jews often define themselves as "religious" Jews so as to distinguish themselves from the other 90 percent (Reformed and Conservative) who are viewed by the Orthodox as ethnic and historical Jews, but who are not following the traditional Jewish religion. Thus, to simplify the discussion of Judaism and modern reproductive technology, it is much easier to concentrate on the more clearly defined "Orthodox" branch of Judaism since it has the most severe set of rules.

Basic Tenets of Orthodox Judaism

The basic and unshakeable tenets of Judaism prior to the Reform and Conservative movements in the past century is that the Torah is the revealed word of God handed down at Mount Sinai 3,500 years ago. The "written Torah" is the first five books of both the Jewish and Christian Bible. Judaism believes that it is not unreasonable to assume that what was witnessed 100 generations (3,500 years) ago was so important in the lives of these desert nomadic people that it has been transmitted accurately from parent to child, and represents the absolute truth of what God expects of us. In fact, the word "Torah" literally means "instructions for living." The Orthodox Jewish view is that life is so complex, challenging, and confusing, that without such a "handbook" so-to-speak, like an instruction manual, it would be impossible to know how to live life in the best possible way. That is why at the stage when humanity was ready to receive these instructions, 3,500 years ago, after Noah had discovered the principles of moral behavior, and after Abraham had discovered the universal validity of monotheism, the world was finally ready for the very specific revelation of the law on Mount Sinai after the exodus from Egypt.

The Torah consists of the classical "written" Torah, which is the first five books of the Bible, that is, the five books of Moses and the "oral" Torah, which is the "Talmud." The Talmud contains the directions that were also given on Mount Sinai to the "children of Israel," but which were too cumbersome and laborious, and too subject to subtle interpretation to be allowed to be "written down." In fact, the oral Torah continued to be added to by religious scholars, rabbis, and sages over the past 3,500 years in the form of legal opinions and disagreements regarding the interpretation of the commandments. Thus, the Talmud consists of rules that were considered to be an oral expansion and clarification of the written Torah composed of the arguments and views and opinions from sages down through the centuries. In early Judaism, it was felt that the oral Torah must not be written down because the very concept of oral Torah allows for re-interpretation of absolute rules and commandments according to new conditions as life changes with the coming centuries. Nonetheless, it was written down after the first century A.D. when it was feared by the rabbis of the time (after the Romans expelled the Jews from Israel) that it might be lost if it were simply left to being handed down orally as it had been in the previous 1,600 years.

The basic tenet of Orthodox Judaism is that this written and oral Torah contains a complete guide to how God expects you to live your life. It is critical that you follow these commandments, and it is critical that when there appears to be conflicts or ambiguities in these commandments, that you use all of your intellectual ability to try to discern from these ambiguities and conflicts what exactly it is that God meant for you to do in every single situation that comes up in your life.

Orthodox Jewish Legal System

The Orthodox Jewish legal system can be viewed as an extraordinary exercise in deductive logic, and can be compared for the sake of clarity to "Euclidean" and "non-Euclidean" geometry. Euclidean geometry, which we all studied in high school is not just a math course about shapes and lines. It is a study in the concept of deductive reasoning. In Euclidean geometry there are a set of six axioms and nineteen postulates, which are basic "obvious" truths from which the entire geometric structure of the world was derived. For example, one of the six axioms is that the "total is equal to the sum of its parts." Axioms are basic truths that are not specific to geometry but to math in general. Postulates are basic truths that are specific to geometry. An example of one of the nineteen postulates is that "the shortest distance between two points is a straight line." From these basic axioms and postulates, with which no one would argue, represent basic general truths, the entire system of Euclidean geometry, involving areas of triangles, squares, polyhedrons, and circles are derived. A complex system whose truth seems incontrovertible could be constructed using deductive logic from these very simple sets of axioms and postulates.

In the same way, the Jewish legal system was derived via logic, extrapolation, and argumentation based on the basic commandments in the Torah that were considered incontrovertible and irrefutable axioms and postulates. The result was a legal system that encompasses every imaginable detail of what one should and should not do, based on Gods primordial directions to mankind from Mount Sinai.

However, Euclidean geometry (as logical and unassailable as it appears to be) has rather unexpected potential deviations if just one of those nineteen postulates is challenged. For example, the nineteenth Euclidean postulate states, "only one line can be drawn through a point which is parallel to another line." That postulate seems to be pretty obvious, but in the nineteenth century, a completely different system of geometry based on the world's being curved rather than a rectangular structure, assumed that if through a point, any number of parallel lines can be drawn parallel to any existing line. This non-Euclidean system of geometry was the basis for much of Einstein's computations of relativity. It is this "risk" that any of the commandments (like postulates) might have been misinterpreted that in Judaism requires constant study, review, and argumentation. The Orthodox Jewish legal system supports this constant questioning process as the only way to attempt to approximate the truth, which Orthodox Jews do believe ultimately derives from Torah.

Major Jewish Themes

The major themes throughout Judaism are that God is one, that life has a purpose, and that purpose is to live a good and moral life. However, life is very confusing and filled with potential conflict. Therefore, the essence of Orthodox Judaism is that only through intense and relentless study involving argument and counter argument via logic and extrapolation can Jews be guided through this confusion into leading the proper life.

Therefore, the Orthodox Jewish essence is that one must study Torah from the earliest years with all of their intellectual might. The purpose is to try to figure out through logic and introspection, debate and counter debate, all based on Torah, what it is that God expects of us. Only through critical study of Torah can Orthodox Jews figure out how to manage every single detail of living.

The Most Important Two Commandments

The first commandment to appear in the Torah is that mankind should be "fruitful and multiply." As a corollary, human life should be preserved above all. For example, if all there is to eat is pork, and otherwise you would die if you did not eat the pork, you are commanded to disobey the injunction against eating pork, so that you can continue to live. The only thing you are not allowed to do to save your life is either to deny the existence of God, or to cause someone else to die. Every other law can be forsaken if otherwise you would die. To either kill yourself or allow yourself to die unnecessarily, or to kill someone else, is strictly forbidden because the most important tenet in Orthodox Judaism is that human life is to be preserved above almost all other laws.

Other examples of Jewish law are that you must say a blessing over every meal and over every single pleasure so as not ever to take anything for granted. The reason for the commandment to say blessings is not because God needs to receive our thank you. The reason that God gives the commandment to say blessings is so that our pleasure in life can be enhanced by never taking the preciousness of life for granted. For example, you must thank God whenever you wake up in the morning for "renewing" your life. You must even remember to say a blessing over your sphincter whenever you are finished going to the bathroom. This may sound humorous and always gets a giggle from the audience. But just think about it. We take our sphincter for granted, unless we have an ileostomy, or incontinence.

As we walk around and live our normal lives, we do not derive any true joy from appreciating how wonderful it is that we have a properly functioning sphincter, unless we remember to say a blessing every time we finish going to the bathroom.

Confusion Which Can Result from Attempting to Follow the "Commandments"

It is well known that Jews must not do any work on the Sabbath so as to remember and be grateful for the creation of the universe. The Sabbath is considered very holy because it is a celebration of our very existence, and it is the most important holiday in Judaism, occurring every single week on the seventh day, the day that God rested from creating the universe. That is the day that Orthodox Jews interface most directly with God, by following the specific commandment not to do any work on the Sabbath. That sounds easy, but how do you define "work"? Rabbis and sages over the past 3,500 years have continually debated this simply to try to figure out what is and is not "work" that is or is not allowable on the Sabbath.

For example, driving your car, even to Synagogue or anywhere else on the Sabbath is considered "work." However, walking twenty or forty miles on Sabbath, if you live that far away, is not considered "work," Lifting a 50-pound weight inside your house is not considered "work," but carrying a single feather outside your enclosed neighborhood, or outside of your house, is considered "work," which is not allowed on Sabbath. The mere flip of a switch, turning on a light bulb is considered "work," whereas serving a meal to forty guests is not considered "work." This is the type of confusion that can result when one sincerely attempts to follow the simplistic commandments of the Torah without having committed oneself to detailed and scholarly questioning. The logical answer has been to consider whatever was not allowable on Sabbath during the building of the tabernacle by Mount Sinai to be defined as "work." Driving a car or turning on a light is considered work because it is the equivalent of starting a fire. Carrying a feather outside of the neighborhood is considered work because transporting from one area to another is not allowed, but rearranging furniture or other items in your house is not considered transport, and is not prohibited in the Torah. What is the point of giving these examples of the difficulties that the most religious Jews have in deciding what actions do or do not conflict with what God expects of us? It is to point out that the Orthodox Jewish views toward IVF (like the Sabbath) and modern reproductive technology has been subject to relentless intellectual scrutiny by some of the most brilliant minds in Judaism, attempting to extrapolate from ancient laws, believed to be handed down directly from God, what is and what is not allowable.

INFERTILITY, IVF AND JUDAISM

The Jewish views on IVF issues are therefore readily deducible. According to the Talmud, the soul does not enter the embryo until forty days. Furthermore, we all have an obligation to have offspring and to "be fruitful and multiply." Therefore, IVF is absolutely obligatory when it is medically indicated in order for a couple to have children. It is not just allowable but it is obligatory. Furthermore, PGD represents no moral or ethical risk because the soul has not yet entered the embryo. Furthermore, selective reduction of a multiple pregnancy is acceptable if its goal is to enhance the possibility of life.

Embryo research to promote life is, therefore, acceptable. Furthermore, not only is therapeutic cloning acceptable but it is an obligation to do any research which can enhance and promote life-saving treatment such as stem cell and cellular replacement therapy.

Commandments in Conflict

The Talmud specifically forbids "cutting the sperm ducts." But yet the Torah insists "be fruitful and multiply." So if we are not allowed to cut the sperm ducts, and yet we are obligated to do whatever we can to have children, what about "MESA" and what about "TESE?" Modern Talmud scholars, universally respected Orthodox Rabbinical minds, have weighed this conflict, and decided that the first commandment "to be fruitful and multiply" takes priority over the commandment not to "cut the sperm ducts." Therefore, MESA and TESE are fully allowable and, in fact, mandatory. However, such a decision, based on a clear conflict between two commandments is referred to as a "leniency." In other words, the rabbi's are not really happy about the prospect of an apparent violation of a Torah commandment, but it is understood that God's intention in the commandment to avoid cutting the sperm ducts was meant to be a corollary to "be fruitful and multiply" and not to be a prohibition against doing whatever you can to "be fruitful and multiply."

Controversial Issues Such as Donor Gametes

Controversial issues such as whether or not donor gametes are allowable have not yet resolved themselves into any clear announcement from rabbinic authorities. The great legal Orthodox Jewish minds are very cautious on this issue. Many Orthodox Jews assume that donor gametes are not allowable and do not even think to engage in detailed, syllogistic scrutiny of this issue. Therefore, most rabbinic authorities generally do not allow either donor sperm or donor eggs. However, there is no clear injunction in the Torah against donor sperm or donor eggs, and there is a clear imperative to "be fruitful and multiply." In fact, the imperative to "be fruitful and multiply" is so strong that prior to modern reproductive technology, divorce (which is generally shunned among Orthodox Jews) would be allowed if the couple were infertile, just to allow them the chance to try via a different marital partner to have children.

Therefore, to solve this issue, the couple has to search "for the right rabbi" who will go through the details of this complex issue with them privately. The greatest and most respected Orthodox Jewish mind of the twentieth century was Rabbi Moshe Feinstein. Unfortunately he has passed away, but his views (however radical seeming) were regarded universally by Orthodox Jews, no matter what their hesitation, as most probably being correct guidelines. His knowledge and his reasoning were considered to be vaster than any other rabbi in the later twentieth century. He never had a chance to make a ruling on donor eggs, but on donor sperm he felt that it was a private matter for the couple to decide, and in certain situations it would be recommended in order to fulfill the first commandment as well as to keep the marriage together. However, despite such an opinion, here is a general "feeling" among Orthodox Jews against donor gametes. However, my discussions with many of the great Talmudic minds would indicate to me (my personal view) that despite the controversy, donor gametes, in special situations, with the right couple, is preferable to going childless, and is acceptable under Jewish law.

Torah and Science Do Not Conflict

Even the most fundamentalist Orthodox Jewish viewpoint is that Torah and science do not conflict. Mankind must use its creative intelligence to resolve conflict and to figure out from the "basic" principles of Torah what is right, and never to be blinded by dogma. A good example is the Orthodox Jewish view of creation and the concept of the Big Bang. Most physicists today believe that the universe is approximately thirteen billion years old. That would seem to conflict with the biblical notion that the universe was created in six days, and on the seventh day, God rested. However, MIT physicists have studied this concept of the Big Bang mathematically using basic principles of the relativity of time and velocity popularized by Einstein.

As an object is proceeding at or near the velocity of light, time slows down dramatically in relation to a fixed observer. Einstein originally postulated that if you were to travel in a spaceship at the speed of light for thousands of years, and then return to earth, you will not have aged significantly, but back on Earth it will be thousands of years later. Time simply gets slower, the faster your velocity in relation to a fixed observer. If God is considered the external observer, and the universe is expanding near the speed of light, then the thirteen billion years which astronomers measure as the age of the universe comes out to approximately six days. Thus, there is no conflict between our observation that the universe is approximately thirteen billion years old, and the traditional biblical view that the universe was created in six days. This is one example of the firm belief in Judaism that science, observation, and study do not, and should not conflict, with religion and spirituality. That is not considered to be God's wish. The Orthodox view of the most respected rabbinic minds is that Torah should be a window to view the universe with an open mind, and should not be a wooden shutter.

THE VIEWS OF THE COPTIC ORTHODOX CHURCH ON THE TREATMENT OF INFERTILITY, ASSISTED REPRODUCTION, AND CLONING

Botros R. M. B. Rizk, M.D., M.A., F.A.C.O.G., F.A.C.S., H.C.L.D., F.R.C.O.G, F.R.C.S.(C)

Professor and Director Division of Reproductive Endocrinology and Infertility

Department of Obstetrics and Gynecology, University of South Alabama, Alabama, USA

Coptic

The Coptic Orthodox church is an apostolic church that is as old as Christendom. The Coptic Orthodox church is rich with her evangilistic and ascetic life, genuine patriotic inheritance, heavenly worship, spiritual rituals, living hymns and beautiful icons. The church is part of Egypt's fabric. One of the statements of His Holiness Pope Shenouda III, Egypt is not a country that we live in, Egypt is a country that lives in us. The word "copt" derives from the Greek Aigyptios "Egyptian" via Coptic kyptaios and Arabic Qibti. Aigyptios derives from hikaptah, house of the Ka (spirit) of Ptah, a most highly revered deity in Egyptian mythology and one of the names for Memphis, the first capital of ancient Egypt (1). The Arabs, upon arriving to Egypt in 640 A.D., called Egypt dar al Qibt (home of the Egyptians) and since Christianity was the official religion of Egypt, the word Qibt came to refer to the practitioners of Christianity as well as to the inhabitants of the Nile Valley (Figure 73.1) (1,2).

Foundation of the Coptic Church by St. Mark

In the first century, Egypt was blessed by the Holy Family's visit (Figures 73.2 and 73.3). There is a strong tradition in Egypt that supports the New Testament story of the Flight into Egypt: Take the young child and his mother and flee into Egypt: (Matt. 2: 13,15); "Behold the Lord rides on a Swift cloud and will come into Egypt" Isaiah 19:1; "Out of Egypt I called my son" (Hosea 11:1); and it is shared by Christians and Muslims alike (3,4). Egypt was a refuge to many people especially during famines. Abraham visited Egypt so did Joseph and Jeremiah. According to tradition, St. Mark (Figure 73.4) brought Christianity to Egypt (5) in the reign of the Roman Emperor Nero in the first century A.D. (1). He preached the Gospel, made his first convert, founded the See, and was martyred in Alexandria.

St. Mark was a Jew from the Levite tribe (6). St. Mark carried two names. His Jewish name, John, means God is merciful and his gentile name, Marcos, the more well known. His Jewish name was used alone in two references in the Acts of the Apostles in Chapter 13, verses 5 and 13 as well as in St. Paul's letter to the Colossians and St. Peter's letter. His two names were used together on three occasions in the Acts of the Apostles.

St. Mark was born in the Cyrene, one of the pentapolis in Libya called Apriatolis (5,6). His mother's name was Mary, one of the Marys who followed the Lord Jesus Christ, and his father was Aristopaul who was a cousin of St. Peter and also a relative of St. Barnabas as mentioned in Colossians 4:10. In Acts, St. Mark is mentioned as a companion of Saul and Barnabas (12:52; 13:13); he is also portrayed as a co-worker of St. Peter, the Apostle to the Jews (12:12) and of St. Paul

732 ▪ B O T R O S R . M . B . R I Z K , S H E R M A N J . S I L B E R , G A M A L I . S E R O U R E T A L . ▪

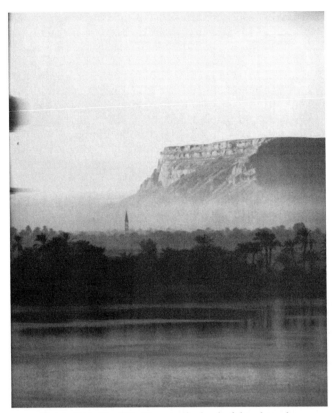

Figure 73.1. The Nile River in the land of the pharoahs.

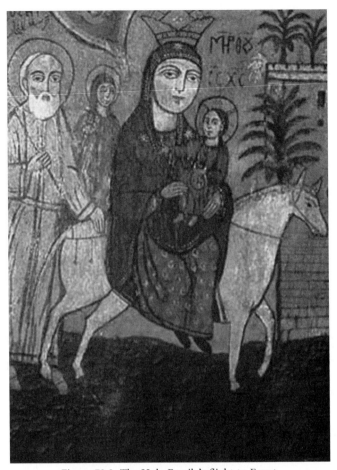

Figure 73.2. The Holy Family's flight to Egypt.

the Apostle to the gentiles (Col 4: 10; 2Tim 4:11). St. Mark preached in Asia, Europe, Antioch, Cypress, Rome, Colossy, and Venice.

According to the historian Eusabius of Pamphylia (fourth century) St. Mark appointed his first convert in Alexandria, the cobbler Anianus, to serve as bishop of Alexandria in his place. Moreover, he ordained three priests Milus, Cerdon, and Primus all of whom became patriarchs of the See of Alexandria. The unbelievers of the city were greatly annoyed by the rapid spread of the Gospel and planned to entrap the evangelist during the Easter celebrations of 68 CE. In the course of the divine Eucharist, the furious mob seized St. Mark, put a rope around his neck, and dragged him through the cities of Alexandria. The following day once again dragged him by the rope until he died (7). Some of the earliest converts to the new faith came from the Jewish community in Egypt which probably represented the largest Jewish population of Jews outside Palestine (1) that existed for more than one thousand years B.C. (8).

The School of Alexandria

Long before the establishment of Christianity in Alexandria, the city was famous for its many schools. By far, the largest school is the "Museum," which was founded by Ptolemy and became the most famous school in the East. In addition, there were the "Serapeum" and the "Sebastion." Each of these three schools had its own huge library. The Museum's library contained 700,000 volumes (9).

Alexandria was the metropolis of Egypt, the flourishing seat of commerce, of Grecian and Jewish learning, and of the greatest library of the ancient world. It was destined to become one

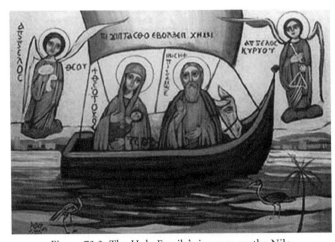

Figure 73.3. The Holy Family's journey on the Nile.

of the great centers of Christianity, the rival of Antioch and Rome.

St. Jerome records that the Christian School of Alexandria was founded by St. Mark himself. He was inspired by the Holy Spirit to establish it to teach Christianity, as this was the only way to give the new religion a solid foundation in the city. The school became the oldest center for sacred sciences in the history of Christianity. In it, the first system of Christian theology was formed and the allegorical method of biblical exegesis was devised.

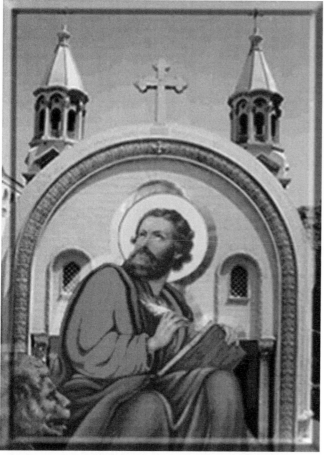

Figure 73.4. St. Mark, the founder of Christianity in Egypt and his Cathedral in Alexandria.

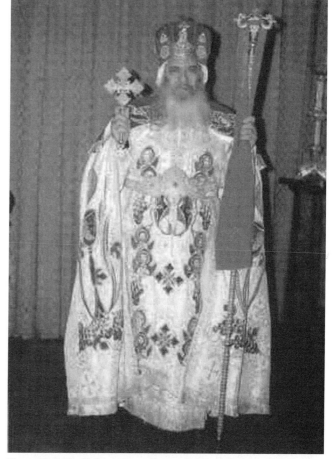

Figure 73.5. His Holiness Pope Shenouda III 117th Pope of Alexandria and Patriarch of the See of St. Mark.

The Orthodox Church's Big Picture in Christianity

If you consider all the Christians in the world, more than 700 million are Catholic and 325 million are Protestants of different denominations and 200 million are Orthodox Christians. However, father Marc Dunaway (1995) states if you are like most Americans, you probably know very little about the Orthodox Church and Orthodox Christianity (10). There are approximately 134 million Christians in the United States: eighty million are Protestant, fifty million are Catholic, and four million are Orthodox. The primary locations of Orthodoxy in the world today are Greece, Russia, Eastern Europe, Egypt, and the Middle East as in Syria, Lebanon, Palestine, and Israel. The Orthodox Church is larger in number than any of the Protestant denominations individually.

The History of the Church

The history of the Church went through different ages. The first was the age of the apostles followed by the age of persecution followed by the age of the ecumenical councils. In a critical moment in Church history, the Church began to be pulled in two directions along the lines of East and West. At that time "East" meant Greece, Asia, Alexandria, and the Middle East and "West" referred to Europe. The causes of this rift were many and complex among which were language and culture, Latin versus. Greek (10). This parting of the ways is known as the "Great Schism."

This was the beginning in the West of what is now called Roman Catholicism and in the East as Orthodox Christianity.

The Coptic Orthodox Church

The Coptic tradition holds that St. Mark heads the list of patriarchs of Alexandria and today's spiritual leader of the Coptic community, His Holiness Pope shenouda III, is 117th Pope of Alexandria, (Figure 73.5). His Holiness the Pope is one of the church's greatest spiritual leaders, theologians, poets and philosophers. He has enriched us with his spiritual lectures, renewed our minds and made the times enjoyable with His great sense of humor. The early history of the Coptic Church is both glorious and tragic (7). It is glorious because of its illustrious children such as the theologians Athanasius and Cyril the Great and the monastic fathers and mothers St. Anthony, St. Pachomias, and St. Syncletica (7) and tragic because of the persecution. Copts regard their Church as the Orthodox Church that held firm to the Nicene Creed as formulated in the first and greatest of the Church councils in 325 A.D. (11). They take pride in the fact that St. Anthony, an Egyptian hermit (Figures 73.6 and 73.7), remains the spiritual father of Christian monasticism (Figures 73.8 and 73.9), and St. Anthanasius, his disciple, was the founder of the Nicene Creed (12). All Christian monasticism by St. Basil, St. Jerome, and St. Benedict stems directly or indirectly from Egyptian monasteries whether by Saint Antony or Saint Pachomias.

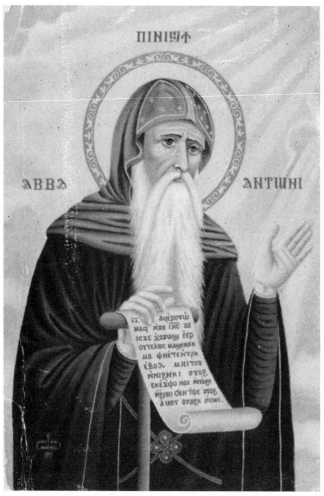

Figure 73.6. St. Anthony, founder of Monasticism.

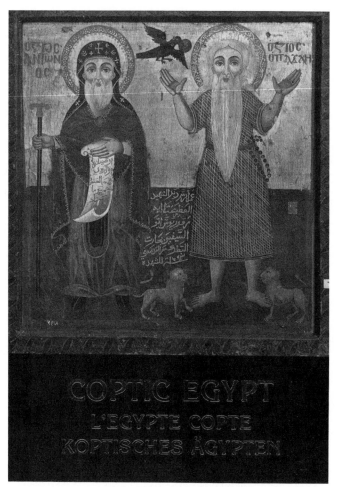

Figure 73.7. St. Anthony and St. Paul depiction of their historic meeting.

Coptic Orthodox Church in the Twentieth Century

The twentieth century has seen a revival of the Coptic Church. The main revival came through the Sunday School Movement and the resurgence of Coptic Monasticism. Coptic Orthodox Christianity has been preached on all the continents during the past four decades by His Holiness Pope Shenouda III. His Holiness ordained more than one hundred bishops in Egypt and several Bishops for the United States in the 1990s. His Grace Bishop Youssef, a beloved and delightful head of the Southern Diocese of the United States kindly revised this manuscript. As he was originally an ENT surgeon he was familiar with medical technology and scientific advances. He worked tirelessly for fifteen years to develop the diocese with grace and in the process built a significant number of churches in Florida and Texas (Figure 73.10).

The First Book on the Christian Opinion on In Vitro Fertilization

The first book on the opinion of the Coptic Orthodox Church on in vitro Fertilization and transfer of embryos was published by His Grace, the late Bishop Gregorios (Figures 73.11 and 73.12), the bishop of theological studies, Coptic culture, and scientific research (13). His book was based on a lecture that he had delivered the year before at the 10th Annual Conference of the College of Medicine, at Ain Shams University in Cairo in

March 1987. The author could personally testify that His Grace Bishop Gregorios was a scholar in different fields of theology and science and represented the ultimate in dedication and purity that could ever be achieved. His book was given to me more than fifteen years ago by Professor Mohamed Aboulghar who started in vitro fertilization in Egypt and sought the opinion of the Coptic Orthodox community as well as the Islamic community. The introduction of his lecture and book starts by ascertaining that the success of in vitro fertilization represents a great success for science by alleviating a great obstacle for married couples wishing to conceive a child. Although having children is not the only reason for marriage, it represents nature's first goal of marriage in all beings including humans. He fully acknowledges that motherhood is the strongest instinct that a woman could have and that having children is the first wish for any mother and certainly infertile women are among the unhappiest people even if they were married to the richest, wealthiest, and most famous. He also acknowledges that the success of in vitro fertilization has brought happiness to thousands of married couples and settled lives among many families. He quoted examples from the Old Testament, painting a picture of how such tragedy could affect family life such as Sara who asked Abraham to marry her maidservant and Rachel and Jacob. He cited Rachel's statement asking Jacob to give her children or she would rather die.

The second chapter focuses on the pitfalls of in vitro fertilization and assisted conception. He emphasized that a key issue

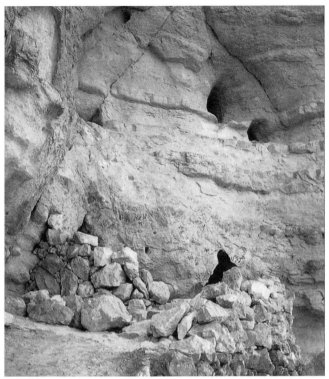

Figure 73.8. The Monastery of St. Anthony on the Red Sea: The world's first monastery.

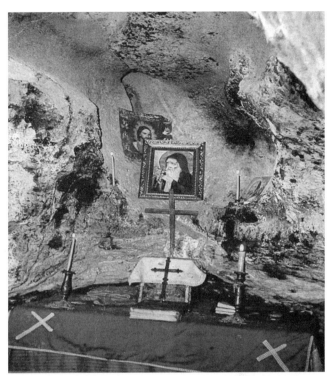

Figure 73.9. St. Anthony's cave in the mountain on the Red Sea.

is the fertilization of a woman's oocyte by her husband's sperm, and extreme accuracy should be exercised in this important issue. He stresses the role of the treating physician in honesty so that there is no question that fertilization has occurred between the husband and wife and not any third party. He acknowledges that in certain situations fertilization might not occur but does not accept that fertilization should be attempted between the wife's oocyte and any other man's spermatozoa, whether it is from a known or an unknown donor. His Grace Bishop Gregorios calls this fertilization incomplete ethically or legally from all aspects because the fruit of the relation between a man and a woman should be from a holy relation.

Another issue that he does not accept is the establishment of embryo banks and the buying and selling of gametes with money. This is fully unacceptable because it brings down the relation of the value of marriage and conception and having children to a low level.

His grace then discusses the difficult issue of surrogate pregnancy and believes that this is an area that has serious consequences. One of those consequences is that the infant may inherit some different psychological or physiological traits of the carrier. He acknowledges that in the past, a mother who died had her child nursed by another woman who could do so and that was a legitimate option in the absence of facilities for feeding. In a later discussion, His Grace Bishop Gregorios denounces surrogacy (14).

In summary, His Grace Bishop Gregorios welcomes and accepts in vitro fertilization only under the circumstances where the oocyte and sperm are taken from the husband and wife and fertilization occurred in vitro with no doubt about gamete mixing. Embryo transfer must be performed to the mother who is the source of the oocytes. All the steps of in vitro fertilization should occur with the approval of the husband and wife, and the treating physician should be alert to the fact that no mixing of gametes

should occur and there should be no doubt in anyone's mind regarding the source of the gametes. He accepted in this lecture that surrogacy is an option when the sperm and oocyte are obtained from the married couple when the wife has lost or does not have the ability to carry a pregnancy as in the case of a woman who has had her uterus removed because of bleeding or cancer. In a later communication, he closed the door on surrogacy even under those rare circumstances (14). In the details of his lecture, he goes through the clinical indications for in vitro fertilization and the steps that should be adhered to from the retrieval of the oocytes until the embryos are transferred to ensure the extreme caution that should be exercised by the couple and the treating physician.

In 1998, His Grace Bishop Serapion of Los Angeles published a series of articles in the El Kiraza journal of which His Holiness Pope Shenouda III is the editor-in-chief (15). His Grace Bishop Serapion (Figure 73.10) who is also a physician by background acknowledges that in vitro fertilization is a legitimate option for couples who cannot achieve a pregnancy by normal means including medical and surgical options. In vitro fertilization is acceptable only if the gametes are from husband and wife. No donor oocyte or spermatozoa should ever be used under any circumstances. Surrogacy is fully unacceptable.

In 1997 His Grace Bishop Moussa, also a medical doctor, published a small book on contraception, in vitro fertilization and cloning, he supported the ethical use of in vitro fertilization using the gametes of the husband and wife. He raised the difficult issue of the fate of the extra embryos and how to handle them (16).

In 2000, His Grace Bishop Moussa published another book on the challenges of the new century, particularly technology, reproduction and organ transplantation. He supported the use of IVF but not donor gametes or third party and condemned cloning. Most importantly, he emphasized the need for honest scientists and clinicians within the church to advise the church on the advances in technology (17).

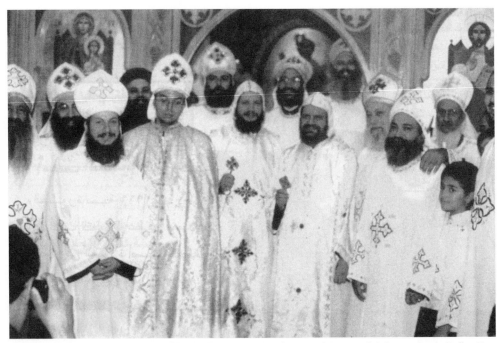

Figure 73.10. Bishop Youssef, Bishop of the Southern Diocese in the United States ordaining a priest in Dallas, Texas.

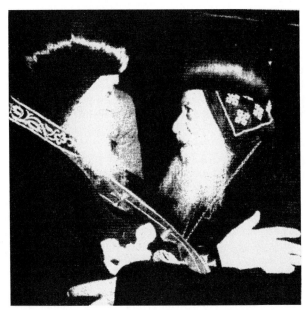

Figure 73.11. His Holiness Pope Shenouda III and His Grace Bishop Gregorios, bishop of scientific research and writer of the first book on in vitro fertilization.

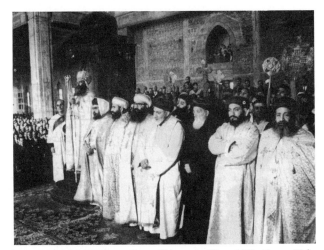

Figure 73.12. His Holiness Pope Shenouda III and His Grace Bishop Gregorios ordaining bishops in 1971.

Sex Selection

Ethicists are divided in two camps: those who feel that sex selection is a choice of couples and those who believe that this would be a biased intervention with negative consequences (16,18). His Grace Bishop Moussa did not support sex selection (17).

Cloning or Somatic Cell Nuclear Transfer

Somatic cell nuclear transfer or cloning is an issue that has divided more ethicists in the Western world (19,20). Cloning could be performed for reproductive reasons. This type of cloning is known as reproductive cloning. To our knowledge, no human being has been successfully cloned. Although it is not impossible, it is extremely difficult to do so. Most medical societies including the American Society for Reproductive Medicine does not accept cloning from an ethical point of view even if it becomes technically possible. Cloning for the production of stem cells is known as therapeutic cloning which is acceptable to some medical societies (19,20). The Coptic Church Los Angeles Diocese has discussed this issue in its Web site. It acknowledges that the goal of stem cell therapy is a nobel goal for millions of peoples. However, it emphasizes that nobel goals should have also nobel means to achieve them. The use of other source of stem cells is therefore advised rather than the use of embryonic stem cells resulting in the destruction of the embryos.

REFERENCES

1. Kamil J. *Coptic Egypt, History and Guide.* American University in Cairo Press. Cairo, Egypt. 1996.

2. Kamil J. *Christianity in the land of the Pharoahs.* The Coptic Orthodox Church Routledge, London. 2002, pp. 1–11.

3. Meinradus OFA. *The Holy Family in Egypt.* The American University in Cairo press. 1986, pp. 15–17.

4. Rev. Fr. Ermia Ava Mina. *The Holy Family in Egypt.* St. Mina Monastery, 1st Edition. St. Mina Press, Cairo, 2000. St. Mina Monastery.

5. His Holiness Pope Shenouda III. St. Mark, the Apostle, Saint and Martyr. 3rd Edition. Ambarouis, Cairo, Egypt, 1996.

6. d'Orlcan Cheneau P. Les Saints d'Egypte. *Jerusalem*, 1923.

7. Meinradus OFA. Coptic Christianity past and present. In: Capuani M (Ed.) *Christian Egypt Coptic Arts and Monuments Through Two Millennia. The Order of St. Benedict Collegeville*, Minesota. pp. 8–20, 2002.

8. Aboulghar M. The Jews of Egypt from Prosperity to Diaspora. *Dar Al Hilal*, 2004. p. 8.

9. Fr. Tadros Y. Malaty. *The School of Alexandria, Before Origen.* Coptic Theological College, Sydney, Australia, 1995, pp. 8–10.

10. Dunaway M. *What is the Orthodox Church? A Brief Overview of Orthodoxy.* Conciliar Press, Ben Lomond, CA, 1995.

11. HG Bishop Bishoy. Ecumenical Councils. The Institute of Coptic Studies, Theology Section. 2003, pp. 1–7.

12. Father Tadros Y. Malaty, Introduction to the Coptic Orthodox Church, 1993. St. George's Coptic Orthodox Church, Alexandria, Egypt.

13. His Grace Bishop Gregorios. The Christian Opinion in In vitro Fertilization and Embryo Transfer. Bisphoric of Higher theological Studies, Coptic Culture and Scientific Research Publications, Cairo, Egypt, 1988.

14. Serour G. Personal Communication.

15. HG Bishop Serapion. The View of the Coptic Orthodox Church on In Vitro Fertilization. Al-Kcraza, Cairo Egypt. 1998.

16. His Grace Bishop Moussa Current medical issues contraception, in vitro fertilization and cloning Youth Bisphorship, cairo, Egypt, 1997.

17. His Grace Bishop Moussa Challenges of the new century Youth Bisphoric, Cairo, Egypt, 2000.

18. Rizk B. Preconception sex selection. American Society for Reproductive Medicine/Middle East Fertility Society Symposium. September, 1999. *Middle East Fertility Society Journal*, 4 (Suppl. 2):14–21.

19. Rizk B. Somatic Cell Nuclear Transfer: Cloning University of South Alabama. *Department of Obstetrics and Gynecology*, Grand Rounds, Dec 17, 2004.

20. Rizk B. Somatic Cell Nuclear Transfer: Cloning. University of Alexandria. Department of Obstetrics and Gynecology 19th Annual Meeting May 5, 2005, Alexandria, Egypt.

ISLAMIC PERSPECTIVES OF ETHICAL ISSUES IN ART

Gamal I. Serour, F.R.C.O.G, F.R.C.S.

Professor of Obstetrics and Gynecology, Director International Islamic Center for Population Studies and Research,

Al-Azhar University, Clinical Director, The Egyptian IVF&ET Center, Maadi, Cairo, Egypt

Science without conscience ruins the soul. It is therefore not surprising that science and religion have been interrelated since the beginning of human history. The past two decades have witnessed the secularization of bioethics. The religious influence on bioethics subsequently declined. Bioethics today is no longer dominated by religion and medical traditions as it used to be in the past. It has become dominated more by philosophical, social, and legal concepts (1). However, in some parts of the world like Middle East, where the three major religions, namely Judaism, Christianity, and Islam emerged, religion still means and influences a lot of behaviors, practices, and policy makings. This also applies to conservative followers and observants of these religions in different parts of the world. The three major religions Judaism, Christianity, and Islam have encouraged procreation, family formation, and child birth through natural conception within the frame of marriage. The Holy Quraan encouraged marriage, family formation, and reproduction. It says: "We did send apostles, before thee, and appointed for them wives and children" (2). In another version it also says "And God has made for you mates (and companions) of your own nature, and made for you, out of them, sons and daughters and grandchildren, and provided for you sustenance of the best" (3). It also refers to the possibility of infertility among some couples as it says "He bestows (children), male or female, according to His will (and Plan), or He bestows both males and females, and He leaves barren whom He will" (4).

ART and Islamic Perspectives

With the advent of assisted reproduction technology (ART) since the birth of Louise Brown in UK on July 25, 1978, it became possible to separate the bonding of reproduction from sexual act (5). ART, whether in vivo or in vitro, enabled women to conceive without having sex. ART made it possible for the involvement of a third party in the process of reproduction whether by providing an egg, a sperm, an embryo, or a uterus. ART opened the way for several other practices including gender selection, preimplantation genetic diagnosis (PGD), genetic manipulation, cryopreservation of gametes, embryos and gonads, cloning . . . etc. This challenged the age-old ideas and provoked ethical debate, which continued since its earliest days (6). An inconsistent attitude was created in many countries all over the world regardless of the religious, cultural, economical, or political background of these countries.

The teaching of Islam covers all the fields of human activity; spiritual and material, individual and social, educational and cultural, economic and political, national and international.

Instruction which regulates everyday activity of life to be adhered to by good Muslims is called Sharia. There are two sources of Sharia in Islam: primary and secondary. The primary sources of Sharia in chronological order are: The Holy Quraan, the very word of God, the Sunna and Hadith, which is the authentic traditions and sayings of the Prophet Mohamed as collected by specialists in Hadith, igmaah, which is the unanimous opinion of Islamic scholars or Aimma and analogy (Kias), which is the intelligent reasoning, used to rule on events not mentioned by the Quraan and Sunna, by matching against similar or equivalent events ailed on. The secondary sources of Sharia are Istihsan, which is the choice of one of several lawful options, views of Prophet's companions, current local customs if lawful, public welfare, and rulings of previous divine religions if they do not contradict the primary sources of Sharia. A good Muslim resorts to secondary sources of Sharia in matters not dealt within the primary sources. Even if the action is forbidden, it may be undertaken if the alternative would cause harm. The Sharia is not rigid. It is flexible enough to adapt to emerging situations in different items and places. It can accommodate different honest opinions as long as they do not conflict with the spirit of its primary sources and are directed to the benefit of humanity (1, 7–9). Islam is a religion of Yusr (ease) not Usr (hardship) as indicated in the Holy Quraan (10). The Broad Principles of Islamic Jurisprudence are permissibility unless prohibited by a text (Ibaha), no harm and no harassment; necessity permits the prohibited and the choice of the lesser harm. ART was not mentioned in the primary sources of Sharia. However, these same sources have affirmed the importance of marriage, family formation, and procreation (2–4, 11, 12). Also, in Islam adoption is not acceptable as a solution to the problem of infertility. Islam gives legal precedence to purity of lineage and known parenthood of all children. The Quraan explicitly prohibits legal adoption but encourages kind upbringing of orphans (13). In Islam infertility and its remedy with the unforbidden is allowed and encouraged. It is essential if it involves preservation of procreation and treatment of infertility in the married couples (7). This is applicable to ART, which is one line of treatment of infertility. The prevention and treatment of infertility are of particular significance in the Muslim World. The social status of the Muslim women, her dignity, and self-esteem are closely related to her procreation potential in the family and in the society as a whole. Childbirth and rearing are regarded as family commitments and not just biological and social functions. As ART was not mentioned in the primary sources of Sharia, patients and Muslim doctors alike thought by seeking ART for infertility treatment, they are challenging God's will trying to make the barren woman fertile, and handling human gametes and embryos. ART was only widely accepted after prestigious scientific and religious bodies and organizations issued guidelines, which were adopted by medical councils or concerned authorities in different Muslim countries and controlled the practices in ART centers.

These guidelines which played a role in the change of attitude of society and individuals in the Muslim World included Fatwa from Al-Azhar, Cairo 1980 (7) and Fatwa from Islamic Fikh Council, Mecca 1984, the Organization of Islamic Medicine in Kuwait (1991), Qatar University (1993), the Islamic Education, Science and Culture Organization in Rabaat (2002), the United Arab Emirate (2002), and the International Islamic Center for Population Studies and Research, Al Azhar University (14–19). These bodies stressed the fact that Islam encouraged marriage, family formation, and procreation in its primary sources. Treat-

ment of infertility, including ART when indicated, is encouraged to preserve humankind within the frame of marriage, in otherwise incurable infertility. The attitude of patients changed from rejection, doubt, feeling of shame, guilt, and secrecy when seeking ART in the eighties to openly asking ART in the nineties. The introduction of the effective ICSI treatment for male infertility played a role in the change of attitude of many couples to ART (9). In family affairs, particularly reproduction, the decisions are usually taken by the couple. However, not uncommonly the husband's decision is the dominating one. Husbands became very enthusiastic about ART. They took the initiative and encouraged their wives to undergo ART treatment for male, female, or unexplained infertility. Today the basic guidelines for ART in the Muslim World are: if ART is indicated in a married couple as a necessary line of treatment, it is permitted during validity of marriage contract with no mixing of genes. If the marriage contract has come to an end because of divorce or death of the husband, artificial reproduction cannot be performed on the female partner even using sperm cells from former husband. The Shi'aa Guidelines has "opened" the way to a third-party donation, via Fatwa from Ayatollah Ali Hussein Khomeini in 1999. This Fatwa allowed third-party participation including egg donation, sperm donation, and surrogacy. The Fatwa is gaining acceptance in parts of the Shi'ite world. Recently, there has been some concern about sperm donation among Shi'aa. All these practices of third-party participation in reproduction are based on the importance of maintaining the family structure and integrity among the Shi'aa family. They are allowed within various temporary marriage contract arrangements with the concerned donors.

Surrogacy

Surrogacy is not permitted for most sunni. The Fatwa of the Fikh council in 1984 allowed surrogacy by replacing the embryos inside the uterus of the second wife of the same husband who provided the sperms. In 1985, the council withdrew its approval of surrogacy (1, 6, 14).

Recently, there had been a debate among Sunni scholars on surrogacy. While some religious authorities thought that it can be permitted, others believed that it should not be approved.

Cryopreservation

The excess number of fertilized eggs can be preserved by cryopreservation. The frozen embryos are the property of the couple alone and may be transferred to the same wife in a successive cycle but only during the validity of the marriage contract (7, 8, 16–18). Whether the couple's preserved embryos could be implanted in a wife after her husband's death was discussed in an international workshop organized by The International Islamic Center for Population Studies and Research, AL Azhar University in 2000. The strict view was that marriage ends at death, and procuring pregnancy in an unmarried woman is forbidden by religious laws, for instance, on children's rights to be reared by two parents, and on inheritance. After due time, the widow might remarry but could not then bear a child that was not her new husband's. An opposing view, advanced as reflecting both Islamic compassion and women's interests as widows, was that a woman left alone through early widowhood would be well and tolerably served by bearing her deceased husband's child, through her enjoying companionship, discharge of religious duties of childrearing, and later support. The Grand Mufti of Egypt (personal communication) stated that permission had once been given for embryo implantation in a wife following her husband's death, based on the circumstances of the particular case. However, this should not be taken as a generalization, and each case should be considered on its own merits (18, 20).

Multifetal Pregnancy Reduction

Multifetal pregnancy particularly HOMP should be prevented in the first place. Should HOMP occur inspite of all preventive measures, then multifetal pregnancy reduction may be performed applying the jurisprudence principles of necessity that permits the prohibited and the choice of the lesser harm. Multifetal pregnancy reduction is only allowed if the prospect of carrying the pregnancy to viability is small. Also it is allowed if the life or the health of the mother is in jeopardy (16, 20–22). It is performed with the intention not to induce abortion but to preserve the life of remaining fetuses and minimize complications to the mother.

Embryo Research

Development of embryo/fetus advances step by step with its morphological development and growth from a clot to a lump of flesh, then boned flesh, and, finally, a fully grown infant (23, 24). Till forty days the embryos in the mother's womb is "a nutfa," then "an alaqa" for an equal period then "a mudgha." The organ differentiation occurs in forty-two days after fertilization. Ensoulment of the fetus occurs after 120 days from fertilization (25). The old threshold of forty days and upward from conception has been brought back to fourteen days because the new embryology has established this embryonic period of cellular activity before which individuation cannot begin (15). Embryo research, for advancement of scientific knowledge and benefit of humanity, is therefore allowed before fourteen days after fertilization on embryos donated for research with the free informed consent of the couple. However, these embryos should not be replaced in the uterus of the owner's of the eggs or in the uterus of any other woman (7, 8, 15, 18). Reflecting the unstructured ethical governance of research in several of the Muslim countries should each country form a national research ethics committee to which any proposed research involving the use of gametes or embryos outside the body shall be submitted for prior review and approval.

Sex Selection

The use of sperm-sorting techniques or PGD for non medical reasons such as sex selection or balancing sex ratio in the family is guarded. These techniques are better alternative to prenatal diagnosis that necessitates abortion for sex selection. Muslims adhere to the view that human life requiring protection commences two to three weeks from conception and uterine implantation (15). Accordingly, decisions not to attempt replacement of embryos produced in vitro on grounds that they show serious chromosomal or genetic anomalies, such as aneuploidy, cystic fibrosis, muscular dystrophy or hemophilia, are accepted. PGD is encouraged, where feasible, as an option to avoid clinical pregnancy terminations for couples at exceptionally high risk (20). More contentious is non medical purposes of sex selection. Arabs more than 1,400 years ago, before Islam, used to practice infanticide for gender selection. The Holy Quraan described this act and condemned it (26, 27). It says: "On God's Judgment Day the

entombed alive female infant is asked, for what guilt was she made to suffer infanticide?" Sex selection technologies have been condemned on the ground that their application is to discriminate against female embryos and fetuses, so perpetuating prejudice against the girl child (28) and social devaluation of women. Such discrimination and devaluation are condemned in the Muslim World. However, universal prohibition would itself risk prejudice to women in many present societies, especially while births of sons remain central to women's well-being. Sex ratio balancing in the family is considered acceptable, for instance, where a wife had borne three or four daughters or sons and it was in her and her family's best interests that another pregnancy should be her last. Employing sex selection techniques to ensure the birth of a son or a daughter might then be approved, to satisfy a sense of religious or family obligation and to save the woman from increasingly risk-laden pregnancies (29, 30). Application of PGD or sperm-sorting techniques for sex selection should be disfavored in principle, but resolved on its particular merits with guidelines to avoid discrimination against either sex particularly the female child (20, 29, 30). It should not be used for selection of the sex of the first child or for selection of one sex only in the family. Also it is only applied to families who have children of only one sex and have intense desire to have one more child of the other sex. The service is only provided after proper counseling with the reproductive medicine physicians, geneticist, social scientist, and psychologist (31).

Pregnancy in the Postmenopause

The possibility of postmenopausal pregnancy in the past before cryopreservation was considered dependent on ovum donation, which was disapproved in principle as it involves mixing of genes (7, 8, 22). Also pregnancy after menopause is associated with increased risks for both mother and child. Accordingly, it was unacceptable in the Muslim World (17). However, with the development of cryopreservation it is now possible to have pregnancy in the postmenopause using one's own cryopreserved embryos or even oocytes and possible in future cryopreserved ovaries. Taking into consideration special care necessary for the safe induction and completion of pregnancy in a woman who was of advanced, or beyond normal, childbearing years and of the easier case where premature menopause affects a woman who would otherwise be of suitable maternal age, and the children's needs of parents likely to survive at least into their midadolescence, research efforts should be concentrated on the prevention of premature menopause and that the postmenopausal pregnancy be permissible to attempt in exceptional cases justified by maintenance of integrity of a child's genetic parentage, the pressing nature of the circumstances, the relative safety to mother and child, and parental capacity to discharge childrearing responsibilities (18, 20).

Cloning

Reproductive cloning for creation and birth of a new person who would be the genetic twin of one born previously is condemned. Research in non reproductive cloning, particularly for stem cell creation, study, and research intended for human benefit is encouraged. Encouragement is not limited by recognition that use of deliberately created embryos is likely to be involved. Study and research were anticipated to have a beneficial impact on reproduction, in that understanding of the origins of genetic defects in embryonic and fetal development would facilitate prevention and correction of defects, and, when prevention or correction were impossible, selection of healthy gametes or embryos (18). Some theologians are sympathetic to consideration of reproductive cloning of cells of a childless sterile man if his wife was willing so to bear the child, to permit discharge of religious duties and relieve family distress and risk of marriage breakdown through the wife's right of divorce. There would be no violation of the rules against third-party involvement or against confusion of lineage. However, the genetic father would be the husband's father, introducing problems of his consent and perhaps of inheritance laws. On balance, it is considered rather premature to recommend department from the prevailing condemnation of reproductive cloning (18, 20).

Allied with stem cell research is the prospect of gene therapy. Progress in somatic cell gene therapy, which alters the genes only of a treated patient, has suffered recent setbacks, and germline gene therapy, which would affect all future generations of a patient's offspring, remains little short of universally condemned and prohibited (32). Genetic alteration of embryos before their cells have reached differentiation, that is, while they are still totipotent, would constitute germline manipulation. Little would be added to reiterate prevailing condemnation. Gene therapy is a developing area that may be used with ART in the future. It is critical that its use be clearly beneficial, focused on alleviating human suffering. The focus on therapeutic applications would exclude purely cosmetic uses and goals of enhancement of non pathological conditions. Alleviation of genetic diseases and pathological conditions alone would exclude such applications as to make people who would be within the normal range of physique, capacity, and aptitude, taller, stronger, more likely to achieve athletic success or to be more intelligent or artistically sensitive or gifted. Gene therapy might be legitimate, not to promote advantage or privilege, but to redeem genetically or otherwise physiologically inherited disadvantage (7, 8, 16).

Conclusions

Physicians providing ART are always concerned about legislations of various practices of ART in countries where they are practicing. However, in many countries legalizations do not exist and physicians follow guidelines issued by prestigious concerned bodies and organizations if they exist.

With globalization, doctors and patients alike are moving around to different parts of the world; it becomes not uncommon that physicians may have to provide medical services to patients with an ethical precepts, which are different from that of their own. However, conscientious objection to offer certain required treatment to patients by their physicians should not deprive them from the right of being referred to other physicians who would provide such treatment. It becomes, therefore, mandatory to be aware of various religious perspectives on various practices in ART.

REFERENCES

1. Serour GI. Ethical considerations of assisted reproductive technologies: a Middle Eastern Perspective. Opinion. *Middle East Fertile Soc J* 2000;5:1:13–18.
2. Sura Al-Ra'd 13:38, Holy Quraan.
3. Sura Al-Nahl 16:27, Holy Quraan.
4. Sura Ai-Shura 42:49–50, Holy Quraan.
5. Steptoe PC, Edwards RG. Birth after the preimplantation of human embryo. *Lancet* 1978;2:366.
6. Scrour GI, Aboulghar MA, Mansour RT. Bioethics in medically assisted conception in The Muslim World. *J Assisted Reprod and Genetics* 1995;12:9:559–565.
7. Gad El-Hak AGH.In vitro fertilization and test tube baby. *Dar El Iftaa*, Cairo, Egypt. 1980;1225:1:115:3213–3228.
8. Gad El Hak AG.E. Serour GI. (ed.) *Some gynecological problems in the context of Islam*. The International Islamic Center for Population Studies and Research. Cairo: Al Azhar University, 2000.
9. Serour GI. Attitudes and cultural perspective on infertility and its alleviation in the Middle East Area. Vaycnna E (ed.) *Current Practices and Controversies in Assisted Reproduction*. Report of WHO Meeting, WHO Geneva 2002, 41–49.
10. Sura Al Bakara 2:185, Holy Quaraan.
11. Hadilh Shareef. Reported by Abou Dawood.
12. Hadilh Shareef. Reported by Bukhary and Muslaam.
13. Sura Al Ahzab 32:4–5, Holy Quraan.
14. Proceedings of 7th Meeting of the Islamic Fikh Council in IVF & HT and AIH, Mecca (1984) Kuwait Siasa Daily Newspaper, March, 1984.
15. Serour GI. *Embryo research. Ethical implications in the Islamic World 2002*. ISESCO, Rabat, Morocco.
16. Serour GI. (ed.). *Ethical guidelines for human reproduction research in the Muslim Worlds. The international Islamic Center for Population studies and Research*. Cairo: Al Azhar University, 1992.
17. Serour GI. (ed.). *Ethical implications of the use of ART in the Muslim World*. The International Islamic Center for Population Studies and Research. Cairo: Al Azhar University, 1997.
18. Serour GI. (ed.). *Ethical implications of the use of ART in the Muslim World: Update*. The International Islamic Center for Population Studies and Research. Cairo: Al Azhar University, 2000.
19. Islamic organization of education, science and culture (ISECO). Ethical reflection of advanced genetic research. Qatar: Doha. February 1993.
20. Serour GI, Dickens B. Assisted reproduction developments in the Islamic World. *International J Gynecol Obstet* 2001;74:187–193.
21. Tanlawi S.Islamic Sharia and selective fetal reduction. *Al Ahram Daily Newsletter*, Cairo: Egypt, 1991.
22. Serour GI. 2002. Medically assisted conception, dilemma of practice and research: Islamic views. GI Serour (ed.). In *Proceedings of the First International Conference on Bioethics in Human Reproduction Research in the Muslim World, IICPSR*. 1992;234–242.
23. Sura E3 Hag 22:5, Holy Quraan.
24. Sura Al Mo'menon 23:14, Holy Quraan.
25. Hadith Shareef Reported by Bokhary and Muslim.
26. Sura Al-Nahl 58–59, Holy Quran.
27. Sura Al-Takwir: 8–9, Holy Quran.
28. Fathalla MF. The girl child. *Int J Gynecol Obstet* 2000;70:7–12.
29. Serour GI. *Transcultural issues in gender selection*. Daya S., Harrison R., Kampers R. (ed.). Recent Advances in Infertility and Reproductive Technology. International Federation of Fertility Societies (IFFS) 18th World Congress on Fertility and Sterility, Montreal 2004.
30. Serour GI. Family Sex and Section. Healy DL (ed.). *Reproductive medicine in the twenty-first century. Proceedings of the 17th World Congress on Fertility and Sterility*, Melbourne: Australia. The Parthenon publishing group 2002;97–106.
31. Serour GI. Ethical guidelines for gender selection: are they needed? *Proceeding in International Conference on Reproductive Disruptions Childlessness, Adoption and Other Reproductive Complexities*, USA; University of Michigan, May 18–22, 2005.
32. El Bayoumi AA, Al Ali K. Gene therapy: the state of the art. Rabat, Morocco: Ethical Reflection of Advanced Genetic Research. In Islamic Educational. *Scientific and Cultural Organization (ESESCO)*, Rabat, 2000.

THE VATICAN VIEW ON HUMAN PROCREATION

Michel Abou Abdallah, M.D.

Chief Consultant, Middle East Fertility Clinic, Beirut, Lebanon

INTRODUCTION

The gift of life which God the Creator has entrusted to man calls him to appreciate the inestimable value of what he has been given and to take responsibility for it: this fundamental principle must be placed at the centre of one's reflection in order to clarify and solve the moral problems raised by artificial interventions on life as it originates and on the processes of procreation. Thanks to the progress of the biological and medical sciences, man has at his disposal ever more effective therapeutic resources; but he can also acquire new powers, with unforeseeable consequences, over human life at its very beginning and in its first stages. Various procedures now make it possible to intervene not only in order to assist but also to dominate the processes of procreation. These techniques can enable man to "take in hand his own destiny," but they also expose him "to the temptation to go beyond the limits of a reasonable dominion over nature" (1). They might constitute progress in the service of man, but they also involve serious risks.

Science and Technology at the Service of the Human Person

God created man in his own image and likeness: "male and female he created them" (Gen 1: 27), entrusting to them the task of "having dominion over the earth" (Gen 1:28). Basic scientific research and applied research constitute a significant expression of this dominion of man over creation. Science and technology are valuable resources for man when placed at his service and when they promote his integral development for the benefit of all; but they cannot of themselves show the meaning of existence and of human progress. Being ordered to man, who initiates and develops them, they draw from the person and his moral values the indication of their purpose and the awareness of their limits.

The rapid development of technological discoveries gives greater urgency to this need to respect the criteria just mentioned: science without conscience can only lead to man's ruin.

Fundamental Criteria for a Moral Judgment

The fundamental values connected with the techniques of artificial human procreation are two: the life of the human being called into existence and the special nature of the transmission of human life in marriage. The moral judgment on such methods of artificial procreation must therefore be formulated in reference to these values.

Advances in technology have now made it possible to procreate apart from sexual relations through the meeting in vitro of the germ cells previously taken from the man and the woman. But what is technically possible is not for that very reason morally admissible. Rational reflection on the fundamental values of life and of human procreation is therefore indispensable for formulating a moral evaluation of such technological interventions on a human being from the first stages of his development.

Teachings of the Magisterium

On its part, the Magisterium of the Church offers to human reason in this field too the light of Revelation: the doctrine concerning man taught by the Magisterium contains many elements which throw light on the problems being faced here. From the moment of conception, the life of every human being is to be respected in an absolute way because man is the only creature on earth that God has "wished for himself" (16) and the spiritual soul of each man is "immediately created" by God; (17) his whole being bears the image of the Creator. Human life is sacred because from its beginning it involves "the creative action of God" (18) and it remains forever in a special relationship with the Creator, who is its sole end (19). God alone is the Lord of life from its beginning until its end: no one can, in any circumstance, claim for himself the right to destroy directly an innocent human being (20). Human procreation requires on the part of the spouses responsible collaboration with the fruitful love of God (21); the gift of human life must be actualized in marriage through the specific and exclusive acts of husband and wife, in accordance with the laws inscribed in their persons and in their union (22).

Respect for Human Embryos

At the Second Vatican Council, the Church for her part presented once again to modern man her constant and certain doctrine according to which "life once conceived, must be protected with the utmost care; abortion and infanticide are abominable crimes" (23). More recently, the Charter of the Rights of the Family, published by the Holy See, confirmed that "human life must be absolutely respected and protected from the moment of conception" (24).

Interventions upon Human Procreation

By "artificial procreation" or "artificial fertilization" are understood here the different technical procedures directed toward obtaining a human conception in a manner other than the sexual union of man and woman. This instruction deals with fertilization of an ovum in a test-tube (in vitro fertilization) and artificial insemination through transfer into the woman's genital tracts of previously collected sperm.

A preliminary point for the moral evaluation of such technical procedures is constituted by the consideration of the circumstances and consequences, which those procedures involve in relation to the respect due the human embryo. Development of the practice of in vitro fertilization has required innumerable fertilizations and destructions of human embryos. Even today, the usual practice presupposes a hyperovulation on the part of the woman: a number of ova are withdrawn, fertilized and then cultivated in vitro for some days. Usually not all are transferred into the genital tracts of the woman; some embryos, generally called "spare," are destroyed or frozen. On occasion, some of the implanted embryos are sacrificed for various eugenic, economic, or psychological reasons. Such deliberate destruction of human beings or their utilization for different purposes detrimental to their integrity and life is contrary to the doctrine on procured abortion already recalled. The connection between in vitro fertilization and the voluntary destruction of human embryos occurs too often. This is significant: through these procedures, with apparently contrary purposes, life and death are subjected to the decision of man, who thus sets himself up as the giver of life and death by decree. This dynamic of violence and domination may remain unnoticed by those very individuals who, in wishing to utilize this procedure, become subject to it themselves. The facts recorded and the cold logic which links them must be taken into consideration for a moral judgment on IVF and ET (in vitro fertilization and embryo transfer): the abortion mentality which has made this procedure possible thus leads, whether one wants it or not, to man's domination over the life and death of his fellow human beings and can lead to a system of radical eugenics.

Nevertheless, such abuses do not exempt one from a further and thorough ethical study of the techniques of artificial procreation considered in themselves, abstracting as far as possible from the destruction of embryos produced in vitro. The present instruction will therefore take into consideration in the first place the problems posed by heterologous artificial fertilization (II, 1–3),* and subsequently those linked with homologous artificial fertilization (II, 4–6).** Before formulating an ethical judgment on each of these procedures, the principles and values which determine the moral evaluation of each of them will be considered.

Heterologous Artificial Fertilization

Why Must Human Procreation Take Place in Marriage?

Every human being is always to be accepted as a gift and blessing of God. However, from the moral point of view, a truly responsible procreation vis-a-vis the unborn child must be the fruit of marriage.

For human procreation has specific characteristics by virtue of the personal dignity of the parents and of the children: the procreation of a new person, whereby the man and the woman collaborate with the power of the Creator, must be the fruit and the sign of the mutual self-giving of the spouses, of their love, and of their fidelity (34). The fidelity of the spouses in the unity of marriage involves reciprocal respect of their right to become a father and a mother only through each other. The child has the right to be conceived, carried in the womb, brought into the world and brought up within marriage: it is through the secure and recognized relationship to his own parents that the child can discover his own identity and achieve his own proper human development. The parents find in their child a confirmation and completion of their reciprocal self-giving: the child is the living image of their love, the permanent sign of their

conjugal union, the living and indissoluble concrete expression of their paternity and maternity (35).

Does Heterologous Artificial Fertilization Conform to the Dignity of the Couple and to the Truth of Marriage?

The desire to have a child and the love between spouses who long to obviate a sterility which cannot be overcome in any other way constitute understandable motivations; but subjectively good intentions do not render heterologous artificial fertilization conformable to the objective and inalienable properties of marriage or respectful of the rights of the child and of the spouses.

Homologous Artificial Fertilization

Since heterologous artificial fertilization has been declared unacceptable, the question arises as to how to evaluate morally the process of homologous artificial fertilization: IVF and ET and artificial insemination between husband and wife. First a question of principle must be clarified.

What Connection is Required from the Moral Point of View between Procreation and the Conjugal Act?

1. The Church's teaching on marriage and human procreation affirms the "inseparable connection, willed by God and unable to be broken by man on his own initiative, between the two meanings of the conjugal act: the unitive meaning and the procreative meaning. Indeed, by its intimate structure, the conjugal act, while most closely uniting husband and wife, capacitates them for the generation of new lives, according to laws inscribed in the very being of man and of woman" (38). This principle, which is based upon the nature of marriage and the intimate connection of the goods of marriage, has well-known consequences on the level of responsible fatherhood and motherhood. "By safeguarding both these essential aspects, the unitive and the procreative, the conjugal act preserves in its fullness the sense of true mutual love and its ordination towards man's exalted vocation to parenthood" (39). The same doctrine concerning the link between the meanings of the conjugal act and between the goods of marriage throws light on the moral problem of homologous artificial fertilization since "it is never permitted to separate these different aspects to such a degree as positively to exclude either the procreative intention or the conjugal relation" (40). Contraception deliberately deprives the conjugal act of its openness to procreation and in this way brings about a voluntary dissociation of the ends of marriage. Homologous artificial fertilization, in seeking a procreation which is not the fruit of a specific act of conjugal union, objectively affects an analogous separation between the goods and the meanings of marriage. Thus, fertilization is licitly sought when it is the result of a "conjugal act which is per se suitable for the generation of children to which marriage is ordered by its nature and by which the spouses become one flesh" (41). But from the moral point of view procreation is deprived of its proper perfection when it is not desired as the fruit of the conjugal act, that is, to say of the specific act of the spouses' union.

2. The moral value of the intimate link between the goods of marriage and between the meanings of the conjugal act is based upon the unity of the human being, a unity involving

body and spiritual soul (42). Spouses mutually express their personal love in the "language of the body, " which clearly involves both "sponsal meanings" and parental ones (43). The conjugal act by which the couple mutually express their self-gift at the same time expresses openness to the gift of life. It is an act that is inseparably corporal and spiritual. It is in their bodies and through their bodies that the spouses consummate their marriage and are able to become father and mother. In order to respect the language of their bodies and their natural generosity, the conjugal union must take place with respect for its openness to procreation; and the procreation of a person must be the fruit and the result of married love. The origin of the human being thus follows from a procreation that is "linked to the union, not only biological but also spiritual, of the parents, made one by the bond of marriage" (44). Fertilization achieved outside the bodies of the couple remains by this very fact deprived of the meanings and the values which are expressed in the language of the body and in the union of human persons.

3. Only respect for the link between the meanings of the conjugal act and respect for the unity of the human being make possible procreation in conformity with the dignity of the person. In his unique and irrepeatable origin, the child must be respected and recognized as equal in personal dignity to those who give him life. The human person must be accepted in his parents' act of union and love; the generation of a child must therefore be the fruit of that mutual giving (45) which is realized in the conjugal act wherein the spouses cooperate as servants and not as masters in the work of the Creator who is Love. In reality, the origin of a human person is the result of an act of giving. The one conceived must be the fruit of his parents' love. He cannot be desired or conceived as the product of an intervention of medical or biological techniques; that would be equivalent to reducing him to an object of scientific technology. No one may subject the coming of a child into the world to conditions of technical efficiency which are to be evaluated according to standards of control and dominion. The moral relevance of the link between the meanings of the conjugal act and between the goods of marriage, as well as the unity of the human being and the dignity of his origin, demand that the procreation of a human person be brought about as the fruit of the conjugal act specific to the love between spouses. The link between procreation and the conjugal act is thus shown to be of great importance on the anthropological and moral planes, and it throws light on the positions of the Magisterium with regard to homologous artificial fertilization.

Is Homologous "In Vitro" Fertilization Morally Licit?

The answer to this question is strictly dependent on the principles just mentioned. Certainly, one cannot ignore the legitimate aspirations of sterile couples. For some, recourse to homologous IVF and ET appears to be the only way of fulfilling their sincere desire for a child. The question is asked whether the totality of conjugal life in such situations is not sufficient to ensure the dignity proper to human procreation. It is acknowledged that IVF and ET certainly cannot supply for the absence of sexual relations (47) and cannot be preferred to the specific acts of conjugal union, given the risks involved for the child and

the difficulties of the procedure. But it is asked whether, when there is no other way of overcoming the sterility which is a source of suffering, homologous IVF may not constitute an aid, if not a form of therapy, whereby its moral licitness could be admitted. The desire for a child – or at the very least an openness to the transmission of life – is a necessary prerequisite from the moral point of view for responsible human procreation. But this good intention is not sufficient for making a positive moral evaluation of IVF between spouses. The process of IVF and ET must be judged in itself and cannot borrow its definitive moral quality from the totality of conjugal life of which it becomes part nor from the conjugal acts which may precede or follow it (48).

Conception in vitro is the result of the technical action which presides over fertilization. Such fertilization is neither in fact achieved nor positively willed as the expression and fruit of a specific act of the conjugal union. In homologous IVF and ET, therefore, even if it is considered in the context of "de facto" existing sexual relations, the generation of the human person is objectively deprived of its proper perfection: namely, that of being the result and fruit of a conjugal act in which the spouses can become "cooperators with God for giving life to a new person" (50). These reasons enable us to understand why the act of conjugal love is considered in the teaching of the Church as the only setting worthy of human procreation. For the same reasons the so-called simple case, that is, a homologous IVF and ET procedure that is free of any compromise with the abortive practice of destroying embryos and with masturbation, remains a technique which is morally illicit because it deprives human procreation of the dignity which is proper and connatural to it. Certainly, homologous IVF and ET fertilization is not marked by all that ethical negativity found in extra-conjugal procreation; the family and marriage continue to constitute the setting for the birth and upbringing of the children. Nevertheless, in conformity with the traditional doctrine relating to the goods of marriage and the dignity of the person, the Church remains opposed from the moral point of view to homologous "in vitro" fertilization. Such fertilization is in itself illicit and in opposition to the dignity of procreation and of the conjugal union, even when everything is done to avoid the death of the human embryo. Although the manner in which human conception is achieved with IYF and ET cannot be approved, every child which comes into the world must in any case be accepted as a living gift of the divine Goodness and must be brought up with love.

What Moral Criterion Can be Proposed with Regard to Medical Intervention in Human Procreation?

The humanization of medicine, which is insisted upon today by everyone, requires respect for the integral dignity of the human person first of all in the act and at the moment in which the spouses transmit life to a new person. It is only logical therefore to address an urgent appeal to Catholic doctors and scientists that they bear exemplary witness to the respect due to the human embryo and to the dignity of procreation. The medical and nursing staff of Catholic hospitals and clinics are in a special way urged to do justice to the moral obligations which they have assumed, frequently also, as part of their contract. Those who are in charge of Catholic hospitals and clinics and who are often religious will take special care to safeguard and promote a diligent observance of the moral norms recalled in the present instruction.

Conclusions

The spread of technologies of intervention in the processes of human procreation raises very serious moral problems in relation to the respect due to the human being from the moment of conception, to the dignity of the person, of his or her sexuality, and of the transmission of life. With this instruction, the Congregation for the Doctrine of the Faith, in fulfilling its responsibility to promote and defend the Church's teaching in so serious a matter, addresses a new and heartfelt invitation to all those who, by reason of their role and their commitment, can exercise a positive influence and ensure that, in the family and in society, due respect is accorded to life and love. It addresses this invitation to those responsible for the formation of consciences and of public opinion, to scientists and medical professionals, to jurists and politicians. It hopes that all will understand the incompatibility between recognition of the dignity of the human person and contempt for life and love, between faith in the living God and the claim to decide arbitrarily the origin and fate of a human being.

In particular, the Congregation for the Doctrine of the Faith addresses an invitation with confidence and encouragement to theologians, and above all to moralists, that they study more deeply and make eves more accessible to the faithful the contents of the teaching of the Church's Magisterium in the light of a valid anthropology in the matter of sexuality and marriage and in the context of the necessary interdisciplinary approach. Thus, they will make it possible to understand ever more clearly the reasons for and the validity of this teaching. By defending man against the excesses of his own power, the Church of God reminds him of the reasons for his true nobility; only in this way can the possibility of living and loving with that dignity and liberty which derive from respect for the truth be ensured for the men and women of tomorrow. The precise indications which are offered in the present instruction therefore are not meant to halt the effort of reflection but rather to give it a renewed impulse in unrenounceable fidelity to the teaching of the Church.

In the light of the truth about the gift of human life and in the light of the moral principles which flow from that truth, everyone is invited to act in the area of responsibility proper to each and, like the good Samaritan, to recognize as a neighbour even the littlest among the children of men (cf. Lk 10: 2 9–37). Here Christ's words find a new and particular echo: "What you do to one of the least of my brethren, you do unto me" (Mt 25:40).

REFERENCES

1. POPE JOHN PAUL II, Discourse to those taking part in the 81st Congress of the Italian Society of Internal Medicine and he 82nd Congress of the Italian Society of Genera! Surgery, 27 October 1980: *AAS*72 (1980) 1126.
2. POPE PAUL VI, Discourse to the General Assembly of the Religious Perspectives in ART United Nations Organization, 4 October 1965: *AAS*57 (1965) 878; Encyclical Populorum Progressio, 13: *AAS*59 (1967) 263.
3. POPE PAUL VI, Homily during the Mass closing the Holy Year,25 December 1975: *AAS*68 (1976) 145; POPE JOHN PAUL II, Encyclical Dives in Misericordia, 30: *AAS*72 (1980) 1224.
4. POPE JOHN PAUL II, Discourse to those taking part in the 35th General Assembly of the World Medical Association, 29 October 1983: *AAS*76 (1984) 390.
5. Cf. Declaration Dignitatis Humanae, 2.
6. Pastoral Constitution Gaudium et Spes, 22; POPE JOHN PAUL II, Encyclical Redemptor Hominis, 8: *AAS*71 (1979) 270–272.
7. Cf. Pastoral Constitution Gaudium et Spes, 35.
8. Pastoral Constitution Gaudium et Spes, 15; cf. also POPE PAUL VI, Encyclical Populorum Progressio, 20: *AAS*59 (1967) 267; POPE JOHN PAUL II, Encyclical Redemptor Hominis, 15: *AAS*71 (1979) 286–289; Apostolic Exhortation Familiaris Consortio, 8: *AAS*74 (1982) 89.
9. POPE JOHN PAUL II, Apostolic Exhortation Familiaris Consortio, II: *AAS*74 (1982) 92.
10. Cf. POPE PAUL VI, Encyclical Humanae Vitae, 10: *AAS*60(1968) 487–488.
11. POPE JOI-IN PAUL II, Discourse to the members of the 35th General Assembly of the World Medical Association, 29 October 1983: *AAS*76 (1984) 393.
12. Cf POPE JOHN PAUL II, Apostolic Exhortation Familiaris Consortio, 11: *AAS*74 (1982) 91–92; cf. also *Pastoral Constitution Gaudium et Spes*, 50.
13. SACRED CONGREGATION FOR THE DOCTRINE OF THE FAITH, Declaration on Procured Abortion, 9, *AAS*66 (1974) 736–737.
14. POPE JOHN PAUL II, Discourse to those taking part in the 35th General Assembly of the World Medical Association, 29 October 1983: *AAS*76 (1984) 390.
15. POPE JOHN XXIII, Encyclical Mater et Magistra, III: *AAS*53 (1961) 447.
16. Pastoral Constitution Gaudium et Spes, 24.
17. Cr. POPE PIUS XII, Encyclical Humani Generis: *AAS*42 (1950) 575: POPE PAUL VI, Professio Fidel: *AAS*60 (1968) 436.
18. POPE JOHN XXIII, Encyclical Mater et Magistra, III: AAS 53 (1961) 447; cf. POPE JOHN PAUL II, Discourse to priests participating in a seminar on "ResponsibJc Procrcation", 17 September 1983, Insegnamcnti di Giovanni Paolo II, VI, 2 (1983) 562: "*At the origin of each human person there is a creative act of God: no man comes into existence by chance: he is always the result of the creative love of God.*"
19. Cf. Pastoral Constitution Gaudium et Spes, 24.
20. Cf. POPE PIUS XII, Discourse to the Saint Luke Medical~ Biological Union, 12 November 1944: *Discorsi e Radiomessaggi* VI (1944–1945) 191–192.
21. Cf. Pastoral Constitution Gaudium et Spes, 50.
22. Cf. Pastoral Constitution Gaudium et Spes, 51: "When it is a question of harmonizing married love with the responsible transmission of life, the moral character of one's behaviour does not depend only on the good intention and the evaluation of the motives: the objective criteria must be used, criteria drawn from the nature of the human person and human acts, criteria which respect the total meaning of mutual self-giving and human procreation in the context of true love."
23. Pastoral Constitution Gaudium et Spes, 51.
24. HOLY SEE, Charter of the Rights of the Family, 4: *L'Osservatore Romano*, 25 November 1983.
25. SACRED CONGREGATION FOR THE DOCTRINE OF THE FAITH, Declaration on Procured Abortion, 12–13: *AAS*66 (1974) 738.
26. Cf. POPE PAUL VI, Discourse to participants in the Twenty-third National Congress or Italian Catholic Jurists, 9 December 1972: *AAS*64 (1972) 777.
27. The obligation to avoid disproportionate risks involves an authentic respect for human beings and the uprightness of therapeutic intentions. It implies that the doctor "above all ... must carefully evaluate the possible negative consequences which the necessary use of a particular exploratory technique may have

upon the unborn child and avoid recourse to diagnostic procedures which do not offer sufficient guarantees of their honest purpose and substantial harmlessness. And if, as often happens in human choices, a degree of risk must be undertaken, he will take care to assure that it is justified by a truly urgent need for the diagnosis and by the importance of the results that can be achieved by it for the benefit of the unborn child himself" (POPE JOI-IN PAUL II, Discourse to Participants in the Pro-Life Movement Congress, 3 December 1982: lnsegnantenti di Giovanni Paolo II, V, 3 [1982] 1512). This clarification concerning "proportionate risk" is also to be kept in mind in the following sections of the present Instruction, whenever this term appears.

28. POPE JOHN PAUL II, Discourse to the Participants in the 35th General Assembly of the World Medical Association, 29 October 1983: *AAS*76 (1984) 392.

29. Cf POPE JOHN PAUL II, Address to a Meeting of. *The Pontifical Academy of Sciences, 23 October 1982: AAS*75 (1983) 37: "I condemn, in the most explicit and formal way, experimental manipulations of the human embryo, since the human being, from conception to death, cannot be exploited for any purpose whatsoever."

30. HOLY SEE, Charter of the Rights of the Family, 4b: *L'Osservatore Romano*, 25 November 1983.

31. Cf POPE JOHN PAUL II, Address to the Participants in the Convention of the Pro-Life Movement, 3 December 1982: Insegnamenti di Giovanni Paolo II, V, 3 (1982) 1511: "Any form of experimentation on the fetus that may damage its integrity or worsen its condition is unacceptable, except in the case of a final effort to save it from death." *SACRED CONGREGATION FOR THE DOCTRINE OF THE FAITH*, Declaration on Euthanasia, 4: *AAS*72(1980) 550: "In the absence of other sufficient remedies, it is permitted, with the patient's consent, to have recourse to the means provided by the most advanced medical techniques, even if these means are still at the experimental stage and are not without a certain risk."

32. No one, before coming into existence, can claim a subjective right to begin to exist; nevertheless, it is legitimate to affirm the right of the child to have a fully human origin through conception in conformity with the personal nature of the human being. Life is a gift that must be bestowed in a manner worthy both of the subject receiving it and of the Religious perspectives ill ART MET'S subjects transmitting it. This statement is to be borne in mind also for what will be explained concerning artificial human procreation.

33. Cf. POPE JOHN PAUL II, Discourse to those taking part in the 35th General Assembly of the World Medical Association, 29 October 1983: *AAS*76 (1984) 391.

34. Cf. Pastoral Constitution on the Church in the Modern world, Gaudium et Spes, 50.

35. Cf. POPE JOHN PAUL II, Apostolic Exhortation Familiaris; *Consortio, 14: AAS*74 (1982) 96.

36. Cf. POPE PIUS XII, Discourse to those taking part in the 4th International Congress of Catholic Doctors, 29 September 1949: *AAS*41 (1949) 559. According to the plan of the Creator, "A man leaves his father and his mother and cleaves to his wife, and they become one flesh" (Gen 2:24). *The unity of marriage, bound to the order of creation, is a truth accessible to natural reason.* The Church's Tradition and Magisterium frequently make reference to the Book of Genesis, both directly and through the passages of the New Testament that refer to it: Mt 19: 4–6; Mk: 10:5–8; Eph 5: 3 I. Cf. ATHENAGORAS, Legatio pro christianis, 33: PO 6, 965–967; ST CIIRYSOSTOM, In Matthaeum homiliae, LXII, 19, I: PG 58 597; ST LEO THE GREAT, Epist. ad Rusticum, 4:

PI. 54, 1204; INNOCENT III, Epist Gaudemus in Domino: DS 778; COUNCIL OF LYONS II, IV Session: DS 860; COUNCIL OF TRENT, XXIV, Session: DS 1798. 1802; POPE LEO XIII, Encyclical Arcanum Divinae Sapientiae: ASS 12 (1879/80) 388–391; POPE PIUS XI, Encychcal Casti Connubii: AAS 22 (1930) 546–547; SECOND VATICAN COUNCIL, Gaudium et Spes, 48; POPE JOHN PAUL II, Apostolic Exhortationamiliaris Consortio, 19: *AAS*74 (1982) 101–1 02; Code 0 Canon aw, Can. 1056.

37. Cf. POPE PIUS XII, Discourse to those taking part in the 4th International Congress of Catholic Doctors, 29 September 1949: AAS 4 (1949) 560; Discourse to those taking part in the Congress of the Italian Catholic Union of Midwives, 29 October 1951: *AAS*43 (1951) 850; Code of Canon Law, Can. 1134.

38. POPE PAUL VI, Encyclical Letter Humanae Vitae, 12: *AAS* 60 (1968) 488–489.

39. Loc. cit, ibid., 489.

40. POPE PIUS XII, Discourse to those taking part in the Second Naples World Congress on Fertility and Human Sterility, 19 May 1956: *AAS*48 (1956) 470.

41. Code of Canon Law, Can. 1061. According to this Canon, the conjugal act is that by which the marriage is consummated if the couple "have performed (it) between themselves in a human manner."

42. Cf. Pastoral Constitution Gaudium et Spes, 14.

43. Cf POPE JOHN PAUL II, General Audience on 16 January 1980: *Insegnamenti di Giovanni Paolo H, III*, 1 (1980) 148–152.

44. POPE JOHN PAUL II, Discourse to those taking part in the 35th General Assembly of the World Medical Association, 29 October 1983: *AAS*76 (1984) 393.

45. Cf. Pastoral Constitution Gaudium ct Spes, 51.

46. Cf. Pastoral Constitution Gaudium et Spes, 50.

47. Cf. POPE PIUS XII, Discourse to those taking part in the 4th International Congress of Catholic Doctors, 29 September 1949: *AAS*41 (1949) 560: *"It would be erroneous. to think that the possibility of resorting to this means (artificial fertilization) might render valid a marriage between persons unable to contract it because of the impedimentum impotentiae."*

48. A similar question was dealt with by POPE PAUL VI, Encyclical Humanae Vitae, 14: *AAS*60 (1968) 490–491.

49. Cf. supra: I, 1 ff.

50. POPE JOHN PAUL II, Apostolic Exhortation Familiaris Consortio. 14: *AAS*74 (1982) 96.

51. Cf. Response of the Holy Office, 17 March 1897: DS 3323; POPE PIUS XII, Discourse to those taking part in the 4th International Congress of Catholic Doctors, 29 September 1949: *AAS*41 (1949) 560; Discourse to the Italian Catholic Union of Midwives, 29 October 1951: *AAS*43 (1951) 850; Discourse to those taking part in the Second Naples World Congress on Fertility and Human Sterility, 19 May 1956: *AAS*48 (1956) 471–473; Discourse to those taking part in the 7th International Congress of the International Society of Haematology, 12 September 1958: *AAS*50 (1958) 733; POPE JOHN XXIII, Encyclical Mater et Magistra, III: *AAS*53 (1961) 447.

52. POPE PIUS XII, Discourse to the Italian Catholic Union of Midwives, 29 October 1951: *AAS*43(1951) 850.

53. POPE PIUS XII, Discourse to those taking part in the 4th International Congress of Catholic Doctors, 29 September 1949: *AAS*41 (1949) 560.

54. SACRED CONGREGATION FOR THE DOCTRINE OF THE FAITH, Declaration on Certain Questions Concerning Sexual ethics, 9: *AAS*68 (1976) 86, which quotes the Pastoral Constitution Gaudium et Spes, 51. Cf. Decree of the Holy Office, 2 August 1929: *AAS*21 (1929) 490; POPE PIUS XII, Discourse to

those taking part in the 26th Congress of the Italian Society of Urology, 8 October 1953: *AAS*45 (1953) 678.

55. Cf. POPE JOHN XXIII, Encyclical Mater et Magistra, III: *AAS*53 (1961) 447.

56. Cf. POPE PIUS XII, Discourse to those taking part in the 4th International Congress of Catholic Doctors, 29 September 1949: *AAS*41(1949) 560.

57. Cf. POPE PIUS XII, Discourse to the taking part in the Second Naples World Congress on Fertility and Human Sterility, 19 May 1956: *AAS*48 (1956) 471–473.

58. Pastoral Constitution Gaudium et Spes, 50.

59. POPE JOHN PAUL II, Apostolic Exhortation Familiaris Cons0l1io, 14: *AAS*74 (1982) 97.

60. Cf. Declaration Dignitatis Humanae, 7.

61. Caed Joseph. Ratzinger (The actual Holy Pope), Instruction on respect for human life in its origin and on the dignity of procreation replies to certain questions of the day, *Given at Rome, from the Congregation for the Doctrine of the Faith*, February 22, 1987, the Feast or the Chair of St. Peter, the Apostle.

74

The Future of Assisted Reproduction

Biljana Popovic Todorovic, Paul Devroey

The past three decades have witnessed revolution in reproductive medicine. Since the birth of Louise Brown in 1978 (1), there has been an expansion in the number of vitro fertilization treatment worldwide. In the first European Register publication (2) 203,893 IVF/ICSI were reported by eighteen European countries, and by 2002, this number rose to 324,238 cycles from twenty-five countries, accounting for almost 60 percent increase of registered cycles (3). In the last World IVF report from 2000, 460,157 cycles were carried out in forty-nine countries, and it was estimated that approximately 200,000 babies were born (4). Although neither European nor World coverage is complete regarding the register data, the expansion of IVF is evident, and the estimate is that more than three million children have been born as a result of assisted reproduction since the beginning.

The driving force of this medical field has always been better treatment outcome. Increasing the efficiency of the treatment is what the future holds for us.

DEFINITION OF SUCCESS

What is the definition of success in assisted reproduction? A debate was started in *Human Reproduction* in 2004, with the suggestion of Min et al., to define success as "BESST – birth emphasizing a successful singleton at term" (5). This sparked discussion of many renowned international groups, and a number of definitions were introduced – healthy lower order birth (6), number of elective single embryo transfers per center (7), and value of cryopreservation programs (8). Danish group suggested that reporting the number of oocytes, implantation rate, and number of deliveries per embryo transfer would cover all steps in ART: stimulation, laboratory, that is, in vitro and embryo transfer/outcome phase (9). Heijnen et al. went a step further and emphasized the need to focus on the whole treatment rather than on single cycle and to report success as singleton birth per started IVF treatment or per given period (10).

All these approaches have a common goal: to increase the efficacy and safety of the treatment on one hand while to decrease the risks on the other.

The future of assisted reproduction lies in this goal, and the accomplishment of it involves optimization of each treatment phase starting with ovarian stimulation through laboratory procedures, selecting the best embryo for transfer, embryo transfer, luteal phase support leading to pregnancy, and the birth of a healthy singleton baby.

OPTIMIZATION OF OVARIAN STIMULATION PROTOCOLS

GnRH Agonists

Ovarian stimulation has come a long way since its first attempts. In an elegant recollection of the past by Professor Howard Jones (11), he looks back at the beginning of IVF and the obstacles encountered on the path of improvement. In 1980, in their center in Norfolk, forty-one aspirations were carried out in a natural cycle, with thirteen transfers and no pregnancy. At the same time in Melbourne, there had been forty-eight transfers following stimulation with clomiphene citrate, resulting in three pregnancies, all of which ended in miscarriages with no term deliveries. By 1981, with ovarian stimulation, there had been no term deliveries anywhere in the world in normal menstruating women with stimulation combined with IVF (12). Jones's group started using Pergonal in 1981 and in their thirteenth attempt were finally successful.

GnRH agonists have changed the course of ovarian stimulation for in vitro fertilization. Since 1984, they have been used to prevent premature surge of LH during controlled ovarian hyperstimulation (13). Profound stimulation regimens have been introduced with a large number of oocytes as the desirable outcome.

Amounting evidence grew with the clinicians experience, causing a shift in the attitudes, from an aggressive approach where a large number of oocytes is considered a criterion of success to a more moderate approach.

What is the optimal number of oocytes retrieved? Increasing number of oocytes gives rise in pregnancy rates, but it eventually levels off (14,15), while side effects and risks continue to increase. OHSS is a well-known short-term risk of COH, with the incidence of 2–5 percent (16). Evidence has arisen showing potential detrimental effect of COH on endometrial receptivity and embryo implantation (17,18). Currently, it is clinically accepted that appropriate ovarian response is achieved with retrieval of five to fourteen oocytes (19).

Figure 74.1 (20) illustrates this concept, from an ideal point of view that patients should be in the high-benefit, low-risk window.

Dutch group has proved this concept in the population of almost 7,500 women, showing that the mean number of oocytes associated with the highest chance of conceiving per embryo transfer (PR/ET) and per started cycle (PR/C) was 13.1 (Fig. 74.2). After this number of oocytes, the pregnancy rates level off

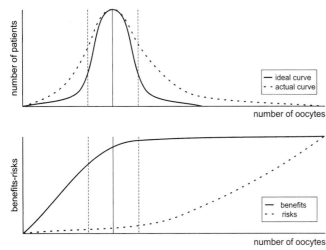

Figure 74.1. Distribution of oocytes, benefits and risks – the present and the ideal situation. Popovic-Todorovic et al. (20).

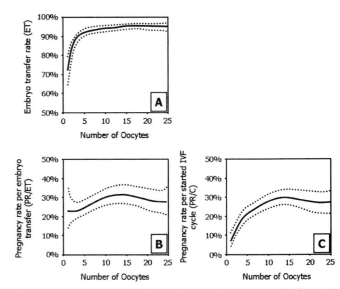

Figure 74.2. Optimum number of oocytes for a successful first IVF treatment cycle. The number of retrieved oocytes (mean with 95 percent CI) in relation to embryo transfer rate (A); pregnancy rate per embryo transfer (B); pregnancy rate per started IVF cycle (C). The optimal number of obtained oocytes to conceive is 13.1. Van Der et al. (21). Reprinted from an article in *Reproductive BioMedicine Online* by Van der Gaast et al., with permission from Reproductive Healthcare Ltd.

and this is not due to the embryo transfer rate since it remains stable at 93–95 percent when four or more oocytes were obtained (21) (Figure 74.2).

In practice, COH is not always "controlled," and a range of inappropriate ovarian responses is often present. At one end of the spectrum, we have inadequate response with retrieval of few oocytes, and increased treatment cancellations, and on the other end, a proportion of exaggerate responses is observed increasing the risk of OHSS. The variability of responses may be due to inherent biological mechanisms in relation to differences in the number of recruitable follicles, follicle sensitivity to FSH, and pharmacodynamics, but it may also be due to factors that may be predicted and at least partially controlled.

During recent years, data have accumulated showing that to some extent we are able to predict ovarian response, investigated factors being age (22), ovarian volume (19,23–27), antral follicle count (19,27–29), evaluation of stromal blood flow (19,28,30), cigarette smoking (31), hormonal markers assessment FSH (32,33), LH (34), inhibin B (35), and AMH (36–38).

How and to what extent is it possible to reduce the incidence of inappropriate responses by administering an appropriate starting dose of FSH?

Starting FSH Doses

Although COH has been in practice for many years, the optimal starting FSH dose has not been established since there have been no randomized controlled trials in the early IVF years (39). After introduction of the rFSH preparations, a number of studies have attempted to define an optimal starting dose (40–44). The doses range from 100 to 250 IU/day, reflecting the range of policies from "friendly IVF" with a minimal dose, to an approach where a large number of oocytes is considered criterion of success. Regardless of the dose used, a variability of responses is present, ranging from one oocyte at retrieval to more than thirty.

Most clinics have opted to use a "standard" dose for a "standard" patient who is below forty years of age, with two ovaries, a normal serum basal FSH, and a regular menstrual cycle. Dose adjustments are common clinical practice, higher doses being given to older patients. The cutoff value for

age is usually thirty-five years, that is, patients aged less than thirty-five years are given 150 IU/day, while those aged less than thirty-five years are started on a higher rFSH dose (usually 225–300 IU/day) (45).

Despite the fact that a lot of research has been carried out in order to establish the predictive factors of ovarian response, they have not been really used in developing dosage nomograms. Firstly, it was done in ovulation induction for PCO patients. The Dutch group has developed a model based on pretreatment clinical and endocrine and sonographic screening characteristics in order to predict FSH threshold dose in normogonadotropic anovulatory infertile women (46). The FSH threshold (75 to >187 IU/day) was determined on the basis of body mass index, presence or absence of resistance to clomiphene citrate, initial free insulin–like growth factor-I, and basal FSH.

There is only one prospective randomized trial that tested the use of a dosage nomogram in 'standard' patients comparing the individual dose, from 100 to 250 IU/day, based on the predictive factors versus a standard dose of 150 IU/day (20). Firstly, a prospective trial was conducted in order to establish the predictive factors of ovarian response in first IVF/ICSI treatment cycle of standard treated with 150 IU/day of rFSH (19). The constructed FSH dosage nomogram consisted of the following parameters: age, antral follicle count, ovarian volume, power Doppler score, and smoking status (19). The nomogram was subsequently tested, and the results showed that an individual dosage regimen in a well-defined first IVF/ICSI cycle standard patient population increased the proportion of appropriate ovarian responses and decreased the incidence of dose alterations during the course of COH. Although the trial was not designed to study a difference in pregnancy rates, higher ongoing pregnancy rate was observed in the individual dose group (20).

A retrospective analysis of eleven randomized phase II–IV trials has been performed in order to define the predictive factors of ovarian response by Howles et al. (47). Predictors were established by scoring their potential influence on a number of dependent variables – fourteen in total, although the primary outcome variable was the number of retrieved oocytes. A dosage calculator based on basal FSH, BMI, age, and antral follicle count is currently being tested.

It is necessary to have this issue further explored; a number of different nomograms have to be tested in prospective randomized trials in order to have tailor-made starting FSH doses already from the first treatment cycle.

GnRH Antagonist Protocols

GnRH antagonists have been introduced recently in ovarian stimulation for pituitary suppression. They compete directly with endogenous GnRH for receptor binding (48), their pharmacological effect being characterized by rapid and reversible blockade of pituitary GnRH receptors, and as such are used to prevent premature LH surges. The clinical acceptance of GnRH antagonists has been slow and mostly due to the initial meta-analysis (49), which has observed 5 percent difference in clinical pregnancy rates. This meta-analysis included five RCTs, and the difference in live birth rate was 3.8 percent higher in agonist cycles, but it is not statistically significant.

Initially, GnRH antagonists were often implemented in poor-prognosis patients, who have already had a number of unsuccessful trials, as was shown by the data from German registry (50). The last meta-analysis showed that among the patients treated for IVF with gonadotropins and GnRH analogues, the probability of live birth does not depend on the type of analogue used (51).

Antagonist protocols are novel compared to more than twenty years of agonist protocols, and optimization progresses with knowledge accumulation. Steroid levels in the antagonist cycles differ from the downregulated levels in the agonist cycles since the antagonist cycle is preceeded by a luteal phase of the natural cycle. It was shown by Kolibianakis et al. (52) that a proportion of patients (5 percent) who exhibit elevated progesterone level at the onset of stimulation have a decreased probability of pregnancy in relation to patients with normal progesterone levels (5 vs. 31.8 percent). This issue needs to be further explored.

There have been only two prospective randomized trials, which compared the use of 150 versus 200 IU/day and 150 versus 225 IU/day in standard patients (53,54). Higher doses yielded more oocytes, but pregnancy rates remained the same. These studies were underpowered to assess the impact of starting dose alterations on the pregnancy rates. Prospective studies establishing predictive factors of ovarian response in antagonist cycles are needed. Furthermore, individual dosing approach has not been explored in GnRH antagonist protocols, and further optimization should evolve in tailor-made dose approach from the first treatment cycle.

Fixed antagonist protocol was introduced empirically on day 6 of stimulation since it was assumed that by that time there would be sufficient production of estradiol, which would induce premature LH rise. In a flexible protocol, onset of administration of antagonist is determined by the follicular size, usually when the leading follicle is 14–15 mm. Meta-analysis of four randomized controlled trials of fixed versus flexible

protocol shows a trend for increased pregnancy rates in the fixed protocol, although the power of the analysis is too low for definite conclusions (55). Another methodological issue is that by day 6, approximately 50 percent of the patients have a follicle of 15 mm (56), and that lowers the chance of detecting an existing difference between the two protocols.

Timing of the antagonist as well as timing of hCG administration require further exploration. Only one trial assessed the impact of delaying hCG and showed that prolongation of follicular phase has a negative impact on pregnancy rates (57). The use of GnRH agonists to trigger final oocyte maturation has a potential benefit in patients at risk for OHSS, but the current evidence suggests that it leads to lower pregnancy rates (58).

There is a need for a number of RCTs to explore further the issues of hormonal assessment at the beginning of the antagonist cycle, fixed or flexible antagonist administration, timing and doses, final oocyte maturation triggering as well as the use of GnRH agonists.

With increased knowledge and experience accumulation of the clinicians, GnRH antagonists will be increasingly used in clinical practice.

OVARIAN STIMULATION, ENDOMETRIAL RECEPTIVITY, AND LUTEAL PHASE

Although ovarian stimulation protocols have evolved, the influence of ovarian stimulation on the endometrial receptivity is not fully understood. Implantation involves a specific interaction of the human blastocyst and maternal endometrium. The window of implantation is defined as the period when the uterus is receptive, and it occurs eight to ten days after ovulation. The importance of the embryo quality has been demonstrated (59), but even when high-quality embryos are transferred (60), the increase in implantation rates levels off. Implantation failure remains the main limiting factor of the success of assisted reproduction.

Priming of endometrium toward the window of implantation is of maternal origin. High implantation and pregnancy rates in oocyte donation cycles irrespective of acceptors' age (61) imply that ovarian stimulation impairs endometrial receptivity in stimulated cycles.

Normal hormonal milieu and a normal endometrium give rise to a functional luteal phase. This is altered by ovarian stimulation at a number of levels. GnRH agonist theoretically could directly interact with GnRH-like peptide receptors in granulosa and theca cells and human endometrium (62). COH induces supraphysiological levels of steroids during follicular phase, resulting in advanced endometrial development regardless of the type of GnRH analogue used. In GnRH agonist cycles, endometrial biopsies taken in the preovulatory phase prior to hCG injection show accentuated proliferative aspects and early secretory changes even before rise in progesterone occurs (63).

Biopsies taken on the day of oocyte retrieval show endometrial advancement in more than 90 percent of the cases, with no pregnancy occurring if the advancement is exceeded by three days (64). These findings were confirmed in GnRH antagonist cycles (65).

Increased sensitivity to progesterone resulting in secretory advancement could be induced by elevated estrogen concentrations (66). Clinical studies in oocyte donation programmes show that increased estrogen levels have a negative impact on implantation rates without affecting the embryo quality (67). Additionally, a step-down regimen improved pregnancy rates (68). Moderate responders exhibit less pronounced endometrial changes compared to high responders (69).

It has been established that corpus luteum support is required following ovarian stimulation and GnRH agonist cotreatment (70,71) due to the prolonged pituitary recovery from downregulation and the lack of support of corpus luteum. Due to the fact that after discontinuation of GnRH antagonists, pituitary recovery occurs within hours (72) it has been speculated that luteal phase support is not needed in GnRH antagonist cotreated cycles. Evidence has shown that this is not the case, and in nonsupplemented GnRH antagonist cycles, luteolysis is induced prematurely and pregnancy rates are severely affected (73).

The series of events leading to a deficient luteal phase include ovarian stimulation per se and removal of granulosa cells during follicular aspiration (74), and a high number of corpora lutea (75) during the early luteal phase could directly inhibit LH release via negative feedback actions at the hypothalamic-pituitary axis (76).

Although there is a lot of heterogeneity in the studies on endometrial morphology in stimulated cycles, a general trend involves endometrial advancement in the peri- and postovulatory period followed by a "normal" aspect of endometrium in the early luteal phase and frequent glandular-stromal dyssynchrony in the mid- and late luteal phase (77). Luteal support is necessary for a regular endometrial development as is shown by normal in-phase endometrial histology, irrespective of the luteal support used (78).

The deleterious effect of ovarian stimulation lies in the elevated steroid levels of the follicular phase, which subsequently cause a chain reaction, leading to a defective endometrium receptivity and an insufficient luteal phase to support embryonic development.

The future of ovarian stimulation must focus on developing milder ovarian stimulation protocols. Introduction of GnRH antagonists allows implementation of this approach with onset of FSH administration later in the follicular phase (79). In a randomized noninferiority effectiveness trial, Heijnen et al. (80) have shown that there is no difference in the cumulative live births between a mild stimulation protocol and a standard stimulation. The question that remains unanswered is what is the optimal ovarian response? In the light of discussed evidence, the definition of success must move to a milder ovarian stimulation, with fewer oocytes retrieved and a more physiological hormonal milieu.

If we alter the hormonal milieu and endometrial receptivity in such a severe way with various ovarian stimulation protocols, cryopreservation programs will play an increasing role in the future. Elective cryopreservation of cleavage embryos in cycles with the risk of OHSS is a well-established clinical entity (81).

Rapidly evolving technologies in the cryopreservation field have allowed development of different treatment approaches in assisted reproduction. In 1985, ice-free cryopreservation of mouse embryos at −196°C by vitrification was reported in an attempted alternative approach to cryostorage (82). Since then, vitrification is steadily becoming the mainstream of assisted reproduction techniques as an alternative cryopreservation method to traditional slow-cooling/rapid-thaw protocols (83).

It can be postulated that implantation rates can be improved by electively freezing the embryos and transferring in a natural cycle where the endometrial receptivity has not been hampered by ovarian stimulation. Although this approach may seem far fetched, evidence is emerging that it can overcome our current treatment limitations. A German group has vitrified all two PN oocytes in patients at risk of developing OHSS, treated with GnRH antagonist protocol where final oocyte maturation was induced with GnRH agonist. All frozen-thawed embryo transfers were performed following spontaneous menses in an artificial cycle where endometrium was primed with transdermal estradiol patches, followed by addition of vaginal progesterone from day 15 onward. In total, nineteen patients underwent twenty-four FT-Ets and the cumulative ongoing pregnancy rate was 36.8% (84).

Endometrial Receptivity

Currently, there is no easily applicable clinical marker of endometrial receptivity. Endometrial biopsy remains the most used method despite its limitations. It is a method established by more than fifty years ago (85), with only infertile patients included in Noyes' criteria, and is a subject of intra- and interobserver variations (86). Furthermore, it shows questionable relationship to endometrial receptivity (87). Most importantly, it is an invasive method and as such cannot be routinely used.

There is an urgent need to establish a clinically useful, applicable in daily routine, marker of endometrial receptivity since all the known markers can be used only for research purposes [pinopodes (88,89), integrins (90,91), leukemia-inhibiting factor (92,93)]. Transvaginal ultrasonography is a noninvasive technique, but the parameters that have been studied so far such as endometrial thickness, endometrial pattern and, endometrial and subendometrial blood flow (94–96) have a low positive predictive value (97,98).

Introduction of three-dimensional ultrasound (99) has opened new possibilities in studying the endometrium. In order to evaluate endometrial receptivity, endometrial volume and subendometrial and endometrial vascularization have been assessed. Regarding the endometrial volume, most studies to date conclude that it does not predict endometrial receptivity (100,101). The reports on the role of endometrial and subendometrial vascularity assessment in predicting pregnancy are conflicting, with some studies finding that endometrial/subendometrial vascularity is increased in conception cycles (102,103), while others found no differences (104). The controversy arises from methodological heterogeneity of the studies, especially due to the timing of ultrasound examination. Since 3D ultrasound is still a novel technique, with growing experience consistency of data will increase.

In the near future, correlation of 3D ultrasonographic data and histological dating of endometrium needs to be established, and if the results are encouraging, a novel clinical marker of endometrial receptivity may be founded.

EMBRYO TRANSFER – HOW, WHEN, AND HOW MANY?

Embryo transfer procedure plays a pivotal role in the success of assisted reproduction. Accumulated evidence shows that a number of factors influence the embryo transfer technique. A recent meta-analysis comparing the use of soft and stiff embryo transfer catheters was in favor of the soft ones regarding the pregnancy rates [odds ratio (OR) 1.34, 95 percent confidence intervals (CI) 1.18–1.54] (105).

Empirically, embryo transfer is performed blindly with the aim to deposit the embryos 1 cm away from the fundus. Recent research has shown that improvement is observed if the distance from the fundus is increased (106,107). In contrast, placement of the embryos in lower segment of uterine cavity may increase the risk of placenta previa (108).

Ultrasound-guided embryo transfer is routine in many infertility centers. A large number of studies has dealt with this issue, and a meta-analysis of four randomized controlled trials has shown increased pregnancy and implantation rates with the use of ultrasound during ET (109). Our own experience is that that there is no outcome difference in ultrasound versus "clinical touch" embryo transfer technique (110).

It has been recognized and clinically accepted that embryo transfer should be performed in atraumatic way, minimizing uterine contractility. A large proportion of IVF patients have persistently high uterine contraction frequency at the time of day 3 transfer. Furthermore, the higher the frequency of uterine contractions, the lower the pregnancy rate (111). The contractility of the uterus decreases toward day 7 following the hCG injection, with the uterus reaching a nearly quiescent status for the day 5 transfer (112).

The future of the procedure will focus on further minimizing this contractility pharmacologically and further defining the correct position for deposition of the embryos.

The day of embryo transfer differs between the centers, and it includes day 2, day 3, and day 5. In the early years, most centers replaced the embryos on day 2 following fertilization, and with the improvement of culture media and laboratory techniques, this has moved to day 3 and in the last couple of years to blastocyst transfer on day 5.

The main disadvantage of transferring cleavage-stage embryos is that current morphological criteria are highly subjective with high inter- and moderate intraobserver variability (113) and in high percentages of the cases do not reflect the euploidy status of the embryo (114). In contrast, the risk of transferring on day 5 is that a number of embryo will not reach the blastocyst stage and there will be increased risk of cycle cancellation. Our group has carried out a prospective randomized controlled trial comparing the day 3 versus day-5 single-embryo transfer in patients younger than thirty-six years. The results showed significantly higher pregnancy and delivery rates among women undergoing transfer of a single blastocyst-stage embryo (60).

Although it is fair to say that presently blastocyst transfer may not be applicable to all patient populations, further research needs to be conducted in different patient populations. High blastocyst pregnancy rates reflect high standards of laboratories, and with further improvement, blastocyst transfer should have wider application in the future.

The leading complication of assisted reproductive techniques is high multiple pregnancy rates, which amounts to 24.5 percent (3,115). Increased perinatal morbidity, maternal complications, and medical costs are too high a price to pay for individuals, society, and medical profession (116).

The milestone in assisted reproduction is the introduction of single-embryo transfer as a strategy to reduce multiple pregnancy rates. Since the only variables predictive of multiple birth are age and the number of good-quality embryos transferred (117), the largest RCT on single-versus double-embryo transfer in women younger than thirty-six years (118), including the frozen-embryo transfer cycle in the SET group, showed that

$1 + 1 = 2$. This means that the cumulative ongoing pregnancy rate in one fresh and one frozen SET was 38.2 percent, which was not significantly different from the 42.9 percent ongoing pregnancy rate in the dual-embryo transfer group (DET). Only one twin birth was registered in the eSET group compared with 33.1 percent in the DET group.

Introducing SET reduces the twinning rate without affecting the pregnancy rates. This trial recognized the paramount importance of a well-functioning freezing program.

Implementation of SET is gaining momentum in some countries, although a large proportion of IVF society is still oblivious to this approach. It has to be recognized that there is a need to have a degree of flexibility over the number of embryo transferred, depending on pregnancy prognosis. The Belgian model recognizes the need for this since it is stratified by age and also by the cycle number, so that lack of success enables an increase in the number of embryos transferred. This legislation was introduced to improve financial access to assisted reproduction treatment and reduce multiple IVF and ICSI pregnancies. It has been estimated that the reduction in costs associated with multiple pregnancies will provide the means for treatment reimbursement. Since July 1, 2003, laboratory costs for IVF and ICSI have been refunded for six cycles in a lifetime for patients younger than forty-three years. For those aged less than thirty-six years, the first two cycles must be SET, but if these fail, cycles three to six can be dual-embryo transfer. For patients aged thirty-six to thirty-nine, the first two cycles can be up to two embryo transfers and cycles three to six can be up to three ET. Patients older than thirty-nine years can have up to three embryos transferred already from first treatment cycle.

In a publication by our group (119), a fifteen-month period was analyzed before and after the legislation was implemented. Overall, the multiple pregnancy rates were reduced from 29.1 to 9.5 percent (all patients) and from 28.9 to 6.2 percent in women younger than thirty-six years. Most twins were observed in the third cycle of patients younger than thirty-six years and in the first three cycles of patients of thirty-six to thirty-nine years. Overall, a significant decline in multiple gestations was mainly observed in the less than thirty-six population. Pregnancy rates were not compromised by the new law. This study also raised the issue for introducing SET for a certain proportion of the thirty-six to thirty-nine year population.

With these results, it is increasingly difficult to accept the rates of multiple pregnancies seen around the world. The financial aspect of the Belgian model clearly shows that the lowering of treatment cost by reducing the incidence of multiple pregnancies provides means for increasing availability of treatment.

EMBRYO SELECTION

The past twenty years have been marked by the immense development in the assisted reproductive techniques. Preimplantation genetic diagnosis (PGD) was introduced to prevent the inheritance of sex-linked diseases, the first successful pregnancy being achieved in 1990 (120).

PGD for aneuploidy screening (PGD-AS, PGS) aims to evaluate numerical chromosomal constitution of the cleavage-stage embryo through removal of a blastomere/s and subsequent analysis by the use of fluorescence in situ hybridization (FISH).

Apparently, approximately a third of all IVF produced embryos is chromosomally abnormal (121,122). In the poor-prognosis IVF population, which includes patients of advanced maternal age (AMA), recurrent implantation failure (RIF), recurrent miscarriage (RM), and testicular sperm extraction, the incidence of chromosomal abnormalities rises to 70 percent (123).

The current morphological criteria for choosing the best embryo for transfer are often unable to allow selection of euploid embryos, that is, morphologically best embryos are aneuploid in 25 percent of the cases (124). The rationale for introducing PGS has been that selection and transfer of euploid embryos would improve implantation and pregnancy rate and decrease miscarriage rate as well as multiple pregnancy rates. PGS is currently being done by an increasing number of infertility centers in the world, and there is a need to assess its effectiveness (124,125).

A large number of comparative studies has investigated the use of PGS in patients of AMA (126–130), RIF (126,127,131,132), RM (122,133,135), and testicular sperm extraction (136,137).

The results have shown initial optimism, but a number of issues have to be addressed in order to interpret the findings and conclusions of different trials.

Certain methodological concerns such as sampling variability (wide array of sample sizes present) and clinical heterogeneity (different study populations, number of blastomeres assessed, number of probes used, methodology used, randomization procedures, etc.) are present in the studies assessing the use of PGS.

In accordance with the methodological concerns, the Cochrane review (138) could only include two randomized prospective clinical trials of Staessen et al. (123) and Stevens et al. (139). There is another small prospective randomized controlled trial by Werlin et al. (140), but it does not provide sufficient data on the methodological quality.

The two randomized controlled trials included in the meta-analysis (138) represent 428 patients, with the majority of patients coming from the study of Staessen et al. ($n = 389$). PGS in the two studies was performed for AMA of thirty-seven years or more in Staessen et al. and more than thirty-five years in Stevens et al. There was no difference in the live birth rate in PGS versus non-PGS group, 11 versus 15 percent, respectively (OR 0.65; 95 percent CI: 0.36–1.19), ongoing pregnancy rate per woman 15 percent in the PGS group versus 22 percent in control group (OR 0.42, 95 percent CI 0.12–1.51).

The trial by Werlin et al. randomized the three categories of patients, AMA, RM, and RIF, to PGS versus non-PGS group. Although this is the only study that randomized recurrent miscarriage patients, 11 versus 8 controls, number of pregnancies 63.6 percent in the study versus 37.5 percent in controls ($P = 0.07$), it is difficult to interpret these results. The sample size was too small, the randomization procedure was not given, and all patients received corticosteroids and low doses of aspirin. Regarding the patients with RIF ($n = 19$, 11 study patients, 9 were controls), number of pregnancies was 20 percent in the study versus 0 percent in the control group.

Furthermore, results of the prospective cohort studies and retrospective studies showed that PGS improves the pregnancy rates, but study design does not allow these results to be used for recommending PGS as a routine procedure.

A recent publication by Munne et al. (141) analyzed 2,279 PGD cycles, which were carried out in patients older than thirty-five years from hundred infertility centers in United States. Majority of the centers had fewer than Thirty cycles per center, 89 of them, while number of cycles per center ranged from 30 to 531 for the remaining eleven centers. In total, 1,886 cycles ended in embryo transfer (82.2%), of which 608 resulted in pregnancy, but only 562 cycles with known pregnancy outcome were included. Results were compared with general IVF population, nondonor fresh cycles, 7,682 from thirty-five to forty years and 1,024 cycles from older than forty years were used as a control group. The mean pregnancy loss for the PGS group (16.7 percent) was significantly lower than for general IVF group (21.5 percent, $P < 0.001$). When stratified for age, in the thirty-five to forty group, rate of pregnancy loss was 14.1 versus 19.4 in the control group ($P = 0.03$), and for patients older than forty, it was reduced from 40.6 percent in the control group to 22.2 percent ($P < 0.001$). Although this trial has a large sample size as such, there was a large heterogeneity in the results of individual clinics, the pregnancy rate varying from 11 to 57 percent.

There have been no RCTs evaluating PGS in couples with NOA and OA, although there is substantial evidence of an increase in aneuplody and mosaicism of embryos derived from azospermic men compared to fertile men (137). Surprisingly, Platteau et al. showed that the aneuploidy frequency in embryos from NOA was 53 percent and in OA 60 percent, despite young age of their female partners.

The results of all these studies confirm high rate of aneuploidies in these patient populations. A recent study of Baart et al. (114) has shown that among young patients, the rate of aneuploidies is 64 percent in embryos that were not selected for transfer.

Although extensive research has been conducted in this field, there is a need for more well-designed randomized prospective trials, which will assess the value of PGS in well-defined patient populations, with delivery of a healthy child as the primary outcome.

Major limitation of PGS is mosaicism, estimate running as high as 50 percent of all the cleavage embryos (142). Mosaicism is the result of presence of euploid and aneuploid cells or distinct aneuplodies on different blastomeres, so that cells analyzed by PGS do not represent genomic content of the rest of the embryo. The mechanisms underlying this phenomenon are mitotic non disjunction and anaphase lagging. Coonen et al. demonstrated that anaphase lagging accounts for 56 percent of the mosaicism in blastocysts (143).

Mosaicism often leads to misdiagnosis, up to 60 percent (144), giving rise to false-positive and false-negative results. It has been argued that removal of only one blastomere is not representative of the embryo and two blastomeres need to be removed. Due to the fact that this removal is not carried in random order, when two blastomeres are analyzed, there is a 25 percent probability of removing both reciprocal daughter cells, resulting in the euploid status of previously mosaic embryo (114). There is also a chance of aggravating existing mosaicism by removal of normal blastomeres (144) and reducing number of healthy embryos for transfer.

It has to be reiterated that the current high incidence of mosaicism after PGS can be an overestimation since the embryos that have been analyzed in majority of the studies are discarded for transfer or cryopreservation. Staessen et al. have shown that in patients of advanced maternal age, the rate of mosaicism is 10.7 percent (123), which is in agreement with the control group for recurrent miscarriage patients, by Pehlivan et al. (131), of 10.8 percent. Although the populations studied are different, mosaicism rate was established in good-quality embryos and as such may be more representative.

There are technical limitations of the procedure itself, which have been acknowledged, namely signal overlapping and signal splitting (145).

Number of probes used varies among different groups; currently, FISH is able to analyze up to ten chromosomes, 1, 7, 13, 15, 16, 18, 21, 22, X, and Y. Irrespective of the number of probes used, not all chromosomes can be assessed by PGS at the moment. Comparative genomic hybridization (CGH) may overcome this since it allows complete chromosomal status assessment, but there are still issues that prevent CGH from being routinely used such as long period of hybridization, necessity of embryo freezing prior to transfer, and inability to distinguish diploid cells from haploid or tetraploid (146). The number of euploid embryos is lower than after FISH analysis, approximately 25 percent (147,148). The first birth following CGH and a modified freezing protocol has been documented by Wilton et al. in 2001 (149).

In conclusion, PGS technique cannot be recommended as a routine clinical procedure. Current clinical evidence shows no benefit in the pregnancy rates in poor-prognosis patients, but lack of well-designed randomized controlled trials hinders definitive conclusions from being made.

Mosaicism of the cleavage embryos remains a great source of misdiagnosis and cannot be overcome by removing two instead of one blastomere.

The most important misinterpretation of the results is linked to the fact that the euploidy status of the blastomere does not correspond to the euploidy status of the embryo due to mosaicism and probably due to the fact that the embryo is self-correcting.

Finally, with the current technology available, including comparative genomic hybridization, screening of blastomeres will not lead to the evaluation of the entire embryo. It is foreseeable that if more randomized controlled trials will be available, the final answer will confirm our interpretation. The future of the embryo selection has to focus on development of new genetic tools for embryo selection.

FINAL CONCLUSIONS

The future developments in assisted reproduction should encompass individualized approach to ovarian stimulation, vitrification, single blastocyst transfer, and development of new tools for genetic testing.

Since ovarian stimulation has a detrimental effect on the endometrial receptivity, development of milder stimulation protocols with tailor-made approach will mark the near future of ovarian stimulation. A fine-tuning should allow synchronization of ovarian folliculogenesis and endometrium. An optimal hormonal milieu needs to be achieved in order to allow harmonious endometrial development with optimal conditions during the implantation window. A step further will be vitrification of all embryos and transfer in a natural or a substituted cycle where the effect of ovarian stimulation on the endometrial receptivity will be completely circumvented.

Overall, the major disadvantage of classical IVF/ICSI is the occurrence of multiple pregnancies, which should be overcome by transfer of one blastocyst.

Embryo selection is in particular a crucial intervention. The main drawback of single or dual blastomere testing is the presence of mosaicism, and although comparative genome hybridization is tempting, it will not solve this problem. Since PGS did not show improved pregnancy rates, future research in this area has to be focused on developing new tools for genetic testing.

KEY POINTS FOR CLINICAL PRACTICE

The future of assisted reproduction should move in the direction of:

- Development of milder stimulation protocols with tailor-made dosing approach.
- Vitrification of embryos and embryo transfer in a natural cycle.
- Transfer of single blastocyst.
- Development of new genetic tools for embryo selection.

REFERENCES

1. Steptoe PC, Edwards RG. Birth after the reimplantation of a human embryo. *Lancet* 1978; 2(8085):366.
2. Nygren KG, Andersen AN. Assisted reproductive technology in Europe, 1997. Results generated from European registers by ESHRE. European IVF-Monitoring Programme (EIM), for the European Society of Human Reproduction and Embryology (ESHRE). *Hum Reprod* 2001; 16(2):384–391.
3. Andersen AN, Gianaroli L, Felberbaum R, de Mouzon J, Nygren KG. Assisted reproductive technology in Europe, 2002. Results generated from European registers by ESHRE. *Hum Reprod* 2006; 21(7):1680–1697.
4. Adamson GD, de Mouzon J, Lancaster P, Nygren KG, Sullivan E, Zegers-Hochschild F. World collaborative report on in vitro fertilization, 2000. *Fertil Steril* 2006; 85(6):1586–1622.
5. Min JK, Breheny SA, MacLachlan V, Healy DL. What is the most relevant standard of success in assisted reproduction? The singleton, term gestation, live birth rate per cycle initiated: the BESST endpoint for assisted reproduction. *Hum Reprod* 2004; 19(1):3–7.
6. Dickey RP, Sartor BM, Pyrzak R. What is the most relevant standard of success in assisted reproduction?: no single outcome measure is satisfactory when evaluating success in assisted reproduction; both twin births and singleton births should be counted as successes. *Hum Reprod* 2004; 19(4):783–787.
7. Land JA, Evers JL. What is the most relevant standard of success in assisted reproduction? Defining outcome in ART: a Gordian knot of safety, efficacy and quality. *Hum Reprod* 2004; 19(5): 1046–1048.
8. Tiitinen A, Hyden-Granskog C, Gissler M. What is the most relevant standard of success in assisted reproduction?: The value of cryopreservation on cumulative pregnancy rates per single oocyte retrieval should not be forgotten. *Hum Reprod* 2004; 19(11):2439–2441.
9. Pinborg A, Loft A, Ziebe S, Nyboe AA. What is the most relevant standard of success in assisted reproduction? Is there a single 'parameter of excellence'? *Hum Reprod* 2004; 19(5):1052–1054.
10. Heijnen EM, Macklon NS, Fauser BC. What is the most relevant standard of success in assisted reproduction? The next step to improving outcomes of IVF: consider the whole treatment. *Hum Reprod* 2004; 19(9):1936–1938.
11. Jones HW Jr. IVF: past and future. *Reprod Biomed Online* 2003; 6(3):375–381.

12. Lopata A. Successes and failures in human in vitro fertilization. *Nature* 1980; 288(5792):642–643.

13. Porter RN, Smith W, Craft IL, Abdulwahid NA, Jacobs HS. Induction of ovulation for in-vitro fertilisation using buserelin and gonadotropins. *Lancet* 1984; 2(8414):1284–1285.

14. de Vries MJ, De Sutter P, Dhont M. Prognostic factors in patients continuing in vitro fertilization or intracytoplasmic sperm injection treatment and dropouts. *Fertil Steril* 1999; 72(4):674–678.

15. Sharma V, Allgar V, Rajkhowa M. Factors influencing the cumulative conception rate and discontinuation of in vitro fertilization treatment for infertility. *Fertil Steril* 2002; 78(1):40–46.

16. Beerendonk CC, van Dop PA, Braat DD, Merkus JM. Ovarian hyperstimulation syndrome: facts and fallacies. *Obstet Gynecol Surv* 1998; 53(7):439–449.

17. Macklon NS, Fauser BC. Impact of ovarian hyperstimulation on the luteal phase. *J Reprod Fertil*Suppl 2000; 55:101–108.

18. Van Der Gaast MH, Beckers NG, Beier-Hellwig K, Beier HM, Macklon NS, Fauser BC. Ovarian stimulation for IVF and endometrial receptivity – the missing link. *Reprod Biomed Online* 2002; 5(3 Suppl. 1):36–43.

19. Popovic-Todorovic B, Loft A, Lindhard A, Bangsboll S, Andersson AM, Andersen AN. A prospective study of predictive factors of ovarian response in 'standard' IVF/ICSI patients treated with recombinant FSH. A suggestion for a recombinant FSH dosage normogram. *Hum Reprod* 2003; 18(4):781–787.

20. Popovic-Todorovic B, Loft A, Bredkjaeer HE, Bangsboll S, Nielsen IK, Andersen AN. A prospective randomized clinical trial comparing an individual dose of recombinant FSH based on predictive factors versus a 'standard' dose of 150 IU/day in 'standard' patients undergoing IVF/ICSI treatment. *Hum Reprod* 2003; 18(11):2275–2282.

21. Van Der Gaast MH, Eijkemans MJ, van der Net JB, de Boer EJ, Burger CW, van Leeuwen FE et al. Optimum number of oocytes for a successful first IVF treatment cycle. *Reprod Biomed Online* 2006; 13(4):476–480.

22. Rosenwaks Z, Davis OK, Damario MA. The role of maternal age in assisted reproduction. *Hum Reprod* 1995; (10 Suppl. 1): 165–173.

23. Lass A, Skull J, McVeigh E, Margara R, Winston RM. Measurement of ovarian volume by transvaginal sonography before ovulation induction with human menopausal gonadotrophin for in-vitro fertilization can predict poor response. *Hum Reprod* 1997; 12(2):294–297.

24. Lass A, Brinsden P. The role of ovarian volume in reproductive medicine. *Hum Reprod Update* 1999; 5(3):256–266.

25. Tomas C, Nuojua-Huttunen S, Martikainen H. Pretreatment transvaginal ultrasound examination predicts ovarian responsiveness to gonadotrophins in in-vitro fertilization. *Hum Reprod* 1997; 12(2):220–223.

26. Syrop CH, Dawson JD, Husman KJ, Sparks AE, Van Voorhis BJ. Ovarian volume may predict assisted reproductive outcomes better than follicle stimulating hormone concentration on day 3. *Hum Reprod* 1999; 14(7):1752–1756.

27. Ng EH, Tang OS, Ho PC. The significance of the number of antral follicles prior to stimulation in predicting ovarian responses in an IVF programme. *Hum Reprod* 2000; 15(9):1937–1942.

28. Kupesic S, Kurjak A, Bjelos D, Vujisic S. Three-dimensional ultrasonographic ovarian measurements and in vitro fertilization outcome are related to age. *Fertil Steril* 2003; 79(1):190–197.

29. Scheffer GJ, Broekmans FJ, Looman CW, Blankenstein M, Fauser BC BC, te Jong FH et al. The number of antral follicles in normal women with proven fertility is the best reflection of reproductive age. *Hum Reprod* 2003; 18(4):700–706.

30. Zaidi J, Barber J, Kyei-Mensah A, Bekir J, Campbell S, Tan SL. Relationship of ovarian stromal blood flow at the baseline ultrasound scan to subsequent follicular response in an in vitro fertilization program. *Obstet Gynecol* 1996; 88(5):779–784.

31. Van Voorhis BJ, Dawson JD, Stovall DW, Sparks AE, Syrop CH. The effects of smoking on ovarian function and fertility during assisted reproduction cycles. *Obstet Gynecol* 1996; 88(5): 785–791.

32. Bancsi LF, Huijs AM, den Ouden CT, Broekmans FJ, Looman CW, Blankenstein MA et al. Basal follicle-stimulating hormone levels are of limited value in predicting ongoing pregnancy rates after in vitro fertilization. *Fertil Steril* 2000; 73(3):552–557.

33. Scott RT, Toner JP, Muasher SJ, Oehninger S, Robinson S, Rosenwaks Z. Follicle-stimulating hormone levels on cycle day 3 are predictive of in vitro fertilization outcome. *Fertil Steril* 1989; 51(4):651–654.

34. Noci I, Biagiotti R, Maggi M, Ricci F, Cinotti A, Scarselli G. Low day 3 luteinizing hormone values are predictive of reduced response to ovarian stimulation. *Hum Reprod* 1998; 13(3):531–534.

35. Seifer DB, Lambert-Messerlian G, Hogan JW, Gardiner AC, Blazar AS, Berk CA. Day 3 serum inhibin-B is predictive of assisted reproductive technologies outcome. *Fertil Steril* 1997; 67(1):110–114.

36. van Rooij IA, Broekmans FJ, te Velde ER, Fauser BC, Bancsi LF, de Jong FH et al. Serum anti-Mullerian hormone levels: a novel measure of ovarian reserve. *Hum Reprod* 2002; 17(12):3065–3071.

37. Fanchin R, Schonauer LM, Righini C, Guibourdenche J, Frydman R, Taieb J. Serum anti-Mullerian hormone is more strongly related to ovarian follicular status than serum inhibin B, estradiol, FSH and LH on day 3. *Hum Reprod* 2003; 18(2):323–327.

38. Penarrubia J, Fabregues F, Manau D, Creus M, Casals G, Casamitjana R et al. Basal and stimulation day 5 anti-Mullerian hormone serum concentrations as predictors of ovarian response and pregnancy in assisted reproductive technology cycles stimulated with gonadotropin-releasing hormone agonist – gonadotropin treatment. *Hum Reprod* 2005; 20(4):915–922.

39. van Hooff MH. The human menopausal gonadotropin (hMG) dose in in vitro fertilization (IVF): what is the optimal dose? *J Assist Reprod Genet* 1995; 12(4):233–235.

40. Out HJ, Lindenberg S, Mikkelsen AL, Eldar-Geva T, Healy DL, Leader A et al. A prospective, randomized, double-blind clinical trial to study the efficacy and efficiency of a fixed dose of recombinant follicle stimulating hormone (Puregon) in women undergoing ovarian stimulation. *Hum Reprod* 1999; 14(3):622–627.

41. Out HJ, Braat DD, Lintsen BM, Gurgan T, Bukulmez O, Gokmen O et al. Increasing the daily dose of recombinant follicle stimulating hormone (Puregon) does not compensate for the age-related decline in retrievable oocytes after ovarian stimulation. *Hum Reprod* 2000; 15(1):29–35.

42. Out HJ, David I, Ron-El R, Friedler S, Shalev E, Geslevich J et al. A randomized, double-blind clinical trial using fixed daily doses of 100 or 200 IU of recombinant FSH in ICSI cycles. *Hum Reprod* 2001; 16(6):1104–1109.

43. Devroey P, Tournaye H, Van Steirteghem A, Hendrix P, Out HJ. The use of a 100 IU starting dose of recombinant follicle stimulating hormone (Puregon) in in-vitro fertilization. *Hum Reprod* 1998; 13(3):565–566.

44. Hoomans EH, Mulder BB. A group-comparative, randomized, double-blind comparison of the efficacy and efficiency of two fixed daily dose regimens (100- and 200-IU) of recombinant follicle stimulating hormone (rFSH, Puregon) in Asian women undergoing ovarian stimulation for IVF/ICSI. *J Assist Reprod Genet* 2002; 19(10):470–476.

45. Tinkanen H, Blauer M, Laippala P, Tuohimaa P, Kujansuu E. Prognostic factors in controlled ovarian hyperstimulation. *Fertil Steril* 1999; 72(5):932–936.

46. Imani B, Eijkemans MJ, Faessen GH, Bouchard P, Giudice LC, Fauser BC. Prediction of the individual follicle-stimulating hormone threshold for gonadotropin induction of ovulation in normogonadotropic anovulatory infertility: an approach to increase safety and efficiency. *Fertil Steril* 2002; 77(1):83–90.

47. Howles CM, Saunders H, Alam V, Engrand P. Predictive factors and a corresponding treatment algorithm for controlled ovarian stimulation in patients treated with recombinant human follicle stimulating hormone (follitropin alfa) during assisted reproduction technology (ART) procedures. An analysis of 1378 patients. *Curr Med Res Opin* 2006; 22(5):907–918.

48. Klingmuller D, Schepke M, Enzweiler C, Bidlingmaier F. Hormonal responses to the new potent GnRH antagonist Cetrorelix. *Acta Endocrinol (Copenh)* 1993; 128(1):15–18.

49. Al Inany H, Aboulghar M. GnRH antagonist in assisted reproduction: a Cochrane review. *Hum Reprod* 2002; 17(4):874–885.

50. Griesinger G, Felberbaum R, Diedrich K. GnRH antagonists in ovarian stimulation: a treatment regimen of clinicians' second choice? Data from the German national IVF registry. *Hum Reprod* 2005; 20(9):2373–2375.

51. Kolibianakis EM, Collins J, Tarlatzis BC, Devroey P, Diedrich K, Griesinger G. Among patients treated for IVF with gonadotrophins and GnRH analogues, is the probability of live birth dependent on the type of analogue used? A systematic review and meta-analysis. *Hum Reprod Update* 2006; 12(6):651–671.

52. Kolibianakis EM, Zikopoulos K, Smitz J, Camus M, Tournaye H, Van Steirteghem AC et al. Elevated progesterone at initiation of stimulation is associated with a lower ongoing pregnancy rate after IVF using GnRH antagonists. *Hum Reprod* 2004; 19(7):1525–1529.

53. Wikland M, Bergh C, Borg K, Hillensjo T, Howles CM, Knutsson A et al. A prospective, randomized comparison of two starting doses of recombinant FSH in combination with cetrorelix in women undergoing ovarian stimulation for IVF/ICSI. *Hum Reprod* 2001; 16(8):1676–1681.

54. Out HJ, Rutherford A, Fleming R, Tay CC, Trew G, Ledger W et al. A randomized, double-blind, multicentre clinical trial comparing starting doses of 150 and 200 IU of recombinant FSH in women treated with the GnRH antagonist ganirelix for assisted reproduction. *Hum Reprod* 2004; 19(1):90–95.

55. Al Inany H, Aboulghar MA, Mansour RT, Serour GI. Optimizing GnRH antagonist administration: meta-analysis of fixed versus flexible protocol. *Reprod Biomed Online* 2005; 10(5):567–570.

56. Kolibianakis EM, Albano C, Kahn J, Camus M, Tournaye H, Van Steirteghem AC et al. Exposure to high levels of luteinizing hormone and estradiol in the early follicular phase of gonadotropin-releasing hormone antagonist cycles is associated with a reduced chance of pregnancy. *Fertil Steril* 2003; 79(4):873–880.

57. Kolibianakis EM, Albano C, Camus M, Tournaye H, Van Steirteghem AC, Devroey P. Prolongation of the follicular phase in in vitro fertilization results in a lower ongoing pregnancy rate in cycles stimulated with recombinant follicle-stimulating hormone and gonadotropin-releasing hormone antagonists. *Fertil Steril* 2004; 82(1):102–107.

58. Griesinger G, Diedrich K, Devroey P, Kolibianakis EM. GnRH agonist for triggering final oocyte maturation in the GnRH antagonist ovarian hyperstimulation protocol: a systematic review and meta-analysis. *Hum Reprod Update* 2006; 12(2):159–168.

59. Liu HC, Jones GS, Jones HWJr., Rosenwaks Z. Mechanisms and factors of early pregnancy wastage in in vitro fertilization-embryo transfer patients. *Fertil Steril* 1988; 50(1):95–101.

60. Papanikolaou EG, Camus M, Kolibianakis EM, Van Landuyt L, Van Steirteghem A, Devroey P. In vitro fertilization with single blastocyst-stage versus single cleavage-stage embryos. *N Engl J Med* 2006; 354(11):1139–1146.

61. Soares SR, Troncoso C, Bosch E, Serra V, Simon C, Remohi J et al. Age and uterine receptiveness: predicting the outcome of oocyte donation cycles. *J Clin Endocrinol Metab* 2005; 90(7):4399–4404.

62. Raga F, Casan EM, Kruessel JS, Wen Y, Huang HY, Nezhat C et al. Quantitative gonadotropin-releasing hormone gene expression and immunohistochemical localization in human endometrium throughout the menstrual cycle. *Biol Reprod* 1998; 59(3):661–669.

63. Marchini M, Fedele L, Bianchi S, Losa GA, Ghisletta M, Candiani GB. Secretory changes in preovulatory endometrium during controlled ovarian hyperstimulation with buserelin acetate and human gonadotropins. *Fertil Steril* 1991; 55(4):717–721.

64. Ubaldi F, Bourgain C, Tournaye H, Smitz J, Van Steirteghem A, Devroey P. Endometrial evaluation by aspiration biopsy on the day of oocyte retrieval in the embryo transfer cycles in patients with serum progesterone rise during the follicular phase. *Fertil Steril* 1997; 67(3):521–526.

65. Kolibianakis E, Bourgain C, Albano C, Osmanagaoglu K, Smitz J, Van Steirteghem A et al. Effect of ovarian stimulation with recombinant follicle-stimulating hormone, gonadotropin releasing hormone antagonists, and human chorionic gonadotropin on endometrial maturation on the day of oocyte pick-up. *Fertil Steril* 2002; 78(5):1025–1029.

66. Jacobs MH, Balasch J, Gonzalez-Merlo JM, Vanrell JA, Wheeler C, Strauss JFIII et al. Endometrial cytosolic and nuclear progesterone receptors in the luteal phase defect. *J Clin Endocrinol Metab* 1987; 64(3):472–475.

67. Simon C, Cano F, Valbuena D, Remohi J, Pellicer A. Clinical evidence for a detrimental effect on uterine receptivity of high serum oestradiol concentrations in high and normal responder patients. *Hum Reprod* 1995; 10(9):2432–2437.

68. Simon C, Garcia Velasco JJ, Valbuena D, Peinado JA, Moreno C, Remohi J et al. Increasing uterine receptivity by decreasing estradiol levels during the preimplantation period in high responders with the use of a follicle-stimulating hormone step-down regimen. *Fertil Steril* 1998; 70(2):234–239.

69. Basir GS, WS O Ng EH, Ho PC. Morphometric analysis of peri-implantation endometrium in patients having excessively high oestradiol concentrations after ovarian stimulation. *Hum Reprod* 2001; 16(3):435–440.

70. Smitz J, Devroey P, Braeckmans P, Camus M, Khan I, Staessen C et al. Management of failed cycles in an IVF/GIFT programme with the combination of a GnRH analogue and HMG. *Hum Reprod* 1987; 2(4):309–314.

71. Akande AV, Mathur RS, Keay SD, Jenkins JM. The choice of luteal support following pituitary down regulation, controlled ovarian hyperstimulation and in vitro fertilisation. *Br J Obstet Gynaecol* 1996; 103(10):963–966.

72. Frydman R, Cornel C, de Ziegler D, Taieb J, Spitz IM, Bouchard P. Prevention of premature luteinizing hormone and progesterone rise with a gonadotropin-releasing hormone antagonist, Nal-Glu, in controlled ovarian hyperstimulation. *Fertil Steril* 1991; 56(5):923–927.

73. Beckers NG, Macklon NS, Eijkemans MJ, Ludwig M, Felberbaum RE, Diedrich K et al. Nonsupplemented luteal phase characteristics after the administration of recombinant human chorionic gonadotropin, recombinant luteinizing hormone, or gonadotropin-releasing hormone (GnRH) agonist to induce final oocyte maturation in in vitro fertilization patients after

ovarian stimulation with recombinant follicle-stimulating hormone and GnRH antagonist cotreatment. *J Clin Endocrinol Metab* 2003; 88(9):4186–4192.

74. Garcia J, Jones GS, Acosta AA, Wright GLJr. Corpus luteum function after follicle aspiration for oocyte retrieval. *Fertil Steril* 1981; 36(5):565–572.

75. Smitz J, Devroey P, Van Steirteghem AC. Endocrinology in luteal phase and implantation. *Br Med Bull* 1990; 46(3):709–719.

76. Fauser BC, Devroey P. Reproductive biology and IVF: ovarian stimulation and luteal phase consequences. *Trends Endocrinol Metab* 2003; 14(5):236–242.

77. Bourgain C, Devroey P. The endometrium in stimulated cycles for IVF. *Hum Reprod Update* 2003; 9(6):515–522.

78. Bourgain C, Smitz J, Camus M, Erard P, Devroey P, Van Steirteghem AC et al. Human endometrial maturation is markedly improved after luteal supplementation of gonadotrophin-releasing hormone analogue/human menopausal gonadotrophin stimulated cycles. *Hum Reprod* 1994; 9(1):32–40.

79. Hohmann FP, Macklon NS, Fauser BC. A randomized comparison of two ovarian stimulation protocols with gonadotropin-releasing hormone (GnRH) antagonist cotreatment for in vitro fertilization commencing recombinant follicle-stimulating hormone on cycle day 2 or 5 with the standard long GnRH agonist protocol. *J Clin Endocrinol Metab* 2003; 88(1):166–173.

80. Heijnen EM, Eijkemans MJ, De Klerk C, Polinder S, Beckers NG, Klinkert ER et al. A mild treatment strategy for in-vitro fertilisation: a randomised non-inferiority trial. *Lancet* 2007; 369(9563): 743–749.

81. Vyjayanthi S, Tang T, Fattah A, Deivanayagam M, Bardis N, Balen AH. Elective cryopreservation of embryos at the pronucleate stage in women at risk of ovarian hyperstimulation syndrome may affect the overall pregnancy rate. *Fertil Steril* 2006; 86(6):1773–177.

82. Rall WF, Fahy GM. Ice-free cryopreservation of mouse embryos at -196 degrees C by vitrification. *Nature* 1985; 313(6003): 573–575.

83. Kuwayama M, Vajta G, Kato O, Leibo SP. Highly efficient vitrification method for cryopreservation of human oocytes. *Reprod Biomed Online* 2005; 11(3):300–308.

84. Griesinger G, von Otte S, Schroer A, Ludwig AK, Diedrich K, Al Hasani S et al. Elective cryopreservation of all pronuclear oocytes after GnRH agonist triggering of final oocyte maturation in patients at risk of developing OHSS: a prospective, observational proof-of-concept study. *Hum Reprod* 2007 22(5):1348–1352.

85. Noyes RW, Hertig AT, Rock J. Dating the endometrial biopsy. *Am J Obstet Gynecol* 1975; 122(2):262–263.

86. Smith S, Hosid S, Scott L. Endometrial biopsy dating. Interobserver variation and its impact on clinical practice. *J Reprod Med* 1995; 40(1):1–3.

87. Murray MJ, Meyer WR, Zaino RJ, Lessey BA, Novotny DB, Ireland K et al. A critical analysis of the accuracy, reproducibility, and clinical utility of histologic endometrial dating in fertile women. *Fertil Steril* 2004; 81(5):1333–1343.

88. Martel D, Frydman R, Glissant M, Maggioni C, Roche D, Psychoyos A. Scanning electron microscopy of postovulatory human endometrium in spontaneous cycles and cycles stimulated by hormone treatment. *J Endocrinol* 1987; 114(2):319–324.

89. Lessey BA. The role of the endometrium during embryo implantation. *Hum Reprod* 2000; 15 (Suppl. 6):39–50.

90. Lessey BA, Ilesanmi AO, Lessey MA, Riben M, Harris JE, Chwalisz K. Luminal and glandular endometrial epithelium express integrins differentially throughout the menstrual cycle: implications for implantation, contraception, and infertility. *Am J Reprod Immunol* 1996; 35(3):195–204.

91. Tavaniotou A, Bourgain C, Albano C, Platteau P, Smitz J, Devroey P. Endometrial integrin expression in the early luteal phase in natural and stimulated cycles for in vitro fertilization. *Eur J Obstet Gynecol Reprod Biol* 2003; 108(1):67–71.

92. Laird SM, Tuckerman EM, Dalton CF, Dunphy BC, Li TC, Zhang X. The production of leukaemia inhibitory factor by human endometrium: presence in uterine flushings and production by cells in culture. *Hum Reprod* 1997; 12(3):569–574.

93. Giess R, Tanasescu I, Steck T, Sendtner M. Leukaemia inhibitory factor gene mutations in infertile women. *Mol Hum Reprod* 1999; 5(6):581–586.

94. Coulam CB, Bustillo M, Soenksen DM, Britten S. Ultrasonographic predictors of implantation after assisted reproduction. *Fertil Steril* 1994; 62(5):1004–1010.

95. Zaidi J, Campbell S, Pittrof R, Tan SL. Endometrial thickness, morphology, vascular penetration and velocimetry in predicting implantation in an in vitro fertilization program. *Ultrasound Obstet Gynecol* 1995; 6(3):191–198.

96. Remohi J, Ardiles G, Garcia-Velasco JA, Gaitan P, Simon C, Pellicer A. Endometrial thickness and serum oestradiol concentrations as predictors of outcome in oocyte donation. *Hum Reprod* 1997; 12(10):2271–2276.

97. Friedler S, Schenker JG, Herman A, Lewin A. The role of ultrasonography in the evaluation of endometrial receptivity following assisted reproductive treatments: a critical review. *Hum Reprod Update* 1996; 2(4):323–335.

98. Pierson RA. Imaging the endometrium: are there predictors of uterine receptivity? *J Obstet Gynaecol Can* 2003; 25(5):360–368.

99. Pairleitner H, Steiner H, Hasenoehrl G, Staudach A. Three-dimensional power Doppler sonography: imaging and quantifying blood flow and vascularization. *Ultrasound Obstet Gynecol* 1999; 14(2):139–143.

100. Schild RL, Indefrei D, Eschweiler S, Vand V, Fimmers R, Hansmann M. Three-dimensional endometrial volume calculation and pregnancy rate in an in-vitro fertilization programme. *Hum Reprod* 1999; 14(5):1255–1258.

101. Yaman C, Ebner T, Sommergruber M, Polz W, Tews G. Role of three-dimensional ultrasonographic measurement of endometrium volume as a predictor of pregnancy outcome in an IVF-ET program: a preliminary study. *Fertil Steril* 2000; 74(4):797–801.

102. Kupesic S, Bekavac I, Bjelos D, Kurjak A. Assessment of endometrial receptivity by transvaginal color Doppler and three-dimensional power Doppler ultrasonography in patients undergoing in vitro fertilization procedures. *J Ultrasound Med* 2001; 20(2):125–134.

103. Wu HM, Chiang CH, Huang HY, Chao AS, Wang HS, Soong YK. Detection of the subendometrial vascularization flow index by three-dimensional ultrasound may be useful for predicting the pregnancy rate for patients undergoing in vitro fertilization-embryo transfer. *Fertil Steril* 2003; 79(3):507–511.

104. Jarvela IY, Sladkevicius P, Kelly S, Ojha K, Campbell S, Nargund G. Evaluation of endometrial receptivity during in-vitro fertilization using three-dimensional power Doppler ultrasound. *Ultrasound Obstet Gynecol* 2005; 26(7):765–769.

105. Buckett WM. A review and meta-analysis of prospective trials comparing different catheters used for embryo transfer. *Fertil Steril* 2006; 85(3):728–734.

106. Oliveira JB, Martins AM, Baruffi RL, Mauri AL, Petersen CG, Felipe V et al. Increased implantation and pregnancy rates obtained by placing the tip of the transfer catheter in the central area of the endometrial cavity. *Reprod Biomed Online* 2004; 9(4):435–441.

107. Coroleu B, Barri PN, Carreras O, Martinez F, Parriego M, Hereter L et al. The influence of the depth of embryo replacement

into the uterine cavity on implantation rates after IVF: a controlled, ultrasound-guided study. *Hum Reprod* 2002; 17(2): 341–346.

108. Romundstad LB, Romundstad PR, Sunde A, von D V, Skjaerven R, Vatten LJ. Increased risk of placenta previa in pregnancies following IVF/ICSI; a comparison of ART and non-ART pregnancies in the same mother. *Hum Reprod* 2006; 21(9):2353–2358.

109. Buckett WM. A meta-analysis of ultrasound-guided versus clinical touch embryo transfer. *Fertil Steril* 2003; 80(4): 1037–1041.

110. Kosmas IP, Janssens R, De Munck L, Al Turki H, Van der EJ, Tournaye H et al. Ultrasound-guided embryo transfer does not offer any benefit in clinical outcome: a randomized controlled trial. *Hum Reprod* 2007;22(5):1327–1334.

111. Fanchin R, Righini C, Olivennes F, Taylor S, de Ziegler D, Frydman R. Uterine contractions at the time of embryo transfer alter pregnancy rates after in-vitro fertilization. *Hum Reprod* 1998; 13(7):1968–1974.

112. Fanchin R, Ayoubi JM, Righini C, Olivennes F, Schonauer LM, Frydman R. Uterine contractility decreases at the time of blastocyst transfers. *Hum Reprod* 2001; 16(6):1115–1119.

113. Baxter Bendus AE, Mayer JF, Shipley SK, Catherino WH. Interobserver and intraobserver variation in day 3 embryo grading. *Fertil Steril* 2006; 86(6):1608–1615.

114. Baart EB, Martini E, van d B I, Macklon NS, Galjaard RJ, Fauser BC et al. Preimplantation genetic screening reveals a high incidence of aneuploidy and mosaicism in embryos from young women undergoing IVF. *Hum Reprod* 2006; 21(1): 223–233.

115. Assisted reproductive technology in the United States: 2000 results generated from the American Society for Reproductive Medicine/Society for Assisted Reproductive Technology Registry. Fertil Steril 2004; 81(5):1207–1220.

116. Pinborg A. IVF/ICSI twin pregnancies: risks and prevention. *Hum Reprod Update* 2005; 11(6):575–593.

117. Strandell A, Bergh C, Lundin K. Selection of patients suitable for one-embryo transfer may reduce the rate of multiple births by half without impairment of overall birth rates. *Hum Reprod* 2000; 15(12):2520–2525.

118. Thurin A, Hausken J, Hillensjo T, Jablonowska B, Pinborg A, Strandell A et al. Elective single-embryo transfer versus double-embryo transfer in in vitro fertilization. *N Engl J Med* 2004; 351(23):2392–2402.

119. Van Landuyt L, Verheyen G, Tournaye H, Camus M, Devroey P, Van Steirteghem A. New Belgian embryo transfer policy leads to sharp decrease in multiple pregnancy rate. *Reprod Biomed Online* 2006; 13(6):765–771.

120. Handyside AH, Kontogianni EH, Hardy K, Winston RM. Pregnancies from biopsied human preimplantation embryos sexed by Y-specific DNA amplification. *Nature* 1990; 344(6268):768–770.

121. Marquez C, Sandalinas M, Bahce M, Alikani M, Munne S. Chromosome abnormalities in 1255 cleavage-stage human embryos. *Reprod Biomed Online* 2000; 1(1):17–26.

122. Rubio C, Simon C, Vidal F, Rodrigo L, Pehlivan T, Remohi J et al. Chromosomal abnormalities and embryo development in recurrent miscarriage couples. *Hum Reprod* 2003; 18(1):182–188.

123. Staessen C, Platteau P, Van Assche E, Michiels A, Tournaye H, Camus M et al. Comparison of blastocyst transfer with or without preimplantation genetic diagnosis for aneuploidy screening in couples with advanced maternal age: a prospective randomized controlled trial. *Hum Reprod* 2004; 19(12):2849–2858.

124. Harper JC, Boelaert K, Geraedts J, Harton G, Kearns WG, Moutou C et al. ESHRE PGD Consortium data collection V: cycles from January to December 2002 with pregnancy follow-up to October 2003. *Hum Reprod* 2006; 21(1):3–21.

125. Donoso P, Staessen C, Fauser BC, Devroey P. Current value of preimplantation genetic aneuploidy screening in IVF. *Hum Reprod Update* 2007; 13(1):15–25.

126. Gianaroli L, Magli MC, Ferraretti AP, Munne S. Preimplantation diagnosis for aneuploidies in patients undergoing in vitro fertilization with a poor prognosis: identification of the categories for which it should be proposed. *Fertil Steril* 1999; 72(5):837–844.

127. Kahraman S, Bahce M, Samli H, Imirzalioglu N, Yakisn K, Cengiz G et al. Healthy births and ongoing pregnancies obtained by preimplantation genetic diagnosis in patients with advanced maternal age and recurrent implantation failure. *Hum Reprod* 2000; 15(9):2003–2007.

128. Montag M, Van dV Dorn C, Van dV. Outcome of laser-assisted polar body biopsy and aneuploidy testing. *Reprod Biomed Online* 2004; 9(4):425–429.

129. Munne S, Weier HU, Stein J, Grifo J, Cohen J. A fast and efficient method for simultaneous X and Y in situ hybridization of human blastomeres. *J Assist Reprod Genet* 1993; 10(1):82–90.

130. Munne S, Magli C, Cohen J, Morton P, Sadowy S, Gianaroli L et al. Positive outcome after preimplantation diagnosis of aneuploidy in human embryos. *Hum Reprod* 1999; 14(9): 2191–2199.

131. Pehlivan T, Rubio C, Rodrigo L, Romero J, Remohi J, Simon C et al. Impact of preimplantation genetic diagnosis on IVF outcome in implantation failure patients. *Reprod Biomed Online* 2003; 6(2):232–237.

132. Wilding M, Forman R, Hogewind G, Di Matteo L, Zullo F, Cappiello F et al. Preimplantation genetic diagnosis for the treatment of failed in vitro fertilization-embryo transfer and habitual abortion. *Fertil Steril* 2004; 81(5):1302–1307.

133. Munne S, Chen S, Fischer J, Colls P, Zheng X, Stevens J et al. Preimplantation genetic diagnosis reduces pregnancy loss in women aged 35 years and older with a history of recurrent miscarriages. *Fertil Steril* 2005; 84(2):331–335.

134. Pellicer A, Rubio C, Vidal F, Minguez Y, Gimenez C, Egozcue J et al. In vitro fertilization plus preimplantation genetic diagnosis in patients with recurrent miscarriage: an analysis of chromosome abnormalities in human preimplantation embryos. *Fertil Steril* 1999; 71(6):1033–1039.

135. Rubio C, Pehlivan T, Rodrigo L, Simon C, Remohi J, Pellicer A. Embryo aneuploidy screening for unexplained recurrent miscarriage: a minireview. *Am J Reprod Immunol* 2005; 53(4): 159–165.

136. Silber S, Escudero T, Lenahan K, Abdelhadi I, Kilani Z, Munne S. Chromosomal abnormalities in embryos derived from testicular sperm extraction. *Fertil Steril* 2003; 79(1):30–38.

137. Platteau P, Staessen C, Michiels A, Tournaye H, Van Steirteghem A, Liebaers I et al. Comparison of the aneuploidy frequency in embryos derived from testicular sperm extraction in obstructive and non-obstructive azoospermic men. *Hum Reprod* 2004; 19(7):1570–1574.

138. Twisk M, Mastenbroek S, van Wely M, Heineman MJ, Van dV Repping S. Preimplantation genetic screening for abnormal number of chromosomes (aneuploidies) in in vitro fertilisation or intracytoplasmic sperm injection. *Cochrane Database Syst Rev* 2006;(1):CD005291.

139. Stevens J, Wale P, Surrey E, Schoolcraft W. Is aneuploidy screening for patients aged 35 or over beneficial? A prospective randomized trial. *Fertil Steril* 2004; 82 (Suppl. 2):249.

140. Werlin L, Rodi I, DeCherney A, Marello E, Hill D, Munne S. Preimplantation genetic diagnosis as both a therapeutic and

diagnostic tool in assisted reproductive technology. *Fertil Steril* 2003; 80(2):467–468.

141. Munne S, Fischer J, Warner A, Chen S, Zouves C, Cohen J. Preimplantation genetic diagnosis significantly reduces pregnancy loss in infertile couples: a multicenter study. *Fertil Steril* 2006; 85(2):326–332.

142. Baart EB, Van Opstal D, Los FJ, Fauser BC, Martini E. Fluorescence in situ hybridization analysis of two blastomeres from day 3 frozen-thawed embryos followed by analysis of the remaining embryo on day 5. *Hum Reprod* 2004; 19(3):685–693.

143. Coonen E, Derhaag JG, Dumoulin JC, van Wissen LC, Bras M, Janssen M et al. Anaphase lagging mainly explains chromosomal mosaicism in human preimplantation embryos. *Hum Reprod* 2004; 19(2):316–324.

144. Los FJ, Van Opstal D, van den BC. The development of cytogenetically normal, abnormal and mosaic embryos: a theoretical model. *Hum Reprod Update* 2004; 10(1):79–94.

145. Munne S, Sandalinas M, Escudero T, Marquez C, Cohen J. Chromosome mosaicism in cleavage-stage human embryos

evidence of a maternal age effect. *Reprod Biomed Online* 2002; 4(3):223–232.

146. Wilton L. Preimplantation genetic diagnosis and chromosome analysis of blastomeres using comparative genomic hybridization. *Hum Reprod Update* 2005; 11(1):33–41.

147. Voullaire L, Slater H, Williamson R, Wilton L. Chromosome analysis of blastomeres from human embryos by using comparative genomic hybridization. *Hum Genet* 2000; 106(2): 210–217.

148. Wilton L, Voullaire L, Sargeant P, Williamson R, McBain J. Preimplantation aneuploidy screening using comparative genomic hybridization or fluorescence in situ hybridization of embryos from patients with recurrent implantation failure. *Fertil Steril* 2003; 80(4):860–868.

149. Wilton L, Williamson R, McBain J, Edgar D, Voullaire L. Birth of a healthy infant after preimplantation confirmation of euploidy by comparative genomic hybridization. *N Engl J Med* 2001; 345(21):1537–1541.